Exploring the
Dimensions of

Human
Sexuality

Fourth Edition

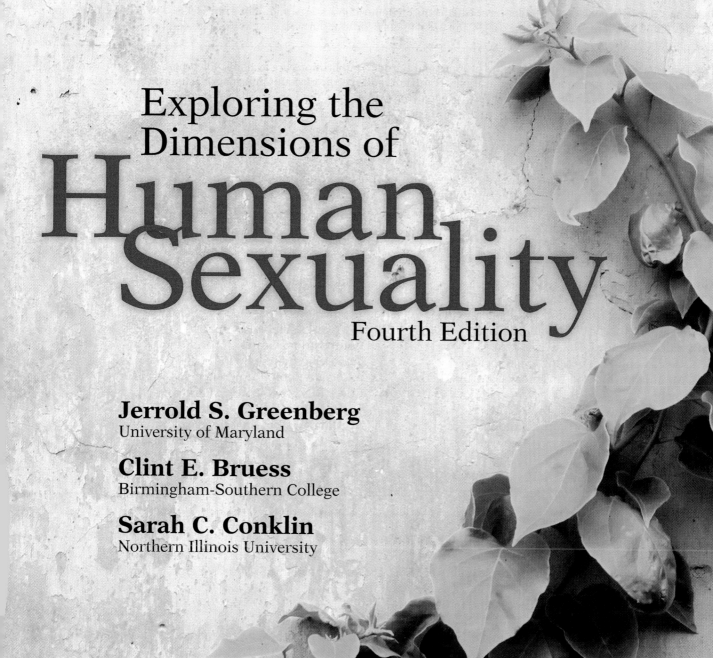

Exploring the Dimensions of
Human Sexuality

Fourth Edition

Jerrold S. Greenberg
University of Maryland

Clint E. Bruess
Birmingham-Southern College

Sarah C. Conklin
Northern Illinois University

JONES AND BARTLETT PUBLISHERS
Sudbury, Massachusetts
BOSTON   TORONTO   LONDON   SINGAPORE

World Headquarters

Jones and Bartlett Publishers
40 Tall Pine Drive
Sudbury, MA 01776
978-443-5000
info@jbpub.com
www.jbpub.com

Jones and Bartlett Publishers
Canada
6339 Ormindale Way
Mississauga, Ontario L5V 1J2
Canada

Jones and Bartlett Publishers
International
Barb House, Barb Mews
London W6 7PA
United Kingdom

Jones and Bartlett's books and products are available through most bookstores and online booksellers. To contact Jones and Bartlett Publishers directly, call 800-832-0034, fax 978-443-8000, or visit our web site, www.jbpub.com.

Substantial discounts on bulk quantities of Jones and Bartlett's publications are available to corporations, professional associations, and other qualified organizations. For details and specific discount information, contact the special sales department at Jones and Bartlett via the above contact information or send an e-mail to specialsales@jbpub.com.

Production Credits

Chief Executive Officer: Clayton Jones
Chief Operating Officer: Don W. Jones, Jr.
President, Higher Education and Professional
  Publishing: Robert W. Holland, Jr.
V.P., Sales: William J. Kane
V.P., Design and Production: Anne Spencer
V.P., Manufacturing and Inventory Control: Therese
  Connell
Acquisitions Editor: Shoshanna Goldberg
Senior Associate Editor: Amy L. Bloom
Senior Editorial Assistant: Kyle Hoover

Senior Production Editor: Carolyn F. Rogers
Associate Marketing Manager: Jody Sullivan
Illustrations: Imagineering Scientific and Technical
  Artworks, Vincent Perez
Composition: Graphic World, Inc.
Text Design: Anne Spencer
Associate Photo Researcher: Jessica Elias
Cover Design: Kristin E. Parker
Cover Image: © Juha Sompinmäki/ShutterStock, Inc.
Printing and Binding: Courier Kendallville
Cover Printing: Courier Kendallville

Chapter 11 is adapted from Debra Haffner, *Beyond the Big Talk*, Newmarket Press, 2001, with permission from the author.

Library of Congress Cataloging-in-Publication Data
Greenberg, Jerrold S.
  Exploring the dimensions of human sexuality / Jerrold S. Greenberg, Clint E. Bruess, Sarah C. Conklin. — 4th ed.
    p. ; cm.
  Includes bibliographical references and index.
  ISBN 978-0-7637-7660-2 (pbk.)
  1. Sex. 2. Sex (Psychology) 3. Hygiene, Sexual. 4. Interpersonal relations. 5. Sexual ethics. I. Bruess, Clint E. II. Conklin, Sarah C. III. Title.
  [DNLM: 1. Sexual Behavior. 2. Reproduction—physiology. 3. Sex. 4. Sexuality—physiology. HQ 21 G798e 2011]
  HQ21.G67118 2011
  306.7—dc22
                    2010000313

6048
Printed in the United States of America
14 13 12 11 10   10 9 8 7 6 5 4 3 2 1

Brief Contents

Contents

Features

Communication Dimensions

Multicultural Dimensions

Global Dimensions

Gender Dimensions

Ethical Dimensions

Preface

The authors of this book feel strongly about the importance of understanding human sexuality as part of a healthy personality. In addition, we have seen numerous positive and negative examples of what can happen when people do or do not understand how human sexuality can be related to human well-being. We have had examples of this kind of outcome with our own children.

Let us start with a positive example. The daughter of one of the authors, the mother of a 14-year-old daughter, lives more than 2,000 miles away. This distance has reduced conversations related to sexuality in recent years. One night a few years ago, she called to discuss a recent incident at her house. She said that her daughter asked about noises she sometimes heard coming from her mom and dad's bedroom. The author's daughter explained that the noises related to her mom and dad enjoying physical contact as part of showing love for each other. Fortunately, she had previously talked with her daughter about physical contact and reproduction so she was able to refer back to that conversation. She asked the author (her dad) for advice about what she should do. He responded that she should feel pleased that her daughter would talk freely with her and ask about the noises. He also said that it was very positive that she had explained physical contact and reproduction to her daughter so she had accurate information that was appropriate for her age. Beyond that, the author simply said that she was on the right track related to the sexuality education of her daughter, and that she should continue to do all she could to keep the lines of communication open related to human sexuality. When the conversation ended, the author felt good that his daughter was comfortable talking about sexuality, and that she was passing along that comfort to her daughter.

When the son of one of the authors was entering fifth grade, school personnel organized a committee of parents to review instructional materials for the sexuality education course. As luck would have it, the author was selected to serve on this committee. At the first committee meeting, he was surprised to learn that the program focused exclusively on reproductive anatomy and physiology. The author asked, with an inquiring tone, "How will you help your students process their feelings regarding sexuality?" The answer was that the reproductive system would be taught just as any other body system would, rather than being highlighted by including discussion of feelings associated with it. At that point the author volunteered to resign from the parent review committee and asked to join the "Digestive System Parent Review Committee." Of course, there was none. That allowed the author to point out that there really is a distinction between education regarding sexuality and education pertaining to health in general and that this distinction needs to be addressed with students. We do so in this book by exploring the varied dimensions of human sexuality.

A final example related to being comfortable studying human sexuality arose on the first day of a recent human sexuality course taught by one of the authors. After introducing the course, the author asked if the students had received any reactions from friends or relatives because they were taking a human sexuality course. After the usual positive and negative reactions were given, one student mentioned an example that was new to the author. The student said that he knew two other students, one male and one female, who also wanted to take the course. However, they did not sign up for the course because they were too embarrassed to have anyone else see that they had filled out the form to sign up for the course. In other words, they were so uncomfortable having someone in the registrar's office see their form that they passed up the opportunity to learn more about human sexuality. The author was almost speechless, but did say that was an excellent example of the need to feel more comfortable learning about human sexuality.

In many regards, human sexuality today does not differ from that of our ancestors' times. In a biological sense, human reproduction occurs the same way as it has throughout history. Religion and culture have long played a role in our sexuality; so has public policy. Nevertheless, a greater awareness now exists of the many dimensions that shape our sexuality.

As long-time sexuality educators, we know that no one aspect of sexuality can be separated from the others, and no one aspect is more important than the others. We have written a text that presents all aspects of sexuality as interconnected and significant. Throughout this text you will find an emphasis on health and well-being based on the assumptions that we are all sexual beings and that sexuality should be viewed in its totality—that is, in terms of its biological, spiritual, psychological, and sociocultural dimensions.

Because we realize that learning best occurs when students are actively involved, we have created a text that goes beyond merely presenting factual knowledge about the varied dimensions of human sexuality. We want students to explore the varied dimensions and see how each affects their personal sexuality.

At the same time, this exploration is facilitated by having accurate and up-to-date knowledge. To help ensure the book's currency, the content in this text has been updated regularly. It was revised for the 2002 update, for the 2004 edition, for the 2007 edition, and now for this 2011 edition. This "up-to-the-minute" aspect of the book is evident in the abundance of 21st-century references cited throughout the text.

The dimensions discussed in the book can be broken down into biological, psychological, and sociocultural categories. Some examples are described here.

Biological Dimensions
Physiology
The basis of understanding sexuality is understanding our bodies' physiology. Factual information lays the foundation of critical thinking; without the facts, you cannot begin to think critically about your sexuality. The greater your knowledge, the more likely you are to take responsibility for your sexual health.

Gender
The physiological differences between genders create the foundation for the development of psychological and social wellness and strongly influence our perceptions of sexual wellness. Gender dimensions is the subject of a full chapter and is also highlighted in boxed features in every chapter.

Psychological Dimensions
Psychology
Developing a positive image of self and sexuality is critical to developing sexual wellness. For example, a positive body image lends itself to overall wellness; a negative self-image can lead to drug abuse (steroids or diet pills) or psychological disorders (anorexia, bulimia, binge eating disorder, or muscle dysmorphia). Body image is so important that we devote a minichapter ("In Focus") to the topic—the most comprehensive coverage in the market!

Spirituality
Religious and spiritual beliefs influence feelings about sexual behavior, premarital sexual activity, adultery, divorce, contraception, abortion—even masturbation. Spiritual issues are discussed in the Multicultural Dimensions boxes and in the opening chapter.

Sociocultural Dimensions
Multicultural Issues
Cultures within the United States and around the world differ in their views of sexuality. From the seminude beaches in the south of France to Middle Eastern Muslim communities where women are covered from head to hand to foot, ours is a world of diversity. Sometimes these diverse behaviors are a part of the culture; other times they are given legal sanction. A good example is the many ways in which abortion is viewed. Such views range from strict prohibition to simply viewing abortion as a method of birth control, such that it is common for women to have as many as four or five abortions. Your ability to respect your sexual partner's cultural beliefs and feelings will result in a higher level of satisfaction for both of you. To help students better understand sexual diversity, almost every chapter contains one boxed example pertaining to a culture within the United States and another example pertaining to a culture from elsewhere in the world.

Ethics
Ethical decision making takes on legal and moral implications in the area of sexuality. The law and the courts have become involved in such far-flung areas as access to abortion clinics, workplace sexual harassment, and ownership of frozen embryos. Moral implications of ethical decisions include sexual coercion and underscore the importance of taking responsibility for your sexual wellness. To emphasize the key role played by ethics in human sexuality, Ethical Dimensions boxes appear in every chapter. Additionally, an entire chapter (Chapter 18, Sexual Ethics, Morality, and the Law) is dedicated to this topic.

Public Policy
Even public policy affects our sexual behavior! The Healthy People 2010 project used health promotion to establish acquired immune deficiency syndrome (AIDS) and sexually transmitted infection (STI) awareness, decrease unwanted teenage pregnancies, and increase the number of women who receive prenatal care. Public policy on free speech continues to allow the uncontrolled distribution of pornographic material on the Internet. Unfortunately, access to proper health care, birth control, and positive sexual role models is often lacking for the poor.

Integration
Integrated Theme
With so many factors influencing our sexual behavior, we have created a striking full-page feature to capture their breadth: Exploring the Dimensions of Human Sexuality, an integrated approach that ties all these strands together. This feature helps students understand how many different aspects affect their sexual health and influence their sexual behavior. Our intention is to help students envision the convergence of the many aspects of sexuality and help them make

sexual decisions that will lead to a lifetime of sexual health and wellness.

Integrated Web Site

Exploring the Dimensions of Human Sexuality also links to the Jones and Bartlett web site (sexuality .jbpub.com/dimensions/4e), where each dimension is presented in greater depth. Students can click on a particular chapter and find self-assessments, exercises, research links, and information that will allow them to explore their own dimensions of human sexuality in greater depth. Integrating the book and web site actively engages the students in the learning process. An "Introduction to Service–Learning" section, which appeared as an appendix in previous editions of this book, will now be available on the web site rather than in the back of the text. *See the Visual Walkthrough on page xviii for an example of this feature.*

Pedagogy

Throughout this book, numerous ways of organizing content are provided to enhance student learning.

In Focus Minichapter on Body Image

We offer a comprehensive look at the concept of body image in a minichapter. It is rare to find so much detail on this subject. Here we discuss how body image affects self-esteem and sexuality; how the quest for a perfect body creates problems ranging from eating disorders to cosmetic surgery and steroid abuse; and how body image affects both genders. There are also three other "In Focus" minichapters: Unexpected Pregnancy Outcomes, HIV and AIDS, and Alternative Sexual Behaviors.

Boxed Feature Program

A carefully designed boxed feature program reinforces the dimensions theme of the textbook with five distinct types of boxes in each chapter: Multicultural Dimensions, Global Dimensions, Gender Dimensions, Communication Dimensions, and Ethical Dimensions. *Please refer to page xviii of the Visual Walkthrough for detailed descriptions of these features.*

Critical Thinking

Exploring the dimensions of human sexuality requires students to think critically about how the multifaceted dimensions relate to them. To that end, we have included critical thinking questions throughout the text to help students reflect on the subject matter and understand its implications for their sexual health.

Critical thinking questions are found in boxes, in photo captions, and in the end-of-chapter section—including application questions related to the chapter-opening story, critical thinking questions about material, and a critical thinking minicase. Critical thinking questions help students recall information and synthesize new material with existing knowledge and stimulate students to make informed judgments about the information provided.

Myth vs Fact and Did You Know. . . Boxes

Students' sexual health and wellness are also influenced by sexual myths and folklore. Many of our brief sidebars are designed to set students straight on such myths. "Did You Know. . ." boxes add whimsical and high-interest information to engage the student further.

Chapter-Opening Story

Each chapter opens with an engaging real-life story that explores the concepts to be discussed in depth in the chapter. Students are drawn into the chapter material with a high-interest case and introduced to the topics that will be discussed. At the end of the chapter, students are asked to relate the chapter's information to application questions about the opening story.

Reviewing the Dimensions of Human Sexuality

Each chapter ends with an interactive feature designed to help students take responsibility for their sexual health and wellness. The "Reviewing the Dimensions of Human Sexuality" activity includes an interactive self-assessment designed to help students understand and clarify their own feelings about sexuality issues presented in that chapter. It also includes discussion questions, application questions pertaining to the opening story, critical thinking questions, a critical thinking minicase, and a self-assessment.

Changes in the New Edition

Throughout this new edition, extensive updates have been made to focus on information and statistics about recent developments. Information from more than 400 new references has been added—almost all of these references dating from the last few years. The lists of suggested readings found at the end of each chapter were updated, as was the "Web Resources" section at the end of each chapter. In addition, a summary was added at the end of each chapter.

There has also been additional reorganization of the book. Chapters were reorganized to promote a more logical flow. For example, Gender Dimensions (previously Chapter 6) is now Chapter 9. Sexual Techniques (previously Chapter 10) is now Chapter 13. Entire sections were moved from one chapter to another. For example, the section on pregnancy and lactation was moved to Chapter 8, Conception, Pregnancy, and Birth; the section on menopause was moved to Chapter 12, Sexuality in Adulthood; and the discussion of the G spot was moved to Chapter 6, Sexual Response and Arousal.

The title of Chapter 16 was also changed—from Atypical Sexual Behavior to Alternative Sexual Behavior. This was done to clarify that sexual behavior comes in many varieties, and to avoid being judgmental about the sexual behaviors in which people choose to participate.

Other examples of changes and updates within selected chapters include the following:

- In Chapter 1, the UNICEF annual report entitled *The State of the World's Children, 2009* is used to illustrate the relationship of medical intervention and the status of women in developing countries to maternal and child health as well as teen pregnancy.

- Chapter 2 contains a new section on evaluating sexuality information on the Internet, in addition to new sections on focus groups and on interpretation of statistics.

- More information is included on breast cancer in men in Chapter 5.

- Chapter 6 now includes a section on the role of culture in sexual arousal.

- Recent contraception methods, availability, and new developments have all been added to Chapter 7.

- In Chapter 8, the section on determining the birth due date using the Nägele's rule and other methods has been expanded, and more information is provided about water birth. A section on psychological and physical adjustments after childbirth has also been added.

- Also in Chapter 8, the discussion of intersexuality (previously referred to as hermaphroditism) has been expanded and updated.

- In Chapter 9, the sections on gender and the workplace, and on gender and advertising, have been updated and greatly expanded.

- Chapter 10 includes expanded discussions of contemporary topics such as statistics related to sexual orientation, gender activism, and sexual orientation and legal issues.

- In Chapter 12, more information is provided about the sexual behavior of college students as well as more information about cohabitation.

- Chapter 13 goes into more detail about the relationship between cervical cancer and HPV, the Gardasil vaccine, and hepatitis B.

- A section on "Keeping It Going" has been added to Chapter 13 to provide guidance for maintaining a satisfying sexual relationship over many years, such as in long-term marriages.

- Chapter 14 contains additional information about what to do if sexual assault occurs and increased information about sexual harassment and college students.

- In Chapter 17, increased information is offered about child prostitution and trafficking of persons.

- The guidance from professional organizations regarding health screenings has been updated to match the latest recommendations. For example, the most current guidance related to breast cancer screening (mammograms) and prostate-specific antigen (PSA) screening is included.

When appropriate, boxed material has been changed and updated throughout the fourth edition of this book. Statistics have also been updated throughout the book: The most current statistics regarding sexually transmitted infections (STIs), adoption, abortion, birth rates, marriage and divorce rates, prevalence of sexual behaviors, and many other categories are presented.

Writing this book has been a service–learning activity for us. We did abundant and thorough research to identify state-of-the-art knowledge and attitudes pertaining to sexuality—and we learned a great deal in doing so. That was the "learning" part of the service–learning equation. The "service" part relates to our interest in helping to enhance the sexual health and wellness of our readers. As such, we hope you find the information we included, the issues we raised and discussed, and the myths we debunked useful as you live and express your sexuality. If that is the case, the time, effort, and energy we have devoted to writing this text will have been well worth that investment.

About the Authors

Dr. Jerrold S. Greenberg

Dr. Jerrold S. Greenberg is Professor Emeritus in the Department of Public and Community Health at the University of Maryland. Dr. Greenberg earned his baccalaureate and masters degrees from The City College of New York and then continued his education at Syracuse University where he earned his doctorate. Dr. Greenberg has taught at Syracuse University, Boston University, and the State University of New York at Buffalo before accepting a professorship at the University of Maryland in 1979. Dr. Greenberg has written over 50 books on such topics as elder care, health, stress management, physical fitness, sexuality, and methods of health education. In addition, he has published over 80 articles in professional journals and in lay magazines. Among Dr. Greenberg's honors are: the University of Maryland Service–Learning Advocate of the Year award for 2003–2004; the American School Health Association's Distinguished Service Award; selection as Alliance Scholar by the American Alliance for Health, Physical Education, Recreation, and Dance; the Presidential Citation, the Certificate of Appreciation, and the Scholar Award of the American Association for Health Education; selection for inclusion in Who's Who in America, Outstanding Young Men of America, and Who's Who in World Jewry. Dr. Greenberg has also served on the editorial boards of the professional journals *Health Education* and *The Journal of School Health;* and as a reviewer for other professional journals. In addition, Dr. Greenberg has conducted stress management workshops for professional, business, and lay organizations throughout the United States.

Clint E. Bruess

Clint E. Bruess is Dean Emeritus of the School of Education and Professor Emeritus of Health Education at the University of Alabama at Birmingham. He is currently Chair of the Division of Education at Birmingham-Southern College. He has coauthored more than 15 textbooks in the areas of human sexuality, sexuality education, personal health, and school health programs. In addition, he has published numerous articles in professional journals and served in elected and appointed positions for the American School Health Association (also a Fellow), American Association for Health Education (also a Fellow), and Society of Public Health Educators.

Sarah C. Conklin, PhD

Sarah C. Conklin, PhD, is Professor and Coordinator of Public Health and Health Education in the School of Nursing and Health Studies at Northern Illinois University. She has taught sexuality classes in middle, junior, and senior high schools, in two seminaries and two universities, and has authored more than 30 scholarly articles and book chapters on sexuality topics. She has contributed to sexuality curriculum development projects in Minnesota, Illinois, Wisconsin, and Wyoming, as well as certificates of graduate study in human sexuality, sexual orientation, and health education. Dr. Conklin serves as a national teacher certification program reviewer for the American Association of Health Education and is an accreditation site visitor for the Council on Education for Public Health.

Acknowledgments

We would like to thank the many reviewers who guided us throughout the various stages of this project. Their voices, criticism, and support have truly made this a better text. We would like to acknowledge Christopher Adamsick for his contributions to the Student Study Guide as well as to the PowerPoints, Instructor's Manual, TestBank, and Web materials for the *Fourth Edition*. His expertise was greatly appreciated. We would also like to thank Dr. Sue Tendy, EdD of the U.S. Military Academy at West Point for her contributions to the material on sexual harassment in the military. Our sincere thanks and appreciation goes to the Jones and Bartlett Health team: Shoshanna Goldberg, acquisitions editor, Carolyn Rogers, senior production editor, Kyle Hoover, senior editorial assistant, and Jody Sullivan, associate marketing manager. We would like to acknowledge the dedication and hard work of these individuals, for without them this project would never have been realized.

This book is dedicated to two of the cutest grandchildren possible: Jonah and Zoe. The joy they bring is unsurpassed.

Jerrold Greenberg
Department of Public and Community Health
University of Maryland

To Susan J. Laing with appreciation for her part in a wonderful relationship.

Clint Bruess
Department of Education
Birmingham-Southern College

With thanks to my parents, LaVonne and the late Burton Souther, who rose to the challenge of nurturing a sexually healthy daughter, and to my lifetime partner, Roger Conklin, who exemplifies a sexually healthy relationship that is unsurpassed.

Sarah C. Conklin
School of Nursing and Health Studies
Northern Illinois University

Reviewers

Veanne N. Anderson, Indiana State University
Betsy Bergen, Kansas State University
Charles Chase, West Texas A&M University
Jeffrey K. Clark, Ball State University
Susan Clark, Ball State University
Terri Clark, Arcadia University
Amanda Collings, University of Massachusetts, Amherst
Dominique Didier Dagit, Assistant Professor of Biology, Millersville University
Mark Doherty, University of Louisiana at Monroe
Judy Drolet, Southern Illinois University, Carbondale
Lyndall Ellingson, California State University, Chico
James Ferraro, Southern Illinois University
Nora Few, University of Illinois at Urbana-Champaign
Mary Rich Goodwin, Brigham Young University
Patricia Goodson, Texas A&M University at College Station

Teri L. Malo, University of South Florida
Susan M. Moore, Western Illinois University
Nancy L. Nygaard, Murray State University
Anthony Parrillo, East Carolina University
Miguel Perez, University of North Texas
Joel B. Piperberg, Millersville University
Catherine Sherwood-Puzzello, Indiana University
Stanley Snegroff, Adelphi University
Susan Sprecher, Illinois State University
Richard Stacy, University of Nebraska at Omaha
Susan Tendy, United States Military Academy, West Point
McKinley Thomas, Augusta State University
Maria Theresa Wessel, James Madison University
Susan Woods, Eastern Illinois University
Donna Videto, SUNY College at Cortland
Emilia Patricia Zarco, University of the Philippines
Mary Rose J. Zink, Wilmington College

A Visual Walkthrough

Exploring the Dimensions of Human Sexuality, Fourth Edition is designed around the central theme that our feelings, attitudes, and beliefs regarding sexuality are continually influenced by our internal and external environments. All aspects of sexuality—biological, spiritual, psychological, and sociocultural—are interconnected and significant. The boxed feature program, additional pedagogy, and ancillaries of this new textbook have been designed around these core concepts.

BOXED FEATURES

Communication Dimensions
These boxes discuss communication issues that arise around sexuality between the genders, partners from different ethnic groups, and others.

Multicultural Dimensions
To better appreciate how various people view sexuality we offer a multicultural boxed feature. These boxes deal exclusively with diversity issues within the United States.

Global Dimensions
Sexuality is viewed very differently outside of the United States. Issues such as divorce in China and international differences in discussing sexuality are discussed in the Global Dimensions boxes.

Gender Dimensions
Issues arising from gender are integrated throughout the text, discussed in detail in the Gender Dimensions chapter, and featured in the Gender Dimensions boxes found in each chapter. Topics covered in these boxes include communication breakdown between genders, responsibility for contraception, and many others.

Ethical Dimensions
The importance of ethics in sexuality is underscored in the Ethical Dimensions box features. This is where topics such as abstinence-only education and the ethics surrounding technological advances are discussed.

Pedagogical Design

Chapter-Opening Pedagogy Each chapter-opening spread gives the reader a glimpse of what is to come with chapter objectives, a list of the Dimensions of Human Sexuality boxed features that will follow, and a list of topics also explored on the companion web site. In addition, a high-interest and engaging real-life story draws students into the chapter material and introduces them to the topics that will be discussed. This opening story is revisited at the end of the chapter in the application questions.

Exploring the Dimensions of Human Sexuality This feature organizes the multifaceted issues in each chapter into biological, psychological, and sociocultural factors. This visual element is integrated with the companion web site where instructors and students can further explore these dimensions.

Reviewing the Dimensions of Human Sexuality This end-of-chapter activity gives students the opportunity to review and apply key chapter concepts. Items in this section include discussion questions, critical thinking questions, and application questions that relate to the chapter-opening story. The Exploring Personal Dimensions section directs students to focus on personal choices and take responsibility for their sexual health and well-being.

Teaching and Learning Aids

Exploring the Dimensions of Human Sexuality Online The companion web site is integrated with the *Exploring the Dimensions of Human Sexuality* feature found in each main chapter of the text and offers four central components:

- Resource links give the instructor the ability to integrate the web into the curriculum.
- Instructor resources such as PowerPoint lecture presentations, a TestBank, and an instructor's manual assist in classroom preparation.
- Student activities such as web exercises and self-assessments involve students in the dimensions of human sexuality in a structured online environment.
- Student study tools like an anatomical review, animated flashcards, crossword puzzles, and practice quizzes offer students the opportunity to review chapter concepts and prepare for exams.

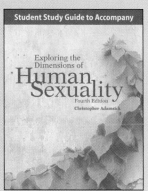

A New Interactive Online Workbook allows students to review chapter topics and assess their own sexuality behaviors in relation to these topics. Exercises and activities include Chapter Summary, Fill in the Blanks, Review the Dimensions, Focus on the Facts, Quick Questions, and Test Your Knowledge.

Visit sexuality.jbpub.com/ dimensions/4e

Instructor's ToolKit CD-ROM offers the instructor maximum flexibility in preparing for class, designing and presenting lectures, and generating tests. The ToolKit features an instructor's manual, PowerPoint lecture presentations, and an image and table bank. Content can be implemented into many of the common distance learning programs. (Available for both PC and Macintosh.)

SPECIAL FEATURES

Myth vs Fact Students' sexual health and wellness are influenced by sexual myths and folklore. Myth vs Fact features common myths associated with the material presented in each chapter along with the fact to dispel each myth.

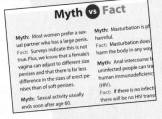

Brief **Did You Know. . .** sidebars add whimsical and high-interest information to further engage the student.

In Focus Minichapters The authors have included focused minichapters which delve into topics that affect students' lives. These take a fully comprehensive look at subjects such as body image, unexpected pregnancy, HIV and AIDS, and atypical sexual behaviors. The concentrated chapters offer today's students a deeper understanding of issues about which they should be informed.

Service–Learning Appendix Although we are all rightfully concerned with our own sexual health and well-being, the authors encourage readers to also recognize the responsibility to contribute to the sexual health of the communities in which they reside. An *Introduction to Service–Learning* appendix, available on the companion web site, gives an overview of the concept of service–learning and suggests specific activities through which the reader can contribute to their community's sexual health. These activities employ a service–learning methodology; that is, students provide service while learning chapter content at the same time.

CHAPTER 1

Introducing the Dimensions of Human Sexuality

FEATURES

Gender Dimensions
The Multifaceted Dimension of Gender

Ethical Dimensions
Should Human Embryos Be Used for Stem Cell Research?

Global Dimensions
A Strong Preference for Sons in India

Multicultural Dimensions
Pregnancy and Health

Communication Dimensions
Talking About Your Human Sexuality Class

CHAPTER OBJECTIVES

1 Identify and discuss the dimensions of human sexuality, including biological, psychological, and sociocultural factors.

2 Discuss the historical aspects of human sexuality, including the sexual revolution, the role of gender, and the role of culture.

3 Apply critical thinking methods to human sexuality.

4 Outline the reasons to study human sexuality, including the steps of the decision-making process.

sexuality.jbpub.com/dimensions/4e

Global Dimensions: Male Genital Mutilation
 and Circumcision Practices
Prostate Cancer
Care from Organizations and Available Publications

INTRODUCTION

L *et us begin our exploration of the many dimensions of human sexuality by examining how they affect the life of one person: Lisa, an 18-year-old college freshman, involved in her first serious—and sexual—relationship. After several months of dating, Lisa experiences the scare of her life: Her period is late. After a few days she purchases a home-pregnancy kit. As she waits until the morning to take the test, she begins to think about the role of sexuality in her life.*

Like most people who grow up in the United States today, Lisa received basic sexuality education in public school. But that brief overview—which Lisa and her friends giggled through—touched only on the physical aspects of reproduction. Nothing prepared her for the emotions she felt during her current relationship, or how her social and cultural upbringing would affect her sexual behavior.

Lisa is a Korean American, a member of a family who respect heritage and tradition. Her parents, a university professor and a homemaker, were born in Korea and had an arranged marriage. The traditional Korean view of sexuality is conservative, and virginity is highly prized for marriage. Although Lisa holds on to many traditional views, she also struggles with the permissive attitude toward sexuality that prevails in the U.S. culture today—an attitude that her boyfriend shares (Brennan, 1999).

An unexpected pregnancy for Lisa would be a major tragedy in her family. Pregnancy outside marriage would shame not only the individual (and make her an "unperson") but also the entire family. Her family could choose to exile her.

Korean Americans tend not to tolerate secrecy by children and exert strict parental control. The Korean culture discourages open discussion of feelings and seeking out of psychological counseling. Thus Lisa is in a crisis because she feels she cannot tell her parents, but she also cannot tell anyone else (who may in turn tell her parents). In fact, Lisa has yet to tell her boyfriend what is upsetting her.

Religion plays a major role in many people's sexuality. For Lisa's parents, whose cultural traditions in Korea can be traced to Confucianism, abortion may be a possibility (as a means of saving face for the family). But many Korean American immigrants are members of fundamentalist Christian groups, who often prohibit abortion. Lisa wonders what she will do if, in fact, she is really pregnant.

Lisa is lucky: She is not pregnant. But Lisa has realized that she has to start taking greater responsibility for her sexual behavior. How can she incorporate the many dimensions affecting her sexuality into her personal sexuality?

This chapter begins our exploration of the many dimensions of sexuality and how they affect our lives.

■ The Dimensions of Human Sexuality

When you think about human sexuality, what do you think of? Some form of physical contact? Human reproduction? Feelings when you see an attractive person? Human sexuality is all that and more. **Human sexuality** is a part of your total personality. It involves the interrelationship of biological, psychological, and sociocultural dimensions.

human sexuality
A part of your total personality. It involves the interrelationship of biological, psychological, and sociocultural dimensions.

The Sexuality Information and Education Council of the United States (SIECUS) defines human sexuality as encompassing the sexual knowledge, beliefs, attitudes, values, and behaviors of individuals. Its various dimensions include the anatomy, physiology, and biochemistry of the sexual response system; identity, orientation, roles, and personality; and thoughts, feelings, and relationships. The expression of sexuality is influenced by ethical, spiritual, cultural, and moral concerns (SIECUS, 2009).

The Alberta Society for the Promotion of Sexual Health (ASPSH) indicates that sexuality means many things: feelings about ourselves, roles we play in society, and reproduction. It is not limited to how we behave sexually. It is the total of our physical, emotional, and spiritual responses, thoughts, and feelings. Sexuality is more about who we are than about what we do (ASPSH, 2009).

Sexuality is a natural part of life. The concepts of human sexuality are learned. From our viewpoint, human sexuality involves at least three dimensions—biological, psychological, and sociocultural. Each dimension has many subdimensions. The interactive relationship of these dimensions describes an individual's total sexuality.

The Interactive Nature of Sexual Dimensions

A complex set of biological, psychological, and sociocultural variables plays a role in all our sexual interactions. The decision to be sexually active is a result of many factors. Sexual arousal is a physiological function. Psychologically, our body image and feelings of self-worth may inhibit getting involved ("I'm not good enough for her"; "I'm not attractive enough for him"). A lack of self-worth may also inhibit arousal. Our culture helps us develop a sense of what is attractive—height, weight, hair style, skin tone. In addition, religious beliefs affect our sexual undertakings, as do legal and ethical considerations. Role models set by family and friends influence us as well.

All these dimensions constantly interact and influence our sexuality. Although we discuss them separately for clarity, remember that almost all sexuality-related decisions we make are influenced by more than one dimension.

Biological Dimension

The basis of understanding sexuality is physiological knowledge about how our bodies work. Factual information lays the foundation of decision making—without the facts, you cannot begin to think critically about your sexuality. The greater your knowledge, the more likely you are to take responsibility for your sexual health.

Until relatively recently, most of the research into human sexuality focused on physiology. For example, a model of the human sexual response cycle, published by the well-known researchers Masters and Johnson in 1966, focused mainly on physiology.

Fisher (1992) emphasizes the genetic aspects of behavior. In her view, humans have a common nature, a set of unconscious tendencies that are encoded in our genes. She believes that although we are not aware of these predispositions, they still motivate our actions. Although she recognizes that culture plays a role in one's sexuality, she also seems to support **essentialism**, the belief that the essence of sexuality is biological.

essentialism
Belief that once the cultural and historical aspects are taken away, the essence of sexuality is biological.

The biological dimension of our sexuality involves our physical appearance, especially the development of physical sexual characteristics; our responses to sexual stimulation; our ability to reproduce or to control fertility; and our growth and development in general. Although human reproductive function does not begin until puberty, human sexual–erotic functioning begins immediately after birth and lasts a lifetime. It is important to realize that biological functioning, as it relates to sexuality, is a part of the natural functioning of human beings. These biological aspects also relate to the other dimensions of sexuality, and all the dimensions work together to produce an individual's total sexuality—which, in turn, is part of the total personality (Bruess & Greenberg, 2009).

The physiological differences between the sexes help to lay the groundwork for the development of psychological and social wellness, and our gender strongly influences our perceptions of sexual wellness. For example, the sexual double standard, in which men are expected to be promiscuous and women are not, is a belief held by many people in the United States. In our human sexuality classes we always ask students to complete the sentences "A man who carries a condom in his wallet is _____" and "A woman who carries a condom in her purse is _____." The man is routinely described as "responsible," the woman as "a slut."

Psychological Dimensions

Although sexual activity is definitely physical, it also involves psychology—our sense of being. The noted

Gender DIMENSIONS

The Multifaceted Dimension of Gender

The first words our parents heard after we emerged from the womb declared our biological gender: "It's a boy!" or "It's a girl!" Our parents bought crib sheets and clothes that were pink or blue to match our gender.

We soon learned the sociocultural meanings of gender: Boys and girls are socialized to play in different styles and usually learn to prefer different sets of toys. Our moms and/or dads tended to do gender-specific chores. Teenage boys are somehow allowed to be sexually active, whereas girls are discouraged from such activities (a concept known as the "double standard").

Psychologically, girls are encouraged to show their emotions, whereas boys learn to suppress emotions. This leads to differing communication styles as well: Females are generally more expressive verbally than males. (Of course, there are many expressive men and inexpressive females. Remember that Lisa in our opening story has been culturally socialized to suppress open discussion of feelings.)

Socially, there are many gender inequalities that will be covered in detail throughout this text. In the workplace, a woman often earns less than a man earns (a concept known as the "wage gap") and often faces a tougher time getting promoted into upper management (a concept known as the "glass ceiling"). After a woman goes home from work, she usually does more household chores (known as the "second shift") than her spouse.

Why are such topics covered in a human sexuality course? Because our gender—who we are as men and women and how we experience ourselves as male and female—is an essential component of our sexuality.

Myth (vs) Fact

Myth: Human sexuality relates mainly to biological functioning.
Fact: Human sexuality includes a biological dimension but also includes psychological and sociocultural dimensions.

Myth: Most people are well informed about human sexuality.
Fact: Unfortunately, most people still have relatively poor knowledge of sexuality. Therefore, many myths about human sexuality still exist.

Myth: Sexual "normality" is similar among various cultures.
Fact: Sexual attitudes and behaviors differ greatly among cultural groups. There is no set standard for "normality."

sexual therapist Dr. Ruth Westheimer has a favorite saying, that sexual behavior "is all between the ears."

A major psychological factor that affects our sexual wellness is body image. A positive body image lends itself to a feeling of overall wellness; a negative self-image can lead to drug abuse (use of steroids or diet pills) or psychological disorders (anorexia, bulimia, binge eating disorder, or muscle dysmorphia). Body image is so important that we have devoted a minichapter to the topic (In Focus: Body Image).

The psychological dimension of sexuality is probably the clearest example of learned aspects of sexuality. Our attitudes and feelings toward ourselves and other people begin to develop very early in life. From the time we are born, we get signals from all around us telling us how to think and act. We learn that some words are "wrong" or "dirty" and that certain parts of our body are "unmentionable." We even learn to be careful about what conversational topics we enter into with certain people. If we feel one way about ourselves but think others would find these feelings unacceptable, we learn to hide our true feelings and to pretend. After all, thinking or talking about sexuality is not a good idea anyway (or so we have learned). Some of us are lucky enough to grow up with a more positive set of experiences. Regardless of whether our experiences are positive or negative, however, our learned responses to them become integral to our sexuality.

Sociocultural Dimensions

The biological and psychological components of sexuality are affected by society and culture. The sociocultural dimension of sexuality is the sum of the cultural and social influences that affect our thoughts and actions.

In contrast to a perception of sexuality's being controlled mainly by biological or genetic character-istics, Tiefer (1995) promotes the idea of **social construction-ism**, which proposes that sexual identities and experiences are acquired from and influenced and modified by an ever-changing social environment. According to social constructionists, people acquire and assemble meanings, skills, and values from the people around them. This dimension of sexuality is the sum of the cultural influences that affect our thoughts and actions, both historical and contemporary. For example, historical influences become evident when one considers roles of males and females as well as certain customs.

social constructionism
The belief that sexual identities are acquired from and influenced and modified by an ever-changing social environment.

Indeed, we are surrounded by social influences on our sexuality. Among the sources of influence are religion, multiculturalism, socioeconomic status, ethics, the media, and politics. We will look at each influence here briefly and will revisit them throughout the text.

Religious Influences

Religious and spiritual beliefs influence feelings about morality, sexual behavior, premarital sexual behavior, adultery, divorce, contraception, abortion, and masturbation.

It is hard to know for sure what influences the attitudes of college students toward many controversial issues, but religion is certainly one of the important influences. It is interesting to note the findings of the UCLA Higher Education Research Institute. Since 1966, this group has done a comprehensive survey of college freshmen.

In 1999 only 40% of freshmen agreed that it is OK for two people who like each other to have sexual intercourse, even if they have known each other for only a short time. In 2001, this percentage increased only slightly, to 41.8%, and in 2002 it was 42.2%. In 2005 it increased a little more, to 46.2%. This represents lower support for casual sexual behavior among the entering class than the all-time high of 52% in 1987. Interestingly, in 2002 this idea was supported by 55.2% of males and 31.7% of females. In 2005 it was supported by 59.8% of males and 35.1% of females. Only half of 1999's freshman class backed efforts to keep abortion legal. This was after a record low figure after 6 years of decline, but in 2001 the proportion increased to 53.9% and in 2002 it was 55%—about equal for males and females. In 2005 it was 53.9%—again about equal for males and females. In 2007 it was 56.9%, and in 2009 it was 58.2%; in both instances it remained about equal for males and females. Support for laws protecting abortion peaked in 1990 at 65% (Characteristics

Romance reality shows have been successful with television viewers. With so many people looking for love, networks have no shortage of candidates, but it remains to be seen whether real romance can blossom in front of the camera. Do you watch romance reality shows? Why do you think society has embraced them? Do you think it's healthy to make a game out of love?

of freshmen, 2001; The nation: Attitudes and characteristics of freshmen at 4-year colleges, 2002; This year's freshmen at 4-year colleges: A statistical profile, 2005; The American freshman: National norms for fall 2007, 2008; This year's freshmen at 4-year colleges: A statistical profile, 2009).

The percentage of freshmen supporting the legal right of gay couples to marry was 57.9% in 2002, 59.3% in 2003, 56.7% in 2005, 63.5% in 2007, and 66.2% in 2009. Interestingly, in 2007 this position was supported by 55.3% of males as compared to

In its infancy, television was reluctant to show a biracial couple. When Lucille Ball and Desi Arnaz proposed the *I Love Lucy* show in the early 1950s, television executives wanted a white actor to play opposite Lucy, fearing problems of showing a white-and-Latino couple. Lucy and Desi were forced to put up $5,000 of their own money to create a pilot, which was, of course, a success.

70.3% of females. In 2009 it was supported by 58.8% of males and 72.4% of females. In 2003, 24.8% said they supported laws prohibiting gay relationships; in 2005, 21.5% believed this; and in 2007, 24.3% did. The percentage who believed married women should confine their activities to the home and family reached a 15-year low of 21.5% in 2002 and was 21% in 2005 (Rooney, 2003; This year's freshmen at 4-year colleges: A statistical profile, 2005; The American freshman: National norms for fall 2007, 2008; This year's freshmen at 4-year colleges: A statistical profile, 2009).

Religion plays a major role in many people's sexuality, including Lisa from the opening story. For Lisa's parents, whose cultural traditions in Korea can be traced to Confucianism, abortion might have been a possibility (as a means of saving face for the family).

Religion can also play a role in use or nonuse of medical services related to sexuality. It can even influence the availability of such services when policies allow service providers to refuse to provide services that are against their personal beliefs. For example, a pharmacist might refuse to sell contraceptives because he does not believe in their use, or a doctor might refuse to perform an abortion because she does not believe abortions are morally appropriate.

Through the years, religiosity (an intense religious belief) has been found to influence the number of sexual partners, the frequency of various forms of sexual behavior, the age at first sexual intercourse, types of sexual behaviors, standards related to sexual activity before marriage, and even marital satisfaction. Religiosity also seems to influence the sexual behaviors of college students. A study conducted at a southeastern university showed that both males and females who reported less frequent worship attendance and weaker religious feelings were more likely to participate in sexual behaviors than those with more frequent worship attendance and stronger religious feelings (Penhollow, Young, & Denny, 2005).

Multicultural Influences

Cultures within the United States differ in their views of sexuality. Your ability to respect your sexual partner's cultural beliefs and feelings will result in a higher level of satisfaction for both of you.

First we must distinguish between ethnic background and ethnicity. A person's ethnic background is usually determined by birth and is related

ethnicity
The degree of identification an individual feels with a particular ethnic group.

to country of origin, native language, race, and religion. **Ethnicity** refers to the degree of identification an individual feels with a particular ethnic group (Harrell & Frazier, 1999).

Our opening story underscores this concept. Had Lisa been pregnant, she would have found herself torn between her parents' strong ethnicity and the individual cultural beliefs and practices that she learned in school and college. Such difficult cultural conflicts might place some people in a position like Lisa's at high risk for potential serious problems.

Cultural influences from citizens of other countries also play a dramatic role in U.S. culture. This is especially important for college students in the United States, because 1 in 10 students is from another country. These students' local cultural understandings of the body, health, and morality shape their use of contraceptive methods and abortion. For example, in the United States, abortion is not viewed as a method of contraception. In some other countries, however, abortion is viewed as a primary method of birth control. Some women from these countries might have as many as four or five abortions. Two other examples of multicultural influences related to Brazil and China follow.

In Brazil, compared with members of evangelical religions, other men are significantly more likely to report having had an extramarital partner and

The cast of the movie *Rent.* Considered revolutionary in the mid-1990s, the story dealt frankly with HIV/AIDS and gay relationships. Such sensitivity has become commonplace in almost all media today.

unprotected extramarital sexual intercourse in the last 12 months. Region of residence is also strongly associated with extramarital sexual activity. Compared with men in southern or central Brazil, those in the north are three times more likely to have had extramarital sexual intercourse and unprotected sexual intercourse in the last year (Hill et al., 2004).

Chinese women whose beliefs and experiences reflect traditional norms limiting gender equality may be at increased risk of being subjected to intimate-partner violence. In 2005, 43% of women said they had been physically or sexually abused by a partner, with 26% experiencing such events during the past year. Several factors suggesting adherence to traditional gender roles were associated with the likelihood of reporting intimate-partner violence. For example, women who had turned down a job because of their partner, women who thought that wife-beating is sometimes justified, and women who believed that a wife has a duty to have intercourse with her husband had elevated odds of having been abused (Xu et al., 2005).

The preceding examples are only a few of the multicultural influences that affect feelings and decisions related to sexuality. Here are some others:

- In Turkey, female virginity is highly valued. Virginity tests are often used, and principals in state schools have the right to expel girls who have had sexual intercourse (Turkey says only virgins can be nurses, 2001).

- In Mexico, hysterectomy is often used to treat cervical abnormalities. This is an example of inadequate knowledge, probably due to multicultural influences (Aldrich et al., 2005).

- In Sweden, a certain degree of openness in thinking about sexuality seems to be prevalent. Teens are more likely to know about sexuality, including contraception. Abortion is available and subsidized by the government at early stages, and parents are likely to know about their children's sexual activities. These attitudes and practices consistently result in lower rates of teen pregnancy and sexually transmitted infections than commonly found in the United States (Caron, 1998).

Socioeconomic Influences
Socioeconomic status and education also influence sexual attitudes and behaviors, at least within the same ethnic group. Examples of this influence include low-income individuals often thinking and acting differently than middle-class individuals, being more likely to engage in sexual intercourse at an earlier age, and having children outside of marriage.

Educational levels also seem to influence sexual behavior. Examples include people with more education masturbating more and people with at least some college education having more sexual partners than those who did not attend college.

Socioeconomic status influences more than just sexual activities. The poor have less access to proper health care, birth control, care during pregnancy, day care for children, and positive sexual role models.

Lisa, from our opening story, is affected by her family's high socioeconomic status. The prevailing indicator of success among second-generation Korean Americans is high academic achievement at prestigious universities, followed by pursuit of professional careers. Lisa's academic performance to this point has reflected this cultural value. An unexpected and unwanted pregnancy would create a major obstacle to achieving the expected success and thus create an added intergenerational cultural conflict.

All people are sexual beings, and our experiences influence our thinking about sexuality.

Ethical Influences
The ethics of sexuality involves questioning the way we treat ourselves and other people. Examples of sexually oriented ethical dilemmas include the following:

- Should I or should I not participate in a certain sexual behavior?
- Is it ethical to use a prostitute?
- Is it ethical not to disclose my full sexual history to a new partner?
- Is it ethical to engage in sexual behaviors with a person who is underage?
- Is it ethical to use a position of power to obtain sexual partners?

Ethical issues are not necessarily the same as legal concerns. For example, prostitution is illegal in the United States except in a few counties in Nevada. However, the ethical question of prostitution would look at the morality of hiring a prostitute—who may be selling her body as a last resort to survive. Also, the age of maturity in your state (the age at which you are deemed legally of age to engage in sexual activity) is probably 16 or 17 years old. Thus, it would be illegal to have a sexual partner younger than that age. However, in Tokyo, Japan, the legal age for girls is 12 years. Is it ethical for you to have a sexual partner who is

of age in the country you are visiting, even if she is very young?

How we consider such questions and ultimately decide what is right and wrong profoundly shapes our sexuality. Ethical decision making underscores the importance of taking responsibility for your sexual wellness. Chapter 18 explores ethical, moral, and legal issues relating to sexuality in detail.

Media Influences
It has long been recognized that the media help shape public attitudes on many topics—especially sexuality, gender roles, and sexual behaviors. The depictions of sexuality we encounter in the media are there mainly to entertain and sell products. Consequently, the media do not provide us with realistic depictions.

Television shows are filled with portrayals of sexual activity and "double-meaning" comments. The music industry has countless sexual images. Listen to the words of many currently popular songs and you will hear the sexual content. Magazines, tabloids, and books contribute to the many sexual themes that bombard us. Next time you are in the checkout line at the supermarket, take a look at the number of magazine covers that relate to sexuality. Numerous advertisements also use sexual themes to sell products. We are told that if we buy the right soap, toothpaste, clothes, or cars we will look sexier and be more attractive.

Some people have argued that, if they would so choose, the media could promote sexual health by communicating accurate information and portraying

¿? Ethical DIMENSIONS

Should Human Embryos Be Used for Stem Cell Research?

In 2005 the National Academies released guidelines for embryonic stem cell research. They were amended in 2007 and 2008. Stem cells are harvested 3 to 5 days after a sperm and egg unite—before implantation in the uterus. Such stem cells have the capacity to develop into almost any type of tissue in the body. Although it is also possible to extract "adult" stem cells from bone marrow, skin, blood, and other types of tissue, adult stem cells have more limited applications than stem cells from embryos. The National Academies developed guidelines because such research is controversial.

Supporters of stem cell research point out that stem cells can be used to treat many human conditions—such as diabetes, Parkinson's disease, and multiple sclerosis. Someday stem cells might even be used to grow spare body parts. Supporters believe researchers should press on to find "cures" for such conditions because the re-

sults could be helpful to so many people. Opponents are strongly against research in which embryos are destroyed. Pro-life groups and others believe government funding should not be provided for such research and that it should not be done at all.

For many years stem cell research has been an important political and ethical issue. Many issues, such as whether a woman should become pregnant to produce stem cells to be used for research, have been heavily debated. Others argue about whether stem cell research results in the taking of a human life.

The guidelines of the National Academies prohibit not only the cloning of human beings, but also payments to egg donors and use of eggs without the donor's informed consent. Debates about stem cell research are likely to continue for years to come.

Source: Stem cells at the National Academies. Washington, DC: National Academies, 2009. Available: http://dels.nas.edu/bls/stemcells.

On the surface, *Sex and The City* seems to present four successful, single women living, loving, and having it all in New York City. Beneath the shoes, clothes, and beautiful faces in beautiful places, some see the show as an insightful commentary on loss, loneliness, and the failure of sexual liberation.

realistic situations. For example, they might show effective communication about sexuality and relationships, interactions as verbally and physically respectful, more examples of responsible sexual activity, more instances where healthy sexual encounters are anticipated and not last-minute responses to the heat of passion, and the importance of having good information and using

contraceptives and condoms to prevent unwanted pregnancies and diseases.

Political Influences

Even public policy affects our sexual behavior. For example, the U.S. government's *Healthy People 2000* and *2010* projects attempt to use health promotion to establish AIDS and sexually transmitted infection (STI) awareness, decrease unwanted teenage pregnancies, and increase the number of women who receive prenatal care. Also, the U.S. constitutional right to free speech allows the uncontrolled distribution of some pornographic material on the Internet.

Even political elections—including choosing elected officials and voting on ballot initiatives—can have a profound effect on policies and on thinking about human sexuality. Consider the political ramifications of election results.

As a result of the 2002 elections, for the first time in decades the same political party (in this case, the Republicans) that occupied the White House also controlled the U.S. House and the Senate. This provided an opportunity for that political party to strongly influence various policy issues, including those related to sexuality. The Republican Party has openly supported limiting the right of women to get abortions. It also has clearly desired to emphasize abstinence from sexual activity as the major way to

Global DIMENSIONS

A Strong Preference for Sons in India In recent years, 47% of women in India reported wanting more sons than daughters, and only 2% preferred daughters. The sex ratio is now about 139 males born per 100 females. Son preference decreased with a decreasing ideal family size. For example, 75% or women who wanted five or more children reported preferring sons over daughters, compared with 67% of those wanting three to four children and 12% of those wanting one to two.

Some people feel that prenatal sex-detection techniques should not be used in India. They are afraid that more women will get abortions if they know at an early stage of pregnancy that the baby is a female. Others feel that prenatal sex selection is acceptable because it allows women to realize their "repressed demand for sons."

Given a cultural situation where sons have been traditionally strongly preferred to daughters, women with no sons have a significantly elevated risk of having their marriage dissolve. Odds of marital dissolution are about 40% higher among women whose only child is a girl than among those who have only a son. For mothers of two children, those with daughters have 70% higher odds of being divorced or separated than those with sons. This holds for women in most demographic, social, and geographic subgroups.

Sources: Bhat, P. N. M., & Zavier, A. J. F. Fertility decline and gender bias in northern India. *Demography, 40, no. 4* (2003), 637–657; and Bose, S., & South, S. J. Sex composition of children and marital disruption in India. *Journal of Marriage and Family, 54, no. 4* (2003), 996–1006.

Even Miss America can be involved in politics related to sexuality.

control pregnancies and STIs among young people. It has gone so far as to provide federal funding for certain types of educational programs only if they emphasize abstinence. It also has not been very supportive of rights for homosexuals.

Many issues in the 2008 elections related to sexuality. There was the first female major party candidate for president. It was announced that the teenage daughter of the female candidate for Vice-President of the United States was pregnant and not married. During the presidential campaign, platforms and debates included discussions about the legality of abortion, rights for homosexuals (including marriage and adoption), stem cell research, and abstinence-only versus comprehensive sexuality education. After Barack Obama was inaugurated as President in 2009, these issues, along with many others, continued to influence politics. Political issues, in turn, continued to influence human sexuality in many ways.

■ Historical–Cultural Influences on Sexuality

Just as many sociocultural influences have affected human sexuality, so have some interesting historical–cultural influences. Because we cannot consider all of them, and because most of these topics are covered in greater depth elsewhere in this text, we briefly focus on some from a historical standpoint—namely, the sexual revolution, control of sexual behavior, conception, contraception, and gender roles. As you read about these historical–cultural influences, think about how you and people you know may have been affected by them.

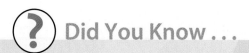
Did You Know . . .

During the first seven to eight decades of the 1900s, there was a steady increase in the rates of premarital sexual intercourse for 15- to 19-year-old students. In 1991, 54.1% had ever engaged in sexual intercourse. The rates then gradually declined, reaching 45.6% in 2001. Since that time, they have again increased to 47.8% in 2007 (49.8% of males and 45.9% of females).

In 2007, the number of teens who have had sexual intercourse increased dramatically with grade level: from 32.8% of ninth graders, to 43.8% of tenth graders, to 55.5% of eleventh graders, to 64.6% of twelfth graders. Nationwide, 7.1% of students had sexual intercourse for the first time before 13 years of age. Overall, the proportion of students who had ever had sexual intercourse was higher among black (66.5%) and Hispanic (52.0%) students than among white (43.7%) students.

Source: Youth risk behavior surveillance—United States, 2007. *Morbidity and Mortality Weekly Report, 57, no. SS-4* (June 6, 2008), 21–23.

Myth vs Fact

Myth: Rates of premarital intercourse increased rapidly in the first 60–70 years of the 20th century.
Fact: There was a rather steady rate of premarital sexual intercourse during the first six to seven decades of the 20th century.

Myth: We have long known that early childhood experiences are important to sexual development.
Fact: It was not until at least the middle of the 20th century that it was recognized that early childhood experiences are important to a child's healthy development.

The Sexual Revolution

No doubt you have heard references to the sexual revolution. The meaning of this term varies according to the speaker; however, it is clear that many changes related to sexuality have occurred in the past 80 to 100 years. Whether there has been an actual revolution—or perhaps an evolution—is for you to decide after considering some facts and observations.

Many people talk about a sexual revolution in reference to rates of sexual intercourse before marriage. Many of our history books would lead us to believe that in the past, Americans were sexually chaste before marriage. If we read between the lines, however, we find that this is not necessarily true. Reiss (1973) informs us that in the late 1700s in Massachusetts, one of three women in a particular church confessed fornication to her minister (the actual number was probably higher yet). The U.S. western frontier society relied heavily on prostitution. The women's liberation movement of the 1870s revealed numerous sexual affairs. And the first vulcanized rubber condom was displayed at the Philadelphia World's Fair in 1876. These are not isolated events, and they should make us question what we think about the sexual purity and innocence of our forebears (Bruess & Greenberg, 2009).

Even out-of-wedlock childbearing may not be more prevalent now than several generations ago. For example, rates of white out-of-wedlock births in 1970 did not differ greatly from those in 1850. However, in 1985 about 25% of U.S. births were to unmarried women, up from about 5% in 1960 (Newcomer, 1990). In 1994 the proportion of children born to unmarried women was 26%, and in 2000 it was 31% (Bachu & O'Connell, 2001).

Studies done between 1920 and 1945 do seem to indicate that the greatest increases in rates of premarital sexual intercourse occurred in the early 1900s (Bell, 1966). This means that the so-called sexual revolution began early in the 20th century and not in more recent years. Many older people who seem so concerned about changes in sexual behavior were in the middle of the sexual revolution themselves. Our best research tells us that approximately 35% to 45% of females and 55% to 65% of males participated in sexual intercourse before marriage during most of the first six to seven decades of the 20th century (Bruess & Greenberg, 2009).

Many changes that influence our thinking about sexuality occurred in the first six to seven decades of the 20th century. For example, as traditional moral viewpoints were questioned, people began to wonder about whether any one standard of morality could apply universally. Social scientists talked about people defining their own morality, while religious leaders often saw morality as determined by an order higher than mere humans.

Several events also occurred during this period that contributed to a trend toward more receptivity to the topic of sexuality. For example, wars exposed many people to other cultures, and the uncertainty of survival contributed to a philosophy of "Live tonight,

Did You Know . . .

During the Middle Ages, some people believed in witches, whom they accused of having sexual relations with the devil. Because that was not generally acceptable behavior, something had to be done about it. Some women who were sexually "loose" were simply ignored, but others were labeled as witches, and witch hunts were common. Women were put on trial, and, if they were found guilty of witchcraft, attempts were made to free them from the devil. This was done by a "laying on of hands" by an appropriate religious leader. If these attempts failed, it was sometimes thought better to kill the witch than to let her live.

Some people thought this performance by Elvis Presley was obscene.

Myth vs Fact

Myth: Contraceptive methods were not available until the 20th century.

Fact: Methods used to prevent pregnancy are as old as recorded history.

for tomorrow we may die." The result was a change in the concept of sexual morality. In addition, there was a rise in the status of women as they became better educated, a more significant part of the workforce, more aggressive, and more active partners in sexual activity.

Rapid improvements in communication and transportation also had a tremendous effect on sexuality. First the telephone became a convenient way to promote interpersonal relationships, and today the Internet provides a means for people to meet, send quick love messages, and stay in touch. Magazines, TV, and films continued to have many sexual themes, and the car became a "bedroom on wheels," providing a way to have private sexual activity.

It became accepted that early childhood experiences are important to the development of young children—including their sexual development. This understanding has had ramifications for sexuality education programs for children of all ages.

Important events that influenced sexuality include the research of Alfred Kinsey in the 1940s and 1950s

related to sexual behavior (see Chapter 2), the first nationwide appearance of Elvis Presley in 1956 (considered obscene by many), and the introduction of the bikini swimsuit in 1959. The lyrics of popular songs became more sexually suggestive, and record smashing by opponents of these songs occurred in an attempt to censor the music.

The 1960s work of William Masters and Virginia Johnson (see Chapter 6) on human sexual response also greatly contributed to our knowledge of how we function sexually and how and why we sometimes do not function. In addition to basic information about sexual functioning, their research provided the foundation for sexual counseling and methods for dealing with human sexual inadequacy.

Increasingly reliable contraceptives, especially the pill (introduced in the United States in 1960), were developed and accepted by large numbers of people. Today many reliable and relatively safe contraceptive methods are available, and the vast majority of married couples use contraception.

In the late 20th century and early 21st century, books, classes, and radio and television programs about sexuality, as well as numerous web sites related to sexuality, became common. The press reports the findings of virtually every new study, and discussions about sexuality in American society are out of the closet and into public forums.

Control of Sexual Behavior

Throughout the history of Western culture, there have been many attempts to control sexual behavior. Most of these are found in moral and legal codes of the time. For example, early Christian moralists taught that because sexual activity outside marriage had a purpose other than **procreation**, it was a sin. Even within marriage, sexual union was lawful only if it was performed for the purpose of begetting children. Almost all medieval theologians emphasized that it was a mortal sin to embrace one's spouse solely for pleasure (Aries & Bejin, 1985, 115).

procreation
Sexual intercourse for the purpose of reproduction.

There were many other religious influences and restrictions. For example, intercourse was objectionable on all fast or feast days, during the days a female was menstruating, for 40 days after childbirth, during pregnancy, and during breastfeeding. Also, intercourse between husband and wife was supposed to take place in the "natural" position, with the wife on her back and the husband on top. All other positions were considered "unnatural."

Many religious people thought that only the lowest type of people engaged in oral–genital sexual activity or anal intercourse. Homosexuality was considered an abomination and punishable by death.

A belief in witchcraft was another means of controlling sexual behavior. Strong feelings, especially lust and passion, were believed to arise from evil spirits, and because women (and not men) inspired lust, some religious leaders saw women as witches or agents of the devil. Witches were tortured, ostensibly to drive the devil out of them, or killed. Bewitchment was said to account for the mysterious and overwhelming emotional effects that women had on men, sometimes driving them to irrational acts. Witch trials were held throughout the Middle Ages, particularly during the 15th century (Sadock, Kaplan, & Freedman, 1973).

In 17th-century England, the Puritan influence was responsible for legislation to prevent amusements such as dancing, singing, and the theater. Women were treated as prostitutes if they wore long hair or makeup. On Sundays any activities not related to worship were banned.

By the end of the 18th century, sexual behavior was subdued and spontaneity inhibited. People conducted their lives very discreetly. Harsh negative attitudes toward same-gender sexual behavior were common during this time, and many people who practiced that behavior were reportedly put to death. So strong were fears and feelings during the period that people who asked for leniency for those convicted of sodomy (which includes almost any sexual behavior one wishes to prohibit) were themselves in danger of persecution. Eighteenth-century studies of sexuality emphasized physiology and generally concluded that excessive sexual activity—specifically, expelling of semen to excess—had debilitating physical consequences.

In the 19th century, during Victorian times, sexual drives were generally repressed. Though it was believed that men had natural and spontaneous sexual desires, women supposedly had dormant sex drives unless subjected to undue excitation. Children, it was believed, had no sexual feelings.

Much was done to protect the people of Victorian times from sexual arousal. Sexual references in literature and general conversation were suppressed, as were most sexual feelings. Masturbation, a particularly repudiated activity, was called the "secret sin," "self-pollution," and the "solitary vice." Devices were even developed to place around the male's penis at night to prevent **spermatorrhea** (more commonly called **nocturnal emissions** or **wet dreams**) (Figure 1.1).

spermatorrhea (wet dreams, or nocturnal emissions)
Emission of semen during sleep.

In the early 20th century, as conservative morality about sexuality diminished and people argued that sexual expression was natural and normal, some secular attempts were made to legislate sexual moral-

(a)   (b)   (c)

FIGURE **1.1** Devices designed to prevent wet dreams. One device caused a bell to ring when erection occurred (a). For some devices, no bell was needed (b and c).

ity. This resulted in censorship, prohibition, and the revival of old statutes against certain sexual behaviors, such as homosexuality, oral–genital relations, and sodomy.

Theoretically, in the United States there is a separation of church and state, but legal debates about such subjects as abortion, access to sexual information and services, homosexuality, and other sexual behaviors have prompted some people to wonder about that separation.

Conception

Much of our information about prehistoric people is obtained by analyzing the remains of their art. In addition, we can make inferences about primitive cultures from the art that exists today. Prehistoric cave paintings indicate that more than 30,000 years ago sexuality was an important part of culture. Some of these stone engravings suggest human intercourse, and some show women and men with exaggerated body parts.

Despite the attention to sexuality in their art and perhaps their religion, prehistoric people apparently did not understand its role in reproduction. Consequently, theorists believe that a number of explanations for childbirth existed. One notion may have

been that children were sent by ancestral deities; sexual intercourse was reserved solely for pleasure. Or a woman became pregnant by sitting over a fire on which she had roasted a fish received from the prospective father. An Australian tribe believed that a woman conceived by eating human flesh. Some cultures thought it was possible for a man to become pregnant (Tannahill, 1980). Some of these theories might seem humorous, but they are really no more peculiar, or at least no more wrong, than such modern superstitions as "You can't get pregnant if you do it only once." By the time of the first written records, however, it appears that humans were aware that they played some part in reproduction, even if they did not know how.

Throughout recorded history, many theories and myths about conception existed. For example, Aristotle theorized that the human fetus resulted from the mixture of menstrual blood and seminal fluid. One hundred years before Aristotle, the Greek poet Aeschylus believed that a child was conceived by a male alone (Where do babies come from?, 1987).

The microscope allowed scientists to see sperm for the first time. In 1677, the Dutch naturalist Anton van Leeuwenhoek described the human sperm discovered by one of his students. Many scientists, however, refused to accept that sperm could be responsible for creating human life. Other scientists claimed they had seen tiny humans inside sperm. This thinking led to the belief that a tiny, fully formed person would not grow until he or she reached the female "nest." At the same time other scientists, known as **ovists**, claimed that the preformed baby was contained in the female and the sperm served only to activate its development. It was not until 1875 that it was demonstrated that the sperm penetrates and combines with the egg (Where do babies come from?, 1987).

> **ovist**
> Adherent to the 17th-century belief that the preformed baby was contained within the female body and that the male's sperm simply activated its development.

It is impossible to know the overall effect of the accurate understanding of conception; however, it would seem that such knowledge was useful to both males and females. The understanding that sexual intercourse could result in conception must have influenced sexual behavior and made it possible to

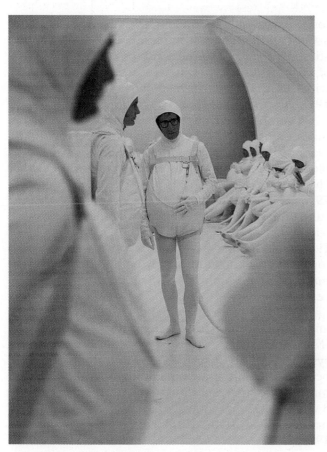

Woody Allen's farcical treatment of sperm cells in *Everything You Always Wanted to Know about Sex…* reflects what was once thought true. When sperm cells were discovered by a magnifying glass in 1677, scientists believed that they saw tiny men (called *animalcules*) inside sperm cells. Other scientists even claimed to see microscopic horses in horse sperm!

have at least some control over whether or not to procreate. The control of reproduction is possible today; throughout most of history it was not.

Contraception

Although the process of reproduction was not understood until relatively recently, **contraception**—methods employed to prevent pregnancy—is as old as recorded history. More than 4,000 years ago Egyptian women used medicated tampons as contraceptives. Lint, moistened in a mixture of acacia tips ground with honey, was placed into the vagina. Many other practices, some of them dangerous, were used in the centuries that followed (*The ecology of birth control*, 1971). Among these were inserting spongy or absorbent fabrics into the vagina or mixing crocodile dung with a paste and inserting the mixture into the vagina. It is said that Persian women placed lemon-soaked sponges in the vagina to prevent pregnancy. It is interesting to note that these methods have some merit. Most of them attempted to form a barrier or alter the acid–base relationship within the vagina. In fact, many of today's contraceptive methods are based on these same principles.

> **contraception**
> Means of preventing pregnancy in spite of sexual intercourse.

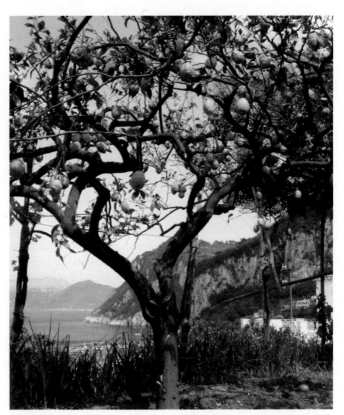

Humans have sought and used contraceptives from the present day to ancient times, when ingredients ranged from lemons to crocodile dung.

The first modern contraceptive device, which was eventually called the condom, appeared in the mid-16th century. It was designed to protect the wearer against the plague of syphilis then spreading throughout Europe. The condom was first made of fine linen, then of animal intestine, and finally of rubber. Even though its original use was for protection from disease, its potential as a contraceptive was quickly noticed (*The ecology of birth control*, 1971).

In the middle of the 19th century, the German physician Mensinga perfected the rubber diaphragm. He believed that women should have equal rights with men and that their lives would be improved by controlling the number of children they conceived. In the United States, the diaphragm was generally unknown until after World War I. Although condoms were not as effective as diaphragms, and although they depended on the male's willingness to use them, they were manufactured in great quantities at the end of the 19th century and thus became cheaper and more available (Bullough, 1976a, 651). Today, 5.5 billion condoms are manufactured in the United States each year.

The idea of the intrauterine device (IUD) was borrowed from an ancient practice of camel drivers, who put a round stone (or an apricot pit, according to some accounts) into the uterus of a female camel to prevent pregnancy on long trips. During the 1920s, a German gynecologist modernized the idea by substituting a ring of surgical silk or silver (*The ecology of birth control*, 1971). It was not until experiments with IUDs were performed in Israel and Japan in 1959, however, that their use became widespread.

A number of effective spermicides appeared on the market at the end of the 19th century. The early ones, marketed in a suppository form, probably worked by blocking the cervix with an oily film. Numerous other chemicals soon appeared on the market (Bullough, 1976a, 651). Foams and jellies were introduced in the early 20th century. Research on an oral contraceptive was widespread in the 1950s, but it was not until 1960 that the first oral contraceptive was approved for public use. It can probably be said that this event marked the beginning of the modern era of contraception.

It was 30 years later, in 1990, that the U.S. Food and Drug Administration approved levonorgestrel (Norplant). This hormonal contraceptive implant system was six capsules 34 mm long, inserted beneath the skin of a woman's upper arm. Its release marked the first time long-term (in this case, up to 5 years) hormonal control of conception was available in the United States (FDA OKs hormonal implant, 1990).

Not necessarily considered a form of contraception, abortion is a means of controlling births. Abortion early in pregnancy was legal in ancient China and Europe. In the 13th century the Roman Catholic church indicated that the soul developed 40 days after conception in males and 90 days after conception in females, and abortion was allowed within those intervals. In the late 1860s the Catholic church declared that life begins at conception; that doctrine led to its abortion ban (O'Keefe, 1995).

Early American law allowed abortion until the woman felt fetal movement, but during the 1860s abortion became illegal in the United States except to save the woman's life. In addition to the religious beliefs of some people, reasons for this included health problems related to crude abortion procedures, the belief that population growth was needed for economic reasons, and maybe a male-dominated political system's response to more women seeking independence and equality (Sheeran, 1987). It was not until 1973 that the U.S. Supreme Court in its famous *Roe* v. *Wade* decision legalized a woman's right to decide to terminate her pregnancy before the fetus could survive independently of the woman's body. Debates about this issue continue.

Gender Roles

"The paramount destiny and mission of women are to fulfill the noble and benign offices of wife and mother. This is the law of the Creator." Words of a time long past? Not quite. This is actually an excerpt from a Supreme Court opinion rendered in the first case tried under the Fourteenth Amendment in 1873. The court's decision upheld the denial of the right of women to practice law (Bardes, Shelley, & Schmidt, 1998).

Historically, the role of the woman as a sexual partner has been to satisfy male needs. In India, for example, women were viewed as nothing without men. In the West, women who enjoyed sexual activity dared not speak of it publicly because of the severe penalties for doing so. Throughout the ages women were viewed as property of men (Spielvogel, 1997). In most societies, if a woman committed adultery, was raped, or lost her virginity, she was considered damaged property. A woman's father or husband could expect to gain compensation for this damage, or, in the case of adultery, he might even kill her and her partner if they were caught (Bullough, 1976b, 677–679).

In many societies men enjoyed a status vastly superior to that of women. This status can probably be accounted for by (1) men's greater physical strength, (2) women's repeated pregnancies in the absence of reliable contraceptive methods, and (3) the ideology that disparity in male and female roles was divinely ordained. Men used their greater physi-

Myth vs Fact

Myth: Open discussion about sexuality will have negative results—people will be more likely to be sexually permissive.
Fact: Healthy communication about sexuality will help people develop into sexually healthy adults—open discussions do not have negative results.

Myth: The relatively open attitudes in thinking about sexuality in Sweden have resulted in higher rates of teen pregnancy and sexually transmitted infections.
Fact: Swedish attitudes and practices related to sexuality have resulted in lower rates of teen pregnancy and sexually transmitted infections.

Myth: Abortion has been illegal throughout most of the history of the United States.
Fact: Early American law allowed abortion until a woman felt fetal movement. In the 1860s abortion became illegal in the United States, but in 1973 the Supreme Court legalized a woman's right to terminate her pregnancy.

Myth: What is sexually arousing to people is very much the same regardless of the culture.
Fact: In different cultures the idea of what is sexually arousing varies a great deal.

cal strength to trap animals and handle livestock, to defend themselves, and to intimidate women. Because women were often pregnant and spent much of their time caring for children, little time was left to alter their inferior status. Those who felt male and female roles had a divine origin saw any attempts to change these roles as antireligious (Murstein, 1974, 566).

The ancient Greeks believed that men were primarily mental and spiritual in their makeup and that women were primarily physical and earthy. Because the Greeks believed the mind and body were separate entities, this meant men had a higher nature and deserved greater privileges. Several centuries later, however, Jesus insisted on the basic equality of the sexes. He opposed Jewish divorce law, which allowed women to be disposed of as property (Nelson, 1978).

Throughout medieval times, women were thought to be inferior to men. Their motives were suspect, they were thought to be sinful, and their female functions were belittled. Some still believed Aristotle's earlier claim that the female was little more than an incomplete male. Both religious and scientific thinking seemed to support these ideas (Bullough, 1976b).

In the early 1800s there were more male children than female children in the western states and territories of the United States. Some researchers have thought this was because nutrition and health of young females were neglected because their labor was not as economically valued. Others have indicated that this imbalance simply occurred because more boys were born in, survived childhood in, or moved to western regions (Courtwright, 1990). This presents another example in which it is difficult to determine the real reasons for the situation.

However, the mid- to late 1800s and the early 1900s witnessed many advances in the status of women in the United States. After the first major organized meeting on the rights of women in 1848, there was a sort of legal emancipation, an opening of work opportunities, and an ideological acceptance of the equality of the sexes. Actual changes in behavior, however, did not keep pace with this verbal acceptance. The average woman was probably more interested in receiving greater respect and consideration, and in receiving the right to vote, than in having equal professional rights. Most articles advocating the causes important to women today were written by highly educated men and women, and probably the majority of Americans were not even aware of these new ideas (Murstein, 1974, 379). Nonetheless, the seeds of the women's rights movement were planted.

The women's suffrage movement began in the late 19th century with the goal of obtaining the right to vote for women. The passage in 1920 of the Nineteenth Amendment to the U.S. Constitution guaranteed women the right to vote. World War II created an environment for increased gender equality. As men were required to leave home for military duty, thousands of women left their traditional roles in the home and took paying jobs for the first time. It was not until the 1960s, however, after many postwar marriages, the baby boom, and continued disappointment about women's roles, that a new movement for gender equality became evident.

Some people had thought that the ratification of the Nineteenth Amendment would end the struggle for women's rights, but this had not happened. In 1963 the Equal Pay Act, which stated that women must receive pay equal to that of men if they perform the same work, was enacted. In 1964 women were included in the protections of the Civil Rights Act. This made it clear that equality of opportunity for women was endorsed by the federal government (Degler, 1980, 442). Still, women today earn an average of less than 90 cents for every dollar men earn.

In 1963 Betty Friedan published *The Feminine Mystique,* which helped create a widespread movement for women's rights. She urged women to

Women did not get the right to vote in the United States until 1920.

make a life for themselves in addition to their homes and families. The case for women's equality was also championed in a number of other books. In 1966 Friedan organized the National Organization for Women (NOW), which has consistently advocated women's rights. By 1970 a number of other organizations that pushed for women's equality were formed, including the Women's Equity Action League and the Women's Political Caucus. So successful was the women's movement that it has been considered "possibly the most lasting legacy of the . . . period of protests" (Degler, 1980, 446).

In recent years many issues related to women's roles have been raised. Women now work in a variety of jobs previously thought to be only for males, and there are more women in positions of authority. Discrimination against pregnant women in the workplace has lessened, many women delay having children to pursue other interests, and there is an increased acceptance of child care while women work. Varied opinions about women's roles continue. Studies about gender and leadership style, gender differences in work, family conflict, gender and the influence of achievement evaluations, gender in the college classroom, among others, continue to provide reams of information about women and their roles and status. But whether we have achieved equality between the sexes is still a matter of debate.

■ Thinking Critically About Human Sexuality

You have probably observed that, when it comes to many topics related to health and sexuality, there are "experts" everywhere. The concept of critical thinking is important to being able to judge the accuracy of what these people say as well as lots of other information you hear related to sexuality. In this case, the word *critical* does not mean being negative or criticizing people or things. It means being careful and somewhat analytical.

In essence, then, **critical thinking** is

> **critical thinking**
> Thinking that avoids blind acceptance of conclusions or arguments and closely examines all assumptions.

Multicultural
DIMENSIONS

Pregnancy and Health

When speaking of culture, sociologists generally refer to the "learned values, beliefs, norms, behaviors, and even material objects that are passed from one generation to the next." Within the culture of the United States, however, are many subcultures—groups of people with shared values within the overall culture. Each subculture has a distinctive way of looking at life that sets it off from the prevalent culture. In the United States, these groups may be defined by ethnicity, age, religion, sexuality, geographical location, and national origin. The Multicultural Dimensions boxes look at varied subcultures within the United States.

The first multicultural issue we explore relates to teen pregnancy in developing countries. In January 2009, UNICEF released its annual report entitled *The State of the World's Children, 2009*. The report pointed out that women in the world's least developed countries are 300 times more likely to die in childbirth or from pregnancy-related complications than are women in developed countries. Put another way, women in developing countries have a 1 in 76 chance of dying from pregnancy or childbirth-related complications, compared with a 1 in 8,000 chance for women in developed countries. A child born in a developing country is almost 14 times more likely to die during the first month of life than a child born in a developed one. Approximately 70,000 young women ages 15 to 19 die in childbirth annually.

It is obvious that better medical intervention is a key to improving the health of mothers and their children. But more than just medical intervention is required: There also needs to be a change in how women are viewed and how things get done to really make a difference. For example, it is essential to have a stable environment that empowers women and respects their rights. Educating girls and women is one of the most fundamental ways to improve maternal and newborn health and benefits both families and societies. Essential interventions will be guaranteed only within the context of improved education and the abolition of discrimination.

Source: The state of the world's children, 2009. New York: UNICEF, 2009.

---

thinking that prevents blindly accepting conclusions or arguments (or headlines) and instead closely examines all assumptions. This includes carefully evaluating existing evidence and cautiously assessing all conclusions (Baron, 1998).

Critical thinking is like scientific methods you may have used in other classes. In practice, it involves guidelines such as these (Baron, 1998):

1. Never jump to conclusions; gather as much information as you can before making up your mind about any issue.

2. Keep an open mind; do not let your existing views blind you to information or new conclusions.

3. Always ask "How?" as in "How was this evidence gathered?"

4. Be skeptical; always wonder about *why* someone is making an argument, offering a conclusion, or trying to persuade you.

5. Never be stampeded into accepting some view or position by your own emotions—or by arguments and appeals designed to play on your emotions.

Not every guideline will apply in every situation, but the important goal is to develop a style of thinking using as many of the guidelines as seems appropriate in a given situation.

Correlation Versus Causation

A research study found that for people 60 years and older, the 62% who drank coffee still enjoyed active sex lives, compared with only 37% of those who were not coffee drinkers (Plotnik, 1993). Does coffee lead to a better sex life for seniors? Or are the two events just coincidental? The study shows a **correlation**, a relationship between two events. But it does not show a **causation**, a relationship in which one event causes the other.

> **correlation**
> A relationship between two events.
> **causation**
> A relationship in which one event causes another event to occur.

It is easy to show that a correlation exists, but correlations do not show cause and effect. There is a high correlation between the winning conference of the Super Bowl and the stock market: When the NFC wins, the stock market goes up in most years; when the AFC wins, the market goes down in most years. In fact, from 1972 to 1985 there was a perfect correlation. However, no scientific study is needed to understand that the Super Bowl does not cause the stock market to go up or down.

Returning to the coffee example, perhaps people older than 60 years old who are in good health enjoy both coffee and sexual activity. However, there does not appear to be a causal link between caffeine use and sexual activity. In contrast, a study showing a correlation between the drug Viagra and an active sex life would appear to have a causal link. So, correlations can sometimes help predict behavior and point to possible causes of behavior. Further studies can help validate the causation.

Being a Good Consumer of Sexual Information

We are bombarded with information—and misinformation—about sexuality issues. In fact, most best-selling newsstand periodicals lure readers with information about "new" sexual techniques or sex surveys. It is important to keep the principles of the scientific method in mind when reading popular literature.

Consider a study that garnered a great deal of media attention: The medical anthropologists Soma Grismaijer and Sidney Ross Singer (2002) surveyed 4,700 women and concluded that their odds of having breast cancer increased the longer women wore bras. Their hypothesis was that the cinching effect of a bra suppresses the lymphatic system below a woman's armpit, blocking an internal network of vessels that are intended to flush toxic wastes from the body. Over time, these toxins accumulate in the breast tissue and create an environment in which cells can turn cancerous.

The results of the survey appear to confirm their hypothesis: Of women who wore bras 24 hours a day, in three of four breast cancer developed; of women who wore bras less than 12 hours a day, in one in seven breast cancer developed; of women who rarely wore bras, in only 1 in 168 did breast cancer develop (Joseph, 1998).

The study appears to have found a *correlation* between length of bra-wearing time and breast cancer. However, few medical scientists would agree that a *causation* exists; many would even question the correlation. First, consider the design of the survey on which the conclusion was based: Participants were not randomly selected, following accepted statistical guidelines. For example, women who have had breast cancer might be more willing to participate in a breast-cancer study. Nor were participants questioned about preexisting breast-cancer risks. In addition, participants answered only 12 questions regarding their bra-wearing habits.

A scientific approach to the correlation of bra use and breast cancer would be to find a large, randomly selected sample of women who wear bras for specific lengths of time each day. The women would need to be prescreened for breast-cancer risk and would need to undergo medical exams before participating. Family history of cancer, age, race, body mass, weight, diet, exercise, alcohol or drug consumption, and other factors would have to be controlled in some manner. A matching control group (not selected by bra-wearing time) would add further validity. The study could follow the women across a long period, perhaps 15 to 25 years.

Thus a critical review of the study quickly calls into doubt the causal factor between bra use and breast cancer. Even the correlation appears to be contrived. However, it does open the door for further studies.

A final point about the scientific method should be made here: When this study first appeared in popular print media, the information provided varied by the source. News media presented the story as provocative and quirky but with powerful opposition voiced by medical doctors and cancer specialists. But one popular "health" magazine reported the study in a way that suggested a causal link—and placed an ad on the opposite page for a "health drug" claiming to lower risk of breast cancer. Always remember to think about why someone is publishing the study. In this case, it was clearly done to help sell a product.

■ Why Study Sexuality?

There are many reasons for studying human sexuality, including obtaining accurate sexual knowledge, clarifying personal values, improving sexual decision making, learning the relationship between human sexuality and personal well-being, and exploring how the varied dimensions of human sexuality influence one's sexuality.

Sexual Knowledge

A major reason for studying human sexuality is to acquire a sound foundation of sexual knowledge. Only knowledge can dispel sexual myths, superstitions, and misinformation that block understanding, inhibit communication, and create confusion. Correct information lays the groundwork for sexual decision making. The greater your knowledge, the more likely you are to take responsibility for your sexual health. Studies have found that college students want specific factual information (probably pertaining to a sexual encounter), as well as the answer to the age-old question, "Am I normal?" (Caron & Bertran, 1988).

The issue of sexual and physical normality underscores the psychological dimensions of human sexuality. It is normal to wonder whether your appearance and/or sexual desires are normal. Many men worry about the size and shape of their penis, and women often worry about the size and shape of their breasts. Learning about the wide variety in appearances, as you will in the anatomy and physiology chapters (Chapters 4 and 5), may help you feel better about yourself. Learning more about sexuality can often increase your sense of personal worth, or **self-esteem**.

self-esteem
Sense of personal worth.

Factual knowledge can also help you interpret sociocultural traditions or myths. History is filled with examples of myths about the biological nature of sexuality. Aristotle, for example, thought that menstrual fluid was the substance from which the embryo was formed, a belief held for centuries. Leonardo da Vinci's anatomical drawings show a tube running from the uterus to the breasts of a woman, depicting the common belief that the menstrual fluid that did not flow during pregnancy was diverted to the breasts to make milk—this in spite of the fact that he had dissected female cadavers and certainly never saw such a tube! The U.S. culture is by no means free of sexual myths, as you will discover throughout this text.

A major issue relating to sexual knowledge involves how to engage in "safer sex." Which activities can lead to the transmission of STIs and HIV? Is your partner, for example, in a high-risk group? What can be done to lower the risk of transmitting STIs and HIV? (These questions will be answered in later chapters.) Does your partner share your knowledge—and concern—about such issues? If not, should you be willing to engage in sexual activity with that person?

Personal Values

A second reason for studying sexuality is to clarify personal sexual **values**, those beliefs to which we attach the most worth. By exploring your own dimensions of human sexuality, you may come to understand the origins and nature of your sexual values, as well as the values of others.

values
Those beliefs to which we attach the most worth.

Remember Lisa from our opening story. She began to understand how sexuality fit into her personal values, especially those involving her family. The values that her family and culture held were very important to Lisa, and she fretted over the prospect of becoming an "unmember" of her family, were she to become pregnant outside marriage.

Responsible Sexual Decision Making

A third reason for studying sexuality is to improve your sexual decision-making skills. Most people have had some sexual experience. A large majority of college students have had sexual intercourse, and almost all have participated in some form of sexual activity. But experience alone does not necessarily provide wisdom or skill in sexual decision making. The study of sexuality provides a sound foundation of sexual information, promotes an understanding of sexual attitudes, and examines a broad range of sexual issues.

For example, assume you were dating Lisa in the opening story. Without an understanding of the many social and cultural factors that influence her sexuality, you would find it hard to understand her

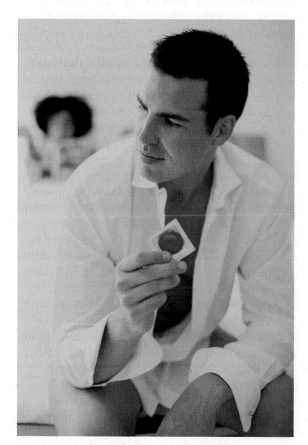
Many values influence sexual decision making.

feelings. Her communication style is restricted by her cultural background, which discourages openly discussing feelings and seeking psychological counseling. Lack of understanding of why Lisa holds in her feelings could lead to a deterioration of your relationship.

Dr. Drew, the dry-witted host of *Loveline*, a radio and TV talk show that answers viewers' sexuality questions, often suggests that listeners think about their actions before they get involved in sexual situations. A frequently occurring situation on the show is that of having sexual activity with a roommate's lover, which callers often claim "just happened." Dr. Drew responds that, in most cases, it does not just happen—the two parties consciously flirt, possibly dress enticingly, and in the end must find a time and place to be alone. Dr. Drew suggests that had the parties stopped to think about the actions they were taking, they could have made the sexually responsible decision not to engage in sexual activity.

A Decision-Making Model
A simple but formal model of the decision-making process consists of the following steps (Bruess & Richardson, 1995).

1. *Recognition.* Only with the recognition of an issue can a decision be made. For example, a couple who consider engaging in sexual intercourse need to recognize the risk of pregnancy, transmission of STIs or HIV, and overstepping of a partner's personal dimensions.

    The best decision making requires defining the issue as precisely as possible: For example, which forms of contraception are acceptable? Which forms are unacceptable? What can be done to promote safer sexual activity? How does my partner feel about this? Which physiological or cultural dimensions might influence my partner's decisions?

2. *Evaluation.* Having recognized a need to make decisions, it is time to gather relevant information, analyze the possible choices, and decide on the best alternative. For example, the latex condom might be a choice for contraception and lowering of the possibility of STI transmission. But the condom also has a lower rate of contraception effectiveness than some other methods. Another choice might be using a contraceptive method with a higher effectiveness rate—such as the pill—combined with a latex condom for STI protection. Further consideration might be necessary if one person is unwilling to use contraceptives because of

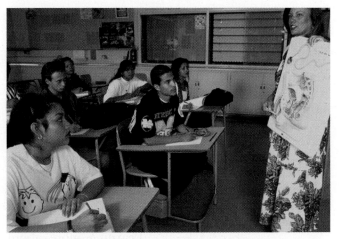
Sound knowledge influences sexual decision making.

religious beliefs. Or perhaps one partner has an allergy to latex condoms (in which case polyurethane condoms could be substituted). The decision to remain abstinent could also be discussed.

3. *Implementation.* When a decision has been reached, the plan needs to be put into action. A decision to combine the pill with latex condoms is not effective unless you can delay intercourse until the woman has received a prescription for the pill and taken it for about a month and the man has purchased latex condoms (and learned how to use them).

4. *Review.* After putting the decision into practice, there should be a periodic review. Are the desired results being achieved, or should another alternative be tried? Perhaps after making the decision, something new is learned about the issues that raises questions about the choice. For example, Lisa's pregnancy scare would likely make her seek out a more effective contraceptive method. If so, the decision-making process can be started again. In fact, you will find yourself renewing the decision-making process throughout your life, according to how your circumstances change. The opening story of the contraception chapter (Chapter 7) illustrates the changes in one woman's contraceptive use throughout her life.

Sexual Health and Wellness

Finally, sexual education can contribute to safer sexual behavior. Given that some sexual behaviors can result in pregnancies and/or the spread of STIs

Communication
DIMENSIONS

**Talking About
Your Human
Sexuality Class**

Expect to find a great deal of interest when you tell people you are taking a class in human sexuality. Inevitably, many of your friends, colleagues, neighbors, and family members will ask, "What are you learning?" How you answer that question says a great deal about your tactfulness, how people perceive your knowledge, and how interestingly and humorously you can present delicate information. We have dealt with this question for years, and here are some suggestions:

- Be careful talking about sexual information at work. One *Seinfeld* episode revolved around Jerry's being unable to remember a new girlfriend's name—except that it rhymed with a female body part. Eventually, he remembers her name is Dolores—which rhymes (sort of) with clitoris. One man embarrassed a sexually inhibited female colleague by describing the episode at work. The woman, who did not know the term *clitoris,* was further embarrassed when the man showed her the definition in a dictionary (in front of several colleagues). She complained to human resources, and he was fired. He sued the company and won a settlement, which is currently in the appeals process. Do not give people sexual information they do not want to hear! As illustrated in the *Seinfeld* case, it is best to change subjects—or even apologize—if someone is uncomfortable with what you are saying. Watch for

nonverbal cues as well. Pressing a point may cost you friends.
- Do not go into detail. Use the KISS method (Keep It Simple and Sincere). If you find the human sexual response cycle (Chapter 6) interesting, discuss it in general terms: "I was surprised to learn that males and females have the same physiological response to sexual activity." If asked further questions, simply arrange for the person to borrow your book.
- Do not gross people out. In general, people do not want to hear sordid stories relating to sexuality. Information on atypical sexual behaviors (In Focus: Alternative Sexual Behavior), female genital mutilation (Chapter 4), or sexual slavery (Chapter 17) is not usually dinnertime conversation. Recognize diversity. In fact, many people will be highly offended by hearing such information.
- Do not be afraid to say something in a straightforward manner. Show comfort with the subject matter by using sexual terminology in a polite, accurate manner. No one will be offended by the use of the word *penis* or *vagina* if used in context—especially if you are answering someone's question.
- Do not lecture. No matter how hard you try (or how sincere you are), you simply will not change friends' sexual behavior by telling them what they are doing wrong.

(including HIV), it is important for people of all ages to understand which practices can result in safer sexual behavior and to incorporate such practices into personal relationships.

Note that although we use the term *safer sex,* no sexual activity can be deemed *perfectly* safe. Although knowing a partner's sexual history, using latex condoms consistently, and avoiding certain sexual behaviors can *reduce* your risk of STIs and HIV, they do not *eliminate* the risk. Condoms can break or be improperly used. Your partner may not wish to disclose a complete sexual history (especially embarrassing or abusive situations). Alcohol can also get in the way of judgment.

Following safer sexual practices does not end with youth. The number of older Americans with HIV/AIDS

is rising steadily. As of 2009, 28% of those diagnosed with HIV were 45 years and older (Centers for Disease Control and Prevention, 2009).

Practicing safer sexual behavior can promote sexual health and wellness, as well as improve self-esteem. The failure to practice safer sexual behavior can result in physiological, psychological, and social trauma. Although many STIs are "curable," some (such as genital herpes) can only be controlled. Knowing that you have herpes or genital warts may lead to lower self-esteem and a reluctance to seek out partners. Contracting HIV would mean a lifetime of treatment to prevent contracting AIDS. An unwanted pregnancy can have devastating results for both the parents and the child. For Lisa, pregnancy outside marriage could have resulted in losing her family.

Throughout this text, we emphasize safer sexual behaviors. We discuss the aspects of safer sexual behavior with each form of contraception in Chapter 7 and with each alternative behavior discussed in a minichapter.

So how do we know if someone is sexually healthy? The Alberta (Canada) Society for the Promotion of Sexual Health lists 17 criteria for sexually healthy individuals. Among the criteria are: appreciate their own bodies, avoid exploitative relationships, interact with both genders in appropriate and respectful ways, demonstrate tolerance for people with different values, decide what is personally "right" and act upon these values, talk with a partner about sexual activity before it occurs, and seek further information about sexuality as needed.

Service–Learning Projects in Your Community

While we focus on how you can develop a healthy and sexually responsible lifestyle, we recognize that all of us also have a responsibility to contribute to the health of our communities. We live in a college community, and in a city, town, or village. We live in a state and in this country. And, of course, we are part of a global community as well. With the knowledge you learn in your sexuality course and by reading this book, you have a unique opportunity to contribute to the sexual health of the communities with which you are associated. One of the best ways to do that is through service–learning. **Service–learning** is an educational method that involves students applying what they learn in their coursework in the community so as to contribute to the welfare of that community. For example, after studying the effects of gangster rap CDs on the sexual attitudes of young people, you might choose to write to local government representatives advocating that warning labels be more explicit on CDs of this nature. Or you might volunteer at a rape crisis center. As a result of our commitment to you, and to help you organize to meet your commitment to your communities, we provide suggestions for sexuality-related service–learning activities on the web site for this book.

service–learning
Educational method that involves students applying what they learn in their coursework in the community to contribute to that community's welfare.

Exploring the
DIMENSIONS
of Human Sexuality

Our feelings, attitudes, and beliefs regarding sexuality are influenced by our internal and external environments. Go to sexuality.jbpub.com/dimensions/4e to learn more about the biological, psychological, and sociological factors that affect your sexuality.

Sociocultural Factors
- Socioeconomic status
- Laws
- Religion
- Culture
- Ethnic heritage
- Media and ad information
- Family, neighbors, and friends
- Ethics

Biological Factors
- Gender
- Genetics
- Reproduction
- Fertility control
- Sexual arousal and response
- Physiological cycles and changes
- Physical appearance
- Growth and development

Psychological Factors
- Emotions
- Experience
- Self-concept
- Motivation
- Expressiveness
- Learned attitudes and behaviors
- Body image

CASE STUDY

Many factors influence our sexuality. Throughout the text we will help you explore the many dimensions of human sexuality. Each chapter will explore how these dimensions interact in a specific instance. For example, consider your physical appearance. At first glance, it appears to be a biological factor, set by genetics. But your body image, or self-concept of your appearance, is psychological. Sociocultural factors also come into play—your perception is influenced by the culture in which you live and conveyed by the media that surround you.

Summary

- Sexuality is part of our personality, and it involves the interrelationship of biological, psychological, and sociocultural dimensions.

- Sociocultural influences include religious influences, multicultural influences, ethical influences, and political influences.

- The sexual revolution had many influences on present thinking about human sexuality.

- Throughout history there have been many attempts to control sexual behavior. Most of these efforts can be seen in the moral and legal codes of the time.

- Throughout recorded history, many theories and myths about conception have existed. It was not until 1875 that it was demonstrated that the sperm penetrates and combines with the egg.

- Methods employed to prevent pregnancy have been used for thousands of years. The condom first appeared in the mid-16th century.

- Abortion in early pregnancy was legal in ancient China and Europe. In 1973 the U.S. Supreme Court legalized a woman's right to decide to terminate her pregnancy.

- There have been changes in gender roles throughout the centuries. In recent years many issues related to women's roles continue to be raised.

- It is important to use sound critical thinking skills when making decisions related to human sexuality.

- Studying human sexuality is important to obtain accurate sexual knowledge, clarify personal values, improve sexual decision making, understand the relationship between human sexuality and personal well-being, and explore how the varied dimensions of human sexuality influence one's sexuality.

Discussion Questions

1. List the three main dimensions of sexuality and their subdivisions, and give examples of each.

2. Trace the historical aspects of human sexuality, including the sexual revolution and the changing roles of gender and culture.

3. Explain a method for critical thinking, and differentiate between correlation and causation. Give examples to back up your answer.

4. Explain the main reasons for studying human sexuality.

Application Questions

Reread the chapter-opening story and answer the following questions.

1. If Lisa were pregnant, what advice would you give her? Consider Lisa's sexual dimensions, including the reaction of her family, her religion, and her communication style.

2. If you were Lisa's lover, how might you respond to the situation? To answer this question, you need to reconcile your sexual dimensions with Lisa's.

3. Do all Korean Americans have the same set of sexual dimensions? How might such dimensions differ, depending on age? Length of time in the United States? Geographic location? Socioeconomic status?

Critical Thinking Questions

1. Consider your own sexuality. Write about how each of the three dimensions affects you. Which has the greatest effect on you? The least? Explain your answers.

2. Use the decision-making model to decide whether to engage in a sexual activity that you have not yet done. Having thought the issue through, would you proceed? Which precautions might you take to promote safer sexual behavior?

Critical Thinking Case

Should an Artificial Womb Be Used?

People often need to focus on ethical questions related to conception. For example, an article in the *New York Times Magazine* by Perri Klass (September 29, 1996, 117–119) reports that Japanese researchers developed a technique called *extrauterine fetal incubation* (EUFI). They took goat fetuses, supplied them with oxygenated blood, and suspended them in incubators that contained artificial amniotic fluid (the fluid that surrounds a fetus in a pregnant woman's uterus) heated to body temperature. So far, the researchers have been able to keep goat fetuses alive for 3 weeks, but they are confident they can extend the length of time and ultimately be able to apply this technique to humans. When they do, we will have an artificial womb. This will allow us to have more control over conception and birth than ever before.

If it were ever possible, should an artificial womb be used for human pregnancies? Which circumstances would warrant the use of an artificial womb for human births? Consider the case in which a woman had fertile eggs but had had her uterus removed as a result of cancer. Should she be able to use EUFI to have a baby? What about the female executive who wants a family but worries that a pregnancy (and postpartum leave) will sideline her career? What about the couple who would otherwise use a human surrogate womb?

Consider further social consequences: Should insurance companies pay for the cost of using the artificial womb? Should the government allot Medicaid money for the socioeconomically deprived who wish to use such a service? Or should such a service be available only to the wealthy?

Exploring Personal Dimensions

Sexuality and Human Relations
A number of internal and external forces in your life influence the decisions you make regarding sexual behavior. What you do may be in harmony with some of these forces and in conflict with others.

Directions
Give a value to the following forces in your life as they pertain to your sexual behavior (i.e., what makes you choose to be sexually active or what makes you refrain from sexual activity). If you are married, apply this tool to a specific sexual behavior such as your degree of fidelity to your spouse or your degree of sexual activity with your spouse.

a = a major force influencing my sexual behavior
b = a moderate force influencing my sexual behavior
c = an insignificant force influencing my sexual behavior

1. Religious influence   a b c
2. Family influence   a b c
3. How it feels when we kiss and hug a b c
4. My own self-image (how I think I look to others) a b c
5. My sense of right or wrong   a b c
6. Radio, television, or movies   a b c
7. How it feels to touch someone   a b c
8. How I learned to act   a b c
9. The way I feel inside   a b c
10. Literature (books, magazines) or music a b c
11. Pleasure   a b c
12. My judgment   a b c
13. My sense of what I should and should not do a b c
14. Friends' influence   a b c
15. Physical stimulation   a b c
16. Introversion or extroversion (how outgoing I am) a b c
17. My morals or values   a b c
18. The expectations/relationship I have with boyfriend/girlfriend (for marrieds, consider friends other than spouse) a b c
19. Fear of, or anticipation of, pregnancy a b c
20. Desire to feel good about myself a b c

Scoring
a = 3   b = 2   c = 1

Total values as follows from top to bottom of the four columns

Column A	Column B	Column C	Column D
1. ____	2. ____	3. ____	4. ____
5. ____	6. ____	7. ____	8. ____
9. ____	10. ____	11. ____	12. ____
13. ____	14. ____	15. ____	16. ____
17. ____	18. ____	19. ____	20. ____
Totals ____	____	____	____

Interpretation
Column A represents the degree to which your morals and values or beliefs influence your sexual behavior and decisions.

Column B represents the degree to which social forces influence your sexual behavior.

Column C represents the degree to which biological factors influence your sexual behavior and decisions.

Column D represents the degree to which psychological forces influence your sexual behavior and decisions.

The relative influences can be compared directly with each other to see which area is the strongest or whether they are equal. You may interpret the results as follows:

11–15   major influence

6–10   moderate influence

1–5   insignificant influence

Suggested Readings

Alberta Society for the Promotion of Sexual Health. *Definitions of sexual health,* 2009. Available: http://www.aspsh.ca/definitions_of_sexual _health.

Bruess, C. E. Sexuality education, in *Battleground schools,* Mathison, S., & Ross, W. eds, Westport, CT: Greenwood/Praeger, 2008.

Bruess, C. E., & Greenberg, J. S. *Sexuality education: Theory and practice,* 5th edition. Sudbury, MA: Jones and Bartlett, 2009.

Edwards, W. M., & Coleman, E. Defining sexual health: A descriptive overview. *Archives of Sexual Behavior, 33, no. 3* (June 2004), 189–195.

Lefkowitz, E. S., Shearer, C. L., & Boone, T. L. Religiosity, sexual behaviors, and sexual attitudes during emerging adulthood. *Journal of Sex Research, 41, no. 2* (Jan 2004), 150–159.

Levine, J. Promoting pleasure: What's the problem? *SIECUS Report 30, no. 4* (April/May 2002), 19–22.

Report of the Task Force on the Sexualization of Girls. Washington, DC: American Psychological Association, 2007.

Rice, S. What does it mean to be healthy? *American Journal of Sexuality Education, 1, no. 2* (2006), 75–82.

Taverner, W. J. Sexual health in prime time. *American Journal of Sexuality Education, 1, no. 4* (2006), 71–82.

Web Resources

For links to the web sites below, visit *http://sexuality .jbpub.com/dimensions/4e* and click on Resource Links.

Sexuality Information and Education Council of the United States
www.siecus.org

Source for the Consensus Statement on Adolescent Sexual Health and other information related to healthy sexuality.

Alberta Society for the Promotion of Sexual Health
www.aspsh.ca

Source for an excellent definition of sexuality.

Think MTV—Relationships & Sex
http://think.mtv.com/Issues/relationshipsexuality

MTV's web site for information related to sexual health.

Sexual Health Network
www.sexualhealth.com/aboutus.php

A network dedicated to providing easy access to sexuality information, education, support, and other resources.

Teens Health
http://kidshealth.org/teen/sexual_health

Designed to help both males and females learn the facts about sexual health.

CHAPTER 2

Sexuality Research

FEATURES

Multicultural Dimensions
The Wyatt Surveys on African American and White Women in Los Angeles

Ethical Dimensions
Permission to Do Research on Sexual Behavior

Global Dimensions
The Liu Report: Sexual Behavior in Modern China

Gender Dimensions
Differences in Research Results

Communication Dimensions
Talking About Sexuality Research Results

CHAPTER OBJECTIVES

1 Describe the various methods used in sexuality research, including the steps in the scientific process.

2 Identify the ethical issues involved in sexuality research.

3 Describe the work of early sexuality researchers, including how they set the stage for modern research.

4 Summarize the contributions of major modern sexuality researchers.

sexuality.jbpub.com/dimensions/4e
Ethical Dimensions: Permission to Do Research on Sexual Behavior
Alfred Kinsey
William Masters and Virginia Johnson
Youth Risk Behavior Surveillance System

INTRODUCTION

You have probably heard the joke, "My mind is made up; don't confuse me with the facts." Unfortunately, when it comes to sexuality research, this attitude too often prevails. For example, a few years ago one of our students mentioned that one of his parents had asked him how his courses were going that term. When he mentioned he was learning about research on human sexuality, there were a few seconds of silence.

He explained that he had been raised in a home where sexuality was not discussed. He asked his parent about the silence, and the answer came back that it was a little difficult to think about research on such a topic. What did the researchers do? How did they do it? Why would they even want to do research on sexuality?

Our student explained that for a few minutes he felt he was the parent while he tried to answer these questions. Fortunately, he had already read the early chapters of his text, so he thought he did a pretty good job.

This is not an isolated instance of lack of understanding, or even of repression, when it comes to sexuality research. For instance, in many places in this text you will find references to the National Health and Social Life Survey (NHSLS). In 1988, a team of researchers at the University of Chicago won a federal government grant competition to conduct an extensive research study on sexual behavior. In 1989, however, conservative members of Congress attacked its research for a number of reasons (Laumann, Michael, & Gagnon, 1994). They said it was a plot by homosexuals to legitimate the normality of gay and lesbian lifestyles; it was an unwarranted intrusion by the government in private matters; it was not needed; it should not be supported with taxpayers' money; and the project staff had an antifamily agenda.

During a federal governmental review, facts about the research were widely misrepresented. It was also claimed that the researchers had published statements that they had not, and statements were taken out of context in an attempt to show that the researchers should not be doing the research. As a result, the previously approved government grant was cancelled. The research was then completed with private funding. Since the study of human sexuality still prompts anxiety and even fear in some people, as well as a hesitancy to talk about the subject with other people, sexuality research can be difficult.

In this chapter we present some of the major 20th- and 21st-century research on sexuality to show you how knowledge about human sexuality is obtained and to discuss some of the findings that researchers believe can aid individuals in accepting and understanding the sexual parts of their personalities. We turn to the findings after identifying some of the methodology used in sexuality research.

■ Research Methods

Research is undertaken to expand our knowledge about specific factors in our environment. Our current knowledge of human sexuality is based on relatively few studies. Perhaps by reading about issues and techniques related to research in general, you will better understand and evaluate the studies we discuss, as well as ask yourself how valid the findings are.

The first task of any researcher, regardless of the subject, is to ask an explicit question. The next is to design a way of gathering the relevant information. In sexuality research the most common methods used are surveys, case studies, and experimental research. Less common is the method of direct observation, a method used more in sexual research clinics but also used extensively in the research of Masters and Johnson (discussed shortly). Each method of research has its advantages and disadvantages, some of which are discussed here.

A good researcher chooses a method according to the particular problem and population being studied. For example, a survey would be used when a large number of responses are desired, as in a study of adolescent behavior. Observation might be desirable when a small number of subjects are involved, as in measuring responses of people who are engaging in a sexual behavior while being electrically monitored.

The Scientific Method

Sexology is the study of sexuality. To study sexuality appropriately, it is necessary to use the **scientific method**—that is, research conducted in an atmosphere free from bias—because it is the most objective way to establish new knowledge in any field. Scientists must always approach research studies without preconceived ideas of what their studies will show. In addition, they cannot have preconceived agendas to show what sexual behavior *should* be. Researchers do not set out to "prove" something but instead conduct research scientifically to discover what *is*—not necessarily just what they want it to be. Researchers follow proper procedures and discover information through research that can then be generalized to the real world outside the study.

> **sexology**
> The study of sexuality.
> **scientific method**
> Research conducted in an atmosphere free from bias.

As we will explain, the scientific method involves the following steps:

1. *Identifying a research question* (which could be based on personal interest or experience, on social concerns, or on the interests of those funding the research, such as government agencies or private industry)

2. *Reviewing the literature*

3. *Formulating a hypothesis (or two or more hypotheses)*

4. *Operationalizing variables*

5. *Collecting data*

6. *Analyzing the data to test the hypotheses*

The scientific method first involves identifying a research question. Not all questions about sexuality lend themselves to scientific research, because many involve subjective values, morals, and philosophical questions. (However, scientific research can provide information that can help us address even these types of questions.)

Second, to inform themselves adequately, researchers must review literature related to the research question. Thus the researchers learn what is already known about the topic, think of ways to conduct the desired research, and possibly even come up with new research questions.

Third, a hypothesis is formulated. A **hypothesis** is a tentative proposal or an educated guess about the results of a research study. It often deals with the relationship between two variables. A **variable** is a measurable event that varies or is subject to change (such as frequency of sexual behavior, use of contraceptives, or amount of alcohol ingested).

> **hypothesis**
> A tentative proposal or an educated guess about the results of a research study.
> **variable**
> A measurable event that varies or is subject to change.

Fourth, operationalizing the variables means specifying how they are going to be measured. For example, some variables, such as gender or income level, are easy to measure. Others, such as sexual desire or satisfaction in a relationship, are not. There are many ways to measure these variables, and the research has to state clearly how this will be done.

Fifth, collecting the data involves using methods such as survey research, case studies, experimental research, and direct observation. Each of these is explained in greater detail shortly.

Sixth, the data are analyzed to test the hypotheses. Data can be analyzed to describe situations, to show a relationship between variables, or to show that one situation causes another. Each of these methods of analysis demands the use of appropriate statistical methods.

Various forms of bias can be problematic. For example, in addition to possible bias of researchers, there could be bias of research subjects. If all subjects are college educated, they will probably be biased. Or, if some subjects are really not willing to participate or to be honest even if they agree to participate, they will also be biased. This type of bias is referred to as **volunteer bias**—characteristics of volunteers that are likely to influence research results.

> **volunteer bias**
> Characteristics of volunteers that are likely to influence research results.
> **generalization**
> The ability to conclude that the same results would be obtained outside the study.

One of the goals of the scientific method is to find information that can be generalized to the real world outside the study. Obviously, when researchers are trying to learn more about human sexuality, they cannot get information from *all* human beings. Therefore, they must study a relatively small group of people from which the results may be generalized to a larger population. **Generalization**, the ability to conclude that the same results would be obtained outside the study, can occur only if all aspects of the scientific method are properly planned, carried out, and controlled as much as possible.

Researchers on Antarctica's Ross Island have noted that female penguins, desperate for stones for their real nest, were willing to engage in "courtship" with an unpaired male penguin in exchange for stones. The penguin expert Eric Bennett decided to try an experiment at the Baltimore Zoo: He dressed up as a penguin and surrounded himself with lots of rocks. Within minutes, female penguins began presenting themselves for courtship. Does Bennett's experiment reflect the scientific method?

population
The group being studied in a research project.
sample
A segment of the larger population.
random sample
A sample that represents the larger population and that is chosen without bias, so that every member of the larger population has an equal chance to be selected.

The **population** is the group being studied in a research project. Usually only a **sample** (a segment of the larger population) participates, because the total population would be too large and unwieldy. A **random sample** represents the larger population and is chosen in a way that eliminates bias. If the sample is selected properly, the researcher can generalize findings to the larger population.

Survey Research

Much information about human sexuality has been obtained by **surveys** asking people about sexual attitudes and experiences. This kind of data can be obtained orally (face-to-face interviews) or in written form (pencil-and-paper questionnaires). Researchers use surveys when information from a large number of people is desired. For example, they might use a survey to find out how people feel about condom advertisements on television.

The **interview** allows the interviewer to explain the purpose and value of the survey, to clarify and explain the questions, and to report answers clearly. However, some individuals may not report their sexual experiences and views honestly because they may be embarrassed to admit particular behaviors and thoughts to a stranger. Also, the subjects being interviewed may be equally embarrassed to admit they do not participate in certain sexual activities.

Questionnaires are less expensive than interviews, which require many people to conduct the interviews. A questionnaire that the subject can fill out at his or her convenience makes many people feel more relaxed and reinforces anonymity; the privacy may also ensure more honest answering. In addition, the questionnaire eliminates the subject's being influenced by the interviewer's facial or bodily gestures.

The major concern with any **self-report data** is that subjects may include inaccuracies. Accuracy is obviously necessary for reliable research. For instance, people often have difficulty recalling past events, and events can become highly embellished or minimized the longer the time between experience and reporting. Recall involves estimating **frequency** and/or **duration** of behaviors, and many people have problems remembering numbers.

survey
Research in which people complete questionnaires or are personally interviewed.
interview
Oral research method designed to gather information.
questionnaire
Written instrument designed to gather information.
self-report data
The respondents' descriptions of something.

frequency
How often something occurs or has occurred.
duration
How long something occurs or has occurred.
case study
In-depth study of individual(s) or small groups.

Case Studies

Case studies are in-depth studies of individuals or small, select groups of individuals. Those under study are generally followed over a period of months or years. Case studies provide a chance to look at specific behaviors or characteristics in great depth. Also, because case studies generally cover a relatively long period, the researcher is able to explore cause-and-effect relationships in detail. For example, much information about sex offenders and people with sexual-response difficulties has been obtained through case studies.

With case studies, however, there is no way to use proper sampling techniques, making it difficult to generalize case-study results to the rest of the population. For instance, how do we know that sex offenders or those receiving treatment for sexual-response problems are like the rest of the population?

Experimental Research

In an **experiment**, behavior can be studied under controlled conditions. A common experimental design is one in which two groups are matched and compared. The groups are identical but for one important difference—the **experimental group** is subjected to a particular event or condition, whereas the **control group** is not. Both groups are observed, and the results are compared to determine whether the experimental condition had an effect. For example, a researcher could compare the responses of different groups of people (perhaps grouped by sex or age) to erotic materials.

Experimental research allows control over variables thought to influence responses or behavior. At the same time, the somewhat artificial setting may influence behavior or response. Merely knowing you are in a study or being in a laboratory might alter your reaction.

experiment
Observation of behavior (or effects) under controlled conditions.
experimental group
In an experiment, the group subjected to a particular event or condition.
control group
In an experiment, the group not subjected to a particular event or condition.

Permission to Do Research on Sexual Behavior

A faculty member at Mercer University in Macon, Georgia, was told by the president of the university that he could not conduct research in the form of a survey of sexual behavior of undergraduate students at Mercer (Wilson, 2002). The president said the project simply was not appropriate at a Baptist institution.

The president was concerned that the survey's explicit questions might offend students and their parents. Even though a 13-member campus review board unanimously approved the survey, top university administrators said that the survey was also subject to their approval. This procedural step had never before been invoked. One of the vice presidents said that such a survey could have negative impacts on admissions and parents' attitudes about the school.

Taking the opposite position, the researchers involved in the study said that better safe-sex programs were needed for Mercer undergraduates, and that a well-done survey about sexual behavior would be a good place to start. The faculty and students working together on the project hoped to publish the results in a scholarly journal. They indicated that preventing them from conducting the survey denied them academic freedom. They were upset that the result was an apparently arbitrary decision of senior administrators.

What do you think? Was it ethical for the researchers to conduct the survey? Was it ethical for the president to tell them they could not conduct the survey? Should the senior administrators have allowed the survey to be conducted even if they did not like the idea of the survey's being done on their campus?

Source: Wilson, R. An ill-fated sex survey, *The Chronicle of Higher Education, 48, no. 47* (Aug. 2, 2002), A10–A12.

Direct Observation

Observation is a method in which subjects are watched in a laboratory, a class, a natural setting, or the workplace. It can be an accurate way to collect sexual information—particularly if the researcher controls the setting. A prime example of observational research has been the human sexual-response research of Masters and Johnson.

observation
Watching subjects in a particular setting.

The major drawback of direct observation is the required expenditure of time and money. In addition, people are likely to be reluctant to perform sexual activity in a laboratory where they are being observed. Some people also question the ethics of participating in observational research either as the researcher or as the subject. When people do feel relatively comfortable and volunteer for observational research related to sexuality, one must always ask whether their sexual responses in such a setting replicate those obtained in the privacy of their normal environment. Another important question is whether people who are comfortable doing this are similar to the majority of people who aren't: Put another way, can the findings be generalized?

Focus Groups

A **focus group** is a form of research where a group of approximately 6 to 10 people are asked about their feelings or attitudes toward a topic and then discuss related issues. For example, the participants might be asked what they think about equal rights for homosexuals and heterosexuals. The leader usually has a focus-group script that guides the discussion (it includes questions, follow-up questions, and other instructions). A typical focus-group session might last for 1–2 hours. It is important to have extensive interchange among the participants to get as many thoughts and ideas as possible from the group. Focus-group members sometimes talk among themselves in reaction to a topic or question from the focus-group leader—with the leader listening and taking notes for analysis later.

focus group
A form of research where a group of 6 to 10 people are asked about a topic and then discuss related issues.

There are arguments both for and against focus groups. Some experts believe they are valuable ways to get important information from a group of people in a relatively inexpensive way. Other experts think they can be very time-consuming, the group cannot possibly be large enough to be a representative sample of the population, and the group can be unduly influenced by the researcher. Traditionally, most focus groups meet in person, but today there are also teleconference focus groups and online focus groups.

Interpreting Statistics

In many kinds of sexuality research, statistics related to the results will be presented. When we hear about statistical results, we have to differentiate between correlation and causation. **Correlation** is a statistical measure that shows how variables are naturally related in the real world. For example, studies might show that youth who watch more television also participate in more sexual behavior. That is interesting information, but it tells us nothing about *why* that relationship exists; it only tells us that the relationship *does* exist.

correlation
A statistical measure that shows how variables are naturally related to each other.

How do we know if the results of a study are accurate? Perhaps the findings just happened to occur in this study, but wouldn't occur in other similar studies. We can use statistics to help us determine how likely it is that the results will also occur in other studies. A number of statistical methods can be used to determine statistical significance. **Statistical significance** refers to the likelihood that a study's results are due to chance. If the results are significant at the .05 level, for example, there is only a 5% chance those results are due to chance. If it has been reported that people who don't use condoms develop HIV to a greater extent than those who do use condoms, and that finding is significant at the .05 level, we can be confident that the difference is attributable to not using condoms rather than to chance. In other words, not using condoms "caused" more people to develop HIV as compared to the rate found among people who did use condoms.

statistical significance
The likelihood that a study's results are due to the relationship uncovered between the study's variables as opposed to chance.

How can you use this information to contribute to your sexual health? When you are deciding whether to engage in a sexual behavior, you can read studies to see if there are statistically significant differences between those who engage in that behavior and those who do not. This will give you confidence that these differences are a result of that behavior, and that you can expect similar results if you decide to engage in that sexual behavior.

Issues in Sexuality Research

Despite the care and planning that go into implementing a research project, the success of a project depends on the cooperation of the subjects. The most difficult task in studying humans is finding a large group who will stay with the project to completion. When mail questionnaires are used, for example, the response rate is generally less than 40% of the total number distributed—and often close to 20%. Interviews are expensive, but the response rate can be high, depending on the interviewer's expertise and awareness. The interviewer must establish rapport with the subjects so that they are not embarrassed, intimidated, or totally unresponsive.

When asked to be surveyed about sexual behavior, many people will refuse, but others will participate. Therefore, those who do participate may be more or less sexually experienced and liberated than those who choose not to take part. This volunteer bias may allow us to draw conclusions from the study results about how some people view sexual matters, but it does not allow us to conclude that people in general behave or believe that way. When people answer surveys or consent to be interviewed, there are always problems of reporting accuracy, ability to recall past experiences as they really occurred, and willingness to be truthful, particularly about sexual matters, when facing an interviewer. Consider, for example, that reporting and evaluating how we feel now are easier than reporting how we felt sometime in the past. In recalling how and where we learned about sexuality or what sexual activities we were involved in as children, we are easily influenced by events that took place in intervening years, by changes in behavior socially defined as normal (or at least permissible), and by our own maturity. Even if subjects want and intend to give honest responses, they may feel reluctant to share the intimate details of their activities with a stranger, worry about the researcher's attitude toward their sexual behavior—particularly in an interview—or be afraid that their responses are not genuinely confidential.

Research on sexuality faces some additional problems. Many conditions affect our sexuality, including broad cultural and social definitions of sexuality roles and proper sexual behavior, as well as characteristics such as ethnic origin, religion, personal experience, and education. Such conditions and their effects may be too complex to measure or control. Also, cooperative subjects may be hard to find, because in our culture people feel anxiety, self-consciousness, and a

Multicultural
DIMENSIONS

The Wyatt Surveys on African American and White Women in Los Angeles

In several places in this book you will see research findings indicating differences in sexual behaviors and attitudes between people of different races. Care is needed when interpreting such findings, because it is often hard to differentiate between what may be a result of racial culture, what may be a result of socioeconomic differences, and what may be random or coincidental. A good example of this is provided by the Wyatt surveys.

Wyatt and her colleagues used Kinsey-style face-to-face interviews to examine the sexual behavior of 122 white and 126 African American 18- to 36-year-old women in Los Angeles. The two samples were balanced in relation to demographic characteristics such as age, education, number of children, and marital status.

Wyatt reported that by age 20, 98% of the people in her study (both white and African American) had experienced premarital sexual intercourse. When social class differences were considered, the ages of first intercourse for African American and white women were similar.

To control for demographic differences between white and African American women, Wyatt limited the subjects to demographically similar (age, education, social class) women. Her sample of African American women then matched the demographic characteristics of the larger African American Los Angeles population. However, because of Wyatt's efforts to use demographically similar groups, the white sample did not match the demographic characteristics of the larger white Los Angeles population because it contained a greater proportion of white women from lower-income families. This is an example of a trade-off in research. Wyatt wanted to be sure her two groups were demographically similar but in doing so ended up with one group that was not demographically similar to its larger population. This is not necessarily bad; however, it illustrates that we must understand what the researchers have done to interpret the results accurately.

Sources: Wyatt, G. E. The sexual abuse of Afro-American and white American women in childhood, *Child Abuse and Neglect, 9*(1985), 5, 7, 19; Wyatt, G. E. Reexamining factors predicting Afro-American and white American women's age at first coitus, *Archives of Sexual Behavior, 18*(1989), 271–298; Wyatt, G. E., Peters, S. D., & Guthrie, D. Kinsey revisited, Part I: Comparisons of the sexual socialization and sexual behavior of white women over 33 years, *Archives of Sexual Behavior, 17*(3, 1988a), 201–209; Wyatt, G. E., Peters, S. C., & Guthrie, D. Kinsey revisited, Part II: Comparisons of the sexual socialization and sexual behavior of black women over 33 years, *Archives of Sexual Behavior, 17*(4, 1988b), 289–332.

reluctance to share private thoughts, experiences, and memories about sexuality. For example, many people would not want to talk about their experiences with forcible sexual behavior. Even talking about whether one masturbates and, if so, how frequently, is not something most people are eager to do.

There can also be some limitations in sexuality research. For example, nonresponse (refusal to participate) can make it difficult to get responses from the desired subjects. Also, self-selection volunteer bias may be a problem. Volunteers for sexuality research may be more sexually experienced and hold more positive attitudes toward sexuality than nonvolunteers. Finally, there may be a demographic bias. As seen in Kinsey's work and even today, it is often easier to get subjects for sexuality research who are white, middle-class, white-collar workers and college students.

Adding to the difficulty of gathering accurate information is the influence of the researcher's own values and biases. The researcher may have very strong opinions about issues in the study and may—perhaps unintentionally—phrase questions in favor of his or her views, emphasize certain words in a face-to-face interview, and/or have certain racial, ethnic, or cultural views that affect rapport with the subjects in the study. Interviewers and writers of questionnaires may have perceptions about the group they are surveying, which can also influence how questions are asked or phrased. When the information is collected and interpreted, the researcher must consciously prevent personal feelings and attitudes from affecting analysis and reporting. For example, a researcher who might be either strongly for or strongly against abortion would need to be very careful when asking questions about abortion and recording the answers of a research subject.

It would be wise to have several researchers with different views work together to check questionnaires and procedures to be sure there is as much **objectivity** as possible—that is, be sure the results

objectivity
Being sure the results are the same no matter who asks the questions or records the answers.

are the same no matter who asks the questions or records the answers.

Ethical Issues in Sexuality Research

Recently there has been increased attention to the need to protect the people participating in any form of human research. Because of the intimate nature of sexual research, the ethical issues involved in this field are particularly important.

An ethical issue of particular concern is obtaining the **informed consent** of participants; subjects of research studies must agree in writing to participate *after* the purposes, risks, and benefits of the study have been explained to them. Consent is obtained to ensure that subjects both understand what the project entails and agree to undergo the experience as described. This requirement protects subjects against physical and psychological abuse by irresponsible researchers and protects researchers against claims that subjects were taken advantage of. Investigators are now required by law to obtain an individual's consent to be subjected to the project as described; those testing minors must also obtain parental or guardian permission.

> **informed consent**
> Document required to participate in a research study after the purposes, risks, and benefits of the study have been explained.

Researchers do not have the right to coerce people to participate in a study, and they must be honest when presenting information about the research. They also have a responsibility to protect the confidentiality of their participants. They must be sure that personal facts can never be connected to a given individual. It is obvious that participants must also be protected from physical and psychological harm. Many methods must be used to guarantee the anonymity of participants and to be sure confidential information is never released.

Human-research review committees commonly exist in government agencies and in universities. These committees must review and approve any research designs and procedures that will use human subjects. Such committees consider the value of the research and compare it to any potential risks to the participants. It can be difficult for committees to decide whether to allow a researcher to carry out a particular study—especially if children are involved. This is one reason why we do not have better information about the sexual thoughts and experiences of young people.

Additional ethical questions arise in studies of the sexual behaviors and attitudes of various racial groups. Some people argue that such research is important to better understanding of diverse feelings and practices. In contrast, others believe that describing sexual behaviors and attitudes according to racial groups contributes to stereotypical thinking.

Another interesting ethical issue arises from the ways that have been developed to measure physiological changes in the vagina or the penis due to sexual stimulation. **Vaginal plethysmography** involves inserting a probe into a woman's vagina to measure increased blood volume, an indication of sexual arousal. Changes in blood volume over time can be charted

> **vaginal plethysmography**
> Insertion of a probe into a woman's vagina to measure changes in blood volume.
> **penile strain gauge**
> A wire or cuff placed around the penis to measure physiological changes over time.
> **plethysmograph**
> A laboratory measuring device that charts physiological changes over time.

with this device. Similarly, a **penile strain gauge** can be used. This is a wire or cuff placed around the penis that is attached to a **plethysmograph**, a laboratory measuring device that charts physiological changes over time and records changes in the girth of the penis as it responds to sexual arousal or loss of arousal.

Plethysmography has been used to see whether a person has certain sorts of sexual interests, such as a sexual interest in children. For example, if it were suspected that a person were sexually attracted to children, the device might provide additional information that could lead to a referral for possible treatment. Following treatment, the device could be used again to see whether the degree of sexual interest in children has decreased. How-

The vaginal plethysmograph is used to measure sexual response by detecting changes in the amount of blood in the vaginal walls. The device is used in sexuality research.

The penile strain gauge is used to measure erectile response by detecting changes in the circumference of the penis. The device is used in sexuality research.

ever, because people can sometimes learn to control their physiological responses, this is not a foolproof test. Also, it would be a mistake to base too many assumptions about a person's future sexual behaviors on one measure of physiological response. Use of penile and vaginal plethysmography is likely to be debated for years to come.

Finally, it is crucial to be sure a test has **validity**—that is, that it tests what it is supposed to test. For example, a sexual-knowledge test must be a good representation of overall sexual knowledge. This might be shown by a comparison to a known good test or by expert ratings.

> **validity, validation**
> Demonstration that tests measure what they are designed to measure.

Most research on sexual feelings, attitudes, responses, and behavior depends on participants' reporting about themselves. Some people believe that sexuality research is useless and meaningless because subjects can lie about their sexual behavior, exaggerate their experiences, or feel too embarrassed to discuss personal sexual matters openly and honestly. Others believe that we need information about sexual matters and must encourage research, even while acknowledging its limitations. Although it is difficult to validate information that people include on a questionnaire or divulge in an interview, validation is frequently done by asking for the same information in another part of the survey or in conversation and cross-checking whether the information given is the same in both instances.

Given the variety of attitudes toward sexuality in our society, the many different opinions concerning moral and ethical issues related to sexuality, and even the disagreement as to whether sexuality should be researched at all, researchers have a difficult job. They must design a scientifically sound study, create confidence in that study, and guarantee their subjects' privacy.

Evaluating Sexuality Information on the Internet

Anyone who uses a search engine to look for information about "sex" or "sexuality" finds so many hits that it is not humanly possible to review all of the sites mentioned. In addition, although accurate and reliable information about sexuality can be found on the Internet, so can a preponderance of information about sexuality that is incorrect or misleading. How can you determine whether information about sexuality found on the Internet is accurate? Here are some suggestions (National Center for Complementary and Alternative Medicine, 2009):

1. *Who runs the site?* Any good web site related to sexuality should make it easy for you to learn who is responsible for the site and its information.

2. *Who pays for the site?* The source of a site's funding should be readily apparent. The funding source can affect what content is presented, how the content is presented, and what the site owners want to accomplish on the site.

3. *What is the purpose of the site?* An "About This Site" link appears on many sites; if it's there, use it. The purpose of the site should be clearly stated and help you evaluate the trustworthiness of the information.

4. *Where does the information come from?* If the person or organization in charge of the site did not create the information, the original source should be clearly labeled. This identification allows others to easily find original sources of information.

5. *What is the basis of the information?* The site should describe the evidence on which the material is based. Facts and figures from valid research should have references. Also, opinions or advice should be clearly set apart from information that is based on research results.

6. *How is the information selected?* Is there an editorial board? Do people with excellent professional and scientific qualifications review the material before it is posted?

7. *How current is the information?* Web sites should be reviewed and updated on a regular basis, and the most recent update or review date should be clearly posted. Even if the information is still accurate, you want to know whether the site owners have reviewed it recently to ensure that it is still valid.

8. *How does the site choose links to other sites?* What is the policy of the web site owner about how links to other sites are established? What are the criteria for the sites that are linked to the web site?

9. *What information about you does the site collect, and why?* Any credible web site should tell you exactly what it will and will not do with personal data gathered about you. Many commercial sites sell data about their users to other companies. Don't sign up for anything you don't fully understand.

10. *How does the site manage interactions with visitors?* There should be a way for you to contact the site owners with problems, feedback, and questions. Information about the terms for using any site services should be readily available as well.

■ Early Sexuality Researchers

As discussed in Chapter 1, we have some information about sexual practices throughout human history. Although not all of the information was gathered in a systematic way, in Western civilization attempts to study human sexual behavior systematically date back at least to the ancient Greeks. Physicians, such as Hippocrates, and philosophers, such as Plato and Aristotle, are the forefathers of sexuality research. They made extensive observations and offered the first elaborate theories regarding sexual responses and dysfunctions, reproduction and contraception, abortion, legislation related to sexuality, and sexual ethics (The Kinsey Institute, 1998).

In Rome, Greek physicians such as Soranus and Galen further advanced sexual knowledge. Their work prompted later Islamic scholars to spend much time on sexual questions. These studies, together with the Greek and Roman manuscripts, became standard texts at medical schools and stimulated a rebirth of anatomical research in the 16th, 17th, and 18th centuries. In the 19th century, new concerns about overpopulation and sexual psychology intensified efforts to study the topic of sexuality. Finally, at the turn of the 20th century, the investigation of sexuality became a legitimate endeavor in its own right (The Kinsey Institute, 1998).

Richard von Krafft-Ebing

Richard von Krafft-Ebing (1840–1902) wrote during a period when Victorian standards strongly suppressed thinking about human sexuality. Because he was a product of this period, and because he was a physician who worked primarily with sexually disturbed people, von Krafft-Ebing's writings (1902) indicated that sexual activity is something to fear.

He supported what we now know as the double standard, whereby men have sexual freedoms that women do not. He may have supported this perspective because of his apparent discomfort with the sexuality of women.

Von Krafft-Ebing's writings had a tremendous influence on many physicians as well as the public. Even though he seemed to be biased and made some false assumptions, his writings convinced some physicians and researchers that the study of sexuality

was legitimate. This helped prepare the way for Ellis and Freud.

Henry Havelock Ellis

Henry Havelock Ellis (1859–1939), an English psychologist and physician who studied human sexuality, grew up in fear of what he had been told about the danger of nocturnal emissions. He was also concerned about his general ignorance of human sexuality. Between 1896 and 1910 Ellis published a six-volume series entitled *Studies in the Psychology of Sex*, which included the following beliefs:

1. Masturbation is common for both sexes.

2. Orgasm in males and females is very much the same.

3. Homosexuality and heterosexuality are a matter of degree.

4. Women do have sexual desire, contrary to Victorian thought.

5. There is no one norm for human sexuality. Thoughts and acts vary among individuals and cultures.

6. There should be sexuality education for both sexes starting at early ages.

7. There should not be laws against contraception or private sexual behavior.

It is clear that Ellis's ideas were controversial and ahead of their time, particularly his support of sexuality education. In fact, some people today still have difficulty accepting his beliefs. Ellis's work influenced the later pursuits of many sexuality researchers and writers.

Sigmund Freud

Sigmund Freud (1856–1939), a psychological researcher, developed theories about human development, personality, and psychopathology that have influenced our thinking today. To develop into a well-adjusted person, according to Freud, one had to progress successfully through a number of psychosexual stages.

Freud viewed sexuality and sexual pleasure as a central part of human life and felt that people naturally sought to have as much pleasure and as little pain as possible. He indicated that sexual activity was natural and that procreation was secondary to pleasure, and he cautioned against severe restrictions on sexual instincts. People, he maintained, could become neurotic if denied natural expression of their sexual instincts.

Freud's theories have influenced thinking about sexuality for the past century.

One of Freud's important contributions was his suggestion that early childhood experiences had strong consequences for adult functioning. Largely because of Freud's work, sexual thoughts and behaviors are still considered to be major influences on contemporary life in general.

Magnus Hirschfeld

Magnus Hirschfeld (1868–1935) was a German physician who started his career in medicine and was soon drawn to the study of human sexuality. He was a transvestite (he coined the word "transvestism") in addition to being a homosexual. He believed that sexual orientation was a naturally occurring trait worthy of scientific study rather than social hostility. He urged homosexuals from all walks of life to come out and get involved in a growing campaign for emancipation. He promoted the idea that sexual honesty was necessary for healthy living.

Hirschfeld produced many books and papers concerning sexuality and succeeded in bringing the discussion of homosexuality into the halls of government as well as the homes of everyday people. As German fascists gained power in the 1920s, however, he was physically attacked at least twice and there were political attempts to suppress his work.

By 1930 he was forced into exile and made his home in France.

Katherine Davis

Katherine Davis (1860–1935) was born in Buffalo, New York, and educated in the United States. She taught high school science for 10 years, then went on to earn a Ph.D. degree in economics in 1900. In 1901 she began working in the field of corrections, and in 1914 became the commissioner of corrections for New York City.

She quickly moved to improve conditions in the penal institutions, then became interested in topics related to the well-being of women. From 1918 to 1928 she was general secretary of the New York Bureau of Social Hygiene board of directors, where she directed research on many topics related to public health. In 1929 she published *Factors in the Sex Life of Twenty-Two Hundred Women*. In addition, she was the author of many articles in professional and popular journals (Women in American history, 2005).

Her survey of married Caucasian women of above-average intelligence, education, and social position revealed some interesting results (History of sex surveys: Factors in the sex life of 2200 women, 2005). For example, contraception (then called "voluntary parenthood") was approved in principle by almost 90% of the respondents and practiced by 73%. Of those who claimed to have "happy" marriages, only one out of four worked outside the home. Based on this fact, the researchers concluded that working was not conducive to marital happiness.

Ninety percent of the married women considered their husband's sex drives to be as strong as or stronger than their own. A little over 3% believed their sex drives were stronger. Masturbation was admitted to by 65% of the unmarried women and 40% of the married women, but 2 out of 3 of these women considered the habit "morally degrading." Slightly more than 50% of the single women said they had experienced "intense emotional reactions" with other women, and over 25% admitted that the relationship involved overt homosexual expression.

Dr. Davis's research included some opinion questions. She found that 39% of the women thought sexual intercourse was necessary for complete physical and mental health, 19% thought a young woman was justified in having intercourse before marriage, 21% thought a young man was justified in having intercourse before marriage, 85% thought married people were justified in having intercourse for reasons other than having children, 63% thought information regarding birth control methods should be available for unmarried people, and 72% felt that it was acceptable for an abortion to be performed.

Clelia Mosher

Clelia Mosher (1863–1940) was born in Albany, New York. She was educated at Stanford University, where in her master's thesis, she debunked a widespread myth of that time: the belief that women breathed differently than men, and were therefore unfit for exercise. Mosher found that this difference was caused by women being laced into tight-fitting corsets, and that there was no reason that they could not otherwise participate in strenuous exercise.

Mosher completed medical school at Johns Hopkins in 1899. In 1923 she wrote a book entitled *Women's Physical Freedom*. She explained her views on women's health, menstruation, and breast care. She promoted a positive view of women's potential and argued against many Victorian attitudes.

Over a period of 30 years, she surveyed Victorian women, most of whom were born about the time of the Civil War, about their sexual lives. This was probably the first known survey of sexual attitudes and behaviors. She gave her nine-page survey to a total of 47 women. Therefore, the sample size was small and the women were not representative of Victorian women in general. Most were faculty wives at universities and also well educated for that era. Even though it was a biased sample, it is noteworthy because it is the only known survey of Victorian women. This was a period when women were not supposed to be sexual. Interestingly, her findings were not published until 1980. Here are some of them:

- Although Victorian women were not supposed to feel sexual desire, 35 of the 47 women indicated that they liked sexual intercourse.

- Thirty-four of the women had experienced orgasms.

- Many of the women indicated that it could be a problem because it took them longer to reach orgasm than their male partner. They said there was a need for men to know about this.

- More than two-thirds of the women used some kind of birth control. Douching was the most common, followed by withdrawal and "timing." Obviously, we do not consider these methods very reliable today. Some husbands used a "male sheath" (a condom), and two women used a "rubber cap over the uterus" (either a diaphragm or a cervical cap). One woman said she used "cocoa butter," but she did not explain why or how.

- Three of the women said that their ideal would be to never have sexual intercourse at all. But most of the women expressed their sexual desires and experienced orgasms. Most seemed to enjoy sexual relations with their husbands.

It is impressive that Mosher was able to accomplish her research at the height of the Victorian era. It seems that she was a talented woman who tried hard to improve the status of women at the same time she was doing groundbreaking research.

■ 20th-Century Sexuality Researchers

The 19th-century model of sexuality and sexual behavior was a medical one. Individuals who differed from the accepted norms were considered ill or, in scientific terms, deviant or pathological; however, little was known about sexual attitudes, behaviors, and activities. There was a dearth of knowledge about human sexuality from the psychological, psychosocial, and physiological perspectives. Research into sexual attitudes and behaviors lacked respectability, and many institutions would not fund or support it. In the 1930s changes in public attitudes in the United States, desire for contraception (both for child spacing and for pop-

Alfred Kinsey and his colleagues were at the forefront of using scientific methodology to study human sexuality. His research, begun in 1938, was revolutionary in that it covered a wide range of sexual activities and applied statistical methods to sexuality research.

ulation control), and a more open interest in the scope of sexual behavior led to greater acceptance of human sexuality as a legitimate field for research.

What follows is an overview of the more prominent research in human sexual behavior during the past 70 or 80 years. Although some of this work was done in the late 1930s, you will find that many of the issues are not very different from those you are concerned with and possibly are experiencing now.

Our overview covers two categories—scientific literature and popular literature. In most instances it is obvious which category applies, but admittedly in a few cases the point is arguable. We hope that a review of these studies will not only add to your sum of information but also help you to expand and develop your sexuality and interpersonal relationships.

Scientific Literature

Alfred C. Kinsey: Establishing Scientific Sex Research

Alfred Kinsey, a biologist and zoologist, joined the faculty of Indiana University in 1920. He gained academic recognition early in his career through his writings in biology. In 1937 Kinsey became the teacher of a newly introduced course in marriage and sexuality education. As his interest in the subject grew, he began to amass information concerning sexual activities and beliefs about sexuality. Dr. Kinsey's scientific background led him to gather facts and statistical data. Kinsey eventually gathered the largest amount of information on human sexuality ever collected.

The interviews conducted by Kinsey and his colleagues covered six ways in which males and females achieve orgasm in our culture: masturbation, nocturnal sex dreams and emissions, heterosexual petting, heterosexual premarital intercourse, homosexual intercourse, and sexual contact with animals. The questions focused on nine major areas: social and economic data, marital history, sexuality education, physical and physiological data, nocturnal sex dreams, masturbation, heterosexual history, homosexual history, and animal contacts. Using these highly specific interviews, Kinsey and his associates collected data from only white males and females. They represented rural and urban areas in each state and a range of ages, marital statuses, educational levels, occupations, and religions. The sample contained a disproportionately high number of better-educated people living in cities. All subjects were volunteers. Kinsey's studies may be the best-known example of survey research related to sexuality, but his sample cannot be viewed as representative of the U.S. population. *Sexual Behavior in the Human Male* (1948) is based on interviews with 5,300 males; *Sexual Behavior in the Human Female* (1953) on interviews with 5,900 females.

Americans had little knowledge about sexual behavior in this culture until Kinsey presented his findings. His conclusions generated a great deal of public reaction. Kinsey concluded that there was a relationship between sexual behaviors and attitudes on the one hand and education and socioeconomic characteristics on the other hand. In males, the lower the educational level, the higher the premarital activity. For women, the findings were the opposite—the higher the educational level, the more likely the premarital activity. He found that those women who had experienced premarital orgasm were more likely to experience marital orgasm. Most of the married females reported orgasm response through coital and noncoital sexual behavior. Only about 2% of women reported a complete lack of sexual arousal. A great many of Kinsey's subjects reported childhood sexual experiences, which reinforced Freud's belief that sexual expression is experienced in childhood. Kinsey concluded from all the data that people are sexual from early childhood through adulthood. Despite its limitations, Kinsey's work was hailed as the first large-scale study of sexual behavior. Some of Kinsey's major findings are described in the following paragraphs.

Masturbation Close to 92% of males in Kinsey's sample stated that they had masturbated at some point in their lives, with the highest incidence reported between 16 and 20 years of age; about 62% of all females reported that they had masturbated. The higher the educational level, the greater the incidence of masturbation in both men and women. In both males and females, the stronger the religious adherence, the lower the incidence of masturbation.

Nocturnal Dreams About Sex Dreams about sex were experienced by both sexes. From the data Kinsey concluded that 70% of females had dreams about sex. About 90% of the females who reported sex dreams had heterosexual dreams with sexual partners they could not identify. About 37% of 45-year-old women had experienced dreams that led to orgasm. The highest incidence of nocturnal emissions was reported by 71% of single males aged 21 to 25 years.

Premarital Intercourse With regard to heterosexual premarital intercourse, Kinsey found that 22% of all adolescent males had experienced intercourse. Among college males 67% had experienced premarital intercourse. Males of lower social class reported greater frequency of premarital intercourse than those of higher social class. Nearly 50% of the females reported premarital intercourse. About two-thirds of the married females reported sexual orgasm before marriage through any one of five techniques: masturbation,

DIMENSIONS

The Liu Report: Sexual Behavior in Modern China

Dalin Liu and associates (1997) interviewed 23,000 Chinese people over a period of 18 months. The nationwide survey about sexual attitudes and behavior, a Chinese "Kinsey Report," was the first conducted in China. Liu reported the following:

1. For high school students, the mean age of first ejaculation was 14.4 years.

2. College students were highest in their masturbation rates (59% for males and 17% for females) as compared to high school students (13% for males and 5% for females), city married subjects (33% for males and 12% for females), and village married subjects (9% for males and 11% for females).

3. Thirteen percent of the college student males and 6% of the college student females had experienced premarital sexual activity. This compared with 22% of the city married men and 16% of the city married women, and 35% of the village married men and 15% of the village married women.

4. Among all groups, college students had the highest proportion of those who had homosexual behavior (8%) as compared to less than 1% of city married subjects and just over 2% of village married subjects.

5. Sexual satisfaction was reported by 55% of married males and 67% of married females.

6. Ninety-five percent of the college students and 67% of the married subjects felt positively about the female's initiating sexual activity. Four percent of the college students and 11% of the married subjects felt negatively about this idea.

7. Fifty-six percent of college students, as compared to 10% of married subjects, approved of extramarital sexual activity. Thirty-nine percent of the college students and 79% of the married subjects felt very negative about extramarital sexual activity.

8. Most Chinese couples engage in little or no foreplay before initiating intercourse. Many wives report some discomfort during intercourse as a result of insufficient vaginal lubrication.

9. Women are more likely than men to initiate divorce proceedings (three of five divorces are requested by women).

Source: Liu, D., Man Lun Ng, Li Ping Zhou, & Haeberle, E. J. *Sexual behavior in modern China.* New York: Continuum, 1997.

---

nocturnal dreams, heterosexual petting, heterosexual coitus, and homosexual contacts. At all social levels, males and females who were devoutly religious reported much less premarital intercourse than nondevout subjects. Kinsey also found that people who married earlier had experienced premarital intercourse at a younger age, and those who married later had begun premarital intercourse at a later age.

Homosexual Activity   Kinsey found homosexual incidence highest in high school males. About 37% of all males had some homosexual experience between adolescence and old age. Twenty-five percent of females aged 30 years and over had been erotically aroused by other females, and 17% had experienced sexual contact with other females. Female homosexual contact was greatest in the college and graduate school groups.

The Kinsey Institute is still operating. It is called the Kinsey Institute for Research in Sex, Gender, and Reproduction and is located at Indiana University. In 2004 Kinsey's life was the subject of a popular movie.

William Masters and Virginia Johnson: The Physiology of Sexual Response

The research efforts and studies of Masters and Johnson are probably the most widely known and cited of all sex-related data. These researchers were the first to observe people's sexual behaviors in a laboratory setting and to identify physiological changes during sexual arousal. William Masters was a gynecologist and Virginia Johnson a psychologist. Together they were the directors of what was the Reproductive Biology Research Foundation in St. Louis and is now the Masters and Johnson Institute. In 1966 they published their data in *Human Sexual Response*, and in 1970 they published *Human Sexual Inadequacy*.

Once the two started their research, they informed university contacts and professionals that they were in search of volunteer study subjects. Of the 1,273 volunteers who initially applied, Masters and Johnson selected 694—276 married couples, 106 unmarried women, and 36 unmarried men. Ninety-eight of the single people had been married previously.

The investigators obtained social and sexual histories for all their subjects, gave them information to explain the studies, and introduced them to the laboratory setting. For experiments involving sexual intercourse, married couples were used as subjects; in studies other than intercourse (such as masturbation and controlled vaginal tests with an artificial phallus), unmarried subjects participated.

Through direct observation, filming, and monitoring with instruments, Masters and Johnson recorded a variety of changes in the physiology of the body in general and in the genitals and reproductive organs in particular. Most of their findings related to physiological responses to sexual arousal that had never before been measured or documented. Their major finding, generally accepted as true since the results were published, was the existence of a cycle of physiological events in response to sexual stimulation. The whole cycle, known as the *human sexual response*, occurs in both sexes in four phases, always in order: excitement, plateau, orgasm, and resolution. (The human sexual response cycle is discussed in detail in Chapter 6.) This research showed that males and females have many similar responses, as well as responses specific to the physiology of each sex. The research of Masters and Johnson now serves as the basis for modern therapy, education, and counseling; cross-disciplinary research; and general information about sexual functioning.

As well developed as it is, Masters and Johnson's research is not without criticism. Some professionals believe that their model of human sexual response ignores psychological and cognitive aspects of arousal. One can only speculate because Masters and Johnson are no longer here to defend themselves. However, it could also be argued that their original model was intended to only demonstrate what happens biologically and that other factors could be considered later. We will never know for sure, but you should realize that criticisms of their work do exist. It is interesting, however, that their second study was expanded to consider a broader range of factors related to human sexual response.

William Masters and Virginia Johnson were the first sexuality researchers to observe people's sexual behaviors in a laboratory setting. Among their many contributions to sexuality research is the human sexual response cycle (Chapter 6).

The second major Masters and Johnson study, *Human Sexual Inadequacy,* was published in 1970. This study of sexual dysfunction (a topic discussed in Chapter 16) put the relationship of the physiology and the psychology of sexual response in sharper focus. Causes of sexual dysfunction, the relationship of the partners who experienced dysfunction, and sexual interaction in general were the concerns of this book. Masters and Johnson defined *sexual dysfunction* as an inability to respond emotionally and physically to sexual arousal. They were able to give a range of dysfunctions, defining six basic types—three for women and three for men. The dysfunctions were also defined in terms of the phases of the sexual response cycle. The physiological, psychological, and emotional (or situational) causes were suggested and defined, with treatment developed to deal with the causes and symptoms presented. Their research has provided a great deal of knowledge of physiological changes that occur in the body during sexual activities.

In 1979 Masters and Johnson published *Homosexuality in Perspective.* This study of the sexual response of homosexuals added much information to the human sexuality literature. The data were gathered by studying the sexual response cycles of 38 lesbian couples and 42 male homosexual couples between 1957 and 1970. The researchers reported that there was little difference between homosexuals and heterosexuals in sexual functioning and response to sexual stimulation. However, homosexuals appeared to communicate with partners more effectively during sexual activity than did heterosexuals. The broadest conclusion reported in this publication was that homosexuality is not a disease and that homosexuals, like heterosexuals, are individuals who have sexual concerns.

Masters and Johnson and You The work of Masters and Johnson affects your sexual life in many ways. Both you and your partner can now better

Myth vs Fact

Myth: Most women prefer a sexual partner who has a large penis.
Fact: Surveys indicate this is not true. Plus, we know that a female's vagina can adjust to different size penises and that there is far less difference in the sizes of erect penises than of soft penises.

Myth: Sexual activity usually ends soon after age 60.
Fact: Most people older than 60 years in relatively good health continue to participate in many forms of sexual activity.

Myth: Masturbation is physically harmful.
Fact: Masturbation does not harm the body in any way.

Myth: Anal intercourse between uninfected people can transmit human immunodeficiency virus (HIV).
Fact: If there is no infection, there will be no HIV transmission. To contract acquired immunodeficiency syndrome (AIDS), a person must first be infected with HIV.

Myth vs Fact

Myth: Most husbands have extramarital affairs.
Fact: The rates may vary in different studies, but the National Health and Social Life Survey reported that 25% of men and 15% of women had extramarital affairs.

Myth: Few women masturbate.
Fact: Most men and women, married and unmarried, occasionally masturbate. About 50% to 68% of females masturbate at least once a month.

Myth: Most normal women have orgasms from penile thrusting alone.
Fact: Different women prefer different kinds of stimulation. Many do not reach orgasm from penile thrusting alone.

Myth: A man cannot have an orgasm without an erection.
Fact: He can have an orgasm even if he does not have an erection.

Myth: Erectile dysfunction (sometimes referred to as "impotence" by the layperson) usually cannot be treated successfully.
Fact: With counseling, medical treatments, surgical treatments, and better sexual knowledge alone or in combination, most instances of erectile dysfunction can be treated.

June Reinisch and Ruth Beasley found these nine myths to be commonly believed. More information about these myths can be found in later chapters in this book and in their book *The Kinsey Institute New Report on Sex* (1991). New York: St. Martin's.

understand your bodies' responses to sexual stimulation. Knowing that you proceed through several identifiable phases during your sexual response cycle (see Chapter 6) will make you and/or any sexual partner more willing to proceed at a sexual pace in synchrony with your physiology. The results will be greater sexual satisfaction and, as we shall see in Chapter 16, less sexual dysfunction. Because of the work of Masters and Johnson and that of others motivated by Masters and Johnson's studies, a person experiencing problems with sexual functioning has access to a whole warehouse of effective sexual therapy modalities. As with the work of Kinsey, the studies of Masters and Johnson not only broke ground for sexual research as a profession, but also produced some very useful information for the general public.

The National Health and Social Life Survey

A University of Chicago research team conducted the first comprehensive survey of adult sexual behavior since Kinsey's research (Laumann et al., 1994). The National Health and Social Life Survey (NHSLS) was designed to assess the incidence and prevalence of a broad range of sexual practices and attitudes within the U.S. population.

When the AIDS epidemic began in the 1980s, experts were not well informed about contemporary sexual practices. Believing that such data might help prevent the spread of HIV, in 1987 an agency within the U.S. Department of Health and Human Services asked for proposals to study adult sexual attitudes and practices. The research team from the University of Chicago was awarded a grant in 1988 to support a survey of 20,000 people.

As mentioned earlier, after 2 years of planning, federal funds for the project were withdrawn. In 1991,

because conservative members of Congress were offended by the idea of using government funds for research on sexual behavior, legislation was passed to eliminate federal funding for such studies.

The research team then obtained funding from several private foundations. They were able to proceed, but with a much smaller sample. After sampling techniques were used to select a representative sample of 4,369 18- to 59-year-old Americans, 79% of the sample agreed to participate. This gave them a sample size of 3,432.

Although they did have a high participation rate, they had been forced to limit their sample size. This resulted in a population that was representative of white Americans, black Americans, and Hispanic Americans; however, there were too few representatives of other groups to provide useful information about them.

The research team trained 220 professional interviewers, and all 3,432 subjects were interviewed face-to-face. The interviewers made sure the respondents understood all questions. The questionnaire also had internal checks to measure consistency of answers and to validate the responses.

You will see references to NHSLS data in other parts of this book, and here are a few examples of findings: (1) Of married persons, 93.7% had had only one sexual partner in the last year as compared with 38% of those never married and not cohabitating; (2) married people were much more likely than

↑♀ Gender
♂♀ DIMENSIONS

Differences in Research Results

When reviewing research results, researchers have historically commonly found relatively large differences between genders in the amount of heterosexual sexual behavior. Even when comparing the amounts for males and females of the same age, it is common to see much higher rates for males than females. The reasons for this are not known, but this situation makes for interesting discussion because one must wonder who the males are having heterosexual behavior with if the numbers are much smaller for females.

Gender differences also often exist when it comes to reasons for first sexual intercourse (Laumann et al.,

1994). For example, among those females who wanted their first vaginal intercourse to happen when it did, just over half the males were motivated by a curiosity about sexual behavior, but a little less than one-quarter of the females were. However, about one-quarter of the males had intercourse because of affection for their partner, whereas 47.5% of the females did it for this reason. Only about 3% of the females said that physical pleasure was their main reason, compared to about four times as many men (12%) who said this.

Watch for these kinds of comparisons as you consider research on sexuality behavior and think about reasons why gender differences might exist.

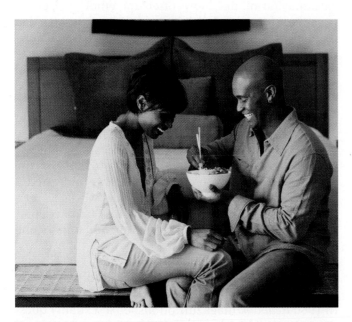

The NHSLS found that married people are much more likely than singles to report being very happy.

singles to report being extremely or very happy; (3) 9.1% of men and 4.3% of women reported engaging in any same-sex activity since puberty (for nearly half of these men the behavior occurred only before the age of 18 years). About 1.4% of the women and 2.8% of the men reported a homosexual identity.

Popular Literature

Shere Hite: Women's Sexuality, Men's Sexuality, and Women and Love

Between 1972 and 1976, when her findings were published in *The Hite Report*, Shere Hite mailed more

than 100,000 60-item essay-type questionnaires to such women's groups as the National Organization for Women, university women's organizations, and women's newsletters. She also placed notices in *The Village Voice, Mademoiselle, Brides, Ms.,* and *Oui* magazines asking women to send for questionnaires. Hite received completed questionnaires from 3,109 women, who expressed their personal feelings about masturbation, orgasm, intercourse, clitoral stimulation, lesbianism, sexual slavery (satisfying males' needs during sexual activity and ignoring their own needs), and the sexual revolution. Many women reported that they experienced orgasm more frequently from clitoral stimulation than from coitus and that they achieved deep orgasm from masturbation. Furthermore, they described a history of orgasm in general. Of the sample, 8% preferred sexual activity with other women, 53% said that they preferred sexual activity with themselves, and 17% preferred no sexual activity at all. Although the question was not directly asked, many women offered the information that they were curious about and might be interested in a sexual encounter with another woman. The majority of older women said that sexual pleasure increased with age, but many respondents older than 45 years reported difficulty in finding new sexual partners.

The findings published in *The Hite Report* were of great interest, for despite the fact that only a relatively small portion of the total female population was reached, no study had previously afforded such large numbers of women the opportunity to express their preferences and desires in matters of sexuality. However, remember that Hite recruited her subjects by inserting a notice in magazines such as *Oui, The Village Voice, Ms.,* and *Mademoiselle.* Rather than

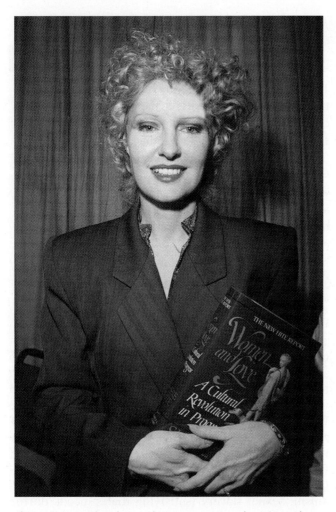

Shere Hite completed several important research projects about sexual behavior.

as indicating strength. Again, because the Hite study of males was anecdotal, it is not considered to be of statistical note.

In 1987 Hite published *Women and Love: A Cultural Revolution in Progress*. After spending 7 years analyzing surveys from 4,500 women, she concluded that women are fed up with men. Despite women's liberation and the sexual revolution, Hite reported that women remain oppressed, and even abused, by men. Four of five women in her study said they still had to fight for their rights within relationships, 87% said that men became more emotionally dependent than women, 92% complained that men communicate with women in language that indicates "condescending, judgmental attitudes," 95% reported forms of "emotional and psychological harassment," 79% said they seriously question whether they should put so much energy into love relationships, 98% wished for more verbal closeness with male partners, 70% of the women married 5 years or more said they had extramarital affairs more often for emotional closeness than for sexual activity, and 87% of the married women said they have their deepest emotional relationship with a woman friend.

Many respectable researchers, both male and female, questioned Hite's findings. Criticisms pointed to a highly self-selected sample—only a 4.5% return from more than 100,000 questionnaires distributed to a variety of women's groups in 43 states—and a likely disproportion of unhappy people, because unhappy people were probably more willing to answer the questions than were happy people. Hite indicated a desire for men to see what women feel works in relationships, but others feared that Hite's book encouraged women to take the easy way out and blame everything on men.

being representative of all women, this small, select group of women is considered to be what is called a biased sample. Hite did not statistically analyze her data; rather, she used what are described as anecdotal reports—essays written by individuals describing their sexual activities and the feelings they experienced.

In 1981 Hite published *The Hite Report on Male Sexuality* using the same anecdotal analysis, this time presenting the views of 7,200 men. Men preferred intercourse to masturbation or oral–genital sexual activity. They were generally unaware that women could achieve orgasm by means other than intercourse. They expressed ignorance of when a female orgasm occurs and expressed anxious feelings about not knowing. Some of the males expressed anger over always being the initiators of sexual activity yet volunteered that sexually aggressive women were difficult for them to deal with. Many men stated that they grew up not being allowed to express themselves emotionally, for the culture demanded that men be strong and showing emotion was not defined

Lorna Sarrel and Philip Sarrel: The Redbook Report on Sexual Relationships

In 1980 *Redbook* magazine published a sexuality questionnaire to which approximately 20,000 women and 6,000 men responded. The questionnaire was primarily concerned with the quality of relationships and the interpersonal communication of couples. More than half of the men (60%) and less than half of the women said that sharing feelings was very important to their relationships. Seventy-five percent of those who answered the questionnaire rated their current sexual relationships as being good or excellent. Fifteen percent reported sexual dysfunction, and these people said that they spoke very little about sexuality with their partner. Of particular interest is the fact that 40% of men and women who were parents said that lack of privacy interfered in some way with their enjoyment of sexual activity. Many individuals accepted sexual activity to satisfy a partner even if

Did You Know...

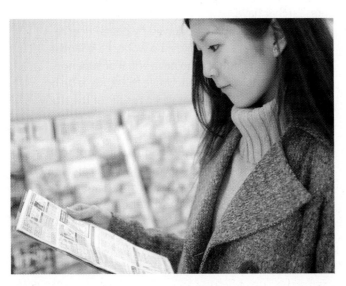

Readers must carefully evaluate information about human sexuality found in popular literature.

they did not want to make love at the time, and half of those who did said they "end up enjoying it."

This study is not indicative of sexual relationships of the population in general, because the readership of *Redbook* in 1980 tended to be youthful, married, better educated, and financially more secure than the general population. However, these people do represent a very large group of our population and they certainly do show an interest in sexual matters, are comfortable with the subject, and possess a willingness to discuss sexuality and interpersonal relationships. It is fair to believe that they did represent many couples in the society (Sarrel & Sarrel, 1980).

June Reinisch and Ruth Beasley: The Kinsey Institute New Report on Sex

The inclusion of a 1991 book within our popular literature section may be debatable, but it is indeed written for the general public. In fact, one of its authors said, "It's a great book to have in the bathroom, when you have time to read bits and pieces. It is designed to be

a 'friendly encyclopedia,' telling readers in question-and-answer format almost everything they wanted to know about sexuality" (Dolan, 1990).

Research from the Kinsey Institute and the results of a Roper poll of 2,000 adults show that knowledge about sexuality is still at a very low level. For example, half of the adults tested did not know that a lubricant such as Vaseline or baby oil can cause microscopic holes in a condom or a diaphragm in as little as 60 seconds. This lack of understanding hardly contributes to safer sex practices.

Of women aged 30 to 44 years, only 55% received a passing grade on the test, and 52% of men in the same age group did. Men answered correctly more often on matters of sexual practices, and women knew more about their own sexual health. People living in the Midwest had the highest scores, and those in the South and the Northeast had the lowest.

Seventeen *Magazine and The Kaiser Family Foundation: SexSmarts Survey on Teen Sexual Behavior*

The latest in a series of surveys of teens aged 15–17 years found that only 1 in 10 teens who have had sexual intercourse discussed his or her sexual plans with parents ahead of time, and more than a third did not tell their parents about their sexual history at all. Forty-eight percent of all survey respondents and 56% of sexually active respondents never talked with a parent about "how to know when you are ready to have sex." Eighty percent of respondents said teens do not discuss sexual issues with their parents because they worry that their parents will disapprove or will assume that they are already participating in sexual behavior if they discuss the subject with them (Kaiser Family Foundation and *Seventeen* magazine release latest SexSmarts Survey on teen sexual behavior, 2002).

Eighty-four percent of all respondents said they had never talked with a health care provider about how to know when one is prepared for sexual behavior. More than two-thirds had not discussed contraception, HIV and AIDS, condoms, or STIs with a health care provider. Nearly two-thirds had spoken with a sexual partner about "what they are comfortable doing

Communication
DIMENSIONS

Talking About Sexuality Research Results

It is not easy to analyze findings of sexual research, and it is common to hear others talking about some "new findings" they just heard about. What if someone tells you about some sexual "research" and some interesting findings? What can you suggest to help the person (and you) analyze whether the research seems sound? Here are some possibilities for questions and conversational points.

- Was the scientific method used? This method does not rely just on testimonials or someone's opinion. It requires proper sampling techniques, accurate measurement and observation, and appropriate statistical analysis of the findings to reach valid conclusions.
- Is the study replicable? One study, taken alone, seldom proves anything. To be valid, one researcher's findings must be repeatable by others.
- Have the research findings been properly used? For example, conclusions based on data from one population may not apply to another population, and the results from animal studies cannot be applied with certainty to humans.

- Were the proper statistics used and were they used correctly? Many people tend to accept statistical data without question, although statistical errors do occur.
- What is the competency of the author or researcher? Does the person have a record of excellent previous research? What kinds of expertise does the author or researcher have?
- Has the research been reviewed by peers? Peer review is the process in which the work of a scientist is reviewed by others who have equal or superior knowledge. It may be done while the study is being developed or afterward, as when results of the study are being considered for publication in a scientific journal.

Even these questions will not guarantee appropriate judgments about the accuracy of sexual research, but it can be very helpful to see whether there are good answers to them. They may also inspire some very interesting conversation.

---

sexually." Fifty-eight percent had never discussed STIs with a partner, 56% had never discussed HIV and AIDS with a partner, and 53% of all respondents and 28% of sexually active teens had never discussed contraception with a partner. Most cited lack of knowledge about sexual issues, fear of what a partner might think, and embarrassment as reasons they do not discuss sexual issues with partners.

NBC News and People Magazine: National Survey of Young Teens Sexual Attitudes and Behavior

NBC News and *People Magazine* had the Princeton Survey Research Associates International conduct a survey of 1,000 young teenagers (ages 13–16) and their parents. The results were reported in 2004 and updated in 2005 (Nearly 3 in 10 young teens sexually active, 2005). Teens were asked about their sexual health, behavior, and attitudes, and parents were asked for their views on the sexual lives of today's teens.

The survey showed that parents and teens have somewhat different opinions on the pressure teens face and their attitudes. For example, 85% of parents strongly or somewhat agreed that "there is a lot of pressure on teenagers to have sex by a certain age,"

compared with 66% of the teens. Forty-seven percent of parents strongly or somewhat agreed with the statement, "for teens oral sex is not as big a deal as sexual intercourse," compared with 75% of teens.

The survey confirmed that teens engage in a wide range of sexual behavior, from kissing to sexual intercourse. For example, 58% of all teens (ages 13–16) reported having "kissed someone romantically," 27% reported having "been with someone in an intimate or romantic way," 21% reported having "touched someone's genitals or private parts," 13% reported having engaged in sexual intercourse, and 12% reported having engaged in oral sex. Among the 12% of all teens who reported having had oral sex, 1% first had oral sex at age 11, 8% at age 12, 19% at age 13, 22% at age 14, 29% at age 15, and 16% at age 16.

As might be expected, older teens (ages 15–16) reported higher rates of sexual behavior. Seventy-two percent had "kissed someone romantically," 41% had "been with someone in an intimate or romantic way," 37% had "touched someone's genitals or private parts," 21% had engaged in sexual intercourse, and 19% had engaged in oral sex.

Parents seemed to underestimate whether their teens had engaged in sexual behavior. When asked

By the time they finish high school, about 62% of females have had sexual intercourse.

think, 75% cited not having met the right person yet, 63% cited religious or moral beliefs, 54% cited worries about what their friends would think, and 49% cited not having had the opportunity as a major or minor reason for their decision.

Among those who had engaged in oral sex, 76% cited "the other person wanted to" as a major or minor reason for their decision, 71% cited having met the right person, 69% cited the belief that "you are still a virgin if you have oral sex," 68% cited not having to worry about pregnancy, 64% cited curiosity, 40% cited wanting to avoid sexual intercourse, 35% cited the belief you can't get STIs from oral sex, 24% cited wanting to avoid being touched or undress, and 21% cited "wanting to be more popular and accepted" as a major or minor reason for their decision.

about their own child, 83% believed he or she had not engaged in sexual activity beyond kissing.

According to the study, many teens were not protecting themselves from pregnancy or STIs. Thirty percent who had oral sex reported "always" using "protection such as a condom" during oral sex, 14% reported using protection "most of the time," 13% "some of the time," and 42% reported "never" using protection during oral sex.

Thirty-six percent of teens who had sexual intercourse used birth control every time, 6% used it "almost every time," 8% used it "most of the time," 7% used it "only sometimes," 1% "hardly ever," and 40% never used birth control.

The survey showed that many factors, from parent's reactions to curiosity to sexual desire, play a role in teens' decisions about sexual behavior. Eighty-two percent of teens who had engaged in sexual intercourse cited having met the right person as a major or minor reason for their decision, 71% cited curiosity, 68% cited sexual desire, 56% cited a hope that it would make their relationship even closer, 34% cited pressure from their partner, and 18% cited a desire "to be more popular and accepted" as a major or minor reason for their decision.

For those who had never engaged in sexual intercourse, 89% cited feeling they were too young as a major or minor reason for their decision, 88% cited "a conscious decision to wait," 86% cited worries about STIs, 85% cited worries about pregnancy, 84% cited worries about what their parents would

■ Examples of Research in the 21st Century

It is almost impossible to count the many research studies related to human sexuality done in recent years. And until these studies stand the test of time, it is difficult to tell which, if any, might become classics. The following is a chronological summary of selected, more recent, research studies.

Studies on Premarital Sexual Attitudes and Behavior Dailard (2001) reported on the findings of the National Longitudinal Study of Adolescent Health (more commonly called the "Add Health Survey"). She indicated that teens' reports of ever having had sexual intercourse increase dramatically with grade level, from

Sexual standards are influenced by culture and gender.

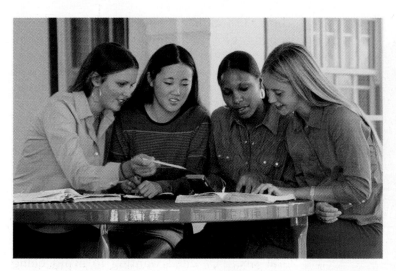

Rates of sexual activity vary with differences in ethnicity.

16% among 7th and 8th graders to 60% among 11th graders. Teenagers who are African American or in low-income or single-parent families are more likely to have had sexual intercourse than their peers. In addition, the Add Health Survey strongly indicates that whether a teenager has ever had sexual intercourse is largely explained by that individual's own sexual history and his or her perceptions about the costs and benefits of having sexual intercourse. In sharp contrast, the data indicate that other major risk behaviors—such as cigarette smoking, drug and alcohol use, weapons-related violence, and suicidal thoughts and attempts—are shaped more by factors such as problems with school or work or the number of friends who regularly smoke or drink.

Dennison and Russell (2005) pointed out that more than 1,000 published reports employed data from the Add Health Study. Findings from these reports indicate that adolescents at the upper and lower ends of the intelligence distribution were less likely to have engaged in intercourse, religiosity reduced the risk of coital debut in both males and females, youth from intact families were less likely to have engaged in intercourse, greater parental involvement was related to a lower likelihood of sex initiation, and most teens had their first sexual experience within the context of a romantic relationship. The average waiting time before engaging in sexual intercourse within these romantic relationships was 5 months. In addition, students who felt connected at school reported later ages at sexual initiation, girls participating in sports tended to delay sexual activity, and students who took abstinence pledges were less likely than nonpledgers to practice safe sex once they became sexually active.

In 2002 the Kaiser Family Foundation reported the results of a national survey of 1,200 adolescents and young adults 13–24 years old (Substance use and risky sexual behavior, 2002). It concluded that for many teens and young adults, alcohol use and drug use are closely linked to sexual decision making and risk taking. Nearly 90% said their peers used alcohol or drugs before having sexual intercourse at least some of the time, and many young people reported that condoms are often not used when people are drinking or using drugs. More than a third of sexually active young people reported that alcohol or drugs had influenced their decisions about sex. Almost as many had "done more" sexually than they had planned while under their influence. As a result, they reported they worried about STIs and pregnancy.

It is interesting that most sexually active teenagers had sexual intercourse for the first time in their parents' homes, late at night (Most sexually active teens first had sex at home, 2002). On the basis of a national survey that had tracked 8,000 children aged 12–16 years since 1997, the study found that 56% of those who had been sexually active said they first had sexual intercourse at their family's home or at the family home of a partner, 12% said at a friend's house, 4% said in a vehicle, 3% said at an outdoor location, 3% said at a hotel or motel, and 10% said at another location. In addition, 42% said they first had sexual intercourse between 10 P.M. and 7 A.M. and 28% said between 6 P.M. and 10 P.M. Only 15% of respondents said they had intercourse for the first time between 3 P.M. and 6 P.M. This study dispels the myth that teens most often have sexual intercourse after school, when parents are at work.

Changes in sexual risk behavior among U.S. high school students (grades 9–12) over a 10-year period were reported in 2002 (Trends in sexual risk behaviors among high school students, 2002). The percentage who reported ever having had sexual intercourse decreased by 16%. In 1991, 56% had participated, but in 2001 only 46% had done so. Also, the overall proportion who had had four or more partners dropped by 24%—from 19% in 1991 to 14% in 2001.

The overall prevalence of "current sexual activity"—defined as having intercourse at any point during the 3 months preceding the survey—did not change between 1991 and 2001. It was reported by about one-third of the respondents. Condom use rose between 1991 and 1999 but had "leveled off" since then. In 2001 about 58% of sexually active teens used condoms, compared to about 46% in 1991. The percentage of sexually active students who had used drugs or alcohol before their most recent intercourse increased 18% between 1991 and 2002.

In 2004, Grunbaum et al. reported on the Youth Risk Behavior Surveillance (YRBS) update.

? Did You Know . . .

Many studies of sexual behavior have examined only whether a person reports ever having had sexual intercourse. When investigating the safety of sexual behavior, it is also helpful to know how often people have participated in sexual intercourse in a recent time, with whom, and which types of sexual practices have been used. For example, we know that teenagers and nonwhite women are at greater risk of contracting HIV than are older women, but teenagers are less consistently sexually active than are older women (Klitsch, 1990). Similarly, nonwhite women are statistically more likely to contract sexually transmitted infections than white women; however, they are less consistently sexually active than white women. Again, researchers need to consider the type of behavior or practice, not just the amount, to determine the degree to which safe sexual behavior is practiced.

They indicated that 47% of high school students (grades 9–12) had had sexual intercourse and 37% of sexually active students had not used a condom at last sexual intercourse. The incidence of sexual intercourse was higher among African American male (74%) and Hispanic male (57%) than African American female (61%) and Hispanic female (46%) students, respectively. It was also higher among 9th-grade male (37%) than 9th-grade female (28%) students. Overall, the incidence of intercourse was higher among African American (67%) than Hispanic (51%) and white (42%) students; higher among African American female (61%) than Hispanic female (46%) and white female (42%) students; and higher among African American male (74%), Hispanic male (57%), and white male (41%) students. Overall, the incidence was higher among 10th-grade (44%), 11th-grade (53%), and 12th-grade (62%) than 9th-grade (33%) students. Nationwide, 7% of students had sexual intercourse for the first time before age 13 years, and 14% had had sexual intercourse during their lifetime with 4 or more partners.

In 2005 Halpern-Felsher et al. reported that ethnically diverse 9th-grade adolescents evaluated oral sexual activity as significantly less risky than vaginal intercourse on health, social, and emotional consequences. They also believed that oral activity is more acceptable than vaginal intercourse for adolescents their own age in both dating and nondating situations, oral sexual activity is less of a threat to their values and beliefs, and more of their peers will have oral sexual activity than vaginal intercourse in the near future. More study participants reported having had oral sexual activity (20%) than vaginal intercourse (14%), and more intended to have oral sexual activity in the next 6 months (32%) than vaginal intercourse (26%).

In 2005, South et al. studied the effect of residential mobility on the timing of first premarital sexual intercourse. They found that adolescents who had recently moved were about one-third more likely than nonmobile adolescents to experience first premarital intercourse. They further found that much of the difference between adolescents who moved and those who didn't in the onset of sexual activity was attributable to the greater propensity for delinquency and weaker academic performance among members of movers' school-based friendship networks.

In 2008, Lescano et al. studied factors associated with anal intercourse among adolescents and young adults. Recent heterosexual anal intercourse was reported by 16% of the 1,348 respondents. Females who engaged in anal intercourse were more likely to be living with a sexual partner, to have had two or more partners, and to have experienced coerced intercourse. For males, only a sexual orientation other than heterosexual was a significant predictor of engaging in heterosexual anal intercourse.

Studies on Ethnic Differences in Sexual Attitudes and Behavior

Only relatively recently have researchers looked at the influence of ethnic differences in sexual attitudes and behavior. Examples of such studies are given in the following discussion.

Ford and coworkers (2001) reported that the sexual partners of white and black adolescents are likely to be similar to them. In contrast, the sexual partners of Latino adolescents and of adolescents of "other" race or ethnicity are more likely to be of a different racial or ethnic group. As adolescents get older, their partners become more heterogeneous.

Cavanagh (2004) studied the sexual debut of girls in early adolescence. She found that among white girls, those who matured early were more likely to have sexual intercourse in early adolescence, and this was partially due to the friendship groups of which they were a part. Early puberty seemed to draw white girls into larger friendship groups characterized by riskier behavior and lower academic achievement. Hispanic girls were similar to white girls in key ways, but different in others. For them, as for whites, both early puberty and friendship group characteristics were closely related to sexual debut, but unlike whites, friendship group characteristics did not mediate the association between early pubertal timing and sexual debut. Early pubertal timing mattered for Hispanics in other ways not captured in the model used in the study. There was also another factor uniquely characterizing Hispanics—the presence of older boys. Interestingly, among African American girls, there were no meaningful associations among early pubertal timing, the friendship group, and sexual debut.

Other studies have shown a variety of ethnic differences related to sexuality. For example, Connell et al. (2004) found that African American groups are more aware of STIs and HIV than either white or Hispanic groups. However, African Americans tend to have a higher percentage of people testing positive for HIV/AIDS (Johnson & Jackson, 2004). The prevalence rate of HIV has been found to be 16% for African Americans, 7% for Hispanics, and 3% for whites (Harawa et al., 2004). Also, Hispanic youth seem to be at a greater risk for experiencing early intercourse than white youth (Adam et al., 2005).

Regarding birth control, use of injectable contraceptives is high among African American women, but not as high among Asian Indian or white women (Burgard, 2004). Knowledge disparities can also be seen when comparing ethnic groups. For example, 41% of Hispanic women and 75% of African American women have heard of emergency contraception as compared to 99% of white women (Chuang & Freund, 2005).

Studies on the Use of Contraception

Ford and colleagues (2001) reported that the less similar adolescents and their sexual partners are to one another—whether because of a difference in

age, grade, or school—the less likely they are to use condoms and other contraceptive methods. The likelihood of having sexual relations with adolescents with different characteristics increases as adolescents get older.

Oncalem and King (2001) reported that many college students either have tried to talk their sexual partners out of using a condom or have had a partner try to dissuade them from condom use. Nearly 14% of women and nearly 17% of men who had engaged in sexual intercourse admitted to having actively tried to dissuade a partner from the couple's using condoms. Thirty percent of men and 41% of women said that a sexual partner had tried to dissuade them. The most frequent reasons cited were (1) that sexual intercourse feels better without a condom, (2) that the woman will not get pregnant, and (3) that the person will not get a sexually transmitted infection.

Related to control of births, in 2002 it was reported that the overall U.S. abortion rate declined throughout the 1990s, but "rose sharply" for low-income women. The abortion rate among U.S. women of childbearing age fell from 24 per 1,000 women in 1994 to 21 per 1,000 women in 2000—an 11% decrease. However, the rate among women earning less than the federal poverty level rose by 25% during this period, and the rate for women earning less than two times the poverty level—or $34,000 for a family of four—rose by 34%. The rate among teens 15–17 years old fell by 40% from 24 per 1,000 girls in 1994 to 15 per 1,000 girls in 2000. The majority (56%) of women who have abortions are in their 20s. Two-thirds have never been married, and 61% have one or more children. More than three-quarters reported having a religious affiliation—43% Protestant, 27% Catholic, and 8% other religions (U.S. abortion rate declines overall but increases among low-income women, 2002).

Grunbaum et al. (2004) reported that nationwide, just over 4% of students in grades 9–12 had been pregnant or gotten someone pregnant (4.9% for females and 3.5% for males). These researchers also indicated that among the 34% currently sexually active adolescents, 63% of them reported that either they or their partner used a condom during the last sexual intercourse. Seventeen percent reported that either they or their partner had used birth control to prevent pregnancy before their last sexual intercourse.

While it may seem obvious, Bruckner et al. (2004) reported that the factor most strongly associated with the risk of pregnancy among young women is contraceptive use, with nonusers being significantly more likely than inconsistent

Adolescents give many reasons why they did not use contraception.

and consistent users to become pregnant. However, these researchers also indicated that adolescents who become pregnant do not sufficiently appreciate the negative consequences, and that prevention programs should target participants' attitudes toward pregnancy. If more positive attitudes toward contraception can be developed, this will help shape effective contraceptive use.

Bancroft et al. (2004) indicated that men with low inhibition of sexual arousal in the face of risk had more partners with whom they had not used condoms and more lifetime "one night stands." Since the correlation between mood and sexual activity is clearly relevant to high-risk sexual behavior, they felt it must be considered when designing behavioral interventions.

While there are many reasons for close involvement between parents and adolescents, Frisco (2005) pointed out an interesting relationship to contraceptive use. Her research showed that parental involvement in education shapes teenagers' attitudes about school and work by encouraging achievement and by providing a home environment that values education. Such parental involvement also increases the odds that young women will use contraception, especially increasing the likelihood of using specific reliable birth control methods.

Manlove et al. (2008) examined a sample of sexually experienced 15- to 19-year-old males to identify factors associated with condom use. They found that Hispanic males and those who did not receive formal sexuality education had lower odds of condom use and/or consistency. African American males and those with more positive attitudes about condoms had greater odds of both using condoms and using them consistently. Males who were older at most recent sexual intercourse, who had an older sexual partner or a casual sexual partner, who were in longer relationships, or who engaged in more frequent sexual intercourse had reduced odds of contraceptive use.

Rose et al. (2009) reported on the validity of female teens' and young adults' self-reported condom use. They used a computer-assisted method to detect the presence of sperm in vaginal fluid for 14 days after unprotected vaginal intercourse. Of the participants who reported sexual intercourse in the past 14 days, 186 reported consistent condom use. However, 63 of them tested positive for the presence of sperm in their vaginal fluid. Therefore, it seems that approximately one-third of the subjects who reported condom use were not giving an accurate response.

Other Representative Studies
Moore (2001) reported that nationally the teen birth rate dropped 22% between 1991 and 2000. Southern and southeastern states had the highest teen birth rates; northeastern and some northern states had much lower birth rates. Interestingly, teens overestimated the number of their peers who had engaged in sexual intercourse. Teens estimated that 38% of their peers had engaged in sexual intercourse by age 15 years, whereas only 25% of girls and 27% of boys had done so.

Similarly, Henshaw (2004) pointed out that after reaching a high of 117 pregnancies per 1,000 females ages 15–19, the U.S. teen pregnancy rate decreased to 84 pregnancies per 1,000 in 2000. The pregnancy rate includes births, abortions, and miscarriages.

A report from the U.S. Centers for Disease Control and Prevention (Martin, Hamilton, & Ventura, 2001) indicated that several factors have contributed to the decline in the teen birth rate. Sexual activity has leveled off, reversing the steady increases over the preceding two decades. Many initiatives have focused on the prevention of pregnancy through abstinence—and many teens have heard the message. Finally, more sexually active teens are using contraception including the more effective newer forms.

Kirby (2001) pointed out that despite declining rates of teen pregnancy, more than 4 in 10 girls become pregnant at least once before age 20, a proportion that translates into nearly 900,000 teen pregnancies per year. When teens give birth, they become less likely to complete school and more likely to be single parents. Their children have less supportive and stimulating home environments, poorer health, lower cognitive development, worse educational outcomes, more behavior problems, and greater likelihood of becoming teen parents themselves. Many teens do not use contraceptives correctly and consistently every time they have sexual intercourse.

Martin et al. (2009) reported that the birth rate for youth ages 15–19 increased 3% in 2006. This interrupted a 14-year period of continuous decline from 1991 through 2005. The teen birth rate had dropped 34% from 1991 to 2005.

The U.S. Surgeon General reported (2001) that almost 775,000 AIDS cases had been reported in the United States since 1981 and that about 900,000 persons were living with HIV. About one-third were aware of their status and were in treatment, one-third were aware and not in treatment, and one-third had not been tested and were not aware. About 40,000 new HIV infections occur each year.

Sternberg (2001) reported that from about 1995 to 1998 new AIDS cases and AIDS deaths dropped because of potent new AIDS drugs. In 1998 they leveled off, and 1998 to 2001 they increased. Reasons for this increase seem to be related to the fact that some people delay getting tested for HIV, AIDS drugs do not work against some strains of HIV, and in some groups there is an increase in risky sexual behavior.

The U.S. Centers for Disease Control and Prevention (HIV/AIDS in the United States, 2008) estimated that 56,300 new HIV infections had occurred in the United States in 2006. Almost three-quarters of the diagnoses were for males. The cumulative number of AIDS diagnoses since 1981 exceeds 982,000, more than 545,000 people with AIDS have died, and more than 436,000 are living with AIDS. Better treatments have led to an increase in the number of persons who are living with AIDS.

In 2002 it was reported that the age at which girls begin menstruating had declined since the 1970s. For African American girls it decreased markedly, dropping by 9.5 months. For white girls it decreased by 2 months. Overall, African American girls on average began menstruating about 3 months earlier than white girls (12.3 years versus 12.6 years) and were 40% more likely than white girls to begin menstruation before age 11 years. The reasons for early menstruation are not well understood (Age at first menstruation continues to decline, especially among African Americans, 2002).

The number of married U.S. teenagers increased by 50% during the 1990s. In 2000, 4.5% of teens were married compared to 3.4% in 1990. The exact reasons for this are not known; however, some people attribute the change to abstinence education and others attribute it to the increased number of immigrants from countries in which teenage marriage is more common (Number of married U.S. teens increased by 50% in 1990s, 2002).

Interestingly, high school- and college-aged Americans indicated stronger support than their parents' generation for some traditionally "conservative" stances, including opposition to abortion. Forty-four percent of survey respondents between 15 and 22 years old said they supported government-imposed restrictions on abortion rights in the United States, whereas 34% aged 26 years and older supported such restrictions (Young Americans more likely than their parents' generation to oppose abortion, 2002).

In 2003 the Henry J. Kaiser Family Foundation released a comprehensive survey of young people about the factors that shape and inform their knowledge and decision making (National survey of adolescents and young adults, 2003). The study involved a nationally representative survey of 1,800 young people aged 13–24 years. The main findings reflected interviews with 1,552 young people between 15 and 24 years of age. More young people reported that sexual health issues are "big concerns" for people their age, more than any other issue. A summary of key findings include the following:

1. Young people report great pressure to participate in sexual activity.

2. One-third of adolescents have participated in oral sexual activity; 1 in 5 are unaware that this behavior can transmit STIs.

Young people say they get a lot of their sexual information from their peers.

3. Pregnancy remains a serious concern for young people, and many have faced pregnancy scares or have been pregnant themselves.

4. Many young people remain reluctant to discuss sexual health issues with partners, family, and health providers.

5. Young people report that alcohol and drugs often play a dangerous role in their sex lives.

6. A surprisingly high number of young people are misinformed about safer sexual activity.

7. While most young people agree that sexual activity without a condom is risky, many young people see sexual activity without condoms occasionally as "not a big deal."

8. When it comes to sex and relationships, young people say they get their information from a variety of places, including their parents, sexuality education, friends, and the media.

9. Young people express a strong desire for more information about sexuality and sexual health.

The study's authors pointed out that in the past decade there has been an increase in the use of condoms among sexually active young people, and a small but significant decline in teen birth rates. However, 10% of the girls between ages 15 and 19 years have become pregnant, nearly two-thirds of the high school seniors have had sexual intercourse, and an alarming percentage of sexually active adolescents and young adults has engaged in unsafe sexual behaviors. Nearly 1 in 4 sexually active young people contract an STI every year, and one-half of all new HIV infections in this country occur among people under the age of 25 years.

Examinations of associations between religiosity and sexual behaviors and attitudes have shown interesting results. In 2004 Lefkowitz et al. found relationships between religiosity (group affiliation, attendance at religious services, attitudes, perceptions of negative sanctions, and adherence to sanctions) and sexuality. They reported that religious behavior was the strongest predictor of sexual behavior. In 2005 research by Penhollow et al. indicated that religiosity variables, especially frequency of religious attendance and religious feelings, were significant predictors of sexual behavior.

In 2004 Vlassoff et al. assessed the costs and benefits of sexual and reproductive health interventions. Their study showed that poor sexual and reproductive health account for a substantial share of the global burden of disease. Their research indicated that the benefits of sexual and reproductive health interventions are far-reaching. For example, in addition to medical benefits, maternal health care lowers death and disability due to pregnancy-related causes, helps families remain intact, enables higher household savings and investment, and encourages higher productivity. Prevention and treatment for STIs and treatments for medical conditions also help reduce social stigma and help parents remain healthy so they are better able to care for and invest in their children. Contraceptives, together with maternal health services, minimize the adverse health effects of unintended pregnancy and high-risk births, including unsafe abortion, hemorrhage, infection, anemia, low birth weight, and malnutrition. These researchers concluded that sexual and reproductive health interventions are a good investment.

In 2004 Denizet-Lewis reported that a number of teenagers are choosing "hookups" or "friends with benefits" over dating. The distinction between hooking up and dating can be unclear, because sometimes one does lead to the other. Hooking up is nothing more than a no-strings sexual encounter. Relatedly, in one state it was found that of the 55% of total 11th graders who engaged in sexual intercourse, 60% said they had done so with a partner who was no more than a friend. The number would likely have been higher if the study had asked about oral sexual activity. Many teenagers have replaced sexual intercourse with oral sexual activity because they think it is definitely not sex ("It's just oral."), and hooking up is definitely not a big deal to them. In a hooking-up relationship, unwritten etiquette indicates that you don't call the person for anything except plans to hook up. You just keep it purely sexual, and that way people supposedly don't have mixed expectations and no one gets hurt. Some

teenagers report that they like the "friends with benefits" arrangements to help keep their emotions in check to avoid getting hurt in a relationship.

In 2005 Mosher et al. reported data from the National Survey of Family Growth. They indicated that, among adults 25–44 years of age, 97% of men and 98% of women had had vaginal intercourse; 90% of men and 88% of women had had oral sexual activity with an opposite-sex partner; and 40% of men and 35% of women had had anal sexual activity with an opposite-sex partner. About 6.5% of men had had oral or anal sex with another man. Eleven percent of women reported having had a sexual experience of any kind with another female.

Koch (2006) reported on women's bodies being a "puzzle" for college men. She found that college men believed women and their bodies are complex "puzzles" that are difficult to understand. The college men also felt ignorance about women's bodies, particularly their genital/reproductive anatomy and menstruation. Confusion over how to deal with women's body image was another major theme. The men believed that women are too concerned about their body image. Most felt that having better knowledge of women's bodies and the experiences they go through would improve their relationships with women.

As electronic devices have played much larger roles in the lives of college students, some issues related to electronic devices and sexuality have arisen. For example, the National Campaign to Prevent Teen and Unplanned Pregnancy and CosmoGirl.com commissioned a survey of teens and young adults to explore electronic activity (Sex and Tech, 2008). The key findings showed that a significant number of teens have electronically sent, or posted online, nude or semi-nude pictures or videos of themselves. Sexually suggestive messages were even more prevalent than sexually suggestive images. Most respondents knew that it was potentially dangerous to post sexually suggestive content, but did it anyway. Many of the teens and young adults said they were pressured by friends to send or post sexual content. Most said it was a "fun and flirtatious" activity.

Research on Sexuality Education

Research has been done to evaluate the effect of sexuality education programs (see Chapter 1). For example, Eisen, Zellman, and McAlister (1990) found that good sexuality education programs help delay the onset of sexual intercourse for teenagers. Those students who were already sexually active and had participated in good sexuality education programs were more likely to have used an effective contraceptive at most recent intercourse. Also, the programs increased the consistent use of effective methods. Along with positive effects on sexual knowledge, good sexuality education programs can have important behavioral effects.

The positive influence of sexuality education on behavior has been verified in many studies. For example, Kirby and Coyle (1994) reported that education programs do not hasten the onset of sexual intercourse and may increase the use of contraception in general and condoms in particular. They indicate that specific programs have delayed the onset of intercourse, increased the use of protection against pregnancy or STIs and HIV, and/or reduced the number of sexual partners. Using appropriate behavior-change theories has enhanced the potential for altering students' risk-taking behaviors.

Kirby (2001a) reported that some sexuality and HIV education programs can delay the onset of intercourse, reduce the number of partners, reduce the frequency of sexual intercourse, increase condom or contraceptive use, and thereby decrease sexual risk taking. Also, some programs that have addressed nonsexual risk or protective factors (such as attachment to family, parental monitoring, and attachment to school) have reduced sexual risk taking. Characteristics of effective programs include the following: (1) They focus on reducing one or more behaviors that lead to unintended pregnancy or STIs; (2) they provide basic, accurate information about the risks of teen sexual activity and about ways to avoid intercourse or use methods of protection against pregnancy and STIs; (3) they provide examples of practice with communication, negotiation, and refusal skills; (4) they continue for a sufficient length of time; and (5) they employ teaching methods designed to involve the participants and induce them to personalize the information.

Some people have promoted "abstinence-only" sexuality education programs that, as the name implies, focus only on the importance of abstinence from sexual activity. Kirby (2002) also reviewed the research results from ten abstinence-only programs selected by the Heritage Foundation as having proof that they reduced sexual activity. Kirby reported that nine of the programs failed to provide credible evidence. The tenth program, called *Not Me, Not Now,* may have delayed the initiation of sexual activity among youth 15 years and younger, but not among those 17 years and younger. It may also have reduced pregnancy rates for youth aged 15–17. However, it could not be determined with certainty that the declines over time were caused by the abstinence-only program, as opposed to other influences in the area. Kirby pointed out that the program—more so than other similar programs—had the strongest evidence so far that it may delay the initiation of sexual activity and even reduce teen pregnancy.

In 2005 Maynard et al. reported first-year findings indicating that students in an abstinence-only program have a more positive view toward abstinence. They were more supportive of abstinence and less supportive of teen sexual activity than students not in the program. They also had an increased awareness of the possible consequences of teen and nonmarital sexual activity.

In 2004 Albert reported on a poll that showed a divide among parents and teenagers on whether comprehensive sexuality education encourages young people to engage in sexual activity. Forty-four percent of the parents said that messages beyond abstinence-only education might encourage sexual activity, but 68% of the teens said that "more information does not automatically translate into more sex." The survey also showed that teenagers most often seek information about sexuality from their parents, but most parents don't believe their kids listen to them. Ninety percent of the parents said they do not know how to discuss sexuality with their children.

Eighty-nine percent of teenagers take a sexuality education class by the time they finish high school. Unfortunately, 46% of them have said such classes fail to teach them how to discuss contraception and STI with their partners and do not address emotional consequences of sexual activity. Almost half of the students said they did not receive enough information in the classes. Many teachers want to do more but are prevented by their school districts from expanding the curricula (Teens unsatisfied with sex ed classes, 2001).

Unfortunately, evaluations of comprehensive sexuality education have tended to focus mainly on whether the programs have helped young people delay sexual activity and prevent unwanted pregnancy and disease (Haffner & Goldfarb, 1998). Other goals, such as helping young people develop an appreciation of their bodies or communicate effectively with peers and partners, are often overlooked. Evaluations of sexuality education need to be improved so they reflect broad program goals. In the meantime, many evaluations have found that high-quality sexuality education programs increase knowledge, clarify values, increase parent–child communication, help young people delay the initiation of sexual intercourse, increase the use of contraception and condoms, do not encourage young people to begin intercourse, and do not increase the frequency of sexual intercourse.

Related to sexuality education, some professionals have promoted virginity pledges. Rosenbaum (2009) found that 5 years after giving pledges, 82% of pledgers denied having ever pledged. Pledgers and nonpledgers did not differ in premarital sexuality activity, sexually transmitted diseases, and anal and oral sex variables. Pledgers were less likely to protect themselves from pregnancy and disease before marriage.

The Future of Sexuality Research

More sexuality research is definitely needed. Not only do we need to have more information on sexual behavior itself, but we also need to explore how we make decisions to engage in sexual activity, how the quality of relationships can be improved, and which factors will be important in helping people achieve sexual satisfaction throughout the life cycle. A variety of cultural and societal factors (age, religion, education) have always affected sexual decision making, but recently a change in societal attitudes toward marriage, divorce, childbearing, and sexual relationships has become evident. The stresses these new attitudes bring to bear on personal relationships need to be explored in the near future.

There are real challenges related to sexuality research. Tiefer (1994), in her presidential address to the International Academy of Sex Research, emphasized three crises facing sexology. First, the media are inundating the public with sexual topics. Second, many people in academic circles still hesitate to accept sexuality research as being as legitimate as other forms of research. Finally, there is a tendency for sexuality research to focus only on medical topics and not on the comprehensive nature of people and society. We have learned a great deal through sexuality research; however, even better research methods are needed to fit together the psychological, the biological, and the sociological aspects of sexuality research.

In closing, Tables 2.1 and 2.2 summarize the sexuality research of selected researchers.

TABLE 2.1 Selected Sexuality Researchers and Their Studies (Grouped by Type of Method)

Author(s)	Date	Title
Interview survey		
Scientific literature		
Kinsey, Pomeroy, & Martin	1948	*Sexual behavior in the human male*
	1953	*Sexual behavior in the human female*
Laumann, Gagnon, Michael, & Michaels	1994	*The social organization of sexuality*
Carolina Population Center	2001	National longitudinal study of adolescent health (The "Add Health Survey")
Karofsky	2001	Parent–teen communication and the initiations of sexual intercourse
Bancroft et al.	2004	Sexual activity and risk taking in young heterosexual men: The relevance of sexual arousability, mood, and sensation seeking
Burgard	2004	Factors associated with contraceptive use in late- and post-apartheid South Africa
Bruckner & Bearman	2004	Ambivalence and pregnancy: Adolescents' attitudes, contraceptive use and pregnancy
Cavanagh	2004	The sexual debut of girls in early adolescence: The intersection of race, pubertal timing, and friendship group characteristics
Connell & Freund	2004	Investigating ethnic differences in sexual health: Focus groups with young people
Harawa et al.	2004	Associations of race/ethnicity with HIV prevalence and HIV-related behaviors
Johnson & Jackson	2004	What is the significance of black–white differences in risky sexual behavior?
U. S. Centers for Disease Control and Prevention (Grunbaum et al.)	2004	Youth risk behavior surveillance system
Adam et al.	2005	Acculturation as a predictor of the onset of sexual intercourse among hispanic and white teens
Chuang & Freund	2005	Emergency contraception knowledge among women in a Boston community

Continued

TABLE 2.1   **Selected Sexuality Researchers and Their Studies (Grouped by Type of Method)—cont'd**

Author(s)	Date	Title
Interview survey		
Scientific literature		
Frisco	2005	Parental involvement and young women's contraceptive use
Halpern-Fisher et al.	2005	Oral versus vaginal sex among adolescents: Perceptions, attitudes, and behavior
South et al.	2005	Residential mobility and the onset of adolescent sexual activity
Popular literature		
Hite	1976	*The Hite report*
	1981	*The Hite report on male sexuality*
	1987	*Women and love: A cultural revolution in progress*
Sarrel & Sarrel	1980	The *Redbook* report on sexual relationships
Reinisch & Beasley	1991	*The Kinsey Institute new report on sex*
Kaiser Family Foundation and *Seventeen* magazine	2002	SexSmarts survey on teen sexual behavior
NBC News and *People Magazine*	2004	National Survey of Young Teens Sexual Attitudes and Behavior
Direct observation		
Scientific literature		
Masters & Johnson	1966	*Human sexual response*
	1970	*Human sexual inadequacy*
	1979	*Homosexuality in perspective*

TABLE 2.2 **Examples of Additional Research**

Author(s)	Date	Title
Oncalem & King	2001	Comparison of men's and women's attempts to dissuade sexual partners from the couple using condoms
Kirby	2001	Emerging answers: Research findings on programs to reduce sexual risk-taking and teen pregnancy
Office of the Surgeon General	2001	The Surgeon General's call to action to promote sexual health and responsible sexual behavior
Ford et al.	2001	Characteristics of adolescents' sexual partners and their association with use of condoms and other contraceptive methods
Kaiser Family Foundation	2002	Substance use and risky sexual behavior: Attitudes and practices among adolescents and young adults
Child Trends	2002	National longitudinal survey of youth (Most sexually active teens first had sex at home, late at night, survey shows)
Kirby	2002	Do abstinence-only programs delay the initiation of sex among young people and reduce pregnancy?
Youth Risk Behavior Surveillance System	2002	Trends in sexual risk behaviors among high school students
Alan Guttmacher	2002	U.S. abortion rate declines overall but increases among Institute low-income women
Centers for Disease Control and Prevention	2002	Age at first menstruation continues to decline
U.S. Bureau of the Census	2002	Number of married U.S. teens increased by 50% in 1990s
University of California–Berkeley	2002	Young Americans more likely than their parents' generation to oppose abortion
Kaiser Family Foundation	2003	National survey of adolescents and young adults: Sexual health knowledge, attitudes, and experiences
Denizet-Lewis	2004	Friends, friends with benefits, and the benefits of the local mall
Henshaw	2004	U. S. teenage pregnancy statistics with comparative statistics for women aged 20–24
Lefkowitz et al.	2004	Religiosity, sexual behaviors, and sexual attitudes during emerging adulthood
Vlassoff et al.	2004	Assessing costs and benefits of sexual and reproductive health interventions
Maynard et al.	2005	First-year impacts of four Title V, Section 510 abstinence education programs
Penhollow et al.	2005	The impact of religiosity on the sexual behaviors of college students
Moshser et al.	2005	Sexual behavior and selected measures: Men and women 15–44 years of age, United States, 2002
Koch	2006	Women's bodies as a "puzzle" for college men: Grounded theory research
Lescano et al.	2008	Correlates of heterosexual anal intercourse among at-risk adolescents and young adults
Manlove et al.	2008	Condom use and consistency among male adolescents in the United States
Sex and Tech	2008	Results from a survey of teens and young adults
Martin et al.	2009	Births: Final data for 2006
Rose et al.	2009	The validity of teens' and young adults' self-reported condom use
Rosenbaum	2009	Patient teenagers? A comparison of the sexual behavior of virginity pledgers and matched nonpledgers

Exploring the
DIMENSIONS
of Human Sexuality

Our feelings, attitudes, and beliefs regarding sexuality are influenced by our internal and external environments. Go to sexuality.jbpub.com/dimensions/4e to learn more about the biological, psychological, and sociological factors that affect your sexuality.

Biological Factors

- The medical model was the focus of sexuality research in the 19th century.
- The sexual response cycle was discovered by the researchers Masters and Johnson.
- Physiological changes in the vagina or penis can be monitored by the vaginal plethysmograph and penile strain gauge, respectively.

Sociocultural Factors

- The gender "double standard" research goes back to the 19th century, when discomfort with women's sexuality prompted such beliefs.
- Education leads to both a later age of first intercourse and a higher likelihood of using contraception at first intercourse.
- Religious adolescents are less likely to participate in sexual intercourse; when they do, they are less likely to use reliable contraceptives.
- Ethical considerations abound in sexuality research.

Psychological Factors

- The NHSLS data found that married people were much more likely than single people to report being extremely or very happy.
- Behaviors and practices, as well as frequency of sexual activity, need to be accounted for in sexuality research.
- Motivation to respond to a sexual research survey may create a bias in the sample.
- Learned attitudes and behaviors may influence answers given on sexuality surveys.

CASE STUDY

It's amazing how many factors are involved in even basic research on sexuality. Political forces have banned the use of government money for research dealing with sexuality, so monies must be provided by private foundations or companies, which may have a political or financial agenda of their own.

Learned behaviors prompt many people to answer questions as they think they should be answered, instead of with the truth, and that tendency can create survey bias. The limited number of people willing to respond to a sexuality survey, especially in lower socioeconomic classes, also hinders researchers.

Finally, cultural, ethnic, and religious biases may hinder researchers from getting the data needed. For example, a survey of sexual behavior based on religious affiliation would do poorly, because many Muslim (the number-two religion in the United States) women would not allow interviews or would do so only with their husband present.

Summary

- The scientific method involves identifying a research question, reviewing literature, formulating a hypothesis, operationalizing the variables, collecting data, and analyzing the data to test the hypothesis.

- Research in sexuality can involve surveys, case studies, experimental research, and direct observation.

- Ethical issues in sexuality research include informed consent, confidentiality, anonymity, and protection of subjects.

- Evaluating information about sexuality found on the Internet is often difficult. We need to ask ourselves important questions, such as the purpose of the site or the source of the information, to better evaluate Internet sexuality content.

- Early sexuality researchers included Richard von Krafft-Ebing, Henry Havelock Ellis, Sigmund Freud, Magnus Hirschfeld, Katherine Davis, and Clelia Mosher.

- In the mid-20th century, Alfred Kinsey did extensive research on sexual attitudes and behavior of males and females.

- The research of Masters and Johnson gave us a great deal of information about human sexual response.

- Many studies have been done to help us know more about premarital sexual attitudes and behavior, teen pregnancy, ethnic differences in sexual attitudes and behaviors, use of contraception, changes in selected statistical relationships, and the effects of sexuality education.

- More sexuality research is definitely needed. Needs include knowing more about how we make decisions about sexual behavior, how to improve the quality of relationships, and which factors will help achieve sexual satisfaction throughout the life cycle.

Discussion Questions

1. Compare and contrast the varied methods of sexuality research.

2. Describe the ethical issues involved in sexuality research, citing examples of each.

3. Who were the early sexuality researchers, and what did they figure out? Is their research still considered valid?

4. List the major modern sexuality researchers and describe their contributions. How has their research changed sexuality?

Application Questions

Reread the story that opens the chapter and answer the following questions.

1. Imagine your parents asked you to explain what sexuality researchers do—and why. Prepare a brief response to their query.

2. Explain which dimensions of human sexuality would influence congressional funding for a study on sexuality. Would representatives from some states be more willing to support sexuality research? Explain your answer.

3. For over a year, allegations of sexual relations between former President Clinton and White House intern Monica Lewinsky rocked the news. Evaluate why, in light of a sexual scandal, the president's approval ratings continued to climb.

Critical Thinking Questions

1. What motivates a person to take the time and effort to respond to a human sexuality research questionnaire? Could that motivation lead to a sample bias?

2. As you will learn in the chapter on sexual arousal and response, Masters and Johnson were not the only team to discover a human sexual response cycle. How is it possible that different research groups obtained different results regarding a physiological response?

3. In 1991, the U.S. federal government pulled support from the NHSLS research project and passed legislation prohibiting the spending of federal funds on sexuality research. Although this was clearly a political move, it raises the question, Why should the government support such research? Put another way, how does sexuality research help the American people?

4. Imagine that you and/or your lover read a popular magazine sex survey that showed that a large percentage of people were doing a sexual activity that you had never tried. Would that motivate you to try something new? Would you encourage your lover to try it? How would you feel if your lover asked you to try it?

Critical Thinking Case

During the 1970s, it was widely reported that Russian track and field athletes were encouraged to have sexual relations the night before a major meet. In fact, reports claimed that those who did so performed better (closer to their potential). Imagine that the coach of your college's track team has just learned this information. He has asked you to design a sexuality research project, using scientific methodology, to prove or disprove the hypothesis that sexual activity leads to improved athletic performance.

Which method(s) of research would give you the best results? Explain why. Is it possible to prove the validity of such a hypothesis? Which other factors might be involved? Which ethical issues might you encounter? How could those issues be overcome?

Exploring Personal Dimensions

Sexuality Research

Mark each of the following statements "true" or "false."

_____ 1. All research completed as part of the National Health and Social Life Survey was financially supported by the U.S. federal government.

_____ 2. The first step in the scientific method is identifying a research question.

_____ 3. A hypothesis is a statement based on research results.

_____ 4. Kinsey's research is an example of survey research.

_____ 5. The research of Masters and Johnson is an example of experimental research.

_____ 6. A plethysmograph is used in the laboratory to measure and chart physiological changes over time.

_____ 7. Most normal women have orgasms from penile thrusting alone.

_____ 8. The Sex and Tech study in 2008 showed that a significant number of teens have electronically sent, or posted online, nude or semi-nude pictures or videos of themselves.

_____ 9. The Liu Report can be correctly referred to as a Chinese National Health and Social Life Survey.

_____10. More than half the U.S. students in grades 9–12 have participated in sexual intercourse.

_____11. Both the proportion of adolescent females in the United States who have experienced sexual intercourse and their likelihood of pregnancy have increased in recent years.

_____12. Good sexuality education programs do not hasten the onset of sexual intercourse and may increase the use of contraception—particularly condoms.

Interpretation

All of the even-numbered statements are true and all of the odd-numbered statements are false. If you were correct on at least 10 statements, you did well. If you were not correct on at least 10 statements, find the correct answers in the chapter. All of the correct answers are in this chapter on sexuality research.

Suggested Readings

Bearman, P. S., Moody, J., & Stovel, K. Chains of affection: The structure of adolescent romantic and sexual networks. *American Journal of Sociology 110, no. 1* (July 2004), 44–91.

Brecher, E. *The sex researchers.* New York: Signet Books, 1969.

Cassell, C. Let it shine: Promoting school success, life aspirations to prevent school-age parenthood, *SIECUS Report 30, no. 3* (February–March 2002), 7–12.

Levine, Judith. *Harmful to minors: The perils of protecting children from sex.* St. Paul, MN: University of Minnesota Press, 2002.

Pomeroy, W. *Dr. Kinsey and the Institute for Sex Research.* New York: Harper & Row, 1972.

Wang, B., Hertog, S., Meier, A., Lou, C., & Gao, E. The potential of comprehensive sex education in China: Findings from suburban Shanghai. *International Family Planning Perspectives 31, no. 2* (June 2005), 63–72.

Zimmer-Gembeck, M. J., Siebenbruner, J., & Collins, W. A. A prospective study of intraindividual and peer influences on adolescents' heterosexual romantic and sexual behavior. *Archives of Sexual Behavior 33, no. 4* (August 2004), 381–394.

Web Resources

For links to the web sites below, visit *http://sexuality.jbpub.com/dimensions/4e* and click on Resource Links.

Information on Marie Stopes, an early sexuality researcher
www.spartacus.schoolnet.co.uk/Wstopes.htm

Contains additional information about an early sexuality researcher.

Society for the Scientific Study of Sexuality: Annual Review of Sex Research
www.sexscience.org

Provides updated information on various sexuality research topics.

The Kinsey Institute Research Program
www.kinseyinstitute.org/research/surveylinks.html

Information about many present and past sexuality research studies.

The Alan Guttmacher Institute: New Research and Analysis
www.agi-usa.org

With emphasis on research related to pregnancy and to abortion, the Guttmacher Institute has information on many sexuality research topics.

Sexuality Information and Education Council of the United States
www.siecus.org

Information and publications on numerous sexuality topics are available from the Sexuality Information and Education Council of the United States (SIECUS).

CHAPTER 3

Sexual Communication

CHAPTER OBJECTIVES

1 Describe the process of sexual communication, including nonverbal communication.

2 Identify barriers to sexual communication, including gender differences, attitudes about sexuality, and sexual language.

3 Discuss techniques for improving sexual communication.

INTRODUCTION

Two for the Road *(1967) is a movie starring Audrey Hepburn as Joanna and Albert Finney as Mark. When they first meet on the road in Europe, Joanna is in a touring girls' choir and Mark is a struggling architect. The film follows their life together—through courtship and marriage, infidelity, and parenthood—all on the road in a variety of cars (hence the title), through a score of time-shifting vignettes.*

The film presents a lovely portrayal of a young couple growing in— and eventually out of—love. It not only shows the life cycle of a 12-year relationship, but also brilliantly portrays how communication changes during that life cycle.

As the couple meets and falls in love at a dizzying pace, conversation flows. It seems there is nothing that Joanna and Mark cannot talk about. They openly share their worlds together, delighting in the pleasure of each other. They communicate with touch, holding hands, kissing, making love (although in a 1967 family movie the lovemaking is only implied).

In one blissful scene, the young lovers are shown to their table in a French restaurant. Joanna and Mark hold hands, giggle, smile, make eye contact while walking across the restaurant. But they notice an older married couple who are eating their dinner. The couple is simply eating— no conversation, no touching, no eye contact. Mark turns to Joanna and suggests, "I guess married people don't talk."

But as their relationship and life change, so does their communication style. In time, Joanna and Mark have experienced life together, and they do not talk about it as much as they used to talk about their lives before they met. The mistakes they made as youths disappear into their sophisticated adulthood. There are no silly mistakes to giggle about anymore.

In time, they begin to know each other so well that each can anticipate what the other is going to say or wants to do. Verbal expression becomes infrequent, because it no longer seems very important.

And their lives change, too: They become parents, and Mark becomes a well-known architect. Children and work decrease the amount of time they have for each other. Again, life changes alter communication styles.

Eventually, Joanna and Mark are back in the same French restaurant, but this time as a married couple—no talk, no touch, no eye contact. A young couple, holding hands and giggling, looks at them; he whispers something in her ear. Joanna and Mark have come full circle—they are the married couple who do not talk!

Of course, one of the pleasures of being in a long-term relationship is that there is such a high level of comfort that sometimes you do not have to talk. Yet the very essence of a relationship is communication. Over time, if you rely on your assumptions about what the other person wants, needs, or thinks, the relationship begins to break down—and knowing what your partner wants all the time can become old hat. As people do in real life, Joanna and Mark fail to bridge the gap between not needing to talk constantly and not communicating.

Joanna and Mark's relationship deteriorates. They meet new people, have affairs—all in an effort to relive those days of carefree expression, of newness and excitement. Eventually the marriage ends; the full cycle of the relationship has been portrayed in less time than it may take you to read this chapter!

Many of you who have had long-term relationships can probably relate to the story of Joanna and Mark. When partners fail to communicate freely about sexuality or other topics, their relationship is bound to be limited—in scope and time. You have a great opportunity to enrich your relationships and sexual experiences when you can communicate with your partner about arousing mind and body experiences, your feelings about each other, and the other's preferences in life and in sexuality.

■ The Process of Communicating Sexually

Effective communication begins with an understanding of how communication works. The basic communication model (Figure 3.1) illustrates the five steps of the communication process. Let us consider how the basic communication model might work in a relationship in which partners are participating in some sexual activity.

First, the sender has an idea. Partner A (the sender) does not want to have sexual intercourse. The nature of the idea is influenced by many factors, such as the context of the situation and the sender's mood, background, culture, and frame of reference. For example, Partner A may be too tired or upset, perhaps it is already too late at night, or perhaps Partner A does not know enough about Partner B. Whatever the reasons, Partner A does not want to participate.

The movie *Two for the Road* (1967) explores the life cycle of a relationship, as well as the way communication changes through the cycle. From your own personal experience, does communication change in a relationship over the long term?

Second, the sender encodes the idea in a message. **Encoding** means converting the idea into words or gestures to convey meaning. Partner A says, "I do not want to have sexual intercourse." A potential problem is that words have different meanings for different people. If misunderstandings result from missed meanings, that process is called **bypassing**. For example, Partner B may think all forms of sexual behavior except sexual intercourse are acceptable to Partner A. It may also be possible that Partner B thinks Partner A is just "saying" this and does not really mean it.

Third, the message travels over a channel. Channels include speech, telephones, fax machines, computers, and written correspondence. In this case, the channel contains speech and gestures. Partner A's voice tones, inflections, and gestures are part of the channel.

Fourth, the receiver (Partner B) decodes the message. **Decoding** means translating the message from its symbol form into meaning. Communication can be successful only when decoding is accurate. Various forms of "noise," however, can distort the message. In its simplest sense, the noise of a crowded room makes hearing difficult. Noise can also be represented by misinterpretation of words, voice tones, or gestures; emotional reactions; or the use of alcohol or other drugs. In our example, after

having several drinks, Partner B hears, "Come and convince me."

Fifth, the receiver responds verbally or nonverbally—this is called **feedback**. Feedback helps the sender know whether the message was received and understood. In view of what Partner B heard, feedback is sent in the form of further sexual advances, because "noise" disturbed the transmission of Partner A's message.

Note that in Figure 3.1 the model provides for continual sending, receiving, and feedback. In our example, it is likely that the feedback provided by Partner B will result in additional communication from Partner A, and so the process continues.

Nonverbal Communication

Nonverbal communication includes all unwritten and unspoken messages. These may be sent intentionally or unintentionally. These silent signals exert a strong influence on the receiver in our basic communication model, but interpreting them can be difficult. For example, does the fact that Person A is looking down indicate modesty or just fatigue? Do crossed arms indicate that a person is unwilling to communicate or that a person feels cold?

The vast majority of message meaning (some experts say

---

encoding
Converting an idea into words or gestures to convey meaning.

bypassing
When misunderstandings result from missed meanings.

decoding
Translating the message from its symbol form into meaning.

feedback
When the receiver responds verbally or nonverbally.

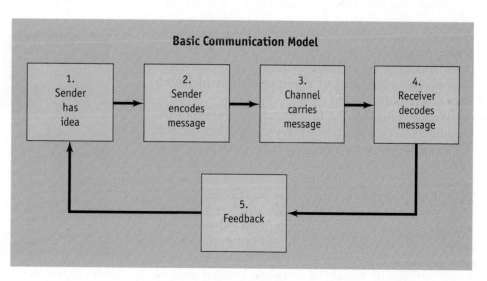

FIGURE **3.1** The basic communication model.

You can show interest in your partner with nonverbal communication. Gazing into each other's eyes, leaning in toward each other, smiling, and touching are all ways of conveying interest in one another.

as much as 93%) (Guffey, 1999) is sent nonverbally. Messages can be difficult to decipher when verbal and nonverbal messages seem to contradict each other. For example, if Person A says it is acceptable to participate in sexual intercourse but then is not very responsive, Person B may have a problem knowing what Person A is really communicating.

When verbal and nonverbal messages conflict, receivers often have more faith in the nonverbal cues than what is said. It is important to recognize the significance of nonverbal communication, but it is unwise to attach a specific meaning to each gesture in every situation.

Note the body posture of your classmates. During an interesting class activity, most of them will probably be leaning or looking toward the lecturer or the center of the group, indicating that they are involved in what is happening. During a boring class, they will probably be leaning away from the lecturer or group. We call this physical behavior *body language*. Communicating by body posture often conveys as much as, or more than, the spoken word. When people feel uncomfortable about expressing their thoughts or feelings verbally, body language may be the only form of communication in which they participate.

We all recognize the importance of communicating nonverbally: We smile when we say hello, scratch our heads when perplexed, and hug a friend to show affection. (We also have an array of body terms to describe our nonverbal behavior: "Keep a stiff upper lip," "I can't stomach him," "She has no backbone," "I'm tongue-tied," "He caught her eye," "I have two left feet," "That was spine-tingling.") We show appreciation and affection, revulsion and indifference with expressions and gestures. We tell people we are interested in them by merely making eye contact and, as the male peacock displays his feathers, we display

our sexuality by the ways we dress and walk and even by the way we stand.

Unfortunately, the nonverbal expression of feelings and thoughts is easy to misinterpret. For example, there is a tendency for people to view their own actions differently from the way their partners view those actions. In addition, people are more likely to notice negative than positive nonverbal behaviors (Manusov & Kerssen-Griep, 1997). There can also be differences in male and female nonverbal communication. Women tend to be more expressive and more skilled at sending and receiving nonverbal messages. Examples include smiling, gazing, having an expressive face, using the hands to communicate, and having an expressive voice. Men tend to be louder and more likely to interrupt and to be more nervous and uneasy about the use of nonverbal messages. Examples include using speech stammers and false starts, interrupting others, having restless feet and legs, interspersing speech with "um" and "ah," speaking loudly, and touching themselves during interactions (Briton & Hall, 1995).

Consequently, to depend on nonverbal communication alone to express yourself sexually is to risk being misunderstood. Furthermore, if your partner is depending on nonverbal communication to express feelings to you, it is up to you to find out—verbally—whether you are getting the right message. Without such a reality check, your partner, although totally failing to connect, might assume that he or she is communicating effectively. For example, imagine that a man and woman on their first date begin hugging, kissing, and caressing each other after a movie. The woman's breathing speeds up, and the man, taking this as a sign of sexual arousal and interest, presses onward. When the woman suddenly pushes free

Misinterpretation of your partner's body language can often lead to conflict in a relationship.

Multicultural DIMENSIONS

Female and Male Subcultures?

Male–female communication is related to gender issues. In the business world males and females seem to be members of different subcultures: Even though meetings in the executive suite increasingly are coed gatherings, there are often real differences in the behavior of females and males.

It could be called the "bad-boy/good-girl" clash. Men seated around conference tables often start acting like adolescents—putting on a show of bravado while trading "witty" put-downs to protect themselves from the pain of criticism. As a prerequisite to success, their culture has taught them to be both self-effacing and self-promoting.

Women, by contrast, have learned from their culture to be earnest perfectionists, eager to show they have done all their homework by explaining every point; yet they are quick to admit mistakes. A woman executive reported seeing this at a meeting where a female colleague began her presentation with many apologies. She told the group that all the information she needed was not available, that she had been rushed, that her slides probably contained typos. She said she was sorry several times but then went on to give a flawless presentation with perfect slides. The man who followed her launched right into his presentation with no apologies whatsoever—and his slides were much less well put together.

Another time the woman executive said she felt frustrated listening to a man who used one incomprehensible acronym after another. Finally, she raised her hand and asked him what one acronym meant. After he explained, the guy sitting next to her leaned over and said, "I'm so glad you asked; I had no idea what he was talking about." She realized that men will not ask questions that make them look uninformed.

Men will, however, take up room at conference tables, spreading out papers, stretching or leaning back, and swiveling around in their chairs. Men are often observed standing up at meetings when they want to make a point or stretching in their seats. Some walk around the room when speaking, asserting their power position.

On average, men talk more at meetings than women, and so their ideas typically are adopted more often. Men also are more comfortable making up things, so if someone asks about a particular financial figure, for example, they may offer one. A woman is more likely to say, "I'm not sure about that." Women give the impression that they do not know what they are talking about, whereas many men seem confident whether they know a little or a lot.

However, it is probably possible to change behaviors and expectations in different cultures. For example, at Eddie Bauer & Co. in Seattle, where half of all managers are women, female executives report a "comfort level" about speaking freely at meetings that they did not feel working at other places. Style differences seem to relate more to job categories than to gender.

Of course, we cannot assume that all males or females will behave exactly as those described do. We also have to remember that possible communication differences are not always a result of being a male or a female. For example, the differences might be related to status rather than gender. The point is that we need to be aware of possible subcultural differences in our personal relationships as well as in our business relationships. Understanding these possible differences can be helpful in improving communication in all relationships.

Source: Hymowitz, C. Men, women fall into kids' roles in meetings, *The Birmingham News* (December 20, 1998), D1–D2.

and complains that the man is too impatient, he is confused. The problem here is one of interpretation rather than incompatibility: The rapid breathing that the man took as a sign of arousal was really a sign of nervousness. If these people had been more effective verbal communicators, they would have been able to clarify the situation in the beginning. Instead they reached a silent impasse, with him confused and her resentful. It can work the other way around, too; both people may want to touch each other but feel too awkward to show it and thus are disappointed.

There are many forms of nonverbal communication. Segal (2008) listed eye contact, facial expression, tone of voice, posture, touch, intensity, timing and pace, and sounds that convey understanding (such as "ahhh," "ummm," and "ohhh") as the most important nonverbal clues. Probably three of the most important forms of nonverbal communication are proximity, eye contact, and touching.

Another name for proximity is *nearness.* Even in our example of students' leaning in the direction of the speaker if they are interested, they are showing

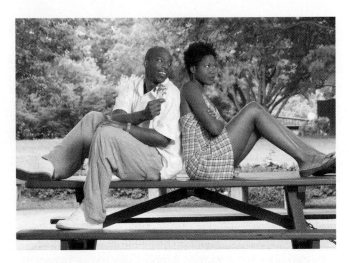

Body position can be a barrier to effective communication.

nearness. Most often, however, proximity refers to the face-to-face distances between people. Although there are differences, in most cultures moving closer indicates increased interest or intimacy, and moving farther away indicates the opposite.

Making eye contact with another person shows interest. This can be true when one is simply listening to another person; however, making eye contact with another person for a little longer than usual can also be a signal of interest in a relationship.

Touching can be very important in a relationship, and it can show interest, intimacy, and emotional closeness. It can range from a slight touch to show concern or connection to the intimate touching associated with sexual relationships. Touch must be used with caution. For example, if someone you do not know very well touches you, that action could be offensive to you. Also, in social and work situations it is important to be careful in using touch to prevent appearing overly intimate and to avoid giving any suggestion of sexual harassment.

Van Wagner (2009) provides some nonverbal communication tips. Here are a few of them:

1. Pay attention to nonverbal signals. This will help improve communication for both the sender and the receiver.

2. Look for incongruent behaviors. When words don't match up with nonverbal signals, people tend to ignore what is said and focus instead on nonverbal expressions of moods, thoughts, and emotions.

3. Use good eye contact. Do not stare fixedly into someone's eyes—but note that failing to look others in the eye makes it seem like there is something to hide.

4. Ask questions about nonverbal signals. If there is confusion about a person's nonverbal signals, it can help to ask questions.

5. Be aware that signals can be misread. A person's overall demeanor tells a lot more than a single gesture.

Barriers to Effective Sexual Communication

The basic communication model is successful only when the receiver understands the message as intended by the sender. In real life, that is hard to accomplish. Consider all the times that you thought you had delivered a clear message, only to be misunderstood. Most messages reach their destination but are disrupted by communication barriers. The most common barriers to successful communication are bypassing, frame of reference, and lack of language and listening skills (Guffey, 1999). To this list we add mind-altering drugs (which include alcohol). Figure 3.2 summarizes ways that barriers play a part in sexual miscommunication.

- *Bypassing:* We all attach meanings to words, but individuals may attach different meanings. Consider the confusion that results if your partner does not want to engage in "sexual relations." You may back off all physical contact. Yet some people—including the former President Bill Clinton—consider sexual relations to refer only to penile–vaginal intercourse. So it is important to understand what meaning your partner attaches to a word.

- *Frame of reference:* Your frame of reference is your unique set of experiences. Your sociocultural upbringing strongly influences your style of communication. A belief in the sexual double standard, in which men pursue women and women "give in" to men, affects the male's frame of reference in our example. As you may remember from Chapter 1's opening story about Lisa, the Korean culture often discourages open discussion of feelings and seeking out of psychological counseling. Thus Lisa was unable to tell her boyfriend of her pregnancy scare.

- *Lack of language skills:* In a new situation, you may not be prepared to communicate effectively. For example, one partner may fear the situation and not know how to communicate effectively that the other's sexual pursuit is unwelcome.

- *Lack of listening skills:* We often listen selectively and interpret messages to our advantage. In our example, the male heard only what he wanted to hear ("Come on and convince me"). He failed to listen to the tone of his partner's voice or look for nonverbal cues.

- *Mind-altering drugs:* Use of alcohol and drugs creates a powerful barrier to communication. More than half of all date rapes involve alcohol. As your inhibitions and ability to communicate clearly fade, so does your ability to control the situation.

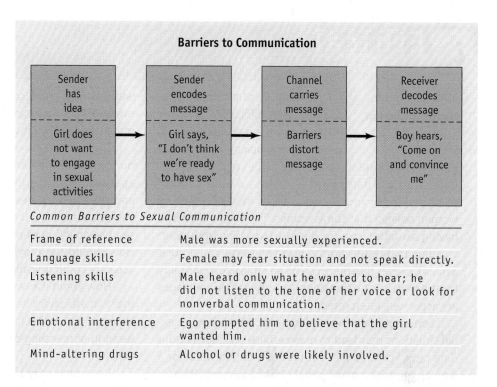

Barriers to Communication

Sender has idea	Sender encodes message	Channel carries message	Receiver decodes message
Girl does not want to engage in sexual activities	Girl says, "I don't think we're ready to have sex"	Barriers distort message	Boy hears, "Come on and convince me"

Common Barriers to Sexual Communication

Frame of reference	Male was more sexually experienced.
Language skills	Female may fear situation and not speak directly.
Listening skills	Male heard only what he wanted to hear; he did not listen to the tone of her voice or look for nonverbal communication.
Emotional interference	Ego prompted him to believe that the girl wanted him.
Mind-altering drugs	Alcohol or drugs were likely involved.

FIGURE **3.2** Common barriers to communication.

Gender Communication Issues

In a popular magazine, Sheidlower (1997) indicated that communication difficulties between the sexes are related to a lack of vocabulary. Men and women are unable to reach a mutual understanding of certain concepts because they cannot describe them to each other. He compares the reality of situations with the words women use in their language ("she-speak"). Here are two examples (***the authors recognize that these examples are quite sexist, but we include them because many people, unfortunately, believe in these stereotypes***):

- "He-speak": A new car has "331 horsepower, five-speed transmission, V-8, four valves per cylinder, dual overhead cam, and a twin turbocharger." "She-speak": "It's red."

- "He-speak": A new amplifier has "twin mono-blocks, low THD, only 40 watts per channel, but it's a small room, so the low-impedance speakers will still work; it'll be expensive if we blow any Gold Aero KT-88 output tubes." "She-speak": "That thing is not going in *my* living room."

Sheidlower's point is that if we want to have high-quality relationships, we have to make an effort. Whether there is really a difference in vocabulary between the genders is for each of us to decide, but we can also do our part to reduce the possibility of a problem of miscommunication.

Gender roles can strongly shape our communication patterns. Because men have traditionally focused on their place in the hierarchy, they tend to be good at public speaking. Women, who have traditionally focused on nurturing relationships, tend to be better at speaking in private. On the emotional level, women tend to be good at verbalizing thoughts and feelings in close relationships. Men, in contrast, tend to be good at dismissing their feelings or keeping them to themselves. For men, expressing feelings does not help determine their status or help them compete in the outside world. It can be helpful to be aware of the context and the power of gender roles to influence what we hear, what we say, and what is the purpose of our communication (Worden & Worden, 1998).

Because emotions are involved in the use of language, remembering that gender differences may affect people's responses to emotion can be helpful. For example, men and women may have subtle differences in their responses to a number of emotions, including anger, sadness, and jealousy (Guerrero, 1998).

Do males and females naturally communicate differently, or are their communication behaviors learned just as other behaviors are? Some people believe that males are socialized to be more assertive and direct, in both verbal and nonverbal communication. Eye contact, body placement, and rough physical contact by males can communicate intention, superiority, and territoriality. Historically, women have generally been

¿? Ethical DIMENSIONS

Ethics, Communication, and Date Rape

One example of potential communication difficulties is sexual behavior on a date. Keeping our basic communication model in mind, let us consider some ethical issues related to communication and date rape.

It has been found that 69% of men and 54% of women believe that some women like to be talked into having sexual intercourse. Because bypassing (misunderstanding that results from a mixed message) can occur if a male believes this, there can be an ethical responsibility for the male or the female to be sure certain messages are accurately interpreted.

Some cultural images of romantic interaction in sexual situations may lead to many ethical questions about date rape. For example, is it part of a dating ritual for a woman to resist a man's initial sexual advances? What is her ethical responsibility to be sure she is sending accurate—and not misleading—messages?

If a woman is drunk or has used other chemical substances that can influence judgment, what is the ethical responsibility of the male in regard to his actions? Should the female have considered the ethics of putting herself (and the male) in that situation in the first place? If she is under the influence of chemical substances, she may send (encode) a message in a way she does not intend.

If a male is drunk or has used other chemical substances that can influence his judgment, the "noise" (see the communication model in Figure 3.2) can interfere with his ability to decode the message being sent accurately. What is his ethical responsibility for accurate communication in this situation?

The feedback being sent is an important part of our communication model. If a woman goes to a man's apartment or invites the man to her apartment for a drink and then participates in heavy petting, do her actions suggest consent? Is it ethical for her to do these things if she has no intent of participating in sexual intercourse? How should she provide accurate feedback so there is accurate communication?

How about if a woman is dressed in revealing clothing? Is it ethical for her to do this if she is not interested in sexual activity? Is it ethical for a man to interpret the wearing of revealing clothing as an invitation for sexual activity?

Date rape may be a result of miscommunication. Following the steps of our basic communication model (sender having an idea, sender encoding the message, message traveling over a channel, receiver decoding the message, and feedback traveling to the sender) and considering how bypassing can occur and how noise can interfere with accurate communication give us many ethical issues related to communication and date rape to consider. Clear communication is needed to help prevent date rape.

Source: Is there a date rape crisis in society? In *Taking sides: Clashing views on controversial issues in family and personal relationships,* 4th ed., Vail, A., ed. Guilford, CT: Dushkin/McGraw-Hill, 1999.

socialized to have a less pronounced presence. They tend, for example, to listen empathetically, communicate and elicit emotions, and process conflict. As a result, a familiar complaint of women in heterosexual relationships is that male partners "never want to talk about things," "aren't sensitive to their needs," and "just don't understand." Conversely, males often wonder how a seemingly innocuous comment could cause their female partner's sudden silence or desire to talk about where the relationship is going. People internalize the values attached to gendered communication to the point that men become used to living within conflict and women prefer the roles of peacemaker and relationship builder. Some people argue that looking at gender exclusively as the source of different communication styles is a mistake and that such elements as upbringing, socioeconomic status,

culture, and ethnicity must be considered within this context (Do women and men communicate differently?, 2003).

Reeder (2005) pointed out that research findings regarding communication differences related to gender are simply contradictory. For example, some studies show men to be more assertive, while others find women to be as assertive or even more assertive than men. When it comes to most communication behaviors, such as leadership style, sociability, or displays of power in intimate relationships, Reeder indicated that academic research reveals little to no difference between genders. Overall, communication research suggests that male–female differences are actually quite small. Gender seems to account for only 1% of the variation in communication behaviors. Other factors play a more significant role, such

Gender DIMENSIONS

Sexual Behavior in Marriage

Listen to this couple in their mid- to late 20s, married 9 years:

Wife: I don't understand him. He's ready to go any time. It's always been a big problem with us right from the beginning. If we've hardly seen each other for two or three days and hardly talked to each other, I can't just jump into bed. If we have a fight, I can't just turn it off. He has a hard time understanding that. I feel like that's all he wants sometimes. I have to know I'm needed and wanted for more than just jumping into bed.

Husband: She complains that all I want from her is sex, and I try to make her understand that it's an expression of love. I'll want to make up with her by making love, but she's as cold as the inside of the fridge. I get mad when that happens. Why shouldn't I? Here I'm trying to make up and make love, and she's holding out for something—I don't know what.

Wife: He keeps saying he wants to make love, but it just doesn't feel like love to me. Sometimes I feel bad that I feel that way, but I just can't help it.

Husband: I don't understand. She says it doesn't feel like love. What does that mean, anyway? What does she think love is?

Wife: I want him to talk to me, to tell me what he's thinking. If we have a fight, I want to talk about it so we could maybe understand it. I don't want to jump in bed and just pretend it didn't happen.

Husband: Talk! Talk! What's there to talk about? I want to make love to her and she says she wants to talk. How's talking going to convince her I'm loving her?

In sexual behavior, as in other matters, the barriers to effective communication are high and the language people use only further confuses and mystifies them. He says he wants to make love, but she says, "It doesn't feel like love." Neither quite knows what the other is talking about; both feel vaguely guilty and uncomfortable, aware only that somehow they're not connecting. He believes that he has already given her a profound declaration of love: He married her and they share a home.

Yet she says, "Just once, I'd like him to love me without it ending up in sex. But when I tell him that, he thinks I'm crazy."

For him, perhaps, it does seem crazy. Sexual activity may be the one way in which he can allow himself the expression of deep feeling. His wife, however, finds it difficult to be comfortable with her feelings in the same area. She keeps asking for something that she can understand and is comfortable with—a demonstration of his feelings in nonsexual ways. He keeps giving her the one thing he can understand and is comfortable with—his feelings wrapped up in a blanket of sex. Thus some husbands and wives find themselves in an impossibly difficult bind, one that stems from the cultural context in which girls and boys grow to adulthood.

We are suggesting that the man's ever-present sexual readiness is not simply an expression of urgent sexual need but is also a complex response to a socialization process that restricts the development of the emotional side of his personality. Conversely, the woman's insistent plea for a nonsexual emotional statement is a response to a process that encourages the development of the emotional side of her personality.

as the type of relationship and the context within which the communication takes place.

Attitudes About Sexuality

Some people are prevented from communicating openly by attitudes learned at home. Some parents "protect" young children from references to sexuality. When as teenagers these children are exposed to talk about sexuality—on the street or at school—they often feel guilty for participating in or eavesdropping on such forbidden conversations. When parents fail to acknowledge our sexuality as children, we should

not be surprised if suppressed feelings permeate our adult sexual lives.

There is a debate over whether men and women have different talking styles (Do men and women speak different languages?, 1999). Some people believe that men have a need for control in their social relationships. During conversations they try to capture the floor, state their issues with forthright clarity, and make decisions confidently. They do not like being interrupted and revel in giving information and advice. By contrast, the argument goes, women are predisposed to being inclusive and nurturing in their conversational style. They wait their turn for the floor and make cooperative decisions after hearing all sides. Women like to keep the conversation flowing, interrupt one another, fill silences, and ask questions. Expressing sympathy and sharing similar feelings are regular elements of women's conversations.

Those who believe that these patterns of communication exist say that the contrasting styles may lead to misunderstanding between men and women in close relationships. Further, to improve rational quality it is necessary to develop understanding and sympathy for differences in the ways men and women talk and to make sincere efforts to listen and appreciate the other's way of speaking. Opponents of this view believe that we must dig deeper than sex differences to understand people's communication problems. Communication may depend more on social status and power of the speaker than on gender.

Deborah Tannen, a professor of linguistics, has written extensively about male and female communication styles. She indicates that many women feel it is natural to consult their partners at every turn, whereas men automatically make more decisions without consulting their partners. This may show a real difference in conceptions of decision making. For example, women expect decisions to be discussed first and made by consensus; however, many men feel oppressed by lengthy discussions about what they see as minor decisions, and they feel hemmed in if they cannot act without talking first. Tannen further indicates that communication is a continual balancing act, juggling conflicting needs for intimacy and independence (Tannen, 1991). Some of Tannen's critics feel that she focuses too much on gender differences and not enough on the similarities between women and men. Whether or not this is true, her work provides important and interesting thoughts for consideration related to communication.

Some writers suggest that men often do not communicate well with women because they have a "fear of intimacy" that is really a fear of rejection. One way to deal with this is for men to learn to talk about their lives more openly, as women have learned to do. Developing their own friendships with other men can help men acquire personal skills that will also improve their relationships with women (Dickson, 2000).

Parent–Teen Communication

An excellent example of the importance of good communication is that between parents and their children—especially their adolescent children. Karofsky (2001) reported a correlation between the level of adolescent–parent communication, as perceived by the teenager, and abstinence from initiation of sexual intercourse. High levels of communication with mothers were most closely associated with abstinence. The

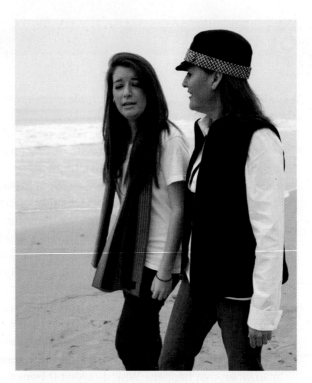

Many teens would welcome communication with their parents about sexuality.

amount of parent–teen communication declined as the teen got older. The authors suggest two possibilities: (1) As communication declined at home, teenagers sought a replacement for intimacy with their parents and then participated in sexual intercourse; or (2) as teenagers became sexually active, they were reluctant to discuss these and other personal issues with their parents, and therefore communication declined.

Dailard (2001) reported that teenagers who feel their parents are warm, caring, and supportive are more likely to delay sexual activity than their peers. Teens who feel highly satisfied with their relationship with their mother are more likely to use contraception and to delay sexual activity and are less likely to have an unplanned pregnancy.

When it comes to communicating with their children about sexuality, many parents consider the task a daunting one, for which they feel ill equipped. Parents often do not have meaningful conversations with sons and daughters because they do not know what to say or how to begin, fearing that talking to children about sexuality may either scare children or encourage them in sexual behaviors at a young age. Most parent–child discussions about sexuality are limited, indirect, and uncomfortable. Yet, parents' failure to provide adolescents with appropriate information and decision-making skills may place teens at risk for negative outcomes such as pregnancy or STI. Only about 15% of adolescents have had conversations about sexuality with their parents. Mothers are more likely than fathers to discuss birth control, adolescent pregnancy, and sexual morality with both sons and daughters (Filomeno, 2002).

Parents and teens also seem to have different estimations of how often they have discussed sexuality (Grunbaum et al., 2004). Forty-two percent of parents said they talked to their teenagers about sexuality and sexual relationships "very often," 43% said they talked "somewhat often," 12% said "not too often," and 2% said "never." In contrast, 11% of teens of those same parents said they talked to their parents about sexuality and sexual relationships "very often," 30% said they talked "somewhat often," 40% said "not too often," and 18% said "never."

Albert (2004) reported that 90% of parents said they did not know how to discuss sexuality with their children. He also pointed out that parents are selling themselves way too short, and that they need to have conversations about sexuality with their children at earlier ages. In fact, 91% of adults and 87% of teens think it would be easier for young people to delay sexual activity and avoid unwanted pregnancy if they could discuss sexuality with their parents.

There are many reasons for good parent–child communication about sexuality. However, the association between parent–child communication and adolescent pregnancy risk remains unclear (Sample lesson plan using JSR, 2005). One difficulty in studying this relationship is that there is little or no agreement between what parents and teens perceive to have communicated between them. Measures of communication content, as well as the frequency, timing, and quality of communication, vary so much across studies that it is hard to establish a pattern of findings.

Because many college students eventually decide to become parents, here are some tips about talking with kids about sexuality (Silverberg, 2008). Perhaps the most important one is to make talking with your children about sexuality a lifelong conversation. Instead of just having a "big sex talk," recognize that many small moments of learning and teaching about sexuality happen throughout a child's development. Also, it is important to be comfortable when it comes to talking about sexuality. Many things, such as reading this book and taking a sexuality class, can greatly help to increase your comfort level with this topic. It is also good to make it OK for your kids to ask about sexuality. All children have such questions, and it helps to create an environment where they feel comfortable asking them. Finally, it is important to use age-appropriate information. A number of excellent resources, such as many of those mentioned throughout this text, are available that can help people understand more about age-appropriate sexuality information.

Sexual Language

One of us was invited to speak with a group of elderly people about sexuality. Proceeding with undaunted courage, he began the session with exercises designed to neutralize the emotional impact of sexual words. He showed slides containing one or two words and instructed the participants to shout in unison the word appearing on the slide. The first slide was shown and the audience shouted *love* with much enthusiasm. Buoyed up by the group's cooperation and interest, he projected the next slide—*hug*. The audience again shook the room with their shouts. From that point on, however, it was all downhill. With each successive word, the decibel level of the voices lowered—no small wonder, considering the remaining words: *kiss, caress, pet, sexual intercourse, oral sex, penis,* and *vagina.* The point was made: People are uncomfortable with sexual language. How can sexual communication be effective if we cannot even speak the language?

When discussing sexual topics, people often find that the words themselves prevent rational, thoughtful, comfortable interaction. Some words evoke such strong emotions—embarrassment, guilt, shame, or anger—that they interfere with thoughtful discourse. Generally, the greater the emotion, the greater the interference.

For example, it may be that the term used influences what a partner hears: "Penis," "dick," and "cock" may all have different connotations for different people. Calling a vagina a "vagina" may sound very clinical to one person, whereas calling it a "pussy" or a "cunt" may sound sexy, dirty, or just fine to someone else. The sexual language used can promote communication and relationships, or it can inhibit them.

■ Techniques for Improving Sexual Communication

As we have discussed, there are many reasons for good sexual communication. One of these includes a need to communicate about desires related to sexual activity. Miller and Byers (2004) interviewed 153 heterosexual couples about their actual and ideal duration of foreplay and intercourse, as well as their partners' desired duration of foreplay and intercourse. Both men's and women's perceptions of their partners' ideal duration of foreplay and intercourse were found to be more strongly related to their own sexual stereotypes than to their partners' self-reported sexual desires. This suggested that people rely on sexual stereotypes when estimating their partners' ideal sexual scripts. Improving communication about sexuality could help eliminate such misperceptions. There are no magical methods for attaining free, open, and

Communication
DIMENSIONS

Clarity in Sexual Communication   In the communication process, the idea sent and the message actually received are ideally the same. But as you likely know from experience, matters do not always work that way. Often, the words chosen, the tone of voice, the body language, or the context in which the message is delivered blurs the true intent of the sender. When you add the ambiguity of sexual language, communicating clearly becomes even more difficult.

Consider former President Bill Clinton and his now-infamous words in a press conference on January 26, 1998: "I did not have sexual relations with that woman—Miss Lewinsky." To President Clinton, "sexual relations" specifically referred to penile–vaginal intercourse, sexual activity in which he and Monica Lewinsky did not participate.

In his own parlance, Clinton was telling the truth. Yet few would agree with him. One reason was the context of the comment—a formal press conference in the White House. Also, the delivery of the comment—with strong body language and tersely delivered words—made it appear that there was no relationship at all between Clinton and Lewinsky.

Now consider how such language ambiguity might affect a newer relationship.

Let us say that you suggest beginning a more "serious relationship" with someone. Your partner responds that the relationship is not ready for "sexual relations." At this point, it is not clear what either party has said. A "serious relationship" could imply having sexual activity, but it could also imply seeing each other more often or not seeing other people. The "sexual relations" comment in the context of an intimate conversation could be construed to refer to any sexual activity.

Thus it is important to be clear in communicating about sexuality with a partner. If you or your partner cannot talk about sexuality, that may be a sign that you are not ready to be involved in a sexual relationship.

A good way to start a conversation is to talk about sexual histories. By starting the conversation and opening it up for participation, you will make it more comfortable for your partner. Talk about sexual activities that you have enjoyed and would like to share with your partner.

Before entering into a sexual relationship, you should talk about any STIs that you or a partner may have had, and any STI and/or HIV testing you have had (and why you had it done). In addition, you should discuss using latex condoms to prevent STI transmission as well as using a contraceptive method to prevent pregnancy.

comfortable communication about sexual topics, but we do have some suggestions.

First, Owen (2008) provides some suggestions to improve the overall atmosphere for communication. She indicates that it is important to realize that one does not know everything. This leads to asking good questions. Also, it helps to ask the right questions. For example, "Is this what you like?" can be a great question that also shows concern about the other person. Being open-minded and nonjudgmental is helpful as well. Maintaining care and trust also leads to better communication. One person is much more likely to open up to another if there is confidence that the information will not be shared with others. Other suggestions for improving communication are found in the following pages.

Planning

One common barrier to good sexual communication is the complete avoidance of the subject by both partners. We suggest that partners set aside time to discuss sexuality as they would any other topic of mutual interest and of significance to their relationship. In setting up a time for such a discussion, it is wise to make the following plans.

1. Make sure you have plenty of time for your discussion. Do not be cut short when one of you has to run off somewhere.

2. Do not allow others to interrupt your discussion by calling you or by barging in on you.

3. Accept all feelings and the right to express these feelings verbally. For example, it is just as appropriate to say, "I feel angry when . . ." as it is to say, "I feel terrific when . . ."

4. Take a risk—really describe your thoughts and needs. Do not expect your partner to guess what they are.

5. Approach the discussion with both people understanding that the goal is to improve your relationship rather than to see who can shock whom.

It can take work to have good sexual communication.

6. Expect changes but not miracles. Sexual communication requires continued dialogue. You might want to seek the help of other family members, friends, peer counselors, members of the clergy, psychologists, sexuality counselors, or others who can contribute to your ability to communicate sexually.

Working to improve your sexual communication will help you and your partner develop a deeper trust, a greater sense of intimacy, and a feeling of adventure about your relationship.

Flooding

A technique for learning to use and become comfortable with sexual language is called **flooding**. In one use of this technique, people stand in front of a mirror, look themselves in the eye, and repeat over and over again the words they feel uncomfortable using. We are not necessarily referring to profanity. We are talking about sexual language. Learning to feel comfortable with these words and being able to use them should be your goals.

> **flooding**
> Experiencing something so frequently that you no longer are aroused by it. This is a technique used to become more comfortable with sexual terminology.

Learning Assertiveness

Some people just have a tough time communicating—period. Inevitably they have trouble communicating sexually. When this is the case, working to improve only the sexual side of communication is a mistake. Therefore, we turn now to a topic that concerns one's ability to express oneself with confidence in all areas—the quality of assertiveness and the means to develop it.

The first step toward grasping what it means to be assertive is to distinguish assertive, aggressive, and nonassertive behaviors. **Assertiveness** means standing up for your basic rights *without violating* anyone else's. **Aggressiveness** means standing up for your basic rights (or more) *at the expense* of someone else's rights. **Nonassertiveness** means *giving up* your basic rights so that other people can achieve theirs.

> **assertiveness**
> Standing up for one's basic rights without violating anyone else's rights.
>
> **aggressiveness**
> Standing up for one's basic rights, but at the expense of someone else's basic rights.
>
> **nonassertiveness**
> Giving up one's basic rights so others may achieve theirs.

For example, an assertive style of verbal sexual communication would be one in which you stand up for your own sexual rights and needs by expressing your wishes, while allowing your partner the same freedom.

Body language, too, can be aggressive, nonassertive, or assertive. Aggressive body language includes a pointing finger, leaning toward the other person, glaring, and using a loud, angry tone of voice. Nonassertive body language is characterized by slumped posture, a lack of eye contact, hand-wringing, hesitant speech, nervous whining or laughing, and not saying or doing what you want to. Assertive behavior, by contrast, entails sitting or standing tall, looking directly at the person you are talking to, speaking in explicit statements with a steady voice, and using the gestures or physical contact that is right for you.

As a first step toward learning to be assertive, consider this formula, developed by Bower and Bower (1976), for organizing assertive verbal responses. The formula, which they call DESC, involves

1. **D**escribing the other person's behavior or the situation as objectively as possible (as in sentences taking the form "When you . . .")

2. **E**xpressing your feelings about the other person's behavior or the situation that you just described (as in statements beginning with "I feel . . .")

3. **S**pecifying changes you would like to see made ("I would like . . ." or "My preference is . . .")

4. **C**hoosing the consequences you are prepared to accept (a) if the situation changes to your satisfaction and (b) if it does not ("If you . . . , I will . . ." or "If you don't . . . , I will . . .")

Using the DESC form, then, let us look at an example of assertive sexual communication: "When you expect me to become sexually aroused in two minutes of foreplay (Describe), I feel as though I'm being used (Express). I would like us to spend more time touching, kissing, and hugging (Specify). If you agree to devote more time to foreplay, I will relax and pay special attention to your sexual needs. If you don't agree to devote more time to foreplay, I won't have intercourse with you (Choose)." Note that our imaginary speaker describes the situation from a personal point of view, expressing his or her own feelings and preferences, as well as the consequences of the listener's choice.

The form of the DESC message just described suggests the philosophical basis of the assertion theory: We are in control of ourselves alone; we have no right to tell others how to behave; we need not tolerate the other person's behavior when it is contrary to our own desires. The basis of assertive behavior is the combination of self-respect with respect for others. One could find no better formula for effective sexual communication.

Expressing Yourself Nonverbally

Words are important, but they do not say it all. Do not be afraid to smile, wink, hug, touch, kiss, or in other ways communicate your affection for another. As we said earlier, in the way you walk, sit, gesture, and so on, you are "talking" to your partner, whether you intend to or not. But you can also consciously use those gestures to help get your message across.

Seeking Information (Listening)

Verify your interpretation of the other person's verbal, and especially nonverbal, communication. Listen actively, and ask whether your understanding of your partner's feelings and intentions is accurate. Listening is often hard and takes real skill. If you want to hear what others say effectively, make sure you are not a

- *Mind reader:* You hear little or nothing as you think, "What is this person really thinking or feeling?"

- *Rehearser:* Your mental tryouts for "Here's what I'll say next" tune out the speaker.

- *Filterer:* Some call this selective listening—hearing only what you want to hear.

- *Dreamer:* Drifting off during a face-to-face conversation can lead to an embarrassing "What did you say?" or "Could you repeat that?"

Sitting close together, touching, and smiling are all ways to show you care. Nonverbal communication is important; expressing feelings in words is also vital.

- *Identifier:* If you refer everything you hear to your experience, you probably did not hear what was said.

- *Comparer:* When you get side-tracked assessing the messenger, you are sure to miss the message.

- *Derailer:* Changing the subject too quickly tells others you are not interested in anything they have to say.

- *Sparrer:* You hear what is said but quickly belittle it or discount it. That puts you in the same class as the derailer.

- *Placater:* Agreeing with everything you hear just to be nice or to prevent conflict does not make you a good listener (Why don't we hear others?, 2005).

The leadership expert Stephen Covey speaks of "attentive" and "empathetic" listening—not the fake or manipulative kind but rather "listening with the intent to understand." Covey speaks and writes about situations related to business; however, the basics of good listening skills apply to intimate relationships as well. Good listeners are rare; most of us have to squelch our natural inclination to talk.

The characteristics of good listeners are as follows:

1. The most visible characteristic is body language—nodding encouragingly, perhaps leaning into the conversation, not glancing around the room or looking for something.

2. Good listeners demonstrate that they are mentally engaged in what the speaker is saying by making brief comments from time to

DIMENSIONS

International Differences in Discussing Sexuality

In many chapters of this book, we have seen examples of international differences related to the topic of human sexuality. One way to gain understanding of these differences is to consider how sexuality education is viewed in some countries. Here are some examples.

1. In Mexico, it is the government's policy to stabilize growth. Family planning is supposed to be implemented by means of education and public services. At the same time, the conservative Catholic church opposes sexuality education.
2. In Chile, sexuality is not a subject that is talked about by family members or in schools.
3. In China, there is virtually no institutional sexuality education. People rely on folklore, sexually explicit materials, and approved marriage manuals for sexuality information.
4. In Denmark, sexuality and social-life education has been a compulsory subject in schools since 1970, and it was a tradition long before then.
5. In Egypt, discussion of sexuality is socially unacceptable. Egypt uses an approach that emphasizes repression rather than education.
6. In Greece, sexuality education does not exist in the school curriculum. Greece is one of the few European countries without sexuality education.
7. In India, sexuality education is not offered in schools because society believes it would "spoil the minds" of children.
8. In Iran, to get a marriage license, couples must take a segregated course in family planning.
9. In Japan, sexuality education in schools (typically focused on reproductive issues) is mandated, beginning at age 10 or 11 years. The Ministry of Education believes that teachers should teach HIV and AIDS prevention to students without mentioning sexual intercourse.
10. In Kenya, the government opposes sexuality education in schools. Young people turn to their peers for sexuality information.
11. In Romania, sexuality education was removed from the schools in the early 1980s. The major sources of contraception and sexuality information are friends, mass media, and health care providers.
12. In Singapore, women are highly ignorant about their bodies, including being unable to locate the vagina. Women complain also of pain during intercourse because of lack of foreplay. Some women who believe they are barren actually turn out to be virgins.
13. In Sweden, sexuality education has been a compulsory subject in schools since 1955. It is well integrated into the school curriculum. In addition, Swedish children receive their first sexuality education at home, from their parents.
14. In Thailand, there are strong taboos surrounding the discussion of sexuality and disease. HIV/AIDS education has been stifled, and many do not know how the disease is spread.
15. In the United Kingdom, sexuality education has been required in secondary schools since 1993. In Northern Ireland, it is not mandated, but it is encouraged in the teaching of health education. In Scotland, jurisdiction over the provision of sexuality education lies with the local education authority. In general, teens report that they believe their parents should be their main source of sexuality information; however, in practice they are more likely to turn to their friends for information.

Although it is difficult to draw definite conclusions from this information, it appears that there can be real differences in the ability of people from various countries to engage in effective communication about human sexuality. For example, think about the differences that are likely to exist between people from Sweden and those from Thailand or from Egypt. Of course, we cannot generalize about all people from any country, because many differences are possible within countries. But these differences can strongly influence communication about sexuality.

Source: Caron, S. L. *Cross-cultural perspectives on human sexuality.* Boston: Allyn & Bacon, 1998.

time and asking focused questions—patiently waiting for the answer before providing one.

3. They listen with the "third ear," seeking to understand those thoughts that are not expressed.

4. They try to understand, rather than first being understood. They try to see the topic of conversation from the speaker's standpoint first. Good listeners push back the urge to express personal opinions until they are asked or until the time is appropriate.

Good listeners show they are mentally engaged.

5. Good listeners have to be trusted. They never repeat confidences and personal problems without consent of the party involved (Listening to understand, 1998).

Hostile settings and other communication hindrances can defeat even the best listeners. Here are a few steps to avoid those pitfalls:

1. Choose the physical environment. Find a quiet, nonthreatening place to talk if you want to ensure true understanding.

2. Cut the interruptions. It can be difficult to communicate if the phone rings or if a person pops in at the door.

3. Recognize differences. People communicate best in different ways. Some of us are primarily auditory, whereas others are visual or "hands-on."

4. Persist. Refuse to believe that you cannot understand another person's message.

Steps Toward Change

Counselors often work with couples to help them improve their communication skills. In summary, the counselor (1) encourages **active listening**; (2) elicits feedback from each partner by asking each to summarize what he or she just heard; (3) facilitates the expression of feelings and thoughts directly and succinctly; (4) requests the use of **"I" statements** (beginning each sen-

active listening
Paraphrasing what someone has said to demonstrate interest and understanding.
"I" statement
Statement that begins with an "I" to express personal feelings.

tence with "I" to express personal feelings better and avoid blaming the other partner) instead of questions; and (5) prohibits interruptions and blaming (Worden & Worden, 1998). These techniques will help all of us communicate much more effectively.

Resolving Conflicts

In relationships—even the best of relationships—conflicts arise. Too often poor communication skills (such as improper listening), a combative or offensive stance geared toward winning rather than communicating, an inability to acknowledge another's point, or a refusal to consider alternative solutions interferes with the healthy resolution of these conflicts. As a result, conflicts threaten the continuation of the relationship and, at the least, tear little pieces from it, potentially leaving the relationship bankrupt. To gain a sense of how these poor communication skills impair effective conflict resolution, consider the following dialogue.

Paul: *Well, Barbara, as you know, I really care for you, and I hope we can continue to develop our relationship. We can't go any further tonight, though, because I'd like you to be tested for HIV.*
Barbara: *Now you ask—right in the middle of this romantic time! Why didn't you say something about this before?*
Paul: *You've got some nerve. You should have realized this is something we need to consider.*
Barbara: *I should have realized? How was I supposed to know you were concerned about HIV status? You never said anything about it.*
Paul: *Why should I take the chance of getting HIV? You're pretty selfish, aren't you?*
Barbara: *I've had it! Either we're going to trust each other and move ahead in our relationship or you can say good-bye right now.*
Paul: *In that case, GOOD-BYE!*

In this example, both Paul and Barbara are trying to win: Paul wants Barbara to have an HIV test, and Barbara wants Paul to have faith and move ahead with their relationship. Neither Paul nor Barbara can possibly win this battle, although they are probably unaware of this. If they proceed with their relationship (including sexual intercourse and other intimate behaviors), Paul will be uneasy because of his concern about HIV. He will probably feel his concerns are not very important to Barbara, will resent her lack of concern, and will have a difficult time participating freely in the relationship.

However, if Barbara agrees to the HIV test, she will feel that Paul did not trust her and "forced" her to take the test. She may also feel he waited to spring the idea on her and wonder why it did not arise earlier.

It becomes evident, then, that regardless of which way they go, one or the other will be resentful. This resentment will probably result in a weakening, or possibly a dissolution, of their relationship. So, no matter who wins, both really lose.

This situation is not totally hopeless, though. Consider the effect on resolving their conflict if Paul and Barbara had communicated as follows:

Paul: *Well, Barbara, as you know, I really care for you, and I hope we can continue to develop our relationship. We can't go any further tonight, though, because I'd like you to be tested for HIV.*
Barbara: *Now you ask—right in the middle of this romantic time! Why didn't you say something about this before?*
Paul: *You feel we should have discussed this earlier?*
Barbara: *Yes, and HIV status is something we both need to be concerned about.*
Paul: *You have a concern about my HIV status, too?*
Barbara: *You bet! And I think it is only fair that we treat ourselves and each other equally in this situation.*
Paul: *You think that it would be a problem if you got the HIV test and I didn't?*
Barbara: *Yes.*
Paul: *Would you be embarrassed if other people knew you had taken the test?*
Barbara: *Yes, I guess I would.*
Paul: *It sounds like my request might have hurt you at least a little?*
Barbara: *Yes, I guess it did.*
Paul: *I'm glad that you also care about our relationship. But HIV is really a serious health problem today, and I am worried about it. And I'm bothered that you didn't understand my concern.*
Barbara: *I guess you do have a reason to be concerned. I'm sorry.*
Paul: *Well, let's see what alternatives we have.*
Barbara: *Maybe I should just go ahead and be tested.*
Paul: *Or perhaps we should both be tested.*
Barbara: *How about agreeing that we will honestly share the results with each other but also that the results are private and not anyone else's business?*
Paul: *That's fine with me. In fact, we don't even need to tell anyone else we took the tests. That is our private matter.*
Barbara: *Would it make sense to agree to take the tests as soon as possible so we both know the results as soon as we can?*
Paul: *That seems sensible, and since your schedule in the next couple of weeks is so busy, I'll be happy to work around your schedule.*
Barbara: *Okay. Remember, though, the next time either of us has concerns or suggestions we need to bring them up as early as possible.*

In this example, Paul took the initiative in resolving his interpersonal conflict with Barbara. He began by employing a technique known as *active listening*, or *reflective listening*. The key to this technique is that the listener paraphrases the words of the speaker to indicate that he or she comprehends the meaning of the speaker's message. The listener tries to pick up on hidden messages and feelings not actually verbalized and paraphrases those as well. For example, Paul understood that Barbara would be embarrassed if other people knew she had taken the test, even though she never explicitly stated that. When Paul was able to understand and listen so well to Barbara—well enough to identify feelings she had not verbalized—Barbara was convinced that Paul cared enough to understand her needs. *Then* Barbara was ready to hear about Paul's needs and became more receptive to his viewpoint. Paul next expressed his opinion and the reasons for his feelings. The point of reflective listening is to enable each participant to acknowledge the other's view and to be less insistent in arguing for his or her own.

The next step in this technique is to propose as many alternative solutions as possible through brainstorming. The result is a win–win, rather than a no-win, situation, reached through a mutual agreement that it is possible to agree. Paul agrees that they both will be tested and that they will treat the testing and the results confidentially. He also shows respect for Barbara's busy schedule and says he is willing to work around it.

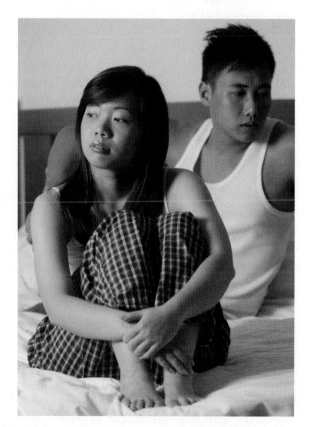

Communication about HIV status can be difficult, but it is very important.

Myth vs Fact

Myth: For most people, good communication comes naturally.
Fact: Although some people may seem to be naturally better than others at communication, good communication is a lot of work for almost everyone.

Myth: Because sexuality is such an open topic today, most people can discuss it rather easily.
Fact: Even though sexuality seems more open, many people still experience much difficulty in talking about sexual topics and personal relationships.

Myth: Communication skills are basically the same in all cultures.
Fact: Although most skills may be quite similar, communicating with people from another culture can be challenging. Even though the language may be the same, communication methods and meanings may greatly differ.

Myth: Because men and women now have the same rights and are equal, they communicate in the same ways.

Fact: Conditions can be slow to change. Even though men and women have equal rights, we still need to be sensitive to differences in learning and motivation related to communication.

Myth: The most important part of communication is the meaning of the words we use.
Fact: It has often been said that "actions speak louder than words." It is also true that nonverbal communication is often more important, and revealing, than words used.

Myth: It is a bad idea to take a risk when trying to communicate with another person. The technique may backfire.
Fact: There are risks in most things we do, and developing and using good communication skills can involve disclosing personal feelings and desires. In a trusting relationship, this should not be too risky.

In addition, Paul and Barbara have improved their relationship *because* of this conflict. The conflict instigates a discussion about their needs and, therefore, provides the opportunity for them to demonstrate their feelings for each other by organizing to satisfy those needs. Instead of threatening the relationship, the conflict has actually improved it.

To reiterate, the steps in this conflict resolution process are as follows:

1. *Active listening:* Reflecting to the other person his or her own words and feelings.

2. *Identifying your position:* Stating your own thoughts and feelings about the situation, and explaining why you feel this way.

3. *Proposing and exploring alternative solutions:* First brainstorming and then evaluating the possibilities.

Although you may feel awkward using this technique initially, and your conversations may seem stilted, with practice it will become a part of your style and will be very effective. The payoffs are huge; do not give up on it.

A similar way to resolve conflict involves four steps (Resolve conflict in four steps, 1995): (1) *Identify the interests* of each person. Ask each person, "What do you want?" Then listen carefully to the answers. (2) *Identify higher levels of interest* by asking, "What does having that do for you?" It is important to understand what each of us really wants. (3) *Create an agreement frame* by asking, "If I could show you how to get X, would you do Y?" X is the person's real interest, and Y is what you want from the person. (4) *Brainstorm for solutions.* Do not just give a solution and expect the other person to accept it. Commitment results from being involved in finding a solution. The solutions must satisfy the interests of all parties.

Giving and Receiving Criticism

Imagine a "sex critic" planned to evaluate your sexual functioning as a movie critic critiques movies! All of us would probably feel threatened, and because of that, our abilities to function normally would most likely be compromised. Well, in a very real sense, our sexual partners are our sex critics. They evaluate what we do in terms of how pleasing it is for both them and us. It would be nice if we could receive our "sex critique" without feeling threatened by it, without feeling that it denigrated our self-esteem. It would also be nice if we were open enough both to give and to receive feedback about our sexual functioning in a way that enhanced our sexual lives and those of our partners. Well, we can learn both to receive and to give criticism in a way that is truly constructive. Here are a few hints:

1. Find a private, relaxing place to discuss thoughts and feelings about your sexual relationship. You do not want to feel uncomfortable in your environment while discussing such a sensitive topic. Feeling uncomfortable will not be conducive to either receiving or giving feedback on such a sensitive issue.

2. Devote sufficient time to such a discussion. It would be unfortunate if you were beginning to communicate well on significant matters just as one of you had to leave.

3. Limit distractions so that your attention is focused on the conversation. Rather than wondering who might overhear you or who might inadvertently hit you in the head with a Frisbee, find a quiet, private place for your discussion.

4. It is probably not wise to do these things just before or just after a sexual encounter. Plan a relaxed time for this discussion.

In addition to these general suggestions, when *giving criticism* try to remember to

1. Begin your comments on a positive note. "You know, when you kiss me I really feel great." Then move to the behavior you would like to change. "I enjoy your touches so much that it would be terrific if you could . . . ."

2. Be specific regarding the change you are recommending. Rather than announcing, "You don't hold me enough," suggest, "When we watch television, I'd really like it if you would put your arm around me."

3. Be aware of the limitations of your partner. Do not expect more than your partner is able to give. To critique something that cannot or will not be changed may harm the relationship. If your partner is slow to arouse, asking him or her to speed up is unrealistic and, we might add, unfair. It is criticism given for no useful purpose.

When *receiving criticism* try to remember to

1. Separate your partner's suggestions and recommendations from your self-worth. You are no less of a person because you might need to adjust some of your sexual behavior. In fact, if you were not open to suggestion, then you might suspect you have a problem.

2. Assume a nondefensive attitude. Rather than attempting to justify your present actions, ask questions to understand the criticism better. Then, if you disagree, you will know why you disagree.

3. If the criticism is too general, ask for specific suggestions to help you make the recommended change. In addition, inquire as to how your partner can help make this change more likely to occur. Ask your partner to participate in remedying the situation or action being criticized.

4. Whether or not you agree with the criticism, thank your partner for being honest enough to express the concern to you. Acknowledge that it is not easy to discuss such matters and you appreciate the opportunity to consider something you have been doing or not been doing that is causing a problem. Encourage future suggestions that have the potential to improve your relationship.

With these recommendations for giving and receiving criticism, your relationship should improve. That is because not only will the specific suggestions lead to actual changes, but the practice of opening

Myth vs Fact

Myth: Being assertive means standing up for your basic rights at the expense of someone else's rights.
Fact: Being aggressive is standing up for your basic rights at the expense of someone else's. Being assertive means standing up for your basic rights without violating anyone else's.

Myth: Conflicts will always get in the way of good relationships.
Fact: It is true that conflicts are a part of life, but if we learn how to deal with them effectively they can help us grow and have better relationships.

up your relationship to discussions of problems will, in itself, help foster a style of communicating that will serve you well in all aspects of your relationship. It will then be easier to discuss matters that bother you, and it will be easier to express emotions such as love, caring, and wonderment. The relationship will improve with this style of communication.

When trying to communicate effectively, it can be helpful to have some ground rules. Silverberg (2009) suggests that talking with a partner about these rules can help in developing your own set of rules. Here are some examples:

1. Check in and check out. At the beginning of the conversation, spend a minute talking about your day and how you are feeling so you know what each person is bringing into the conversation. It can also help to take a minute at the end of the conversation to say how it went.

2. Define safety for yourselves and to each other. Discuss what is needed to feel safe so partners can talk honestly and openly.

3. Listen without interrupting. This can be a hard rule to follow, but it is a very important one.

4. Respect differences in interests and desires. If one person exposes personal information, the other person should consider that a compliment, even if the desire is not something he or she is interested in doing.

5. Bring a sense of goodwill to the conversation. Neither partner should be trying to intentionally hurt the other or be mean to the other.

6. Anyone can call time-out at any time. To have a safe conversation, partners need to feel they can stop the conversation at any time. This doesn't mean that one partner should storm out in the middle of a sentence, but

rather that either partner can ask for a time-out to end the conversation at that time with the agreement to pick it up at a later point.

Final Thoughts on Sexual Communication

In this chapter we have discussed the importance of word meanings, nonverbal communication, cultural and personal backgrounds, and attitudes toward communication about sexuality. We have also seen that there are many ways to improve our ability to communicate significantly but that doing so usually takes a great deal of effort.

At the same time, however, to be effective, communication must be truthful. In practice, this is often not the case. For example, lying is common in relationships involving college students (Saxe, 1991). The majority of these lies (41%) were about relations with other partners. In another study, respondents said they did not regard their lies as serious, did not plan them, and did not worry about getting caught. They averaged about two lies each day (DePaulo et al., 1996).

Communication difficulties may even increase the level of risk—especially for females. Rickert and associates (2002) reported that about 20% of women believe they never have the right to stop foreplay, including at the point of intercourse; refuse to have sexual intercourse, even if they have had intercourse with that partner before; make their own decisions about contraception, regardless of their partner's wishes; ask their partner whether he has been examined for STIs; or tell their partner that they want to make love differently or that he is being too rough. Moreover, more than 40% of young women believe that they never have or only sometimes have the right to tell a relative they are not comfortable with being hugged or kissed in certain ways. These findings show that some young women may be unable to communicate their sexual beliefs and desires clearly and are therefore at risk for undesired outcomes.

Finally, it is interesting to note what a number of leading sexologists have said about communication. They were asked to relate the most important information they had learned about sexuality over the years. Here are some of the ideas they expressed about communication (Haffner & Schwartz, 1998):

1. It is hard to be honest about past sexual experiences with a new partner.

2. Some sexual secrets—unless they pose a health threat—are better left unshared.

Appropriately giving and receiving criticism will enhance communication in a relationship.

3. Nonverbal communication often works better than words in bed.

4. Talking during sexual activity—sharing fantasies, using forbidden words—can be very sexy.

5. Couples who have nothing to say to each other in restaurants are usually married—and they may be in trouble.

6. Open, honest communication is the most important foundation for a relationship.

7. You cannot underestimate the value of humor.

8. After humor, consideration is the second most important ingredient in a sexual relationship. Most people appreciate a sensitive and thoughtful partner.

9. Most people are not comfortable talking about sexual issues.

10. Consent requires communication.

11. It is better to talk about sexual feelings, desires, and boundaries in relationships.

12. Talking about scenes in movies or books can sometimes be a good way to communicate what you like in sexual behavior and relationships.

Exploring the
DIMENSIONS
of Human Sexuality

Our feelings, attitudes, and beliefs regarding sexuality are influenced by our internal and external environments. Go to sexuality.jbpub.com/dimensions/4e to learn more about the biological, psychological, and sociological factors that affect your sexuality.

Sociocultural Factors
- Media strongly influence sexual communication.
- Gender affects style of communication.
- Sexuality education may increase confidence.
- Cultures influence communication style.
- Religion may influence the sexual activities in which one participates.
- Family and peers set an example of sexuality.

Biological Factors
- Physiological reactions—such as blushing or erections—are nonverbal means of communicating sexual attraction.
- Alcohol or drugs can distort the communication process.
- Physical touching can indicate interest, intimacy, and emotional closeness.
- Hearing loss over time can inhibit communication and frustrate a partner.

Psychological Factors
- Emotions can overwhelm the ability to communicate.
- The role of the double standard in thinking may alter the communication process.
- Ego may get in the way of listening to a partner.
- Self-image and body image may distort communication.

CASE STUDY

Your ability to communicate sexually plays an important role in your sexual wellness and self-image. Your capacity to discuss sexual histories, contraceptives, and safer sexual activities can help prevent unwanted pregnancy and transmission of STIs and HIV.

From a psychological standpoint, a positive self-image as a communicator gives you confidence. A negative self-image may hinder your ability to ask for dates, to ask for sexual activities that you like, or to ask for safer sexual activities.

Sexual communication is influenced by virtually all social and cultural phenomena, including religion, ethnic heritage, language, family traditions, peers, geographical region, and even mass media.

Gender plays a pervasive role: Men and women communicate in different styles and express emotions differently.

Consider the confusion of sexual language: If your partner suggested that you were not close enough to engage in "sexual relations," you might back off any type of physical contact. It is important to talk with your partner to make sure each of you understands what the other wants.

Summary

- The process of communication consists of having an idea, the sender encoding a message, sending the message over a channel, the receiver decoding a message, and the receiver providing feedback.

- Nonverbal communication includes all unwritten and unspoken messages. It is a very important part of effective communication, but it can also be easy to misinterpret.

- Barriers to communication include bypassing, the frame of reference, lack of language skills, lack of listening skills, and use of mind-altering drugs.

- There are many things that parents can do to improve communication about sexuality with their children, including making conversations about sexuality ongoing, knowing individual comfort levels, and making it acceptable for children to ask about sexuality.

- Communication can be improved by planning, using flooding, learning assertiveness, using effective nonverbal communication, and using good listening skills.

- Counselors often help people improve their communication skills by encouraging active listening, eliciting feedback from each partner, facilitating the expression of thoughts directly, using "I" statements, and not allowing interruptions and blaming.

- It can be helpful to establish ground rules to help promote good sexual communication. Examples include listening without interruption and respecting differences in desires and interests.

Discussion Questions

1. Describe the steps of the communication process. Explain how they would work in discussing specific relationship or sexuality issues.

2. What are the barriers to effective sexual communication? How can they be overcome?

3. How can you improve your communication abilities? Which techniques would work best for you? Which would not work for you? Explain why.

Application Questions

Reread the chapter-opening story and answer the following questions.

1. If you were teaching this course, and Joanna and Mark were students, what information would you want them to leave with from your course?

2. The changes in communication style across the life cycle of the relationship can enhance or harm it. For example, anticipating what your partner wants can lead to a strengthened relationship, but it can also lead to deterioration of communication. What could Joanna and Mark have done to maintain interest in their relationship? (You may want to think about what successful couples you know do to stay happy.)

Critical Thinking Questions

1. Should sexual partners communicate all they think and feel so that they can better respond to each other's needs? Or should sexual partners be selective in relating their innermost thoughts and feelings? Explain why or why not. Would your opinion change from situation to situation?

2. You are excited about an upcoming first date when you overhear a conversation describing your date as someone who has had many sexual partners in the past. You have no idea whether the information is correct. Later, on your date, your partner implies a willingness to engage in sexual activity. Although you like the person and are sexually attracted, you are unable to forget what you overheard. How can you open the discussion of sexual histories without offending your date?

3. On the last episode of MTV's *Road Rules Latin America* (1999), all five of the campers (three males and two females) climb naked into a Jacuzzi as a final "gathering of friends." In real life, if you climbed naked into a Jacuzzi with some "close friends," what kind of sexual message might that be sending? What if you climbed into the Jacuzzi with just one other person whom you wanted to get to know better?

Critical Thinking Case

The following is a true date-rape case that occurred at Georgetown University in the mid-1990s. Kim and Mark (names changed) decided to go to the senior black-tie dance together. Both had agreed beforehand that it would not be a "real date." But during the long evening of drinking and dancing, their plans changed.

They met at 8:30 and went to two parties, the dance, and a bar before returning to Mark's apartment at about 4:00 A.M. Kim had lost her key and had agreed to go back to his apartment. "I decided I wouldn't mind kissing him." They kissed, undressed, and climbed into his bed. Kim said later that she had frequently shared a bed with her previous boyfriend without having sexual intercourse and assumed she could do the same with Mark. When Mark asked whether he should get a condom, Kim said they did not know each other well enough to have sex. At that point, the stories diverge.

Kim said she told Mark, "I've never had sex before, and I don't want to have it on a whim." Then, "all of a sudden, he was on top of me, forcing himself into [me]. . . . I kept trying to push him off with my hands and squirming around, and I kept saying I didn't want to have sex."

Mark said in an affidavit that she was "kissing me and thrusting her pelvis against me. . . . At no time during our sexual activity did I use any kind of physical force against Kim. Nor did I threaten Kim verbally."

How could communication have gone so awry? Consider the dimensions of human sexuality as you explain what went wrong. Then describe what could have been done to prevent the incident.

Exploring Personal Dimensions

Measure Your Assertiveness

Indicate how characteristic or descriptive each of the following statements is of you by using the code given.

+3 very characteristic of me, extremely descriptive

+2 rather characteristic of me, quite descriptive

+1 somewhat characteristic of me, slightly descriptive

−1 somewhat uncharacteristic of me, slightly nondescriptive

−2 rather uncharacteristic of me, quite nondescriptive

−3 very uncharacteristic of me, extremely nondescriptive

_____ 1. Most people seem to be more aggressive and assertive than I am.

_____ 2. I have hesitated to make or accept dates because of "shyness."

_____ 3. When the food served at a restaurant is not done to my satisfaction, I complain about it to the waiter or waitress.

_____ 4. I am careful to avoid hurting other people's feelings, even when I feel that I have been injured.

_____ 5. If a salesperson has gone to considerable trouble to show me merchandise that is not quite suitable, I have a difficult time saying no.

_____ 6. When I am asked to do something, I insist upon knowing why.

_____ 7. There are times when I look for a good, vigorous argument.

_____ 8. I strive to get ahead as well as most people do.

_____ 9. To be honest, people often take advantage of me.

_____ 10. I enjoy starting conversations with new acquaintances and strangers.

_____ 11. I often don't know what to say to attractive persons of the opposite sex.

_____ 12. I will hesitate to make phone calls to business establishments and institutions.

_____ 13. I would rather apply for a job or for admission to a college by writing letters than by going through personal interviews.

_____ 14. I find it embarrassing to return merchandise.

_____ 15. If a close and respected relative were annoying me, I would smother my feelings rather than express my annoyance.

_____ 16. I have avoided asking questions for fear of sounding stupid.

_____ 17. During an argument I am sometimes afraid that I will get so upset that I will shake all over.

_____ 18. If a famed and respected lecturer makes a statement that I think is incorrect, I will have the audience hear my point of view as well.

_____ 19. I avoid arguing over prices with clerks and salespeople.

_____ 20. When I have done something important or worthwhile, I manage to let others know about it.

_____ 21. I am open and frank about my feelings.

_____ 22. If someone has been spreading false and bad stories about me, I see him or her as soon as possible to "have a talk" about it.

_____ 23. I often have a hard time saying "no."

_____ 24. I tend to bottle up my emotions rather than make a scene.

_____ 25. I complain about poor service in a restaurant and elsewhere.

_____ 26. When I am given a compliment, I sometimes just don't know what to say.

_____ 27. If a couple near me in a theater or at a lecture were conversing rather loudly, I would ask them to be quiet or to take their conversation elsewhere.

_____ 28. Anyone attempting to push ahead of me in a line is in for a good battle.

_____ 29. I am quick to express an opinion.

_____ 30. There are times when I just can't say anything.

Scoring

To score this scale, first change the signs (+ or −) to the opposite for items 1, 2, 4, 5, 9, 11, 12, 13, 14, 15, 16, 17, 19, 23, 24, 26, and 30. Next, total the plus (+) items, then total the minus (−) items, and, last, subtract the minus total from the plus total to obtain your score. This score can range from −90 through zero to +90. The higher the score (closer to +90), the more assertively you usually behave. The lower the score (closer to −90), the more nonassertive is your typical behavior. This particular scale does not measure aggressiveness.

Source: Rathus, S. A. A 30-item schedule for assessing assertive behavior, _Behavior Therapy, 4_ (1973), 398, 406. Copyright © 1973 Academic Press, Orlando, FL.

Suggested Readings

Baxter, L. A. Family communication environments and rule-based social control of adolescents' healthy lifestyle choices. _Journal of Family Communication, 5, no. 3_ (July 2005), 209–214.

DeVore, E. R., & Ginsburg, K. R. The protective effects of good parenting on adolescents. _Current Opinions in Pediatrics, 17, no. 4_ (August 2005), 460–465.

Gossett, J., & Bellas, M. You can't put a rule around people's hearts . . . can you? Consensual Relationship policies in academia, _Sociological Focus, 35, no. 3_ (August 2002), 267–284.

Hinchliff, S., Gott, M., & Galena, E. "I daresay I might find it embarrassing": General practitioners' perspectives on discussing sexual health issues with lesbian and gay patients. _Health & Social Care in the Community, 13, no. 4_ (July 2005), 345–353.

Owen, C. The importance of sexual communication. suite101.com, July 2008. Available: http://improving-relationships.suite101.com.

Rosenfeld, S. M. Psychosocial correlates of sexual communication. _Dissertation Abstracts International: Section B: The Sciences & Engineering, 65, no. 9-B_ (2005), 4849.

Segal, J. Nonverbal communication. _Helpguide Newsletter_ (October 2008). Available: http://www.helpguide.org/mental/eq6_nonverbal_communication.htm.

Silverberg, C. How to talk with your kids about sex. About.com Sexuality, March 2008. Available: http://sexuality.about.com/od/sexeducationforparent1/a/talk_sex_kids.htm?p=1.

Silverberg, C. Sexual communication ground rules. About.com Sexuality, January 2009. Available: http://sexuality.about.com/od/improvingsexcommunication/a/ground_rules.htm.

Somers, C. The sexual communication scale: A measure of frequency of sexual communication between parents and adolescents. *Adolescence, 38, no. 149* (Spring 2003), 43–56.

Sprecher, S. Sexual satisfaction in premarital relationships: Associated with satisfaction, love, commitment, and stability, *Journal of Sex Research, 39, no. 3* (August 2002), 190–196.

Tannen, D. *You just don't understand.* New York: Morrow, 1990 (also available in paperback from Ballantine, 1991).

Van Wagner, K. Top 10 nonverbal communication tips. About.com Psychology, 2009. Available: http://psychology.about.com/od/nonverbalcommunication/tp/nonverbaltips.htm.

Web Resources

For links to the web sites below, visit *http://sexuality.jbpub.com/dimensions/4e* and click on Resource Links.

Planned Parenthood: Educator's Update
www.plannedparenthood.org

Gives ideas that can help communication between parents and their children.

BBC Health: Sexual Communication
www.bbc.co.uk/health/conditions/mental_health/support_sexual.shtml

Emphasizes points for good communication such as expressing affection, finding a mutual vocabulary, communicating likes and dislikes, and negotiating and compromising.

Double Your Dating: Sexual Communication Workbook
www.freewebs.com/maestro_mr/SCW.pdf

Gives hints about many aspects of sexual communication within relationships.

MindTools: Improve Your Communication Skills
www.mindtools.com/page8.html

Contains numerous articles related to communication skills in many different situations.

Queendom: The Land of Tests
www.queendom.com/tests/access_page/index.htm?idRegTest=683

You can find out how your interpersonal skills rate by taking a Communication Skills Test.

CHAPTER 4

Female Sexual Anatomy and Physiology

CHAPTER OBJECTIVES

1 Name and describe the parts of the female reproductive system, to include external and internal genitalia.

2 Discuss the role of breasts in sexual arousal and response, as well as in the reproductive function of lactation.

3 Explain the role of hormones as they pertain to sexuality.

4 Describe what occurs during menstruation, to include menarche, the menstrual cycle, and problems associated with each.

5 Cite various diseases that can affect the female reproductive system and the self-care procedures, as well as medical treatments, associated with these diseases.

sexuality.jbpub.com/dimensions/4e

Global Dimensions: Female Genital Mutilation
Amenorrhea
Breast Cancer

INTRODUCTION

O ne of the authors of this text was sitting at his desk preparing for an upcoming class. On the desk were diagrams of the female and male reproductive systems, colored pictures with various parts differentiated from others by different pastel colors and shading. Before long, a colleague walked into the office. The visitor was a professor of educational administration and the proud recipient of a baccalaureate degree in mathematics, a master's degree in counseling, and a doctorate in educational administration. In short, this was an educated man, one on whom students and family relied and whose opinions were accorded the respect someone of his stature deserves. As he entered the office, he glanced at the desk and was fascinated with the reproductive system diagrams. When he inquired as to their purpose, he was told that they were to be used in a sexuality education class to help students learn about their sexual organs. It was then that he sheepishly admitted his own ignorance about the structure and function of the reproductive system. For the next 20 minutes, he and his colleague proceeded to discuss the reproductive systems of females and males, referring to the diagrams on the desk.

The only surprising aspect of this incident was the openness with which this educated man admitted his ignorance. In general, people know less about themselves, both physically and psychologically, than they know about cars or ecology or sports or politics or contemporary musicians or any of the hundreds of topics people care about or find fascinating. The less we know about our bodies, the less well equipped we are to keep them healthy. The more we know, the more choices we have and the better decisions we can make. Appropriate health maintenance should be valued similarly by males and females, and both genders need to adopt certain behaviors, such as periodic medical screenings, to *maintain their health. However, men's and women's reproductive health issues are not the same.*

The purpose of this chapter and the next is to describe the anatomy of the female and male reproductive systems as a step toward creating a comprehensive picture of human sexuality.

■ The Female Reproductive System

Both females and males have external and internal genitals, or reproductive organs. We begin with the external female genitals and progress inward.

The External Genitals

The external female genitals are the mons pubis, labia majora, labia minora, clitoris, vestibule, and urethral opening (Figure 4.1). All of these organs together are called the **vulva**.

The Mons Veneris
The **mons pubis** (also called the **mons veneris**, or **mount of Venus**) is the rounded, soft area above the pubic bone that becomes covered with hair at puberty. Since the mons contains numerous nerve endings, it can be sexually stimulated.

vulva
The female external genitalia.

mons pubis (mons veneris, mount of Venus)
The rounded, soft area above the vaginal opening that becomes covered with hair at puberty.

The Labia Majora
The **labia majora** (major lips) are two large folds of skin whose main function is to protect the external genitalia. Unless the labia majora are spread apart, the other external genitalia are not visible. The outer surfaces of the labia majora also grow hair after puberty, and the inner surfaces remain smooth. Within the tissue of the labia majora are smooth muscle fibers, nerves, and vessels for blood and lymph.

The Labia Minora
The **labia minora** (minor lips) are two folds of skin lying inside the labia majora. Loaded with blood vessels and nerve receptors, the labia minora and their upper part, the clitoris, are very sensitive to stimulation. During sexual arousal, blood fills the labia minora, causing them to spread, making the vagina more accessible. Within the labia

labia majora
Two large folds of skin whose main function is to protect the external genitalia and the opening of the vestibule (defined later).

labia minora
Two folds of skin lying inside the labia majora, which contain numerous blood vessels and nerve receptors.

Mons veneris

Clitoral hood

Clitoris

Labia minora

Hymen

Vaginal orifice (introitus)

Urethral orifice

Vestibular bulb

Labia majora

Perineum

Anus

FIGURE **4.1** Female external reproductive organs.

Female Genital Mutilation in Various Parts of the World

Female genital mutilation has been used throughout the world as a means of diminishing sexual stimulation. The result, the argument goes, is that fewer women participate in sexual intercourse outside marriage and fewer women engage in masturbation. Female mutilation can take several different forms. The most simple form is *circumcision,* whereby the clitoral hood is removed. In a *clitoridectomy,* the clitoris itself is surgically removed. Genital *infibulation* is the most complex procedure: The clitoris and the labia minora are removed, and both sides of the vulva are scraped raw and then stitched together. When the tissue grows together, only a small opening remains through which urine and the menstrual flow pass. During these procedures, it is unusual for sterile instruments to be used. Most of the time razor blades or broken glass is used to do the cutting, without the benefit of pain-reducing medications or disinfectants. Therefore, as you might imagine, aside from causing psychological trauma, female mutilation can result in serious medical complications. The combination of infections, bleeding, and pain can cause shock, gangrene, and even death.

Female mutilation is common in some African, Middle Eastern, and Asian countries. In fact, one study found that 97% of married women in Egypt had had some form of genital mutilation performed on them (El Hadi, 1997)— this in spite of the World Health Organization (WHO) and the United Nations Children's Fund (UNICEF) 1980 joint plan to lobby leaders of countries in which female mutilation is common to work toward eliminating this practice. A new statement, with wider United Nations support, was then issued in February 2008 (World Health Organization, 2008). Numerous other organizations and governments have publicly opposed female genital mutilation, even though the tendency is to avoid interference in cultural practices of sovereign countries. Grass-roots organizations, such as the Kenyan women's organization Maendeleo ya Wanawake, and Tostan in Senegal, have also sprung up around the world with the goal of eliminating female genital mutilation. These groups conduct educational campaigns encouraging women to break the generational cycle of female genital mutilation by preventing their daughters from experiencing it. Even so, WHO estimates that between 100 million and 140 million girls and women worldwide have been subjected to female genital mutilation. Estimates are that 91.5 million girls and women older than 9 years in Africa are currently living with the consequences of female genital mutilation. An estimated 3 million girls in Africa are at risk of undergoing female genital mutilation every year. More than 80% in Eritrea, Guinea, Mali, Egypt, Sudan, and Ethiopia have experienced genital manipulation and between 60% and 85% in Mauritania, Chad, Kenya, and Burkina Faso (UNICEF, 2005).

minora lie **Bartholin's glands**. The glands slightly lubricate the labia during coitus (intercourse).

The Clitoris

The **clitoris** is the most sensitive structure in the female body. This small organ contains two spongy bodies, the **corpora cavernosa**, that have the capacity to fill with blood during arousal. (The penis, a similar organ, contains spongy bodies that react to arousal in a similar way.) During sexual stimulation, the corpora cavernosa fill with blood, causing the clitoris to become erect. Popular knowledge about the sensitivity of the clitoris has led males to seek out and stimulate it to arouse their female sexual partners. (Here is a case in which knowledge can have either a positive or a negative effect on sexual relationships. Men who carefully and delicately stimulate the clitoris may sexually arouse their partner, but those who rub incessantly will only irritate the clitoris and thereby irritate their partner. We discuss sexual-arousal techniques in more detail in Chapter 6.)

The clitoris is covered by the **clitoral hood**. As can be seen in Figure 4.1, the hood is attached to the labia minora. One function of the clitoral hood is to protect the glans of the clitoris. When we discuss the male reproductive organs, we will observe that the foreskin of the penis protects the glans penis in a similar way.

Knowing about the anatomy of the reproductive system

Bartholin's glands
Small glands located within the labia minora that secrete a few drops of fluid during sexual arousal.

clitoris
The structure located at the upper part of the labia minora that is homologous to the penis and is very sensitive to stimulation.

corpora cavernosa
A cavernous structure located within the clitoris and the penis that fills with blood during sexual excitement, causing erection.

clitoral hood
The skin covering the clitoris.

Many variations exist in the female external genitals.

offers guidance for sexual functioning, and the relationship of the clitoris, the clitoral hood, and the labia minora provides a case in point. During sexual excitement, the clitoris retracts under the clitoral hood. Therefore, stimulating the clitoris requires pulling back the clitoral hood, pulling the labia majora upward, or putting pressure on the hood or clitoris itself. For example, during sexual intercourse, the clitoris can be stimulated if the penis is positioned correctly. One position that will stimulate the clitoris is called "riding high." With the female lying on her back, the male places his penis into the vagina so that its upper shaft rubs on the clitoris. Another option is for the penis to be pressed, thrusting downward, on the lower part of the labia minora so as to create downward movement of the hood and its contact with the clitoris. Many women, however, require additional manual stimulation of the clitoris to cause orgasm during intercourse.

The Vestibule
When the clitoris is erect and the labia minora spread, the urethral and vaginal openings (called the **vestibule**) become visible.

The Urethral Opening
The urethral opening, where urine is excreted, is not generally considered a part of the reproductive system in females, although there is some evidence that women who do experience something akin to ejaculation do so through the urethra.

The Hymen
The **hymen**, a thin connective tissue containing a relatively large number of blood vessels, covers the opening of the vagina in women who have an intact hymen. The function of this tissue is unknown. Hymens vary in shape and size: A hymen may surround the vaginal opening (an **annular** hymen), bridge it (a **septate** hymen), or form a sievelike covering (a **cribriform** hymen) (Figure 4.2).

Normally all forms of hymens have openings that are large enough to permit menstrual flow or the insertion of a tampon or a finger but that are usually too small to permit an erect penis to enter without the hymen's tearing. His-

vestibule
The area containing the vaginal and urethral openings.

hymen
A thin connective tissue covering the opening of the vagina.

annular
Type of hymen that surrounds the vaginal opening.

septate
Type of hymen that bridges the vaginal opening.

cribriform
Type of hymen that creates a sievelike covering for the vaginal opening.

Annular hymen   Cribriform hymen   Septate hymen

FIGURE **4.2** The various types of hymens.

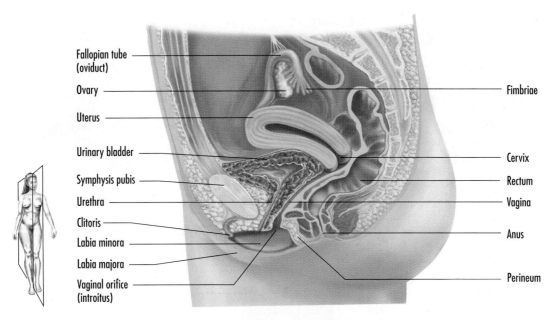

Fallopian tube (oviduct)

Ovary

Uterus

Urinary bladder

Symphysis pubis

Urethra

Clitoris

Labia minora

Labia majora

Vaginal orifice (introitus)

Fimbriae

Cervix

Rectum

Vagina

Anus

Perineum

FIGURE **4.3** Organs of the female reproductive system.

torically the presence of an intact hymen was considered proof that a woman had never had intercourse. But the hymen can be ruptured by accident or by normal exercise, as well as by intercourse, so a tear in the tissue is not a reliable indication that a woman is no longer a virgin. The rupturing of the hymen during first intercourse generally does not result in a great deal of pain and bleeding, although some people expect it to do so. Pain is usually related to muscular tension due to anxiety or to entry of the penis into the vagina before the vagina is sufficiently lubricated; care and attention can ordinarily prevent it. A few drops of blood may be noticeable.

The Internal Genitals

The female internal genitals consist of such structures as the vagina, uterus, fallopian tubes, and ovaries. These structures of the female internal genitalia, as well as relevant surrounding structures, are depicted in Figures 4.3 and 4.4.

The Vagina
The **vagina** is a hollow, tunnel-like structure, about 4.5 inches (11.4 centimeters) long, that opens outward to the vestibule and at the opposite end into the uterus. The vagina has several reproductive functions: It surrounds the penis and receives its ejaculate during intercourse, serves as the route of exit for the newborn, and provides an exit for menstrual flow. When the vagina is empty, its lips and walls are in contact, but during childbirth the vagina can expand wide enough for the baby to pass through, and during intercourse it can both expand and close tightly enough on a penis to provide sexual satisfaction. Soft transverse folds in the

vaginal wall enable the vagina to expand, and muscle fibers within the walls enable it to contract, as they do in orgasm. No muscles surround the vaginal entrance (the **introitus**); however, the **pubococcygeal** and **bulbocavernosus muscles** that support the vagina can be voluntarily contracted so as to intensify sexual responsiveness by forcing the vaginal walls to close on the penis. Exercises to help women develop greater control of these muscles (called **Kegel exercises** after their proponent) are frequently recommended by sexual counselors (Kegel, 1952). To learn to control the pubococcygeal muscles, try the following:

1. Insert a finger into the vagina and contract muscles in that area until you feel the vagina squeeze the finger.

2. Practice squeezing and then relaxing these muscles—first slowly, then rapidly.

3. Practice the preceding exercise about three times daily until you feel you have voluntary control of the pubococcygeal muscles.

vagina
A hollow, tunnel-like structure of the female internal genitalia whose reproductive functions are to receive the penis and its ejaculate, serve as a route of exit for the newborn, and provide an exit for menstrual flow.

introitus
The vaginal entrance.

pubococcygeal muscle
A muscle that encircles the vagina and supports it.

bulbocavernosus muscle
A muscle that encircles and supports the vagina.

Kegel exercises
Exercises to help women develop greater control of muscles supporting the genitalia.

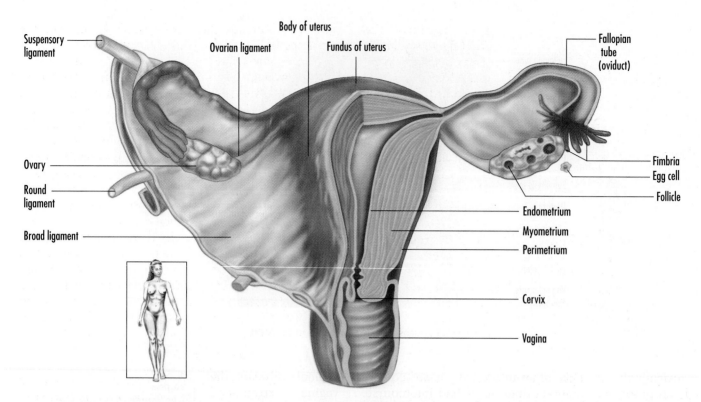

FIGURE **4.4** An anterior view of the female reproductive organs showing the relationships of the ovaries, fallopian tubes, uterus, cervix, and vagina.

FIGURE **4.5** The location of the Grafenberg spot.

The Grafenberg Spot

One would think that after centuries of studying the human body and its sexual nature there would be little room for disagreement regarding its function. Not so. The existence and the effect of the **Grafenberg spot (G spot)** provide a case in point.

The stimulation of an area along the anterior (front) wall of the vagina, several inches into the vaginal canal and just below the bladder, appears to be sexually exciting for many females. This area is known as the Grafenberg spot, named after Ernest Grafenberg, the gynecologist who first noted its erotic potential (Figure 4.5) (Grafenberg, 1950). The presence of glands in this area has been known for some time (Skene, 1980), and it is these glands—called **Skene's glands**—through which a type of ejaculate is expelled in some women when they experience orgasm by stimulation of the G spot (Grafenberg, 1950; Sevely & Bennett, 1978; Addiego et al., 1981; Belzer, 1981; Perry & Whipple, 1981; Zaviacic et al., 1988).

Others maintain that there is no one particular spot in the vagina that is more sensitive than others to stimulation. For example, the noted sexual therapist Helen Singer Kaplan believes there are many spots within the vagina that are sexually arousing, and the G spot is merely one of those (Kaplan, 1983). Masters and Johnson agree with Kaplan; they report that only 10% of the women they studied "had an area of heightened sensitivity in the front wall of the vagina or a tissue mass that fit the various descriptions of this area" (Masters, Johnson, & Kolodny, 1985). Although some women reported sensitivity in the front wall of the vagina, a study by Alzate and Londono (1984) could not locate a specific spot such as that described by Grafenberg. Heath (1984) found an area of erotic sensitivity and concluded that it is larger than previously described: about the width of the middle two fingers and at least two-thirds the length.

The Female Prostate
That glandular tissue exists in the area of the G spot is not debatable. The pathologist Robert Mallon (1984) conducted autopsies on women and found evidence of this glandular tissue, as did Heath (1984). Both of these researchers found prostate-like glandular tissue in the front wall of the vagina. When the substances within these glands were analyzed, they were found to contain fluids similar to those found in the male prostate. Hence, some sexuality experts have concluded that there are a female prostate (the Skene's glands) and a female ejaculate. Further evidence for a female ejaculate is offered by Addiego and colleagues (1981), who analyzed the fluid expelled by females at the time of orgasm and found it to contain an enzyme (prostatic acid phosphatase, or PAP) characteristic of semen. However, when Goldberg and associates (1983) studied this ejaculate, they concluded that it was similar to urine. Alzate and Hoch (1986) also found ejaculate secreted through the urethra. To complicate matters further, a study conducted by Belzer and associates (1984) concluded that the ejaculate obtained from women contained significantly more prostatic acid phosphatase than did their urine.

Obviously, further study is needed to confirm the existence of a female ejaculate beyond any doubt.

That some women expel a fluid from the vagina during orgasm has been demonstrated. The prevalence of this phenomenon remains unknown. Whether this fluid is similar to that of the male prostate is a matter of much research and debate. What is not discussed or researched, however, is the concern first expressed by the Boston Women's Health Collective (1998) regarding the possibility that the G spot orgasm will become a new "ideal" for the sexually liberated woman. It would indeed be unfortunate if this new ideal created pressure on women who do not experience erotic feelings when the Grafenberg spot is stimulated and, therefore, perceive themselves to be inadequate sexually. When the media popularize sexual information, as they did with the Grafenberg spot, often education is needed to remind the public about the many paths to sexual fulfillment. This is particularly true today.

The Uterus
At the top of the vagina lies the **uterus**, a pear-shaped hollow organ with muscular walls. Its function is to nurture the developing embryo and fetus. Except during pregnancy, the uterus is about 3 inches (8 centimeters) long, 3 inches wide at the top, and 1 inch (2.5 centimeters) thick. The uterus extends into the vagina at its **cervix**; the actual opening to the uterus in the cervix is called the **os**. The upper two-thirds of this cavity is called the **corpus**, and the top end is called the **fundus**. Most uteruses tilt forward (that is, they are *anteflexed*) over the bladder; approximately 20% tilt backward (*retroflexed*) (Figure 4.6). Women with retroflexed uteruses are more likely to experience discomfort during menstruation and may have more difficulty in inserting a diaphragm as a result of the angle of the cervix. Contrary to widespread belief, however, the ability to conceive is in no way affected by the position of the uterus.

The uterus consists of three layers. The outermost layer, the **perimetrium**, is very elastic, enabling the uterus to accommodate a growing embryo during preg-

FIGURE **4.6** Various positions of the uterus: (a) retroflexed and (b) anteflexed.

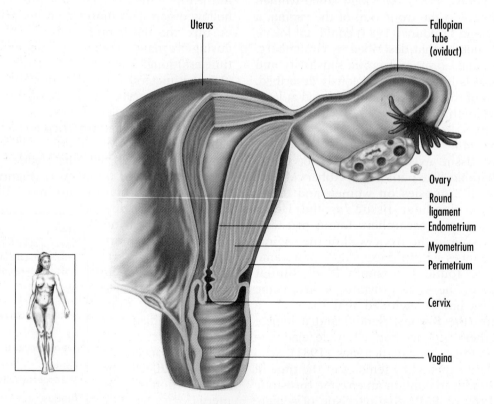

FIGURE **4.7** Layers of the uterine wall.

nancy. The middle layer, the **myometrium**, consists of smooth muscles, whose ability to contract helps push the newborn through the cervix and into the vagina (which during childbirth acts as the birth canal). The innermost layer of the uterus is the **endometrium**. This layer is loaded with blood ves-

sels and can therefore provide the nourishment necessary to sustain a developing fetus. It builds up and partly sloughs off as the menstrual flow in every menstrual cycle, unless fertilization takes place. Figure 4.7 depicts the anatomical relationships of the three layers of the uterus.

myometrium
The middle layer of the uterus, consisting of smooth muscle that aids in the pushing of the newborn through the cervix.

endometrium
The innermost layer of the uterus, to which the fertilized egg attaches and by which it is nourished as it develops before birth, which is partly discharged (if pregnancy does not occur) with the menstrual flow.

fallopian tubes (oviduct)
The routes through which eggs leave the ovaries on their way to the uterus, in which fertilization normally occurs.

ovary
A structure of the female genitalia that houses ova before their maturation and discharge and that produces estrogen and progesterone.

Graafian follicle
A part of the ovary from which a mature egg ruptures, allowing the corpus luteum to develop in the location where the egg was released.

corpus luteum
A yellowish structure that develops in the Graafian follicle at the discharge of an ovum and that produces progesterone and estrogen.

progesterone
A hormone secreted by the corpus luteum signaling the endometrium to develop in preparation for a zygote.

estrogen
A hormone produced by the ovaries whose level in the blood helps control the menstrual cycle.

fimbriae
The fingerlike ends of the fallopian tubes that catch the ova when they are discharged from the ovaries.

The Fallopian Tubes and the Ovaries

At the fundus, the uterus opens into the two **fallopian tubes** (we will use this more common name, although **oviduct** might be more appropriate). At the other end of each tube is an **ovary**, the organ that produces and stores the *ova*, or eggs. When a female is born, each of her ovaries contains approximately 40,000 to 400,000 eggs. Every egg has the potential to be fertilized by a sperm to become an embryo. After the girl reaches puberty, one of these eggs is usually discharged through the wall of one of her ovaries during each menstrual cycle. The egg develops inside a capsule called a **Graafian follicle** and is discharged when it has matured. The discharged egg, now matured and freed from its capsule and the ovary, is ready to be fertilized by a male's sperm. When the follicle ruptures to discharge its egg, the empty follicle, now a yellowish structure called the **corpus luteum**, secretes a hormone (**progesterone**) that signals the endometrium to prepare for a fertilized egg. Progesterone and **estrogen**, another hormone produced by the ovaries, play significant roles in menstruation, birth, growth, and aging.

When the ovum is discharged from the ovary, it is directed into the fallopian tubes. As shown in Figure 4.4, these tubes serve as routes for ova to reach the uterus. The newly released ovum is caught by the fingerlike end of the fallopian tube, called a **fimbria**, and is guided into the cone-shaped open end of the tube. If fertilization takes place, it usually takes place there.

Whether fertilized or not, the ovum continues on its journey through the tube, moved along in a sweeping motion by tiny hairlike structures called **cilia**. The destination of the fertilized ovum is the endometrium in the uterus, where it becomes attached and continues its development. An unfertilized ovum also travels to the endometrium, then disintegrates, and eventually is expelled through the vagina, along with some of the endometrium, in the process called *menstruation*. (Once an ovum is expelled, the menstrual cycle is completed. Soon an ovary will discharge another mature egg and the process will begin again.)

It should be noted that occasionally a woman may produce more than one egg per cycle, thereby becoming prone to multiple births. Fertility drugs, which may result in multiple births, are suspected of causing the maturation of several eggs per cycle. Sometimes the fertilized egg may attach in the abdominal cavity or the fallopian tube rather than in the uterus. This is termed an **ectopic pregnancy**. Ectopic pregnancies are discussed in Chapter 8.

cilia
Hairlike structures that guide objects, such as ova, moving past them.

ectopic pregnancy
The attachment and development of the zygote in a location other than in the uterus.

mammary glands
Milk-secreting glands located in the female breast.

prolactin
A pituitary hormone that stimulates the production of milk from the mammary glands.

areola
The darkened part of the breast immediately surrounding the nipple.

■ The Breasts

Although the female breasts are not reproductive organs, they do have significance in sexual arousal and response, and they serve an important reproductive function in providing milk for the newborn infant. Each breast contains about 15 to 20 clusters of milk-secreting structures called **mammary glands** (Figure 4.8). Each of these mammary gland clusters has an opening to the nipple, where the milk ducts open. The stimulation of the newborn's sucking on the nipple causes the pituitary gland to secrete a hormone called **prolactin**, which in turn stimulates the production of breast milk.

Most of the breast is fat and connective tissue. Except for small muscles in the area of the nipple and **areola** (the darkened skin around the nipple), there are no muscles in the breast. Because the breast is muscle-free, exercises to increase breast size are ineffective. Over the years the breasts may hang lower than normal if the ligaments are stretched by lack

FIGURE **4.8** The female breast.

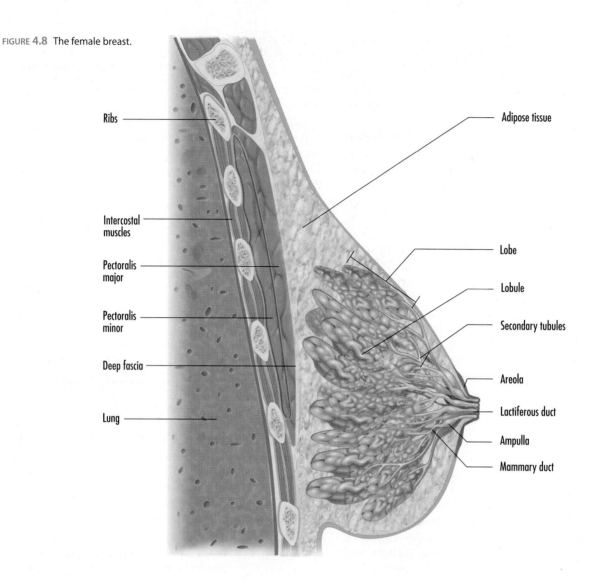

Ribs

Intercostal muscles

Pectoralis major

Pectoralis minor

Deep fascia

Lung

Adipose tissue

Lobe

Lobule

Secondary tubules

Areola

Lactiferous duct

Ampulla

Mammary duct

of support or by jostling (for example, not wearing a bra while jogging).

The nipples—of men as well as women—are richly supplied with nerve endings that respond with pleasurable sexual feelings when stimulated. During sexual arousal the nipples become erect. The size of the breasts or their shape is not related to sensitivity. Women with either small or large breasts may be equally sexually stimulated by the fondling of the breasts. Though some have characterized our society as making a fetish of large breasts, preferences in breast size and shape vary from individual to individual. It should be noted, however, that although breast size varies, extent of glandular tissue is comparable in all women's breasts. Because the amount of glandular tissue is the same, women with small breasts produce the same amount of breast milk after childbirth as women with larger breasts and are therefore as successful breastfeeding their babies as are women with larger breasts.

Our society has so emphasized breast size that many women have their breasts reconstructed. In

the past, liquid silicone was injected to enlarge the breast, but approximately 60% of women experienced problems such as infection, deformity, or exceptional hardness of the breast. More recently, silicone pouches containing saline solution have been implanted to reshape the breast. However, in 1992, in response to reported breakage of the pouches, the Dow Chemical Company, the largest manufacturer of silicone pouches, stopped manufacturing them and agreed to pay for their removal for women who so desired. The most recent research, however, indicates that silicone implants are not the health issue previously thought. In a study of the research related to silicone breast implants, the Institute of Medicine (a subgroup of the National Academy of Sciences) found no convincing evidence that chronic disease was more likely to develop in women with silicone breast implants than women without implants (Reuters, 1999). Furthermore, during a lawsuit against breast implant manufacturers, a federal judge appointed a panel of scientists to study the issue and report their findings

The size and shape of breasts vary among women.

TABLE 4.1	Functions of the Female Reproductive Organs

Organ	Function
Ovary	Production of egg cells and female sex hormones
Fallopian tube	Conveying of egg cell toward uterus; site of fertilization; transport developing zygote to uterus
Uterus	Protection and sustaining of life of embryo and fetus during pregnancy
Vagina	Conveying of uterine secretions to the outside of body; receiving of erect penis during sexual intercourse; transport of fetus during birth process
Labia majora	Enclosing and protection of other external reproductive organs
Labia minora	Formation of margins of vestibule; protection of openings of vagina and urethra
Clitoris	Organ richly supplied with sensory nerve endings associated with feeling of pleasure during sexual stimulation
Vestibule	Space between labia minora that includes vaginal and urethral openings
Vestibular glands	Secretion of fluid that moistens and lubricates vestibule

to the court. The court-appointed panel found no convincing evidence that silicone breast implants cause disease of the immune system as alleged in the lawsuit (Schwartz, 1998). The Food and Drug Administration also approved silicone-gel implants for breast enhancement in 2003 (Kaufman, 2003). Silicone pouch implants are still regularly used in breast reconstruction for women who have had a radical mastectomy due to cancer of the breast.

We also need to be concerned about other health issues regarding the breast, such as cancer of the breast. (We discuss this in greater detail later in the chapter.) Suffice it to say here that women need to perform regular breast self-examinations and obtain periodic medical checkups by a health professional to make sure that any abnormalities are identified early, thereby increasing the likelihood that treatment will be successful and as non-invasive as possible.

Table 4.1 reviews the functions of the female reproductive organs.

▨ The Hormones

What happens at the sight of an attractive person in a skimpy bathing suit? If the stimulus is suf-ficiently interesting, it can result in the first stages of sexual response—for example, increased heart rate, vaginal lubrica-tion, and erection of the penis or clitoris. How does the visual image result in these physical changes? The chain of events is rather complex. It starts with the **hypothalamus**, a struc-ture in the brain that, either through direct nerve pathways or through chemicals called **releasing factors**, can instruct various body parts to func-tion. The hypothalamus might be said to serve as a bridge between external stimuli and physiologi-cal responses. But let us go back to the bathing suit. Two things happen: (1) When the individual perceives the external stimulus as sexually excit-ing, the hypothalamus "tells" the pituitary gland to secrete its hormones, and (2) these chemicals stim-ulate the adrenal gland to secrete its hormones and the testes and ovaries to secrete their hormones. These secretions change the blood flow (producing vasocongestion), the heart rate, breathing, vaginal moistness, and so on.

hypothalamus
A structure in the brain that controls the pituitary gland and is directly con-nected by nerve pathways to various organs of the body.

releasing factors
Chemicals released from the hypo-thalamus that affect the function of various body parts.

hormone
A chemical substance secreted by a ductless gland, which is carried to an organ or tissue where it has a specific effect.

endocrine glands
Glands that secrete their products into the bloodstream.

pituitary
The "master gland," an endocrine gland located at the base of the brain that stimulates the other endocrine glands to produce their hormones.

gonadotropins
Sexual hormones secreted by the pituitary that stimulate the gonads to produce their hormones.

gonads
The male testes and the female ovaries, which produce gonadotropin hormones responsible for the development of secondary sexual characteristics.

follicle-stimulating hormone (FSH)
A hormone, secreted by the anterior portion of the pituitary gland, that "instructs" the ovaries to prepare an egg to be released from a follicle.

luteinizing hormone (LH)
A hormone, secreted by the anterior portion of the pituitary gland, that stimulates ovulation.

interstitial-cell-stimulating hormone (ICSH)
A hormone, secreted by the anterior portion of the pituitary gland in males, that stimulates the production of sperm.

androgens
Male sex hormones.

spermatocytes
Cells that develop through several stages to form sperm.

testosterone
The male sex hormone produced in the testes that is responsible for the development of male secondary sexual characteristics.

menarche
The time when a female begins her first menstrual cycle, usually at 8 to 16 years of age.

menstruation
The cyclical emission of the blood-enriched endometrium when pregnancy does not occur.

These powerfully acting **hormones** are chemical substances that influence organs and tissues. They are produced by **endocrine glands**, glands that secrete their products into the bloodstream. The thyroid, for example, secretes a hormone that travels to the heart and increases the heart rate. The adrenal gland secretes the hormone adrenalin, which travels to the bronchial tubes of the lungs and dilates them. As we have just seen, the secretions of several glands are involved in sexual response.

The **pituitary**, a pea-shaped gland located at the base of the brain, serves as a sort of master gland to the others in the system. It stimulates the other glands to release their hormones. The front part of the pituitary secretes three sexual hormones, called **gonadotropins**, which act on or stimulate the **gonads** (the testes and ovaries). The gonads are also endocrine glands, and they produce their own hormones. The three gonadotropins are **follicle-stimulating hormone (FSH)**; **luteinizing hormone (LH)**, often called the **interstitial-cell-stimulating hormone (ICSH)** in males; and prolactin (produced only during pregnancy and breastfeeding). Once stimulated by these gonadotropic hormones, the gonads produce their own hormones: estrogens, progesterones, and androgens. The adrenal gland also secretes androgen directly.

In women, estrogens and progesterones regulate the menstrual cycle, with estrogens important in producing vaginal lubrication. Although estrogens and progesterones have no known function in men, the presence of too much estrogen in the male body can lower interest in sexual activity and may result in enlargement of the breasts. **Androgens** affect the sex drive of both men and women: The presence of too much causes excessive sexual appetite, the presence of too little androgen decreases sexual interest. FSH stimulates cells in the seminiferous tubules (called **spermatocytes**) to produce sperm.

Despite the fact that hormones account for and influence sexual differences, males and females produce the same hormones. Estrogens and progesterones are considered female hormones and androgens male hormones, but both males and females produce all three. They do differ in the amounts they produce, however. For example, males have levels of the strongest androgen (**testosterone**) 10 times those of females, and females have significantly more estrogens than males. Obviously, too, males and females differ in the organs activated by the hormones. Long before we begin to think about hormones and our sexuality, hormones have already had significant effects.

Menstruation

At some time during puberty, a girl reaches **menarche**; that is, she has her first menstrual cycle. Then, and cyclically thereafter unless she is pregnant, blood (actually the blood-enriched endometrium) is discharged (or flows) from her uterus through her vagina for several days. The Latin origin of the word **menstruation** is *mensis,* meaning "month," because the menses, or periods, supposedly occur monthly. Actually they are not so predictable. Between menarche and menopause, when menstruation ceases, a woman's menstrual cycle may stabilize in a 28- to 30-day pattern (20- to 40-day cycles are also quite normal), or it may never stabilize. Cycles may vary in length from period to period, or they may be stable for a long time, fluctuate, and become stable again. Menstruation has been called the "curse," the "monthly sickness," and worse, but it is a normal physiological response to hormonal activity.

Menarche

The reason menstruation begins when it does is not exactly known. One hypothesis relates to the increase in body fat at puberty as a result of hormonal secretions. Evidence for this hypothesis can be found in long-distance runners. Many women who jog long distances lose considerable weight and body fat. It is not uncom-

amenorrhea
The absence of menstruation in a woman who should be menstruating.

mon for such women to experience secondary **amenorrhea**; that is, they no longer menstruate regularly. In fact, some experts estimate that as many as 50% of women runners experience a cessation of menstruation (Reynolds, 1997). In addition, women suffering from anorexia nervosa—a condition in which the woman is so preoccupied with being thin that she eats very little and loses a great deal of body weight and fat—often lose their periods. In truth, though, no one really knows why women joggers or anorexics cease to menstruate, and, at least for the joggers, there appears to be more going on than just a loss of body fat. Other studies have found that many thin female joggers continue to menstruate, and many heavier ones do not.

Menstrual Physiology

The menstrual cycle begins when the pituitary gland secretes two hormones: FSH, which stimulates the growth, or "ripening," of follicles in the ovary; and LH, which stimulates the ovary to release one egg, that is, to *ovulate*. Once the egg is released, the area from which it was released (the Graafian follicle) becomes a yellow body (corpus luteum). The Graafian follicle secretes the hormone estrogen, and the yellow body secretes progesterone and estrogen. Progesterone causes the lining of the uterus to thicken and store nutrients in preparation to receive, implant, and nourish a fertilized egg, called a **zygote**. If the egg is not fertilized, the yellow body degenerates and thus becomes unable to secrete progesterone any longer. The lack of progesterone is a signal to expel the unneeded endometrium. This tissue, which is gradually shed over the course of a few days, is the menstrual flow. The cycle is then ready to begin anew.

Phases of the Menstrual Cycle

Figures 4.9 and 4.10 depict the roles of hormones in the menstrual cycle and its phases. The first phase is termed the **proliferative phase**. It is during this phase that FSH production is increased by the

zygote
A fertilized egg.

proliferative phase
The first part of the menstrual cycle, during which FSH production is increased and the follicles are maturing.

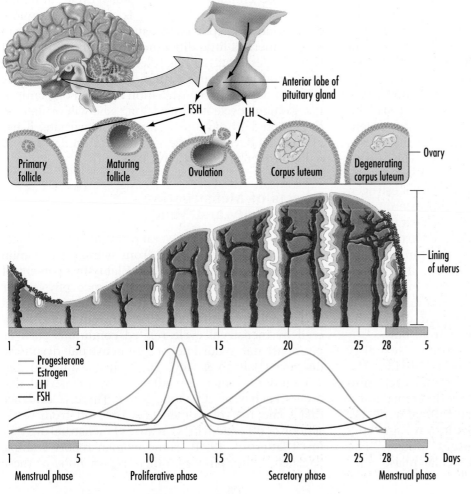

FIGURE **4.9** Hormones from the hypothalamus control the release of hormones from the pituitary gland, which in turn regulates production of ova and sex hormones from the ovaries. Note how the rise and fall of the hormone level is related to the building up and sloughing off of the uterine lining.

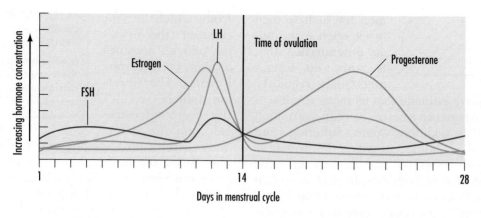

FIGURE **4.10** Changes in relative concentrations of hormones during ovulation and menstruation.

pituitary gland, which in turn stimulates the follicles in the ovaries to mature. The follicles then can produce estrogen, which causes the endometrial lining of the uterus to thicken and prepare for the implantation of the zygote. The pituitary then increases production of LH in response to the elevated levels of estrogen in the bloodstream, causing one follicle to prepare to expel an ovum (the Graafian follicle), and the proliferative phase proceeds until ovulation.

The **secretory phase** of the menstrual cycle begins once ovulation occurs and entails continued secretions of LH, which stimulate the development of the corpus luteum. The corpus luteum secretes progesterone, causing further thickening and engorgement of blood of the endometrium. If implantation does not occur, the pituitary shuts down production of FSH and LH, causing degeneration of the corpus luteum. The result is a decrease in the secretions of estrogen and progesterone.

The next phase of the menstrual cycle is the **menstrual phase**, in which the endometrial lining of the uterus is sloughed off as the menstrual flow.

Some sexuality experts divide the menstrual cycle into three different phases: the **follicular phase**, **ovulation**, and the **luteal phase**. The follicular phase coin-

cides with the menstrual and proliferative phases, ovulation is marked by the discharge of the ovum from the Graafian follicle, and the luteal phase is the same as the secretory phase. This categorization pertains to changes in the ovaries, whereas the previous categorization refers to changes in the uterus.

As noted in Figure 4.10, in a 28-day cycle ovulation occurs on day 14, with the menstrual flow lasting for 4 days. The great variation in the menstrual cycle—among women and even in any one woman—should be emphasized. The 28-day cycle, although often spoken of as *the* cycle, is not very common. Furthermore, in spite of menstrual cycles' differing in length, there is little difference in the luteal phase of these cycles. That is, regardless of the length of the menstrual cycle, once ovulation occurs, it basically takes 14 days until menstruation begins. For example, if a woman's cycle is 42 days long, she will ovulate on day 28, and 14 days later she will menstruate; if her cycle is 30 days long, she will ovulate on day 16 and will still menstruate 14 days later.

Effects of Menstruation on the Body and Mind

Menstruation can have several physical and emotional effects, which vary greatly from woman to woman and from one cycle to another. Eighty-five percent of women of reproductive age experience physical or emotional changes associated with their menstrual cycle, and approximately 40% of women are bothered by menstrual cycle–related conditions such as premenstrual syndrome or premenstrual dysphoric disorder (Ballagh & Heyl, 2008). It is estimated that 2.5 million women are affected by menstrual disorders each year (Clayton, 2008). There is evidence that some 10% of women take time off from work, school, or other activities because of menstrual discomfort (Patterson, 1990). Some women report cramps, backaches, and pimples; others report none of these

secretory phase
The second part of the menstrual cycle, during which ovulation occurs and the production of LH stimulates the development of the corpus luteum.

menstrual phase
The part of the menstrual cycle during which the endometrial lining is sloughed off as the menstrual flow.

follicular phase
The part of the menstrual cycle during which menstruation occurs and the pituitary increases the production of FSH so the follicles mature: a combination of the menstrual and proliferative phases.

ovulation
The part of the menstrual cycle when the ovum is discharged from the ovary.

luteal phase
The same phase of the menstrual cycle as the secretory phase, which includes ovulation and the production of LH from the corpus luteum.

Menstruation can affect a woman's body and mind. Cramps and backaches can occur, as well as feelings of nervousness or depression. Different women are affected differently by menstruation—some women have minor symptoms whereas others have symptoms that are more severe.

symptoms. Some women report feeling depressed, bloated, nervous, or weak, and others do not.

Whether a woman experiences any of these effects—be they physical or emotional—may be a function of what she expects to experience. Evidence for this hypothesis does exist. For example, when researchers conducting studies of menstruating women inform the women of what the study is about, women report more of these symptoms than when they do not know what is being studied (Brooks, Ruble, & Clark, 1977; Ruble & Brooks-Gunn, 1979). Because many of these symptoms cannot be objectively measured, what a woman expects to feel may create a self-fulfilling prophecy. That is not to say women do not experience real discomfort; rather, the mind may affect the amount of discomfort experienced.

Stress researchers have determined that the mind–body connection is a real one. That is, with certain actual illnesses and diseases, either the mind affects the body so as to prepare it to become ill or the mind changes the body in a way that makes the illness worse than it might otherwise be (Greenberg, 2009). Other factors that might influence menstrual symptoms include diets too high in saturated fats, a lack of regular exercise, and work in extremely cold environments (Greenwood, 1986; Barnard et al., 2000).

The preceding discussion is not meant to negate the real physical and emotional effects of menstruation. For example, depending on one's age, and whether one has given birth to a child or not, cramping associated with menstruation can vary. Teenagers and perimenopausal women—those in the period between the beginning of menopause and the complete cessation of a woman's period—report worse cramping than is usual, whereas women who have given birth to a child report less cramping.

Menstrual Problems

Several conditions associated with menstruation require special attention. Among these conditions are dysmenorrhea, amenorrhea, and premenstrual syndrome.

Dysmenorrhea

Painful menstruation is termed **dysmenorrhea**. Many women experience some discomfort and pain during some menstrual cycles, and other women experience discomfort and pain regularly. It has been estimated that 70% to 90% of menstruating women have some degree of menstrual problems on a regular basis (Sommerfield, n.d.). Women may experience severe abdominal cramping, a bloated feeling, headaches, backaches, and nausea. An estimated 10% to 15% of women experience menstrual pain each month severe enough to prevent normal daily function at school, work, or home (www.drkoop.com).

The cause of **primary dysmenorrhea**—that is, pain during menstruation—is not specifically known. Many health practitioners identify the cause as **prostaglandins**, substances produced by body tissues that act as hormones. Prostaglandins, which are found in unusually high amounts in women with dysmenorrhea, cause the muscles in the uterus to contract. This contraction causes pain and cuts off some of the blood supply (with its oxygen) to the uterus, thereby causing more discomfort.

dysmenorrhea
Painful menstruation.

primary dysmenorrhea
Painful menstruation, the cause of which is unknown.

prostaglandins
Hormonelike substances produced by body tissue that may cause dysmenorrhea.

To treat primary dysmenorrhea, physicians sometimes prescribe antiprostaglandin medications such as naproxen (Aleve), Anaprox, or Ponstel. These medicines inhibit the production of prostaglandins and relieve pain, dizziness, headache, nausea, vomiting, and irritability in many women. Many women who do not use prescription drugs find aspirin or ibuprofen helpful in relieving pain (these also somewhat inhibit prostaglandin production). Other remedies proposed for dysmenorrhea include eating more fish and vegetables and less animal fats and taking calcium, vitamin B, and magnesium supplements. Drinking plenty of fluids has also been recommended, because it seems that when the body is dehydrated, the hormone vasopressin is secreted. Vasopressin conserves body fluids, an effect that is not what a woman feeling bloated needs. Oral contraceptives can also help relieve menstrual pain by eliminating ovulation and thereby decreasing the amount of prostaglandin produced (American College of Obstetricians and Gynocologists, 2006). In addition, placing a heating pad on the abdomen, lightly massaging the abdomen with the fingertips (effleurage), drinking warm beverages, taking a warm shower, doing waist-bending exercises, having an orgasm, and walking may alleviate some menstrual pain.

Secondary dysmenorrhea is painful menstruation caused by some other identifiable condition. For example, **endometriosis** (a condition in which endometrial cells attach and develop on some body tissue other than the uterus) can cause secondary dysmenorrhea, as can pelvic inflammatory disease, uterine tumors, and blockages of the opening to the uterus (the os). In these cases, treatment consists of finding and removing the cause of the menstrual pain, which may require surgery or medication.

Amenorrhea

Amenorrhea is the absence of menstrual flow. If a woman has never menstruated and is 18 years or older, her condition is called **primary amenorrhea**. If menstruation ceases after menarche, the condition is called **secondary amenorrhea**. Amenorrhea may be caused by pregnancy, malfunctioning of the ovaries, cysts or tumors, disease, hormonal imbalance, poor nutrition, or emotional distress. It may also be caused by strenuous exercise of the sort done by runners and young

secondary dysmenorrhea
Painful menstruation caused by some identifiable condition such as endometriosis.

endometriosis
The growth of the endometrium uterine lining at a location other than in the uterus.

primary amenorrhea
A condition in which a woman of age 18 years or older has never menstruated.

secondary amenorrhea
A condition in which a woman has ceased menstruating after menarche.

dancers (Koutedakis & Jamurtas, 2004; Torstveit & Sundgot-Borgen, 2005). The causes of amenorrhea in physically active women are not known. Some experts hypothesize that exercising women experience a decrease in body fat that may contribute to the cessation of their periods, as it does in anorexic women. Lower body fat may interfere with production of the amount of estrogen needed to menstruate. Among female athletes, amenorrhea is quite common (Mayo Clinic, 2007a), and it is suspected the cause is a combination of low body fat, the stress upon the body as a result of strenuous physical exercise, and the psychological stress associated with competition. Although the actual cause of amenorrhea in female athletes is difficult to determine, it does not follow that some physical condition does not exist in any one woman—athlete or not—that can be identified as the cause of her menstrual problem. It is advised that women whose menses cease consult their physicians to discuss any conditions or illnesses that are treatable.

The fear of pregnancy also has been known to create enough anguish and anxiety in sexually active women to cause a cessation of menses. Fearing pregnancy, many couples wait with bated breath for the evidence that the woman is not pregnant—menstruation. A slight delay in her period (not unusual) makes the woman anxious about the possibility of an unwanted pregnancy. Her anxiety can then further delay menstruation or create amenorrhea. Thus a vicious cycle develops that only a pregnancy test or the menstrual flow can break. Any woman who has been sexually active and has missed more than one period should have a pregnancy test.

Premenstrual Syndrome

Some women experience mood changes and other physical and emotional discomforts just before their menstrual periods. This condition is referred to as **premenstrual syndrome (PMS)**. In fact, more than 150 disorders have been associated with premenstrual syndrome; some of the more common ones are depression, tension, anxiety, mood

premenstrual syndrome (PMS)
Marked mood fluctuation during the week before menstruation, accompanied by physical symptoms.

swings, irritability or anger, difficulty in concentrating, lethargy, weight gain, fluid retention, bloating, breast soreness, joint or muscle pain, nausea, vomiting, and headaches (Mayo Clinic, 1998a). It has been estimated that at some time during their reproductive years 75% of women experience PMS (Mayo Clinic, 2007b).

Premenstrual syndrome was described by Katharina Dalton, a leading researcher in the treatment of PMS, in *Once a Month* (1979): "Once a month with

TABLE 4.2 **Premenstrual Symptoms**

The American Academy of Family Physicians (2004) lists the following symptoms of PMS:

• Acne	• Feeling irritable or tense	• Tender and swollen breasts
• Bloated abdomen	• Feeling tired	• Trouble concentrating
• Constipation	• Feeling anxious	• Trouble sleeping
• Crying spells	• Headache	• Swollen hands or feet
• Depression	• Joint pain	• Wanting to be alone
• Fast heartbeat	• Mood swings	• Weight gain
• Feeling hungry	• Not feeling as interested in sex	

Source: American Academy of Family Physicians. PMS: What you can do to ease your symptoms. *Family Doctor Org.* (2004). Available: http://familydoctor.org/141.xml?printxml.

monotonous regularity, chaos is inflicted on American homes as premenstrual tension and other menstrual problems recur time and again with demoralizing repetition." Reading this, many women found solace in the fact that other women had similar experiences each menstrual cycle. It is undeniable that many women do experience something akin to PMS fairly regularly (see Table 4.2).

There is no laboratory test or other sure way to diagnose premenstrual syndrome. Doctors rely on the woman's menstrual history, often requesting that patients keep a diary of the onset, duration, and the nature and severity of symptoms for at least two menstrual cycles. If symptoms such as those cited are present in the week before a woman's period, subside as her period starts, and are absent the week after her period, she is diagnosed as having PMS. This diagnosis is important not only to determine the treatment to recommend but also to help screen out other conditions commonly confused with PMS, such as contraceptive side effects, dysmenorrhea, eating disorders, substance abuse, depression, and other psychiatric disorders (Ransom & Moldenhauer, 1998).

There have been numerous theories about the causes of PMS. These are described in the following list, along with the recommended treatment based on the theory of causation.

1. *Prostaglandins.* As a woman's uterine lining begins to shed during the menstrual cycle, prostaglandins (hormones) are released into her bloodstream. As the prostaglandins build up, they cause the uterine walls to become tense and to contract, resulting in cramping. As with dysmenorrhea, antiprostaglandin medications are recommended, such as aspirin, acetaminophen (for example, Tylenol or Datril), naproxen (Aleve), or ibuprofen (Motrin, Advil, or Nuprin).

2. *Progesterone.* Progesterone builds up during the menstrual cycle, causing PMS symptoms. Antiprogesterone medications are recommended to alter the menstrual cycle (speeding or delaying the onset of bleeding).

3. *Natural opiates.* Women experience a drop in the level of the neurotransmitter beta-endorphin, which is manufactured in the brain the week before the menstrual flow. This neurotransmitter has been described as the body's natural opiate in that it alleviates pain and generally makes you feel good. Treatment involves administering the drug naloxone, which maintains high levels of beta-endorphins.

4. *State of mind.* The symptoms of PMS are the result of brain activity—that is, the mind. Moods, perceptions, thoughts, ideas, self-confidence, and self-image are "choreographed" by the brain premenstrually. Treatment, therefore, entails counseling and other means to help women change their states of mind.

Other treatments include the following:

1. Birth control pills to stop ovulation.

2. Medications such as injectable medroxyprogesterone acetate (Depo-Provera) to stop ovulation and menstruation temporarily in severe cases.

3. Antidepressants in lower dosages than usually prescribed for depression, such as fluoxetine hydrochloride (Prozac), sertaline hydrochloride (Zoloft), paroxetine hydrochloride (Paxil), and venlafaxine hydrochloride (Effexor), if symptoms are mainly emotional.

4. A vegetarian diet.

5. Naturopathic medicine that includes lifestyle and dietary changes and may consist

? Did You Know...

When the American Psychiatric Association included PMS in its *Diagnostic and Statistical Manual of Mental Disorders IV* as an illness, terming it **late luteal phase dysphoric disorder (LLPDD)**, some people objected to the potential negative economic and social impact for all women. They believed it promoted a view of women as unreliable and unstable. However, others were grateful that women could then collect health insurance for treating PMS and that research would be focused on the condition.

late luteal phase dysphoric disorder (LLPDD)
A type of premenstrual syndrome in which mental and emotional symptoms occur the week before menstruation. This is the name given to that condition by the American Psychiatric Association.

of nutritional supplements, botanical medicines, homeopathy, Chinese medicine, acupuncture, hydrotherapy, manipulation, physical therapy, or minor surgery (Phalen, 2000b).

In addition, the following is recommended (Mayo Clinic, 2007b):

1. Maintain a healthy body weight.

2. Lower the intake of salt and salty foods, especially before the period, to reduce fluid retention and bloating.

3. Avoid alcohol before the period to minimize depression and mood swings.

4. Avoid caffeine, such as in coffee, cola, and tea, to reduce moodiness, tension, and breast tenderness.

5. Increase the intake of carbohydrates such as breads, potatoes, cereals, vegetables, and rice.

6. Exercise regularly to enhance the sense of well-being.

7. Reduce stress by getting plenty of sleep, practicing a relaxation technique regularly, and trying yoga or massage.

Premenstrual Dysphoric Disorder

As many as 10% of women experience premenstrual symptoms so severe they cannot maintain their daily routines (Mayo Clinic, 2008). Some experts believe this is a result of a condition they term *premenstrual dysphoric disorder* (PMDD). PMDD has been described as a supercharged PMS, and is cited in the *Diagnostic and Statistical Manual of Mental Disorders, Fourth Edition*. PMDD's symptoms include

- A marked depressive mood

- A decreased interest in usual activities

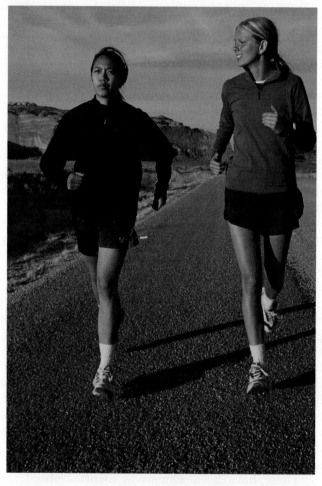

Exercising regularly and maintaining a healthy body weight are two strategies that are recommended to help women limit the severity of their menstrual and premenstrual symptoms.

- Lethargy, fatigability, or lack of energy

- Hypersomnia (falling asleep when not wanting to) or insomnia (difficulty falling asleep)

There is disagreement among women's health specialists about whether PMDD should be categorized as a "mental disorder." Some believe that classifying menstrual problems as a mental disorder stigmatizes women. As one psychologist argued: "It's a label that can be used by a sexist society that wants to believe that women go crazy once a month" (Daw, 2002).

Ethical DIMENSIONS

Should PMS Be Used as an Excuse for Socially Unacceptable Behaviors?

In 1980 and 1981, in two separate trials, British courts set free two women who admitted to murder because they were judged to suffer from PMS. In the first case, a barmaid, Sandie Smith, stabbed another barmaid during a fight. Testimony proved Smith had a history of violent outbursts that, when subsequently treated, were controlled with injections of progesterone. In the other case, Christine English purposely drove her car into her lover after an argument. English, too, was able to prove that she suffered from PMS and that she had menstruated a few hours after the murder. Both women were judged to have "diminished responsibility" and had their charges reduced to manslaughter. They were then released contingently on their getting treatment for their PMS.

Some people believe that PMS is so unsettling a condition that the physical discomfort and the emotional changes can understandably make a woman irritable, angry, hostile, and prone to do things she might not otherwise do. Given an incident to provoke such a reaction, even violent acts can be performed without the woman's really being responsible for them. These women should be encouraged to seek treatment for their illness rather

than be regarded as criminals. They should be treated with compassion rather than imprisoned. Advocates of this position would contend that these women are not in control of their decisions and should, therefore, be excused for their actions.

Others argue that murder is never excusable. If women are allowed to offer PMS as a defense, then any ill person can use a similar defense. That would allow antisocial behavior to occur without any punishment or societal sanctions. Anarchy would result. Women, or other sick people, could (short of committing murder) sign contracts and not be held responsible for them, could steal items from stores and not be prosecuted for that theft, and could even sexually abuse children without fear of reprisal. Opponents of this PMS defense conceive of an unmanageable situation if PMS sufferers, or any other group of ill people, are not held accountable for their actions.

If you were a judge, would you rule that "diminished responsibility" was a justifiable defense for women who experienced PMS? What other behaviors would you allow to be excused by PMS? What other physical or emotional conditions would you allow to be similarly used to explain people's actions?

Others believe a PMDD classification acknowledges women's feelings and focuses researchers' attention on developing medications to help premenstrual women. The medications now used to treat PMDD are fluoxentine (Sarafem), sertraline HTL (Zoloft), and paroxetine HCl (Paxil) (U.S. Department of Health and Human Services, 2007a).

Endometriosis
Sometimes tissue resembling the inner lining of the uterus (the endometrium) is found outside the uterus. This condition is known as *endometriosis*. Endometriosis is found most often on the lining of the pelvic cavity, the ovaries, the rectum, and the colon, and in the uterus and on the bladder. Sometimes it is also found on the small intestine, liver, spleen, and lymph nodes. Endometriosis is, unfortunately, not an uncommon occurrence. In fact, it affects 5.5 million women and girls in the United States and Canada, and millions more worldwide (Endometriosis Association, 2005). Although it can affect all women, endometriosis is most common among 25- to 30-year-olds,

and it has also occurred in girls as young as 11 years of age.

The causes of endometriosis are not known, although there are several theories. One theory holds that pieces of the endometrium somehow find themselves in the fallopian tubes and are transported into the pelvic cavity. This is called *retrograde menstruation*. The endometrium pieces then adhere to one another to form adhesions, which cause pain. Another theory is based on the realization that in the early stages of fetal development there are but a few cells present and that these cells eventually differentiate into different tissue. This theory posits that perhaps cells outside the uterus, for some unknown reason, take on the function of cells in the endometrium. Still another theory argues that endometrial cells are transported through the bloodstream or through the lymph system to sites elsewhere in the body. Finally, some researchers believe that endometriosis is caused by a breakdown in the function of the immune system, resulting in an inability to destroy endometrium cells that manage to leave the uterus.

Myth vs Fact

Myth: The menstrual cycle is 28 days long and does not fluctuate in length for any one woman.
Fact: The most prevalent menstrual cycle happens to be 30 days long. Even so, the cycle varies greatly from woman to woman and even for any one woman.

Myth: Women are usually emotionally "low" premenstrually and emotionally "high" at ovulation.
Fact: This has not been conclusively determined. There are conflicting research findings and criticism of the methodology researchers have employed to answer this question.

Myth: Women's work activity needs to be adjusted during their periods.
Fact: Though this myth has been used to support job discrimination practices against women, there is no evidence that women cannot function normally in their jobs when menstruating.

Myth: Women should not swim or exercise as usual during their periods.
Fact: With the usual hygienic practices used by women, there are no known physical reasons for not exercising as usual. For some women, iron supplementation may be necessitated by the iron lost in the menstrual blood, but that precaution is a simple one.

Myth: Women's sexual desire is at a peak just before and just after menstruation.
Fact: For some women and for some cycles this may be true. However, sexual desire involves more than one's physical condition—the nature of the relationship, the setting, one's comfort with sexuality, one's health, and so on—so that expecting sexual desire to be determined solely by the menstrual cycle is unrealistic.

Women who acquire endometriosis usually experience a great deal of pelvic pain. This pain most often occurs just before or during menstrual bleeding, and usually abates after bleeding ceases. Pain may also be experienced in the lower back or lower abdomen and may be associated with urination. Fatigue and/or bloated feelings may occur, there may be blood in the urine and/or heavy menstrual bleeding, and diarrhea or constipation may result. In addition to causing these uncomfortable symptoms, endometriosis can lead to serious health consequences. For example, scar tissue can form and result in infertility. Or, adhesions can connect organs such as the uterus, fallopian tubes, ovaries, and intestines.

Endometriosis is treated in several ways, depending on the severity of the symptoms and the location of the tissue. Laparoscopic surgery—in which two small incisions are made in the abdomen through which is inserted a viewing instrument to perform the surgical cut—can be helpful in identifying the existence of endometrial tissue outside the uterus and determining its location. Then the tissue can be surgically removed before the procedure is completed. Sometimes the tissue has spread so extensively that the surgeon needs to open the abdomen to remove it rather than merely inserting a laparoscope. This procedure is called a *laparotomy*.

In addition to surgery, there are medications that result in lower levels of estrogen than normal and, therefore, alleviate much of the pain associated with endometriosis. Some of these drugs are synthetic hormones that stop the ovaries from producing estrogen, causing cessation of menstruation. These are known as *gonadotropin-releasing hormone analogues (GnRH analogues)*. Another drug sometimes used is a synthetic hormone derived from testosterone (Danazol). More frequently, oral contraceptives are prescribed to prevent ovulation and reduce (when estrogen and progestin are used in combination) or eliminate menstrual bleeding. Finally, relief from pain may be obtained temporarily with ibuprofen or other analgesics (pain relievers).

The Menstrual Cycle and Sex

Many researchers have searched for a relationship between sexual interest and the time of the menstrual cycle. Findings of these studies have, for the most part, been contradictory (Bullivant et al., 2004). Some researchers report that women are more interested in sex just *before* menstruation (Kinsey, Pomeroy, & Martin, 1953), and others find them most interested *during* menstruation (Friedman et al., 1980). Still others report the *middle* of the menstrual cycle to be the most sexually active (Adams, Gold, & Burt, 1978) or the time just *after* the menses to be when most sexual fantasizing occurs (Matteo & Rissman, 1984). Several other studies have not found the midcycle

Did You Know . . .

If a couple decides to engage in sexual intercourse when the woman is menstruating, they should realize that transmission of HIV is probably more likely at this time of the menstrual cycle than at any other. That is because of the blood present and the probability that some of that blood will have contact with an opening (albeit microscopic) into the body. If HIV is in that blood, it can infect the sexual partner. The "safer sex" practice of refraining from sexual intercourse while a woman is menstruating is usually overlooked. From the woman's perspective, participating in coitus while menstruating can facilitate HIV entry into her body.

related in any way to heightened sexual arousal (Slob et al., 1991; van Goozen et al., 1997).

Some researchers describe two peaks during the menstrual cycle: just before menstruation and just after. Gold and Adams (1981) proposed an interesting explanation for why these parts of the menstrual cycle are associated with heightened sexual arousal. They suggest the anticipation of a lack of sexual intercourse while they are menstruating leads women to want to "get all they can" before they begin menstruating, and the actual deprivation during menstruation leads women to "want to make up for lost time."

When are women most sexually aroused? The answer to this question probably varies from one woman to another and, in addition to menstrual physiology, depends on such factors as one's lover, the setting, and numerous psychosocial factors such as the woman's comfort with her body, her level of self-esteem, and her religious and cultural beliefs regarding menstruation.

Although there are no medical reasons to refrain from coitus during menstruation (if one or both partners are HIV-negative, see the Did You Know box on previous page), many couples do so. At least one study found over half the men and women surveyed believed couples should not engage in sexual intercourse when the woman is menstruating (Research Forecasts, 1981). According to a 1996 study, 16 percent of women 20 to 37 years of age reported that they had had sexual intercourse during their last menstrual period (Tanfer & Aral, 1996). Some people refrain from coitus during menstruation because of religious taboos. For example, in Orthodox Judaism menstruating women are considered unclean and are supposed to sleep in a separate bed. When they are through menstruating, Jewish women are supposed to cleanse themselves in a ritual bath called a *mikvah*. Others refrain from sexual intercourse during menstruation because of the potential messiness. Still others refrain because of the physical discomfort they feel—bloating, cramping, or fatigue. And, finally, there are women who are ashamed of their menstrual flow and prefer to keep it a private matter not shared with anyone. A couple who refrains from sexual intercourse during menstruation should be comfortable with their decision, whatever the reason; likewise, a couple who decides to engage in coitus during this time should be comfortable with their decision.

A couple who decide to engage in sexual intercourse during the menstrual period can take several actions to make that experience as enjoyable as possible. First, they should discuss any concerns they may have—for example, the potential messiness or any religious inhibitions. Second, the woman can wear a diaphragm or cervical cap to hold back the menstrual flow. Because the menstrual fluid can sometimes irritate the penis, the man should wear a condom (a good idea anytime coitus occurs). With these simple actions, coitus during menstruation can be a positive and rewarding experience.

Menopause

Usually between the ages of 40 and 55 years, women produce progressively less estrogen and progesterone, as an effect of aging on the ovaries. Whereas the pituitary continues to produce FSH and LH, the ovaries can no longer respond to these pituitary hormones as they once could. This decrease in estrogen and progesterone occurs over approximately a 5- to 10-year period and results in a cessation of menstruation. The period when these changes take place is called the **perimenopause**, or the **climacteric**; when menstruation has not occurred for a year, we call that **menopause**. Menopause is discussed in detail in Chapter 12.

> **perimenopause (climacteric)**
> The period just before menopause when the production of estrogen and progesterone is decreasing, usually a 5- to 10-year period.
>
> **menopause**
> The time when a woman's menstrual cycle ceases, usually between 40 and 55 years of age.

Sexually Related Diseases: Self-Care and Prevention

Some diseases are not transmitted by sexual activity but do affect sexual organs. These are termed sexually related diseases (SRDs). Advances in chemical and surgical treatment of diseases of the sex organs have improved 5- and 10-year survival rates and made restoration of function more attainable than ever before. Maintaining reproductive health means following safer sexual practices, paying attention to your body, monitoring it for certain signs, using the specialized health services available, and seeking information—from organizations and publications—on issues related to reproductive health. Successful treatment of SRDs generally depends on early diagnosis of potential problems.

The Female Reproductive System

Self-care and disease prevention activities for the female involve many of the sexual organs, including the breasts, cervix, uterus, ovaries, and vagina.

The Breasts

The most common breast disorders are cancer, cystic mastitis (mammary dysplasia), fibroadenoma, nipple discharge, and breast abscess. Most of these disorders occur only in women, but men are susceptible to breast cancer too.

Breast Cancer   The breast is the leading site of cancer in American women and the second major cause of cancer death (the first is lung cancer). At the time of this writing, it is estimated that 182,460 new cases of **breast cancer** will have been diagnosed in women in 2008, and 1,990 cases will have been diagnosed in men (American Cancer Society, 2008a). After increasing about 4% per year in the 1980s, breast cancer incidence rates have leveled off. Still, 40,480 women and 450 men will probably have died of breast cancer in 2008. And yet, death rates from breast cancer continue to decline, especially among younger women. The 5-year survival rate for localized breast cancer increased from 72% in the 1940s to 98% in 2008. If the cancer has spread regionally, however, the 5-year survival rate drops to 84%, and, if the cancer has spread to distant locations (metastasized), the survival rate drops to 27%. Eighty percent of women diagnosed with breast cancer survive 10 years, and 89% survive 5 years.

> **breast cancer**
> The most common type of cancer in women.

No specific cause of breast cancer is known, but epidemiological studies have identified certain risk factors that predispose women to breast cancer. One of these risk factors is age. As women get older, the risk increases. The risk is also higher in women who have a family history of breast cancer, who experienced an early menarche or a late menopause, who recently used oral contraceptives or postmenopausal estrogens, and who never had children or had the first live birth at a late age. Other suspected risk factors are a diet high in fat, although a large-scale 1999 study calls this relationship into question (Holmes et al., 1999); exposure to pesticides and other selected chemicals; alcohol consumption; weight gain; and physical inactivity. In addition, two new genes that appear to make women susceptible to breast cancer have been discovered, BRCA1 and BRCA2. However, only 5% to 10% of breast cancers are thought to be inherited, and only 5% of breast cancer patients were found to have the gene BRCA1 or BRCA2. One study found that 75% of women in whom breast cancer develops have no identifiable risk factor other than gender and age (Hortobagyi, McLelland, & Reed, 1990). This makes it especially important for all women to learn breast self-examination and to have regular breast examinations by a physician.

Breast self-examination (BSE) is a self-care procedure women can adopt. Although medical specialists actively check for breast cancer in routine examinations, some experts believe that checking one's own breasts every menstrual cycle increases the chances of early detection. The technique is simple. If cancer is present, the earlier it is diagnosed, the better the chance for survival.

It is recommended by several organizations that women over the age of 40 years get a mammogram annually. Younger women should have annual clinical breast exams every 3 years.

In April 1987 a committee of the United States Public Health Service (which had been established to recommend those medical procedures with demonstrated effectiveness and those without) caused concern among cancer prevention specialists by citing BSE as a procedure whose value had not been clearly shown. The committee was charged with reviewing the scientific evidence for many medical screenings and examination procedures and eliminating those that contributed to the increasing cost of health care. As such they decided that BSE was not employed by enough women and cancers not found in enough quantity to warrant public health campaigns to encourage women to perform the examination. Other cancer experts, who argued that BSE does not cost a woman any money and that it can uncover early treatable cancers, recommended that women ignore the committee's finding and continue doing monthly BSEs. Canadians have also weighed in on this issue. The Canadian Task Force on Preventive Health Care (Baxter, 2001) studied the benefits and harms associated with breast self-examinations and found no evidence of effectiveness and evidence of harm. The harm included an increase in the number

> **breast self-examination (BSE)**
> A periodic self-care procedure that involves feeling the breast for any abnormalities. The test is performed once every menstrual cycle or every month after menopause.

Gender
DIMENSIONS

Breast Self-Examination

By regularly examining her own breasts, a woman may notice any changes that occur. The best time for breast self-examination (BSE) is about a week after your period ends, when your breasts are not tender or swollen. If you are not having regular periods, do BSE on the same day every month.

1. Lie down with a pillow under your right shoulder and place your right arm behind your head.
2. Use the finger pads of the three middle fingers on your left hand to feel for lumps in the right breast.
3. Press firmly enough to know how your breast feels. A firm ridge in the lower curve of each breast is normal. If you are not sure how hard to press, talk with your doctor or nurse.
4. Move around the breast in a circular, up-and-down line, or wedge pattern (a, b, c). Be sure to do it the

6. If you find any changes, see your doctor right away.
7. Repeat the examination of both breasts while standing, with one arm behind your head. The upright position makes it easier to check the upper and outer part of the breasts (toward your armpit). This is where about half of breast cancers are found. You may want to do the standing part of the BSE while you are in the shower. Some breast changes can be felt more easily when your skin is wet and soapy.

For added safety, you can check your breasts for any dimpling of the skin, changes in the nipple, redness, or swelling while standing in front of a mirror right after your BSE each month.

same way every time, check the entire breast area, and remember how your breast feels from month to month.
5. Repeat the exam on your left breast, using the finger pads of the right hand. (Move the pillow to below your left shoulder.)

(a)   (b)   (c)

of physician visits for the evaluation of benign breast lesions and significantly higher rates of benign breast biopsy findings. As a result, the Canadian Task Force recommended that women not perform breast self-examinations. The American Cancer Society (2007a) takes a neutral stance, stating in their guidelines that breast self-exam is an option for women starting in their 20s. More recently, after conducting an extensive review of the research literature, the U.S. Preventive Services Task Force (2009) concluded there were more risks than benefits associated with breast self-exams and, therefore, recommended against teaching women how to perform breast self-examination.

If choosing to perform BSE, for best results, perform the exam when the skin is wet or moist—after showering or after applying body lotion. Menstruating women should perform this test 1 week after their period; postmenopausal women should check their breasts at least once a month. All women should check their breasts visually in the mirror and by means of this exam. Consult a gynecologist if you find a lump, a thickening, or any other unusual feature. These symptoms may include pain in the breast, discharge from the nipple, a change in the character of the nipple itself, or changes in the character of the breast.

In addition, the American Cancer Society, the American Medical Association, and the National Comprehensive Cancer Network recommend that women have regular breast examinations by a physician. These examinations include both **clinical breast exams** and **mammography** screening, depending on a woman's age and medical history. A clinical breast exam is similar to BSE, except that it is conducted by a physician trained to detect any abnormalities. It is suggested that women aged 20 years and older have a clinical breast examination regularly, preferably every 3 years between ages 20 and 40 years and annually thereafter. However, the U.S. Preventive Services Task Force also questioned the value of clinical breast exams (2009).

Mammography is also recommended. A mammogram is an X ray of the breast that often allows physicians to detect breast lumps before they would be palpable by a physician (see Figure 4.11). It is agreed that women older than age 40 years should have a mammogram annually. However, whether women in their 40s or women over 74 years old receive benefit from mammograms has been called into question by the U.S. Preventive Services Task Force (2009). (See Table 4.3.) The American Cancer Society reports that in 2005, 66% of women aged 40 years and older had had a mammogram within the previous 2 years, a decline from 70% in 2000 (American Cancer Society, 2007b). Obviously, we have a long way to go in educating women about the need to get mammograms and the benefits they can expect.

There is increasing interest in using breast magnetic resonance imaging (MRI) as a screening test for breast cancer. The use of MRI to detect breast cancer is being studied at the time of this writing. Some studies have shown that MRI is associated with higher false-positive rates. Thus women who are screened with MRI may have more unnecessary surgical biopsies. At the present time, it is still undetermined whether the increase in cancer detection achieved with MRI, in conjunction with the as-yet-undemonstrated decrease in death rates as a result, conveys enough of a benefit to warrant recommendations for wider use of this technology, given the large increase in false-positive rates and the possibility of overdiagnosis (National Cancer Institute, 2008a).

When breast cancer is suspected, a **biopsy** is performed. In a **needle biopsy** a fine needle is inserted into the tumor and fluid or cells are withdrawn. If the lump dissipates as soon as fluid is obtained, the lump is confirmed as a cyst and generally no further procedure is needed. An **open biopsy** is a minor surgical procedure during which tissue of the tumor is removed and

clinical breast exam
A breast examination conducted by a physician to detect any abnormalities.

mammography
An X ray of the breasts to detect any abnormality before it is visible or palpable.

biopsy (open biopsy)
Usually referred to as an open biopsy, a minor surgical procedure during which tissue of a tumor is removed and examined for presence of cancer.

needle biopsy
Insertion of a needle into a lump in a breast to see whether fluid (which indicates a cyst rather than a tumor) can be removed.

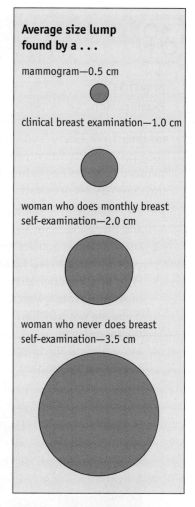

Average size lump found by a . . .

mammogram—0.5 cm

clinical breast examination—1.0 cm

woman who does monthly breast self-examination—2.0 cm

woman who never does breast self-examination—3.5 cm

FIGURE **4.11** The sizes of breast masses detectable by mammography, physical examination, and self-examination illustrate the importance of screening mammography in the early detection of breast cancer.

TABLE 4.3 **Breast Cancer Screening Controversy**

In November of 2009, the U.S. Preventive Services Task Force issued new guidelines regarding breast cancer screening. These guidelines generated a good deal of discussion with some experts and organizations agreeing and others disagreeing with the task force. The recommendations of the task force and several other organizations are summarized below.

Procedure	Organization(s)	Recommendation
Breast Self-Exams	USPSTF	Not recommended
	American Cancer Society	Optional
	American Medical Association	Recommended
	National Comprehensive Cancer Network	Recommended
	Canadian Task Force on Preventive Services	Not recommended
	American College of Obstetrics and Gynecology	Optional
	World Health Organization	Not recommended
Clinical Breast Exams	USPSTF	Not recommended
	American Cancer Society	Recommended
	American Medical Association	Recommended
	National Comprehensive Cancer Network	Recommended
	Canadian Task Force on Preventive Services	Not recommended
	American College of Obstetrics and Gynecology	Optional
	World Health Organization	Not recommended
Mammograms	USPSTF	Only for ages 50–74
	American Cancer Society	For age 40+
	American Medical Association	For age 40+
	National Comprehensive Cancer Network	For age 40+
	American College of Physicians	Optional for age 40+
	Canadian Task Force on Preventive Services	For age 40+
	American College of Obstetrics and Gynecology	For age 40+
	World Health Organization	Only ages 50–69

Given the variance in these recommendations, it is suggested that women discuss the best screening procedures for their individual circumstances with their physicians considering such factors as their family history, health status, and age.

Source: U.S. Preventive Services Task Force. Screening for breast cancer: U.S. Preventive Services Task Force recommendation statement. *Annals of Internal Medicine, 151* (2009), 716–726.

---

carcinoma
A type of cancer emanating from epithelial cells.

metastasis
Spread of cancer from a primary site to other parts of the body.

lumpectomy
Removal of a lesion, benign or malignant.

mastectomy
Removal of the breast and/or other tissue. *Simple:* Removal of only the breast (sometimes with removal of lymph nodes under the arm). *Modified radical:* Removal of the breast, lymph nodes, lining of the chest muscle, and sometimes part of the chest wall. *Radical:* Removal of the breast, lymph nodes, and chest muscle.

chemotherapy
Use of chemicals (medication) to treat disease; may be oral, intravenous, intramuscular, or topical.

examined for possible cancer (**carcinoma**).

Patients who have breast cancer are classified in terms of stages. These stages are determined by the characteristics of the tumor and the lymph nodes and whether **metastasis**—spread of the cancer to other body sites—has occurred. Treatment naturally depends on the stage of the cancer. The treatment of breast cancer may involve **lumpectomy**, in which only the breast lump and lymph nodes under the arm are removed, usually followed by radiation therapy; **mastectomy**, in which the breast and lymph nodes under the arm are removed; **chemotherapy**, treatment with drugs; **radiation therapy**; and **hormone therapy**. There are three kinds of mastectomy: *simple mastectomy,* in which the whole breast

radiation therapy
A form of treatment for cancer that uses carefully directed radiation to destroy cancer cells.

hormone therapy
Form of treatment for cancer that uses hormones to combat cancer cell growth.

is removed, sometimes along with lymph nodes under the arm; *modified radical mastectomy*, the most common form of mastectomy, in which the breast, many of the lymph nodes under the arm, the lining over the chest muscles, and sometimes part of the chest wall are removed; and *radical mastectomy* (also called the *Halstead radical mastectomy*), in which the breast, chest muscles, and all lymph nodes under the arm are removed. Radical mastectomy used to be the most frequently performed operation for breast cancer but now is used only when the tumor has spread to the chest muscles.

For patients with no lymph node involvement, hormone therapy may be prescribed as a preventive measure against recurrence of cancer. The most commonly used hormones are tamoxifen and special "designer estrogens," which may be administered for 5 years. There presently remains a question regarding the increased risk of development of cancer of the uterus for women on hormonal therapy. For early-stage breast cancer, long-term survival rates after lumpectomy plus radiation therapy are similar to survival rates after modified radical mastectomy, and, therefore, this less invasive procedure is being used more often—except for those women who choose not to experience the side effects of radiation and thus choose mastectomy.

We live in a society in which breast size and shape are mistakenly seen as contributing greatly to a woman's sexuality. Thus a woman who loses a breast through amputation can be devastated. Many women who have had mastectomies, whether or not they are sexually active, suffer feelings of loss, fear of rejection, and, of course, fear of the cancer's recurrence. Community support systems such as the Reach to Recovery Project of the American Cancer Society (ACS) and the Breast Referral Service, founded by Rose Kushner, who herself recovered from a mastectomy, give invaluable support to women in adjusting to the treatment of their cancers. The involvement of lovers or husbands and children is of great importance, because all of them, not just the woman, must

Multicultural DIMENSIONS

Breast Cancer More Deadly in African Americans

Although breast cancer develops more often in white women, African American women are more likely to die of it (American Cancer Society, 2008a). Researchers and epidemiologists have been perplexed as to why. It was originally assumed that this difference was due to the disproportionately high number of African American women who live in poverty, resulting in lack of access to health care. That, in turn, would lead to later diagnosis and, consequently, less effective treatment. However, having studied this dilemma for several years, scientists have concluded that, although poverty status plays a role (it is estimated that poverty accounts for approximately 50% of the cause), biology is significantly involved. Tumors in African American women are just more virulent.

Evidence for this conclusion can be found in a study that compared African American and white women who belonged to health maintenance organizations (HMOs) in which health care was readily available (access to mammograms and other medical care). Still, the African American women HMO members had larger and more advanced tumors when diagnosed. The suspicion was that these tumors grew faster, and that is why at the time of diagnosis they were larger and more advanced.

Research also indicates that African American women do not wait any longer to seek medical diagnosis when identifying a breast abnormality than do white women. Consequently, that is not a significant variable in the difference in tumor size or death rates between African American and white women.

A review of research of breast cancer in African American women published in the *New York Times* (Kolata, 1994) summarized what is known about this situation. Cited are several studies in which tumors in African American women were found to be more actively dividing than those in white women, and more lacked hormone receptors and had tissue features indicative of unfavorable diagnosis.

Although it is wise for all women to perform breast self-examinations on a regular basis and to obtain regular medical examinations, given what we know about tumors in African American women, it is particularly prudent for them to do so.

After mastectomy.

After reconstructive surgery after mastectomy.

adjust to her changed appearance and emotional sensitivity. Breast reconstruction after a mastectomy is also available. It offers a woman a more normal appearance and often eases her acceptance of the change in her body. This option should be discussed with the surgeon before breast surgery, if possible.

Reconstructive breast surgery can create a breast-like structure by using saline (salt) water encased in a silicone pouch that is implanted under a woman's skin and chest muscle.

Cystic Mastitis Also called *chronic cystic mastitis, fibrocystic condition,* and *mammary dysplasia* (cell change), **cystic mastitis** is the most common breast condition. It is usually found in women 40 to 60 years of age (California Pacific Medical Center, 2008). Because cystic mastitis is uncommon in postmenopausal women, it is believed to be related to estrogen activity. In cystic mastitis small and large cysts form in the breast tissues. The cysts are generally filled with fluid and may have to be drained frequently. Sometimes the cysts must be removed. Studies have concluded that "fibrocystic breasts" occur frequently in women and are not associated with significant increases in risk for breast cancer (Cady, 1986; Deckers & Ricci, 1992). One research report indicated a possible link between cystic mastitis and coffee, tea, cola, and chocolate consumption. On the basis of this study, some practitioners recommend that women decrease or eliminate the consumption of these products. But because this treatment approach has not been tested by using randomized double-blind studies, medical researchers and practitioners have questioned its validity.

cystic mastitis
Known also as fibrocystic disease, a condition characterized by fluid-filled lesions (cysts) that are tender and believed to be related to estrogen activity.

Fibroadenoma **Fibroadenoma** is a benign (noncancerous) tumor that may develop in white women in their early 30s and in black women somewhat earlier (there are no data on other groups). The tumor is usually firm, round, and somewhat movable. Generally the treatment is surgical removal.

Nipple Discharge A discharge from the nipples of women who are not nursing can be due to cystic mastitis, to a small benign tumor (called a *papilloma*) in a duct leading to the nipple, or to an uncommon condition *(ectasia)* in which the ducts of the breast enlarge and distend, allowing fluid to accumulate and escape. Occasionally the use of hormones—such as oral contraceptives and postmenopausal estrogen supplements—can cause nipple discharge, which should cease when the drugs are discontinued. Any discharge from the nipples should be checked by a physician.

Breast Abscess Generally **breast abscesses** (infections) are seen in nursing women, but they occur in nonnursing women as well, and in either case should be treated by a physician. Redness, swelling, or a tender, painful mass is symptomatic of breast infection. If the infection is not stopped, an abscess can develop. These are usually treated by incision and drainage, antibiotics, or both.

The Cervix
Rates of **invasive cervical cancer**, which involves deep-tissue layers of the cervix and sometimes spreads to other organs, have decreased steadily

fibroadenoma
A benign (noncancerous) tumor that is firm, round, and somewhat movable.

breast abscess
Infection of the breast characterized by redness, swelling, and a painful or tender mass.

invasive cervical cancer
Cancer that has invaded a wide area of cervical tissue.

over the past several decades. This decline is attributed to the increase in Pap smear screening, which leads to early detection and subsequent early treatment. Still, an estimated 11,070 cases of invasive cervical cancer were diagnosed in 2008 with 3,870 deaths (National Cancer Institute, 2008b), in spite of a steady decline in death rate from cervical cancer since 1982. Cervical cancer death rates declined for African Americans more rapidly than for whites. However, in 2005 the mortality rate for African American women (4.7 per 100,000) was twice as high as it was for white women (2.3 per 100,000). The 5-year relative survival rate for the earliest stage of invasive cervical cancer is 92%. The overall (all stages combined) 5-year survival rate for cervical cancer is about 72% (American Cancer Society, 2008b).

Although the exact cause of cervical cancer is unknown, several factors can put you at risk. Among these are having your first intercourse at an early age, having multiple sex partners, having many pregnancies, having a mother who took diethylstilbestrol (DES) while pregnant with you, and having a sexually transmitted infection caused by the human papillomavirus (HPV).

The American Cancer Society (2008b) recommends a **Pap smear** be performed annually with a pelvic exam in women who are, or have been, sexually active or who have reached the age of 18 years. After three consecutive annual exams have normal findings, the Pap test may be performed less frequently at the discretion of the woman and her physician. Pap smear screening is a simple procedure that involves swabbing a small sample of cells from the cervix, transferring these cells to a slide, and examining them under a microscope. Regular gynecological screening is advised for all women, particularly because early cell changes in the cervical tissue do not present symptoms a woman can recognize herself—although invasive cervical cancer sometimes does cause a bloody discharge between periods and/or bloody spotting after intercourse. Unfortunately, data indicate that not enough women are getting regular Pap tests. In 2003, only 79% of women had a Pap smear within the past 3 years (National Center for Health Statistics, 2006).

Other procedures have been developed to screen for cervical cancer. One of these is called *PapSure* (Redfran, 2002). This procedure involves a visual inspection of the cervix using a scope and a blue chemical light, and is performed in conjunction with a traditional Pap smear. Another cervical cancer detection test is the experimental *LUMA Cervical Imaging System* (McMillan, 2004). In this procedure, the cancerous tissue absorbs light differently than healthy tissue,

> **Pap smear**
> A test of the tissue of the cervix for cervical cancer (named after its founder, Dr. Papanicolaou).

showing possible problematic areas. Certainly, even more advanced screening techniques will be developed in the coming years.

Treatment for invasive cervical cancer generally consists of surgery and radiation, or both. Ninety percent of patients survive 1 year after diagnosis, and 73% survive 5 years. When detected at an early stage, invasive cervical cancer is one of the most successfully treated cancers, with a 5-year survival rate of 92% for cancers that have not spread. Unfortunately, only 57% of invasive cervical cancer in white women and only 49% in African American women are diagnosed at this stage. Again, this points to the value of getting a Pap test regularly (American Cancer Society, 2008b).

At the time of this writing, it was estimated that 40,100 cases of cancer of the uterus, most often of the endometrium, would be diagnosed in 2008. Incidence rates of uterine cancer have varied since the mid-1980s. In 2005, the incidence rate for white women was 24.3 per 100,000, and 20.3 per 100,000 for African American women (National Cancer Institute, 2008c). Although incidence rates are higher among white women than African American women, the relationship is reversed for mortality rates: African American women have mortality rates that are nearly twice as high as rates among white women.

Estrogen is the major risk factor for uterine cancer. Women who choose estrogen replacement therapy to combat the effects of menopause, who are administered tamoxifen to prevent breast cancer or its recurrence, who experience an early menarche, who have a late menopause, who never have children, or who do not ovulate have been shown to be at increased risk. Conversely, pregnancy and the use of oral contraceptives appear to provide protection against uterine cancer.

The Pap test is rarely effective in detecting uterine cancer early. It is with this realization that the American Cancer Society recommends that women older than 40 years have an annual pelvic exam and that women at high risk have an endometrial biopsy at menopause and periodically thereafter. Early warning signs include uterine bleeding or spotting; pain is a later symptom. Treatment, which depends on the stage of the cancer, consists of surgical removal of the uterus and/or ovaries, radiation therapy, hormonal therapy, and chemotherapy. The 5-year survival rate is 95% if the cancer is discovered at an early stage, when it is contained regionally. Survival rates for whites exceed that for African Americans.

The Ovaries

Ovarian cysts and tumors can occur when a female is any age. A cyst is an abnormal cavity that is filled with fluid. The most common ones are called **functional cysts**; these occur on the follicle or corpus luteum and are usually caused by the failure of the follicle to rupture and discharge the egg. Generally they are small and not particularly significant. They usually disappear spontaneously within a month or two.

Dermoid cysts are common in young women. They contain hard, fatty material, and sometimes remnants of teeth. These are believed to be embryonic in nature and are considered benign. Most ovarian cysts and tumors are usually benign, but if they cause symptoms such as pain, tenderness, and internal bleeding, they can require surgery. Because there is always the possibility of future problems, such as malignancy, a woman should remain under medical supervision once cysts or tumors have been diagnosed.

In the **Stein–Leventhal syndrome** the ovaries become enlarged and have cysts on them. Infertility and secondary amenorrhea also result. This condition affects one in ten women of childbearing age and is the most common cause of female infertility. Although its causes are not specifically known, genes are thought to be one factor because women experiencing this condition tend to have a mother or sister with it as well. Researchers also think insulin could be a cause given that Stein–Leventhal syndrome affects the ovaries and ovulation (U.S. Department of Health and Human Services, 2007b). Symptoms include infrequent menstrual periods, no menstrual periods, and/or irregular bleeding; infertility; increased hair growth on the face, chest, stomach, back, thumbs, or toes; and pelvic pain. Treatment may include birth control pills; medications such as Clomid and Serophene to stimulate ovulation; surgery ("ovarian drilling") that involves puncturing the ovary and administers an electrical current to destroy a small portion of the ovary; and lifestyle changes (eating a healthy diet, exercise, and weight loss) to improve the body's use of insulin. Most patients respond to therapy, and frequently fertility is restored to normal.

Ovarian cancer killed an estimated 15,520 American women in 2008. In fact, ovarian cancer causes more deaths than any other cancer of the female reproductive system. An estimated 21,650 new cases of ovarian cancer were diagnosed in 2008, amounting to 3% of all cancers among women. One of the reasons ovarian cancer is so deadly is that its symptoms are "silent": They may go unnoticed until late in development. Rarely does abdominal swelling occur and even more rarely abnormal vaginal bleeding. Stomach gas, discomfort, and distention that cannot be explained by other causes may indicate a need to have a thorough medical examination with ovarian cancer in mind.

Risk factors include never having children, being older (ovarian cancer occurs more frequently in women in their 80s), and having had certain other cancers such as colon and endometrial cancers. As with all cancers, early detection is important. Pelvic exams are most valuable, because Pap tests rarely are effective in uncovering ovarian cancer. In 2000 a new technique using sonography was developed that has the potential of diagnosing ovarian cancer earlier than is presently possible. This new method, *transvaginal ultrasonography,* was able to diagnose stage 1 ovarian cancer in 59% of women, whereas other methods could detect only 30% of these stage 1 cancers (Sato et al., 2000). Treatment can include surgical removal of one or both of the ovaries and/or the fallopian tubes (called a *salpingo-oophorectomy*) and the uterus (*hysterectomy*). If disease is detected early and the tumor is small, only the involved ovary is removed. This consideration is especially important to young women who want to have children. Radiation therapy and chemotherapy are also used in the treatment of ovarian cancer. The 5-year survival rate varies by the stage when diagnosed. If cancer is diagnosed and treated early, the survival rate goes up to 93%. Unfortunately, only 19% of cases are detected in their localized stage. Five-year survival rates vary from 18% to 93% depending on the stage of the cancer.

The Vagina

Normal vaginal secretions are odorless, and the acidity of the vagina helps it to cleanse itself. Nevertheless, some women choose to cleanse the vagina by **douching**—that is, by rinsing with water or a vinegar and water solution. A vaginal douche, the value of which has been questioned, is not recommended and can be harmful if not done correctly. Damage can occur in two main ways: (1) Improper insertion of the douching material may actually damage the tissue, resulting in an increased chance of infection; (2) the chemical balance of the vagina can be altered, affecting contraceptive function. For instance, if a woman is using a spermicidal cream or

functional cyst
An ovarian cyst that occurs on the follicle or corpus luteum, usually caused by the failure of the follicle to rupture and release an egg.

dermoid cyst
A type of benign ovarian cyst commonly found in young women.

Stein–Leventhal syndrome
Reproductive malfunction in women; a syndrome of endocrine origin that involves ovarian cysts, amenorrhea, and infertility.

ovarian cancer
Cancer of the ovaries; it causes more cancer deaths than any other cancer of the female reproductive system.

douche
Cleansing of the vagina by inserting a nozzle that secretes a recommended cleansing substance, a controversial procedure.

unusual discharges, abdominal pain, or open sores on your genitalia.

Toxic Shock Syndrome (TSS)

In the late 1970s several young women died of a previously little-known disease called **toxic shock syndrome (TSS)**. The toxins that cause this syndrome are produced by the *Staphylococcus aureus* bacteria, which may grow in the vagina and are absorbed by the body. These toxins enter the bloodstream and cause high fever (above 102°F), nausea, vomiting, diarrhea, a rapid drop in blood pressure, and sometimes aching muscles and peeling skin on the palms and feet. The exact mechanism of transmission is unknown. The syndrome appears to be linked to the use of tampons—particularly those made of superabsorbent material. It is thought that the presence of the tampon in the vagina for a prolonged period (6 hours or more) may provide an environment conducive to proliferation of the toxin-producing bacteria. When some tampons are inserted into the vagina, small irritations of the vaginal mucosa may occur and promote entry of the bacteria.

> **toxic shock syndrome (TSS)**
> A syndrome caused by *Staphylococcus aureus* bacteria in which symptoms include high fever, nausea, vomiting, diarrhea, and a drop in blood pressure; a potentially fatal syndrome that has been linked with the use of superabsorbent tampons.

It is recommended that superabsorbent tampons not be used because they pack the vagina tightly, prevent air circulation, and allow bacteria to proliferate. It has also been suggested that women using other types of tampons leave them in place for no longer than 2 hours and not use them at all during the night while sleeping.

Toxic shock syndrome has been seen in both genders among postsurgical patients, burn victims, and patients with boils and abscesses. Nonmenstrual cases constitute about half of all reported cases (Nemours Foundation, 2007).

Care from Medical Specialists

All health-related specialists agree that you should report any unusual signs or symptoms related to the reproductive system to a specialist in women's reproductive health—a **gynecologist** or a gynecological nurse practitioner. Furthermore, the American College of Obstetrics and Gynecology recommends that women have a routine gynecological exam every year, even when no signs or symptoms appear. Routine checkups, usually

> **gynecologist**
> A physician specializing in women's reproductive health.

Sexual health begins with routine self-exams.

other form of spermicide as a means of contraception, douching may destroy its effectiveness.

Smegma, a cheeselike substance secreted by the glans penis of males, may have effects on women's health. A female engaging in coitus with a male who has not washed away smegma could be subjecting herself to vaginal infections. There is also some concern that smegma may contribute to cancer of the cervix. It seems prudent, therefore, for sexually active women to make sure that their male sexual partners engage in the routine hygiene care necessary to remove smegma. Although it may be embarrassing, this may be a small price to pay for the prevention of vaginal infection and cervical cancer. Signs of sexually transmitted infections should also be given attention. Make sure to check your vulva routinely. See a health care provider if you have conducted on a special table with the woman's knees up and her feet in stirrups, consist of the following procedures:

1. An inspection of the external genitals for any irritations, discolorations, unusual discharges, or other abnormalities.

2. An internal check for cystoceles (bulges of the bladder into the vagina) and rectoceles (bulges of the rectum into the vagina). The examiner also looks for pus in the Skene's glands and for the strength of the pelvic and abdominal muscles. He or she also tests urine control by asking the patient to cough while checking to see whether urine flows involuntarily.

3. An inspection of the vagina and cervix by means of a **speculum**, a plastic or metal instrument that is inserted into the vagina to hold the walls apart during the examina- tion (Figure 4.12). (At this point and throughout the remainder of the examina- tion, if you are interested in seeing your genitals and watching the exam, ask the examiner to set up a mirror for you and to point out the various organs. If the exam- iner is not sympathetic to this request, you

speculum
A metal (or plastic) instrument that is inserted into the vagina to hold the walls apart, allowing for medical examination.

might consider looking for another practi- tioner.) The examiner will look for anything unusual, such as lesions (sores) or inflamma- tion affecting the vagina or cervix. Next the practitioner will scrape a tiny amount of tis- sue from the cervix by using a small wooden instrument called a *spatula*. This tissue will be used for the Pap smear. *If requested by the patient,* the smear can also be tested for signs of gonorrhea.

4. A bimanual examination (Figure 4.13). By sliding the index and middle fingers of one

Speculum and spatula.

FIGURE **4.12** Medical examination with speculum and spatula in place.

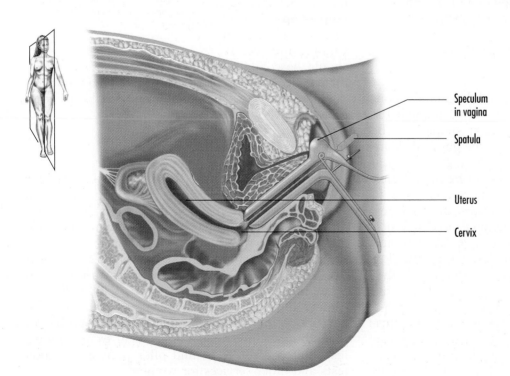

Speculum in vagina

Spatula

Uterus

Cervix

FIGURE **4.13** Bimanual examination.

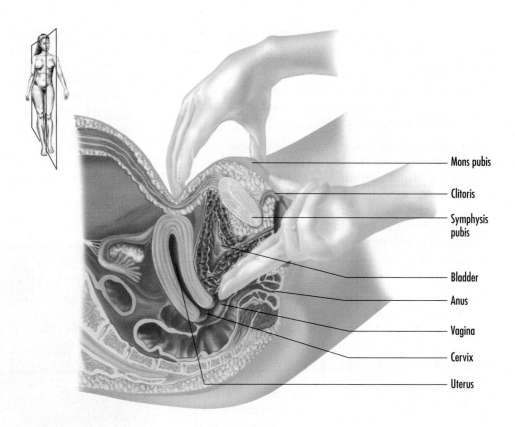

- Mons pubis
- Clitoris
- Symphysis pubis
- Bladder
- Anus
- Vagina
- Cervix
- Uterus

hand into the vagina and pressing down on the abdominal wall from the outside, the examiner feels for the uterus, fallopian tubes, and ovaries to determine their position, their size, and the presence of pain or inflammation. The examiner may also examine the internal genitals by inserting one finger into the rectum and another into the vagina.

5. An examination of the breasts for lumps or thickenings.

Two additional points should be noted about the routine gynecological exam. First, although the checkup may be uncomfortable, it should not be painful. Second, before beginning the physical examination, the practitioner should take a gynecological history. Noted on the history should be information regarding the regularity, flow, and any changes in the menstrual cycle; any pregnancies, miscarriages, or abortions; all birth-control methods used; the incidence of breast cancer in close female relatives; and whether the woman's mother took the drug DES during her pregnancy with the patient—that is, whether the patient is a "DES daughter." DES is a drug that was given in the 1940s and 1950s to women with a history of miscarriage. It is no longer used for miscarriages, because it has been found that vaginal cancer is more prevalent in DES daughters than in other women (Kaufman, 2000; Herbst, 1972), that DES sons

may also experience higher than expected infertility rates (Gill, Schumacher, & Bibbo, 1977), and that women who took DES have breast cancer in greater numbers than non-DES women. If the patient's mother did take DES, a periodic **colposcopy**, a check for changes in the vagina and cervix, should be conducted. The examiner uses an instrument called a *colposcope* to view the vagina for abnormal tissue growth. The examiner might also perform a biopsy.

> **colposcopy**
> An examination of the vagina and cervix using an instrument—a colposcope—to detect abnormal tissue growth.

Care from Organizations and Available Publications

For women, the ACS, the National Organization for Women, the March of Dimes, the National Women's Health Network, women's health centers and clinics, as well as local organizations of women who have had breasts removed due to cancer are but a few of the groups devoted to improving women's reproductive health. These groups function in various ways: Some publish written material, others lobby for legislation and funds, and still others provide social support for women with reproductive health problems. In addition, clinics conduct medical examinations, test and care for STIs, and offer premarital blood tests and other services for women.

Exploring the
DIMENSIONS
of Human Sexuality

Our feelings, attitudes, and beliefs regarding sexuality are influenced by our internal and external environments. Go to sexuality.jbpub.com/dimensions/4e *to learn more about the biological, psychological, and sociological factors that affect your sexuality.*

Sociocultural Factors

Sociocultural factors interact with biological factors to influence health.

- Socioeconomic status influences prenatal care and nutrition.
- Ethnic heritage influences health. African American women tend to get a more virulent form of breast cancer, resulting in a higher death rate. Jewish women are genetically at risk for scoliosis (curvature of the spine).
- Culture influences women's health. Fear of Western medicine prevents some immigrants from seeking treatment at early stages of a problem.
- Laws can affect what health insurance is required to cover. Because women are underrepresented in public office, their needs are sometimes overlooked.
- Media and ads that present ultrathin women as ideals can influence the eating patterns and health of women.

Biological Factors

When a sperm with an X chromosome meets an egg (all of which have X chromosomes), a female will develop. Biological factors continue to influence development throughout life.

- Genetic coding affects physical appearance, including height; coloration of skin, hair, and eyes; breast size; and many aspects of health.
- Female physical appearance changes at puberty, when the lean-body-mass-to-fat ratio changes from about 5:1 to about 3:1, signaling the body to commence menarche.
- Hormonal changes affect mood.
- At menopause, lower estrogen levels increase a female's risk for heart attack.

Psychological Factors

Psychological factors interact with other factors and can influence health.

- Women tend to have nearly twice the rate of depression of men.
- Teen women with low self-concept have a higher probability of having an unwanted pregnancy and birth.
- Expressiveness of emotions helps women stay mentally and physically healthy.
- Learned attitudes and behaviors about gender roles can prevent a woman from fulfilling her potential.
- Body-image problems in women can lead to long-term disorders, such as bulimia and anorexia nervosa.

CASE STUDY

The physiological development of a female starts when a sperm with an X chromosome fertilizes an egg. But socioeconomic status of the mother influences whether prenatal care is received, good nutrition will be available, and medical help will be sought. If the mother smokes, drinks, or abuses drugs during pregnancy, the fetus will be affected.

A woman's physiology is further altered during puberty and menopause. The increased fat content at puberty negatively affects many women's body image, which in turn negatively affects self-concept.

Unable to control the changes taking place within her body, the pubertal girl sometimes resorts to controlling the one thing she can control: food intake. Dieting is common, but excessive food control, or self-induced vomiting after meals, can result in a serious eating disorder.

Summary

- The external female genitals (the vulva) consist of the mons pubis, labia majora, labia minora, clitoris, vestibule, and urethral opening.

- The clitoris is protected by the clitoral hood and is very sensitive because it contains many nerve endings.

- The internal female genitals consist of the vagina, uterus, fallopian tubes, and ovaries.

- In the vagina, the outer one-third contains the most nerve endings. As a result, the length of the penis is generally irrelevant to sexual satisfaction. Furthermore, the vagina contracts around an object inserted in it, making the width of the penis also generally irrelevant to sexual satisfaction.

- The uterus consists of three layers: the perimetrium, which is elastic, thereby enabling the uterus to stretch during pregnancy; the myometrium, which is made up of smooth muscle, thereby helping to push the baby through the cervix; and the endometrium, which is loaded with blood vessels, thereby providing the nourishment needed to sustain a developing fetus.

- Hormones control menstruation. Follicle-stimulating hormone (FSH) stimulates the ovary to ripen an ovum, luteinizing hormone (LH) signals the Graafian follicle to release the ripened ovum, estrogens signal the pituitary gland to release LH, and progesterone released by the corpus luteum prepares the uterus for implantation of the fertilized ovum.

- Menstrual problems include dysmenorrhea (painful menstruation), which can be either primary or secondary; amenorrhea (a lack of menstruation); and premenstrual syndrome (menstruation associated with bloating cramping, fatigue, depression, headache, and other symptoms).

- The breast is the leading site of cancer in women, and breast cancer is the second leading cause of cancer deaths among women. Breast care consists of breast self-exams, annual clinical breast exams, and mammograms as recommended. In addition, women should have annual gynecological exams and Pap smears as recommended.

Discussion Questions

1. List and describe the parts of the female reproductive system, including external and internal genitalia.

2. Compare the roles of breasts as child nurturer and sexual organ.

3. Describe how hormones react to sexual stimuli and make a person aroused.

4. Which physiological changes occur in a woman's body during the menstrual cycle? What are the resulting psychological effects?

5. For which diseases of the reproductive system is a woman at risk? How can she prevent these diseases?

6. Describe the self-care and preventive medicine that a woman should practice to ensure her sexual health.

Application Questions

Reread the anecdote that opens the chapter and answer the following questions.

1. How could you use your understanding of the parts of the human body to improve your sexuality? Is such knowledge as important as the ability to communicate or to understand the diverse needs of a partner? Put another way, would an expert on sexuality be a better lover?

2. Describe how you feel when you look at anatomical drawings of genitalia. Do you feel sexually excited? Embarrassed? Bored? Explain why you feel that way.

Critical Thinking Questions

1. Some women argue that only another woman can really understand the feelings and sensations that a woman feels, that male gynecologists are likely to discount some female concerns, and that it is easier to talk with another woman than a man about their sexual health. Others may argue that medical competency and compassion are not limited by gender. Should a gynecologist be a woman? Explain your answer.

2. If you look at the women on TV, in movies, and in magazines, the pervasive image is clear: lean and busty. Yet the psychologist G. Terence Wilson, an eating disorder specialist, points out that a woman cannot be lean and have large breasts—it is not biologically possible. As a woman loses fat, her breasts reduce in size. Should a woman who finds herself lean and flat get breast implants or regain weight so her breasts will be larger? Explain your answer.

Critical Thinking Case

As discussed in the chapter, some researchers believe that onset of menarche occurs on the basis of body composition—namely, when a woman reaches a certain percentage of body fat. It also appears that amenorrhea (cessation of menstruation) occurs in women athletes with low body fat and in women with anorexia nervosa.

Consider the negative connotations associated with body fat in our society, especially as portrayed in the mass media. What reaction might prepubescent girls have to learning that they will gain body fat and then reach menarche? How could middle and high school students be taught in a positive manner about the body composition changes associated with the onset of menarche? Would such knowledge lead young girls to diet to prevent menarche?

One final question: A very athletic person in your dormitory tells you that she has heard about the relationship between body fat and amenorrhea. She tells you that she does strenuous aerobic exercise as a means of what she calls "natural birth control." What would you tell her?

Exploring Personal Dimensions

For Women Only

Taking charge of self-care and prevention greatly increases your chance of achieving sexual health and wellness. If you are a female, for the following statements, circle YES or NO. Then fill in the dates to help you keep track of your self-care activities. Males will have their chance to answer similar questions in Chapter 5.

I do breast self-examinations monthly.   YES   NO
    My last breast exam was on _____.
    My next breast exam is due on _____.

I do vaginal self-examinations on a   YES   NO
regular basis.
    My last vaginal exam was on _____.
    My next vaginal exam is due on _____.

I have regular gynecological   YES   NO
examinations.
    My last gynecological exam was on _____.
    My next gynecological exam is due on _____.

I have regular Pap smears.   YES   NO
    My last Pap smear was on _____.
    My next Pap smear is due on _____.

I have regular mammograms   YES   NO
(if applicable).
    My last mammogram was on _____.
    My next mammogram is due on _____.

I keep track of my menstrual cycle.   YES   NO
    My last period began on _____.
    My next period is due on _____.

I practice safer sexual activities.   YES   NO

I understand that vaginal intercourse   YES   NO
during menstruation increases the risk
of transmitting HIV.

I have a family medical tree listing   YES   NO
diseases.

I discussed my family's medical   YES   NO
history with my doctor.

Suggested Readings

Anatomical Chart Company. *Female reproductive system: Anatomy and pathology chart.* Skokie, IL: Author, 2003.

Carlson, K. J., Eisenstat, S. A., & Ziporyn, T. D. *The new Harvard guide to women's health.* Cambridge, MA: Harvard University Press, 2004.

Gaudet, T., & Spencer, P. *Consciously female: How to listen to your body and your soul for a lifetime of healthier living.* New York: Bantam Books, 2004.

Minkin, M. J., & Wright, C. V. *A woman's guide to sexual health.* New Haven, CT: Yale University Press Health & Wellness, 2004.

Minkin, M. J., & Wright, C. V. *The Yale guide to women's reproductive health: From menarche to menopause.* New Haven, CT: Yale University Press, 2003.

Morris, D. *The naked woman: A study of the female body.* New York: St. Martin's Press, 2007.

Staff of Boston Women's Health Book Collective. *Our bodies, ourselves: A new edition for a new era.* New York: Simon & Schuster, 2005.

World Health Organization. *Mental health aspects of women's reproductive health: A global review of the literature.* Geneva, Switzerland: World Health Organization, 2008.

Web Resources

For links to the web sites below, visit *http://sexuality.jbpub.com/dimensions/4e* and click on Resource Links.

Female Reproductive System
www.training.seer.cancer.gov/anatomy/reproductive/female

Diagram of the female reproductive system with links providing more information. Links include ovaries, genital tract, external genitalia, female sexual response and hormonal control, and mammary glands.

Network for Excellence in Women's Sexual Health
www.einet.net/review/37764-600702/NewShe_Network_for_the_Excellence_of_Women_s_Sexual_Health.htm

Web site in which Drs. Laura Berman and Jennifer Berman provide links to obtain information about sexual dysfunctions, sexual aging, menopausal health, incontinence, gynecology, and other sexual health issues. Articles on timely topics also appear on this web site.

National Woman's Health Network
www.womenshealthnetwork.org

The National Women's Health Network seeks to improve the health of women by developing and promoting a critical analysis of health issues in order to affect policy and support consumer decision making. The Network aspires to a health care system that is guided by social justice and reflects the needs of diverse women. On the web site, women's health information and resources, as well as health alerts, are provided.

National Women's Health Information Center
www.4women.gov

A web site maintained by the U.S. government that provides resources and information about women's health issues. Includes health topics, health organizations, statistics, publications, and other links.

Society for Women's Health Research
www.womenshealthresearch.org

The Society for Women's Health Research is a non-profit organization whose mission is to improve the health of women through research, education, and advocacy. The society encourages the study of sex differences between women and men that affect the prevention, diagnosis, and treatment of disease. The information provided on this site is designed to support, not replace, the relationship that exists between a woman and her doctor.

CHAPTER 5

Male Sexual Anatomy and Physiology

FEATURES

Global Dimensions
Male Genital Mutilation and Circumcision Practices

Ethical Dimensions
What Are a Dead Man's Rights?

Communication Dimensions
Should Physicians Have to Provide Care Regardless of Their Personal Values or Moral Convictions?

Multicultural Dimensions
PSA Cancer Screening

Gender Dimensions
Testicular Self-Examination

CHAPTER OBJECTIVES

1 Name and describe the parts of the male reproductive system to include the external and internal genitalia, including the pathway of the sperm.

2 Discuss the role of hormones in males as they enter puberty.

3 Cite various diseases that can affect the male reproductive system and the self-care procedures, as well as medical treatments, associated with these diseases.

sexuality.jbpub.com/dimensions/4e

Global Dimensions: Male Genital Mutilation and
   Circumcision Practices
Prostate Cancer
Care from Organizations and Available Publications

INTRODUCTION

*A*n economics professor recently told me that a father had come in to talk about his son's mediocre academic performance. The father asked for a second chance for his son, explaining that "too often he thinks with his other head." Of course, this is not the first time I had heard this suggestion that men "think with their penises."

The notion goes back to the fifth century. In the Greek comedy Lysistrata, *the women of the city decide to withhold sex from their men until all wars are ended. The men quickly put their civic pride aside in favor of their women—thinking with their "other heads," no doubt!*

However, today's man may think more about his penis than with it. And the great obsession seems to be size. In the mid-1900s a national sex survey found that men thought the average length of a penis was 14 inches; women thought it was 12 inches. However, the average length is really about 6 inches!

Magazines like Penthouse Forum *do not help, either. Chock-full of large appendages—10 inches here, 8 inches there, a "foot long" here, as "thick as his arm" there—the stories are meant to present fantasy, not reality.*

The writer Susan Minot provides an interesting perspective in her short story "Lust."

> Tim's was shaped like a banana, with a graceful curve to it. They're all different. Willie's like a bunch of walnuts when nothing was happening, another's as thin as a thin hot dog. But it's like faces; you're never really surprised.

As you will read in this chapter, for all the worry that men may feel, it is quite natural for men's penises to vary considerably, just as their faces do.

The Male Reproductive System

As females do, males have both external and internal genital organs. Figure 5.1 depicts a side view of the male external and internal genitalia, and Figure 5.2 shows a view from the rear. We begin our study of the male reproductive system with the external genitals.

The External Genitals

The male external genitals are the penis and the scrotum.

The Penis

The **penis** is a male sexual organ consisting of the root, the shaft, and the glans. As we have mentioned, penis size concerns many students, who often ask about the "average-size penis." As a *general* guideline, the average penis is about 2–5 inches long when relaxed (flaccid) and about 4–7 inches long when erect. When sexually aroused, the penis becomes stiff and enlarged (erect) because its tissues fill with blood. The penis shaft is attached to the body by its root. The head of the penis is called the **glans penis**. The glans contains the urethral opening, or **meatus**, where both seminal

penis
Structure of the male external genitalia consisting of the root, shaft, and glans; also contains the urethra, through which urine is excreted.

fluid (which contains sperm) and urine are passed. Marking the end of the glans is a raised ridge called the **coronal ridge**, or **corona**. The coronal ridge helps to form a seal with the walls of the vagina during sexual intercourse. Below the corona the body, or shaft, of the penis begins. Although the entire penis is sensitive and sexually excitable, the glans and corona are particularly sensitive; in fact, they are the most sensitive parts of the male anatomy.

Historically penis size has been a matter of fascination. The **Kamasutra**, an ancient Indian book on erotica, classified men according to penis size in three categories: hare-men (erect penises of approximately 4.5 inches [11 centimeters]), bull-men (erect penises of approximately 6.75 inches [17 centimeters]), and horse-men (erect penises of approximately 9 inches [23-centimeters]). Other sources correlated penis size with personality traits or with the size of some other part of the body. Penises that are short when **flaccid** gain more size during **erection** than those that are longer when flaccid.

glans penis
The head of the penis.

meatus
The opening of the urethra in the head of the penis, where both seminal fluid and urine are passed.

coronal ridge (corona)
The raised ridge where the glans penis ends and the penile shaft begins.

Kamasutra
Ancient sex manual from India.

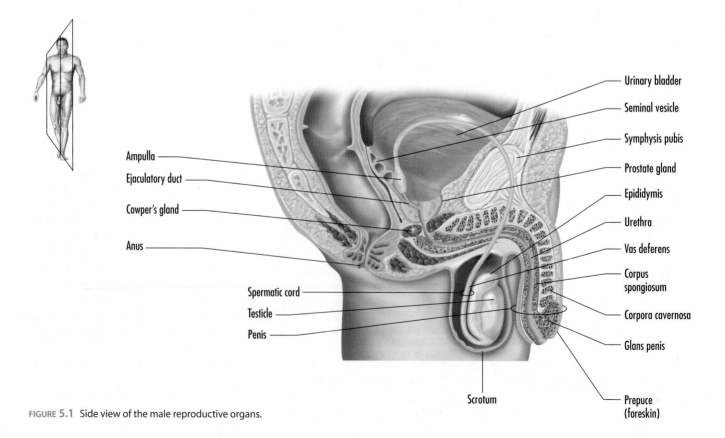

Urinary bladder
Seminal vesicle
Symphysis pubis
Prostate gland
Epididymis
Urethra
Vas deferens
Corpus spongiosum
Corpora cavernosa
Glans penis
Prepuce (foreskin)

Ampulla
Ejaculatory duct
Cowper's gland
Anus
Spermatic cord
Testicle
Penis
Scrotum

FIGURE 5.1 Side view of the male reproductive organs.

FIGURE **5.2** Posterior view of the male reproductive organs.

flaccid
The relaxed, unerect state of the penis.

erection
The extension of the penis and its engorgement with blood when the male is sexually stimulated.

Thus, although flaccid penises may differ significantly in length, erect penises are of similar lengths (Jamison & Gebhard, 1988). One way this has been described is that some men are "showers" and others are "growers" (Haffner & Schwartz, 1998).

Two contradictory views regarding penile size flourish in our time: "The larger the penis, the more satisfied the sexual partner" and "Sexual partners don't care about the size of a man's penis." It is not clear which is nearer the truth. Because the vagina adapts to the penis regardless of its size, some people have argued that size is unrelated to the sexual satisfaction of the female. However, part of our response to another's body is visual, and it seems reasonable to assume that if people have preferences for breasts of certain sizes and shapes, so might they react differently to penises of different shapes and sizes. None of these preferences has anything to do with function unless it causes anxiety. The vagina contracts around the penis, regardless of its width or circumference. Furthermore, the inner two-thirds of the vagina has very little sensitivity. Both of these facts lead most authorities to conclude that penile width or length is unrelated to sexual satisfaction. Some people do, however, report preference for penises of a certain width or length. Whether these preferences are physiological or psychological is unknown at this time.

Just as women can strengthen the pelvic musculature with Kegel exercises, so can men strengthen

Many variations exist in the size and shape of the male genitals.

the muscles surrounding the penis. Because these muscles are usually contracted only during ejaculation, they tend to be weak. By strengthening the muscles surrounding the penis, men may experience more satisfying orgasms and maintain better control of ejaculation. To do male Kegel exercises (National Kidney and Urologic Diseases Information Clearinghouse, 2007):

1. Identify the right muscles by imagining that you are trying to stop yourself from passing gas or urinating. Squeeze the muscles you would use. If you sense a "pulling" feeling, those are the right muscles for pelvic exercises.

2. Do not squeeze other muscles at the same time or hold your breath. Also, be careful not to tighten your stomach, leg, or buttock muscles. Squeezing the wrong muscles can put pressure on your bladder control muscles. Squeeze just the pelvic muscles.

3. Pull in the pelvic muscles and hold for a count of 3. Then relax for a count of 3. Repeat, but do not overdo it. Work up to 3 sets of 10 repeats.

4. Start doing your pelvic muscle exercises lying down. This position is the easiest for doing Kegel exercises because the muscles then do not need to work against gravity. When your muscles get stronger, do the exercises sitting or standing. Working against gravity is like adding more weight.

5. Be patient. Do not give up. It takes just 5 minutes, 3 times a day. Your ejaculatory control may not improve immediately, but most people notice an improvement in approximately 1 month.

Circumcision

The glans penis is covered by a **foreskin** (sometimes called the **prepuce**). For hygienic, cultural, or religious reasons, the foreskin is sometimes surgically removed. Removal of the foreskin—called **circumcision**—is more usual in the United States than in European countries. Circumcision takes place in the hospital approximately 2 days after birth or, if performed according to Jewish custom, 8 days after birth. In addition to Judaism, the Muslim faith requires circumcision. Figure 5.3 shows how circumcision is performed.

> **foreskin (prepuce)**
> The covering of the glans penis, which is removed during circumcision.
>
> **circumcision**
> The surgical removal of the foreskin covering the glans penis.
>
> **smegma**
> A cheeselike substance secreted by the glans penis that must be removed from below the foreskin of uncircumcised males to prevent irritation and/or infection.

Hygiene also provides a rationale for circumcision. Several preputial glands—glands that secrete hormones only after puberty—are located in the foreskin and under the corona (Tyson's glands). These glands secrete an oily substance that, if not removed from under the foreskin, can combine with dead skin cells to form a cheesy substance called **smegma**. If this smegma is not regularly removed from under the foreskin, it becomes granular and irritates the glans penis, causing discomfort and possibly infection. Removing the smegma requires washing the glans penis. This becomes more difficult if the foreskin is not removed, because it has to be retracted manually to expose the glans.

Since 1971, the American Academy of Pediatrics (AAP) has released several statements noting that there is no medical reason for circumcision. As a result, circumcision rates in the United States dropped from a high of 95% of newborn males in

FIGURE **5.3** Methods of performing circumcision. (a) In this method, a piece of plastic is placed over the glans, and the foreskin is stretched over the plastic and trimmed off. (b) In this method, the foreskin is carefully cut "freehand" and then stitched.

(a)

(b)

the mid-1960s to an estimated 58% in 1987 (Rovner, 1990). However, in 1990, the Academy (Brower, 1989) reversed its position, citing advantages based on the work of Dr. Thomas Wiswell and colleagues (1985). Wiswell found that uncircumcised infants were 10 times more likely to have urinary tract infections than circumcised babies. Wiswell also reported that of 50,000 cases of cancer of the penis over a 50-year period, only 10 occurred in circumcised men.

However, not everyone agrees with the AAP's 1990 position. For example, Smith and colleagues (1987) found no difference in rates of urinary infections, and other researchers have reached similar conclusions over the years (Samuels & Samuels, 1983; Wallerstein, 1980). More recently, however, AAP has advised that the benefits of circumcision are not significant enough to recommend it as a routine procedure (American Academy of Pediatrics, 1999). This policy was reaffirmed by the AAP in 2005.

But another argument attempts to justify circumcision: The foreskin interferes with sexual stimulation because it serves as a barrier to the glans penis. There are no data to support this argument and, in fact, logic would indicate otherwise. The foreskin retracts when the penis becomes erect, and the glans penis is, therefore, able to be stimulated just as it is for the circumcised male. Furthermore, some people have argued the opposite: That is, if the glans is not usually protected by a foreskin, it may become insensitive because of its repeated contact with clothing. Therefore, the circumcised penis may, in fact, be *less* sensitive than the uncircumcised penis. Neither viewpoint is conclusive.

Still other reasons have been offered to justify circumcision. For example, uncircumcised males may be at greater risk of penile cancer, and their female sexual partners may be at greater risk of vaginal infections, cervical cancer, genital warts, and other sexually transmitted infections. However, for every study that supports these concerns, there appear to be studies that refute them.

There are more reasons for not being circumcised. First is concern about the trauma the infant experiences. Because infants cannot be administered general anesthesia or pain-relieving narcotic agents, circumcision is often performed without the benefit of anesthesia. To respond to this concern, some physicians inject a local anesthetic directly into the penis in an attempt to diminish or eliminate the pain associated with circumcision. Another issue is the risk of infection, hemorrhage, emotional trauma, and other effects associated with any surgical procedure.

Yet, there is agreement among medical experts that when the foreskin is so tight that an erection hurts or pain is experienced during sexual intercourse, removal of the foreskin is recommended. This condition is known as **phimosis**. As of this writing, the Centers for Disease Control and Prevention and the American Academy of Pediatrics appear ready to change their recommendations regarding circumcision. Both organizations are about to recommend circumcision citing new evidence that the benefits outweigh the risks and disadvantages.

To summarize, here are reasons parents might consider circumcising their son:

phimosis
Condition resulting when penile erection causes pain because the foreskin is too tight.

- They are Jewish or Muslim. Infant circumcision is part of these religious traditions.

- If the father is circumcised, parents might want their son's penis to be like his father's penis.

- Parents do not want to have to teach their sons to clean their foreskins.

- Circumcised men have a lower incidence of urinary tract infections.

- Some uncircumcised men have problems as they grow up, for example, pain during intercourse, requiring circumcision during adulthood. This is much more painful and dangerous than newborn circumcision.

- The rate of cancer of the penis, though extremely rare, is higher in uncircumcised men.

- Uncircumcised men may be more susceptible to sexually transmitted infections.

Here are reasons parents might not want to circumcise their son:

- Circumcision is not part of their cultural tradition.

- Circumcision is painful for infants.

- If the father is not circumcised, parents might want their son's penis to be like his father's penis.

- As with any surgery, circumcision poses some risks. In rare cases (less than two times in 1,000) infection or even damage to the penis occurs.

- They think circumcision is not natural. Boys are born with penises with foreskins; their intact penises should be left alone.

- Circumcision is done without the infant's permission. This should be an adult choice.

- The child is ill at birth. Circumcision should never be done on a sick or medically unstable infant.

The Scrotum
The other external structure of the male reproductive system is the **scrotum**, which is located below

Global DIMENSIONS

Male Genital Mutilation and Circumcision Practices

Around the world and throughout history there have been many societies that have practiced male genital mutilation. For example, castration, the removal of the testes, was common in ancient Rome; eunuchs, castrated men, dressed as women and became priests. Islamic societies are forbidden by the Koran to castrate men. Yet they used men castrated by the Christians as keepers of the harem, because they posed no threat of engaging in sexual activities. In addition, boys were castrated in the Middle Ages in Europe to maintain their soprano singing voices after puberty.

In some societies in the Pacific, men are circumcised, but the foreskin is not totally removed; instead, it is slit lengthwise and folded back. This is called *supercision*. Sometimes the foreskin is stretched tightly over a piece of bamboo, and then the incision is made. Circumcision is often associated with entry into manhood in these cultures and is usually celebrated with a ceremony of some sort.

scrotum (scrotal sac)
A sac of skin that contains the testes and spermatic cords.

testes
Male gonads contained within the scrotal sacs that produce sperm cells and the male sex hormone testosterone. Singular form: testicle.

spermatic cord
The cord from which the testicle is suspended that contains the vas deferens (defined later), blood vessels, nerves, and muscle fibers.

the penis. The scrotum is a sac of skin containing the **testes** and the **spermatic cords**. It comprises two layers: the outer layer, which is covered with hair and sweat glands, and the inner layer (called the *tunica dartos*), which contains muscle and connective tissue. This organ regulates the temperature in the testes by drawing them up toward the body when the body is cold and letting them hang lower, away from the body, when it is hot. As a consequence the temperature of the testes is always approximately 5.6°F (3.1°C) cooler than the internal body temperature. This temperature-control function is necessary for the production of viable sperm. The scrotum also contracts when the inner thigh is stimulated or when it is chilled. This effect, is due to the contraction of the cremasteric muscles located in the spermatic cord, which is known as the *cremasteric reflex.*

The Internal Genitals

The male internal genitals contain numerous organs housed within the penis, the scrotum, and the pelvis (refer again to Figure 5.1).

The Urethra
The **urethra** is a tube through the penis that begins at the bladder and ends at the meatus. Its function is to provide a route for both semen and urine to exit the body. **Urine** is a waste product of the body that is stored in the bladder until it is expelled through the urethra. **Semen**, which is discussed later in this section, contains **spermatozoa**, or **sperm**, as well as other substances.

urethra
The tube through which the bladder empties urine outside the body and through which the male ejaculate exits.

urine
The body-waste product stored in the bladder and eliminated through the urethra.

semen
The male ejaculate, which contains sperm and other secretions.

spermatozoa (sperm)
The mature male sperm cell.

The Corpora Cavernosa and the Corpus Spongiosum
In addition to the urethra, the penis contains three spongy bodies: two **corpora cavernosa** and the **corpus spongiosum**, which are structures filled with networks of blood vessels and nerves. It is these columns of tissue, which

Myth (vs) Fact

Myth: Whereas females can strengthen their pelvic muscles, thereby exercising better control of their sexual response, there is not much males can do.
Fact: Males can strengthen their pelvic muscles also. They can perform Kegel exercises to strengthen the muscles surrounding the penis, thereby achieving more satisfying orgasms and maintaining better control of ejaculation.

Myth: There is no medical reason for males to be circumcised.
Fact: Recommendations regarding circumcision have changed over the years. More recently, it has been suggested that uncircumcised males may be at greater risk of penile cancer and that their female partners may be at greater risk of reproductive health problems. However, circumcision poses the risk of infection, hemorrhage, emotional trauma, and other conditions. Whether to be circumcised is a decision that needs a great deal of consideration.

Myth: Breast cancer affects women; men do not have to worry about contracting it.
Fact: Men can also contract breast cancer. In 2008 approximately 1,990 new cases of breast cancer were diagnosed, and 450 men died of it.

Myth: The ejaculate is made up predominantly of sperm.
Fact: The ejaculate, semen, consists mostly of seminal vesicle and prostate gland secretions. The volume of sperm is approximately the size of a pinhead.

Myth: A male with a small flaccid penis has much to worry about.
Fact: First, small flaccid penises tend to expand more during erection than do large flaccid penises. Second, the nerve endings in the vagina are in the outer third, making the length of the penis somewhat superfluous, at least as far as sexual satisfaction is concerned.

fill with blood during sexual arousal, that make the penis grow hard and erect. During ejaculation the muscle surrounding the corpus spongiosum (the bulbocavernosus muscle) contracts and forces semen outward through the urethra.

The Testes
As mentioned, the testes (Figure 5.4) are suspended in the scrotal sac by spermatic cords, the **vas deferens** (through which sperm leave the testes), blood vessels, nerves, and muscle fibers. The testes produce sperm (about 50,000 every minute) and **testosterone**, a male sex hormone generally responsible for male secondary sexual characteristics

corpora cavernosa
A spongy body in the penis that contains a network of blood vessels and nerves.

corpus spongiosum
A spongy body in the penis that contains a network of blood vessels and nerves.

vas deferens
The duct, through which sperm stored in the epididymis (discussed later) is passed, that is cut or blocked during vasectomy.

testosterone
The male sex hormone produced in the testes that is responsible for the development of male secondary sex characteristics.

Organs

Testicle vertical cross section

Seminiferous tubules horizontal cross section

FIGURE **5.4** Testicle cross section.

seminiferous tubules
The structures located within the testes that actually produce the sperm.

spermatogenesis
The manufacturing of sperm in the seminiferous tubules.

interstitial cells
The cells (sometimes called Leydig's cells) between the seminiferous tubules, where testosterone is produced.

vasa efferentia
The duct through which sperm produced in the seminiferous tubules travel to the epididymis.

epididymis
The location where sperm are stored in the testes and where nutrients are provided to help the sperm develop.

(for example, deep voice, facial hair, and body hair). Within each testicle are approximately 1,000 **seminiferous tubules**, which are responsible for producing sperm, in a process called **spermatogenesis**. The cells between the seminiferous tubules, called **interstitial cells**, produce testosterone.

Once sperm are produced in the seminiferous tubules, they travel through the **vasa efferentia** to the **epididymis**, where they are stored and nourished for up to 6 weeks.

The Pathway of the Sperm

A mature sperm is about 0.0024 inch (0.0060 centimeter) long, with a head, neck, midpiece, and tail. The normal sperm contains 23 chromosomes. Each sperm contains a sex chromosome that determines the sex of the

ampulla
The enlarged portion of the vas deferens where sperm are provided nutrients from the seminal vesicles; also, the part of the fallopian tube of women containing the cilia.

seminal vesicles
Two sacs of the male internal genitalia that secrete nutrients to nourish sperm.

motility
The ability to move spontaneously, which is required for fertilization.

offspring. Sperm can be stored for up to 6 weeks in the epididymis before proceeding up the vas deferens to the **ampulla** (an enlarged portion of the vas deferens). Here in the ampulla the sperm receive more nutrients from the **seminal vesicles**, two sacs, each about 2 inches (5 centimeters) long, that secrete a substance believed to activate the sperm's **motility** (ability to move spontaneously).

 Did You Know . . .

1. Testosterone causes bones to thicken and for this reason is sometimes administered to elderly people who have osteoporosis.

2. Excessive concentrations of sex hormones are metabolized primarily in the liver, with the products excreted in the bile and urine. Consequently, people with liver disorders experience the effects of excessive sex hormones (for example, the development of excessive body hair, development of breasts, or aggressiveness).

3. Sex hormones stimulate growth, thereby explaining the rapid growth that occurs during puberty. However, they also stimulate ossification (hardening) of the epiphyseal disks (a band of cartilage at the end of the bone), which causes bones to stop growing. Because estrogens produce greater effects on the disks than androgens, females stop growing earlier than males.

With sufficient sexual stimulation, the ejaculatory process begins. Fluid from the **prostate gland** mixes with the sperm and with the secretions of the seminal vesicles, further aiding sperm motility and prolonging sperm life. The prostate fluid is an alkaline medium that offsets the acidity in the vagina that would otherwise kill the sperm. The **Cowper's glands**, two pea-sized glands adjacent to the urethra, empty into the urethra another alkaline fluid, which serves to neutralize the acidity caused by the urethra's transport of urine. The Cowper's glands secretions are the tiny droplets that sometimes appear on the tip of the penis before ejaculation. This secretion may contain some sperm left over from a previous ejaculation; therefore, it can cause pregnancy to occur even if the penis is withdrawn before ejaculation.

Ejaculation itself is the expulsion through the penis of semen, the mixture in which the sperm are carried. Ejaculation results from muscular contractions of the glands and ducts of the reproductive system. The expelling of semen is usually accompanied by **orgasm**, the climax of a growing complex of pleasurable sensations. Both the ampulla and seminal vesicles contract, as does the bulbocavernosus mus-

cle surrounding the corpus spongiosum in the penis. The ejaculated semen contains sperm (the volume is about the size of a pinhead) and about a teaspoonful of secretions from the seminal vesicles, the prostate gland, and the Cowper's glands. Approximately 300 million sperm are expelled in a single ejaculation. According to some authorities, semen contain at least 20 to 35 million sperm per cubic centimeter in a male who is fertile—that is, able to fertilize an ovum.

During ejaculation a valve at the bladder's entrance closes to prevent urine from entering the urethra.

Table 5.1 reviews the functions of the male reproductive system.

Hormones

At some time during puberty, boys become capable of reproduction. This capability is accompanied by the ability to ejaculate, although initially the male's ejaculate does not contain mature sperm. The cause of male reproductive capacity is the increased secretion of androgens, followed by the development of secondary sex characteristics. Accompanying male reproductive capacity, and also a result of increased androgen production, is a heightened interest in sex. This can be considered double jeopardy, because an increase in sexual appetite in a person newly capable of fertilizing an ovum can create problems—such as unplanned pregnancy or frustrated **libido**. The majority of both males and females seem to adjust to this new condition and pass through this

> **prostate gland**
> A structure of the male internal genitalia that secretes a fluid into the semen before ejaculation to aid sperm motility and prolong sperm life.
>
> **Cowper's glands**
> Two pea-sized glands adjacent to the urethra that secrete a lubricating fluid before ejaculation.
>
> **ejaculation**
> The ejection of semen from the penis during orgasm.
>
> **orgasm**
> The peak release of sexual tension, accompanied by sensory pleasure and involuntary rhythmic muscular contractions; ejaculation in the male.

> **libido**
> Sexual desire, or drive.

TABLE 5.1	Functions of the Organs of the Male Reproductive System
Organ	**Function**
Testes	
Seminiferous tubules	Produce spermatozoa
Interstitial cells	Produce and secrete male sex hormones
Epididymis	Stores and allows maturation of spermatozoa; conveys spermatozoa to vas deferens
Vas deferens	Conveys spermatozoa to ejaculatory ducts
Ejaculatory ducts	Receive spermatozoa and additives to produce seminal fluid
Seminal vesicles	Secrete alkaline fluid containing nutrients and prostaglandins
Prostate gland	Secretes alkaline fluid that helps neutralize acidic seminal fluid and enhances motility of spermatozoa
Cowper's gland	Secretes fluid that lubricates urethra and end of penis
Scrotum	Encloses and protects testes
Penis	Conveys urine and seminal fluid outside the body; acts as the organ of copulation

Ethical DIMENSIONS

What Are a Dead Man's Rights? The Center for Bioethics at the University of Pennsylvania documented 25 cases in which sperm were taken from dead men and preserved by deep-freezing. Furthermore, a survey of 273 fertility centers in the United States identified 82 requests for taking sperm from dead men, of which 25 had been honored. It is possible to remove sperm up to 24 hours after death, and the person most often making the request is the widow. However, there also are records of social workers and even an intensive care nurse who made such a request.

Who has a right, if anyone at all does, to have such a request honored? Only the spouse, or a parent as well?

Should men have the right to decide whether they will have children and with whom, even after they are dead?

Should sperm taken from dead men be used by women unrelated to them, whose husbands do not produce viable sperm? Who else should have access to this sperm?

Should the sperm be sold and the proceeds go to the man's family? What should be done with the frozen sperm if the dead man's family decides not to use them?

These are tough decisions that should be guided by ethical principles, which you will study in Chapter 18.

---

phase of life unscarred. Unfortunately some do not, as evidenced by the high rate of pregnancy in unmarried teenage girls.

During puberty, increased testosterone level leads to growth of the penis, prostate, seminal vesicles, and epididymis. The reason males cannot ejaculate before puberty is that the prostate and seminal vesicles are not functional until they are "turned on" by the increased level of testosterone. Late-developing boys (15 to 16 years old) have been found to experience less sexual activity during adolescence than do early developers (Kinsey, Pomeroy, & Martin, 1948; Masters, Johnson, & Kolodny, 1982, 169). This difference has been attributed to the effect of testosterone on increasing the sexual appetite in males. No long-lasting effect on sexual behavior has been reported, however.

Hormone Therapy

Hormone therapy is sometimes administered to men. For instance, testosterone supplements are sometimes administered to treat erectile dysfunction in older men (although testosterone levels are not low in all men who have trouble maintaining erection). Sometimes this treatment for erectile dysfunction is effective; other times it is not. The reason for this inconsistency is unclear; however, it is safe to say that the complex nature of sexuality makes it only partially responsive to hormone treatment. Testosterone supplements may not have much effect when personality, past experiences, the sexual partner, effectiveness in communication, setting, and so on, continue to have negative effects.

■ Self-Care and Prevention

Male reproductive care is as specialized as female reproductive care. Men should learn proper hygiene and methods of monitoring their reproductive health. When problems arise, males should consult their own medical specialists (internists or urologists). As with females, there are many organizations and publications that focus exclusively on issues of male reproductive health.

 Did You Know . . .

Androstenedione is the supplement that Mark McGwire made famous during his 70-home-run season. Touted as an artificial steroid, it was said to raise testosterone levels. But researchers at the University of Iowa found that it did not raise testosterone levels or increase strength. A side effect was lower levels of "good" cholesterol (high-density lipoproteins),

raising the risk of heart disease. Preliminary results of a further study by the Harvard researcher Hoel Finkelstein for Major League Baseball showed that androstenedione raised estrogen levels in men—and could result in breast enlargement!

Source: Body-building aid questioned, *CBSNews@aol.com* (June 3, 1999).

Communication
DIMENSIONS

Should Physicians Have to Provide Care Regardless of Their Personal Values or Moral Convictions?

One month before George W. Bush's presidency was to end, he finalized a regulation allowing health professionals to refuse to provide any medical service they objected to on moral grounds (Meckler, 2008). This "right of conscience" regulation was interpreted to mean that abortion, family planning, providing prescriptions for emergency contraception (the "morning after pill"), giving certain information or advice, or any other service the medical provider deemed immoral—even referrals for such services—could be withheld from the patient.

Those favoring such a regulation argue that no one—not even a health professional—should be required to behave in a manner that the person considers immoral. Furthermore, if the patient is denied a medical service, there will always be other medical staff willing to provide the desired service. Lastly, medical providers should not face the threat of being fired or losing a promotion because they refuse to do something they believe to be against their religious or moral beliefs.

Those opposed to the "right of conscience" regulation believe that because medical providers are licensed by the state, they are obligated to serve the medical needs of *all* citizens of that state. They also argue that the rule sacrifices the patient's health to the religious belief of the providers (Savage, 2008). Furthermore, not providing a medical service requested by a patient, and not referring the patient to another health care provider from whom those services could be obtained, is doing harm to the patient and, therefore, is itself immoral and unethical.

Would you support a "right of conscience" regulation or would you advise President Obama to overturn it? What reasoning would you use when making this decision?

Breast Cancer in Men

Cancer of the breast occurs in men as well as women, although it is considered rare. An estimated 1,990 new cases of male breast cancer were diagnosed in 2008, and 450 men died of it that same year (American Cancer Society, 2008a). Breast cancer is seen in men as early as their 30s. Although this cancer is rare, men are wise to examine their breasts for lumps. The procedure is the same for men and women (see Chapter 4).

It appears that several factors are related to the development of breast cancer in men. Among these are obesity, a lack of regular physical activity, and tobacco use (Brinton et al., 2008). Also, African American males have a higher incidence of breast cancer than do white males (Nahleh et al., 2007). In addition, as with women, breast cancer is more prevalent in men who carry the BRCA1 and BRCA2 genetic mutations (Tai et al., 2007). Another cause of concern is that male breast cancer is associated with a higher incidence of prostate cancer, suggesting careful screening for prostate cancer should be performed in men with breast cancer (Lee & Jones, 2008). In one large-scale study (Nahleh et al., 2007), male breast cancer patients survived an average of 7 years as compared to 9.8 years for female breast cancer patients. However, males in this study were diagnosed with breast cancer at a more advanced stage and with more lymph node involvement compared to the female patients. Furthermore, the male patients were diagnosed at a mean age of 67 years, whereas the female patients were diagnosed at a mean age of 57 years.

Treatment for male breast cancer is similar to that of female breast cancer with one major difference: The psychological and emotional consequences of breast removal are not as significant for males as for females. Consequently, men seldom need counseling or a cosmetic means of disguising breast-tissue removal.

The Prostate

An important self-care procedure involves the prostate gland. The symptoms of **prostatitis** (inflammation of the prostate) are pain in the lower back, pain in defecation, pain during a rectal exam, and pus in the urine. Prostatitis usually affects younger men and can be cured with antibiotic drugs. If you experience these symptoms, consult a physician.

prostatitis
Infection of the prostate gland.

An estimated 186,320 new cases of prostate cancer were diagnosed in the United States in 2008, and an estimated 28,660 men died of it that same year. Prostate cancer is the second leading cause of cancer deaths in men in the United States (lung cancer is the first). Between 1989 and 1992,

During a rectal digital exam, the physician feels for the size and texture of the prostate gland in an attempt to discover any abnormalities that need follow-up evaluation.

prostate cancer rates increased dramatically, probably because of the use of a blood test developed to identify an antigen produced when prostate cancer is present. The blood test measures the presence of prostate-specific antigen (PSA). Since 1993, prostate cancer incidence rates have declined. It should be pointed out that prostate cancer incidence rates are one and one half times as high for African American men as they are for white men. The reason for this difference is not known, but some experts have conjectured that diets high in fat and/or the presence of a gene that may make the prostate more susceptible to the effects of testosterone may be the cause.

There are several factors that place a man at risk of development of prostate cancer. One of these is age. As a man gets older he becomes more suscep-

tible to prostate cancer, although the cancer may have been present at a younger age but not fully developed. More than 70% of prostate cancers are diagnosed in men who are older than 65 years of age. Heredity is suspected of playing a role in perhaps 5% to 10% of cases.

Signs and symptoms include weak or interrupted urine flow; the need to urinate frequently, especially at night; blood in the urine; pain or burning when urinating; and persistent pain in the lower back, pelvis, or upper thighs. However, some of these symptoms may be caused by an enlargement of the prostate, which is common as men age, without the presence of a tumor. This condition is called *benign prostatic hyperplasia (BPH)* and can be treated with medications. The only way to distinguish BPH from prostate cancer is by a medical examination that includes a

Multicultural DIMENSIONS

PSA Cancer Screening

There is disagreement among health care specialists about the advisability of men obtaining PSA screening for prostate cancer. The U.S. Preventive Services Task Force is hesitant to recommend PSA screening for most young men and, in particular, recommends against screening for men 75 years of age or older. By comparison, the American Cancer Society recommends annual screening for men 50 years of age and older. To further complicate matters, the American Medical Association and several other respected medical organizations suggest that clinicians discuss the potential benefits and known harms of PSA screening with their patients, and consider their patients' preferences rather than routinely ordering PSA screenings.

One ethical principle guiding this kind of decision making is *paternalism* (see Chapter 18). Medical care providers who are advocates of paternalism argue that they are experts in health and, therefore, know more than their patients. It follows, then, that they can make a more in-

formed and appropriate medical decision than can their patients. As a result, they are reluctant to discuss the pros and cons of screening *with* their patients and more comfortable making these decisions *for* their patients. This feeling of paternalism becomes even more pronounced when patients are minorities, or poorly educated. Given that some studies have found African American males are less knowledgeable about prostate cancer screening than white males (Chan et al., 2003; Barber et al., 1998), in spite of their higher incidence and mortality rates, the paternalism argument takes on added validity for some health care providers.

It seems to your authors that all men deserve to be informed about medical procedures available to them. After all, it is the patient—not the health care provider—who has to live with the outcomes of these procedures. If there is potential harm associated with PSA screening, we believe the patient should know that before consenting to the procedure.

---

digital rectal examination (DRE)
A rectal examination whereby a physician inserts a finger into the rectum of a male patient to check for any abnormalities of the prostate.

digital rectal examination (DRE), PSA blood test, and biopsy of the prostate. On June 12, 1997, the American Cancer Society published updated guidelines for prostate cancer screening (American Cancer Society, 1997). The guidelines state, "Both prostate specific antigen (PSA) and digital rectal examination (DRE) should be offered annually, beginning at age 50 years, to men who have a life expectancy of at least 10 years. Men at high risk (African American men and men with a family history of one or more first-degree relatives diagnosed with prostate cancer at an early age) should begin treatment at age 45." The reason a 10-year life expectancy is cited is that prostate cancer is usually a slow-growing cancer; thus it is thought prudent for men to refrain from having treatment if they are not expected to live long enough to benefit from that treatment. These men would likely die of some other condition before the prostate cancer killed them. An abnormal PSA test result is one with a value above 4 ng/mL (some suggest above 2 ng/mL), which would then lead to follow-up evaluation and subsequent

procedures. These may include a biopsy of tissue extracted from the prostate gland.

In 2008, the U.S. Preventive Services Task Force, which evaluates medical screenings and makes recommendations regarding those screenings, published new guidelines for the use of the PSA test. It stated that men age 75 years of age and older should not be screened for PSA because the length of time one would die of prostate cancer is greater than 10 years, and a 75-year-old man's average life expectancy is only 10 years. Therefore, older men should not be subjected to the test, as it could lead to other medical procedures. For men younger than 75 years, the Task Force states, "Current evidence is insufficient to assess the balance of benefits and harms of screening." The harms referred to relate to unnecessary medical screenings. The reasoning behind these recommendations pertains to the lack of evidence of the validity of PSA screening when a cutoff score of 4.0 ng/mL is used, as was standard practice. To respond to the lack of sensitivity of the screening at a score of 4.0 ng/mL, lowering the score to 2.5 ng/mL has been increasingly used. However, lowering the score leads to more false positives and, therefore, subjects men to more unnecessary biopsies and other medical procedures. Furthermore, two recent large-scale, long-term studies have concluded that PSA screening does not affect the prostate cancer death rate (Andriole et al., 2009; Schroder et al., 2009). The researchers found that the rate of death from prostate cancer was very low and did not differ significantly between the group of men who were screened and the group of men who were not.

Recognizing the controversy and lack of clear guidance, most major medical organizations recommend that clinicians discuss the potential benefits and known harms of PSA screening with their patients, and consider their patients' preferences rather than routinely ordering PSA screening. Among these organizations are the American Academy of Family Physicians, American College of Physicians, American College of Preventive Medicine, and American Medical Association. In contrast, the American Urological Association and the American Cancer Society recommend digital rectal examinations and PSA screening to men annually beginning at age 50 years.

If cancer is suspected, treatment consists of surgery, radiation, and/or hormonal therapy and chemotherapy if the cancer is in a late stage. However, because there is significant potential for serious side effects of these treatments (such as erectile dysfunction and/or incontinence), if the cancer is classified as low-grade and/or at an early stage, careful observation over a period without immediate treatment (called "watchful waiting") may be advised.

Eighty-five percent of all prostate cancers are diagnosed while still localized, and these patients have a 100% 5-year survival rate. During the past 20 years, the 5-year survival rate for all prostate cancers increased from 67% to 97%. Seventy-nine percent of men with prostate cancer survive 10 years, and 57% survive 15 years.

The Testes

Testicular cancer is the most common form of cancer in men during late adolescence and early adulthood. Most cases occur in men aged 15 to 40 years. It is estimated that about 8,090 new cases of testicular cancer were diagnosed in 2008 and that 380

Sexual health begins with routine self-exams.

men died of testicular cancer that year (American Cancer Society, 2008a). The testicular cancer risk is four times greater

> **testicular cancer**
> Cancer of the testicles; the most common form of cancer in men aged 29 to 35 years.

for white men than it is for African American men. The rate has doubled among white Americans in the past 40 years and has remained the same for African Americans.

Among the risk factors for testicular cancer are undescended testes (cryptorchidism). Approximately 14% of cases of testicular cancer occur in men with a history of cryptorchidism. Other risk factors include a family history of testicular cancer, certain occupations (miners, oil and gas workers, leather workers, food and beverage processing workers, janitors, and utility workers), cancer of the other testicle, and infection with HIV. Testicular cancer is not related to injury or to vasectomy.

Treatment consists of surgery, radiation therapy, and/or chemotherapy. Surgery involves removal of the testicle. A cut is made in the groin, and the spermatic cord and the testicle are withdrawn from the scrotum through the opening. This procedure is called a *radical inguinal orchiectomy*. Depending on the stage of

Gender
DIMENSIONS

Testicular Self-Examination

To examine your testicles, first take a hot shower or bath so that the testicles hang farther outside the body than usual. Check each testicle in turn, rolling it gently between the thumb and the index and middle fingers to search for any small, hard lumps or swelling (testicular lumps are usually painless). The scrotal skin should feel firm but not too hard (somewhat like an earlobe). Call any lumps, swelling, hardness, or other unusual features to a physician's attention.

the cancer, some lymph nodes may also be removed. With only one testicle removed, the patient remains fertile. However, if two testicles need to be removed, the patient will no longer be able to produce sperm. Another side effect of the surgery is the possibility of damage to the nerves that control ejaculation. Damage to these nerves may also cause infertility. Men who still wish to have biological children can store sperm in a sperm bank for use after the surgery.

Treatment is highly effective if the cancer is diagnosed early. Seven-time Tour de France winner, bicyclist Lance Armstrong, is a good example. He even won the Tour de France several times after being treated for testicular cancer. Ninety-five percent of stage 1 cancers can be cured, 90% to 95% of stage 2 cancers can be cured, and approximately 70% of stage 3 cancers can be cured. The lower the stage number, the earlier the cancer was diagnosed.

Self-examination of the testicles can lead to early detection of problems (see the accompanying Gender Dimensions feature). Any lumps, masses, or thickened areas may be symptoms of abnormality, not always cancerous; however, because the statistics show high incidence of malignancy of testicular tumors, medical diagnosis and consultation are imperative. As with other forms of cancer, early diagnosis increases your chance of survival.

The Penis

Penile discharges of pus, painful urination, itching, or sores or warts on the genitals may indicate the presence of a sexually transmitted infection. Also, as suggested earlier in this chapter, men should make sure that smegma is washed away daily to prevent irritation or infection in themselves and their partners. For circumcised males, keeping the penis smegma-free is easy, involving rolling only a little of the remaining foreskin out of the way during normal showering. Uncircumcised men have to be more careful, pulling back the foreskin and washing the glans and the inside of the foreskin.

Bicycle Riding and Sexual Health

The area between the penis and the anus is called the perineum; it is where the perineal nerve is located. Researchers have found that the perineal nerve is compressed during bicycle riding of three hours per week or longer and that blood flow to the area can be impaired as a result (Huang, Munarriz, & Goldstein, 2005). That can lead to numbness in the penis and perineum and is associated with the onset of erectile dysfunction (Marceau et al., 2001). Erectile dysfunction—the inability to achieve penile erection—is discussed in detail in Chapter 16.

The possibility that this problem might occur does not mean, however, that men should not ride bicycles for protracted periods of time. A minor adjustment in the bicycle saddle can prevent this condition. The bicycle saddle should be changed from the traditional one with a protruding nose to no-nose saddle (Lowe, Schrader, & Breitenstein, 2004). In a study of bicycle police officers, who spend a considerable amount of time riding their bicycles, a no-nose saddle was found to reduce perineum pressure and decrease symptoms (Schrader, Breitenstein, & Lowe, 2008).

Care from Organizations and Available Publications

Several organizations aid men in caring for their reproductive health: The American Cancer Society publishes brochures and pamphlets describing self-examinations of the breasts and testicles; local health departments operate clinics providing medical examinations, testing, and care for STIs, premarital blood tests, and counseling about birth control and sexual problems. Other organizations, such as the National Cancer Institute, keep track of the incidence and frequency of diseases related to reproductive health. And still other organizations, such as the Health Research Group, a nonprofit group devoted to studies to improve health care, conduct research to prevent and treat various conditions affecting the male reproductive system.

Exploring the
DIMENSIONS
of Human Sexuality

Our feelings, attitudes, and beliefs regarding sexuality are influenced by our internal and external environments. Go to sexuality.jbpub.com/dimensions/4e to learn more about the biological, psychological, and sociological factors that affect your sexuality.

Biological Factors

When a sperm with a Y chromosome meets an egg, a male offspring will develop. Biological factors continue to influence development throughout life.

- Genetic coding affects physical appearance, including height; coloration of skin, hair, and eyes; muscularity; and many aspects of health.
- Physiological changes result at puberty from the hormone testosterone, which in turn affects muscle development and body size. Testosterone also increases aggression and leads to increased rates of heart attacks.
- Toward middle age, testosterone levels begin to drop, resulting in decreased muscle mass, increased fat, and a reduced sex drive.

Sociocultural Factors

Sociocultural factors interact with biological factors to influence health.

- Laws affect what conditions health insurers must cover. Several states in 1998 passed laws requiring Viagra to be covered as a prescription.
- Religion may affect the decision as to whether to circumcise the penis.
- The cultural bias allowing men to be sexually permissive can compromise a man's sexual health and wellness.
- Ethnic heritage influences health; for example, African American males tend to have higher levels of stress and heart disease than white males.
- Media and ads portray the ideal man with extreme muscularity, achievable only with tremendous work and, in many cases, illegal steroids.
- Family, neighbors, and friends often reinforce gender stereotypes.
- Behavior proscribed by society as illegal can influence health; for instance, a man can compromise his health by using anabolic steroids.

Psychological Factors

Biological and sociocultural factors combine to influence psychological factors.

- Body image and self-concept are enhanced for many men through exercise and competitive sports.
- In men who suppress their emotions, increased levels of stress can result.
- Learned attitudes and behaviors about gender roles can lead to unhealthy lifestyles for men.

CASE STUDY

The physiological development of a male starts when a sperm with a Y chromosome fertilizes an egg. More male than female pregnancies occur, but because male fetuses are weaker, a greater number of miscarriages result. Also, more male infants die than do female infants.

Socioeconomic status of the mother determines whether prenatal care is received, appropriate prenatal and postnatal nutrition is available, and medical help is sought. If the mother smokes, drinks, or abuses drugs during pregnancy, the fetus can be adversely affected.

A man's physiology is altered during puberty. The increased testosterone levels result in greater muscularity and a slimmer body. But testosterone also causes increased aggression.

Male gender roles are often hard for many men to uphold and can result in unhealthy behaviors. Repression of emotions also results in increased stress.

Summary

- The male external genitals consist of the penis and the scrotum. The penis contains the urethra, through which urine and the ejaculate is omitted; the scrotum houses the testes.

- Surgical removal of the foreskin (prepuce) is called circumcision. Over the years there have been differing views on the necessity for circumcision. In some cultures and religions, circumcision is recommended and, therefore, frequently performed.

- The male internal genitals contain numerous structures. The urethra is the tube through which the ejaculate is ejected. The corpora cavernosa and corpus spongiosum fill with blood during sexual arousal, resulting in erection of the penis. Sperm are produced in the seminiferous tubules in the testes, stored in the epididymus, and travel out of the testes through the vasa efferentia.

- The ejaculate consists of secretions from the prostate gland, the seminal vesicles, and sperm. It travels through the vas deferens to the urethra, where it is eventually ejected through the meatus of the penis.

- During puberty, boys become capable of reproduction. This is a result of increased secretion of androgens, followed by the development of secondary sex characteristics. Males are not capable of reproduction before puberty because the prostate and seminal vesicles are not functional until they are activated by the increased production of testosterone that occurs during puberty.

- Males are susceptible to a variety of reproductive system illnesses and conditions. Among these are breast cancer, inflammation of the prostate (prostatitis), enlargement of the prostate (benign prostatic hyperplasia), and prostate cancer.

- Males should regularly care for their reproductive systems. These measures include screenings as appropriate, medical examinations by health care providers, testicular self-exams, and behaviors to prevent illnesses and diseases (for example, eating a nutritional diet, maintaining the recommended weight, exercising regularly, and adjusting the bicycle seat if one is a bicycle rider).

Discussion Questions

1. Name and describe the parts of the male reproductive system, including external and internal genitalia.

2. Explain how the increase and decrease of testosterone level affect the male reproductive system, including physiological and psychological effects.

3. Describe the self-care and preventive practices that a man should use to ensure his sexual health.

Application Questions

Reread the story that opens the chapter and answer the following questions.

1. The phrase "Most men think with their penis" clearly derives from the belief that hormones (physiology) control the man, and not vice versa. Do you believe this is correct? Or do sociocultural and psychological factors help balance a man's thinking?

2. The notion of penis size has generally been shown in research to be of little importance to women. Why does size continue to be a matter of jokes and of apprehension among men?

3. Can the male concern with penis size be compared to a woman's concern about her breast size? (After all, more than 100,000 women have breast enhancements each year.) If men could get relatively safe penis-enlargement surgery, do you believe that many would?

Critical Thinking Questions

1. In many schools throughout the country, sexuality education classes mention the concept of menstruation in a mixed-gender goup. But the real discussion of menstruation occurs only in the follow-up "girls only" groupings. Consider whether boys should be taught about menstruation. Without factual knowledge, how can boys comprehend the physical and emotional issues surrounding menstruation? How can they be prepared for safer sexual practices during menstruation if they have not learned about it? Finally, how would you explain menstruation to a group of fifth-grade boys?

Critical Thinking Case

Dad has not been feeling like himself lately. He is unusually tense and easy to upset. It may be due to his lack of sleep. He goes to bed at the same time he always has, but he wakes up often in the middle of the night to urinate. When you ask him about it, he says that he really does not excrete a great deal of urine, just enough to relieve the feeling of having to urinate. As you try to help Dad, answer the following questions.

1. What are some possible causes of Dad's waking up often in the middle of the night to urinate?

2. What would you suggest Dad do about his dilemma? How could you help facilitate his taking this action?

3. What other reproductive system health issues would you expect Dad to encounter as he gets older? What can he do to prevent or postpone the occurrence of these conditions? What can he do to respond to them as they arise?

Exploring Personal Dimensions

For Men Only

Taking charge of self-care and prevention greatly increases your chances of achieving sexual health and wellness. For the following statements, circle YES or NO. Then fill in the dates to help you keep track of your self-care activities.

I do testicular self-examinations   YES   NO
monthly.
    I did my last testicular exam on _____.
    My next testicular exam is due on _____.

I have regular physician's examinations.   YES   NO
    My last physician's exam was on _____.
    My next physician's exam is due on _____.
    My physician perfoms a digital   YES   NO
    rectal exam.

I practice safer sexual activities.   YES   NO

I have a family medical tree listing   YES   NO
diseases.

I discussed my family's medical history   YES   NO
with my doctor.

Suggested Readings

Bostwick, D. G., Crawford, E. D., Roach III, M., & Higano, C. (eds.). *American Cancer Society's complete guide to prostate cancer.* Atlanta, GA: American Cancer Society, 2004.

Bubley, G. J., & Conkling, W. *What your doctor may not tell you about prostate cancer: The breakthrough information and treatments that can help save your life.* New York: Warner Books, 2005.

Fisch, H., & Braun, S. *The male biological clock: The startling news about aging, sexuality, and fertility in men.* New York: Free Press, 2004.

Gilbaugh, J. H. *Men's private parts: A pocket reference to prostate, urologic and sexual health.* New York: Simon & Schuster, 2002.

Madaras, L., Sullivan, S. (illustrator), & Madaras, A. *What's happening to my body? A growing-up guide for parents and sons.* New York: Newmarket Press, 2001.

Peate, I. *Men's sexual health.* Chichester, UK: Whurr Publishers, 2003.

Scardino, P. T., & Kelman, J. *Dr. Peter Scardino's prostate book: The complete guide to overcoming prostate cancer, prostatitis, and BPH.* North Stratford, NH: Avery Publishing Group, 2005.

Spark, R. F. *Sexual health for men: The complete guide.* New York: Perseus Publishing, 2000.

Taguchi, Y., & Weisbord, M. (ed.). *Private parts: An owner's guide to the male anatomy.* Toronto, Canada: McClelland & Stewart/Tundra Books, 2003.

Web Resources

For links to the web sites below, visit *http://sexuality.jbpub.com/dimensions/4e* and click on Resource Links.

Male Reproductive System
www.training.seer.cancer.gov/anatomy/reproductive/male

Diagram of the male reproductive system with links providing more information. Links include testes, duct system, accessory glands, penis, and male sexual response and hormonal control.

National Cancer Institute
www.cancer.gov

A federal government web site providing information about cancer, including prostate and testicular cancers. Includes links to cancer topics, clinical trials, cancer statistics, research and funding, and current news pertaining to cancer.

American Cancer Society
www.cancer.org

A resource for all matters pertaining to cancer, including prostate and testicular cancers. Includes links to types of cancers, making informed treatment decisions, statistics, resources, and recent news.

The Male Health Center
www.malehealthcenter.com

An Internet education site providing information about male health. Included is information about sexual dysfunction, male sexual health problems, sexually transmitted infections, sexual hormones, and sexual aging issues.

Men's Health Network
www.menshealthnetwork.org

Men's Health Network (MHN) is a nonprofit educational organization comprised of physicians, researchers, public health workers, individuals, and other health professionals. MHN is committed to improving the health and wellness of men through education campaigns, partnerships with retailers and other private entities, workplace health programs, data collection, and work with health care providers to provide better programs and funding for men's health needs.

CHAPTER 6

Sexual Response and Arousal

CHAPTER OBJECTIVES

1 Describe the role of the brain in sexual response, including the hormones involved and the role they play.

2 Describe the four phases of the Masters and Johnson sexual response cycle, as well as other theoretical models of sexual response.

3 Describe the physiology of orgasm in both males and females, differentiating between the different types of orgasm.

sexuality.jbpub.com/dimensions/4e

The Brain and Sexual Response
Aphrodisiacs
The Masters and Johnson Sexual Response Cycle

INTRODUCTION

*B*rian was sitting in his social studies class paying more attention
to the attractive Tanya than to the teacher's lecture. Since he had
entered high school he found himself more and more interested
in girls, whose presence distracted him from his school work at times
that were inappropriate. It was during one of these times that his social
studies teacher asked Brian to identify a particular geographical region on
the map in the front of the room. This was a problem for two reasons,
both related to Tanya. First, Brian had no idea where that geographical
region was, and, second, Brian's infatuation with Tanya and the accompanying fantasies resulted in Brian's having an erection. Now, erections
are not something that high school students, or anyone else for that matter, choose to display before peers, so understandably Brian was embarrassed. What was he to do?

This has happened to many high school males, who somehow manage to use textbooks to shield their erections or find some excuse to
delay walking to the front of the room until "it is safer." Some high
school girls and older females also experience sexual excitement that
results in an erection, in this case of the clitoris. Yet, they are not as
vulnerable as males to being exposed because clitoral erection is not evident through women's clothes. Women also experience vaginal lubrication when sexually excited, but this too is not readily identifiable when
one is dressed.

If this reaction has happened to you, perhaps you wondered whether
you are "normal"—you are. Perhaps you discussed this concern with your
close friends. Most of us probably did not discuss it with our parents.
That would have been too embarrassing. Maybe you read about these
reactions in a magazine or saw them depicted in a movie. Unfortunately,

too many young people rely on these sources for information about sex— and magazines and movies often relay misconceptions and misinformation. But how were you to know that? Where else could you go? Whom else could you speak with?

This chapter provides the information you may have wondered about since that time when your body first responded sexually. Included is a description of the typical human sexual response and the means of eliciting that response. Our goal is to help you establish and maintain a satisfying and effective sexual relationship when you decide you are ready for one. We begin with the study of the usual human sexual response.

■ Sexual Arousal and Response

When unaroused, the penis is flaccid; the skin of the scrotal sac is wrinkled, thin, and loose; and the testes hang down from the body. In females, the labia are thin and enclose the vestibule, the clitoris extends from under the clitoral hood, the inner part of the vagina remains elongated, and the nipples of the breast are not erect.

After sexual excitement diminishes, these structures return to their prearoused state. This takes some time, which varies from person to person.

Sexual pleasure and satisfaction are both psychologically and physiologically based. Without the subjective feeling of pleasure, physiological arousal will not occur. For example, if you dislike the body odor of your partner, it will be difficult for you to develop an erection if you are a male or lubrication of the vagina if you are a female. As we shall soon see, pleasurable sexual stimulation will lead to an identifiable sexual response cycle. Knowing what this response cycle is can help you view your sexuality as a normal part of your functioning, for it suggests that sexual responses can be understood, predicted, and studied in the same way that other physiological processes can. Furthermore, learning to discern and distinguish your own bodily responses can enable you to pay attention, tell your partner about your responses, and thus increase your enjoyment.

How the Mind and Body Control Sexual Response

When a person becomes sexually aroused, several different parts of the body work together to create the psychological feeling of arousal and the accompanying physiological reactions. When Brian fantasized about Tanya, his brain, glands, nervous system, circulatory system, and reproductive system were only some of the bodily parts involved. Before we discuss the particular response to sexual stimulation, let us look more closely at what happens between the body and mind on such occasions.

The Brain: The Master of the Body

As with most vital functions, the brain is a key player during sexual arousal (Greenberg, 2009). It is the brain that interprets the stimulation—be it visual, olfactory, or other—and begins the process of "activating" other body parts.

The brain includes two major components: the **cerebral cortex** (the upper part) and the subcortex (the lower part). Figure 6.1 shows the structures of the brain and their locations. The subcortex includes the cerebellum (coordinates body movements), the medulla oblongata (regulates heartbeat, respiration, and other such basic physiological processes), the pons (regulates the sleep cycle), and the diencephalon. The diencephalon has many purposes, including the regulation of the emotions. It is made up of the thalamus and hypothalamus. The thalamus relays sensory impulses from other parts of the nervous system to the cerebral cortex. The hypothalamus, a key structure in sexual arousal, is the primary activator of the autonomic nervous system, which controls basic body processes such as hormone balance, temperature, and the constriction and dilation of blood vessels.

The **limbic system**, called the "seat of emotions," con-

cerebral cortex
The part of the brain called the *gray matter* that controls higher-order functioning such as language and judgment.

limbic system
The part of the brain referred to as the "seat of emotions," which produces emotions in response to physical and psychological signals.

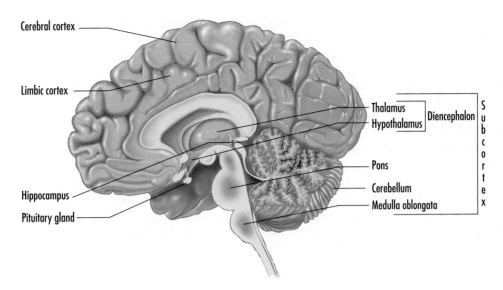

FIGURE **6.1** Many areas of the brain are involved in interpreting and determining each person's reaction to sexual stimulation.

sists of the thalamus and hypothalamus (the diencephalon) and other structures important in sexual arousal. The limbic system is connected to the diencephalon and is primarily concerned with emotions and their behavioral expression. The limbic system is thought to produce such emotions as fear, anxiety, and joy in response to physical and psychological signals.

The cerebral cortex (called the *gray matter*) controls higher-order abstract functioning, such as language and judgment. The cerebral cortex can also control more primitive areas of the brain. When the diencephalon recognizes fear, for instance, the cerebral cortex can use judgment to recognize the stimulus as nonthreatening and override the fear.

Last is the **reticular activating system (RAS)**. In the past, cortical and subcortical functions were considered dichotomized; that is, human behavior was thought to be a function of one area of the brain or the other. Now, brain researchers believe that neurological connections between the cortex and subcortex feed information back and forth. This network of nerves, the RAS, can be considered the connection between mind and body. The reticular system is a kind of two-way street, carrying messages perceived by the higher-awareness centers to the organs and muscles and also relaying stimuli received at the muscular and organic levels up to the cerebral cortex. In this manner, a sexually stimulating touch can generate physiological responses.

reticular activating system (RAS)
A network of nerves that connect the cortex and the subcortex—the connection between mind and body.

The Brain and Sexual Response

When you encounter a sexual stimulus of whatever kind, this message is passed to the brain via nerves. Once it reaches the brain, the message passes through the reticular activating system either from or to the limbic system and the thalamus. The limbic system is where emotion evolves, and the thalamus serves as the switchboard, determining what to do with the incoming messages. Next, the hypothalamus is activated and, in turn, activates the autonomic nervous system and the endocrine system through messages sent via nerves or substances released into the bloodstream.

All of this is generalized, of course. No two people are exactly the same, so no two people should be expected to react in exactly the same manner to sexual stimulation. First, what one person finds sexually arousing, another might not. As a result, one person might experience erection or vaginal lubrication when seeing pictures of people engaged in sexual activities, whereas another person might be "turned off" by this material. Second, because of illness or injury, some typical responses may be precluded for some people. For example, a male with a spinal cord injury might not be able to achieve an erection in spite of what might usually be sexually arousing for others. Furthermore, some people have little control over apparently involuntary responses; however, other people are able to exercise some control. For example, although ejaculation is considered an involuntary response to sexual stimulation, we know that people can learn to control (that is, delay) ejaculation should they choose to. So, in general, there is a great deal of variation in sexual response, even though there are certain typical means of reacting to sexual stimulation.

The Autonomic Nervous System

The autonomic nervous system consists of the sympathetic nervous system and the parasympathetic nervous system. These "subnervous systems" connect to various parts of the body through nerves. Consequently, as sexually arousing stimuli are experienced, messages are sent via the nerves to body parts, instructing them to react. The heart rate increases, muscles tense, perspiration occurs, and the mind starts racing. In addition, certain arteries are instructed to open (dilate) and allow more blood to flow through. That is why, for instance, the penis and the clitoris become erect. Arteries in these structures dilate, allowing blood to flow to the area; the nerves instruct veins to constrict, thereby holding the blood in that one place. The result is erection. The increase of blood to the genital area, called *engorgement,* also creates pressure on the walls of the vagina, resulting in vaginal lubrication. Furthermore, muscles contract as a result of messages sent through the nerves that make up the autonomic nervous system. For men, for example, contractions of the Cowper's gland, the seminal vesicles, and the prostate gland result in fluids being secreted into semen; contractions of the abdominal muscles and the muscles surrounding the reproductive organs are experienced by women.

The Role of Hormones in Sexual Arousal

The endocrine system is responsible for the secretion of hormones that travel to various body parts, instructing them how to behave. For example, when you are "stressed out," hormones are deposited into the bloodstream by the pituitary, adrenal, thyroid, and other glands and transported around the body, resulting in an increase in heart rate, muscle tension, blood pressure, and perspiration.

Sexual arousal works similarly. When you encounter a sexually arousing stimulus, your endocrine system is activated; hormones are secreted and changes occur in your body. That is what happens when someone fantasizes about a sexual experience. The fantasy translates into a sexual response that depends on the release of hormones that target certain body parts and bodily functions.

As we discussed in Chapters 4 and 5, sexual hormones are produced in the testes and ovaries. Testosterone, an androgen produced predominantly in the interstitial cells of the testes in men and in the ovaries in women (although a small amount is also produced in the adrenal glands), affects sexual interest, or *libido.* The more testosterone, the greater the interest in sex. Conversely, the less testosterone, the less interest in sex. As discussed in Chapter 5, Islamic societies once used castrated men to watch the women in the harem because their lowered interest in sex made them no threat to the women.

Recognizing the influence of testosterone on sexual interest, and in an attempt to enhance sexual satisfaction, some people turn to chemical aids. One of these "aids" is the substance used by the baseball player Mark McGwire during his record-breaking home run season. Popularly referred to as "andro," androstenedione was marketed as a dietary supplement; thus it was not regulated by the U.S. Food and Drug Administration (FDA). Athletes employ androstenedione to help them recover from weight-training workouts. Chemically, androstenedione is a steroid hormone "and a near cousin of testosterone" (How experts view andostenedione, 1998). The association with testosterone was enough to convince some people to use it to enhance sexual satisfaction. The problem with doing so is twofold: (1) The amount of testosterone may not be sufficient for the desirable effects, and (2) its use may result in harmful side effects, especially over the long term. Among other potential side effects, steroid use can lead to liver cancer, mood swings, hair growth, masculinization in women, and atrophied testes in men. In spite of these problems, androstenedione's possible effects on sexual arousal seem to override good judgment for some people hell-bent on making their sex lives ever richer.

The Role of Culture in Sexual Arousal

Whereas sexual arousal involves a physiological reaction to sexual stimulation, that reaction depends on the interpretation of the stimulant. For example, penis and clitoral erections are physiological responses to something interpreted as sexually stimulating. And yet, what someone finds sexually stimulating in one culture may have just the opposite reaction in another culture. For example, one culture might value a "full-bodied" woman, whereas another might value thinness. Furthermore, perceptions of what is sexually stimulating may differ within the same culture over time. In the United States, for instance, the actress Marilyn Monroe was a sexual icon in the 1950s. Today, she would probably be viewed differently because we now place a higher value on thinness than we did back then.

Subcultures also may have different perceptions of what is sexually stimulating. One of your authors' graduate students conducted a study of what African Americans and Caucasians considered to be the ideal body type. Research subjects were given silhouettes to evaluate. Whites reported that a thinner silhouette was more attractive, whereas African Americans stated a more full-figured body type was more desirable.

In some Muslim societies, women are required to be covered from head to toe. In contrast, in many Western societies, scantily clad women evoke a sexual response. In some subcultures, pornographic material is sexually stimulating while in others it is considered disgusting.

Thus, although sexual stimulation is a physiological process, it has a cultural and societal component to it that starts the physiological reaction in the first place.

■ The Masters and Johnson Sexual Response Cycle

The research of Masters and Johnson (1966) revealed a great deal about human sexuality. One of their major contributions was their description of the four phases of the human sexual response.

Excitement Phase

During the first phase of the Masters and Johnson **sexual response cycle**, the *excitement phase*, sexual stimuli result in a number of specific changes in the bodies of men and women. Heart rate, blood pressure, and muscle tension all increase. Blood engorges the abdominal area, resulting in an increase in penile and clitoral erection, as well as an increase in size of the labia minora, vagina, and nipples. The testes move closer to the body, and the scrotal skin thickens and tightens during the excitement phase. In women, vaginal lubrication occurs, and the labia majora spread and separate so as to make the vestibule more accessible. Some of these structures also deepen in color as a result of the increased blood to the area. The engorgement of blood is also responsible for the darkening of the skin on the chest and breasts called the *sex flush*. Although the sex flush occurs in both genders, it is more common in women and occurs in all ethnic groups, although it may be more evident in whites than in people of color.

Transudation is the process resulting in vaginal lubrication. When a female is sexually aroused, blood flows into the area surrounding the walls of the vagina in a process called *vasocongestion*. The pressure of the increased blood causes a seepage of moisture from the spaces between the cells. This moisture crosses the vaginal lining, first appearing as droplets. Eventually the fluid builds up in sufficient quantity to moisten the entire inner walls of the vagina. The amount of moisture may even be enough, depending on the woman's position, to leak out of the vagina and lubricate the labia and introitus.

The excitement phase may be short or last for several hours. The longer it lasts, the more variability occurs. For example, changes in the penis and the vagina vacillate over time during an extended excitement phase, so that the penis may occasionally become less erect, and vaginal lubrication may diminish periodically as well. The exciting aspect of excitement (pun intended) is the great variability among people. Some respond quickly; others need more time. Some favor moving to the next phase quickly; others desire more time. Some focus on their own reactions and feelings and satisfaction; others are more concerned with the partner's satisfaction. Furthermore, any one person may experience the excitement phase differently from one sexual encounter to another.

Plateau Phase

The second phase of Masters and Johnson's sexual response cycle is called the *plateau phase*. During the plateau phase, excitement becomes enhanced. Heart rate quickens, blood pressure rises, muscle tension increases, and breathing is faster. In men, Cowper's gland secretions may result from muscular contractions. The penis becomes fully erect, and the testes move closer to the body cavity. In women, the clitoris retracts under the clitoral hood; the inner two-thirds of the vagina fully extends, forming a "tenting" effect and creating a receptacle for semen; and the outer third of the vagina engorges with blood, forming the orgasmic platform. Although the plateau phase usually lasts but a few minutes, there are reports of more intense orgasms by people who have purposefully extended the plateau phase. And yet, orgasm is not the necessary follow-up to plateau. Although for men the loss of erection is unlikely once plateau is reached, in women as we shall soon see, reaching the plateau phase may be sufficient for sexual satisfaction.

Orgasm Phase

The *orgasm phase* for males consists of two stages: the *emission stage* and the *expulsion stage*. During the emission stage, muscular contractions of the vas deferens, the seminal vesicles, and the prostate gland create a buildup of semen in the urethral bulb located at the base of the penis. At the same time, the external urethral sphincter contracts, holding in the semen. Concurrently, the internal urethral sphincter contracts, thereby preventing semen from entering the bladder (a condition known as *retrograde ejaculation*) and urine from entering the urethral bulb where the semen has

sexual response cycle
The sequence of physiological and psychological reactions as a result of sexual arousal.

transudation
The process of vaginal lubrication resulting from engorgement of blood that creates pressure that forces moisture to seep from the spaces between the cells.

accumulated. The accumulation of semen in the urethral bulb creates a sensation of imminent and inevitable ejaculation, which usually lasts only a few seconds. Soon the second stage, expulsion, occurs.

During the expulsion stage, the **internal urethral sphincter** remains contracted, so urine and semen do not mix. However, the **external urethral sphincter** relaxes, and muscles surrounding the urethral bulb and the urethra contract, with the result that the accumulated semen is expelled from the urethral opening. Although there is some variation from one person to another, males generally experience intense sensations during the first couple of contractions and less sensation during later contractions. The degree of sensation appears also to be related to the amount of semen expelled.

> **internal urethral sphincter**
> The valve that prevents urine from entering the urethra and sperm from entering the bladder during ejaculation.
>
> **external urethral sphincter**
> The valve that closes during the emission stage, resulting in a buildup of semen, and that opens during the ejaculation stage, allowing semen to be expelled.
>
> **orgasmic platform**
> The narrowing of the outer third of the vagina during orgasm caused by contractions of the muscles in that area.

In women, the orgasm phase also consists of muscular contractions and intense sensations. The pelvic muscles that surround the vagina, in particular those that make up the **orgasmic platform**, contract 3 to 15 times, each contraction lasting less than 1 second. Other weaker and slower contractions follow. In addition, uterine contractions occur, beginning from the top of the uterus and proceeding downward.

In both males and females, other changes occur during orgasm. For example, heart rate increases dramatically, blood pressure rises, and breathing becomes rapid and shallow. Muscles throughout the body contract, and perspiration is evident. And an intense, pleasant psychological feeling associated with the release of sexual tension afforded by orgasm occurs.

Resolution Phase

During the *resolution phase*, there is a return to the unaroused state. In males, there is a decrease in the size of the penis as the erection is lost. This occurs in two stages: The first lasts about 1 minute as the blood exits the corpora cavernosa; the second takes several minutes as the blood leaves the corpus spongiosum. This is a result of the opening of the veins in the penis, which allows blood to be removed from the area. The testes become smaller and move down from the body cavity, and the scrotal skin becomes thinner and looser.

In women, muscles relax, and the uterus, vagina, and labia return to their unaroused positions and color.

As a result of the uterus's returning to its unaroused position, the cervix lowers into the seminal pool. If sperm is present in the seminal pool, the cervix is likely to have contact with them, and fertilization is possible. If one is trying to become pregnant, then the woman should lie on her back after intercourse to encourage this contact. Of course, the best way to prevent pregnancy if engaging in sexual intercourse is to use some method of contraception.

In addition to the preceding changes, during the resolution phase the clitoris returns from under the clitoral hood and the sex flush dissipates. In both males and females, heart rate, blood pressure, and breathing rate return to normal, and muscle tension decreases. Males then experience a **refractory (recovery) period** during which they are incapable of another orgasm. This period may be only several minutes for young males but is usually longer in older males. Females, however, are capable of having **multiple orgasms** before needing to recover.

> **refractory (recovery) period**
> The time needed by males for recovery between orgasms.
>
> **multiple orgasms**
> Orgasms that occur without the need for a refractory, or recovery, period.
>
> **sex flush**
> A darkening of the skin of the neck, face, forehead, or chest during sexual stimulation.
>
> **myotonia**
> Muscle tension occurring during sexual arousal.
>
> **hyperventilation**
> Deep and rapid breathing that occurs during sexual excitation.
>
> **tachycardia**
> An increase in heart rate that occurs during sexual activity.
>
> **vasocongestion**
> Increased blood flow to an area of the body, which occurs in the pelvic area during sexual arousal.

Females and males have many sexual responses in common, as well as many that differ. One of the differences is that males need a refractory period in which to recover before being capable of another orgasm, whereas females do not.

Gender
DIMENSIONS

Male–Female Differences in Sexual Response

There are many similarities and many differences in how males and females respond to sexual arousal. Masters and Johnson found the following similarities in the response cycle of men and women:

1. *Nipples.* Both males' and females' nipples become erect and wider in diameter when sexually stimulated.
2. *Sex Flush.* Males and females both experience a darkening of the skin of the neck, face, forehead, or chest during sexual stimulation, known as the **sex flush**. This darkening of the skin is a result of the accumulation of blood in these areas.
3. *Muscle Tension.* Commencing during the plateau phase and involving the legs, arms, abdomen, neck, and face, muscle tension (**myotonia**) appears in both sexes. During orgasm, muscles of the abdomen, chest, and face are also tensed. After orgasm, during the resolution phase, there is a release of all muscular tension in both sexes.
4. *Breathing.* During sexual excitation, both sexes experience deep and rapid breathing, called **hyperventilation**.
5. *Heart Rate.* Heart rate increases from a normal resting rate of about 72 up to 180 or more beats per minute during orgasm are not unusual in either sex. Such an increase is termed **tachycardia**.
6. *Blood Pressure.* Blood pressure rises in both males and females during sexual excitation.
7. *Perspiration.* Approximately one-third of both males and females perspire after orgasm.
8. *Blood Flow.* Increased blood flow to the pelvic area results in clitoral and penile erection and vaginal lubrication. This increased blood flow is termed **vasocongestion**.
9. *Orgasm.* During orgasm there is a rapid contraction of muscles in both sexes, with a relaxing of the muscles after orgasm.

The following listing describes the differences in the sexual responses of males and females:

1. *Nipples.* Whereas females are most likely to experience nipple erection during the excitement phase, males usually experience it during the plateau phase. Further, female nipple erection appears to disappear soon after orgasm (although this is an illusion caused by the swelling of the areolae), whereas male nipple erection is often obvious long after.
2. *Sex Flush.* Whereas males experience sex flush only in the plateau phase, in females sex flush can occur either late in the excitement phase or in the plateau phase. And though it may occur on the neck, forehead, and chest of both males and females, the sex flush occurs over the lower abdomen, thighs, lower back, and buttocks of females only.
3. *Muscle Tension.* In females, muscular tension causes an increase in the length and width of the vagina and expansion of the diameter of the cervix. In males, it causes elevation of the testes; that is, they are moved closer to the body by the contraction of muscles supporting them.
4. *Breathing.* Hyperventilation has different effects on males and females. After orgasm, males must wait for hyperventilation to diminish before being able to have another orgasm or even to achieve another erection; this period while breathing slows is referred to as a *refractory period*. Females, however, may have another orgasm before hyperventilation subsides—that is, without a refractory period and without entering a resolution phase. Consequently some females are capable of many orgasms in a short period.
5. *Blood Pressure.* Blood pressure increases somewhat more in males than in females. In males systolic blood pressure has been found to increase 40 to 100 mm Hg and diastolic blood pressure 20 to 50 mm Hg during sexual stimulation. In females the increase ranges from 30 to 80 mm Hg systolic and 20 to 40 mm Hg diastolic.
6. *Perspiration.* In men, sweating is usually limited to the soles of the feet and palms of the hands. Women are more likely to perspire over the back, thighs, chest, and sometimes the trunk, head, and neck.
7. *Orgasm.* Women are more likely than men to be multiorgasmic. Further, orgasm for the woman usually lasts longer than for men. The disagreement about female ejaculation was discussed in Chapter 4; it is sufficient to say here that, at the very least, female ejaculation does not occur as often during orgasm as does male ejaculation.

Each of us, male and female, progresses sequentially through the preceding four phases if we experience orgasm. Clearly, many body processes are involved during sexual activity, and each phase of the response affects the body somewhat differently. Even if we do not reach the orgasmic phase, we may pass through the earlier phases. For example, you may be engaged in sexual stimulation and quickly reach the excitement phase. The plateau stage may occur next, but—just your luck—the telephone rings and your excitement dissapates when you find out a loved one needs your help.

In studying the sexual response cycle in males and females, Masters and Johnson found both startling differences and amazing similarities. Knowing how females and males compare and contrast sexually is important to reinforcing the notion that we all have much in common while still preserving our differences.

If any of these responses is new to you, do not be surprised. You probably do not know everything about your digestive functions or nervous system, for instance, so why would you know everything about your sexual responses without studying them? The next time you are sexually aroused (either physically or by thoughts or fantasies), stop for a moment and attempt to identify the responses just discussed—or reflect now on some past sexual experience. Remember, no two of us are exactly alike. Consequently you may not experience all the sexual responses as we have described them. This is to be expected. Generally, though, you will find that your sexual responses are similar to the ones described.

Figure 6.2 depicts the typical male sexual response according to Masters and Johnson. Males start with the excitement phase, move to the plateau phase, proceed to have an orgasm, and then either move through the resolution phase, in which they return to the prearoused state, or to a refractory period (a part of the resolution phase), during which they recover from the orgasm and prepare themselves for another orgasm. Masters and Johnson found this pattern to be standard, although men report variations on this model.

Females were described by Masters and Johnson as being more varied in their sexual responses. Figure 6.2 also shows this variability. Pattern (a) is similar to the male pattern with a progression from excitement to plateau to orgasm and then resolution, except that it depicts a female's ability to have multiple orgasms without a refractory period. Pattern (b) shows the woman's progressing from excitement to an enhancement of this excitement during the plateau phase and then moving directly to resolution (bypassing orgasm). This pattern implies that women may be sexually satisfied without experiencing an orgasm. Pattern (c) depicts another possible female sexual response cycle in which there is no definitive plateau phase but a rapid escalation to orgasm and a very quick resolution.

Figures 6.3 and 6.4 summarize changes that occur in males and females during the four phases of the Masters and Johnson sexual response cycle.

(a) Phase of Sexual Response Cycle for Males

Time

(b) Phase of Sexual Response Cycle for Females

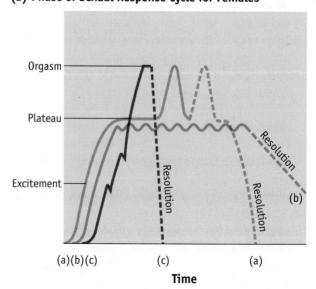

Time

FIGURE 6.2 According to Masters and Johnson, the male sexual response cycle (a) is much more predictable than is the female response cycle (b), and females can have a similar response to males—that is, moving through the four phases and experiencing orgasm—or can maintain the plateau phase without orgasm. Females can also be multiorgasmic without experiencing a refractory period.

(a) Unaroused State

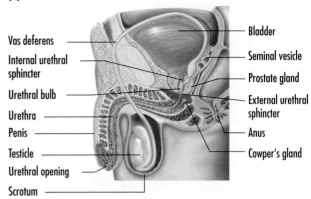

Vas deferens

Internal urethral sphincter

Urethral bulb

Urethra

Penis

Testicle

Urethral opening

Scrotum

Bladder

Seminal vesicle

Prostate gland

External urethral sphincter

Anus

Cowper's gland

■ **(b) Excitement Phase**

Urethral opening dilates slightly

Partially aroused penis becomes erect

Scrotal skin thickens and tightens

Testicles begin to engorge and move closer to the body

■ **(c) Plateau Phase**

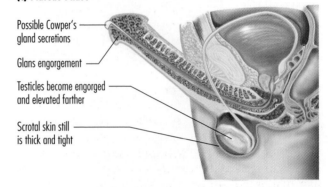

Possible Cowper's gland secretions

Glans engorgement

Testicles become engorged and elevated farther

Scrotal skin still is thick and tight

■ **(d) Orgasm Phase: Emission Stage**

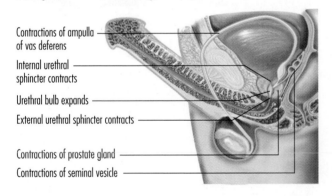

Contractions of ampulla of vas deferens

Internal urethral sphincter contracts

Urethral bulb expands

External urethral sphincter contracts

Contractions of prostate gland

Contractions of seminal vesicle

■ **(e) Orgasm Phase: Expulsion Stage**

Semen expelled

Internal urethral sphincter stays contracted

Contractions of urethra

External urethral sphincter relaxes and opens

Contractions of muscles around base of penis

Contractions of rectal sphincter

■ **(f) Resolution**

Rapid partial decrease in size of penis; then slow return to unaroused state and size

Testicles become smaller and move down from the body

Scrotal skin thins and becomes more loose

FIGURE **6.3** Male sexual response cycle, in detail.

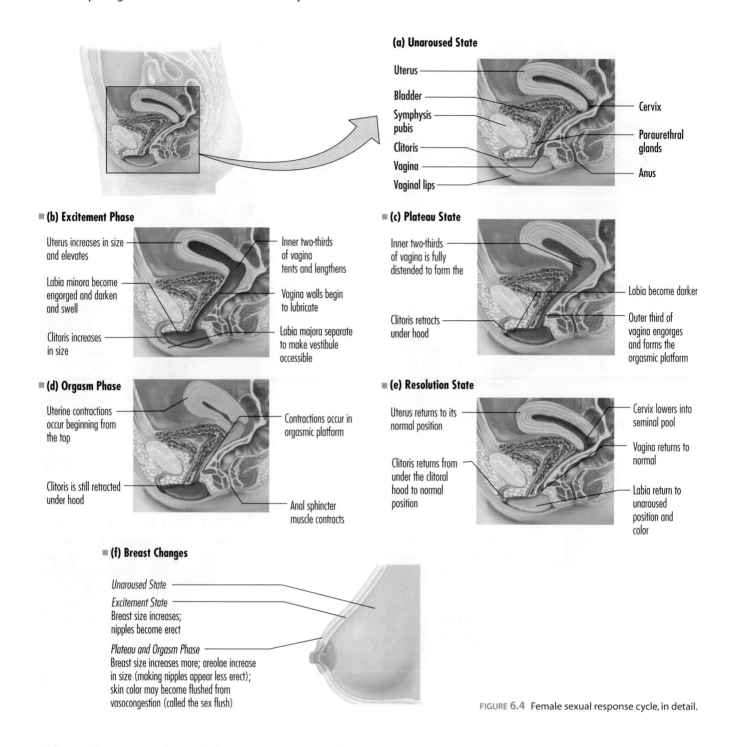

(a) Unaroused State

Uterus

Bladder

Symphysis pubis

Clitoris

Vagina

Vaginal lips

Cervix

Paraurethral glands

Anus

■ (b) Excitement Phase

Uterus increases in size and elevates

Labia minora become engorged and darken and swell

Clitoris increases in size

Inner two-thirds of vagina tents and lengthens

Vagina walls begin to lubricate

Labia majora separate to make vestibule accessible

■ (c) Plateau State

Inner two-thirds of vagina is fully distended to form the

Clitoris retracts under hood

Labia become darker

Outer third of vagina engorges and forms the orgasmic platform

■ (d) Orgasm Phase

Uterine contractions occur beginning from the top

Clitoris is still retracted under hood

Contractions occur in orgasmic platform

Anal sphincter muscle contracts

■ (e) Resolution State

Uterus returns to its normal position

Clitoris returns from under the clitoral hood to normal position

Cervix lowers into seminal pool

Vagina returns to normal

Labia return to unaroused position and color

■ (f) Breast Changes

Unaroused State

Excitement State
Breast size increases; nipples become erect

Plateau and Orgasm Phase
Breast size increases more; areolae increase in size (making nipples appear less erect); skin color may become flushed from vasocongestion (called the sex flush)

FIGURE 6.4 Female sexual response cycle, in detail.

Other Theoretical Models of Sexual Response

Other models descriptive of the human sexual response have been proposed. These models are the product of years of experience in sexual counseling and therapy.

Kaplan's Triphasic Model

Originally, the noted sex therapist Helen Singer Kaplan (1974) proposed a biphasic model of the human sexual response. That model conceptualized sexual response as having two identifiable phases. The first phase involved vasocongestion of the genitals, and the second phase consisted of the reflexive muscular contractions of orgasm. Kaplan argued that the two phases were each controlled by a different part of the nervous system: vasocongestion, by the parasympathetic nervous system, and orgasm, by the sympathetic nervous system (both are components of the autonomic nervous system). Furthermore, she explained, different structures are involved in each of these phases: the blood vessels for vasocongestion and the muscles for orgasm. Kaplan gave other justifications for the biphasic model, but space limits our discussion to the justification that derived from Kaplan's observations in her professional practice. Kaplan noted that the interference with vasocongestion resulted in erection problems in the male, whereas different sexual dysfunctions (premature ejaculation and retarded ejaculation) were the result of orgasm impairment. In some females, normal vasocongestion and sexual excitement were experienced in spite of the presence of orgasm problems. Because problems with vasocongestion were quite different from and mutually exclusive with problems with orgasm, Kaplan believed the biphasic model to be valid.

Over the years Kaplan's biphasic model evolved into a triphasic one. Kaplan (1979) now conceptualizes human sexual response as consisting of a **desire phase**, an **excitement phase**, and a **resolution phase**. During her practice as a sex therapist Kaplan has found that sexual dysfunctions fall into one of these three categories and that these categories are separate and distinct (that is, it is possible to function well in one or two phases while having problems in another). The unique component of Kaplan's triphasic model is the desire phase—a psychological prephysical sexual response stage. Masters and Johnson's model ignores this part of the sexual response.

Sexual desire is not always present during sexual activity, however. Sometimes a person may engage in sexual activity to satisfy his or her partner rather than because he or she feels desire. A speaker in one of our sexuality classes described how when his wife complains of some ache or pain (or the proverbial headache) when he is interested in sex, he asks where she feels bothered. When he finds the spot, he gently massages that area, soon turning the massage into a sensual experience. Shortly, he relates, the desire phase is reached.

desire phase
The first stage of the sexual response cycle, as described in Helen Singer Kaplan's model, which consists of psychologically becoming interested in sex before any physical changes occur.

excitement phase
The second stage of Kaplan's model of sexual response, which consists of physiological arousal and changes and, possibly, orgasm.

resolution phase
A stage of the sexual response cycle consisting of a return to the pre-aroused state.

Zilbergeld and Ellison's Model
Another model of human sexual response consists of five components. The therapists Bernie Zilbergeld and Carol Ellison (1980) were concerned that Masters and Johnson's model ignored the cognitive and subjective

aspects of the sexual response, while focusing exclusively on the physiological aspects. They argued that the subjective elements of sexual desire and sexual arousal were omitted from the Masters and Johnson model. *Sexual desire* is defined in this five-component model as the frequency with which a person wants to engage in sexual activity; *sexual arousal* is defined as how excited one becomes during sexual activity. The five components of this model are as follows.

1. Interest, or desire
2. Arousal
3. Physiological readiness (for example, erection or vaginal lubrication)
4. Orgasm
5. Satisfaction (one's evaluation of how one feels)

As with Kaplan's model, Zilbergeld and Ellison's model allows for sexual dysfunctions that pertain to desire although other responses may be normal. Consequently, this component can be isolated from the other components for treatment by a sex therapist. One might describe the triphasic and five-component models as being more inclusive of the psychological aspects of the sexual response, whereas the Masters and Johnson model is more concerned with the physiological aspects.

Walen and Roth's Model
The contribution of Walen and Roth (1987) relates to the inclusion of perception as the beginning of the sexual response. They argue that without perceiving a potential stimulus as sexually exciting, no sexual response is elicited. Further, they state that a stimulus that is sexually arousing in one situation may not be in another situation. For example, having one's genitals fondled in private may be arousing, but having one's genitals fondled in public may only be embarrassing.

Further, Walen and Roth's model of sexual response includes people evaluating the situation and their response to it to determine if everything is going according to plan. They might evaluate the amount of vaginal lubrication, the presence of penile erection, or heavy breathing. Expecting these to occur and finding that they have occurred validates that the encounter is progressing as expected. The partners can then relax and enjoy the situation, thereby becoming more sexually aroused. However, determining things aren't going as planned can interfere with the sexual response as we try to decide what the problem is and how to solve it. The result might be an inability to have an orgasm, or even to just enjoy the sexual encounter. Recognizing that evaluating one's performance or the situation too critically can interfere with sexual arousal, Walen and Roth advise not placing too high an expectation on performance, not spending too much time observing what is occurring, and relaxing and being fully involved in a manner that will enhance sexual arousal and the enjoyment of the sexual encounter.

Thayton's Model

Wiliam Thayton (2002) is a Baptist minister, and the model of sexual arousal he developed, understandably, has a spiritual and theological perspective. Thayton acknowledges that sex is pleasurable. He proposes that God intended for humans to respond to sex with pleasure and to enjoy the blessing of sexual arousal. Thayton offers evidence of this view by stating that Jesus never preached that sexual pleasure was sinful or to be avoided, in spite of advocating self-denial in other areas of life. Therefore, Thayton concludes that spirituality, sexuality, and love are bound together in God's creation of people who are sexual by nature. As a result, when one is sexual, one is also spiritual. However, love is an important component in this mix for Thayton. Love is the glue that binds sexuality, spirituality, and pleasure. After all, he argues, love allows us to be one with the universe and what is more spiritual than that?

Lastly, Thayton considers sex researchers as sexual guides, just as clergy and theologians are spiritual and religious guides. They all study their area of expertise to understand it better, and then communicate their findings and recommendations to the public at large.

Basson's Model

Basson (2000) is a sex therapist and, as such, her model of sexual response stems from her experience in treating sexual disorders. Basson has no argument with the models offered by Masters and Johnson or Kaplan. However, like Walen and Roth, she believes that how one perceives and interprets a situation is an important component of sexual response. Basson states that feeling positive toward one's partner is necessary for sexual arousal to occur. If one hates one's partner or doesn't trust one's partner, sexual arousal will not occur.

Basson also believes there is a difference in sexual response between males and females. In females, she argues, emotions and intimacy are important precursors of sexual response. Whereas sexual response begins with desire or arousal in males, Basson believes it begins with intimacy in females. In other words, women desire being close to their partners, whereas men desire a physical release of sexual tension. Once women feel intimate toward their partners, desire and arousal are then possible. In fact, Basson believes that intimacy leads to arousal, which

in turn leads to desire. Desire creates greater intimacy, which then results in even more arousal and desire. All along the way, though, there are interpretations and evaluations of what is occurring, similar to the recognition of perceptions in the Walen and Roth model. These interpretations and evaluations affect intimacy, arousal, and desire.

Orgasm is a possible result of this cycle, but not a necessary one for women to feel sexually satisfied, which is the key for Basson. Some people may experience orgasm but not feel the sexual encounter was satisfying. Others may not experience orgasm but feel the encounter was extremely satisfying. Basson believes that should be the goal of the encounter—being satisfied, not orgasm.

Erotic Stimulus Pathway

An important contribution to our knowledge of sexual response is that of the Erotic Stimulus Pathway (ESP) theory of David M. Reed (Haffner & Stayton, 1998). The ESP theory enhances our understanding and ability to treat sexual dysfunctions. Reed divides the sexual response cycle into four phases that correspond to those of Kaplan and Masters and Johnson. For many people, these phases are learned developmentally. Figure 6.5 compares the Masters and Johnson model with the Reed model.

In the *seduction phase* a person learns how to get aroused sexually and how to attract someone else sexually. Seduction translates into memories and rituals. For example, adolescents may spend much time on personal appearance, choice of clothes, and mannerisms, all of which can enhance positive self-esteem if the adolescents like the way they feel. If the adolescents feel good about the way they look and feel, then attracting another person will be much easier. As the adolescents get older, these positive feelings are translated into sexual desire and arousal. These seductive techniques are stored in memory and can be activated later on in life.

In the *sensations phase*, the different senses can enhance sexual excitement and ideally prolong the plateau phase. The early experiences of touch (holding hands, putting arms around a loved one) become very important. The sense of vision (staring at a loved one, holding an image of him or her when absent) is a way of maintaining interest and arousal. Hearing the loved one in intimate conversation or over the telephone becomes very important. Hearing the sounds of a partner responding to sexual stimulation can be titillating. The smell of the loved one, either a particular scent he or she wears or the sexual smell, produces additional excitement. Finally, the taste of a food or drink or the taste of the loved one becomes important to memory and fantasy. All these senses

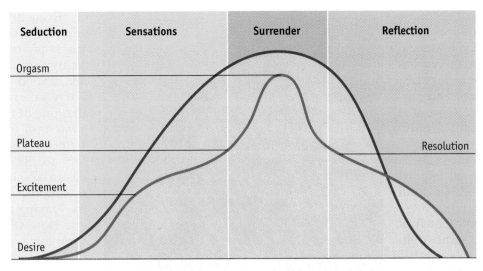

FIGURE **6.5** Sexual response curve. *Source:* Masters, et al., 1966; Kaplan, 1979.

Many senses can evoke a sexual response. The soft touch, kiss, sight, or smell of a partner can be quite sexually stimulating.

extend the excitement into a plateau phase, which makes one want to continue the pleasurable moment over a longer period. These seduction and sensation experiences are the psychological input to the physiology of sexual response. They are the precursors to sexual climax and orgasm.

In the *surrender phase,* orgasm is a "psychophysiological surprise." The psychodynamic issues surrounding orgasm are power and control. Persons with orgasmic dysfunction may be in a power struggle with themselves or with their partners or with the messages received about sex. Overcontrol or undercontrol can affect orgasmic potential and the ability to allow all of the passion to be expressed.

In the *reflection phase,* meaning is given to the experience. Whether the sexual experience is interpreted as positive or negative may determine the desire for subsequent sexual activity—at least with that sexual partner, under those circumstances, or with those behaviors. Recognize, though, that not every sexual experience can be, or should be, a "10." As the authors have heard it expressed, "Sometimes sex is a four-course gourmet meal, and sometimes it's like having cereal for dinner. Most of the time it's like having hamburgers or chicken. When it's cereal, you have to remember that there are better times ahead."

Aphrodisiacs: Seeking the Ultimate in Sexual Pleasure

An *aphrodisiac,* named after the Greek goddess Aphrodite, the goddess of love, is any substance that arouses sexual desire and/or enhances sexual response. For centuries people have searched for a safe and effective aphrodisiac without much luck. This search has led to "Spanish fly" (*cantharidin*), which results in irritation of the urinary tract. Now, is that sexually arousing? It has led to substances to make one "horny," such as ground-up rhinoceros horns or elephant tusks, which just do not work. Oysters, clams, and even the testicles of bulls ("prairie oysters") have been tried without the desired effect.

Even toxic substances have been ingested in the hope of enhancing sexual desire and response; *amyl nitrate* is one of these substances. Amyl nitrate is designed for use by heart patients to reduce chest pain. Its container is "popped" open when chest pain occurs; thus the containers are often called "poppers." Amyl nitrate became popular among some gay men as an aphrodisiac because it facilitated anal intercourse by relaxing the anal sphincter muscle. Although it does dilate blood vessels in the brain and genitals, resulting in warmth in the abdomen and pelvis, facilitating erection, and possibly prolonging orgasm, it is also associated with disturbing side effects. For example, amyl nitrate can cause dizziness, headaches, and fainting and can even result in death in extreme cases.

Bupropion (acquired under the brand name Wellbutrin) and L-dopa are other substances that have been ingested for their aphrodisiac effects. Bupropion is an antidepressant drug, and L-dopa is a drug used for treating patients with Parkinson's disease. Both of these drugs act on the brain receptors that produce dopamine and so can increase libido. However, unsupervised use of a drug that affects the brain is dangerous; it must be monitored by a physician and prescribed for a specific medical purpose.

Alcohol and *marijuana* have also been ascribed aphrodisiaclike qualities. However, if they work at all, they diminish judgment and make people feel less stress about sex. That may be good, or that may be bad. A decrease in inhibitions may result in high-risk sexual behaviors (such as vaginal or anal intercourse without a condom) that may transmit a sexually transmitted infection (STI) or cause an unwanted pregnancy. Furthermore, alcohol is a central nervous system depressant that can interfere with sexual arousal rather than enhance it. Marijuana can distort perceptions and make one think that the sexual experience continued longer than it really did. Both of these substances can lead to problems in the short run and over prolonged use; in addition, marijuana is illegal.

One substance that appears to have potential as an aphrodisiac is *yohimbine hydrochloride*, from the sap of a West African tree, the yohimbine tree. Yohimbine has been reported to aid some men with erectile dysfunction to achieve and maintain an erection for a long-enough period to engage in sexual intercourse (Senbel & Mostafa, 2008). However, it does not work for all men with erectile dysfunction, and whether it enhances the sexual response of other men is unknown.

For centuries, people have searched for substances that arouse sexual desire and/or enhance sexual response. Many substances have been proposed to be aphrodisiacs, even chocolate. However, most of these substances either do not work or have disturbing side effects. Still, the search continues.

Even drugs that inhibit sexual desire have been the focus of researchers for many years. These drugs are called *anaphrodisiacs*. For years, rumor has had it that one of these substances, *potassium nitrate*, known as *saltpeter*, is used by the military to diminish the sexual desire of soldiers and is used in summer camps to control the "raging urges" of teenagers. However, all that potassium nitrate does is increase the need to urinate; some people obviously think that is enough to interfere with sex.

Yet some drugs do interfere with sexual response. These tend to be central nervous system depressants such as opiates (for example, heroin), tranquilizers, antihypertensive medications, antipsychotic and antidepressant drugs (such as Prozac), and, surprisingly to many people, nicotine, which constricts blood vessels and decreases vasocongestion in the genitals.

■ Orgasm

Our nonsexual lives tend to be goal oriented. We may have goals to graduate from college, to become established in a good career, or to live in a large house. It should be no surprise that goal orientation has invaded our sexual lives as well. For too many of us, orgasm becomes the goal of almost all of our sexual behavior. We forget about the pleasure that can be derived from sexual activity that does not lead to orgasm, and we forget that the communication and the quality of our relationships can be enhanced through sexual activity that does not result in orgasm. The question "Did you come?" tends to be as much a part of the sexual experience as removing one's clothes.

Orgasmic Sensation

The feelings that accompany orgasm are quite different from the physiological responses and may even contradict what we know is occurring physiologically. For example, women may experience a physiologically intense orgasm (a dozen or so measurable

Global DIMENSIONS

Aphrodisiacs and Tigers: A Strange Mix

Some of the most expensive aphrodisiacs in the world are made from parts of male tigers. The most prized and valuable aphrodisiacs are made from the tiger's penis—often made into a soup! Less expensive "love potions" are made from everything else down to the tiger's crushed bone. Such aphrodisiacs are extremely popular, predominantly in Asian countries.

The net result is that the last several thousand of the world's tigers are endangered—and all for naught. As with many other aphrodisiacs, no physiological sexual response results from ingesting tiger parts.

To help debunk the myth of the tiger as aphrodisiac, the Wildlife Conservation Society hired a Singapore ad agency to create the ad shown here. The TV ad (intended for an Asian audience) shows mating tigers. The voice-over reads, "The last 5,000 tigers in the world are being killed. All because some men believe that eating tiger penis will give them legendary sexual prowess. Perhaps they too can make love for a full 15 seconds."

What psychological effects might such an "aphrodisiac" have in a country where there is a long-standing cultural belief that it works? Might the ability to pay a great deal of money for such an aphrodisiac have a psychological boosting effect? Will the ad help to "destroy the myth," as it claims? Explain your answer.

muscular contractions) but report the orgasm to be of mild intensity, or they may experience a mild orgasm physiologically (four muscular contractions) but report the sensation of an intense orgasm. The reason for this discrepancy lies in the understanding that sexual experience is interpreted by the mind as well as the body. When the relationship is a healthy one, sexual partners may experience a great deal of pleasure from a mild orgasm because the experience was shared and made them feel closer. Other factors such as mood, expectations, and the setting can also affect one's subjective judgment regarding the intensity of the orgasm.

Generally, sensations from orgasms are experienced similarly by males and females, but there are exceptions (Silverberg, 2008). In women, there is a highly pleasurable feeling that usually begins at the clitoris but quickly spreads to the whole pelvic area. The genitals often feel warm and tingly, and then a sensation of throbbing in the lower pelvis may be noticed. In men, the experience is also highly pleasurable. They usually experience warmth, pressure, and sometimes a throbbing during the moment when they have reached the "point of no return" (that is, ejaculatory inevitability), at which point men cannot prevent ejaculation. In many men, ejaculation itself is experienced as a sensation of pumping.

The similarity of male and female orgasms was vividly demonstrated by two studies involving college students (Proctor, Wagner, & Butler, 1974; Wiest, 1977). In these studies, students wrote descriptions of their orgasms, and these descriptions were analyzed by a group of experts. The experts could not distinguish between the male and female descriptions, and the researchers concluded that males and females experience similar sensations as a result of orgasm. Although males and females do not generally differ in the sensations they report accompanying orgasm, orgasms *do* differ. That is, an individual may experience an orgasm today that is either more or less intense than one yesterday, and one person may experience orgasms generally more intensely than another person. These differences are not a function of gender; rather, a less pleasurable experience may be a result of guilt, shame, embarrassment, an uncomfortable setting, frustrations with the sexual partner, hostility, distrust, low self-esteem, or other factors.

Controversies About Orgasm

Several controversies surround the topic of orgasm.

Types of Orgasm

First, experts disagree about the types of orgasms that exist. In the early 1900s, Freud theorized there were two different types of female orgasm: the clitoral and the vaginal. He viewed the clitoral orgasm as an immature sexual response that women outgrew. Because he considered the clitoris to be a stunted penis, Freud believed the clitoral orgasm was an expression of masculine sexuality rather than feminine sexuality. If at adolescence the woman had not transferred her erotic focus from the clitoris to the vagina, Freud believed that psychotherapy was in order. When Freud's theory was operationalized, surgical removal of the clitoris (**clitoridectomy**) was actually performed on girls who were too clitorally focused, as determined by their masturbating by stimulating the clitoris.

Masters and Johnson's (1966) research identified but one type of orgasm. Regardless of the point of stimulation—clitoris or vagina—and regardless of the method of stimulation—penile insertion or vibrator—Masters and Johnson reported the same physiological occurrences during orgasm. However, Masters and Johnson did report a difference in the sensations of orgasm that depended on whether they were a result of coital or noncoital activities. They found orgasms from coitus to be less intense than orgasms from noncoital means. This finding was validated by Hite (1976), who found the clitorally stimulated orgasm to be more intense than the orgasm from coitus. Hite also found the coital orgasm to be more diffused throughout the body than was the locally intense clitoral orgasm.

To complicate matters further, other researchers (Singer & Singer, 1972) have reported three distinct types of orgasms: vulval, uterine, and blended. Singer and Singer included emotional satisfaction as a consideration in their research. **Vulval orgasm** is the same as the orgasm described by Masters and

clitoridectomy
Surgical removal of the clitoris.

vulval orgasm
An orgasm in a female that includes the contractions of the orgasmic platform, which is not sexually satisfying and, as a result, allows another orgasm to occur almost immediately.

Communication
D I M E N S I O N S

Discussing Sexual Desires

Communicating sexual desires is embarrassing for many people. After all, sex is not something we are taught to talk about openly. The irony for many of us is that we are taught at a very young age that sex is so "dirty" that we should save it for someone we love. Does not make much sense, does it? Of course, sex is not dirty, although it may make sense to refrain from certain sexual activities altogether and to engage in others only when you are ready. When the time is right, if we could share what we find sexually arousing with a partner, we would be that much more satisfied. To help you along in this process, we have prepared the following guidelines. We recognize, though, that not all of you have chosen to engage in sexual activities with a partner. Still, these guidelines will be useful if and when you decide the time is right for you to do so.

- Speak about what you like sexually at times in which you are not engaged in sexual activity. This allows for a conversation that can be more rational than one carried on while emotions are running high.
- Be specific. State what you like and how you like it, what you dislike and why you dislike it.
- Ask your partner to do the same. Let your partner know that you want to please him or her as well as yourself. If your partner realizes you are concerned about his or her pleasure, he or she will be more likely to be concerned about your pleasure.
- During sex, let your partner know how you feel about what he or she is doing. Reinforce the behaviors you like by letting him or her know they are pleasing.
- Do not hesitate to refrain from any sexual activity you find unpleasant, uncomfortable, or distasteful. When doing so, explain your reasons to your partner.

Remember, you can have a more satisfying sexual relationship, when you are ready to do so, by being able to communicate freely about sex and what you find pleasurable and what you find displeasing.

---

uterine orgasm
An orgasm in a female that can occur only in the presence of penile penetration and that involves a woman's holding her breath just before orgasm and then exhaling when the climax occurs.

blended orgasm
An orgasm in a female in which there are contractions of the muscles in the outer third of the vagina as well as breath holding; a combination of the vulval and uterine orgasms.

Johnson and includes contractions of the orgasmic platform; however, the vulval orgasm is not sexually satiating, and therefore another orgasm can be experienced immediately. A **uterine orgasm** can occur only in the presence of vaginal penetration and involves a woman's holding her breath just before orgasm and then exhaling when the climax occurs. In contrast to the vulval orgasm, the uterine orgasm is sexually satiating and is therefore usually followed by a refractory period. The **blended orgasm** is a combination of these two; that is, there are contractions of the outer third of the vagina as well as breath holding. These researchers make it clear that no one form of orgasm is better than another, just different.

How many forms of orgasm are there? As with other areas of human sexuality, there is disagreement. The important point is that orgasm can be conceptualized as merely a physiological reaction to sexual stimulation or as a complex of interactions between partners (the setting, the mood, and a host of other variables). To consider an orgasm as solely a bodily reaction is to ignore the interactive nature of the human mind and the human body and the impossibility of separating them. Without a mind to realize that sexual stimulation is, in fact, stimulating, there is no orgasm.

Recognizing Orgasms

At the beginning of the sexuality classes we teach, we ask students to write questions they would like answered before the semester ends. A common question asks how a man can recognize when his female partner is faking an orgasm. The women in the class are astute enough to know that when their male partners ejaculate, they experience orgasm. What they do not usually know is that sometimes orgasm can occur without an ejaculate—for example, in men with disease of the prostate or in prepubescent boys. Men, however, want to know how to recognize that their partners are sexually satisfied.

This question has several implications that deserve some attention. First, it expresses a concern for the woman's sexual satisfaction. On the surface, that appears to be healthy; however, it is our experience that when asked by men, this question is more

Myth (vs) Fact

Myth: It is easy to tell when a male has an orgasm because the ejaculate gives it away.
Fact: Although it is usually true that a male will ejaculate during orgasm, this is not always the case. Males may have an orgasm without ejaculating.

Myth: During the plateau phase of the Masters and Johnson sexual response cycle, conditions remain pretty much the same.
Fact: Although Masters and Johnson chose to call the second phase of the sexual response cycle the *plateau phase,* changes do occur. What occurred during the excitement phase is intensified during the plateau phase.

Myth: Whereas women can be multiorgasmic, men cannot.
Fact: Although it occurs relatively infrequently, some men do report needing very little time before being able to have another orgasm.

Myth: Males and females differ tremendously in their responses to sexual excitation.
Fact: There certainly are many differences between males and females in their responses to sexual excitement. Still, there are many similarities as well.

Myth: The clitoris can be stimulated easily during sexual intercourse.
Fact: Relatively early in the sexual response of women, the clitoris retracts under the clitoral hood. Therefore, it is not easily accessible to touch and/or stimulation unless the clitoral hood is purposefully pulled back.

related to a man's ego than to a woman's satisfaction. That is, if the male can "give" the woman an orgasm, he must be a good lover. Another interpretation of this question could be that men are afraid their female sexual partners might fake orgasms. A woman may fake an orgasm to meet her partner's expectation, to feed her partner's ego, to end the sexual encounter, to present herself as "normal," or to meet the "goal."

Beyond the fact that faking an orgasm is dishonest and deceitful, it may lead your partner to think that something unsatisfying to you was great and should be repeated the next time. However, if what a partner does is pleasurable but does not result in a climax, that might be enough. If so, why not tell your partner? Sexual activity can be enjoyed for itself without being directed toward the goal of orgasm.

Men are also prone to faking orgasms if they are unable to achieve one. When a man has been drinking alcoholic beverages, for example, and cannot reach the orgasmic phase, he might feel threatened by how this may be interpreted by his partner. Will his partner think he is less than a real man? Will his partner think he is sexually dysfunctional? Will his partner think he does not find him or her sexually attractive? Some men believe it is easier to fake an orgasm than to allay these fears.

Whether a man or woman fakes orgasm regularly, the person would be well advised to discuss

¿? Ethical DIMENSIONS

Should Sexual Enhancements Be Used to Increase Sexual Arousal?

How far should people be allowed, or encouraged, to go in their search for sexual satisfaction and sexual arousal? Some people argue that anything that does not negatively affect another person is appropriate to enhance sexual arousal. They believe the use of X-rated videotapes, sexually explicit written material, and erotic clothing is within the bounds of acceptability. They also suggest that engaging in sexual relations with a number of different people can provide the experience necessary to reach one's sexual potential. Further, any physical barriers to sexual arousal should be eliminated at any cost. So if a man has blockage of the penile arteries, he should undergo bypass surgery to provide the penis with the blood it needs to become erect. And if there is damage to the penis as a result of an accident, options should include Viagra, artificial penises, surgery to implant rods in the penis to provide an erection, or penis transplantation

(from someone who has recently died—similar to heart, kidney, and other organ transplantation).

Others believe that enhancing sexual arousal is appropriate, but only within certain limits. They argue that sexually explicit material is pornographic and/or obscene. Its use is unacceptable for any reason, and it should be outlawed. Furthermore, altering the body "merely" for sexual purposes goes against nature, is therefore "unnatural," and should not be tolerated. Sexual arousal should be enhanced through improving the relationship between the couple, and that can be accomplished only in a marriage, and one in which the spouses remain sexually faithful to each other. Only then, advocates of this view argue, can the couple engage in "lovemaking" as opposed to "sexmaking," because sex without love can never achieve the level of arousal that sex with love can.

What do you think? What is appropriate and what is inappropriate when trying to enhance sexual arousal?

Global DIMENSIONS

Age of First Intercourse

A study by the London International Group (1998) found that men and women worldwide are starting to engage in sexual intercourse at ever earlier ages. The study queried 10,000 sexually active adults from 14 developing and developed countries. The average age at first intercourse was 17.4 years (down slightly from the previous year's 17.6 years). However, there was a great deal of variability from country to country. For example, the average age at first intercourse in the United States was 15.8 years, whereas it was 19.0 years in Hong Kong. In a subsequent study, average age at first intercourse was 16.8 years in Kenya, 19.0 years in Bolivia, 18.8 years in Brazil, 18.6 years in Guatemala, and 22.8 years in the Philippines (Population Reference Bureau, 2000). Differences also occurred in the frequency of intercourse. Whereas the average adult reported engaging in coitus 112 times a year, French and Americans reported more frequent intercourse (151 and 148 times per year, respectively) than did men and women from Hong Kong and Thailand (77 and 69 times per year, respectively). In addition, 40% of Americans wanted coitus more often, whereas only 7% of Mexicans expressed that desire.

 Did You Know . . .

An ancient Indian philosophy rebelled against the tenets of organized religion that restricted sexual practices. *Tantra* taught that sexuality was a doorway to the divine and that earthly pleasures were sacred acts. Becoming more popular in Western culture, *tantric sex*, seeks to teach means of pleasuring one's lover and connecting with him or her fully, rather than simply to achieve an orgasm. It is seen as a dance with no beginning or end, and the goal is to be in the present moment. One of the outcomes of tantric sex, however, is to extend orgasm and to enjoy multiple orgasms. Among the tantric sex techniques are these (Painter, 2009):

- Welcoming love (making time for each other), creating an inviting atmosphere (for example, candles and flowers), and dressing provocatively
- Using ritual for intimacy (for example, bathing together)
- Experimenting with erotic touch
- Maintaining a deep level of intimacy (for example, gazing into each other's eyes)
- Keeping it slow
- Varying positions
- Pumping the pubococcygeal (PC) muscles
- Stimulating the clitoris and labia during sex
- Stimulating the G spot (see Chapter 13), called the sacred spot in tantra

the situation candidly with his or her partner. Such a discussion can often result in a closer relationship and the understanding that setting up sexual performance goals is self-defeating. Some women do not reach orgasm, some have an orgasm once during intercourse, and some are multiorgasmic. Some men do not reach orgasm, some have an orgasm once during intercourse, and some are multiorgasmic (although some recovery time between orgasms is necessary). For people of either gender who do not reach orgasm, pleasure from coitus can still be attained. Rather than asking, "Did you come?" we should ask, "What did I do that you liked?" "How can I pleasure you more?" "How can we feel more intimate?" "How can we improve our relationship?"

Simultaneous Orgasm

Another question students often ask is how they and their partners can achieve an orgasm together. Unfortunately, some couples have as an ideal a choreographed orgasmic release, timed so that it occurs at the same time for both partners. Not only is this difficult to achieve, but concentrating on this goal detracts from the enjoyment of the coital experience. As long as each person is satisfied, the exact timing of the orgasm is of no particular importance. Although simultaneous orgasm is an undeniably exciting event, it is only one of a wide range of satisfying sexual patterns.

Exploring the
DIMENSIONS
of Human Sexuality

Our feelings, attitudes, and beliefs regarding sexuality are influenced by our internal and external environments. Go to sexuality.jbpub.com/dimensions/4e to learn more about the biological, psychological, and sociological factors that affect your sexuality.

Biological Factors

- Sexual arousal and response are physiological reactions to sexual stimuli.
- Masters and Johnson showed that some aspects of the human sexual response cycle are similar in men and women; however, differences exist.
- The body releases hormones when a person is sexually stimulated.
- Physical disabilities, injuries, or illness may alter the ability to respond to sexual stimuli.
- Male testosterone levels decline with age, affecting sexual response.
- Drugs, alcohol, and some aphrodisiacs may alter sexual response.

Sociocultural Factors

Biological factors are influenced by sociocultural and psychological factors. For example, some people are turned on by pornography; others are turned off.

- Religious beliefs influence our feelings about sexuality in general.
- Culture and ethnic heritage influence what we find sensual or attractive.
- Media and ads influence the types of sexual stimulation to which we react.
- Family, neighbors, and friends provide information about and influence our sexuality.
- Ethical decisions must be made regarding how far you and your partner are willing to go to achieve sexual arousal.

Psychological Factors

- Our feelings toward our partner influence the sexual response derived.
- Our level of experience influences our response to sexual stimuli.
- Learned attitudes and behaviors include discovering the stimuli to which we respond.
- Body image influences our self-concept. The better we feel about ourselves, the sexier an image we portray to others.

CASE STUDY

Although the human sexual response cycle is a physiological pattern, many factors influence the ways individuals actually experience the stages. Physical differences, including age, illness, injuries, and disabilities, may alter the response. Illicit drugs, alcohol, and aphrodisiacs also may alter the physical sensation we experience. Some drugs, such as Viagra, may enhance the response cycle.

The stimuli that we react to differ with culture and ethnic group, media exposure, even hygiene. Education and religious beliefs may also have an effect; a person who feels guilty about sexuality may have a more repressed reaction.

Finally, our self-image and our feelings about our partner greatly influence sexual response and arousal. Many people believe that happy times—experiencing a loving relationship, being successful professionally, and so on—make for better sex.

Summary

- When a sexual stimulus is encountered, a message is sent via nerves to the brain. Upon reaching the brain, the message passes through the reticular activating system either from or to the limbic system and the thalamus.

- During sexual arousal, the autonomic nervous system is responsible for sending signals through nerves that result in blood vessels in the penis and clitoris dilating. The effect of the dilation is that these structures become engorged with blood and, consequently, become erect.

- Sexual hormones are produced in the testes and ovaries and affect many different sexually related functions. For example, testosterone affects sexual interest, also known as libido.

- Masters and Johnson described the human sexual response cycle as consisting of four phases: excitement, plateau, orgasm, and resolution. Kaplan described the human sexual response cycle as being triphasic: desire, excitement, and resolution.

- The female sexual response cycle is more varied than the male sexual response cycle. Females sometimes experience a sexual response cycle similar to males except they are more capable of having multiple orgasms without having to pass through a refractory period. In addition, females can move from the excitement phase to the plateau phase and, without having an orgasm, return to resolution; they can also experience rapid escalation from excitement to orgasm without passing through a plateau phase.

- Orgasm is the release of sexual tension resulting in muscular contractions and, at least in males, ejaculation. In most males, orgasm is followed by a refractory (recovery) period in which orgasm is not possible. In many females, orgasm can occur without a refractory period.

- Orgasm in females is preceded by the uterus increasing in size and elevating, the inner two-thirds of the vagina lengthening and expanding, lubrication of the vaginal walls, engorgement of blood in the outer third of the vagina, and retraction of the clitoris under the clitoral hood.

- In males, orgasm is a two-stage process: emission and expulsion. Emission involves contractions of the vas deferens, seminal vesicles, prostate, and external and internal urethral sphincters. Expulsion consists of relaxation of the external urethral sphincter, contractions of the urethra and muscles at the base of the penis and the anus, and the expulsion of the ejaculate from the penis.

Discussion Questions

1. Describe the reaction of the mind and the body when one is aroused by a sensual stimulation. How might artificial hormones or aphrodisiacs alter the response cycle? How would alcohol or other mood-altering drugs affect the cycle?

2. Compare and contrast the Masters and Johnson human response cycle with the models proposed by Kaplan, Zilbergeld and Ellison, and Reed. Why does the Masters and Johnson model continue to attract the most attention?

3. Explain how understanding types of orgasms and recognizing orgasms could lead to a better sexual relationship.

Application Questions

Reread the story that opens the chapter and answer the following questions.

1. Assuming that Brian and Tanya start dating, which visible signs of sexual arousal (aside from erection) might Tanya detect in Brian? Which signs might Brian detect in Tanya?

2. Do you think Brian's feelings about Tanya might differ if he met her after gym class and she reeked of sweat? Explain.

Critical Thinking Questions

1. Laurie Cabot, a well-known practicing witch, often suggests that love potions or spells do work. She writes that a "spell is a thought, a projection, or a prayer." Thus Cabot implies that the psychological effort that you put into a spell can produce a physiological response. Given this idea, would a love potion work? Put another way, would the extra attention you lavish on someone make that person more attracted to you?

2. The drug Viagra positively affects sexual response, especially in older men. However, increased sexual response is accompanied by higher blood pressure and a faster heartbeat—which has resulted in heart attacks and some deaths. Explain why 30 million U.S. males have been willing to take this risk, albeit a small one. Also consider why their partners would want them to risk their health for sexual pleasure.

3. *Baywatch* was one of the most-viewed TV shows in the world, with more than 1 billion viewers per week. Apply what you learned in the chapter to explain why.

Critical Thinking Case

It has been argued that too much emphasis is placed on orgasm and not enough on the total sexual experience, including talking and nongenital touch. Because sexual intercourse is a way of expressing love for another, the argument proceeds, the emphasis during the experience should be on the total relationship, the love expressed, whole-body sensations, and the feeling of closeness. Concentrating exclusively or primarily on the orgasm is self-defeating and narrows one's experience of sexuality.

In contrast, some people believe that sexual intercourse (or mutual masturbation or oral–genital sex) certainly includes all of the above but, in addition, has a culmination—orgasm. This culmination is so satisfying and, given effective sexual therapy, so available that it should be sought. Although sexual intercourse and other modes of sexual expression can be satisfying without orgasm, an orgasmic conclusion certainly adds to the experience and satisfaction.

What do you think? Why?

Exploring Personal Dimensions

Sexual Stimuli

Once the senses encounter sexual stimuli, the brain takes over, deciding how to respond. You become sexually aroused, although you may decide, for many reasons, not to act on that sexual arousal. Which of the following sexual stimuli do you find arousing? If you have a partner, which does your partner find arousing? More importantly, with which stimuli do you share sexual arousal?

	YOU		YOUR PARTNER	
SIGHT				
Sexually explicit videos	Y	N	Y	N
Sexually explicit magazines	Y	N	Y	N
Romantic movies	Y	N	Y	N
Books	Y	N	Y	N
Lingerie	Y	N	Y	N
Skin	Y	N	Y	N
TOUCH				
Satin sheets	Y	N	Y	N
Leather	Y	N	Y	N
Massage	Y	N	Y	N
Scratching	Y	N	Y	N
SMELL				
Perfume (or cologne)	Y	N	Y	N
Flowers	Y	N	Y	N
Scented candles	Y	N	Y	N
TASTE				
Kissing	Y	N	Y	N
Oral sexual activities	Y	N	Y	N
Whipped cream	Y	N	Y	N
SOUND				
Whispering	Y	N	Y	N
Moaning (or groaning)	Y	N	Y	N
Music	Y	N	Y	N
Silence	Y	N	Y	N

What other sexual stimuli can you think of?

Suggested Readings

Bakos, S. C. *The orgasm bible: The latest research and techniques for reaching more powerful climaxes more often.* Beverly, MA: Quiver, 2008.

Barbach, L. *For yourself: The fulfillment of female sexuality.* New York: New American Library, 2000.

Barbach, L. *For each other: Sharing sexual intimacy.* New York: New American Library, 2001.

Bodansky, S., & Bodansky, V. *The illustrated guide to extended massive orgasm.* Alameda, CA: Hunter House, 2002.

Bodansky, V. *To bed or not to bed: What men want, what women want, how great sex happens.* Alameda, CA: Hunter House, 2005.

Carrellas, B., & Sprinkle, A. *Urban tantra: Sacred sex for the twenty-first century.* Berkeley, CA: Celestial Arts, 2007.

Chance, R. S. To love and to be loved: Sexuality and people with disabilities. *Journal of Psychology and Theology, 30* (2002), 195–209.

Chia, M., Chia, M., Abrams, D., & Abrams, R. C. *The multi-orgasmic couple: Sexual secrets every couple should know.* New York: HarperCollins, 2002.

Keesling, B. *Sexual pleasure: Reaching new heights of sexual arousal and intimacy,* 2nd ed. Alameda, CA: Hunter House, 2004.

Lacroix, N. *Tantric sex and lovemaking.* London, UK: Lorenz Books, 2008.

Stanway, A., & Geary, J. *The art of sensual loving.* Emeryville, CA: Avalon Publishing Group, 2003.

Taylor, S. *101 sex positions: Steamy new positions from mild to wild.* Berkeley, CA: Amorata Press, 2008.

Web Resources

For links to the web sites below, visit *http://sexuality.jbpub.com/dimensions/4e* and click on Resource Links.

Wikipedia, the Free Encyclopedia
http://en.wikipedia.org/wiki/Masters_and_Johnson

Description of the history of the Masters and Johnson team approach to sexual therapy. Also included are discussions of the four-stage model of sexual response, sexual response in the aging male and female, sexual dysfunction, and criticisms of the Masters and Johnson approach to sexual therapy.

Sinclair Intimacy Institute
www.bettersex.com/sexdata

The Sinclair Intimacy Institute is an online sexual health encyclopedia. It regularly consults with sexual health experts, many of whom serve on the Sinclair Advisory Council, to provide an accurate and up-to-date sexuality dictionary, covering more than 270 sexuality-related terms; access to additional sexual health online resources to further research sexual topics of interest; and answers to frequently asked questions.

SexTutor.com
www.sextutor.com

Sex Tutor offers accurate, clearly written, helpful sex advice on such topics as anal sex, cunnilingus, fellatio, female ejaculation, female masturbation, male masturbation, kissing, sex positions, prolonging sex, adult toys, and others.

iVillage.co.uk: The Website for Women
http://iVillage.co.uk/relationships/sex

Provides articles discussing various sex-related topics for women. Among these topics are sexual dilemmas, hot sex, talk about sex, sex and health, oral sex, orgasms, bedroom basics, and others.

Global Oneness: Sexual Arousal—Causes of Human Sexual Arousal
www.experiencefestival.com/sexual_arousal_-_causes_of_human_sexual_arousal

A selection of articles related to various aspects of human sexual arousal.

FEATURES

Ethical Dimensions
Abstinence-Only
Versus Comprehensive
Sexuality Education

Communication Dimensions
Condom Use and
Consistency: Talking
About Condom Use

Multicultural Dimensions
Ethnic and Age
Differences in Access
to Emergency
Contraception

Gender Dimensions
Gender Equality in
Contraception Use

Gender Dimensions
Margaret H. Sanger: A
Woman of Influence

Global Dimensions
Emergency
Contraception: How
Is NOR-Levo in France
Different from Plan B
in the United States?

Global Dimensions
Unmet Need for
Contraception in
Developing Countries

CHAPTER OBJECTIVES

1 Discuss the reasons to use contraceptives, ways to choose a contraceptive, and the difference between perfect use and typical use.

2 Evaluate the nonprescription methods of contraception, including the effectiveness, the reversibility, and the advantages and disadvantages of each. Explain why some have higher rates of user effectiveness than others.

3 Evaluate the prescription methods of contraception, including the effectiveness, the reversibility, and the advantages and disadvantages of each. Explain why some have higher rates of user effectiveness than others.

4 Discuss the viability of future contraceptive methods. Consider the impact of gender issues, pharmaceutical industry costs for litigation, federal regulation compliance, and FDA approval.

sexuality.jbpub.com/dimensions/4e

Ethical Dimensions: Abstinence-Only Versus Comprehensive
  Sexuality Education
Emergency Contraception
The Future of Contraceptives

INTRODUCTION

*T*hroughout life, people's use of and need for contraceptives change. The case history of Susan presents a typical contraceptive user. During her first sexual encounter at age 18 years, Susan's high school boyfriend used withdrawal.

During her freshman year at college, she began a steady sexual relationship with Jack. Because she was in a monogamous relationship and did not have to worry about sexually transmitted infection (STI) transmission, Susan began to use oral contraceptives (the pill). After she had difficulty remembering to take her pill every day, Susan switched to injectable medroxyprogesterone acetate (Depo-Provera). Every 3 months she would receive her birth-control shot at a clinic.

After she and Jack broke up, she was abstinent for a year—the most foolproof method of contraception available. Susan graduated from college and was fitted with a diaphragm; she also used condoms with her two partners.

By age 25 years she married Stephen and had levonorgestrel (Norplant) inserted into her upper arm. The Norplant releases a steady stream of contraceptive into the reproductive system and is effective for up to 5 years. When the company producing the implants withdrew them from the market, she had the Norplant removed. At her doctor's suggestion, she switched to a non-hormone-based contraceptive (foam and condoms) for 3 months before trying to conceive a child.

After the birth of her first child, she was fitted with an intrauterine device (IUD). Two years later it was removed when she planned to conceive a second child. After the birth of their second child, Stephen had a vasectomy. After several follow-up tests to assure that no sperm were left in his ejaculate, Susan and Stephen enjoyed monogamous, unprotected sex.

Five years later, Susan and Stephen divorced. As one of her first acts as a newly divorced woman, Susan had a laparoscopy—a method of female sterilization. Although she could not become pregnant, she also began to practice safer sex and insisted that her partners wear latex condoms.

In other words, it is possible for a woman to use nearly every contraceptive method available during her more than 30 years of fertility. The method may change, depending on where she is in the life cycle.

This chapter reviews the currently available methods of contraception, their effectiveness, and their advantages and disadvantages.

■ Contraception

Contraception is the prevention of conception. You may already have thought hard about the consequences of such decisions as whether to become pregnant, have an abortion, or adopt a child. If you

> **contraception**
> Means of preventing pregnancy.

have considered or do consider such matters, you will understand how significant contraception can be to your life. Many babies are born each year to mothers who are too young or too emotionally immature to raise them well, or to mothers who are too old to carry a fetus to term without a high probability of a birth defect. Many pregnant teenagers and their sexual partners never finish their schooling because of the need to support and care for their child. Some couples who marry in response to pregnancy are soon divorced. Married couples who have already raised children may find yet another pregnancy a threat to their economic and psychological health. Managing this financial burden, as well as dealing with the time and energy necessary to care for an infant, can be as harmful to them—though perhaps in different ways—as to teenagers. But clearly the economic burden a child entails can present problems for people in various age groups and income levels.

Contraceptive and condom use should be routine for sexually active young people and adults unless they are seeking pregnancy *and* they are in a mutually monogamous relationship. Yet, too many people use contraception inconsistently or ineffectively. The result is that the United States has a higher rate of unintended pregnancies than all other developed countries. Currently, it is estimated that every year 1 in 20 American women has an unintended preg-

nancy (Finer & Henshaw, 2006). Researchers know that many factors increase one's motivation to use contraception. These factors include the following:

- Ability to communicate with a partner
- Cost and accessibility of a method
- Frequency of sexual intercourse
- Motivation to avoid pregnancy
- STI concerns and risks
- Contraceptive's side effects
- One's attitudes and openness about sexuality (Frost, Darroch, & Remez, 2008; Hatcher et al., 2007)

Ask yourself these questions as you read this chapter: Am I ready to have sexual intercourse? Am I committed to avoiding pregnancy myself or preventing a partner's pregnancy at this time? Am I committed to avoiding passing on a sexually transmitted infection? Am I committed to using a contraceptive method every time I have intercourse? Is my partner? If the answer to any of these questions is no, ask yourself another question: What will I do when a pregnancy occurs? Remember, almost 9 in 10 heterosexual couples who do not use a contraceptive method become pregnant within a year.

Contraceptive Effectiveness

We begin our discussion of contraception methods with a warning: The effectiveness of each method is difficult to determine precisely, so you should consider the rates cited for each method as being *approximations only*. Also note that for each method we provide both the percentage of women experiencing an unintended pregnancy during the first year of contraceptive method use when the method is used perfectly (consistently and correctly) and the percentage when it is used typically (Trussell, 2007).

In the latter setting, mistakes are often made—for example, a condom may be put on incorrectly. Consequently, **typical use** is always less effective than **perfect use**. A good contraceptive method is one that limits the gap between the way it is prescribed to be used and the way it is actually used. As can be seen in Table 7.1, there is usually a vast difference between these two measures of contraceptive effectiveness.

Use is measured by the number of women in 100 who will become pregnant during the first year of use of the particular method. Table 7.1 shows the effectiveness of varied methods of contraception.

Contraception Versus Safer Sex

Couples today need to discuss how they will prevent both pregnancy and transmission of STIs (see Chapter 15). Many of the most effective methods of preventing pregnancies—oral contraceptives, hormonal implants, sterilization—provide *no* protection against STIs. The IUD, which is highly effective at preventing pregnancies, is not recommended for women who have either gonorrhea or chlamydia (WHO, 2008). The male condom provides the best protection available against sexually transmitted infection but has a lower rate of effectiveness against pregnancy. There are three ways to achieve maximal effectiveness against both STIs and pregnancies relative to sexual intercourse: abstain from all types of intercourse, use a condom and a spermicide together, or use a condom and a hormonal contraceptive together. Because STIs pose a threat to the future fertility and health of college students, and because emergency contraception (EC) and abortion are available, many experts recommend that if only one method is used, it should be a condom.

■ Nonprescription Methods

Abstinence

People define **abstinence** in different ways: For some it means no sexual contact of any kind; for others it means no **penetrative behaviors**, including penile–

vaginal intercourse, oral sex, or anal intercourse. Many adolescents, young adults, and adults choose to abstain. People choose abstinence for a variety of reasons:

typical use
The ability of a method of contraception to prevent pregnancy as actually used at home by people not being monitored.

perfect use
The ability of a method of contraception to prevent pregnancy as measured by consistent and correct use.

abstinence
Avoidance of any type of sexual intercourse.

penetrative behaviors
Any behavior whereby penetration occurs—for example, penile–vaginal intercourse, oral sex, or anal intercourse.

- Their religion teaches that sexual intercourse is appropriate only in marriage.

- They are not in a loving, committed relationship.

- They do not have a partner.

- They want to avoid the risk of pregnancy or STI.

- The relationship they are in is not ready for the intimacy of intercourse.

- They are not ready for intercourse.

- They are ill or their partner is ill.

- They or a partner have been exposed to an STI.

- They feel that a sexual relationship would complicate their life.

Choosing abstinence does not necessarily mean forgoing sexual pleasure. There are many ways to give and receive sexual pleasure without the risks of sexual intercourse. These include deep kissing, massages, fondling, dancing, masturbating alone, masturbating together, and showering together.

However, for these activities not to end in intercourse, couples must communicate their desire not to have sexual intercourse in any form and must agree to stick to sexual limits.

Effectiveness
Abstinence is the only 100% effective method of fertility control and STI prevention—if the couple or individual is truly committed to remaining abstinent. Actual user effectiveness rates are unknown. A popular saying is that vows of abstinence fail much more frequently than condoms do; people say that they are practicing abstinence but have intercourse in spite of their intention. Communication and commitment are essential. Because abstinence has never had the scientific scrutiny given other methods to determine user or typical use effectiveness, there are no data to make a fair comparison between abstinence effectiveness and other methods. Proponents of abstinence may cite typical use of various contraceptive methods to demonstrate their risk of failure and yet claim the perfect use effectiveness rate of abstinence as 100%. Such a

TABLE 7.1 **Contraceptive Effectiveness: Rates of Unintended Pregnancies per 100 Women**

Method	Consistent and Correct (Perfect) Use	As Commonly Used (Typical Use) (U.S.; Trussell, 2007)	As Commonly Used (Typical Use) (Developing Countries; Cleland & Ali, 2004)
Implants (Implanon)	0.05	0.05	—
Male sterilization (vasectomy)	0.1	0.15	—
Levonorgestrel IUD (Mirena IUS)	0.2	0.2	—
Female sterilization	0.5	0.5	—
Copper-bearing IUD (ParaGard copper T)	0.6	0.8	2
LAM (lactational amenorrhea method)[1]	0.9	2	—
Injectables			
Combined monthly	0.05	3	—
Progestin only	0.3	3	2
Combined pill and progestin-only pill	0.3	8	7
Combined patch (Evra Patch)	0.3	8	—
Combined vaginal ring (NuvaRing)	0.3	8	—
Condom[2]			
Male	2	15	10
Female (Reality)	5	21	—
Fertility awareness-based methods			
Ovulation method[3]	3	—	—
Two-day method[3]	4	—	—
Standard days method[3]	5	—	—
Diaphragm with spermicide	6	16	—
Sponge			
Nulliparous women[4]	9	16	—
Parous women[5]	20	32	—
Withdrawal	4	27	21
Spermicides[6]	18	25	—
Cervical caps			
Nulliparous women[4]	9	16	—
Parous women[5]	26	32	—
No method[7]	85	85	85

Key

0–0.9	1–9	10–25	26–32
Very effective	Effective	Moderately effective	Less effective

1. LAM is a highly effective, *temporary* method of contraception. However, to maintain effective protection against pregnancy, another method of contraception must be used as soon as menstruation resumes, the frequency or duration of breastfeeding is reduced, bottle feeding is introduced, or the baby reaches 6 months of age.
2. Without spermicides.
3. The ovulation and 2-day methods are based on evaluation of cervical mucus. The standard days method avoids intercourse on cycle days 8 through 19.
4. Pregnancy rate for women who have never given birth.
5. Pregnancy rate for women who have given birth.
6. Foams, creams, gels, vaginal suppositories, and vaginal film.
7. The percentages becoming pregnant in columns (2) and (3) are based on data from populations where contraception is not used and from women who cease using contraception in an effort to become pregnant. Among such populations, approximately 89% become pregnant within 1 year. This estimate was lowered slightly (to 85%) to represent the percentage who would become pregnant within 1 year among women now relying on reversible methods of contraception if they abandoned contraception altogether.

Sources: Adapted from Trussel, 2007; Cleland & Ali, 2004.

comparison is inappropriate from a public health perspective unless perfect use effectiveness rates are used for the other methods (for example, male condom, 98%; withdrawal, 96%) (Dailard, 2003).

Reversibility
Abstinence does not affect fertility.

Advantages and Disadvantages
Abstinence is an excellent method of fertility control and STI prevention. It is free, you always have it with you, there are no side effects, and no one's parents will be upset if you use it! It is 100% effective but only if you use it every time and only if your partner is equally committed to its use. Just as with any method, one should occasionally reconsider whether it is still the method of choice. Research demonstrates how difficult it is to practice abstinence consistently over time. One study showed that 60% of college students who pledged virginity had broken their vow to remain abstinent until marriage. Such a high risk of failure would be concern enough, but another study showed that teens who promised to abstain from sex until marriage were more likely to have unprotected sex when they broke their pledge than those who never made such a promise. Perhaps strategies to promote abstinence are actually increasing the risks for people when they eventually become sexually active (Dailard, 2003). For that reason, it is particularly important for anyone using abstinence as a contraceptive method to choose a different method *before* they stop using abstinence.

Ethical DIMENSIONS

Abstinence-Only Versus Comprehensive Sexuality Education

For more than three decades, "abstinence-only-until-marriage" was the government-sanctioned approach to reducing U.S. rates of teen pregnancy and STIs. More than $1 billion in federal and mandated state matching grants supported sexuality education (some say "values education" is a more appropriate label) that restricts or ignores the effectiveness of contraceptives and safer-sex behaviors (Santelli et al., 2009).

Recently, the tide may have turned, as continued funding was hotly debated before a House Oversight Committee in 2008. A panel of public health experts and researchers testified that evidence to support the effectiveness of these programs is lacking. In fact, a study published in the January 2009 issue of *Pediatrics* (Rosenbaum, 2009) found that teens signing virginity pledges are just as likely to engage in sexual behavior as those who do not sign such pledges. Moreover, they are less likely to use contraception, are less likely to get tested for STIs, and may have STIs for longer periods of time when they do break their pledges. Two other major studies, Mathematica findings (Trenholm et al., 2007) and *Emerging Answers 2007* (Kirby, 2007), demonstrated that the evaluated abstinence education programs have no statistically significant beneficial impact on the sexual behavior of young people; in fact, strong evidence does not exist that *any* abstinence program delays initiation of sex, hastens return to abstinence, or reduces the number of sexual partners.

Given these findings, it is not surprising that many leading health professional groups have raised serious ethical concerns about U.S. support for abstinence-only sexuality education programs. Policy apprehension is based on questionable science, medical inaccuracies, withholding health- and life-saving information, and being antithetical to informed consent and free choice (SIECUS, 2008a). Concern at the state level is evidenced by the trend to no longer accept and match funding that supports abstinence-only education programs (SIECUS, 2008b). Within Congress, Responsible Education About Life (REAL) Acts have been introduced in both the House and Senate. This change in direction matches what Americans say they want for their children. A 2005–2006 nationally representative survey of U.S. adults, published in the *Archives of Pediatrics and Adolescent Medicine* (Bleakley, Hennessy, & Fishbein, 2006), demonstrated strong support for comprehensive sexuality education (favored by 82% of those polled); 68% favored instruction on how to use a condom; only 36% supported abstinence-only education.

The goal underlying this fundamental change is to make sure that young people have the information and skills they will need to make healthy choices about sexual behavior. If adolescents are sexually active, or will be shortly, they need information to protect themselves. Where there is a need to know, medically incomplete is medically inaccurate (Boonstra, 2009).

Continued

Ethical DIMENSIONS

Abstinence-Only Versus Comprehensive Sexuality Education—cont'd

Abstinence Versus Sex Education

Abstinence-Only Education, as Defined by 1996 Federal Law

According to Title V of the Social Security Act, an eligible abstinence education program is a program that

(A) has as its exclusive purpose, teaching the social, physiological, and health gains to be realized by abstaining from sexual activity;

(B) teaches abstinence from sexual activity outside marriage as the expected standard for all school-age children;

(C) teaches that abstinence from sexual activity is the only certain way to avoid out-of-wedlock pregnancy, sexually transmitted diseases, and other associated health problems;

(D) teaches that a mutually faithful monogamous relationship in the context of marriage is the expected standard of human sexual activity;

(E) teaches that sexual activity outside of the context of marriage is likely to have harmful psychological and physical effects;

(F) teaches that bearing children out of wedlock is likely to have harmful consequences for the child, the child's parents, and society;

(G) teaches young people how to reject sexual advances and how alcohol and drug use increases vulnerability to sexual advances; and

(H) teaches the importance of attaining self-sufficiency before engaging in sexual activity.

Sex Education, as Defined by the Responsible Education About Life Act

According to the Responsible Education About Life Act, a sex education program is a program that

(1) is age appropriate and medically accurate;

(2) stresses the value of abstinence while not ignoring those young people who have had or are having sexual intercourse;

(3) provides information about the health benefits and side effects of all contraceptive and barrier methods used—

    (a) as a means to prevent pregnancy; and

    (b) to reduce the risk of contracting sexually transmitted disease, including HIV/AIDS;

(4) encourages family communication between parent and child about sexuality;

(5) teaches young people the skills to make responsible decisions about sexuality, including how to avoid unwanted verbal, physical, and sexual advances and how to avoid making verbal, physical, and sexual advances that are not wanted by the other party;

(6) develops healthy relationships, including the prevention of dating and sexual violence;

(7) teaches young people how alcohol and drug use can affect responsible decision making; and

(8) does not teach or promote religion.

Source: Boonstra, H. D. Advocates call for a new approach after the era of "abstinence-only" sex education. *Guttmacher Policy Review, 12* (Winter 2009), 6–11. Retrieved June 17, 2009, from www.guttmacherinstitute.com/pubs/gpr/12/1/gpr120106.pd.

Withdrawal

Withdrawal is probably the oldest contraceptive method on record. In the Bible, Onan practices withdrawal, or **coitus interruptus**, so as not to impregnate his brother's widow. To practice withdrawal, the couple has vaginal intercourse until the man feels that he is about to ejaculate. He withdraws his penis and ejaculates away from the woman's vulva.

> **withdrawal**
> Removing the penis from the vagina before ejaculation.
>
> **coitus interruptus**
> The Latin term for *withdrawal,* which means "interrupted intercourse."

Effectiveness

Many people assume that withdrawal is an ineffective method of contraception. However, many contraceptive experts believe that withdrawal is an underrated method. It is about as effective as most barrier methods. When practiced correctly, the rate of efficacy for withdrawal is 4 pregnancies per 100 per year. When practiced incorrectly, the rate of efficacy lowers to 27 pregnancies per 100 per year (WHO, 2008).

Many people have been taught that preejaculate fluid might contain sperm. However, preejaculate fluid is a neutralizing solution produced by the Cowper's glands (see Chapter 5). Zukerman and Orvieto (2007) studied 12 subjects who all had sperm in routine semen analysis; none of their preejaculatory samples contained sperm. Therefore, the researchers concluded that the failure of coitus interruptus as a contraceptive method is probably due to late withdrawal (after emission and onset of ejaculation) because preejaculatory fluid secreted at the tip of the urethra during sexual stimulation did not contain sperm.

To quote the authors of *Contraceptive Technology* (Hatcher et al., 2007), "Withdrawal is definitely better than using no contraceptive at all." If the man does not withdraw in time and the woman is at a fertile point in her cycle, emergency contraception should be considered (covered later in this chapter).

Advantages and Disadvantages

Withdrawal is free, always available, and relatively easy to use. It has no medical side effects, and it encourages male involvement.

The major disadvantage to withdrawal is that some men, particularly young men, do not recognize impending ejaculation and thus ejaculate inside their partner, putting her at risk of pregnancy. Thus it has a relatively high failure rate among typical users and does not adequately protect against STIs. However, it may reduce the risk of fluid-borne infection. Some couples report that withdrawal reduces the sexual pleasure of the woman and intensity of orgasm of the man. It requires the man to think about what is happening during intercourse.

Male Condom

Condoms are one of the oldest contraceptive methods (Hatcher et al., 2007). Today most condoms are made of **latex**, a synthetic form of rubber. About 5% of condoms are made from the intestines of lambs; these are known as *skin* or *lambskin* condoms. Skin condoms, because they are more porous than latex condoms, do not provide protec-

> **condom**
> A sheath that covers the penis.
>
> **latex**
> A synthetic rubber.

A wide variety of condoms are available in various colors, sizes—even flavors. Only latex condoms have been shown to prevent transmission of STIs and HIV; animal skin condoms do not. Condoms should be used in every act of intercourse, from start to finish.

> **polyurethane**
> A type of plastic.

tion against many STIs and are not recommended for that purpose.

In 1997, the U.S. Food and Drug Administration (FDA) approved the first condom made of **polyurethane**, a type of plastic. Initial studies show that polyurethane condoms are as effective as latex condoms for both contraception and STI prevention but more comfortable to use (Kalichman & Cherry, 1999). Subjectively, consumers expressed significantly greater preference for the polyurethane condom over latex in regard to appearance, lack of smell, likelihood of slippage, comfort, sensitivity, natural look, natural feel, and overall (Rosenberg et al., 1996).

There are more than 100 brands of condoms available in the United States today. The U.S. Centers for Disease Control and Prevention provides the following directions for the consistent and correct use of condoms. Individuals who use condoms to prevent unwanted pregnancies and STIs must understand the meaning of *consistent* and *correct* condom use.

CONSISTENT USE

- Use a condom with every act of sexual intercourse, from start to finish, including penile–vaginal intercourse, oral intercourse, and anal intercourse.

CORRECT USE

- Store condoms in a cool place out of direct sunlight (not in wallets or glove compartments). Latex will become brittle as a result of changes in temperature, rough handling, and age. Do not use damaged, discolored, brittle, or sticky condoms.

- Check the date on the condom carefully. If it is an expiration date, do not use the condom beyond that date. If it is a date of production, the condom may be used for several years beyond that date (2 years for spermicidal condoms, 5 years for nonspermicidal latex condoms) (Zieman et al., 2007).

Communication
DIMENSIONS

Condom Use and Consistency: Talking About Condom Use

Except for withdrawal, condoms have the greatest gap between perfect use (98% effectiveness) and typical use (82.6%–90% effectiveness) of all the contraceptive methods (see Table 7.1). Because this method is popular and its use is increasing (the rate of condom use at first sex increased from 22% in the 1970s to 67% in 2002), factors associated with its use and consistency are important to know (Guttmacher, 2008). Among teens, high rates of both STIs and unintended pregnancy could be reduced with condom use. A study examining condom use patterns among sexually experienced male adolescents, age 15–19, found multiple domains of influence. Those who had formal sex education, had positive attitudes about condoms, were younger, had a partner close in age, and were committed to a relationship had greater odds of correct and consistent condom use. Recommendations include providing programs with targeted services that address condom use attitudes and that help teens negotiate condom use decision making with sexual partners (Sonenstein, 2008). The following scenario could be helpful.

You are on your third date in a nice restaurant with a new friend. You are attracted to each other; on the last date, you spent a pretty hot half hour kissing and touching each other. You are pretty sure that you are ready to have intercourse and are hoping that your new friend feels the same way. But how do you know? And, how do you bring up condom use?

The waiter just delivered dessert. Dinner is coming to an end. Your date says, "Hmmm, do you want to come back to my room?" You say, "I think there are a few things we need to talk about first."

Here's how a successful discussion about condoms with a new partner might go.

CHRIS: I really like you. I've been fantasizing a lot since our last date about us having sex.

PAT: Me, too. But, it's important to me that we use condoms and practice safe sex.

CHRIS: Of course. I always use condoms. And because I was hoping you were interested too, I bought some today.

PAT: I bought some today, too! How about we skip dessert?

But of course, it is not always that easy (although it should be). Chris might have said, "I hate condoms." Here are some ways that Pat might answer.

1. "Not with me you won't. I've learned how to make condom use really fun. I hope you want me to show you."
2. "I'm really sorry to hear that. I would never have sex with someone unless he used a condom."
3. "Tell me which condoms you've used. Maybe we can try a different brand or type."
4. "Well, it looks as if we have an important decision to make. We can agree not to have any kind of intercourse and just mess around. Or, we can just be friends. But, I won't have intercourse with you without a condom."

Condom use with a new partner is essential until you have both been tested for STIs and have decided to be monogamous. Remember, "A man who doesn't want to use a condom with you probably didn't use one with his last partner either" (Haffner & Schwartz, 1998).

- Carefully open the condom package—teeth or fingernails can tear the condom.

- Use a new condom for every act of sexual intercourse.

- Put on the condom after the penis is erect and before it touches any part of a partner's body. A man who is uncircumcised must pull back the foreskin before putting on the condom.

- Put on the condom by pinching the reservoir tip and unrolling it all the way down the shaft of the penis from head to base (see Figure 7.1). If the condom does not have a reservoir tip, pinch it to leave a half-inch space at the head of the penis in which semen can collect after ejaculation.

- Withdraw the penis immediately if the condom breaks during sexual intercourse, and put on a new condom before resuming intercourse. When a condom breaks, use spermicidal foam or jelly and speak to a health care provider about emergency contraception.

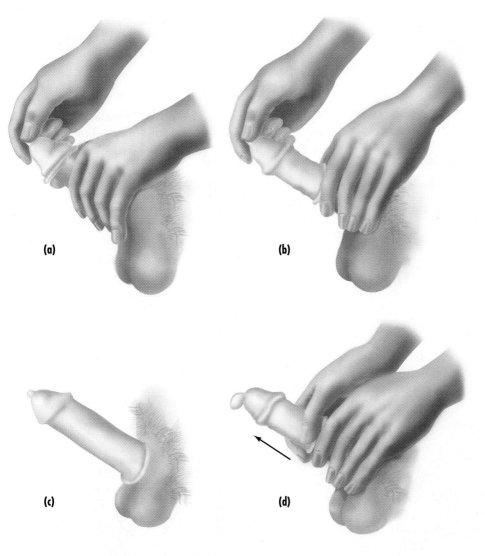

(a)   (b)

(c)   (d)

FIGURE **7.1** If you have never used a condom, you should practice before the first time you use one during sexual intercourse. To put a condom on: (a) Put on the condom by pinching the reservoir tip and unrolling it all the way down the shaft of the penis. (b) Be sure that there are no air bubbles, which could cause the condom to break. (c) The condom should have extra rubber at the top and should be unrolled to the very base of the penis. (d) After ejaculation, be sure to withdraw the penis with one hand holding the rim of the condom so that it does not accidentally slip off or leak.

- Use only water-based or silicone-based lubrication with latex condoms. Use oil-based lubricants such as cooking/vegetable oil, baby oil, hand lotion, or petroleum jelly only with polyurethane condoms. Spermicidal condoms are no longer recommended, although spermicides do not damage latex.

- Withdraw the penis immediately after ejaculation, while the penis is still erect; grasp the rim of the condom between the fingers, and slowly withdraw the penis (with the condom still on) so that no semen is spilled.

- Check for breakage; dispose of condom (Zieman et al., 2007).

Effectiveness
Condoms are very effective: Only 5% of couples using a condom correctly and for every act of intercourse become pregnant in the first year of use. It is 79% effective in typical users. The major reason condoms fail is that people forget to use them for each act of intercourse. Breakage, slippage, or leakage can also reduce effectiveness. Condom fit may be a factor. Do not use lubricant inside a condom or use one that is too large; it may slip off. If the condom is too small, breakage or reduced sensation may be a problem. Condoms are also highly effective at preventing the spread of HIV, gonorrhea, chlamydia, and trichomoniasis (Zieman et al., 2007).

Advantages and Disadvantages
Advantages of condoms include the following: They are relatively inexpensive, they are easy to obtain, they do not require a visit to the doctor, they may help a man control ejaculation, they provide protection from STIs (with consistent use, risk of HIV transmission is reduced 10-fold), and they have none of the unhealthy side effects associated with some of the other methods of contraception. Finally, condom use takes some of the burden of birth control off women. As the women's movement works toward female–male equality, more and more women seek to share the practice of birth control with their partners.

Posters have been part of media campaigns to raise awareness and overcome societal taboos about condom use. The South Australia Health Commission developed this one. In many countries the effort to increase condom use acceptance is central to AIDS prevention programs.

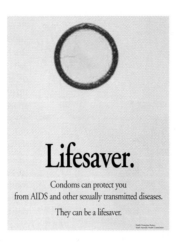

Lifesaver.

Condoms can protect you from AIDS and other sexually transmitted diseases.

They can be a lifesaver.

The major disadvantage is that many men complain that condoms reduce sensitivity and spontaneity. Trying different brands can improve sensation, and putting the condom on as foreplay can make it more fun. Another potential problem is a latex allergy or reaction to spermicide. About 2% to 3% of Americans are allergic to latex and another 14% are latex

sensitive. Polyurethane condoms (Durex-Avanti or Trojan-Supra) or the female (Reality) condom (see below) are alternatives (Zieman et al., 2007).

Female Condom

A recent vaginal barrier is the **female condom** (Figure 7.2). The female condom appeared on the market in the United States in 1993. The Reality Female Condom is a loose-fitting sheath made of polyurethane with rings on both ends. One ring covers the cervix; the other ring remains outside the vagina and partially covers the vulva. A new version of the female condom, the FC2, was approved by the U.S. Food and Drug Administration (FDA) in March 2009. Although it looks similar to its predecessor, it is made from synthetic rubber, making it cheaper to produce. The FC2 is also less noisy during use. In addition to cost, complaints about squeaky noises were among the factors that slowed acceptance of the original version. For now, the price

female condom
A polyurethane or synthetic rubber sheath with flexible inner and outer rings worn inside the vagina.

FIGURE 7.2 Inserting a female condom. (a) Photo of a female condom. (b) The inner ring is squeezed for insertion and the sheath inserted into the vagina similarly to a tampon. (c) With the index finger, push the inside of the inner ring as far as it will go. Make sure the sheath is not twisted during insertion. The outer ring should remain outside the vagina. (d) Hold the outer ring in place while inserting the penis, making sure the penis is inserted into the condom and not next to it. Be careful when removing the condom to ensure semen does not spill out.

Multicultural
DIMENSIONS

Ethnic and Age Differences in Access to Emergency Contraception

Background Information

Emergency contraception (EC) includes any method used after intercourse to prevent pregnancy. None of the current methods is an abortifacient and none disturbs an implanted pregnancy. There are currently three methods in widespread use worldwide:

- High-dose progestin-only contraceptive pills (POPs)—Plan B
- Thirteen brands of combined oral contraceptive pills (COCs)—Yuzpe method
- Copper IUD insertion (Paragard)

An estimated 51,000 pregnancies were averted by EC use in 2000, accounting for 43% of the decrease in abortions since 1994. Only the two hormonal methods (oral contraceptive pills) are utilized to any significant degree in the United States.

Research Findings

- Studies have found women getting EC in advance are not more likely to have unprotected sex.
- Women in EC studies often underutilize EC. Inconvenience and fear of the side effects were reasons for nonuse cited in one study.
- A recent review found increased access to EC enhanced use but did not decrease pregnancy rates.
- EC is an appropriate backup option for adolescents. Having EC available does *not* make teens less likely to use regular contraception or more likely to have unprotected sex.

Accessibility

In August 2006, the U.S. FDA ruled that Plan B can be provided from behind the counter (i.e., directly from the pharmacist without a prescription) for people ages 18 and older. At the time of this writing, the states with EC available directly from pharmacies for people of any age are Alaska, California, Hawaii, Maine, Massachusetts, Montana, New Hampshire, New Mexico, Vermont, and Washington. In 34 countries, EC is available directly from pharmacies (Zieman et al., 2007).

Equal Access?

In California, EC is available without a prescription to females younger than 18 through pharmacy access. Timely access to this method of contraception is critical to reduce the rate of unintended pregnancy among adolescents. One study was designed to explore barriers adolescents might face and differences in access to EC by age, ethnicity, and region.

In 2005–2006, researchers posing as English- and Spanish-speaking females—who said they either were 15 and had had unprotected intercourse last night or were 18 and had had unprotected sex 4 days ago—called 115 pharmacies in California. Each pharmacy received one call using each scenario; a call was considered successful if the caller was told she could come in to obtain the method. Statistical measures were used to assess differences between subgroups. In-depth interviews with 22 providers and pharmacists were also conducted, and emergent themes were identified.

Thirty-six percent of all calls were successful. Spanish speakers were less successful than English speakers (24% versus 48%), and callers to rural pharmacies were less successful than callers to urban ones (27% versus 44%). Although rural pharmacies were more likely to offer Spanish-language services, Spanish-speaking callers to these pharmacies were the least successful of all callers (17%). Spanish speakers were also less successful than English speakers when calling urban pharmacies (30% versus 57%).

Interviews suggested that little cooperation existed between pharmacists and clinicians and that dispensing the EC method at clinics was a favorable option for adolescents. Adolescents face significant barriers to obtaining emergency contraception, but the expansion of Spanish-language services at pharmacies and greater collaboration between providers and pharmacists could improve access (Sampson et al., 2009).

is about 60 cents compared to less than 4 cents for mass-distributed male condoms, a difference that is an issue in the developing world (Crary, 2009).

The female condom is like the male condom in that it can be used only for one act of intercourse. It is unlike the male condom because it can be inserted up to 8 hours before intercourse, although it may not be comfortable for everyday wear. Female and male condoms should *not* be used together because they can stick together and dislodge each other.

Effectiveness

The female condom has effectiveness rates similar to those of the diaphragm and cervical cap. For perfect users, it is 98% effective in preventing pregnancies. In typical users, studies have found it to be 85% effective. As noted by the Planned Parenthood Federation of America (2003), although it is not as effective as the male condom, the female condom is a valuable option for women who want to prevent STI or unintended pregnancy.

Advantages and Disadvantages

This method is available without prescription, is controlled by the woman, can be inserted in advance of intercourse, and is a safe alternative for people with latex allergy or sensitivity. Its disadvantages include somewhat difficult insertion requiring practice for new users and noise during intercourse that may be distracting. The noise can be reduced with additional lubricant, however.

Contraceptive Sponges

The Today contraceptive sponge is made of polyurethane foam (latex-free) and is prefilled with Nonoxynol 9 spermicide (discussed in the next section) that is continuously released into the vagina during use. The sponge acts both as a mechanical barrier to sperm migration into the cervical canal and as a chemical agent by applying spermicide directly to the cervix. It is not reusable. The sponge is sold over the counter, without the need for a prescription (three sponges for $14.99). When used as a primary method, this barrier method should be coupled with counseling to have EC pills on hand at home.

This contraceptive method was originally introduced in 1983. The manufacturer stopped distributing the product over a dispute not related to its quality or efficacy. In spring 2009, the new, exclusive distributor of the Today Vaginal Contraceptive Sponge for the United States, Canada, and European Union announced that the sponge has been relaunched through three major drug store chains in the United States (Mayer Laboratories, 2009).

Effectiveness

When the sponge was introduced originally, its perfect-use failure rate in the first year of use was 9% to 11%; the typical-use failure rate in the first year was not much different, at 13% to 16% (Edelman, 1987). A more recent review found pregnancy rates during 1 year of sponge use to be in the range of 17% to 24% as compared to 11% to 13% for the diaphragm (Kuyoh et al., 2003). Table 7.1 reports that the sponge is twice as effective for women who have never given birth (nulliparous women: perfect

The contraceptive sponge is a one-time use method combining a barrier that prevents sperm from entering the cervix with a chemical spermicide.

use 9% and typical use 16%) as for those who have given birth (parous women: 20% perfect use and 32% typical use).

Advantages and Disadvantages

The contraceptive sponge method is controlled by the woman, is active immediately after placement, can be inserted several hours before sexual intercourse to permit spontaneity, can remain in place for multiple acts of intercourse up to 24 hours, and is entirely reversible. This female-controlled barrier method may reduce risk of cervical infections, including gonorrhea, chlamydia, and pelvic inflammatory disease, but offers no protection against HIV infection.

Some disadvantages are that the sponge requires placement prior to genital contact, which may reduce spontaneity of sex; some women do not like placing their fingers or a foreign body into their vagina; the sponge does not provide protection against HIV and some STIs as a result of the presence of Nonoxynol 9 as the spermicide; the couple must use condoms if they are considered to be "at risk"; failure rates are higher than with hormonal contraception; odor may develop if the sponge is left in place too long; and severe obesity or arthritis may make insertion or removal of the sponge difficult. No cases of toxic shock syndrome have been reported, but theoretically the risk may be increased if this method is left in too long or used during menses. An increase in uterine tract infections is another possible complication (Zieman et al., 2007).

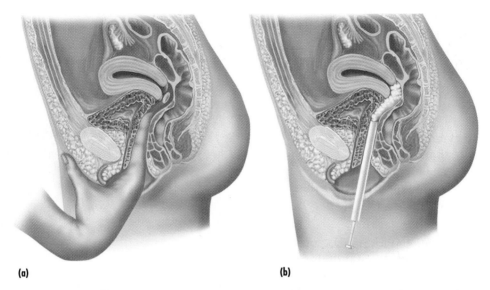

(a)   (b)

FIGURE **7.3** (a) Read the instructions for use of suppositories carefully and follow them. Be sure to wait the proper time for the suppository to dissolve. (b) Insert the plastic applicator into the vagina as far as possible to make sure that the foam covers the cervical opening, and press the plunger.

Spermicides

A **spermicide** kills and/or immobilizes sperm on contact and acts as a cervical barrier, thereby preventing their movement toward an egg (Figure 7.3). Spermicides are available as vaginal creams, films, foams, gels, suppositories, sponges, and tablets. Foams and creams are placed against the cervix by means of a plastic applicator. Spermicidal films (small squares coated with spermicides) and suppositories are inserted manually high into the vagina. Most spermicides must be inserted within 1 hour of intercourse, and some are not effective for the first 10 to 15 minutes after insertion. Users should read the packet insert instructions carefully.

> **spermicide**
> Chemical detergent compound that immobilizes or kills sperm on contact; as a barrier, prevents sperm from entering the uterus through the cervical os.

Effectiveness
The perfect use effectiveness rate of spermicides is 82%, meaning that only 18% of women using spermicides perfectly would become pregnant in 1 year. However, they have a high user effectiveness rate (about 71%). Just as for condoms, their ineffectiveness is probably due to inconsistent use of spermicide with every act of intercourse or incorrect use (for example, putting it in too soon or too late). However, the good news is that using condoms and spermicides *together* provides contraceptive protection almost as effective as that of oral contraceptives. The bad news is that few couples use both methods simultaneously.

Reversibility
Spermicide use has no effect on future fertility.

Advantages and Disadvantages
There are many advantages to spermicide use. They are easy to use, are available at drug stores and supermarkets without a prescription, and do not require partner involvement.

The major disadvantages of spermicides are the relatively high failure rates for both perfect use and typical use as well as the recent reversal in recommendations involving **Nonoxynol 9**. It is the major spermicidal ingredient sold over the counter in the United States. Although several other spermicides (menfegol, benzalkonium chloride, sodium ducosate, and chlorhexidine) are used in products available in Canada and in Europe, these compounds are not available in the United States.

> **Nonoxynol 9 (N-9)**
> The major spermicidal ingredient in U.S.-made products.

Women are advised to avoid products with Nonoxynol 9 because several studies showed vaginal irritation due to this spermicide, actually increasing the possibility of acquiring HIV and other STIs from an infected partner. As a result, a coalition of experts, women's health, and AIDS organizations was called together by the World Health Organization (WHO) and the U.S. Centers for Disease Control and Prevention (CDC) to make recommendations. The coalition did not ask manufacturers to withdraw all products containing N-9 from the market, but rather to stop adding N-9 to condoms and sexual lubricants. The CDC published the following conclusions in 2002:

- N-9 is not effective against HIV or other STIs and, when used vaginally multiple times a day, can cause genital lesions—a condition that may increase a woman's risk of acquiring HIV.

- Even at low doses, N-9 can cause massive, short-term damage to the rectal epithelium (lining), thereby increasing an individual's risk of contracting HIV and other STIs during anal intercourse.

- Although noncondom contraceptive products containing N-9 are moderately effective in preventing pregnancy and safe when used infrequently (no more than once a day), condoms lubricated with a small amount of N-9 are no more effective in preventing pregnancy than are lubricated condoms without N-9 (Boonstra, 2005).

On its own initiative, the U.S. FDA proposed new labeling for over-the-counter stand-alone vaginal contraceptives and spermicidal products that address the N-9 issue. Stand-alone spermicides include gels, foams, films, or inserts containing N-9 that are used by themselves for contraception. The final rule requires manufacturers of these products to include a warning stating that the chemical N-9 does not provide protection against infection from HIV (the virus that causes AIDS) or other STIs. The FDA issued the rule in an effort to correct misconceptions that N-9 protects against STIs, including HIV infection. The agency believes the warning will empower consumers to make better-informed decisions about the use of these products, and will better protect the public health. Finally, it issued the rule to provide a clear, consistent message—that N-9 may actually facilitate transmission of the disease for those who are at risk for HIV/AIDS. The final rule is consistent with the FDA's draft guidance for N-9 use with condoms (FDA, 2007).

Fertility Awareness Methods

You may have heard this riddle: Q: What do you call people who practice rhythm? A: Parents.

Natural family planning (NFP) is also known as **fertility-awareness methods**, or the *rhythm method*. There are several fertility-awareness methods: the *calendar method, ovulation method,* and *symptothermal method.* Each of these methods is based on the identification of the days in the woman's menstrual cycle when she is most likely to be fertile and the avoidance of intercourse during those days (natural family planning) or use of a barrier method or withdrawal during those days (**fertility-awareness-combined methods**).

CycleBeads are used as part of the standard days method. Using a string of 33 colored beads, women keep track of their cycle. When used correctly, the efficacy rate is 5 pregnancies per 100 per year.

Fertility-awareness methods are based on the knowledge that there are only about 6 days in a cycle during which a woman can become pregnant. The ovum lives less than 1 day; sperm can live up to 5 days inside the woman's genital tract (Zieman et al., 2007).

People interested in using these methods need to see a trained educator for help in learning to observe, chart, and recognize the woman's fertility signs and patterns. It is estimated that it requires 4 to 6 hours to learn fertility-awareness methods so that they can be used effectively (Zieman et al., 2007). For that reason, detailed instructions are not included in this text.

People using the **calendar method**, first developed in the 1930s, keep track of the woman's menstrual cycles for several months and then, with the help of a trained person, determine which days she is most likely to ovulate. It is the least effective of the fertility-awareness methods; even with perfect use, there is a 9% chance of becoming pregnant.

Ovulation methods are much more effective. Women can chart their **basal body temperature** or their cervical secretions or both. Basal body tem-

fertility-awareness-combined methods
Calculation of a woman's fertile times and use of a barrier or withdrawal on fertile days.

calendar method
Charting of the length of a woman's periods for several months to determine the days she is most likely to be fertile.

ovulation methods
Observation of signs of ovulation to calculate fertile days.

basal body temperature
A woman's body temperature immediately upon waking.

natural family planning (NFP)
Calculation of a woman's fertile times and abstention from intercourse on fertile days.

fertility-awareness methods
Methods used to determine fertile days.

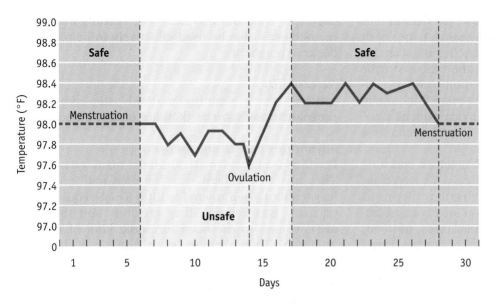

FIGURE **7.4** The basal body temperature method of contraception involves charting a woman's body temperature each morning to determine when unprotected sexual intercourse is safe. Once the basal body temperature has risen for three consecutive days, she can assume that ovulation has taken place and that the rest of the days in that menstrual cycle are safe for unprotected intercourse.

Gender
DIMENSIONS

Gender Equality in Contraception Use

During most of human history, contraception was a male responsibility. The only methods available were the condom and withdrawal. Oral contraceptives became available in 1961, and many women were elated. They could now control contraceptive use and thus their risk of becoming pregnant. The pill was effective, was easy to use, and did not require partner participation. Many men who came of age during the 1960s and 1970s never thought much about contraception.

In the 1990s, the HIV/AIDS epidemic and the epidemic of STIs once again shifted the responsibility. Men who are not in monogamous committed relationships now have to use condoms on a regular basis. But many women are unwilling to rely on condoms for pregnancy prevention because they are only 85% effective in preventing pregnancies in typical users. Some men are unwilling to use condoms once they find out that their partner is using the pill. And many men do not like to use condoms, claiming that they reduce sensitivity and sensation.

Heterosexual couples today need to negotiate how they will prevent an unwanted pregnancy *and* how they will protect themselves against STIs. Couples need to discuss who has primary responsibility for contraception. They need to address such questions as, Who will buy the condoms? Who will pay for contraception? Should the man accompany the woman to the clinic visit? And, perhaps most important, what will they do if an unplanned pregnancy occurs?

There are ways that couples can share the responsibility for contraceptive and condom use. Men can remind their partners to take their pills or check their IUD strings. They can learn to insert the diaphragm or female condom as part of foreplay. Women can learn to place the condom on the man's penis as part of foreplay. Contraceptive use and safer sex practices can truly be a shared responsibility.

perature is a person's temperature upon awakening. Temperatures usually drop immediately before ovulation and then rise sharply during and after ovulation (Figure 7.4). Thus a woman takes her temperature by using a specially calibrated **basal body thermometer** before she gets up each morning. The temperature is then charted on a monthly graph, and after 3 days of elevated temperature, it is considered safe to have intercourse without the risk of pregnancy.

Cervical secretions can also be monitored and charted. After menstruation, cervical secretions

basal body thermometer
A special thermometer used to measure changes in basal body temperature.

cervical secretions
Normal fluids from the cervix that change consistency during the month.

are scant. As estrogen levels increase, cervical mucus becomes thick and cloudy. When estrogen peaks at midcycle, the secretions become clearer, stretchy, and slippery. In fact, at ovulation, the mucus can be stretched 2 to 3 inches between the thumb and forefinger. After ovulation, the secretions become thick again, and some women may notice a cervical mucus plug. At this point, it is considered safe to have intercourse without worrying about pregnancy.

The **symptothermal method** involves checking both basal body temperatures and cervical secretions and charting them to identify fertile periods (begins as soon as cervical secretions are noticed) and nonfertile times (beginning the fourth day after the last day of wet, clear, slippery mucus—post ovulation). When this method is used perfectly, only 2% of women become pregnant, making it as effective as the most effective prescription forms of contraception.

> **symptothermal method**
> A combination of natural family-planning methods, in which both temperature and signs of ovulation are observed and charted.

Costs involve training and supplies (such as special digital basal body thermometer, cycle beads, and charts) (Zieman et al., 2007).

Effectiveness

Natural family-planning methods can be highly effective methods of contraception. If they are used perfectly, only 1% to 9% of women using these methods in a year have an unintended pregnancy. The symptothermal method is the most effective natural family-planning method; using a calendar alone is only 75% effective in typical use. Fertility-awareness methods can also be used effectively to help couples become pregnant.

Reversibility

Natural family-planning methods stop preventing pregnancies as soon as they are discontinued.

Advantages and Disadvantages

Fertility-awareness methods have many advantages. They are an excellent way for men and women to learn about their own fertility. They require both partners' involvement, they are free, and they may alert women to the need for some kind of medical attention. Their primary disadvantage is that they provide no protection against STIs, cervical mucus techniques may be complicated by vaginal infections, and the couple must be vigorously committed to abstaining from intercourse during fertile times. If the couple is not rigorous about charting cycles or has intercourse during fertile periods, pregnancy is likely to occur.

■ Prescription Methods

Oral Contraceptives

There are several different types of **oral contraceptives (OCs)**. In fact, since oral contraceptives were introduced, there have been 63 brands that included 39 unique formulations

> **oral contraceptive (OC)**
> A daily pill taken to prevent ovulation.

CONTRACEPTIVE TIMELINE

Ancient Practices—Coitus interruptus (the withdrawal method) was first mentioned in the Biblical Book of Genesis (Genesis 38:8).

1564—The earliest published description of the "condom" was by the Italian anatomist Gabriel Fallopius in 1564. The term "condom" was likely derived from the Latin word *condus*, meaning "receptacle" (Birth control, 2009).

1873—State and federal legislation, collectively referred to as the Comstock Laws, prohibited the importation or mailing of obscene matter. Obscene matter included contraceptive products as well as information about those products.

1350 B.C.—As one of the earliest forms of the condom, Egyptian men may have placed linen sheaths on the penis before intercourse. It is difficult to determine the accuracy of this claim; this time period covers prehistorical events, and evidence suggests that Egyptians worshipped the god of fertility (Youssef, 1993).

1840 through 1870s—Paralleling Charles Goodyear's vulcanization of rubber in the first half of the 19th century, the rubber condom became a popular choice of contraception. Other rubber-made contraceptive products, such as the earliest intrauterine devices, douching syringes, and diaphragms, were referred to as "womb veils" (Birth control, 2009; *Timeline*, 2002).

1879—Margaret H. Sanger was born Maggie Louise Higgins (*Timeline*, 2002)

1881—Surgical occlusion of the fallopian tubes (e.g., the first female sterilization) was performed by an Ohio surgeon (Birth control, 2009).

Gender DIMENSIONS

Margaret H. Sanger: A Woman of Influence

In 1931, the futurist H. G. Wells said Margaret H. Sanger (1879–1966) started the most influential movement of all time (Lehfeldt, 1967). In 1998, she was recognized among the 100 most important people of the 20th century by *Time* magazine. Today, early in the 21st century, her life concerns health disparities due to poverty, the burdens of unintended pregnancy, and women's access to safe methods of birth control—are still problems, but are now recognized public health priorities. In her lifetime, Margaret Sanger was a catalyst for contraceptive research, an emancipator of women, and a practicing nurse among the marginalized and poor who eventually became known as the woman who established the American birth-control movement.

Margaret H. Sanger was born in 1879, the sixth child of a working-class, Irish Catholic family in New York. As a young nurse tending to the poor on the Lower East Side, Sanger witnessed the severe illness and even death that women suffered when attempting self-induced abortions (Hymowitz & Weissman, 1978). Seeing such tragedy combined with "revolting conditions," where extreme poverty and child labor added to the misery, moved Sanger to find the "secret" of preventing unwanted pregnancies (Lehfeldt, 1967).

The barriers she faced were huge. At first, Sanger began in earnest by writing her radical journal *The Woman Rebel* as well as the *Family Limitation* pamphlet. Even though she did not give instructions regarding specific methods for contraception, the Comstock Laws' definition of "obscene, lewd, lascivious" matter was cited to have her arrested and eventually jailed (Jensen, 1981). Sanger temporarily fled to Europe, where she was introduced to the various contraceptive technologies currently available, as well as several European benefactors and professionals who championed her cause, including British sexologist Havelock Ellis. Based on these experiences, Sanger believed that the diaphragm, along with spermicidal jellies, were the secrets to having a simple, cheap, harmless contraceptive that could be used throughout the world (Lehfeldt, 1967).

In the latter part of Sanger's career, she concentrated on the development of new contraceptive technologies—specifically oral contraceptives. Through the Planned Parenthood Foundation, she arranged for the first grant supporting investigation of progestinal compounds for the purpose of contraception. She obtained additional funding for the scientists who would later be recognized as the inventors of the oral contraceptive (Lehfeldt, 1967). Although she received neither the Nobel Peace Prize nor the Presidential Freedom Award for which she was nominated, she was successful in searching for safe, effective forms of birth control, offering the leading voice in the development of oral contraceptives, as well as providing the foundations for Planned Parenthood.

20th Century—*Hormones,* from the Greek *hormaô,* meaning "stir up" or "incite," were isolated (e.g., estrogen). This development opened the door for the hormonally based methods of contraception in the latter half of the 20th century (Birth control, 2009).

1916—Sanger opened the first birth control clinic in the United States. Ten days after the opening, the clinic was raided, all birth control devices were confiscated, and Sanger was arrested and jailed (Hock, 2007).

1950s and 1960s—Strong arguments were made for the acceptance and use of oral contraceptives. Factors included advancements in hormonal/synthetic research, growth in pro-contraceptive sociopolitical movements, and federal government policy decisions supporting an individual's right to personal privacy.

1914—Pioneer Margaret Sanger published the first major statement on birth control and contraception in her pamphlet *Family Limitations* (Jensen, 1981). She coined the term "birth control" and challenged women to use the term from the pages of her radical journal *The Woman Rebel* (Timeline, 2002).

1923—Sanger opened the first legal birth control clinic in the United States (*Timeline,* 2002).

1936—In the *United States v. One Package of Japanese Pessaries,* the court ruled that contraceptives could be sent through the mail if they were to be intelligently employed by conscientious physicians for (1) the purpose of saving life or (2) promoting the well-being of their patients (Birth control, 2009). This decision marked a reversal of one of the last surviving Comstock Laws (Hock, 2007)

1951—The Roman Catholic Church sanctioned the use of the rhythm method, but remained opposed to any other form of birth control, including "the pill." Pope Paul VI issued the encyclical *Humanae Vitae* ("Of Human Life") in 1968 as the authoritative guide for birth regulation among many Catholics (Catholic Church, 1968).

Continued

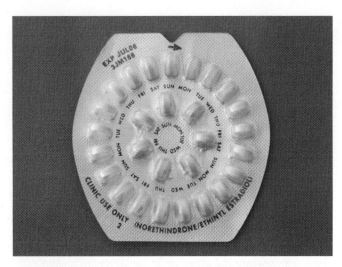

Although oral contraceptives are effective in preventing pregnancy, they offer no protection against STIs or HIV. For protection against pregnancy and STIs, try combining the use of oral contraceptives and latex condoms.

in the United States alone (Gerstman et al., 1996). These different pills can be categorized as monophasic formulations, in which all the active pills contain the same amount of hormone, and multiphasic formulations, in which the active pills throughout the cycle contain varying amounts of progestin and/or estrogen. The monophasic formulation accounts for the majority of the oral contraceptive market, with the combined pill being much more widely used than the minipill (Gerstman et al., 1996; Zieman et al., 2007).

The **combined pill (COC)**, used since the 1960s, contains both estrogens and progestin (synthetic progesterone). To use the combined pill, a woman ingests the first pill in the packet and takes a pill each succeeding day. Most packets contain 28 pills, but some contain only 21. The 28-pill packets contain 7 pills that have no benefit other than convenience: That is, the woman need not remember to stop taking her pills and then resume taking them 7 days later—as is required if using the 21-day packets. Usually menstruation occurs on the 23rd or 24th day (2 or 3 days after the last pill containing a hormone is ingested). In 2003, the FDA approved a long-acting version of the combined pill called Seasonale. It has 84 consecutive hormone-containing pills followed by 7 placebo pills, resulting in only 4 menstrual periods per year rather than the monthly periods associated with traditional pill cycles. With this method, however, there is increased risk of unexpected breakthrough bleeding, especially in the first months of use (Zieman et al., 2007; WHO, 2008).

> **combined pill (COC)**
> Oral contraceptive containing estrogen and progestin.

The combination pill's estrogen signals the brain's hypothalamus to prevent the pituitary gland from producing FSH and LH; the progesterone also inhibits LH production. Ovulation is suppressed. This suppression mimics the changes that occur in pregnancy.

The progestin-only pill was introduced in 1972. In spite of its lack of estrogen (high dosages of which were found to be related to physical complications),

CONTRACEPTIVE TIMELINE—cont'd

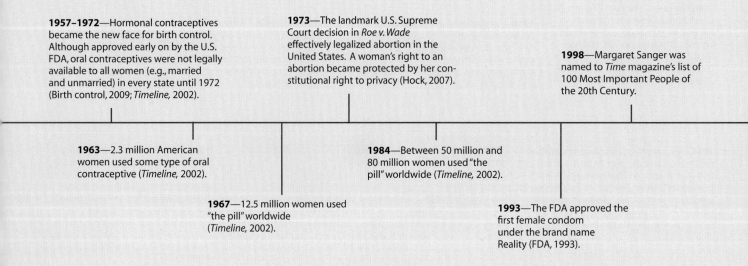

1957–1972—Hormonal contraceptives became the new face for birth control. Although approved early on by the U.S. FDA, oral contraceptives were not legally available to all women (e.g., married and unmarried) in every state until 1972 (Birth control, 2009; Timeline, 2002).

1973—The landmark U.S. Supreme Court decision in Roe v. Wade effectively legalized abortion in the United States. A woman's right to an abortion became protected by her constitutional right to privacy (Hock, 2007).

1998—Margaret Sanger was named to Time magazine's list of 100 Most Important People of the 20th Century.

1963—2.3 million American women used some type of oral contraceptive (Timeline, 2002).

1984—Between 50 million and 80 million women used "the pill" worldwide (Timeline, 2002).

1967—12.5 million women used "the pill" worldwide (Timeline, 2002).

1993—The FDA approved the first female condom under the brand name Reality (FDA, 1993).

minipill (POP)
A progestin-only pill.

the **minipill (POP)** never achieved a great deal of popularity, and the percentage of women using it remains relatively low to this day. To use this type, a woman takes a pill on the first day of menstruation and every day thereafter. Because progestin is included in every pill, the hormone is ingested daily. With minipills, approximately 40% of women still ovulate (40% do not ovulate, and 20% sometimes ovulate). However, even if fertilization occurs, the progestin inhibits implantation. Moreover, the progestin causes the cervical mucus to inhibit to some degree the sperm's movement and ability to penetrate the ovum. Minipills are appropriate for women who cannot use estrogen.

The chemical composition of oral contraceptives has changed over the years in response to research on their effects and side effects. The typical amount of estrogen in early birth control pills was 0.1 milligram (mg). In 1968, fewer than 1% of the estimated 54 million retail prescriptions for oral contraceptives contained less than 0.5 mg of estrogen. In 1988 approximately 82% of the estimated 57 million retail prescriptions for oral contraceptives contained less than 0.5 mg of estrogen. In the 1970s it was found that use of the higher-dosage pills (more than 0.5 mg) was related to cardiovascular complications. Today those higher-dosage pills are still available and used by women with specific medical problems such as uterine bleeding and endometriosis. However, most oral contraceptives using estrogen now contain between 0.20 and 0.35 mg.

Myth vs Fact

Myth: Birth control pills cause cancer.
Fact: Birth control pills are very safe. Although there may be a slightly increased short-term risk of being diagnosed with breast cancer, it is believed that this is due to (1) detection bias (more breast exams and more mammography) or (2) promotion of already-present cancer cells. In the long term, women who have taken birth control pills have a 25% reduction in risk for benign breast disease. Furthermore, the pill is protective against other cancers such as ovarian and endometrial cancer as well as death from colon cancer. Thus women using the pill are less likely to contract cancer than women who have never been on the pill.

Myth: You need to take a break from the pill.
Fact: Women can stay on oral contraceptives as long as medical side effects do not develop. There is no need to take a break.

Myth: All condoms protect against STIs.

Fact: Only latex and polyurethane condoms protect against STIs. Animal skin condoms provide no protection against STIs.

Myth: Condoms protect against all STIs.
Fact: Condoms are highly effective at preventing the spread of such diseases as HIV infection, syphilis, and gonorrhea. They do not provide protection against genital warts, crabs, or lice, which can be transmitted through contact with the pubic hair or other parts of the genitals that are not covered by the condom.

Myth: Withdrawal is not a method of birth control.
Fact: Withdrawal is about as effective as barrier methods. It is much better than using nothing.

Myth: Once a person has had intercourse, he or she can no longer practice abstinence.
Fact: Abstinence is always a choice. Many teens, college students, and adults choose abstinence even though they have already had sexual intercourse.

1999—The FDA approved the emergency contraceptive Plan B by prescription only. Although emergency contraceptives had been available since the 1970s, Plan B found a new generation of consumers.

1999—Wal-Mart refused to sell the "morning-after pill" with the brand name Preven (Canedy, 1999). Under mounting pressure, Wal-Mart began to sell the emergency contraceptive Plan B in 2006 (Barbaro, 2006).

2007–2009—Unlike "the pill," new forms of hormonal contraceptives (injectables, implants, patch, ring) were introduced that either reduce or eliminate a woman's menstrual period altogether.

2008—Four federally funded longitudinal studies showed abstinence-only sex education is associated with (1) no significant impact on teen sexual activity, (2) no differences in rates of unprotected sex, and (3) some impacts on knowledge of STIs and perceived effectiveness of condoms and birth control pills (Trenholm et al., 2007).

2009—Pending legal challenges were dropped in the federal court, making Plan B available on an over-the-counter basis to women 17 and older, and to women younger than age 17 by prescription only.

Regardless of which pill is used, a backup method of contraception should be employed for the first 7 days of pill use and as a precaution if a pill is forgotten for 2 or more days in a row. If a pill is forgotten one day, that pill should be taken immediately and the next pill taken as regularly scheduled. A backup method should also be used any time a woman uses antibiotics, such as tetracycline or penicillin, which reduce the effectiveness of the pill.

It is a good idea for a woman using oral contraceptives to have regular medical exams. Most physicians require a visit 3 or 6 months after a woman starts OCs, followed by an annual exam thereafter. There is no medical reason for a woman to "take a break" from pill use (WHO, 2008).

Effectiveness

Apart from abstinence, sterilization, and hormonal injections, oral contraceptives provide the most effective means of preventing pregnancy. Only 3 in 1,000 women using oral contraceptives becomes pregnant in 1 year of perfect use. Among typical users—for example, some who forget to take their pills as directed—as many as 8% become pregnant in the first year.

It cannot be overemphasized that oral contraceptives provide *no* protection from STIs. Unless you are in a 100% monogamous relationship with a partner who has been tested for STIs and HIV, a condom must be used for each act of intercourse.

Reversibility

Some women who have been on the pill may require slightly more time to become pregnant than women using other methods. Therefore, clinicians generally recommend that women plan 3 months off the pill before they begin to try to conceive. However, oral contraceptive use does not affect future fertility.

Advantages and Disadvantages

Birth control pills have been reported as being 92% effective as actually used and 99.7% effective if used correctly all the time (Zieman et al., 2007). Besides being effective, the pill does not necessitate interrupting sexual activity. An added benefit for some women is that it helps to regulate the menstrual cycle. Birth control pills are available in the United States only by prescription from a physician, because they have other effects as well. For example, the combination pill may enlarge the breasts, may reduce acne, often eliminates mittelschmerz (a sensation of abdominal pain that sometimes occurs during ovulation), and reduces menstrual cramps. For estrogen-related problems with the combination pill, the progestin-only pill is recommended, because it contains no estrogen, and its low pro-

gestin dosage is thought to reduce adverse effects that progestin might otherwise cause.

Combined pills are very safe. In addition to protecting a woman against pregnancy, they lower a woman's risk of ovarian cancer, endometrial cancer, breast masses, and ovarian cysts. They also lessen menstrual blood loss, cramps, and acne. Their primary disadvantage for sexually active college students is that they provide *no* protection against STIs, including HIV.

Symptoms can develop after use of the pill, even after some time. Abdominal pain, chest pain, shortness of breath, headaches, eye problems such as blurred vision, and severe leg pain are examples of such symptoms. If any of these is encountered, call the doctor. Other possible side effects exist. For example, the combination pill has been associated with a greater risk of circulatory system diseases, including heart attacks and strokes. If a woman is obese, diabetic, or hypertensive, the risk of circulatory system diseases is greatly increased. These women should use a different method (Zieman et al., 2007). Smoking is also a factor. The American College of Obstetricians and Gynecologists (ACOG) found that, among approximately 10 million users of oral contraceptives, 500 women die each year. The death rate would even be lower if heavy smokers, especially those older than 35 years, did not take the pill. This death rate is about 10 times lower than a woman's chance of death from an automobile accident or from childbirth. In addition, women with liver function problems, hypertension, circulatory problems, heart disease, breast cancer, asthma, varicose veins, or migraine headaches should avoid using oral contraceptives (Zieman et al., 2007).

There has been considerable debate over the years about whether oral contraceptive use can lead to breast cancer. After more than 50 studies and 50 years, most experts believe that pills have little, if any, effect on the risk of developing breast cancer. The Women's Care Study of 4,575 women with breast cancer and 4,682 controls found no increased risk for breast cancer among women currently using pills and a decreased risk of breast cancer for those women who had previously used pills. Use of pills by women with a family history of breast cancer was not associated with an increased risk of breast cancer, nor was initiation of pill use at a young age. Breast cancers diagnosed in women currently on pills or women who have taken pills in the past are more likely to be localized (less likely to be metastatic). By the age of 55, the risk of having had breast cancer diagnosed is the same for women who have used pills and those who have not. While there are still unanswered questions about pills and breast cancer, today, four decades after their arrival on the contraceptive scene, the overall conclusion is that pills do not cause breast cancer. "Many years after stopping oral contraceptive use, the main effect may be protection against metastatic disease" (Speroff & Darney, 2005, cited in Zieman et al., 2007).

Emergency Contraception

Condoms sometimes slip or break; women forget more than two contraceptive pills in a row; the man ejaculates too close to the vulva even though he withdraws; a couple vowing abstinence has intercourse anyway. For all these cases, **emergency contraception** is now available. In addition, emergency contraception is available in cases of rape or incest.

> **emergency contraception**
> The use of oral contraceptives after unprotected sex has occurred at midcycle.

Oral contraceptive pills have been used for emergency contraception (EC) since the 1960s. Various amounts of ordinary combined (estrogen and progestin) birth control pills can be prescribed and cut the chance of pregnancy by 75%.

Alesse, Aviane, Cryselle, Enpresse, Jolessa, Lessina, Levlen, Levlite, Levora, Lo/Ovral, Low-Ogestrel, Lutera, Lybrel, Nordette, Ogestrel, Ovral, Portia, Quasense, Seasonale, Seasonique, Tri-Levlen, Triphasil, and Trivora have all been declared safe and effective for use as EC by the FDA. Unlike Plan B, which contains progestin only, combined oral contraceptive pills may cause nausea because they contain estrogen. If antinausea medication is *not* taken prior to the first dose of EC (which is recommended if nausea has been a problem in the past), it may be taken after the first dose, should nausea be severe or should vomiting occur. Antinausea medication such as meclizine hydrochloride is recommended because it has a 24-hour duration of action. It is available over the counter as Bonine and as Dramamine 2. Other medications to prevent nausea may be prescribed instead (Zieman et al., 2007).

The only dedicated product (intended specifically for emergency contraception) marketed in the United States is a progestin-only kit called Plan B. Taking the two pills (containing Levonorgestrel) within 120 hours (5 days) after having unprotected sex reduces the risk of pregnancy by 89%. However, the sooner the pills are taken, the greater the chances that pregnancy will be avoided. If a woman is already pregnant or becomes pregnant following the use of emergency contraception, there are no documented negative impacts on fetal development.

Another FDA-approved method is insertion of an intrauterine device (Copper T/ParaGard IUD) that

Take the first tablet as soon as possible within 72 hours of unprotected sex.

In recent years, there has been a movement toward making emergency contraceptives available without prescription. Outside the United States, more than 50 emergency contraceptive products are specifically packaged, labeled, and marketed. Levonorgestrel-only ECPs are available either over the counter or from a pharmacist without having to see a clinician in 50 countries. On August 24, 2006, the FDA approved Plan B for nonprescription sale to women and men age 18 and older.

The label for Plan B says to take one pill within 72 hours after unprotected intercourse and another pill 12 hours later. However, recent research has found that both Plan B pills can be taken at the same time. Research has also shown that all of the oral contraception pills (in the prescribed amounts for EC) are effective when used within 120 hours (5 days) after unprotected sex (http://ec.princeton.edu/questions/dose.html).

reduces the pregnancy risk by 99% and can be left in place to provide continuous contraception for up to 10 years. However, all women are not equally good candidates for IUD use, especially those at risk for STIs (NOT-2-LATE.com, 2009).

How emergency contraception prevents pregnancy depends on the day of the menstrual cycle on which the pills are taken. Several mechanisms are possible—inhibition of ovulation, prevention of fertilization, or interference with implantation. It is important to differentiate that, unlike the **abortifacient** RU-486, emergency contraception does not disrupt an implanted fertilized ovum (Zieman et al., 2007).

> **abortifacient**
> A medical method that causes an embryo or fetus to die.

Knowledge and access are critical barriers that keep emergency contraception from being widely used. Yet, research has clearly demonstrated that access does not increase sexual behavior nor does it diminish use of other methods of contraception (Zieman et al., 2007).

Some university clinics offer emergency contraception as part of their reproductive health services.

If they do not, there is a toll-free number that has been set up in the United States to help women find clinics and doctors who will prescribe emergency contraception. It is 1-888-NOT-2-LATE.

Effectiveness

With Plan B (emergency contraception with progestin-only pills), effectiveness studies indicate that failure rates were not significantly greater if taken at day 5 versus day 3. Failure rates when taking both pills at once (1.5%) were almost the same as if single pills were taken 12 hours apart (1.8%). Both pills may be taken at once with no increase in nausea (15%) or vomiting (1%). Pretreatment with an anti-emetic an hour before taking the first pill should be considered if the patient has a history of past problems with nausea. On average, using Plan B as emergency contraception reduces the risk of pregnancy by 89%. This means that if 100 women had unprotected sex during the second or third week of their cycle, about 8 would become pregnant. If the same 100 women used Plan B, only 1 would become pregnant (Zieman et al., 2007; NOT-2-LATE.com, 2009).

Advantages and Disadvantages

The advantage to emergency contraception is that it is the only method available if unprotected intercourse has occurred when fertility is likely. Emergency contraception should not be used as a regular method of contraception. It is significantly less effective than other methods, and its long-term use has not been studied. It also provides no protection against STIs. Because EC has no impact on existing pregnancies, there is no need to test for pregnancy before taking the first dose. However, if menses do not occur within 21 days, a pregnancy test should be done. Another method of contraception should be used following EC (Zieman et al., 2007).

The Combined Contraceptive Patch

In December 2000, Johnson and Johnson applied for approval to market the first contraceptive patch. In March 2003, the patch became available to women seeking a method of contraception that released a steady delivery of hormones over time.

Similar to the use of the nicotine patch, users wear it on the lower abdomen, buttocks, or upper arm. The patch is about the size of a matchbook and delivers a combination of estrogen and progestin through the skin. Each patch is used for 7 days, but contains sufficient hormone for 9 days; then it is removed and discarded. Patches are worn for 3 weeks, followed by a patch-free week to allow menstruation to occur.

Effectiveness

The patch is approximately as effective as birth control pills. It is 99.7% effective when used perfectly; for typical use it has a 92% user effectiveness rate. Some clinicians recommend using another method if the

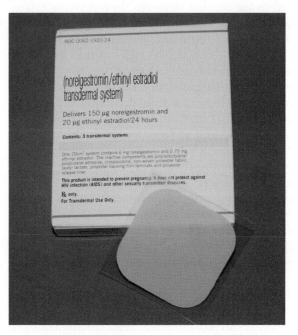

Ortho Evra is the first birth control patch approved by the FDA. Although the patch contains hormones similar to those in combined birth control pills, the patch needs to be changed only once a week, minimizing the margin of error and subsequent decreased effectiveness that is often the case with oral contraceptives.

patient weighs over 198 pounds. The patch prevents pregnancy by preventing ovulation, thickening the cervical mucus, and suppressing endometrial growth (Upadhyay, 2005).

The FDA suggests that women who use or are considering the contraceptive patch work with their health care providers to balance the potential risk related to increased estrogen exposure against the risk of pregnancy (FDA News, 2005). This view would concur with that of researchers who compared the user-effectiveness and cost-effectiveness of the contraceptive patch and the combined oral contraceptive pill. They found both methods to be highly effective in preventing pregnancy with perfect use. Therefore, differences were due to user-effectiveness. The difference was greatest in the youngest age group (15–19 years) for whom the annual probability of pregnancy was 13.1% with combined oral contraceptives and 7.5% for the contraceptive patch. As the age group increased, the probabilities of pregnancy decreased for both methods and the differences between methods also decreased. For example, in the 30–34 age group, the rates were 4.8% and 4.1% for the pill and the patch, respectively. In summary, the researchers view the contraceptive patch as a regimen that holds promise for improving correct use and thus reducing the risk and cost of pregnancy because it requires only 3 weekly applications per month compared with 21 days of active pill taking (Sonnenberg et al., 2005).

Advantages and Disadvantages
This method is comparable to combined pills in menstrual advantages. It adheres well to the skin. The Ortho Evra patch is light colored, but a smaller, clear patch is in the late stages of development. Although weight is a restricting factor, age is not. Compliance among teens is good. Disadvantages include breakthrough bleeding and spotting in about one-fifth of users, lack of STI protection, and visibility on the skin. The primary side effects of the patch are headache, nausea, and site reactions, which were experienced by 20% of users in clinical trials (Contraceptive patch, 2001; Zieman et al., 2007).

Combined Injectables

Combined injectables—that is, injectable contraceptives that contain both a progestin and an estrogen—are gaining new attention among family planning clients and providers. Combined formulations are generally injected once a month compared with once every 2 or 3 months for progestin-only injectables such as norethindrone enanthate (NET-EN) and depot-medroxyprogesterone acetate (DMPA/Depo-Provera). Compared with progestin-only injectables, combined injectables disturb vaginal bleeding patterns less and allow earlier return to ovulation after women discontinue use.

While even the newer combined injectables have been on the market for years, they have become more widely known and used in recent years because new safety and effectiveness data have become available. The U.S. FDA approved Lunelle, although it is currently not available in the United States. WHO accelerated the development of Cyclofem for use in developing countries in response to requests from India, Mexico, and other countries in the 1970s for a safe and effective monthly injectable. Today Cyclofem is available in 18 countries, mostly in Latin America and Asia. Another monthly injectable, Mesigyna, is also supported by WHO and is now available in 36 countries (Updahyay, 2005).

Depo-Provera is another form of a progestin-only contraception method. It is a shot that is given every 12 weeks. Depo-Provera suppresses ovulation by inhibiting production of FSH and LH.

> **Depo-Provera (DMPA)**
> An injectable progestin-only contraceptive.

Effectiveness
Depo-Provera is even more effective than the pill. In 1 year, only 0.3% of women using Depo-Provera become pregnant. And because it is an injection, there is no chance that a typical user can use it incorrectly, unless she does not return in 3 months for her next shot. Many couples prefer Depo-Provera because its use is not related to intercourse activity.

Reversibility
Fertility may resume immediately after 13 weeks has passed since the last injection. However, studies show that women generally do not conceive for an average of 10 months after the date of the last shot (Zieman et al., 2007). In contrast, women who stop using combined injectables can become pregnant as soon as 6 weeks after their last injection (Upadhyay, 2005).

Advantages and Disadvantages
Depo-Provera is easy for a woman to use, simply requiring that she return to the clinic every 3 months. It is not used during coitus, and it is one of the most effective methods of preventing pregnancies.

Depo-Provera has few practical disadvantages. Women do need to have injections every 3 months, which may be difficult for some to schedule. Some women report minor weight gain, and many report changes in their periods. Some women have no periods on Depo-Provera; some have frequent bleeding. Spotting between periods is common in the first months of use. The major disadvantage to Depo-Provera is that it provides no protection against STIs.

Implants

Implants are small plastic rods or capsules that are inserted into the nondominant upper arm of a woman by her health care provider. This contraceptive method helps to greatly reduce the risk of pregnancy by releasing the hormone progestin. Subsequently, the implant works by (1) thickening the cervical mucus, which blocks the sperm from meeting the egg, and (2) disrupting the menstrual cycle and preventing ovulation (WHO, 2008). Depending on the brand of implant, implants last anywhere from 3 to 7 years. They may be replaced immediately following the end of life of the previous implant. Implants are available under the brand names Implanon, Norplant, Jadelle (Norplant II), and Sinoplant. Currently, Implanon is the only implant available in the United States. It is considered effective for at least 3 years.

Effectiveness

The efficacy rate for implants is less than 1 pregnancy per 100 users per year. However, some evidence suggests that the effectiveness of Implanon decreases for women who weigh more than 130% of their ideal body weight. As with all implants, the risk of pregnancy increases slightly after the first year of use and continues during its lifespan (WHO, 2008).

Reversibility

Implants are considered a reversible form of birth control, as the woman returns to normal fertility once the implant is removed.

Advantages and Disadvantages

Implants are safe for nearly all women, including women who cannot take estrogen. Irregular bleeding (e.g., between 6 and 12 months) is the primary side effect, but is not harmful. Once the implant is in place, very little maintenance by the user is required. The disadvantages include unpredictable or irregular menstrual bleeding, hormonal side effects (of which headache is most common), and lack of STI protection (Zieman et al., 2007).

Intrauterine Devices and Systems

Intrauterine devices (IUDs) and **intrauterine systems (IUSs)** are reversible methods of contraception. They are synthetic devices that are inserted by a medical provider into the uterus to prevent pregnancy (Figure 7.5). Currently only one IUD and one IUS are available in the United States. The ParaGard Copper-T 380A is also labeled for use as an emergency contraceptive and can remain in place for 10 years. During that time, women experience regular menstrual cycles that may even involve heavier flow or more cramping than prior to insertion of the IUD. Minera is a levonorgestrel-releasing intrauterine system (LNG-IUS) introduced in 2000 that is labeled for 5 years of effectiveness. This method reduces or may eliminate menstrual flow over time, although some initial irregular spotting or breakthrough bleeding may occur after insertion of the device (Ramchandran & Salem, 2008).

The intrauterine copper contraceptive works primarily as a spermicide, immobilizing sperm so they rarely reach the fallopian tube, to prevent fertilization. Evidence suggests that IUDs do not work after ferti-

> **intrauterine device (IUD)**
> Synthetic device that is inserted into the uterus to prevent the sperm from fertilizing the ovum.
>
> **intrauterine system (IUS)**
> Synthetic device placed in the uterus that releases a continuous amount of hormone (levonorgestrel) to prevent ovulation, fertilization, or implantation.

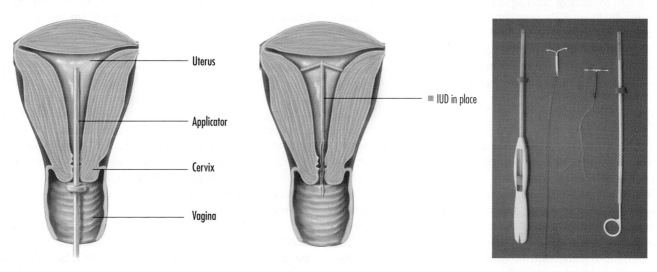

FIGURE 7.5 The IUD is inserted past the cervix into the uterus. Before insertion, the length of the uterus is measured with an instrument called a *sound*. Upon insertion, the arms of the IUD gradually unfold. Once the inserter is removed, the threads attached to the IUD are clipped to extend into the vagina through the cervical opening.

lization and therefore are not abortifacients. The hormone levonorgestrel in the IUS operates somewhat differently. It causes cervical mucus to thicken so sperm cannot enter the upper reproductive tract to reach an ovum. Changes in uterotubal fluid also restrict sperm movement. Finally, the endometrium is altered to prevent implantation. In the first years of use, this method is also shown to inhibit ovulation in some users (Zieman et al., 2007).

IUDs are a highly effective method of birth control and are a good alternative to hormone-based methods. Although worldwide IUD use has increased steadily, use in the United States rapidly declined as IUD-related product liability litigation peaked in the 1980s. This concern was compounded by the perceived risk of pelvic inflammatory disease. Recent studies confirm the safety and efficacy of IUDs for the great majority of women (Doyle et al., 2008). Misperceptions about potential infertility also help explain the low U.S. rates of IUD use in general and particularly among women who have never had children. Nevertheless, well-designed studies have found that former IUD users are no more likely than other women to be infertile (Doll, Vessey, & Painter, 2001; Grimes, 2000; Hubacher et al., 2001). Additionally, 72% to 96% of women conceived within 1 year of having their IUD removed; this rate is comparable to levels among women who never used contraception (85%) (Ramchandran & Salem, 2008; Zieman et al., 2007).

Effectiveness
The IUD/IUS is one of the most effective contraceptive methods. Because compliance is not an issue, actual-use efficacy and perfect-use efficacy are nearly the same. For the ParaGard IUD with copper, the pregnancy rate has been less than 1 pregnancy per 100 women each year. The Mirena IUS, which contains the progestin levonorgestrel, has contraceptive efficacy comparable to female sterilization (0.01%). In addition to preventing pregnancy in general, the progestin-releasing system (Mirena or LGN-IUS) reduces the chances of ectopic pregnancy, which is the leading cause of pregnancy-related death (Doyle et al., 2008). Women are advised to check the strings to assure the IUD is still in place; not doing so accounts for the minor difference in effectiveness rates.

Reversibility
Once the IUD is removed, fertility resumes immediately. Compared to possible detrimental effects of various hormonal contraceptives (oral contraceptives, implants, injectables) on subsequent fertility, the use of LNG-IUS does not affect conception rate; all users in one study conceived within 1 month of discontinuation of the IUS (Backman et al., 2004).

Myth vs Fact

Myth: Providing birth control to young people encourages them to have sexual relationships. **Fact:** There are no studies that indicate that young people who have access to family-planning methods are more likely to have sexual intercourse. They are more likely to use contraception.

Myth: You can borrow a friend's diaphragm in a pinch. **Fact:** Diaphragms are fitted to an individual woman. You cannot borrow another woman's diaphragm.

Myth: If you roll on the condom the wrong way, reverse it and put it on the right way.

Fact: Microscopic tears can occur when you roll on a condom. Throw it out and start with a new one.

Myth: There is nothing you can do but hope and pray if you forget to use your method. **Fact:** If you forget to use a method, there is emergency contraception available. It must be used within 120 hours (5 days) of the act of unprotected intercourse. Call a provider near you or 1-888-NOT-2-LATE.

Advantages and Disadvantages
The IUD/IUS is an excellent method for most women. In addition to being highly effective, it is easy to use and has no systemic side effects.

A major advantage of the IUD is that once inserted it remains in place, so planning before intercourse is unnecessary. (When it is in place, a string attached to the IUD emerges through the cervix. The woman feels for the string to make sure the IUD is present, because it is possible for it to pass out of the uterus with the menstrual flow or at other times. The device can also be removed by a physician by means of this string.) Other advantages include probable protection against endometrial cancer and possible protection against cervical cancer, its availability for women who cannot use hormonal methods, a rapid return to fertility, convenience as a single insertion that provides 5–10 years of protection depending on the type, cost-effectiveness in terms of the greatest net benefit of any contraceptive if used for more than 2 years, high level of user satisfaction, and use of one type (ParaGard) as emergency contraception.

In terms of disadvantages, the copper ParaGard IUD may cause increased monthly blood loss (menorrhagia) and possibly anemia due to lowered hemoglobin levels in some users. Conversely, the progestin-delivering Mirena (LNG-IUS) actually increases hemoglobin levels over the years of usage by reducing or eliminating menstrual flow (amenorrhea). This method requires an office procedure for both insertion and removal; both can be uncomfortable. Some protocols recommend a chlamydia/gonorrhea check before insertion, as these STIs could lead to the development of pelvic inflammatory disease (PID) as a consequence of the insertion process. This contraceptive method offers no protection from HIV or other STIs. Expulsion of the device, either obviously with cramping or bleeding, or silently without the user's awareness, places the woman at risk for pregnancy. The likelihood of expulsion declines over time, but women who have expelled one IUD have about a one in three chance of expelling another (Doyle et al., 2008; Zieman et al., 2007).

Women who receive extensive counseling on the possibilities of amenorrhea and bleeding problems, occurrence of PID, hormonal adverse effects, and expulsion of the device and risk of pregnancy are significantly more likely to be very satisfied with this method. Modest weight gain could be viewed as a hormonal effect, except that women not using contraception experience virtually the same weight gain (Inki, 2007).

Diaphragm

When in place, the **diaphragm** prevents the sperm from traveling through the uterus and up the fallopian tubes to fertilize an egg, and it holds sper-

A diaphragm is a barrier method of contraception that can be used repeatedly with spermicidal cream or jelly. It requires a physician to fit the diaphragm initially.

micide against the cervix (Figure 7.6). The diaphragm is a shallow rubber, or synthetic rubber, cap surrounding a flexible metal ring that covers the cervix.

diaphragm
Shallow rubber cap that covers the cervix and prevents sperm from entering the uterus.

Diaphragms are available in several sizes and styles. Because the diaphragm's purpose is to prevent sperm from going beyond the vagina, its size and shape are very important. If the diaphragm does not fit exactly right, a chance exists that sperm can bypass this barrier. Clearly, using someone else's dia-

FIGURE 7.6 Procedure for inserting a diaphragm: (a) Before inserting the diaphragm, coat the rim and cup with a spermicidal cream or jelly. (b) Squeeze the rim of the diaphragm together between your thumb and index finger. (c) Insert the diaphragm into the vagina with the rim facing up and push it toward the small of your back. As you let go of the diaphragm, it will spring open. Continue to guide it to your cervix with the tips of your fingers. (d) Be sure to check that the diaphragm completely covers the cervix.

phragm is a poor idea. Diaphragms are fitted by a clinician and refitted after women give birth or gain or lose a significant amount of weight. Fit should also be checked during the yearly gynecological exam, and the diaphragm should be replaced every 2 years or with any signs of wear or damage.

The diaphragm must remain in place for at least 6 hours after intercourse, and spermicide must be added for *each* act of intercourse. This combination of requirements, besides increasing effectiveness, allows the male and female to share the responsibility for contraception. (Diaphragms should be removed at least once every 24 hours to reduce the risk of toxic shock syndrome.)

Effectiveness
When inserted properly and used with spermicide, the diaphragm is theoretically 94% effective and 84% effective as actually used. Some studies suggest that spermicides may prevent some STIs, and thus the diaphragm may help prevent STIs. Other studies indicate that they may cause abrasions in the vaginal walls that could increase susceptibility to STIs. The contraceptive effectiveness of diaphrams without a spermicide containing Nonoxynol 9 (N-9) has been insufficiently studied. However, this combination should be assumed to decrease effectiveness. Women infected with or at high risk for HIV, however, should *not* use spermicides containing N-9. Conversely, routine use of N-9 by women not at high risk of HIV does not pose any known increased risk (WHO, 2008; Zieman et al., 2007).

Reversibility
The diaphragm does not affect fertility (except when it is in place).

Advantages and Disadvantages
The major advantages of the diaphragm are that it is highly effective if used correctly and consistently, is easy to learn to use, and has no systemic side effects unless latex allergy is involved. Some couples make diaphragm insertion part of foreplay. The man can insert it into the woman's vagina before intercourse.

One disadvantage of the diaphragm is that it must be inserted before intercourse and inserted properly, requiring the woman or couple to plan ahead. Some women are not comfortable touching their genitals and therefore find diaphragm use uncomfortable. Diaphragms provide only limited protection against certain STIs, so condoms must also be used to prevent STI transmission. In addition, some users may experience an increased risk of urinary tract infections. Oil-based lubricants should not be used with diaphragms as they erode the rub-

ber. Odor may develop if the diaphragm is left in place for more than 24 hours. Severe arthritis or obesity may make insertion or removal difficult. A reaction to latex or superficial cervical erosion may cause vaginal spotting or discomfort in some women (Zieman et al., 2007).

Cervical Cap

The **cervical cap** is a silicone rubber, latex-free, dome-shaped device that covers the cervix and holds spermicidal cream or jelly. It is similar to, but smaller than, the diaphragm; is meant to stay in place longer; and is slightly less effective than the diaphragm (Figure 7.7). In 1988, the FDA approved the sale of cervical caps in the United States, although they have been used in Europe for decades. Currently, the FemCap is available through Planned Parenthood, in the United States.

> **cervical cap**
> Shallow silicone rubber device, smaller than a diaphragm, that covers the cervix to prevent sperm from entering the uterus.

The cervical cap can be left in place for 48 hours. However, it must be removed during menstruation to allow the menstrual flow to leave the body.

Although the cap is made in different sizes, not all women can use it because of the variation in shapes and sizes of cervixes.

Effectiveness
Overall, the cervical cap and the diaphragm have similar rates of effectiveness. Theoretical effectiveness of the cervical cap ranges from 91% to 74%. The cap is much more effective in women who have never been pregnant (nulliparous women). User effectiveness for the cap is 84% for nulliparous women compared to only 68% in women who have been pregnant. As with the diaphragm, spermicide used with the cervical cap may provide some protection against some STIs, but it may increase susceptibility to others. In nonmonogamous couples, condoms should also be used to prevent STI transmission. The same precautions and uncertainties regarding the use of N-9 apply to cervical caps (Zieman et al., 2007).

Reversibility
The cap does not affect fertility (except when it is in place).

Advantages and Disadvantages
The cap is easy to use and has no systemic side effects unless spermicide sensitivity is present. Many women like the fact that it can be kept in place for up to 48 hours and that spermicide use for additional acts of intercourse is optional.

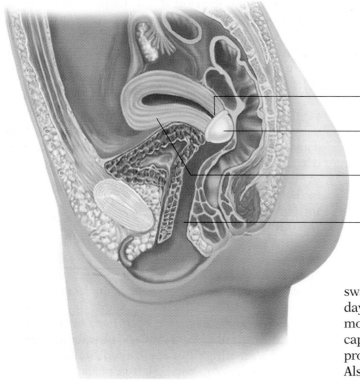

Cervix

Cervical cap
encircling cervix

Uterus

Vagina

FIGURE 7.7 It is important that your cervical cap is always inserted correctly. You should practice inserting before using the cap during sexual intercourse.

There are also disadvantages associated with use of the cap. The cervical cap may occasionally irritate the cervix, may cause an unpleasant odor or vaginal dryness, and has the potential for becoming dislodged during coitus. It can also cause toxic shock syndrome if it is not removed regularly.

Combined Vaginal Ring

The NuvaRing provides protection from pregnancy by emiting ethinyl estradiol (the estrogen component) and etonogestrel (the progestin component) daily for 21 days. In contrast, low-dose estrogen contraceptive pills contain slightly more estrogen, and other contraceptive pills contain almost twice as much estrogen. Additionally, with oral contraceptives, there is a daily spike in hormone levels when the pill is

NuvaRing is a flexible, transparent, odorless ring that is about as big as a silver dollar and is inserted into the vagina, where it continuously releases low doses of estrogen and progestin that prevent pregnancy. Heralded for its convenience, NuvaRing leaves even less room for error than the contraceptive patch.

swallowed, followed by a gradual drop throughout the day. In contrast, the ring provides a steady rate of hormone release. Whereas the diaphragm and cervical cap must be positioned correctly to provide maximal protection, NuvaRing cannot be inserted incorrectly. Also, it comes with a timer to use as a reminder of when it needs to be replaced. Even if it is not removed immediately, protection remains for 35 days. NuvaRing costs approximately the same as a cycle of pills in pharmacies and requires a prescription to be purchased.

Effectiveness

NuvaRing is an effective hormonal contraceptive with many advantages. It has a theoretical or perfect-use effectiveness rate of 99.7%. Because once it is in place there is nothing else to do (contrasted, for example, with oral contraceptives, which require remembering to take a pill), effectiveness is greatly enhanced. User effectiveness is not yet established but is expected to be approximately 94% (Zieman et al., 2007).

Reversibility

Fertility is not affected after NuvaRing is removed.

Advantages and Disadvantages

NuvaRing contains the lowest serum levels of estrogen and progestin in any combined hormonal method, thereby decreasing the risks associated with synthetic estrogens. In addition, the ring does not require any daily action, as does taking a pill each day. All that is required is replacement of the ring after 21 days or 1 month. With this method, privacy is maintained; there is no visible patch or pill package. Another advantage compared to combined oral contraceptive pills is the presence of regular withdrawal bleeding. Because this assures women of the absence of pregnancy, it may result in greater acceptance of NuvaRing as an effective contraceptive method (Sarkar, 2005). Furthermore, the vast majority of women cannot feel the ring when it is in place and report being satisfied with this method of contraception.

As with all methods of contraception, there are also disadvantages associated with NuvaRing. The risk of synthetic estrogen is not eliminated; it is merely reduced. Therefore, as advised by the manufacturer, smokers and those susceptible to blood clots should not use the ring. Further, 14% of users experienced vaginitis (Redfearn, 2002), and 25% of men felt the ring during intercourse, although most reported they did not perceive that to be a problem. If necessary, it can be removed for up to 3 hours without losing its effectiveness. Another disadvantage of the ring for women who are uncomfortable touching their genitalia is the need for the user to insert it manually through the vagina. These women may prefer another contraceptive method that does not entail touching the genitalia. In addition, NuvaRing does not offer any protection against STIs (Zieman et al., 2007).

Permanent Methods

Sterilization
Sterilization is a form of contraception that renders a person biologically incapable of reproducing. Men and women both may choose to be sterilized—made infertile—because they have all the children they want or because they do not want to have children. Women in ill health, perhaps those with serious heart conditions, may choose to prevent life-threatening pregnancies and births. Couples may choose not to have children if their genetic makeup, when passed to their offspring, would be likely to result in birth defects (for example, sickle-cell anemia or Tay-Sachs disease).

Individual methods of sterilization for men and women are described shortly. Contraceptive choices vary markedly with age. By age 35, more women rely on sterilization than on the pill. Of all women aged 40–44 who practice contraception, 50% have been sterilized and another 18% have a partner who has had a vasectomy. If both male (9.2%) and female (27%) sterilization percentages are combined, then sterilization (36.2%) exceeds oral contraceptives (30%) as the leading contraceptive method of choice (Guttmacher, 2008).

> **sterilization**
> A procedure that makes a person biologically incapable of reproducing.

Effectiveness
Male and female sterilization is highly effective. In the first year after sterilization, only 1 woman out of every 1,000 sterilized becomes pregnant, and only 1 in every 2,000 sterilized men causes a pregnancy.

Reversibility
According to Hatcher and colleagues (2004, p. 144), regarding fertility after vasectomy, a "man must accept that vasectomy is irreversible and permanent. Microsurgical techniques of reversal [**vasovasectomy**] now result in return of sperm to ejaculate in over 90% of men, but in pregnancy rates of only 50% or above. Reversibility rates decrease as time since procedure increases. Important factors for reversal are skill of the microsurgeon, length of time from vasectomy, presence of antisperm antibodies (man), partner's fertility, and manner in which the vasectomy was performed (amount of vas removed or cauterized)." In other words, although sterilization may be reversible, it should be considered a permanent method.

> **vasovasectomy**
> Reversal of a vasectomy, so that sperm can be ejaculated.

Advantages and Disadvantages
Sterilization is only for people who are certain that they do not want more children and who are fertile. Both female and male sterilizations have the same advantages. They are permanent, highly effective (99.9%), are cost-effective, lack side effects, do not interfere with intercourse, and are very safe. Their primary disadvantage is they provide no protection against STIs.

Male Sterilization
In men, sterilization entails interruption of the vas deferens in a procedure called a **vasectomy** (Figure 7.8). Vasectomy became popular as a method of contraception in the late 1960s and early 1970s. In 1971, a peak of 701,000 vasectomies were performed in the United States (Association for Voluntary Sterilization, 1982). The interest in vasectomy was a result of several factors, including concern about the health hazards of the oral contraceptive and extensive promotion by several national organizations (Association for Voluntary Sterilization, Planned Parenthood Federation of America, and Zero Population Growth). In addition, the medical community announced its support for

> **vasectomy**
> Cutting or cauterizing of the vas deferens to prevent sperm from being ejaculated; a means of sterilization.

FIGURE **7.8** Vasectomy.

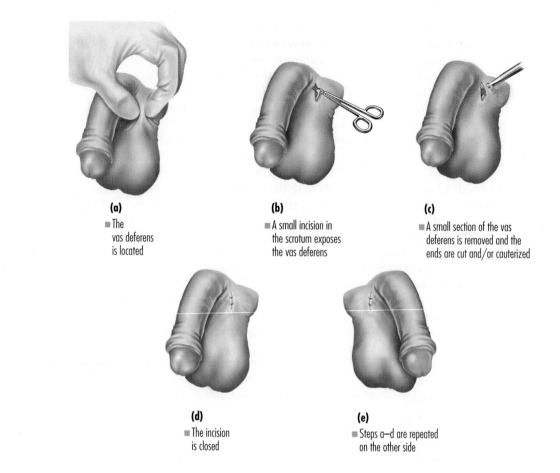

(a)
■ The vas deferens is located

(b)
■ A small incision in the scrotum exposes the vas deferens

(c)
■ A small section of the vas deferens is removed and the ends are cut and/or cauterized

(d)
■ The incision is closed

(e)
■ Steps a–d are repeated on the other side

vasectomy as a contraceptive method that was safe and effective.

Despite acceptance among the medical community, vasectomy continues to be an underused method. To determine factors that might influence men to choose or reject this method, a study was undertaken to determine characteristics of men receiving vasectomies in the United States. The results demonstrate that in spite of great racial, ethnic, and socioeconomic diversity, those men seeking vasectomies are a fairly homogeneous group. Low-income and minority men seem to lack relevant information and access to services. By recognizing these underserved groups, program providers and managers may be able to help reduce the large difference in utilization of vasectomy among men of different races, ethnicities, and income groups. This could also help close the gap between male and female sterilization rates (Barone et al., 2004).

Vasectomy is a simple, minor surgical procedure that takes about 30 minutes. A small opening is made in the scrotum, and the vas deferens is severed. This severing blocks sperm from entering the ejaculate, because it has no route out of the testes. Clips and plugs can also be used to interfere with the vas deferens passageway; the most widely used technique involves cutting the vas and sealing off its ends (by suturing or cauterization). Vasectomies

are done under local anesthesia and require minimal care afterward. Vasectomized men are instructed to avoid hard work or strenuous exercise for several days, to wear a scrotal support for a week, and to apply ice and take mild painkillers for postoperative discomfort. As soon as the man feels ready, he may resume sexual intercourse.

Unlike female sterilization, a vasectomy does not provide immediate infertility. Sperm may still be stored in the urethra or elsewhere in the reproductive tract and may not be expelled for 10 weeks or more. The amount of time required to expel this sperm depends partly on the frequency of ejaculation. For this reason, men are asked to return to the physician twice after the vasectomy with a semen specimen to be tested for the presence of motile sperm. Until the absence of sperm is verified, a condom, diaphragm, or other method of contraception is required to prevent conception. Usually two consecutive negative sperm analysis results are required before a backup method of contraception is no longer necessary.

Female Sterilization

Female sterilization takes several forms; the goal is to prevent the egg from moving down the fallopian tube to be fertilized by a sperm. Currently, most female sterilization procedures involve tubal ligation, in which the woman's fallopian tubes are surgically cut or blocked by applying clips, rings, or heat. The two most common surgical approaches are the minilaparotomy and laparoscopy. These approaches require skilled medical professionals and sterile conditions. Local or general anesthesia is also required. The newer approaches not involving surgery can increase access to sterilization (Upadhyay, 2005).

A recent approach to transcervical sterilization called Essure is a nonsurgical method using a spring-like device (microcoil) inserted through the uterus into each fallopian tube. This causes gradual tubal blockage over a 3-month period by encouraging local scar tissue growth with polyesther (PET) fibers. At 5 years, effectiveness is 99.74%. However, Essure is unlikely to be introduced in developing countries soon because of the high cost and complexity of the insertion instruments (New Contraceptive Choices, 2005; Zieman et al., 2007).

Minilaparotomy

A **minilaparotomy**, sometimes called a *minilap*, requires a small incision just above the pubic hairline. An instrument is then inserted into the cervix to move the uterus and pull each fallopian tube into the incision. Part of the tube is taken out of the incision, where it is blocked by **ligation**, clips, or rings and then replaced in the abdomen. This procedure takes about 20 minutes, and the woman can usually leave the medical setting in 2 or 3 hours. Because the incision is very small (about 3 cm), few complications develop.

> **minilaparotomy**
> Female sterilization procedure that involves a small incision in the abdomen through which the fallopian tubes are pulled so they can be blocked.

> **ligation**
> The tying of the fallopian tubes to prevent the sperm–egg union.
>
> **laparoscopy**
> Female sterilization procedure that involves inserting a narrow viewing instrument—a laparoscope—through an incision in the abdomen and then performing ligation or applying clips or rings to block the fallopian tubes.

Laparoscopy

A **laparoscopy** involves inserting into the abdomen a narrow stainless steel tube with fiber-optic cylinders that transmit light (Figure 7.9). This tube is called a *laparoscope*. Two types of laparoscopes can be used. With one, the physician can insert forceps and other instruments through the tube itself; therefore, only one incision is necessary. With the other type of laparoscope, two incisions are required because the tube does not permit other instruments to be inserted through it. Ligation by electrocoagulation (high-frequency electrical current) or application of clips or rings can take place during this procedure to prevent the passage of the egg.

Transcervical Methods

Other sterilization techniques that do not involve surgery are undergoing testing. These techniques per-

(a) Cross section

(b) Front view

Laparoscope

Fallopian tube

Cauterized

Tied and cut

Fallopian tube

Ovary

Uterus

FIGURE **7.9** Female sterilization by laparoscopic ligation. (a) Cross section: The tubes are located using a laparoscope and cut, tied, or cauterized through a second incision. (b) Front view: The tubes after ligation.

Emergency Contraception: How Is NOR-Levo in France Different from Plan B in the United States?

NOR-Levo is the same postcoital pill as Plan B. Each is a progestin-only emergency contraceptive. Introduction of NOR-Levo in France in 1999 led quickly to a change in the country's constitution; by 2002 NOR-Levo could be distributed free in middle and high schools. Minors can also obtain NOR-Levo free of charge in pharmacies without parental consent. Adult women can be reimbursed up to 65% of the cost of NOR-Levo by insurance. No adverse effects of NOR-Levo have been reported. The interest in emergency contraception has created "more open discussion among pharmacists, nurses in schools, and across all society about what to do to prevent pregnancy and sexually transmitted disease" (AGI, 2003). France has one of the lowest abortion rates in the world: 12 per 1,000 women aged 14–44 (AGI). Among teenagers aged 15–19, there are 10.9 abortions per 1,000 women.

Contrast the above picture with the Plan B story in the United States. Approved at the end of the 1990s, Plan B distribution is spotty at best. Many pharmacies do not stock Plan B. No high schools or middle schools give it to students. And Plan B may cost anywhere from $10 to $100. The hoops women must jump through to obtain Plan B increase the time from unprotected sex until Plan B is taken or lead to its not being used at all. In contrast to France, where discussion of emergency contraception has fos-tered increased discussion (and presumably use) of other contraceptives, controversy over emergency contraceptive pills has fueled debate in Kentucky and Ohio over how pills, minipills, and Depo-Provera injections work, jeopardizing the availability of these traditional contraceptives in the public family planning clinics of northern Kentucky.

The result? Abortion rates in U.S. teens aged 15–19 years are three times higher in the United States than in France (29.2 versus 10.2 per 1,000 teens), and pregnancy rates in U.S. teens are 4 times higher in the United States than in France (86.6 versus 20.2 per 1,000 teens).

What is wrong with this picture? What seems to underscore the differences in how the United States and France approach teen sexuality—specifically, how they approach sexual intercourse in teenagers—is the word "responsibility."

Parents, teachers, and community leaders in France and throughout Europe seem to be able to express the sentiment: "A teenager who is having intercourse must be responsible about this potentially dangerous activity."

Why is it that we can say to a 20-year-old who is drinking illegally: "If you drink, don't drive." Or a parent can say to his or her child: "If you drink, call me and I'll come get you."

So NOR-Levo and Plan B are exactly the same drug, but France and the United States are as different as night and day in the access women have to this drug.

Source: Hatcher, R. A., Zieman, M., et al. *A pocket guide to managing contraception.* Tiger, GA: Bridging the Gap Foundation, (2004), 74.

---

manently prevent pregnancy by blocking the fallopian tubes through the vagina and the uterus. Some methods are FDA approved and on the market in the United States (Essure). Others, such as the Adiana procedure that involves blockage using a porous plastic matrix implanted into a superficial lesion in each fallopian tube, are in review for FDA approval. Both of these methods require skilled use of an expensive hysteroscope for insertion and follow-up X ray or ultrasound imaging 3 months after insertion (New Contraceptive Choices, 2005).

Nonsurgical Female Sterilization
Quinacrine is a permanent, nonsurgical method of female sterilization that is currently undergoing safety evaluations, toxicology studies, and clinical trials. Small pellets containing quinacrine are inserted into the uterus through the cervix; the pellets dissolve and the liquid flows into the fallopian tubes and obstructs them (Quinacrine sterilization, 2002). Because of its

profound implications for permanent contraception worldwide, quinacrine has been extensively studied, frequently in poorer nations. Because of its role as a mutagen, it has been implicated as a potential carcinogen, though this has never been definitively established. In fact, quinacrine has been used as an antimalarial agent in more than 100 million people since the 1930s with no associated increases in cancers. Nor have there been any reports of birth defects that would indicate teratogenic potential in more than 130,000 quinacrine sterilizations.

The most attractive feature of this form of sterilization from a world health perspective is cost; the inserter and pellets cost less than $1 per sterilization (Greenberg, 2008).

Reversibility
As with male sterilization, female sterilization should generally be considered irreversible. Although surgical techniques can be successful in opening up the

fallopian tubes, highly skilled surgeons and modern microsurgical equipment are required and are very costly. Therefore, women seeking sterilization must expect it to be permanent because reversal is costly and failure rates are high. In vitro fertilization may be possible but many cannot afford this procedure and it is not always successful (Zieman et al., 2007).

■ The Future of Contraceptives

Research to find better methods of contraception continues. The perfect method of contraception, which will probably never exist, would:

1. Be 100% effective

2. Be very inexpensive (or even free)

3. Have no side effects

4. Be reversible

5. Involve no remembering to do something

6. Be convenient (not messy)

7. Prevent STIs

8. Be religiously and morally acceptable

9. Not interrupt sexual behaviors

During the 1990s, several new methods were approved for use in the United States. These included the female condom, nonlatex male condoms, Norplant, Depo-Provera, and Lunelle. New research continues, most involving extensions and improvements of current methods. However, several of the new methods (and some old standbys) were removed from the market. It seems the driving influence behind business decisions to withdraw a product are based on costs—profit and loss—rather than its safety and efficacy. Two researchers drew the following conclusion. "A mechanism and resources must be devised to retain accessibility of useful contraceptive products when their sponsors discontinue marketing them for business reasons. There are women who would happily choose a long-acting subdermal contraceptive implant or a combined estrogen/progestin injectable product . . . if they were again made available on the U.S. market" (Gardner & Miller, 2005). The contraceptive methods now being researched include the following:

1. *Male contraceptive methods:* Hormonal contraception for men that works by using testosterone or a combination of testosterone with progestin to suppress sperm production. This method involves monthly or bimonthly injections or use of an implant (Upadhyay, 2005). In trials in China, only 1 man in 100 fathered a child while on the injections. Still, experts

Latex dams (top) are used to prevent the spread of STIs. Spray-on contraception (bottom) is a new way to supply a preset dose of hormones.

say that more trials are needed to check safety, especially because previous attempts to develop an effective and convenient male contraceptive have encountered problems over reliability and side effects (BBC News, 2009). However, another viewpoint on the development of male contraceptives claims they will perpetually remain 5 to 10 years away, primarily due to money. Another conjectured barrier is the misperception that men are not interested in these kinds of contraceptives and women will not trust men to use them. Neither of those assertions is supported by the data (Goodman, 2008).

2. *BioRing:* A new vaginal ring that releases multiple types of non-hormonal agents and microbicides, which would prevent conception

as well as sexually transmitted HIV infection (Moscicki, 2008). This is a new approach to birth control and STI prevention; it is suitable for women who are averse to current methods, who cannot tolerate hormone-derived active agents, or who have allergies to latex condoms. The vaginally inserted ring contains multiple antiviral drugs that prevent HIV infection and are time-released over a period of up to 28 days. The compounds allowing the vaginal ring to prevent conception do so by arresting sperm motility, raising vaginal mucous viscosity, and sustaining vaginal acidity at a level sperm cannot survive. They are natural materials already approved by the FDA (Rodgers, 2009).

3. *Nesterone:* A spray-on contraceptive containing synthetic progestin that can be delivered transdermally and is appropriate for breast-feeding women. The spray-on approach is a new technique for transferring a preset dose of fast-drying hormones onto the skin where it is almost instantly absorbed. It slowly diffuses into the bloodstream over a 24-hour period. Advantages include lower or equivalent cost compared to other hormone-based methods, as well as being easy, convenient, and discreet to use. If estradiol (a form of estrogen) is added to the hormone formulation, this would be the first non-oral contraceptive delivering natural estradiol. The transdermal approach could make the risk of blood clots four times lower than it would be with oral delivery (Acrux, 2009; Lewcock, 2007; Population Council, n.d.; Updahyay, 2005).

DIMENSIONS

Unmet Need for Contraception in Developing Countries

What is unmet need?

If a woman is not using any method of contraception, either modern or traditional, she has unmet need if she is married and in a consensual union, or never married and sexually active; able to become pregnant; and does not want a child in the next 2 years or wants to stop childbearing.

How extensive is unmet need?

• In 53 developing countries surveyed, 15% of married women aged 15–49 had unmet need for contraception, and 7% of never-married women in 36 countries had unmet need.

• Approximately 71 million married women are at risk of an unplanned pregnancy in 53 countries, as are 4.2 million never-married women in 36 countries. Without access to contraceptive services and supplies, millions of these women will become pregnant unintentionally each year.

• Unmet need in sub-Saharan Africa declined less than 10% between 1990–1995 and 2000–2005. By contrast, unmet need declined by a third or more in the other three regions surveyed.

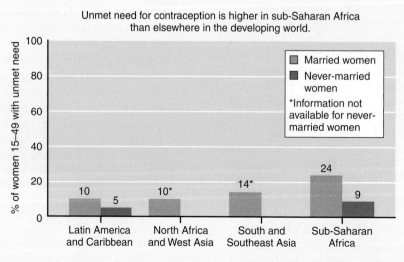

Unmet need for contraception is higher in sub-Saharan Africa than elsewhere in the developing world.

Global
DIMENSIONS

Unmet Need for Contraception in Developing Countries—cont'd

Who are the women with unmet need?

- In most developing countries, women who are rural, uneducated, poor, and married are more likely to be at risk for unplanned pregnancies than are urban, educated, or nonpoor married women. In sub-Saharan Africa, however, there is no single pattern of unmet need.
- In many countries, women who have had more than three children tend to have higher levels of unmet need as compared to women who have never had a child or who have had one to three children.
- Variations in unmet need reflect patterns of social and economic development. Women who are urban and nonpoor are first to want smaller families and have unmet need. Eventually, this desire extends to rural and poor women as well, increasing their unmet need.

Why do women not use or discontinue using contraceptives?

- The most prevalent reason is that women do not believe they are at risk of becoming pregnant.
- Lack of access and concerns about methods account for a third of the nonuse.
- Among never-married women, infrequent sexual activity and belief they should be married before seeking contraception accounts for nonuse and discontinuation.

Many are not using a method because they think they will not get pregnant or they are concerned about health or side effects.

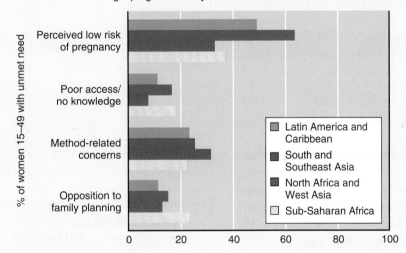

Recommendations for meeting unmet need:

- Focus on places where the gap between fertility desires and contraceptive practice is greatest—many countries in sub-Saharan Africa.
- Enhance effectiveness by including counseling and education to clarify issues of health and side effects.
- Ensure as many options are available as possible; help women match their method with their needs.
- Improve both contraceptive technologies and access to them.

- Promote societal receptivity to contraceptive use to help women overcome cultural and social barriers to achieving their desired family size.

Source: Facts about unmet need for contraception in developing countries: Guttmacher Institute in brief, May 2007; data from Sedgh, G., Hussain, R., Bankole, A., & Singh, S. Women with an unmet need for contraception in developing countries and their reasons for not using a method. Occasional Report, 37. New York: Guttmacher Institute, 2007.

Exploring the
DIMENSIONS
of Human Sexuality

sexuality.jbpub.com/dimensions/4e

Our feelings, attitudes, and beliefs regarding sexuality are influenced by our internal and external environments. Go to sexuality.jbpub.com/dimensions/4e to learn more about the biological, psychological, and sociological factors that affect your sexuality.

Sociocultural Factors
- Socioeconomic status affects contraceptive availability and use.
- Laws and government regulations limit contraceptive approval and availability.
- Religion affects contraceptive decisions, limiting some couples to natural family planning.
- Media and ad information can affect both contraceptive choice and brand choice.

Biological Factors
- Gender may affect contraceptive decision making. Males have only the option of condoms or vasectomy available; women have to deal with the fact that only they can become pregnant.
- STIs and HIV can be prevented only through strict use of latex condoms, abstinence, or 100% monogamy.
- Natural family planning relies on using physiological cycles and changes to monitor ovulation.
- Hormones such as estrogen and progesterone prevent the pituitary gland from producing FSH, without which the ova do not develop in the ovaries.

Psychological Factors
- Experience may determine the contraceptive you choose.
- Emotions often get in the way of practicing contraceptives and safer sex.
- Learned attitudes and behaviors affect your willingness to negotiate contraceptive use and practice safer sex.
- Your self-concept may influence whether you negotiate contraceptive use with your partner or simply accept what your partner desires.

CASE STUDY

When choosing a method of contraception, you must consider the effectiveness, side effects, convenience, cost, and protection from STIs and HIV. However, your partner's willingness to use the same method also comes into play, because contraceptives are ineffective if not used properly over time.

Many factors influence your contraceptive use. Legally, the federal government regulates which contraceptives you can buy in the United States. Socioeconomic status also is a factor, because most contraceptives are neither free nor covered by all types of health insurance. Also, people of higher socioeconomic status have greater access to prescription contraceptive methods and are more likely to receive more education about contraceptive methods.

Religion also plays a role in contraceptive choice, because some religions only officially sanction natural family-planning methods. Communication skills also are involved as you negotiate your contraceptive use with a partner.

Summary

- Contraception is used to avoid unplanned pregnancy. User motivation accounts for much of the variability in the effectiveness of different methods.

- Perfect use of a contraceptive method reflects the number of pregnancies likely to occur among 100 women in a year's time if the method is always used consistently and correctly. Often typical use effectiveness is less because of human error.

- Except for abstaining from sexual intercourse, condom use (male or female) is the only readily available and widely used contraceptive method that protects against sexually transmitted infections (STIs).

- Of the non-prescription methods, both abstinence and withdrawal are free, always available, and theoretically easy to use with no side effects. However, in practice, both methods have low effectiveness because intentions and practice don't always match.

- More than 100 brands of male condoms are available. All materials protect against pregnancy if used consistently and correctly; latex and polyurethane both protect against many STIs, but lambskin condoms do not. Female condoms, made of either polyurethane or synthetic rubber, are more costly.

- The vaginal contraceptive sponge and spermicides in the form of gels, foams, films, and inserts all use Nonoxynol-9; the FDA has mandated a warning label that this spermicide does not protect against HIV or other STIs and may actually increase risk among susceptable women.

- Fertility awareness methods depend on tracking a woman's fertile time using the calendar, basal body temperature, cervical secretions, cycle beads, or combinations; effectiveness can be high but requires careful record keeping.

- Prescription methods are for females; they include combination oral contraceptive pills containing both estrogen and progestin to suppress ovulation and mimic pregnancy, progestin-only pills, and other mechanisms to deliver hormones such as the patch, injections, implants, and vaginal rings.

- Emergency contraception (EC) is a hormone-based method used effectively (up to 120 hours or 5 days) after intercourse to prevent pregnancy. None of the current methods is an abortifacient and none disturbs an implanted pregnancy. Plan B is available in the United States over the counter to those 18 and over and in some states to anyone; a generic version has FDA approval.

- Intrauterine devices are highly effective and reversible. The ParaGard IUD can be used for EC and then can remain in place for up to 10 years; the Mirena IUS delivers a hormone that reduces or eliminates menstrual flow and is effective for up to 5 years.

- Diaphragms and cervical caps are barrier methods that are clinically fitted to cover a woman's cervix and used in combination with a spermicide to prevent sperm from entering the uterus.

- Sterilization for males and females is a permanent method of contraception that is almost 100% effective and widely used among adults over age 35 who are fertile but certain they do not want more children.

Discussion Questions

1. List six key considerations in choosing a contraceptive method, and rank their relative importance. Which method did you use to rank their importance?

2. Describe the nonprescription methods of contraception. Discuss the relationship issues that affect the choice of these methods.

3. Describe the methods of contraception requiring prescriptions. Which types of information should be disclosed to a doctor when making a selection?

4. Discuss the varied methods of female and male sterilization. Should the possibility of reversibility be part of the decision process?

Application Questions

Reread the chapter-opening story and answer the following questions.

1. Discuss how Susan altered her contraception use in light of her changing lifestyle. Which other contraceptive methods could she have used at each point? Which suggestions would you have for her?

2. If Susan had a family history of diabetes, high blood pressure, or breast cancer, how would her choices of contraceptive be altered?

3. Consider Stephen's decision to have a vasectomy. Although it may have seemed the perfect method for him at the time—married, monogamous, finished with childbearing—it also leaves him without the ability to father more children, should he remarry. In light of this, should men routinely postpone sterilization until a later age—just in case? Or should they have sperm frozen for the future?

Critical Thinking Questions

1. Assume that you began a relationship with a partner who wanted to use natural family planning because of religious convictions. What advantages and disadvantages would that hold for you from a contraceptive and safer sex standpoint? Answer this question from both male and female viewpoints.

2. The prescription methods of birth control are all female based. What role, if any, should the male partner have in the decision to use these methods?

Critical Thinking Case

Ben and Allie, both age 25 years, had been dating for 6 months and using latex condoms as their contraception method. Because their relationship was monogamous and increasingly dedicated, they had talked about switching to a different method but had never taken the time to discuss the options and how they would fit their lifestyle.

Then one evening, a condom broke. Allie pulled out the calendar on which she mapped her period, but the news was bad: It was right around the time of ovulation. Although committed to one another, they were not prepared to face the possibility of parenthood.

First consider what Allie and Ben should do immediately. Then outline some options for the couple's future, so that they do not face this situation again.

Exploring Personal Dimensions

Choosing a Contraceptive

There is no such thing as a 100% safe, 100% convenient, 100% easy-to-use contraceptive. Every contraceptive has advantages and disadvantages. People need to weigh these advantages and disadvantages for themselves.

Some questions that people need to ask themselves are as follows:

1. *Effectiveness.* What are the relative effectiveness rates for each method considered? How important is it to prevent pregnancy now? Is using abortion as a backup acceptable to you and your partner, or is an unplanned pregnancy acceptable at this time?

2. *Side effects.* Are you a good candidate for this method? Will you experience adverse side effects? Do you have a medical condition that should prevent you from using this method?

3. *Convenience.* Is this method easy for you to get? Is it easy to use? Will you use it every time?

4. *Cost.* Can you afford it? Does your campus health center provide it? Does your insurance cover it?

5. *STI protection.* Are you in a monogamous relationship? Are you sure? Do you have more than one partner? Do you know your partner's HIV status? Are you willing and committed to using a condom in addition to this method?

6. *Partner.* What does your partner think about this method? Will he or she want to use it every time? Do you want contraception to be a shared responsibility, or is it yours alone?

Suggested Readings

Boston Women's Health Collective. *Our bodies, our selves: New edition for a new era,* 8th ed. New York: Simon & Schuster, 2005.

Chaker, A. M. College students face rising birth-control prices: Drug makers end discounts long offered to school clinics; Privacy vs. parents' insurance. *Wall Street Journal,* July 26, 2007. Available at: http://online.wsj.com/public/article/SB118540828452878301-lTd0IYJ1cx_JPjy5dHVQAMwfGRw_20080725.html?mod=rss_free#printMode.

Chesler, E. *Woman of valor: Margaret Sanger and the birth control movement in America.* New York: Simon & Schuster, 2007.

Guttmacher Institute. *Perspectives on sexual and reproductive Health,* 2009. Available at: http://www.guttmacher.org/archive/PSRH.jsp.

Rooney, K. The high price of campus birth control. *Time,* 2007. Available at: http://www.time.com/time/specials/2007/article/0,28804,1651473_1651472_1650461,00.html.

Web Resources

For links to the web sites below, visit *http://sexuality.jbpub.com/dimensions/4e* and click on Resource Links.

The Emergency Contraception Web Site: NOT-2-LATE.com
http://ec.princeton.edu/questions/dose.html

This web site is operated by the Office of Population Research at Princeton University and by the Association of Reproductive Health Professionals. Funding is provided by the William and Flora Hewlett Foundation. This web site provides accurate information about emergency contraception derived from the medical literature. This web site has no connection whatsoever with any companies that manufacture or sell emergency contraceptives.

Guttmacher Institute: Resources—Contraception
www.guttmacher.org/sections/contraception.php

The Guttmacher Institute helps advance sexual and reproductive health worldwide through research, policy analysis, and public education. Its web site takes a comprehensive look at contraception in the United States and abroad. As such, it provides access to media kits, fact sheets, state policies, policy articles, research articles, reports, statistics, slide shows, and audio clips.

Planned Parenthood: Health Topics—Birth Control
www.plannedparenthood.org/health-topics/birth-control-4211.htm

Planned Parenthood provides a broad, up-to-date list of safe and effective methods of birth control for both women and men. Covering methods from sterilization to withdrawal and from intrauterine devices to emergency contraception, its web site describes how the contraceptive works, what the advantages and disadvantages of using the method are, and what research says about its effectiveness, safety, and reversibility.

Planned Parenthood: Health Topics—Speaking of Sex (Podcast)
www.plannedparenthood.org/health-topics/speaking-of-sex.htm

Speaking of Sex is Planned Parenthood's award-winning podcast and videocast that takes a fun, yet informative look at sexuality and its important role in our life and relationships. Available since 2006, the *Speaking of Sex* podcasts cover a wide range of topics, including hormonal contraception, the history of contraception, emergency contraception, and what contraception means to the average person on the street. The podcasts/videocasts are available as a free subscription from Apple iTunes as well as via direct download from Planned Parenthood.

CHAPTER 8

Conception, Pregnancy, and Birth

FEATURES

 Global Dimensions
Childbearing Rituals

 Communication Dimensions
Communicating About Pregnancy

 Gender Dimensions
Fathers and Childbirth

 Multicultural Dimensions
Differences in Infant Mortality

 Ethical Dimensions
Surrogate Mothers

CHAPTER OBJECTIVES

1 Explain what happens during the process of conception and implantation.

2 Explain what happens developmentally to the mother and embryo and fetus during the three trimesters of a pregnancy.

3 Describe the concept of prenatal care, and discuss the options for birth attendants and place of birthing.

4 Explain the many behaviors that can affect pregnancy outcomes, including use of drugs, diseases, and Rh incompatibility.

5 Identify maternal health problems that may be experienced during pregnancy.

6 Describe the physical and emotional reactions common during the three stages of giving birth.

7 Cite the causes of infertility, and describe various methods of treating it.

 sexuality.jbpub.com/dimensions/4e
Birthing Alternatives
Nutrition and Weight Gain
Breastfeeding

INTRODUCTION

*M*ary was in her late 30s when she and her husband, Rich, decided to have another child. For a while, they did not expect to be successful. Month after month of unprotected intercourse resulted in no pregnancy. They began to think they might have waited too long.

Finally, all their efforts paid off. Mary's period was late, and an at-home pregnancy kit confirmed their hopes. Mary immediately set up a doctor's appointment to confirm the pregnancy. When she received the positive results, she set up a series of prenatal care appointments with her obstetrician.

At the first appointment, Mary checked out well. The doctor wanted her to have a sonogram—just as in her previous pregnancies. But, because Mary was now older than 35 years, the doctor also wanted her to undergo amniocentesis to check the fetus for potential congenital abnormalities.

Mary had the sonogram and was told everything was fine. She had amniocentesis during the 16th week of pregnancy. The doctor called and scheduled an appointment to discuss the results, and Mary and Rich knew that prospects were not good.

The doctor explained that the test detected abnormal results, which could indicate a number of conditions—including mental retardation of the child. The doctor explained the problems of raising a mentally challenged child to the stunned couple and suggested they discuss whether to continue the pregnancy.

Mary and Rich pondered what to do. They believed this would be their last chance to have a child. And Mary, although very much in favor of a woman's right to choose to have an abortion, did not want to do so.

Although Mary and Rich knew in their hearts from the start that they wanted the baby, they were both still nervous as the due date neared. Mary went into labor. Because of the questions raised by the amniocentesis, the baby was to be delivered in an operating room; extra support staff stood by just in case.

The attending obstetrician delivered the baby and announced, "The first one is a bouncing baby boy." Now Rich and Mary were really stunned—what do you mean, "the first one"? Within a few minutes, the fraternal twin was delivered. Both children were born without any birth defect.

At the first follow-up appointment with her doctor, Mary wanted to know why she was not told she was pregnant with twins. The doctor said that during the sonogram, the one child must have been hidden behind the other. Because there was no indication of twins, the amniocentesis abnormalities were not attributed to a twin pregnancy.

In spite of Rich and Mary's experience, most conceptions and birth deliveries proceed as planned. Still, others result in unique circumstances, as did Rich and Mary's. In this chapter we discuss the usual and the unusual aspects of conception, pregnancy, and birth.

Creating a New Life

After the man ejaculates, the sperm move through the cervical mucus into the uterus, reaching the fallopian tube within about 5 minutes. Propelling movements of the uterus and fallopian tubes help the sperm to move. Also, prostaglandin, a hormone found in semen, may intensify uterine contractions—not felt by the woman—and shorten the sperm's travel time. Sperm stay alive in the female reproductive tract for 24 to 72 hours. During the first 24 hours after ejaculation, they are at a peak level of health and fertility. The egg's peak fertile period lasts 8 to 12 hours, though an egg can be fertilized for up to 24 hours after ovulation.

Most frequently the millions of sperm in the ejaculate meet an egg in one of the fallopian tubes. For egg and sperm to unite, at least one sperm must penetrate the transparent outer layer of the egg. The sperm secretes an enzyme, hyaluronidase, that dissolves this outer layer, allowing the sperm to enter and fertilize the egg. The union of the egg and the sperm is called **conception**, and the product of that union is called a **conceptus**. At this point the sex of the potential offspring has already been determined by the absence or presence of a Y chromosome in the sperm. It is also possible, though not certain, that the number of offspring has been determined (more than one conceptus may have been conceived).

Implantation

Once the egg is fertilized, the conceptus is known as a **zygote**. The one cell of the zygote begins to divide even as it travels down the fallopian tube on its way to implant itself in the uterus. One cell divides into two cells, the two become four, and so cell division continues. By a week after concep-

Although many sperm cells may reach the egg cell, usually only one will fertilize it.

conception
The union of the sperm and ovum; also called *fertilization*.

conceptus
The fertilized ovum; the product of conception.

zygote
A fertilized egg.

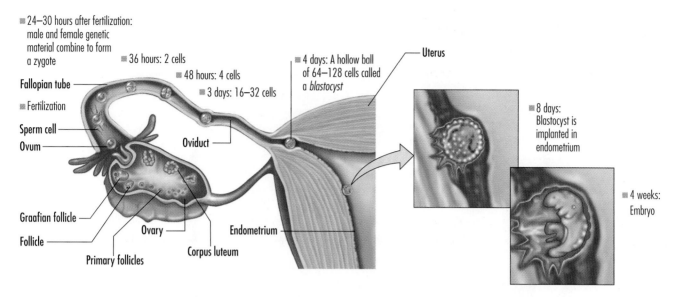

FIGURE 8.1 Following the ovum from ovulation through fertilization and implantation. After being ruptured from the ovary, the ovum is fertilized within the fallopian tube. It then travels to the uterus, where, as a blastocyst, it is implanted on the endometrium (lining) of the uterus.

tion, the zygote is a hollow ball of 100 cells. At this point it is termed a *blastocyst*. Now two layers of cells begin to form. The inner layer of cells will become the **embryo**; the embryo is the zygote from the time of implantation through the first 8 weeks of development. The outer layer of cells, called *trophoblasts*, secretes enzymes that erode the uterine lining so that the blastocyst can attach itself to the endometrium 7 or 8 days after fertilization (Figure 8.1). After implantation these trophoblasts and other cells proliferate and eventually form the placenta, the umbilical cord, and the amniotic sac, a membrane filled with **amniotic fluid**, which surrounds the developing fetus and embryo by the end of the eighth week and absorbs shocks (Shier, Butler, & Lewis, 2003).

Immediately after implantation, the embryo begins receiving nourishment from the endometrial tissue of the mother. Progesterone acts on this tissue to produce the necessary nutrients—glycogen, proteins, lipids, and some minerals. The embryo is nourished from this source for 8 to 10 weeks until the placenta has developed sufficiently to take over.

The **placenta** is a disc-shaped organ that attaches to the uterine wall and is connected to the fetus by the **umbilical cord**. Together the placenta and the umbilical cord (which is attached to the baby at the navel and to the

mother at the placenta) form the lifeline between the mother and the fetus. Nutrients, oxygen, and chemicals pass through the walls of the placenta to the fetus. Waste from the fetus is returned to the mother's blood. The placenta, which by the end of the pregnancy will reach a diameter of 8 inches (about 20 centimeters), contains two sets of blood vessels (Figure 8.2). Fetal circulation occurs within the fetus and the inner part of the placenta, while the mother's circulation flows in the walls of the uterus and the uterine side of the placenta. The fetus's blood flows through two umbilical arteries to the placenta and back from the placenta to the fetus by one vein. One important function of the placenta is to keep the blood systems of the mother and child separated from each other. It does this even though the placenta has *permeability*—that is, it allows some substances to pass between mother and fetus. Throughout the pregnancy, besides allowing nourishment and waste to pass between mother and child, the placenta helps to keep bacteria away from the fetus and allows antibodies (disease fighters) to cross to the fetus. These antibodies make the baby immune to diseases to which the mother is immune for about 6 months after birth.

As the embryo develops, the placenta secretes the hormone **human chorionic gonadotropin (HCG)**. This hormone is detectable through blood tests 8 days

embryo
The developing fetus during the 2 months after conception.

amniotic fluid
The fluid inside the amniotic sac in which the fetus floats; it acts as a shock absorber, maintains the fetus at a constant temperature, and serves as a nutrient.

placenta
An organ of interchange between mother and fetus; oxygen, nutrients, and waste are exchanged through its cells.

umbilical cord
The lifeline between mother and fetus, which contains two arteries and one vein. Food, oxygen, and chemicals are transported to the child through the arteries, and waste is returned to the mother through the vein.

human chorionic gonadotropin (HCG)
The hormone that appears in the blood and urine, providing evidence that a pregnancy has occurred.

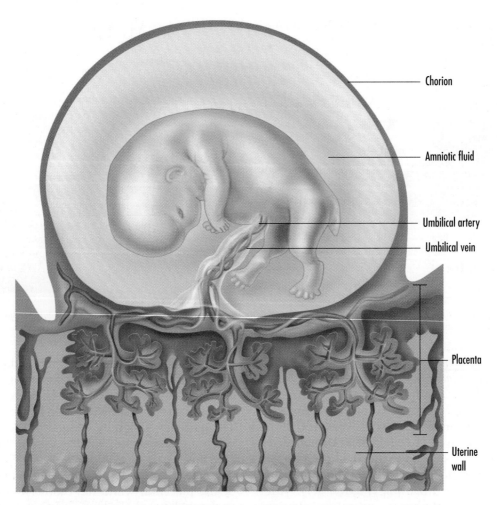

Chorion

Amniotic fluid

Umbilical artery

Umbilical vein

Placenta

Uterine wall

FIGURE 8.2 The embryo and placenta as they appear during the seventh week of development.

after fertilization, just as the blastocyst is implanting, and its presence confirms pregnancy. HCG reaches its maximal level 7 weeks after fertilization and its lowest level about 9 weeks later (16 weeks after fertilization). The function of HCG is to keep the corpus luteum of the ovum alive so that it can continue to secrete estrogen and progesterone. Estrogen and progesterone maintain the uterine endometrium, which nourishes the early pregnancy. By about the 11th week of pregnancy, the placenta itself secretes enough progesterone and estrogen to maintain the pregnancy, and the corpus luteum dies.

Pregnancy

In the preceding section we focused on the developing zygote almost as if it were a being apart. But the development of a new person involves physiological changes in two human beings: the forming fetus and the mother. Let us back up now to account for the change in a woman after an egg is fertilized within her body.

After conception a woman is in a state of pregnancy, which lasts for the time the fetus takes to develop. This period can vary, but the time span from the last menstrual period to the birth of the baby is usually 9 calendar months (10 lunar months, 40 weeks, or 280 days). Most women deliver their babies within 2 weeks of the predicted date, sometimes called the **expected date of confinement (EDC)**. About 4% deliver on the exact date. The EDC is calculated by a formula called *Nägele's rule:* Establish the first day of the last normal menstrual period, add 7 days, and subtract 3 months from this date. The date is the EDC. Nagele's rule is based on a 28-day cycle, however, and, as we have noted, not all women have this cycle. Therefore, a medical practitioner will calculate each patient's EDC to the best of his or her ability, adapting the rule as necessary. At the point at which the fetus has the optimal chance for sur-

> **expected date of confinement (EDC)**
> Due date for normal pregnancy that is usually estimated by Nägele's rule.

vival outside the uterus, the pregnancy has reached term, or completion.

Ectopic Pregnancy

An **ectopic pregnancy** is characterized by implantation of the blastocyst in a site other than the uterus. The rate of ectopic pregnancy has increased sixfold since 1970 and is now the main cause of maternal morbidity (illness) and mortality in the first trimester (Sepillian & Wood, 2007).

Women 30 years of age and older and African American women are at a greater risk for ectopic pregnancy. It has been hypothesized that rates are higher for African American women because they also have higher rates of **pelvic inflammatory disease (PID)**.

> **ectopic pregnancy**
> The development of the zygote in a location other than the uterus.
>
> **pelvic inflammatory disease (PID)**
> Infection of the reproductive organs, particularly the uterus, fallopian tubes, and pelvic cavity.

Several major risk factors that are believed to predispose one to an ectopic pregnancy have been identified (American Pregnancy Association, 2006). These include PID, sexually transmitted infections (STIs), previous ectopic pregnancies, abdominal surgery, use of either an intrauterine device (IUD) or oral contraceptives at the time of ovulation, and maternal cigarette smoking at the time of conception.

It is essential that an ectopic pregnancy be diagnosed quickly. According to the Centers for Disease Control and Prevention, all women should be aware of the signs and symptoms of ectopic pregnancy (*Female sterilization: Risk of ectopic pregnancy after tubal sterilization fact sheet*, 2005). Women of reproductive age should seek medical advice immediately if they experience pelvic and abdominal pain and a lack of menstruation accompanied by vaginal spotting or bleeding. These symptoms indicate the possibility of ectopic pregnancy. Ultrasound can confirm the presence of an ectopic pregnancy by 6 weeks' gestation, facilitating treatment that is the least destructive and costly.

Confirming Pregnancy

The signs of pregnancy known long before our current methods of testing were available are divided into three categories: presumptive, probable, and positive. Because many of the signs and symptoms of pregnancy may also be attributed to other conditions, medical practitioners proceed with caution to avoid a wrong conclusion. Emotional, endocrine, or systemic conditions can cause symptoms identical to the early signs of pregnancy.

Myth vs Fact

Myth: The peak period for sperm and egg to be fertilized is 1 week after they are released.
Fact: The peak period for sperm is about 24 hours after ejaculated, and the peak period for the egg is approximately 12 hours after release.

Myth: The egg is fertilized by the sperm in the uterus.
Fact: The egg–sperm union occurs in the fallopian tube.

Myth: Obstetricians are very accurate at predicting the date of delivery.
Fact: Only approximately 4% of women actually deliver on the expected date of confinement; most women do deliver within 2 weeks of their predicted due date.

Myth: To protect the fetus, pregnant women should refrain from exercising during their pregnancy.
Fact: Pregnant women can exercise without causing harm to the fetus. However, they should follow the exercise guidelines of the American College of Obstetrics and Gynecology.

Myth: As long as drugs are available over the counter, a pregnant woman can feel safe taking them.
Fact: All drugs have the potential to cause harm to fetuses. Therefore, pregnant women should refrain from taking all medications without the advice of their doctors.

Presumptive Signs
Presumptive signs and symptoms are those that may indicate pregnancy but that may occur when a woman is not pregnant. The presumptive signs and symptoms include missed menstrual periods, nausea and vomiting, a tingling feeling in the breast (*mastodynia*), increased urinary frequency, some weight gain, fatigue, a rise in the basal body temperature, some skin changes, slight abdominal enlargement, and some vaginal discoloration and discharge. It is important to note that not all pregnant women experience all these symptoms.

Probable Signs
Probable signs and symptoms include the presumptive symptoms plus enlargement of the abdomen and the uterus, some painless uterine contractions, *ballottement* (at 16 to 20 weeks, bimanual examination gives the physician an impression that a floating object is in the uterus), and *uterine souffle* (a rushing sound, which the physician hears through a stethoscope placed on the woman's abdomen). Uterine souffle in pregnant women is caused by blood filling placental blood vessels and spaces.

Positive Signs
What are conventionally called the positive signs of pregnancy are not present until the 17th week after conception. There are three of these signs, any one of which can confirm a pregnancy: fetal heartbeat, which can be monitored at 17 to 18 weeks; active

DIMENSIONS

The Couvade Syndrome

Around the globe, men whose partners are pregnant are experiencing sympathetic pregnancy symptoms. Called the *couvade syndrome*, it has been verified in men in America, Europe, and Asia (Khanobdee, Sukratanachaiyakul, & Gay, 1993). Cases have been reported across cultures, continents, and centuries (Polinski, 2009). Symptoms include indigestion, increased or decreased appetite, weight gain, diarrhea or constipation, headache, and toothache. Onset is usually during the third gestational month. Symptoms generally resolve with childbirth (Budur, Mathews, & Mathews, 2005). The exact cause of these symptoms is not known. Symptoms typically occur during the late stages of the first trimester, with an increase in symptoms during the late stage of the third trimester. Studies report between 11% to 65%

of men experience sympathetic pregnancy symptoms (Masoni, Maio, Trimarchi, de Punzio, & Fioretti, 1994).

Katherine E. Wynne-Edwards and Anne Storey studied the couvade syndrome to determine the biological changes that occur in men experiencing sympathetic pregnancy symptoms (Polinski, 2009). What they found was fascinating. When examining the saliva and blood of men whose partners were pregnant, they found increased levels of the hormones prolactin (involved in breast milk production), estradiol (a form of estrogen), and cortisol (related to the stress response), and a decreased level of testosterone (a male hormone associated with aggression) (Being a Dad . . ., 2000). The conclusion was that men experience hormonal changes similar to changes experienced by their pregnant spouses.

fetal movement, at about the fifth month or between the 20th and 24th weeks; and palpation of the abdomen, by which the practitioner can detect the fetus. X ray would reveal a fetal skeleton, but this procedure is rarely used, because it can harm the developing fetus.

Women today do not need to wait months to confirm a pregnancy, and for the health of both the woman and the developing fetus it is best not to do so. Echography or ultrasonography (which measures sound waves as they pass through tissues of various densities, each returning its own echo) can be done as early as 4 weeks, and laboratory tests on urine and blood samples can now be done as early as 8 days after conception.

Pregnancy Tests

Pregnancy is confirmed by the presence of the hormone human chorionic gonadotropin (HCG), which is found in the blood and urine if a pregnancy exists. Currently the most frequently used laboratory test has the intimidating name of *beta subunit HCG radioimmunoassay*. This test measures the HCG in a blood sample and can confirm pregnancy, as mentioned earlier, about 8 days after conception occurs.

Two other laboratory pregnancy tests currently in use are the slide test and the test tube test. The slide test is a urine test that can be performed 2½ weeks after a missed menstrual period. Results are obtainable in about 1 or 2 minutes. The test tube test is performed, at the earliest, 2½ weeks after a missed menstrual period. In both the slide and tube tests, urine is mixed with a chemical reagent. The slide test is less sensitive and the blood test more sensitive to the presence of HCG.

Home pregnancy testing is also available. Commercial test kits that measure the presence of HCG in urine can be used as early as the day menstruation should have started. When used according to directions, they are considered to be quite accurate. The problem is that accurate use of a test by an inexperienced person can sometimes be difficult. Nervousness, possible misreading of directions, and improper handling of the kit's components can lead to inaccurate results. Often people feel the tests should be repeated. This can increase the cost considerably and still does not guarantee accurate findings. If one has a choice, a professional laboratory procedure is preferred. Professional testing is done by private, health-department, clinic, and hospital laboratories.

Due Date and Delivery Date

As mentioned earlier, to determine the approximate due date, obstetricians use what is called Nägele's rule. They identify the first day of the last period, count back 3 months, and then add 7 days. For example, if the first day of the last missed period was January 1, 2009, the approximate due date would be October 8, 2009. If the pregnancy exceeds 38 weeks and more urgently after 40 weeks, concern for the health of the fetus may necessitate inducing labor (Greenfield, 2004). Pregnancies of that length are associated with a higher risk of infant mortality and injury to the mother and baby (Bruckner, Cheng, & Caughey, 2008). In addition, induction may be recommended if there is a maternal illness such as high blood pressure, diabetes, or uterine infection.

Labor can be induced in several ways. One method involves the intravenous administration of pitocin, an artificial version of the hormone oxytocin. Generally, the amount is increased every 15 to 30 minutes until a good contraction pattern is achieved. Induction can also occur by the administration of prostaglandin gels or suppositories. These are used when the cervix is not favorable, meaning that it is dilated less than 3 centimeters, is hard, posterior, not effaced, or barely effaced, or any combination of these characteristics (Weiss, 2009). Another method of inducing labor is to artificially rupture the membrane ("breaking the bag of waters"). Lastly, some midwives or other holistic providers practice *natural induction,* which may include use of herbs, castor oil, or other agents to stimulate or advance a stalled labor.

■ Fetal Development

Prenatal development is commonly regarded as having two stages: the **embryonic stage** (from the Greek *embryo,* "to swell"), which lasts 2 months, and the **fetal stage** (from the Latin *fetus,* "the young one"), which lasts from the beginning of the third month—when the fetus begins to look human—to birth (Figure 8.3). The 9-month pregnancy, however, is commonly viewed as consisting of three 3-month developmental periods called **trimesters**.

embryonic stage
The stage of prenatal development that includes the first 8 weeks of pregnancy.

fetal stage
Period from the ninth week of pregnancy to birth.

trimester
A 3-month period of the 9-month pregnancy, which is typically divided into three trimesters.

By the beginning of the eighth week of development, the embryonic body has recognizable human features.

The First Trimester

During the first trimester, weeks 1 through 12, most of the embryo's physiological systems and body parts begin to form. At the end of the first month, the embryo is about 0.25 inch (0.6 centimeter) long. By this time, three cell layers have formed: the *ectoderm* (outer layer), from which the skin, sense organs, and the nervous system will grow; the *mesoderm* (middle layer), from which the muscular, circulatory, and excretory systems will form; and the *endoderm* (inner layer), from which the digestive system, glandular systems, and lungs will develop.

At the end of the second month, the embryo is about 1¼ inches (3 centimeters) long and weighs 1/30 ounce (0.9 gram). The head represents almost half the embryo's total bulk. Facial features such as eyes, ears, nose, lips, and tongue are visible, and the forehead is prominent because of the brain size (Figure 8.4).

When the third month begins, as mentioned, the developing child is called a **fetus**. At the third month the fetus, afloat in the amniotic fluid, is 3 inches (7.6 centimeters) long and 1 ounce (2.8 grams) in weight. It can move, but its motions are not yet felt by the mother. The fingers and toes have nails, and the genitals can be seen as male or female. By the end of the first trimester, the fetus is a miniature human. During the next two trimesters, organs mature and general growth occurs.

fetus
The developing child from the ninth week after conception until birth.

The Second Trimester

During the fourth month, the first month of the second trimester, the greatest amount of fetal growth

FIGURE 8.3 Major changes in fetal development from the 3rd week after conception through the 10th week.

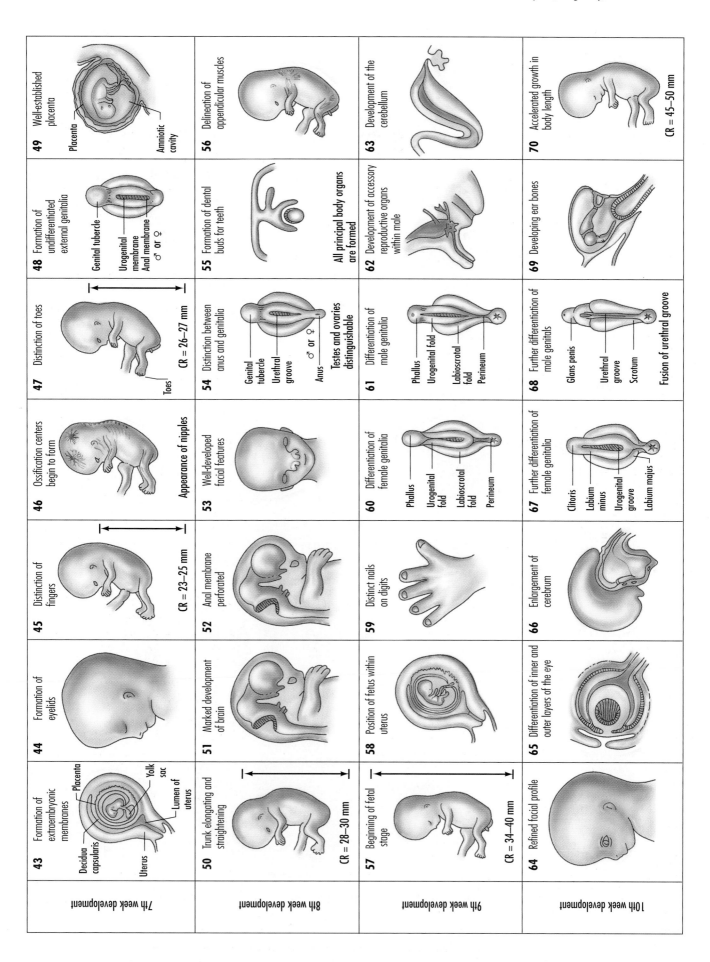

43 Formation of extraembryonic membranes

Placenta
Decidua capsularis
Uterus
Yolk sac
Lumen of uterus

44 Formation of eyelids

45 Distinction of fingers

CR = 23–25 mm

46 Ossification centers begin to form

Appearance of nipples

47 Distinction of toes

CR = 26–27 mm

Toes

48 Formation of undifferentiated external genitalia

Genital tubercle
Urogenital membrane
Anal membrane
♂ or ♀

49 Well-established placenta

Placenta
Amniotic cavity

7th week development

50 Trunk elongating and straightening

CR = 28–30 mm

51 Marked development of brain

52 Anal membrane perforated

53 Well-developed facial features

54 Distinction between anus and genitalia

Genital tubercle
Urethral groove
Anus
♂ or ♀

Testes and ovaries distinguishable

55 Formation of dental buds for teeth

All principal body organs are formed

56 Delineation of appendicular muscles

8th week development

57 Beginning of fetal stage

CR = 34–40 mm

58 Position of fetus within uterus

59 Distinct nails on digits

60 Differentiation of female genitalia

Phallus
Urogenital fold
Labioscrotal fold
Perineum

61 Differentiation of male genitalia

Phallus
Urogenital fold
Labioscrotal fold
Perineum

62 Development of accessory reproductive organs within male

63 Development of the cerebellum

9th week development

64 Refined facial profile

65 Differentiation of inner and outer layers of the eye

66 Enlargement of cerebrum

67 Further differentiation of female genitalia

Clitoris
Labium minus
Urogenital groove
Labium majus

68 Further differentiation of male genitals

Glans penis
Urethral groove
Scrotum

Fusion of urethral groove

69 Developing ear bones

70 Accelerated growth in body length

CR = 45–50 mm

10th week development

Actual size

4 weeks

5 weeks

6 weeks

7 weeks

FIGURE **8.4** In the fifth through seventh weeks of development, the embryonic body and face start to develop a humanlike appearance.

occurs. The fetus is now 6 inches (15 centimeters) long, the lower body is growing increasingly larger, and the head is now one-third the length of the body. The fetus moves and can suck, and its motion, called **quickening**, is felt by the mother. During the fifth month, the halfway point of the pregnancy, the fetus weighs about 1 pound (454 grams) and is about 12 inches (30 centimeters) long. It sleeps and wakes and has a preferred body position. During the sixth month the fetus grows about 2 inches (5 centimeters) and gains another pound. By this point the fetus's eyes are formed, it is sensitive to light, and it can hear uterine sounds. The skin is wrinkled and covered with fine hair. Though development is well under way, a baby born at this stage probably would not survive. By the end of this trimester, refinement of body features has occurred, movement is stronger, and further growth has been achieved.

> **quickening**
> Movements of the fetus felt by the mother; usually occurs about the fourth month of pregnancy.

The Third Trimester

During the period of the third trimester, the baby positions itself more or less for birth. The most common fetal position, or *presentation*, is head down (Figure 8.5).

As a fat layer is laid underneath the skin, the fetus takes on a more babylike form. By the end of the seventh month, it is generally agreed, the baby can live outside the uterus, although babies have survived when born much earlier and cared for in neonatal intensive care units. By the end of the eighth month, the fetus weighs about 5 pounds and 4 ounces (2,384 grams) and is about 20 inches (51 centimeters) long. During the eighth and ninth months, skin redness lessens and wrinkles begin to disappear as the fetus begins to gain about $1\frac{1}{2}$ pound (227 grams) a week. The nails reach the end of the fingers and toes and the fetus's actions become limited because of its tight fit in the uterus. As birth becomes imminent, in the 38th to 40th weeks, the head is 60% of its full size, the fine body hair has about disappeared, and the skin becomes smoother

- Uterus
- Pelvic bones
- Vaginal canal

■ Head down with baby's chin on chest

■ Head extended, face presentation

■ Head down, brow presentation

■ Frank breech, baby's legs over abdomen (most common breech presentation)

■ Incomplete foot presentation

■ Transverse, with shoulder presentation

■ Full breech, baby cross-legged in mother (most infrequent presentation)

FIGURE **8.5** Fetal positions.

Communication
DIMENSIONS

Communicating About Pregnancy

Although it is not routinely discussed, most women do not have an easy time with pregnancy: Morning sickness, continual tiredness, and new physical sensations may bring about momentary feelings of "Did I do the right thing?" This is balanced against society's view of happy pregnant women, who work until the last days of pregnancy and always smile.

From our experience, pregnant women who talk to other women who have been pregnant gain a great sense of relief. They find that their experience is not unique. Few women go through a "perfect" pregnancy. Ironically, women who have been pregnant usually wait for the pregnant woman to discuss an issue before opening up about their experience.

But pregnant women who talk to those who have not had children (a group that includes men) are often chided for their complaining. One pregnant woman recently said that after she had morning sickness at work—every day for weeks on end—most colleagues would smile and remind her of how "lucky" she was. Any complaining during lunch or breaks was met with reproachful glares—how dare she have a negative thought about the fetus inside her! She soon learned to keep her feelings to herself.

Explain why people have such a hard time talking about pregnancy. Is it because it is the result of sexual activity? Or because of the special roles that young children play in our society?

and is now covered with a waxy protective substance called the *vernix caseosa*.

During this last trimester, the fetus will have reached a weight and size that prepare it to live independently of the mother. The baby is ready for delivery and birth.

Bearing a Healthy Infant: Prenatal Choices

Staying as healthy as possible is the pregnant woman's chief responsibility to her developing child. Pregnancy is a time of great change: Both physical and psychological factors affect the health and well-being of an expectant mother and her developing child. Many choices must be made by expectant parents, including whom to seek out for advice during pregnancy, where the birth will take place, and what health-enhancing lifestyle modifications they can make throughout the pregnancy. In the sections that follow, we discuss the many decisions facing today's expectant parents.

Birth Attendant Options

Even though pregnancy is a normal physiological event, there is still no question that a woman's general health affects not only her own experience of pregnancy but also the health of her developing child. The best advice for a healthy pregnancy is supervision by a health practitioner trained to give prenatal (prebirth) care. Thus, the selection of a health professional who will advise during the pregnancy and serve as the birth attendant during labor and delivery is an important decision that should be made by the expectant parents early in the pregnancy.

In the United States all physicians are trained in medical school in the procedures involved in pregnancy and birth. Generally, however, the family-practice specialist (a newer term for general practitioner) and the **obstetrician** are the primary providers of pregnancy care. The obstetrician has had specialized advanced training in this area. Many women physicians specialize in obstetrics, and a considerable number of pregnant women purposely seek women obstetricians. Some women feel that a female physician is more empathetic and understanding of the variety of body changes that occur during pregnancy and delivery. There is the possibility that the female physician has experienced parturition (the process of giving birth), and many pregnant women find this reassuring and relaxing.

Midwifery has also been used in the United States. Historically, Ameri-

obstetrician
A physician who specializes in the care of pregnant women and the process of childbirth. Because these physicians are also gynecologists, they are often referred to as obstetrician–gynecologists or OB–GYNs.

midwifery
The practice by nonphysicians of assisting in the process of pregnancy and childbirth. Lay midwives are not trained health care professionals; nurse midwives are registered nurses who have received advanced training and often certification in the techniques of the birthing process.

can midwives were laypeople who helped with birth deliveries. Today nurse–midwives are registered nurses (RNs) or certified nurse–midwives (CNMs) who receive advanced training in childbirth processes. Many states require nurse–midwives to pass a national certification exam given by the American College of Nurse–Midwives to be licensed.

Whereas midwife-attended births steadily increased from less than 1% in 1975 to 8% in 2004, the rate has remained constant since then in this country (Martin et al., 2009). In 2006, 8% of births in the United States were attended by midwives—94% of whom were CNMs. Most midwife-attended births occur in hospitals (93%).

Nurse–midwifery is often chosen by families who consider birthing to be a natural process that does not require highly technological interventions. Nurse–midwives routinely practice in freestanding birth centers and in hospitals. Some nurse–midwives work with an obstetrician present at the delivery; some work alone but have an affiliation with an obstetrician who is on call for problem deliveries. Some nurse–midwives assist in home deliveries with a physician present or on call.

Increasingly couples are planning their deliveries, making decisions that suit them, and choosing birth attendants and facilities to match their needs.

Birthing Alternatives

To receive the kind of care they want before, during, and after delivery, future parents should investigate the birthing alternatives available in their area as soon as possible. Often the choice of a birth attendant is tied to the setting in which that birth attendant chooses to or is allowed to practice. Currently in the United States there are three major settings where labor and delivery typically occur: hospitals, the home, and freestanding birth centers. Each setting has advantages and disadvantages that should be considered by prospective parents.

Hospital Birth

Not many years ago most babies were born in hospital delivery rooms with the mother heavily drugged and the father barred from participating. Nowadays expectant parents often have a wide range of choices regarding the kind of delivery they will experience in the hospital setting.

Perhaps the most marked change is the increased participation of fathers in the birth of their children. Even in traditional births, fathers are now allowed to be present in the delivery rooms of many hospitals, and in less conventional setups fathers often participate—perhaps by helping to hold the newborn as it emerges from the birth canal or by cutting the umbili-

Many hospitals encourage fathers to participate in the birth of their children. Some even allow the father to hold the newborn as it emerges from the birth canal, or to help cut the umbilical cord.

cal cord (under guidance, of course). This trend reflects a new appreciation for the role of fathers in child rearing. Although long considered "women's work," childbearing and raising are increasingly being recognized as joint undertakings, involving father and mother equally. The benefit of this new trend is that fathers share openly not only in the work and responsibility of parenting but also in the joys and satisfactions. Many believe that this form of "male liberation" results in sounder father–child relationships and that strong father–infant bonds begin, as do mother–child bonds, at the moment of birth.

Most traditional hospital maternity facilities consist of separate rooms for labor, delivery, and recovery. Physicians, usually obstetricians, serve as the primary birth attendant, with assistance from nurses. Emergency equipment and trained personnel are quickly accessible should the need arise. **Analgesics** and **anesthetics** are options typically available only in this setting. High-risk pregnancies especially benefit from technological advances found in the hospital setting.

Although traditional labor and delivery rooms are still the standard in many hospitals, some hospitals provide the option of a more homelike birth setting for their clients. Typically this takes the form of a **birthing room**, which is attached to a labor

analgesics
Substances that decrease pain locally, such as topical creams.

anesthetics
Substances that elicit unconsciousness and thereby relieve pain.

birthing room
A homelike birth setting now available in some hospitals.

(a)

(b)

Many hospitals now offer a birthing room alternative (a) in addition to the traditional hospital delivery room (b).

and delivery suite and is often run by nurses and nurse midwives. The birthing room is decorated in a homelike style, often including soft lighting, wallpaper, a rocking chair, and a private bath. Mothers labor, deliver, and recover in one room with a support person, such as a spouse or other family member, present. Regulations regarding the use of a birthing room vary from one hospital to the next, and not uncommonly birthing rooms are used only for low-risk pregnancies. Couples interested in using a hospital birthing room need to find out whether this option is available at local hospitals and whether they are likely candidates for its use.

Home Birth

Home birth with a nurse–midwife is another birth alternative. Home birth is an option for only the healthiest women, and nurse–midwives are trained to screen out women who might be at risk of complications during labor and delivery. For low-risk women, studies have found home birth to be as safe as hospital delivery (Johnson & Davis, 2005). Home birth candidates are watched closely during pregnancy for signs of possible risk. Nevertheless, the safety of home birth is debated in this country (Reinberg, 2005).

If a couple chooses the home birth option, the midwife or physician—though relatively few physicians support home birth—goes to the couple's home and delivers the baby in a previously selected room. Children and other family members may be present. Currently only about 1% of women in the United States choose to have their babies at home (Martin et al., 2009).

Freestanding Birth Centers

The birth center is a birthing alternative available to prospective parents that represents a compromise between the traditional hospital delivery, character-

ized by medical intervention, and the controversial option of home birth. Birth centers are facilities that offer a homelike birth experience outside a hospital setting. Most birth centers are licensed by the state and are often run by nurse–midwives. Typically, birth centers limit their clientele to low-risk pregnancies. Women are monitored throughout the pregnancy by a nurse–midwife and may be referred to a hospital for delivery if complications arise during the prenatal period. Some emergency equipment is available in birth centers, and most birth centers are located in close proximity to a hos-

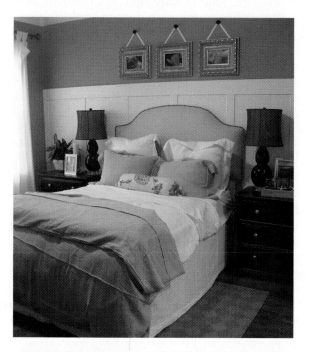

Many hospitals have built plush birthing centers to attract patients to this highly profitable area. Consumers have many options to choose from and should shop around and ask people they know for referrals before making a final selection.

pital for ready access if medical care is needed. It has been estimated that approximately 13% of women who begin delivery at a birth center are transferred to a hospital setting to complete the delivery (Reinberg, 2005).

Prenatal and postnatal care are provided by the birth center's staff, and this continuity of care is a major benefit offered by birth centers. Freestanding birth centers are family oriented, encouraging family participation throughout the prenatal period. Couples are active participants in designing their personal birth plan, and family members are allowed to stay near the mother during labor and delivery.

Additionally, the infant remains with the mother after delivery. Although birth centers have increased in popularity and availability, they are not available in every city or even every state. Couples who wish to use a birth center must investigate the availability of this birth alternative in their community.

Nowadays it is acknowledged that childbirth is an emotional experience as well as a physical one—and not just for the mother and child but for the father as well. The many birthing options available reflect this perspective and make responsible decision making by expectant parents increasingly important. If a birthing center option is chosen, a center that is accredited by the Commission for the Accreditation of Birth Centers (CABC) should be selected. In addition, some states regulate birth centers; therefore, only those facilities sanctioned by the state should be considered.

Prenatal Care

Traditionally, **prenatal care** consists of monitoring fetal development, screening for high-risk pregnancy, and educating those involved about pregnancy and childbirth. For most normal pregnancies 10 to 12 prenatal care visits, beginning at about the 6th week of pregnancy, are optimal.

> **prenatal care**
> Care given to an expectant mother before the birth of her child that typically consists of monitoring fetal development, screening for high-risk pregnancy, and providing education for pregnancy and childbirth.

For a high-risk pregnancy more frequent visits may be necessary. Studies show that the risk of very low birth weight increases when women do not receive comprehensive prenatal care.

The prenatal evaluation begins, as most medical visits do, with the taking of a personal health history, relevant social and emotional factors, employment of the parents, conditions of their work environment, and the stability of their relationship itself. The practitioner is usually interested in knowing what sort of support system the woman and her new child will have, for many factors—both medical and nonmedical—can

affect the well-being of a pregnant woman and her child. Additionally, a series of laboratory tests is usually completed at the first prenatal examination. These laboratory tests normally include examination for hemoglobin levels, glucose or protein in the urine, evidence of a current syphilis infection, antibodies for rubella (German measles), and blood type and Rh determination (discussed shortly). An examination of the cervix is also done at this time.

A family history is taken as well. Is the woman on her own—and thus possibly facing much stress and financial anxiety—or does she live with the baby's father? Is the father involved in the pregnancy? Is the baby wanted or unwanted? Was the pregnancy planned or unexpected? All these factors can place stress on the mother, and thus they have a bearing on her prenatal care. The medical practitioner overseeing her care will—or should—take an interest in these matters from the start. On the basis of this medical and social history, the practitioner will also determine how much information the expectant parents lack, what sort of guidance they need to adapt to the pregnancy, and, of course, what sort of delivery they favor. When pregnancy is concerned, the practitioner–client relationship is unique. If the couple, and particularly the mother, feel misgivings about their first choice, seeking another practitioner early in the pregnancy is highly advisable.

Nutrition and Weight Gain

Maternal nutrition directly affects fetal growth and development. The developing fetus depends on the mother for nutrition and can deplete her supply of necessary nutrients. For example, the mother usually needs iron supplements to prevent anemia. Iron is a major component of hemoglobin, which carries oxygen to the cells of both mother and baby. Protein influences tissue building in both the mother and baby and contributes to maintaining a healthy placenta and uterus. Vitamins ensure better resistance to infection, influence energy level, and aid in the absorption of calcium. Calcium is needed by the mother to prevent muscle irritability and by the baby to allow bone growth. Trace minerals, such as zinc and cobalt, build enzymes that influence chemical actions. The food intake of the mother fuels the development of the baby and directly influences the baby's weight gain (Table 8.1).

Among the most important nutrients to obtain during pregnancy is folate (a B vitamin), which helps prevent serious abnormalities of the brain and spinal cord. Lack of folate also may increase the risk of preterm delivery, low birth weight, and poor fetal growth. Folate obtained through vitamin supplements is called folic acid. At mentioned, other necessary nutrients

TABLE 8.1   Daily Dietary Allowances Recommended by the Food and Nutrition Board

Dietary Allowance	Pregnant	Lactating
Protein (g)	71	71
Fat-Soluble Vitamins		
Vitamin A (μg RE)	770	1,300
Vitamin D (μg)	5	5
Vitamin E (mg [α = TE] TE)	15	19
Vitamin K (μg)	90	90
Water-Soluble Vitamins		
Vitamin C (mg)	85	120
Thiamine	1.4	1.4
Riboflavin (mg)	1.4	1.6
Niacin (mg NE)	18	17
Vitamin B_6 (mg)	1.9	2.0
Folate (μg)	600	500
Vitamin B_{12} (μg)	2.6	2.8
Minerals		
Calcium (mg)	1,000	1,100
Phosphorus (mg)	700	700
Magnesium (mg)	350	310
Iron (mg)	27	9
Zinc (mg)	11	12
Iodine (μg)	220	290
Selenium (μg)	60	70

RE = retinol equivalents
TE = tocopherol equivalents
NE = niacin equivalents
Source: Excerpted with permission from *Dietary reference intakes for energy, carbohydrate, fiber, fat, fatty acids, cholesterol, protein, and amino acids (macronutrients)*. National Academy of Sciences. Washington, DC: National Academies Press, 2005.

include calcium for strong bones and teeth, protein for growth and repair of body tissue, and iron.

Even if they eat healthfully, women may miss out on key nutrients. A daily prenatal vitamin, ideally starting 3 months before conception, can compensate for any missed nutritional needs. In addition, health care providers may recommend special supplements for women who follow a strict vegetarian diet or who have chronic health conditions (Mayo Clinic Staff, 2007b).

In the past it was the fashion in prenatal care to place pregnant women on strict regimens to prevent them from gaining more than about 20 pounds. Obese patients were even put on weight-reduction programs. New attitudes suggest that dieting during pregnancy can be harmful in that breakdown of fat produces toxic substances (called *ketones*) that can impair the mental and physical development of the fetus. Current recommendations for a healthy weight gain during pregnancy vary with the prepregnancy weight of the mother (Mayo Clinic Staff, 2007b; National Academy of Sciences, 2004). Those mothers who were considered by their physician to be at a normal weight before conception should gain between 25 and 35 pounds. Those women who were underweight should gain slightly more (28 to 40 pounds); those who were overweight before pregnancy should gain less weight (15 to 25 pounds) (Figure 8.6). As has been noted in this discussion, extra nutrients are needed in pregnancy, and a wide variety of foods is needed to provide them.

Exercise During Pregnancy

The safety of aerobic exercise during pregnancy has been questioned (Magann, 2002; Walling, 2002). Special concern has been voiced about the effects of such exercise on the developing fetus, especially in respect to potential fetal distress, intrauterine growth retardation, fetal malformations, and prematurity (Artel & Wiswell, 1986). Studies to date indicate, however, that exercising is safe for both the pregnant woman and the fetus. It has been suggested that women who exercise during pregnancy benefit from a greater sense of well-being and control over their changing bodies (Morris & Johnson, 2005). Other benefits include a lessening of the physical discomforts of pregnancy and an enhanced postpartum recovery (ACOG, 2003).

To ensure the safety of both the mother and the developing infant, pregnant women should follow the exercise guidelines of the American College of Obstetrics and Gynecology (ACOG, 2003). ACOG states that women can enjoy a much broader range of physical activity during pregnancy than previously believed. Whereas the ACOG guidelines previously took a more cautious approach to exercise during pregnancy, findings from more current research studies have led to their new guidelines. Now ACOG recommends that pregnant women engage in 30 min-

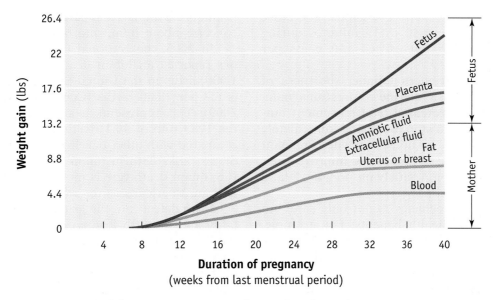

FIGURE **8.6** Pattern and components of maternal weight gain during pregnancy.

utes or more of moderate exercise on most, if not all, days of the week. The exceptions to this recommendation include proscriptions against scuba diving (due to the risk of fetal decompression sickness) and activities that carry a risk of abdominal injury (ice hockey, kickboxing, soccer, or horseback riding). In addition, women with high-risk pregnancies should consult with their physicians before engaging in exercise.

Before exercising during pregnancy, a woman should consult her physician or nurse–midwife. There are certain conditions, such as cardiac disease, a history of three or more spontaneous abortions (miscarriages), or abnormal bleeding, that are contraindications to exercise during pregnancy. If a woman has been sedentary before her pregnancy she should not attempt to take up a strenuous aerobic exercise program. A walking program or a program designed specifically for pregnant women would be most appropriate in this case (BabyCenter, 2006). For those women who wish to continue their aerobic exercise program while pregnant, certain modifications should be made. In the past, it was thought that, regardless of her level of fitness, a pregnant woman should not exercise aerobically for longer than 15 minutes at a time. Strenuous activity lasting longer than 15 minutes was thought to significantly raise maternal core body temperature and lead to nervous system damage in the fetus (Sussman & Levitt, 1989). We now know this is not accurate (Larsson, 2005). Core temperature does not increase significantly and this is no reason for pregnant women to avoid exercising.

Regular intake of fluids during exercise and consumption of adequate calories daily (usually an additional 200 to 300 calories) are essential

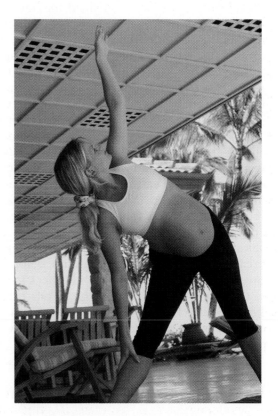

There is no reason that pregnant women should not maintain an exercise regimen. In fact, the American College of Obstetrics and Gynecology recommends pregnant women engage in 30 minutes or more of moderate exercise on most days.

for maintaining a safe exercise program. Pregnant women should not start or stop exercising suddenly; gradual warm-up and cool-down periods of 5 to 10 minutes are recommended. Proper clothing, especially a support bra and good athletic shoes, should be worn during exercise sessions. The pulse should be checked every 10 to 15 minutes during exercising and should not exceed 140 beats per minute.

If a woman experiences fatigue, shortness of breath, dizziness, nausea, uterine contractions, pain, vaginal bleeding, or decreased fetal movement during exercise, she should stop exercising immediately and call her physician or nurse–midwife. Pregnant women who follow these guidelines improve their chances of experiencing a satisfying pregnancy and delivering a healthy baby.

Exercise during pregnancy is not only safe, but can also have many health benefits. For example, prenatal exercise can help prevent preeclampsia, a leading cause of maternal and fetal morbidity and mortality (Weissgerber, Wolfe, & Davies, 2004). Exercise has also been found to decrease low back pain, a common condition in pregnant women (Garshasbi & Faghih, 2005). And, as discussed earlier, exercise during pregnancy can have beneficial mental health benefits, such as an improved sense of well-being. Recognizing these and other health benefits, 66% of pregnant women have been found to engage in leisure-time physical activity (Evenson, Savitz, & Huston, 2004). The most common activities include walking, followed by swimming laps, weight training, gardening, and aerobics. This is not surprising given that 95% of women believe that participating in prenatal exercise is helpful (Krans et al., 2005). Even vigorous exercise during and after pregnancy has been found to be safe and is recommended for top competitive athletes (Kardel, 2005). Among the many benefits are a more rapid return to competition and a physically active lifestyle.

Exercise programs designed especially for pregnant women can be found in many communities. Before joining, however, a pregnant woman should check to make certain that the program follows the ACOG exercise guidelines just described. For women in communities without such programs, ACOG has developed videotape programs that can be used at home.

■ Threats to Having a Healthy Infant

Mothers- and fathers-to-be often worry about whether their baby will be born healthy. In our technological society we are exposed to a larger number of risks to healthy pregnancy than ever before. Exposure to chemicals and radiation at the work site and in the home, lifestyle factors such as cigarette smoking and other drug use and abuse, and exposure to infectious agents are just some of the factors currently posing a risk to bearing healthy children. Although the great majority of infants are born healthy, both public

health professionals and parents-to-be have legitimate concerns about infant morbidity and mortality.

In 2005, the National Center for Health Statistics reported an infant death rate of 6.9 deaths per 1,000 births in the United States. The 2009 estimate is 6.3 per 1,000 births (Central Intelligence Agency, 2009). This represents a significant decrease from the 1988 rate of 10.1 deaths per 1,000 births. Still, compared with other developed countries, the United States ranks 28th in infant deaths. Additionally, the U.S. infant death rate is more than twice as high for African Americans as for whites.

Birth defects are the leading cause of infant mortality and the fifth leading cause of years of potential life lost in the United States. It is estimated that approximately 130,000 infants are born with a major birth defect in this country every year. Many of these babies die during their first year of life. Birth defects are the leading cause of death during the first year of life (March of Dimes, 2006a). The vast majority of children with birth defects, however, must cope with a range of defects throughout their lives.

A new branch of research called **teratology**, which searches for the cause of birth defects, has emerged in recent years. Presently teratologists estimate that 5% to 6% of birth defects are caused by chromosomal defects, another 8% to 10% are caused by mutant genes, and 6% to 10% are related to environmental causes such as toxic chemicals and drugs (Dowie, 1990). For the remaining 70%, the cause is unknown.

> **teratology**
> The study of causative factors of birth defects.

Birth defects are one of the important causes of infant death in the United States; the second leading cause of infant deaths is low birth weight. Low birth weight, which is considered to be a birth weight of less than 5 pounds, 8 ounces, and very low birth weight (less than 3 pounds, 4 ounces) substantially increase an infant's chances of dying during the first year of life. This is especially true for African Americans, for whom low birth weight is the leading cause of infant death in the United States.

There are two types of low birth weight. The first involves infants who are born prematurely (before 36 weeks of gestation) and are thus underweight. A second type of low birth weight is known as *intrauterine growth retardation* (IUGR). These infants are born full term, but they are underdeveloped. Risk factors associated with low birth weight include younger (less than 18 years) and older (greater than 45 years) maternal age, high parity (having given birth to a large number of babies), poor reproduction history (especially a history of low birth weight), low socioeconomic status, low education levels, late or no prenatal care, low pregnancy weight gain, low prepregnancy weight, smoking, and substance abuse (U.S. Department of Health and Human Services, 2000).

Research into the causes and prevention of birth defects and low birth weight is greatly needed. Yet there is much we already know about preventing these conditions. Reducing these risk factors is the focus of our attention here.

Drugs and Other Substances

Any drug taken by a pregnant woman can potentially pass through the placenta to the fetus. If the drug (whether medically prescribed or self-prescribed) affects the mother in some way, it will also affect the developing baby. A danger of taking drugs during pregnancy is that an adult dose can be an overdose for a fetus. The liver of the fetus cannot metabolize drugs as can the adult liver, and the unchanged drug can affect the fetus differently from the mother. Furthermore, drugs can alter the metabolism of the mother, influence hormones in the bloodstream, and affect placenta functioning.

Over-the-Counter Drugs

Many Americans are polydrug users. *Over-the-counter drugs (OTCs),* sold legally without a prescription, are widely used for self-medication purposes. The use of many OTCs causes special concerns for pregnant women. Because of the extensive number of OTCs available, it is beyond the scope of this chapter to provide a complete review. The safest course of action for pregnant women is to avoid self-medication and OTC drugs until their use is approved by the physician or midwife acting as birth attendant.

Cigarette Smoking

Cigarette smoking has been identified as the most toxic harmful exposure during pregnancy (Cornelius & Day, 2000); unquestionably it is harmful to the unborn baby. Still, worldwide, less than 50% of pregnant women manage to stop smoking (Ducret, 2005). In general, smoking during pregnancy is associated with lower birth weights, higher rates of spontaneous abortion, structural changes in and decreased functioning of the placenta, and higher perinatal mortality rate (the perinatal period encompasses the time from 28 weeks of pregnancy to 1 to 4 weeks after birth). In addition, there is a greater risk of ectopic pregnancy (DeKeyser-Boccara & Milliez, 2005). After birth, the infants of mothers who smoke are at a greater risk for childhood illnesses, especially respiratory disorders.

Infants born to smoking mothers weigh less than infants born to nonsmoking mothers. As we mentioned, infants weighing less than 2,500 grams

Cigarette smoke is one of the most toxic substances for fetuses and newborns. Smoking before birth exposes the fetus to a range of health risks, including low birth weight and birth defects. Smoking after birth exposes the infant to breathing problems and other health risks.

(5 pounds, 8 ounces) at birth are classified as low-birth-weight infants and have greater mortality rates. Only 7% of nonsmoking pregnant women's babies are born at low birth weight, whereas 12% of smoking pregnant women give birth to low-birth-weight babies (U.S. Census Bureau, 2002). Yet approximately 25% of women arrive at the end of their pregnancies without having stopped smoking (Contal et al., 2005). The cause of low birth weight in infants of smoking mothers, although not proved, may be oxygen deprivation. Because carbon monoxide combines more readily with hemoglobin (oxygen carriers in the blood) than does oxygen, and because cigarette smokers inhale carbon monoxide, the hemoglobin may be transporting more carbon monoxide and less oxygen than normal to the fetus (Marret, 2005). It is also possible that nicotine reduces placental blood flow, because it is a powerful constrictor of blood vessels, thereby lowering birth weight. The cyanide in smoke might also cause vitamin depletion. To detoxify the cyanide, the mother's body uses more vitamin B_{12} and essential sulfur amino acids, thus depriving the fetus of these nutrients. If smoking is stopped even by the end of the second trimester of pregnancy, birth weights have been shown to approximate those of infants born to nonsmokers

(March of Dimes, 2008). Furthermore, tobacco use is associated with periodontal disease. Maternal periodontal disease, in turn, is a risk factor for preterm deliveries and preterm low birth weight (Boutigny, Boschin, & Delcourt-Debruyne, 2005).

Marijuana

The research needed to establish the effect of a mother's marijuana use on the fetus is currently under way. Preliminary results suggest that there are many potential dangers involved in using marijuana while pregnant.

Tetrahydrocannabinol (THC), the primary psychoactive agent in marijuana and other cannabinoids, can pass through the placental barrier and affect the ability of the placenta to function.

Animal studies have indicated that marijuana is a teratogen (an agent capable of causing birth defects). Many researchers who specialize in the study of birth defects now cautiously assume that any substance capable of causing birth defects in animals is potentially hazardous to humans as well (Dowie, 1990).

Research has found a clear relationship between marijuana use by pregnant women and their offspring. Development of the brain (Fernandez-Ruiz et al., 2004; Suárez et al., 2004; Wang et al., 2004), nervous system (Smith, Fried, Hogan, & Cameron, 2004), and heart (Williams, Correra, & Rasmussen, 2004) in utero are all negatively affected when a pregnant woman uses marijuana. In addition, a significant reduction in birth weight occurs (Shankaran et al., 2004; Hurd et al., 2005). Not surprisingly, children born to women who used marijuana while pregnant experience effects long after birth. For example, they have poorer memories and more difficulty processing information (Kalant, 2004). They also have lower reading and spelling scores, and teachers' evaluations of their performance are lower (Goldschmidt et al., 2004).

Alcohol

It is estimated that 14% of pregnant women in the United States drink alcohol while they are pregnant (Alcohol consumption among women, 2004). Percentages of pregnant drinkers are even higher among some groups of women, such as smokers and the unmarried. Although the overall percentage of pregnant women who consume alcohol appears to be decreasing significantly, this trend is not seen in women with a high school education or less, or in younger women (age 18 to 24 years).

Alcohol consumption by pregnant women is one of the leading causes of mental retardation in the United States (Centers for Disease Control and Prevention, Fetal alcohol spectrum disorders, 2006). To date, there is no consensus as to the amount of alco-

hol necessary to damage a fetus. Alcohol crosses the placental barrier and can affect fetal cells and tissues, as well as interfere with a pregnant woman's ability to maintain a successful pregnancy (Zhang, Sliwowska, & Weinberg, 2005). Furthermore, offspring of women who ingested alcohol during their pregnancies have been found to have a less effective immune system, thereby subjecting them to a greater risk of infections and the effects of stress (Zhang et al., 2005; Gauthier et al., 2005). In addition, attention-deficit hyperactivity disorder (ADHD) occurs more frequently in girls whose mothers report heavy alcohol ingestion during their pregnancies (Knopik et al., 2005). Another condition, dyslexia, is also related to prenatal alcohol exposure (Coffin et al., 2005). Alcohol's effects on the fetus's brain creates cerebellum information-processing deficits that appear to be the reason for the development of dyslexia. Consequently, pregnant women are advised to refrain from drinking alcohol altogether.

A particular pattern of deformity with mental impairment that occurs in offspring of these drinkers has been labeled the **fetal alcohol syndrome (FAS)** and more recently referred to as **fetal alcohol spectrum disorders (FASD)**. Infants suffering from FAS may have unusual facial features, such as small eye slits; deep epicanthic folds (a fold of skin from the eyelid to the inner corner of the eye, giving it a slanted effect); upturned nose; a thin, flattened upper lip; and a flattened or decreased groove in the upper lip. They may also have heart defects, dysfunctions of the central nervous system, or growth deficiency.

> **fetal alcohol syndrome (FAS)**
> Impaired psychological and physical characteristics common in infants born to alcoholic women.
>
> **fetal alcohol spectrum disorders (FASD)**
> The full spectrum of birth defects that are caused by prenatal alcohol exposure.

No safe level of alcohol consumption during pregnancy has been established (American Pregnancy Association, 2008). In fact, a review of studies concluded that even small amounts of alcohol ingested during pregnancy resulted in offspring who were slightly shorter and weighed slightly less than children of mothers who did not ingest alcohol during their pregnancies (Fackelmann, 2002). Although it is problematic extrapolating research findings in animals to humans, it is still worth noting that rat pups exposed to alcohol in utero were more likely to have breast cancer as adults than rat pups not exposed to alcohol in utero. The Surgeon General of the United States recommends that pregnant women avoid use of alcohol during any stage of pregnancy, because it can increase the risk of prematurity, low birth weight, and congenital defects.

Cocaine

The Centers for Disease Control and Prevention (2003) reports on the prevalence of cocaine use, and this report is not reassuring. In fact, cocaine use starts at a young age. For example, 7.2% of ninth graders reported having used cocaine at least once in their lives. This figure increased as students got older so that by their senior year in high school, 12.1% report having used cocaine at least once. And, contrary to some people's stereotype of the typical cocaine user, white Americans report using cocaine twice as much as do African Americans, although African Americans have more cocaine-related emergency room episodes. In 2002, for instance, there were 199,198 cocaine-related emergency room visits, of whom 49,305 were white males, 52,463 were African American males, and 15,881 were Hispanic males. In addition, 29,736 were white females, 27,089 were African American females, and 7,841 were Hispanic females (National Center for Health Statistics, 2004).

Cocaine use by pregnant women is associated with higher rates of miscarriage, low birth weight, stillbirth, birth defects, premature labor, and long-term mental defects in the child exposed to cocaine in utero (March of Dimes, 2006b). More recent research has identified cocaine use by pregnant women to be associated with their children exhibiting significant behavioral problems (Savage et al., 2005), especially aggression (Estelles et al., 2005; Nordstrom et al., 2005). In addition, the offspring of cocaine-using pregnant women develop an inferior attention span and impulsivity (Noland et al., 2005), exhibit poor school performance (Hurt et al., 2005), and poor motor performance (Miller-Loncar et al., 2005). Even the relationship between mother and child suffers. Researchers have found that women who used cocaine during their pregnancies were less sensitive to their infants and that mother–infant interactions during the first year of life were affected (Minnes et al., 2005). However, other researchers have found that the offspring's intelligence and school readiness were not affected (Pulsifer et al., 2004; Frank et al., 2005). Babies born to cocaine-using mothers may be born with an addiction to cocaine themselves and be subjected to a range of health risks, even death. We call these babies *crack babies*, named after crack cocaine, which is smoked rather than snorted. Research also indicates that the testes may be damaged in male fetuses exposed to cocaine, and both male and female infants may have chromosomal abnormalities caused by such exposure (Cocaine and pregnancy, 1991). Further research is needed to determine the effects of cocaine on the developing fetus.

Heroin and Other Narcotics

The common narcotics (or opiates) in use today are heroin, morphine, codeine, paregoric, hydramorphone hydrochloride (Dilaudid), laudanum, meperidine, and a synthetic narcotic, methadone. With the exception of heroin, which is outlawed, these drugs are used in medical practice for specific reasons under close supervision. For the discussion of drugs and pregnancy, we are referring to deliberate drug abuse—the street-drug use or abuse of narcotics.

Use of and addiction to heroin and the other opiates in a pregnant woman result in a narcotized fetus who must go through withdrawal. The mother's withdrawal from heroin while pregnant can lead to fetal death. Rapid withdrawal of the mother during the first trimester may result in miscarriage and result in life-threatening fetal distress if done during the third trimester. The experience of withdrawal after birth is very stressful for a newborn infant.

Heroin use during pregnancy has also been associated with jaundice, respiratory distress syndrome, low birth weight, growth retardation, birth defects, and infant death (March of Dimes, 2006b).

Steroids

Steroids are prescribed drugs such as sex hormones and other specific chemicals (cortisol and prednisone) used to treat kidney inflammations, joint inflammation, and tissue damage caused by rheumatic fever and other serious diseases. They can cross the placenta and cause fetal distress.

Diethylstilbestrol (DES)

DES is a synthetic nonsteroid estrogen first prescribed in the 1950s to prevent miscarriage. In 1971 it was discovered that DES caused a specific vaginal cancer in some female offspring of women who took the hormone during their pregnancy before the 18th week of gestation. Additionally, approximately 35% of exposed women exhibit benign vaginal epithelial cell changes. There is also a risk of problems with fertility and pregnancy. Male offspring are possibly vulnerable to infertility and prostatic problems.

Birth Control Pills

Studies of children of women who took oral contraceptives during pregnancy (before the pregnancy was known) have led medical experts to suspect that the pill increases the risk of heart and limb defects. Women who take oral contraceptives are advised to discontinue them for a few months before they attempt to conceive to ensure that the body's hormones are in natural balance before a pregnancy begins.

Diseases

Certain diseases can be passed from mother to fetus, but their significance varies with the stage of pregnancy. No matter how severe or how innocuous a disease might be in the pregnant woman, the effect on the fetus depends on the stage of fetal development at the time. Common diseases that can be transmitted to the fetus with harmful consequences follow.

German Measles (Rubella)

The disease rubella is most harmful to the fetus in the first trimester (the effect is almost nil after the third or fourth month). If a pregnant woman contracts rubella early in her pregnancy, there is an 80% chance her baby will be born with a birth defect (Centers for Disease Control and Prevention, 2005). Common effects on the infant include hearing loss or deafness, eye defects, mental retardation, and behavioral problems. Death sometimes occurs shortly before or after birth. To prevent rubella and its effects, it is recommended that women who have not had rubella be vaccinated well before they decide to conceive. Additionally, vaccines should be given to children at 15 months of age, because children are the major sources of rubella infection of pregnant women.

Diabetes

Diabetes is an insulin deficiency that affects sugar metabolism and that can influence fetal weight and complicate delivery. Infants of diabetic women may have a high birth weight (10 pounds or more) and a higher than average mortality rate.

Staying as healthy as possible is the pregnant woman's chief responsibility to her developing child. Many choices must be made by expectant parents, including which health-enhancing lifestyle modifications, such as following a healthy diet, they can make throughout the pregnancy.

Human Immunodeficiency Virus

A fetus can become infected when the human immunodeficiency virus (HIV) crosses the placenta of an infected woman or during the birth process, when the infant might have contact with the mother's infected blood during delivery. It is currently estimated that about 26% of infants born to HIV-positive mothers will also be HIV-positive and may contract AIDS. Acquired immune deficiency syndrome (AIDS) is a viral disease characterized by depression of the immune system and the presence of certain opportunistic infections and malignancies. However, with the administration of zidovudine, formerly azidothymidine (AZT), or in combination with nevirapine (3TC) to the mother during pregnancy and in infants shortly after birth, this number can be decreased to 8.3% (March of Dimes, 2005).

Syphilis

The STI syphilis is a common cause of stillbirth and can infect a fetus when the spirochetes cross the placenta. The infected fetus may show signs of syphilis at birth or may appear normal until adolescence, when signs of late syphilis appear. The fetus is unaffected if the mother receives penicillin before the fourth month.

Gonorrhea

This STI affects the eyes as the baby passes through the vagina and can, by transmission through the placenta, eventually cause a form of arthritis.

Herpes Genitalis

Herpes genitalis is an STI caused by the herpes simplex virus (HSV). If lesions are present on the genitals of the mother at the time of delivery, the virus can be absorbed by the baby, causing encephalitis, inflammation of the brain, and possible death. Less commonly, the fetus may be infected through the placenta while still in utero. A woman with a history of genital herpes will be followed closely from 32 weeks of gestation until delivery. If herpes lesions are present on her genitals, delivery will be by cesarean section.

Chlamydia

The STI chlamydia is caused by the intracellular parasite *Chlamydia trachomatis*. Infants born to mothers with chlamydia infections have a 70% chance of acquiring either inclusion conjunctivitis (an eye infection) or chlamydial pneumonia during delivery. All pregnant women should be screened for chlamydia at their first prenatal visit. The infection is easily treated with erythromycin stearate.

Genital Warts

Genital warts, another STI, are caused by the human papillomavirus (HPV). Infected mothers may transmit HPV to the fetus in utero or during the birth process. Genital warts have been found in children born to HPV-infected women. More common in infected infants, however, is respiratory papillomatosis, which causes hoarseness and respiratory distress. This is a lifelong illness that often requires multiple operations. If a pregnant woman has genital warts that are large, they may interfere with the birth process, requiring a cesarean delivery. Because of HPV's long latency period, many women may not know they are infected. Unfortunately, reliable screening tests are expensive and not routinely employed (Division of Sexually Transmitted Diseases, 2002).

Rh Incompatibility

The **Rh factor** is a substance in the blood of about 85% of the population. If the Rh factor is present, the person's blood type is Rh positive (Rh+); if it is not present, the blood type is Rh negative (Rh−).

A problem in pregnancy exists when an Rh− mother is pregnant with an Rh+ child, a child who has inherited the positive factor from the Rh+ father. The mother's body develops anti-Rh agglutinins, antibodies to the presence of the Rh+, similar to the antibodies that fight disease. These anti-Rh antibodies enter the fetus and cause its red blood cells to clump together—that is, agglutinate. During the first such pregnancy, the mother's body does not develop many agglutinins. However, in subsequent pregnancies her body develops the anti-Rh agglutinins rapidly, and the babies of these pregnancies may be born anemic and jaundiced, with red blood cells and hemoglobin below normal. Treatment is accomplished by transfusion of the newborn infant with Rh− blood to stop the destruction of the red blood cells. In time the Rh− cells are replaced with the Rh+ cells that the baby's body normally makes. However, this condition can be prevented if the woman is administered the drug RhoGAM within 72 hours after a delivery or an abortion. RhoGAM neutralizes antibody formation.

> **Rh factor**
> The presence of Rh agglutinogens (antigens) in the blood, which indicates that a person is Rh positive, whereas its absence designates the person as Rh negative.

Testing for Disorders

Amniocentesis is the drawing of fluid from the amniotic sac for the purpose of diagnosing fetal abnormalities (Figure 8.7). The procedure cannot be safely performed until the 16th week of pregnancy. A **sonogram**, or ultrasound, picture is taken to show the outline of the fetus so that the needle used will not touch the baby. Under sterile conditions and using a local anesthetic, a physician inserts a long needle through the abdominal and

> **amniocentesis**
> Withdrawal by syringe of amniotic fluid to determine the presence of fetal abnormalities.
>
> **sonogram**
> A diagnostic picture revealing the fetal outline. In ultrasonography, sound waves are bounced off the fetus. With a scanner, the image is then projected onto a computer screen, revealing whether certain defects are present.

FIGURE **8.7** Amniocentesis is a test for fetal abnormalities that involves withdrawing amniotic fluid and inspecting the cells contained within it.

uterine walls into the amniotic sac and withdraws up to 20 milliliters (2/3 ounce) of fluid. The fluid, which contains cells sloughed off by the fetus, is analyzed for a variety of fetal abnormalities. The test analysis takes 10 days or longer. Chromosomal disorders, genetically induced metabolic disorders, sex-linked diseases, and genetics-linked inherited conditions can be determined by this procedure. Maternal age older than 35 years carries a higher risk of chromosomal disorders (such as Down syndrome), and amniocentesis is recommended for these pregnant women. The sex and exact age of the fetus can also be determined by means of this procedure, although amniocentesis is rarely performed for these reasons alone because it always entails some risk to the fetus. Even though the procedure is performed under sterile conditions, there is always the risk of introducing infection into the uterine environment, inducing miscarriage, or damaging the fetus.

A newer technique for prenatal detection of genetic defects, **chorionic villi sampling (CVS)**, has been approved by the Food and Drug Administration. The procedure is performed ideally at 8 to 10 weeks into the pregnancy. The chorion is the outermost protective covering of the growing embryo. The villi are threadlike, vascular (containing blood) protrusions growing on the outer surface of the chorion. In the procedure a plastic catheter is passed through the vagina into the uterus to these villi. Ultrasound is used to guide the insertion of this catheter. About 30 milligrams (0.001 ounce) of tissue is suctioned and then studied. Chromosome analysis can be done the same day; that is a significant advantage over the 2- to 3-week wait often required for amniocentesis analysis, particularly if pregnancy termination is desired. Also, if an abortion is needed, a first-trimester abortion is less risky to the mother than is one done in the second trimester. However, certain defects, such as neural tube defects, cannot be detected by this technique. If such a problem is suspected, amniocentesis must be performed. In a study comparing CVS with amniocentesis it was concluded that CVS is a safe and effective technique for early diagnosis of genetic abnormalities (Lewis, 1990). Nevertheless, CVS does carry a slightly higher risk of miscarriage than amniocentesis (1.3% and 0.5%, respectively).

Another prenatal screening test is available for detection of fetal abnormalities early in pregnancy. Maternal serum alpha-fetoprotein (MSAFP) testing is a blood test, performed at 16 to 18 weeks of pregnancy, to detect neural tube defects such as spina bifida (an open spine) and anencephaly (lack of higher brain structures). Abnormal levels of MSAFP also indicate several other conditions, such as twin pregnancy, ventral wall (heart) defects, Down's syndrome, and fetal demise. This test, however, is a screening test that detects *potential* problems; it is *not* a diagnostic test that can confirm these conditions with certainty. Abnormal levels of MSAFP are an indication that a diagnostic test such as amniocentesis should be performed. MSAFP could be an important screening test for pregnant women aged 35 years and older. If such a pregnant woman, who would normally be placed in a high-risk category, had the MSAFP test and it indicated a low risk for fetal abnormalities, it could spare her from having amniocentesis (with its inherent risk of miscarriage).

> **chorionic villi sampling (CVS)**
> A technique for prenatal detection of genetic defects that involves removal of some of the villi growing on the outer surface of the chorion and examining their chromosomes.

■ Maternal Health Problems During Pregnancy

About 20% of all pregnant women and their babies are "at risk." When a practitioner deems a pregnancy to be a high-risk one, the label indicates that the mother and/or child could suffer some adverse effects during pregnancy, labor, or delivery. The mother's health, economic status, and access to medical care, as well as the genetic history of both parents, influence the risk status of the pregnancy. The mother's age, too, has a major effect: Those younger than 18 years and older than 40 years are at greatest risk. About 60% of maternal deaths in pregnancy and childbirth in the United States are due to hemorrhage, infection, preeclampsia, eclampsia, and convulsions.

Hypertension

Blood pressure that is above normal while the heart is contracted or relaxed, or both, is the condition called *hypertension*. Women who have a history of hypertension or who become hypertensive in pregnancy need attentive medical supervision, but their condition by no means precludes a successful pregnancy.

Hypertensive conditions induced by a pregnancy have been traditionally called the **toxemias of pregnancy**. Despite the term, however, these conditions are not caused by toxins—poisons—circulating in the blood, as some people believe. Toxemias are also called *preeclampsia* and *eclampsia*. **Preeclampsia** is pregnancy-induced hypertension accompanied by swelling of the face, neck,

> **toxemias of pregnancy**
> Hypertensive conditions, subdivided into preeclampsia and eclampsia.
>
> **preeclampsia**
> Pregnancy-induced hypertension; symptoms include swelling of the face, neck, and upper extremities; and excess levels of protein in the urine.

and upper extremities. These body parts swell when tissues retain too much fluid. Proteinuria, an abnormal amount of protein in the urine, is another symptom of preeclampsia. The term **eclampsia** refers to the preeclampsia events, plus convulsions or coma, which can be fatal. At present the causes of preeclampsia and eclampsia are unknown.

It is important to state that edema—swelling of the tissues—does not always indicate an abnormal condition in pregnancy. In fact, it is quite common among pregnant women. There is more than one type and cause of edema in pregnancy.

Nausea and Vomiting

Although the exact cause is unknown, the nausea and vomiting common to early pregnancy are thought to be caused by hormonal changes. **Morning sickness** is the usual term applied to these conditions, because the nausea often occurs early in the day and dissipates relatively quickly. Small meals, avoidance of strongly flavored foods, and eating of toast and jelly before moving around in the morning are suggested. As the body adjusts to the pregnancy, the nausea and vomiting disappear.

Severe, continuous vomiting in pregnancy (*hyperemesis gravidarum*) can be serious. Dehydration, loss of electrolytes, and dietary insufficiency can result and threaten the pregnancy. Bed rest and sedation are frequently necessary, and, in extreme cases, hospitalization and intravenous feeding are required. The treatment usually includes a search for the physiological or psychological causes, because most practitioners favor limiting the use of medication in pregnancy.

Hemorrhoids

Hemorrhoids are varicose veins of the anal area. They are caused by the same pressures that create varicose veins in the legs. The increased flow of blood to the pelvic area during pregnancy results in added pressure of blood flow, which stresses the inelastic veins. In an effort to accommodate the increased blood flow, the veins are stressed, resulting in swelling, pain, and bleeding. The usual treatment employs sitz baths (a bath in which only the hip area is immersed) and topical creams. A pregnant woman who has hemorrhoids should tell her practitioner and allow him or her to prescribe treatment.

Other Conditions

A number of conditions frequently associated with pregnancy, although not serious, are often irritating. **Chloasma**, or the "mask of pregnancy," is a usually yellow to brown patch of skin pigmentation that appears on the faces of white women. The mask is thought to be caused by hormonal action that increases the number of pigment cells. Estrogen and progesterone can also produce these skin changes, as can ultraviolet light. When the pregnancy ends, the chloasma disappears.

Stretch marks, also more common in white women than in others, are visible white streaks in the skin of the abdomen and breasts, which enlarge during pregnancy. They are thought to be caused by a weakening of fibers in the tissue under the skin. It is believed that some people have a predisposition to this condition. In most instances stretch marks do not disappear, although they may fade or lighten in time.

Hair loss sometimes occurs because of an increase in hormone production. It is temporary when it does occur, and as long as no significant health problems exist, normal growth recurs within 6 months after delivery.

Reddish branchlike vascular "spiders" in the neck, chest, face, and arms are due to high estrogen levels and vascular weakness. Small capillaries under the skin surface break, and uneven streaks become visible on the surface. These streaks also fade, but in some women they do not disappear completely.

During the last few months of a pregnancy, weak and slow contractions of the uterus occur. Known as **Braxton-Hicks contractions**, these contractions become more frequent as the pregnancy proceeds. Some researchers consider this a means through which the uterus practices for labor.

■ Childbirth

Parturition, derived from a Latin term meaning "to produce," is the process of giving birth. It begins with **labor**—contractions of the uterus, a gradual opening of the cervix, and purposeful bearing down by the woman—and ends in **delivery**—the expulsion of a child and

(a) Early first-stage labor

(b) Later first-stage labor: the transition

(c) Early second-stage labor

(d) Third-stage labor: delivery of afterbirth

FIGURE **8.8** Childbirth: The stages of labor. (a) First stage: The cervix is dilating. (b) Late first stage (transition stage): The cervix is fully dilated, and the amniotic sac has ruptured, releasing amniotic fluid. (c) Second stage: The birth of the infant. (d) Third stage: Delivery of the placenta (afterbirth).

the placenta. Sometimes women experience what is called *false labor*. False labor, common in late pregnancy, is characterized by brief uterine **contractions**, sometimes accompanied by mild back and abdominal pain and involving no changes in the cervix. **True labor** is characterized by (1) regularly spaced contractions of the uterus that gradually gain in intensity, (2) thinning and **dilation** (gradual opening) of the cervix, and (3) descent of the presenting part of the fetus into the vagina (Figure 8.8). The presenting part of the fetus is that part of its body that can be felt through the cervix during a vaginal examination. Usually the cervix begins to soften and dilate a few days to a few weeks before the actual delivery time.

> **contraction**
> The shortening or tension of uterine muscles during labor.
>
> **true labor**
> Characterized by regularly spaced contractions of the uterus, thinning and dilation of the cervix, and a descending of the presenting part of the fetus into the vagina.
>
> **dilation**
> In childbirth, the gradual opening of the cervix during labor.

Labor

Labor takes place in three distinct stages—at least from an obstetrician's point of view. Stage I is the period from the onset of labor to the point at which the cervix is fully dilated; that is, when the cervix is opened to 4 inches (10 centimeters) across. The average length of the first stage in a first pregnancy is 8 to 12 hours, but it often lasts up to 20 hours. Stage II is the period from full cervical dilation through the birth of the child. This stage can last from a few minutes to 2 hours in a normal delivery, though the longer time is most common. Stage III is the period from the infant's birth to delivery of the placenta, or **afterbirth** (usually taking up to half an hour).

> **afterbirth**
> The delivery of the placenta.

Labor usually begins with the first of the contractions that will mark the whole of the first stage. Often the contractions are irregular at first and of unequal length. But in true labor, they eventually occur in a settled pattern: for example, contractions of 30 to

Gender DIMENSIONS

Fathers and Childbirth

One of us vividly remembers driving his wife to the hospital when she went into labor and being met by a very accommodating nurse. She took us immediately into the labor room, an area in which women could scream and shout and kick. The comfort I was able to offer my wife was not immediately acknowledged—she had other things on her mind—but was nonetheless helpful and appreciated in retrospect. Yet, when it came time for her to deliver our son, my wife was wheeled into the delivery room and I was escorted to the waiting room. That was how it was done in those days.

Since then, more and more fathers are accompanying the mothers of their babies into the delivery room and observing the birth. Some even view the birth through a camera lens as they try to capture the moment for posterity. In this way they feel involved in all phases of childbirth and, some research indicates, develop a greater sense of closeness—bonding—with their children as well as with their spouses.

Although this trend may be welcomed by most men, it places a burden on others. Akin to the pressure on women to work outside the home or to have a "natural childbirth delivery," the one-model-fits-all approach ignores those men who prefer not to be in the delivery room. Some men may feel squeamish about medical procedures and fear fainting during the delivery, and others may feel uncomfortable observing their partners in pain. Which types of accommodations could a hospital or birthing center provide for fathers who do not feel comfortable attending a delivery?

---

40 seconds occurring every 2 to 3 minutes. Along with the onset of contractions, a **bloody show** occurs—the disintegration of the mucus plug at the cervix. Usually the **amniotic sac** (the "bag of waters") ruptures spontaneously near the beginning of labor, experienced as either a rush or trickle of fluid through the vagina. Sometimes, however, contractions increase, but the amniotic sac remains unruptured; in such cases the attending physician or midwife breaks the sac. In some situations in which labor is overdue or dilation is progressing poorly, the drug oxytocin (Pitocin) is used to start labor or to increase the frequency of the contractions.

The medical attendants monitor the heartbeat of the fetus regularly by placing a stethoscope on the mother's abdomen, and they perform vaginal examinations periodically. In addition, an **electronic fetal monitor** is used to assess fetal heart rate. The doctor attaches an electrode to the woman's abdomen, and electrocardiographic impulses are transmitted to paper, giving a tracing (a reading) of the fetal heartbeat. Fetal heart rate can be influenced by such conditions as uterine contractions, problems with the placenta, and problems with the umbilical cord.

If anesthesia is used to reduce or eliminate the pain of contractions, it is administered late in the first stage or in the second stage. We discuss some of the choices women have regarding anesthesia later in the chapter.

Delivery

It is considered good medical practice for the physician or midwife to control the delivery to prevent a too sudden or too forceful ejection of the baby. The goal is to prevent injury to the central nervous system of the baby or injury to the mother's perineum, the area between the vulva and the anus.

Sometimes there is a need to enlarge the vaginal opening to permit the baby to pass through and to prevent the mother's tissue from tearing. In this event an incision is made into the perineum, a procedure called an **episiotomy**. Although in the past episiotomy was performed routinely in all hospital births, recently many physicians and midwives have been challenging the need for routine episiotomies, making the incision only when absolutely necessary (ACOG, 2003).

The usual delivery is divided into three phases: delivery of the head, of the shoulders, and of the body

bloody show
The expelling of the mucus plug (often streaked with blood) that has closed off the cervix during pregnancy.

amniotic sac
A fluid-filled membrane that surrounds the developing infant in the uterus.

electronic fetal monitoring
A technique used during labor whereby a physician places an electrode on the woman's abdomen to monitor the fetal heart rate for signs of fetal distress.

episiotomy
Incision between the vulva and anus to enlarge the vaginal opening at the time of birth.

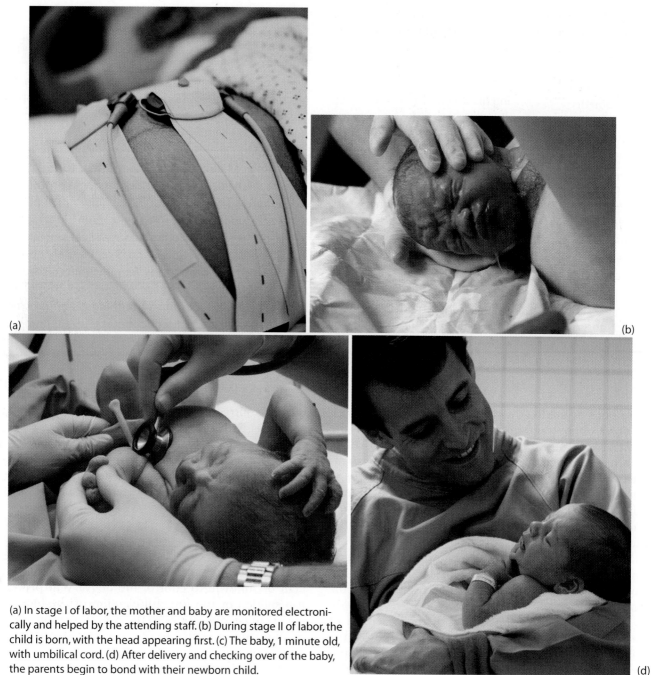

(a) In stage I of labor, the mother and baby are monitored electronically and helped by the attending staff. (b) During stage II of labor, the child is born, with the head appearing first. (c) The baby, 1 minute old, with umbilical cord. (d) After delivery and checking over of the baby, the parents begin to bond with their newborn child.

crowning
The presentation of the baby's head at the vaginal opening.

breech delivery
A delivery in which the infant is born with another body part first, rather than head first. This form of delivery can be hazardous for both mother and infant.

and legs. **Crowning** is the presentation of the baby's head at the vaginal opening, or introitus. In a **breech delivery**, the baby presents the hip, body, shoulder, and head, in that order. Though rare, a breech delivery can be hazardous to the mother or baby, or both, for several reasons. The membranes can rupture prematurely, predisposing the mother to infection; because the buttocks of the baby do not conform to the contours of the lower uterus, labor can be prolonged; manipulation of the baby is more involved than in a head presentation; and lacerations may occur in the cervix, vagina, and perineum, possibly causing infection or hemorrhage. A breech delivery can be hazardous to the baby in that the umbilical cord may separate or be compressed between the baby and the inner wall of the uterus, depriving the baby of oxygen; intracranial hemorrhage can occur because of stress on the head as it is delivered last; and injuries to the head, neck, and upper arms can occur during manipulations of delivery. Each breech delivery is managed according to its need.

Under certain conditions in which resistance inhibits the normal delivery mechanism, a forceps delivery may be necessary. Such conditions include the mother's exhaustion, cardiac or pulmonary problems, or illness; fetal distress; or certain obstetrical conditions (such as certain positions of the baby's head). The forceps is a tool designed to deliver the baby's head and is used to gain traction and to rotate the baby. A forceps must be used carefully, however, because it exerts force and can cause fetal damage.

After delivery of the baby, the umbilical cord is clamped and cut.

Delivery of Placenta

The third stage, delivery of the placenta and the membranes, usually occurs about 5 minutes after the baby is born. When the placenta emerges—again through contractions of the uterus—the doctor or midwife examines it carefully to be sure it is completely smooth. If the placenta is not smooth, it is likely that some placental tissue has remained in the uterus. Any tissue left behind may cause uterine bleeding or infection. If contractions stop before the placenta is expelled, manual techniques or injection are used to facilitate its delivery. If an episiotomy has been performed, it is repaired after the placenta is delivered.

Drugs Used in Childbirth

Expectant parents must grapple with the question of whether drugs will be used during delivery. Decisions about drugs in childbirth require some homework, because many kinds of drugs are available, all having different effects. Anesthetics inhibit perception, not just of pain but of touch and all other sensations, in the mother. General anesthetics not only affect the mother but also cross the placental barrier and reach the fetus. Most are central nervous system depressants and can act as such on the fetus. Some general anesthetics are used in pain-reducing concentrations, in which case they are less powerful depressants. These are usually inhaled. Among them are continuous nitrous oxide and enflurane.

Whereas general anesthetics put the individual to sleep, local anesthetics and local and regional analgesics (reducers of pain perception) inhibit feelings and sensations in specific parts of the body. They can be used to reduce pain without placing the fetus in jeopardy. Hypnosis is an example of what is called an **obstetrical analgesia**, a nondrug pain reliever.

A local anesthetic injected around the nerves in a given spinal area reduces sensory feeling in a specific area of the body. A local anesthetic is generally administered during the later part of the first stage of labor and during all of the second stage. Single or multiple injections are administered via a catheter into the spinal area. Drugs commonly used for local pain relief include tetracaine, lidocaine, and bupivacaine. Different areas of the pelvic region are anesthetized by different procedures. **Saddle blocks**, or **epidural blocks**, anesthetize the area of the buttocks, perineum, and inner thigh (the area that literally sits on a saddle). In a **paracervical block**, injections are given at positions around the cervix.

Drugs have been used successfully and safely during labor for many years. Therefore, their use is not cause for alarm. Still, as with all drugs, there are potential, though minimal, risks. Spinal anesthesia, for example, can cause headache, nausea and vomiting, and a drop in blood pressure. A reduction in blood pressure can reduce the oxygen supply to the baby and can change the fetal heartbeat.

Because pregnancy is a 9-month experience, expectant parents have plenty of time to discuss alternatives. Talks with the physician or midwife, with friends who have used different methods, and, most important, with each other will yield a well-thought-out decision.

Natural Childbirth

Drug-free childbirth gained support in the latter part of the 20th century, particularly as the adverse effects of some drugs on the newborn were discovered. This mode of giving birth is **natural childbirth**—or *prepared childbirth*, as it is sometimes called, because it involves education and practice. Electing to have a natural delivery often means that both parents are more involved in the pregnancy than they would be in a more traditional approach.

Within the natural childbirth movement, a number of specific options exist. The movement began early in the 1930s with Dr. Grantly Dick-Read, an English physician. He developed a method of childbirth with no anesthetics or analgesics and

---

obstetrical analgesia
A nondrug pain reliever used in delivery (e.g., hypnosis).

saddle (epidural) block
An anesthetic used during childbirth that blocks pain sensations in the buttocks, perineum, and inner thigh.

paracervical block
An anesthetic used during childbirth that blocks pain sensations in the pelvic area, in which injections are given at positions around the cervix.

natural childbirth
Drug-free childbirth; sometimes called *prepared childbirth*.

? Did You Know . . .

Some women choose to give birth immersed in a pool of water as a way to relax, alleviate pain, and minimize the need for medications during childbirth (Waterbirth International, 2008). The baby receives oxygen via blood passing through the placenta, so the fact that birth occurs under water is not a cause of concern, some argue. Data do indicate that giving birth in a pool of water decreases the need for pain-relieving medications (Cluett et al., 2004). Water births are usually attended by a midwife and are recommended only for women with low obstetric risk (MIDIR, 2005). Although more research is needed, one study comparing 3,617 water births to 5,901 land births over a 9-year period found that water birth resulted in women having lower blood loss, less pain, less perineal trauma, and fewer neonatal complications requiring transfer to a neonatal intensive care unit; maternal and neonatal infection rates were the same for both groups (Geissbuehler, Stein, & Eberhard, 2004). Another study of 1,355 water births conducted over a 5-year period reported that women who gave birth in water had fewer episiotomies, had a shorter first stage of labor, and required lower levels of analgesia; no differences in rates of infection, aspiration pneumonia, or birth weight were observed (Thoni & Moroder, 2004). Even so, researchers have concluded that questions regarding the efficacy and effectiveness of water birth remain unanswered and that more valid evidence is needed (Grunebaum & Chervenak, 2004).

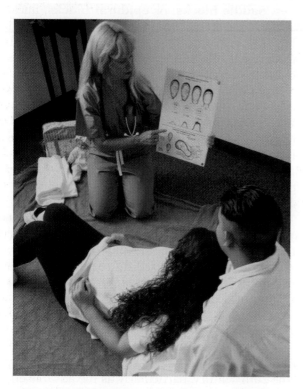

Natural, or prepared, childbirth involves both of the prospective parents being educated in techniques—exercise and breathing techniques among them—to decrease the likelihood that anesthetics will be required during childbirth.

published his approach in *Childbirth Without Fear*. At the heart of his method were techniques for relaxing tension to reduce the pain of labor. In 1950 a Russian named Velvoski published a work on his theory of psychoprophylaxis, which was taken up in France by Fernand Lamaze. Psychoprophylaxis is based on the premise that with the aid of a supportive coach (usually a husband, but any concerned, interested adult friend can play this role), a woman who has positive attitudes can reduce the stress and tension of parturition and relax the pelvic muscles. The objective is to reduce the pain of labor to the point where painkilling drugs become unnecessary. Exercise and breathing techniques are integral to what has come to be called the **Lamaze method**. The woman and her coach attend classes together once a week for approximately 6 to 8 weeks before the expected delivery date. Both adults participate in the birth process, with the coach guiding the mother in performing the exercises appropriate to the stage of labor.

Lamaze method
An approach to childbirth in which exercise and breath control are central to reducing anxiety and discomfort.

With this approach the woman receives both emotional support and coaching, particularly during the delivery itself. As was noted earlier, an effort to include the father has many advantages, particularly regarding his relationship to the newborn. Because some men may feel frightened or uncomfortable at the prospect of being present at a birth, a couple must discuss the option thoroughly. Does the man eagerly look forward to participating? Is the woman willing to undergo a natural birth without her partner present and perhaps with another coach? As do most other aspects of reproductive behavior, the natural childbirth option requires free and open communication between partners.

Although natural childbirth can be extremely satisfying, it is important to realize that natural methods are not suited to every pregnancy. The mother's health, as well as her pain threshold, will influence the decision. It is particularly important for expectant parents to realize that even when they have made the decision to have a drug-free delivery, the woman may decide during labor that she needs something for pain. In such a case the mother may be given a mild tranquilizer. Women ought not to feel guilty about asking for drugs in labor. Natural childbirth is not a contest!

Cesarean Section

Cesarean section (C-section) is the delivery of the fetus and placenta through an incision in the walls of the abdomen and uterus. The procedure is performed when a delivery through the vagina would be of risk to mother or to baby. Presently, the most common reasons for C-sections are difficulty in delivery, repeat cesarean births, breech presentation, or fetal distress (Cesarean section, 2005). C-sections are also performed if the mother has an STI that can be transmitted to the baby during a vaginal delivery, if the baby is too large to pass easily through the vaginal canal and opening, and if a vaginal delivery will cause potential harm to the mother because of certain illnesses (such as diabetes). In 2006, C-sections accounted for 31.1% of all deliveries in the United States (Martin et al., 2009). This is an all-time high and a jump of 3% from 2005. Some experts perceive the increased rate of C-sections as beneficial. They point to the possibility of fetal and maternal death from childbirth, and ruptured uteruses. The effects of labor and delivery on women's bodies are also reasons C-sections have increased. In particular, this concern revolves about "pelvic floor" disorders, such as muscles, ligaments, and other tissues being stretched and damaged, resulting in urinary and/or fetal incontinence. "Twenty to 30 percent of women become incontinent after a single vaginal delivery," states the director of female pelvic medicine and reconstructive surgery at Loyola University Medical Center in Chicago (Stein, 2002). If C-sections can prevent these disorders, all the better, they argue. In addition, C-sections may alleviate anxiety because women know they do not have to endure hours of painful labor and delivery. C-section rates also have increased, proponents argue, because women are having babies at older ages and, therefore, having more complications. Finally, the increase in weight of Americans in general has led to an increase in the number of overweight mothers who carry bigger babies, for whom vaginal delivery is much more risky.

Opponents of the increasing use of C-sections argue it is the result of obstetricians' being concerned about malpractice lawsuits. That is one reason, these opponents argue, that women who have had previous

> **cesarean section (C-section)**
> Surgical intervention to deliver the fetus, placenta, and membranes through an incision in the walls of the abdomen and uterus.

The number of cesarean sections has increased among Americans in recent years. Some argue that this is the result of fear of lawsuits on the part of obstetricians, whereas others believe it is less traumatic for the mother than the strains of natural childbirth and is best for the newborn. Whether C-sections are performed too often is still being debated by the experts.

C-sections are increasingly finding that their doctors and hospitals refuse to participate in a vaginal delivery with them. In addition, fees are higher for C-section deliveries than they are for vaginal deliveries, and those suspicious of physicians believe this fee structure difference is one of the prime reasons for the high number of cesarean sections. Furthermore, those opposed to increases in C-section deliveries point out the risks of any surgery. These risks can be avoided, they believe, if a woman has vaginal delivery. As with many issues of sexuality, the appropriate use of cesarean sections is a matter of debate at the current time.

There are disadvantages to having a C-section. It is expensive; the mother needs a recuperative period that may interfere with her caring for her baby; there is scarring of the uterus; and there is the possibility, though slight, of hemorrhage or infection. It must be pointed out, however, that many babies and mothers would die without surgical intervention. Cesarean intervention is an alternative delivery method to be considered in certain complicated situations.

Premature Birth

When a child is born before the normal gestation period is completed but still has a chance of surviving, its birth is regarded as **premature**. In 2006, 13% of all babies born in the United States were

> **premature**
> Type of birth in which an infant is born before the complete term of gestation but late enough in the pregnancy that it has a chance to survive.

premature (Martin et al., 2009). A premature infant is usually between 28 and 34 weeks gestation, although some are as young as 24 weeks. These infants generally weigh less than 5.5 pounds (2,500 grams). Of the 250,000 "preemies" born annually, about 100,000 weigh less than 3.3 pounds (1,500 grams).

Prematurity is caused by many factors. One common cause is a maternal age younger than 16 years or older than 40 years. Other causes include maternal malnutrition, cigarette smoking and alcohol consumption, inadequate prenatal care, and a history of a previous premature delivery.

The premature baby is born before some of its body systems can perform adequately. The respiratory system in particular is immature in these babies. They may forget to breathe and may have difficulty in moving the air through the respiratory tract. Sometimes their lung surfaces are unable to work with the necessary amounts of oxygen needed for survival because of immaturity of the lungs. These infants are usually placed in incubators, which are special cribs with controls to monitor temperature and oxygen levels. Because oxygen is necessary to sustain life, on the one hand, and because an excess of oxygen can cause eye damage (retrolental fibroplasia [RLF]), on the other hand, oxygen levels must be carefully controlled. A device has been developed that, when put on the baby's skin, can measure blood oxygen levels continuously.

Premature infants often have difficulty swallowing and digesting food, so they require special intravenous feedings. Small amounts of breast milk are fed to the baby as he or she begins to mature, both for nutrition and for the antibodies provided by the milk. Chemical tests that can detect some metabolic problems are used in the monitoring techniques.

Neonatal intensive care is the name given to the medical specialty of premature infant care. It is costly because it requires the talents of trained specialists and special equipment. Given this care, however, most premature babies develop

neonatal intensive care
A medical specialty that focuses on the care of premature infants.

normally and catch up to their peers somewhere between the end of the first year and the third year. The investment to child, family, and ultimately society certainly justifies the time and costs involved.

Psychological and Physical Adjustment After Childbirth

Psychological reactions after childbirth can occur. One of these reactions is depression, called *postpartum depression*. It is not unusual for women to have the "blues" after childbirth, in which they experience mood swings; feel sad, anxious, or overwhelmed; or have crying spells, loss of appetite, or trouble sleeping. These symptoms usually go away after a few days or a week. When they persist or include thoughts of hurting the baby or oneself, or having no interest in the baby, postpartum depression may exist.

Hormonal changes may trigger symptoms of postpartum depression. During pregnancy, levels of the hormones estrogen and progesterone increase greatly. In the first 24 hours after childbirth, these hormones' levels quickly return to normal. Researchers think this major change in hormone levels may lead to depression, similar to the way smaller hormone changes can affect women's moods before their periods. Levels of thyroid hormones (thyroxin) may also drop after giving birth. Low levels of thyroxin can cause symptoms of depression (U.S. Department of Health and Human Services, 2009).

Certain factors may increase a woman's risk of developing postpartum depression. These include a personal history of depression or another mental illness, a family history of depression or another mental illness, lack of support from family and friends, anxiety or negative feelings about raising the child, problems with a previous pregnancy or birth, marriage or money problems, stressful life events, young age, and substance abuse. Women who are depressed during pregnancy have a greater risk of depression after giving birth.

The two common types of treatment for depression are talk therapy and medication. Talk therapy involves talking to a therapist, psychologist, or social worker to learn to change how depression makes one think, feel, and act. Medication includes a variety of antidepressant medicines.

Physical changes also occur after childbirth (Schuler & Curtis, 2009). Women who have given birth will experience a discharge of blood, called *lochia*, that occurs as the lining of the uterus is shed. The discharge gradually turns from bright red to pink or brown and finally to yellow or white before it stops. It is heavy at first but becomes lighter with time. It should stop altogether by the time of the 6-week postpartum check-up.

There may also be pain between the vagina and the rectum (*perineum pain*). This discomfort is caused by the stretching, tearing, or cutting of the area that allowed for delivery of the baby. If the woman received an episiotomy, the area where the incision was made may be quite painful, but it will heal very quickly.

Uterine contractions, termed *afterpains*, may occur for several days after the birth, signaling that the uterus is shrinking to its prepregnancy size. Women may also experience engorged and sore breasts as milk begins to flow into the breasts. The best way to treat this condition is by breastfeeding often. Cold compresses and a supportive brassiere may also help.

Incontinence may also occur; emptying the bladder frequently can help alleviate this problem. Constipation, uncomfortable bowel movements, and hemorrhoids are also physical changes that often occur after childbirth. However, it is advisable for the woman not to strain during a bowel movement so as to limit damage to abdominal organs and tissue. Drinking plenty of fluids, eating bran and prunes, and taking stool softeners can all help.

Breastfeeding

To ready the breasts for producing milk (**lactation**), glandular tissue and ducts proliferate during pregnancy as a result of the placenta's secretion of estrogen, progesterone, and **lactogen**. These developments account for the increase in breast size in pregnancy. Large amounts of estrogen and progesterone secreted by the placenta prevent milk production before birth, but after the placenta is delivered, both estrogen and progesterone levels drop significantly, and the level of the pituitary hormone prolactin rises. Prolactin secretion activates the breast cells to produce milk. A second pituitary hormone, **oxytocin**, acts as a stimulant for the breasts to eject milk.

Twenty-eight to 48 hours after delivery, the lactation process begins. For the first 3 or 4 days, a thin, yellowish liquid called **colostrum** is secreted by the breasts. Colostrum is a high-protein substance containing many antibodies. Actual milk production begins between the fourth and seventh days, and by the seventh day mature milk production begins. The infant's sucking stimulates nerve cells in the nipples; the mother's brain receives the message and stimulates the pituitary to secrete oxytocin, which in turn stimulates ejection of milk from the breasts. When the milk is forced out, the mother feels a tingling sensation known as a **letdown** about 30 to 60 seconds after suckling begins. This feeling is produced by a neurogenic reflex that is necessary for adequate milk supply to reach the infant. Continued milk supply is dependent on sucking.

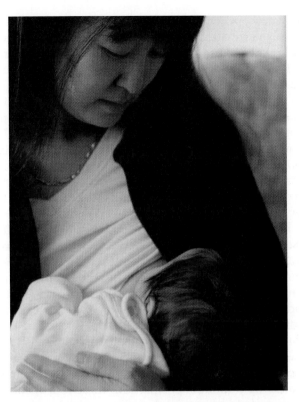

Breastfeeding conveys many benefits to both the newborn and the breastfeeding mother. Breastfeeding provides newborns with uncontaminated nutrients and antibodies against infection. It also helps the mother's uterus return to its nonpregnant shape and postpones the return of menstruation.

The infant's demand regulates the breasts' supply. When the baby sucks longer, the breasts produce more milk to meet the increased demand. When the baby sucks less, milk production decreases.

Breastfeeding benefits the baby by providing a diet of balanced, uncontaminated nutrients and antibodies against disease. The breastfeeding mother benefits, too. Nursing helps the uterus to return to its nonpregnant shape and postpones the return of menstruation (although it is not a sufficient contraceptive by itself). In addition, breast cancer rates are lower for mothers who breastfeed. A study of more than 50,000 women from 30 different countries found that each year a mother breastfed reduced her risk of breast cancer by 4.3% (Collaborative Group, 2002). Furthermore, data analyzed from the Women's Health Initiative found that women who reported breastfeeding for more than 12 months were, even many years later, less likely to develop hypertension, diabetes, high serum cholesterol, and cardiovascular disease than nonbreastfeeding women (Schwarz et al., 2009). But probably most important, breastfeeding encourages the close attachment, or **bonding**, of infant

lactation
Production of breast milk.

lactogen
A hormone that stimulates the production of milk, the principal one being prolactin.

oxytocin
A pituitary hormone that stimulates the breasts to eject milk so that breastfeeding may occur after childbirth.

colostrum
The yellow fluid secreted by the breasts just before and after childbirth until milk production begins.

letdown
The tingling sensation in the breasts when milk is forced out about 30 to 60 seconds after the infant begins to suckle.

bonding
A sense of close emotional attachment.

and mother. Perhaps not incidentally, breast milk is less expensive than formula milk. Because of these multiple benefits, the American Academy of Pediatrics and the U.S. federal government recommend breast-feeding over formula feeding.

The American Academy of Pediatricians recommends that mothers breastfeed throughout the infant's first 6 months of life and up to a year if desired by mother and child (American Academy of Pediatricians, 2005). Yet, researchers in a national study found that although 83% of survey respondents initiated breast-feeding right after birth, the percentage who breastfed declined rapidly to 50% at 6 months and to 24% at 12 months (Grummer-Strawn, Scanlon, & Fein, 2008). The federal government reports even lower figures. In 2004, the government reported that only 11% of women exclusively breastfed their infants for the first 6 months of their lives (Centers for Disease Control and Prevention, 2007a). In addition, other researchers found that in the early postpartum period, nearly half of the mothers surveyed fed their infants breast milk fewer than 8 times a day, which is below the range of 8 to 12 feedings per day typically included in common advice. By 3 months postpartum, three-fourths of the mothers fed breast milk less frequently than is commonly advised (Shealy et al., 2008).

Support for breastfeeding mothers is provided by organizations such as La Leche League and numerous books and articles. Such support is necessary in view of the inconvenience that accompanies breastfeeding, especially for employed women, and because some people regard it as old-fashioned or improper in public.

Some women do not produce sufficient milk to breatfeed. This may be the case with mothers who smoke cigarettes, for example. Others may not want to breastfeed because it is inconvenient or for other reasons. These women can also bond with their babies by holding them closely while bottle feeding. If inconvenience is the only issue, mothers can use a breast pump to extract milk that is stored for use by fathers or caregivers during bottle feeding.

■ Sexual Activity During Pregnancy and After Delivery

Some, perhaps many, pregnant couples are afraid to have intercourse for fear of hurting the fetus. The frequency and kinds of sexual activity that are safe during and after pregnancy are determined both by personal preference and by health. A woman with no medical problems can continue to have the kind of sexual and sensual life she had before pregnancy (Figure 8.9). Even for healthy women, though, changes in body size and sense of comfort might dictate alterations in sexual habits. In advanced pregnancy some couples tend to replace intercourse with manual stimulation.

When certain physical conditions are present, however, coitus might add risk to the pregnancy. For example, when spotting, bleeding, pain, or past history of spontaneous abortion is present, a medical practitioner should decide whether intercourse is permissible. In healthy women, orgasmic contractions are not harmful to the fetus and will not initiate labor.

Sexual feelings can change during pregnancy. A woman's desire may be influenced by her personal involvement with the baby late in pregnancy, her individual personality, her attitudes about sexuality, her feelings about her physical appearance, and so on. Here again, the necessity for free-flowing sexual communication, both trustful and honest, cannot be stressed enough.

FIGURE **8.9** Pregnancy need not mean the end of sexual intercourse.

**Differences in
Infant Mortality**

Infant mortality comprises deaths occurring within the first year of life. The good news is that the infant mortality rate continues to decline. Whereas in 1983 it was 10.9 per 1,000 live births, in 2009 the infant mortality rate was 6.3 per 1,000 live births (Central Intelligence Agency, 2009).

The bad news was that the infant mortality rate for African Americans is still much higher than that for other subgroups in the population. In 2005, the white infant mortality rate was 5.7 per 1,000 live births, but the African American infant mortality rate was 13.3 per 1,000 live births. The reasons for the high rate among African Americans are many and varied; poverty is foremost. Poverty rates are proportionately higher among African Americans than among whites. Consequently, African Americans cannot as readily afford health care, proper nutrition, and other services and behaviors that are conducive to birth of healthy babies. For example, whereas 86% of white mothers began prenatal care during the first trimester, only 76% of African American mothers did. And, though only 3.0% of white mothers began prenatal care either during the third trimester or not at all, 5.7% of African American mothers began prenatal care late or not at all (National Center for Health Statistics, 2008).

To respond to this infant mortality rate gap between African American and white Americans, communities have instituted educational campaigns encouraging early prenatal care, particularly targeted at African American populations. Some of these programs rely on public service advertisements in newspapers, on signs on buses, or as messages over radio or television. Other programs employ women who live in the targeted communities to identify pregnant women, meet with them, and encourage them to see a health care provider. Still other programs employ a combination of these and other methods in conjunction with free or low-cost health care to help pregnant moms be healthier and deliver healthier children.

Intercourse after delivery depends on many factors: whether there were complications during and after delivery, whether a C-section was performed, and of course, whether the woman is comfortable, particularly after a difficult delivery. Most obstetricians prefer that couples delay intercourse until after the first postdelivery examination, which usually takes place 4 to 6 weeks after delivery. This is to be sure that the vulva has healed if there was a tear or an episiotomy and to allow time to discuss the choice of a method of birth control.

Couples should be sure to resume contraception before sexual intercourse after childbirth. Despite the fact that breastfeeding delays the return of menstruation, that alone is not a dependable form of birth control.

■ Hormonal Influences on Prenatal Development: Becoming Male or Female

The process of becoming a male or a female is a complicated one, involving chromosomes and hormones. As we have mentioned, a key influence on sex determination is the presence or absence of a Y chromosome.

Normal Sexual Differentiation

In the uterus, the fertilized egg always develops as if it were going to be female. If a Y chromosome is present, however, a male develops. Although the process by which the Y chromosome results in the development of testes is not completely understood, it appears that the body produces a substance called *H-Y antigen* that initiates this process. The testes then begin to form where ovaries might have otherwise been. If no Y chromosome is present, ovaries develop instead. This process of gonadal development, termed *sexual differentiation* (Figure 8.10), does not start until the beginning of the second month after conception.

Gonadal development is significant because the gonads produce their own hormones, which, in turn, affect the development of other structures in the reproductive system. For example, the fetal testes produce testicular hormones (androgens) that instruct the body to develop the vas deferens and other male reproductive structures. In addition, the fetal testes produce a "defeminizing hormone" called *Mullerian inhibiting hormone (MIH)* (or *Mullerian inhibiting substance [MIS]*), which prevents the reproductive tissue from forming a uterus and fallopian tubes. In females the absence of testicular hormones allows the tissue to form female reproductive structures (the labia, uterus, fallopian tubes, and others).

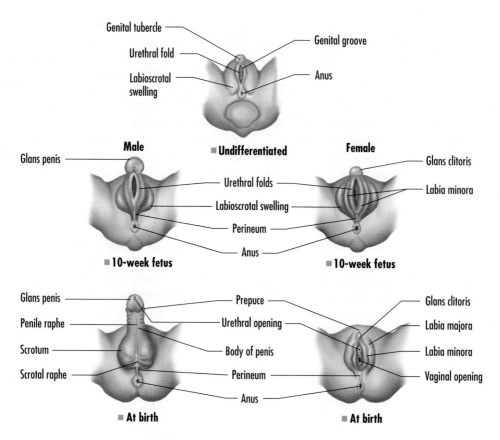

FIGURE **8.10** Prenatal development of external genitalia.

The tissue from which the reproductive organs develop is part of one of a pair of embryonic ducts. One of these, the *Mullerian duct,* develops into the female reproductive organs. The other, the *Wolffian duct,* develops into the male reproductive organs after the Mullerian duct degenerates as a result of MIH secreted from the testes. By the fourth month after conception, the gender of the fetus is clearly identifiable by the external genitalia.

The presence or absence of androgens determines whether a particular piece of tissue becomes a penis or a clitoris, a prostate gland or a Skene's gland, a Cowper's gland or a Bartholin's gland, or a scrotum or a labia majora. Structures that develop from the same tissue in this way are called **homologous** structures (see Table 8.2).

The differentiation of the male and female brain is called *brain dimorphism.* Although this is a relatively new scientific endeavor, we do know that brain differentiation may extend into the first few days or weeks after birth. Interestingly, it appears that brain differentiation is *ambitypic*; that is, it allows for the coexistence of both masculine and feminine nuclei

homologous
Organs that differ but that developed from the same tissue—for example, the glans penis and clitoris.

and pathways in some, if not all, parts of the brain. What this means is that the female can demonstrate masculine behavior and the male can demonstrate feminine behavior.

Variance of Sexual Differentiation

The description of sexual differentiation assumes that everything goes according to plan, and it usually does. However, once in a while something goes wrong. In fact, it is possible for the genetic sex, or *genotype* (the chromosomes); the gonadal sex, or *phenotype* (testes or ovaries); and the internal sexual structures (uterus, fallopian tubes, prostate gland, and vas deferens) to differ. For example, a person with two X chromosomes can have a penis and an empty scrotum (no testes), two ovaries, a uterus, and fallopian tubes—yet still feel and act male. Conversely, it is possible for a female to grow up feeling feminine but have an X and a Y chromosome, two testes, and some internal male sexual structures (Money, 1987b).

This latter condition, in which an X and a Y chromosome are present but the tissues are insensitive to the testosterone produced by the fetal testes, is called the *testicular feminizing syndrome.* This is the most common form of **intersexuality** (formerly referred to

TABLE 8.2 Homologous Structures

Female	Male
Clitoral glans	Penile glans
Clitoral shaft	Penile shaft
Clitoral hood	Penile foreskin
Labia majora	Scrotum
Labia minora	Bottom of penile shaft
Ovaries	Testes
Bartholin's gland	Cowper's gland
Skene's gland	Prostate gland

intersexuality
A condition in which a person has reproductive organs of both sexes.

as hermaphroditism), a condition in which organs of both sexes are present. Intersexuality can also develop by the secretion of an excessive level of androgen from the adrenal gland of a female fetus. This condition is called *adrenogenital syndrome*. In addition, intersexuality has resulted from administration of a synthetic hormone (progestin)—a practice that is now banned but was previously used to prevent miscarriages.

Some experts differentiate between true intersexuality and *pseudointersexuality*. True intersex, which is very rare, is characterized by the presence of both ovarian and testicular tissue (sometimes called *ovotestes*). Pseudointersexuals have gonads that match their chromosomes (testes if they are XY or ovaries if they are XX), but their other reproductive structures may be mixed. This is a much more common form of intersexuality. Either type of intersexuality is treated with hormonal therapy, surgery, and counseling.

An activist organization has formed to represent the interests of intersexuals. The Intersex Society of North America's web site (www.isna.org) states that ISNA "is devoted to systemic change to end shame, secrecy, and unwanted genital surgeries for people born with an anatomy that someone decided is not standard for male or female."

Other problems with sexual differentiation can be traced to the chromosomes. For example, in a condition called *Turner's syndrome*, which is caused by the presence of only one X chromosome (instead of two), the female fetus may be born with swollen hands and feet, be sterile, and remain short. In another condition, *Klinefelter's syndrome*, caused by an XXY genetic makeup, boys appear normal until puberty but then do not develop the normal secondary sex characteristics (discussed later) and often require testosterone injections throughout life.

Still another problem associated with sexual differentiation is called an *inguinal hernia*. The testes descend into the scrotum through a structure called the *inguinal canal*. This normally occurs by the seventh month of fetal development. If the inguinal canal does not close properly after the testes descend or if it opens up afterward, it is possible for the intestine to move down the canal and enter the scrotum. An inguinal hernia can be corrected surgically.

If the testes do not descend down the inguinal canal, as occurs in about 2% of male newborns, the condition is called *cryptorchidism* (more commonly called *undescended testes*). Usually the testes will descend during early childhood or by puberty. If they do not, however, either surgery or hormonal therapy is necessary for two reasons: (1) Testes in the abdomen are at too high a temperature to produce viable sperm, and if they are left undescended, infertility is likely to result; and (2) there is a greater risk of testicular cancer if testes are left undescended.

■ Infertility

Infertility, or the inability to reproduce, can cause great emotional anguish for people who want children. This unhappiness, accompanied by tension, frustration, and even resentment, can damage the health and the marriages of infertile couples. The situation may be further complicated by an inability or unwillingness to adopt a child. It is important to add, however, that while adoption may relieve the stress of wanting to raise children, it may not eliminate the stress related to infertility.

infertility
The inability to reproduce.

More than 5 million people of childbearing age experience infertility. Primary infertility is defined as inability to conceive despite having unprotected intercourse for at least 1 year. Secondary infertility is defined as inability to conceive despite having unprotected intercourse for at least 1 year and having previously conceived (Hatcher et al., 2004). It is estimated that 10% to 15% of couples experience primary infertility.

Women and men can both contribute to infertility. Infertility is caused by the woman's problem in 35% of cases, by the male's problem in 35% of the cases, and by both the woman and the man in 20% of cases. In 10% of cases, there is no discernible reason for the infertility.

Causes of Infertility

Among the leading causes of infertility in women are untreated gonorrhea and chlamydia infections. These may cause tubal occlusion in women and chronic

Ethical
DIMENSIONS

Surrogate Mothers Some couples who attempt to conceive children cannot. In some cases, the cause is a lack of viable sperm. In other cases, the problem is a blockage of the fallopian tubes, which prevents the sperm–ovum union. In still other cases, the woman does not produce an ovum to be fertilized or, because of some medical condition, cannot carry a fetus in her uterus until delivery. In the latter circumstance, the woman's ovum can be fertilized by her partner's sperm outside the womb and implanted in the uterus of another woman, a *surrogate womb*. However, when a woman does not produce ova for fertilization, sometimes another woman's egg is fertilized by her partner and develops in that other woman's uterus. Upon delivery, the baby becomes the child of the father and his partner rather than of the father and the woman

whose eggs and uterus were used for 9 months or so. The woman whose eggs and uterus were used is the biological mother, referred to as a *surrogate mother*.

When surrogate motherhood occurs without complications, it provides for everyone's needs. However, every once in a while, circumstances requiring creative solutions develop. For example, what do you think should happen if the surrogate mother does not want to give up the child after delivery? (Maybe she develops an attachment to the baby, or her situation has changed and she now wants a child of her own.) What should happen if the father and his partner do not want to accept the baby? (Maybe the baby has a birth defect, the couple has separated or divorced, or they just changed their minds about wanting children.) Each of these situations has actually occurred. What is your opinion?

cervicitis, both of which produce subfertility. In men, these diseases, if untreated, can cause epididymitis, leading to blocked sperm ducts and poor semen quality. Sexually active college students can help protect themselves from infertility by using condoms, practicing safer sex behaviors, and getting regular testing for STIs.

STIs are not the only diseases that affect fertility. About 1% of men become infertile after mumps. People with sickle-cell disease have higher infertility rates. Several drugs may inhibit sperm production or sperm function, including antimalarial drugs, antihypertensives, and calcium-channel blockers.

Health and lifestyle can affect fertility. For example, in men, chronic stress may interfere with the production of certain hormones needed to produce sperm; diets low in vitamin C, selenium, zinc, and folate (a vitamin B) can affect sperm, as can obesity (Mayo Clinic Staff, 2007a). Cigarettes, alcohol, cocaine, and marijuana are all associated with lower sperm count and poor sperm quality in men, as is use of recreational drugs such as narcotics and barbiturates. Anabolic steroids, which are taken by some men to enhance muscular strength and growth, can result in the testes decreasing in size and sperm production decreasing. Age also affects sperm production and quality (Fisch, 2009). Lastly, pesticides and other chemicals (for example, herbicides and insecticides) can result in lower sperm production.

In women, recreational drugs can inhibit ovulation, as can cigarette smoking and alcohol use. Age

is also a factor in infertility for women (Younis et al., 2009). The older the woman is, the more likely she is to be infertile. Women are most fertile in their mid-20s; by the time a woman is 40 years old, she has a 50% decreased fertility rate and a two to three times greater chance of miscarriage (Toner & Flood, 1993).

Finally, in some couples, a lack of knowledge about anatomy, physiology, and reproduction leads to infertility. These couples may not know when conception is most likely to occur, they may not have intercourse frequently enough to conceive, and they may not know how to time intercourse. The ovum is alive for less than 1 day; sperm can live as long as 5 days inside the woman. Couples must have intercourse before ovulation to maximize the possibility of pregnancy.

Treatment for Infertility

Infertility can be successfully treated. At least half of people with infertility who receive treatment are ultimately able to conceive.

Fertility may be enhanced with some simple techniques. For example, having the woman lie on her back for an hour after coitus to aid sperm in traveling up, rather than out of, the vagina or even having more frequent intercourse, especially near the time of ovulation, can be enough to allow some couples to conceive. In addition, the man-on-top coital position increases the chances of conception because the cervix drops into the seminal pool. Placing a pillow under the woman's buttocks may also help prevent sperm from escaping out of the vagina. Identifying the time of ovulation and having sexual intercourse near that time can enhance the chance of conception as well, because the ovum is available for impregnation for only a short period. Trying to conceive often, in the most conducive position to conception, cannot result in pregnancy if there is no egg to fertilize.

For many couples, these simple techniques are not enough. Other procedures have thus been developed to enhance fertility. In all cases, however, the first step is an examination to determine why a couple is unable to conceive. At present several basic infertility screening procedures are used in this examination phase:

1. *Semen analysis.* The man is asked to masturbate and collect the ejaculate in a container. The ejaculate is then examined to determine the number of sperm present, the sperm's motility, and the amount of fructose (nourishment for the sperm) in the semen.

2. *Basal body temperature (BBT) recordings.* The woman is required to record her body temperature (with an oral or BBT thermometer) daily. The decrease in estrogen production as ovulation nears causes the basal temperature to drop about 0.3 degree. When ovulation occurs, basal temperature rises about 0.6 degree as a result of the corpus luteum's production of the hormone progesterone. Thus a physician can determine whether ovulation is occurring normally by monitoring the basal temperature.

3. *A fuller evaluation of ovulatory function.* A *biopsy* (microscopic examination of excised tissue) of the endometrium is performed. The secretions that progesterone produces in the endometrium are studied to provide further information regarding the normality of the woman's ovulation.

4. *Tubal patency tests.* Dye is projected through the fallopian tubes and observed by X ray to detect any blockage; this test is also called a *hysterosalpingogram.*

5. *Postcoital examination.* Two to 4 hours after the couple has had sexual intercourse, the cervical mucus is examined microscopically. The physician checks for several conditions of the cervical mucus that can be fatal to sperm (for example, too much viscosity or too little salt). The sperm are counted and their ability to travel determined, because the more motile the sperm, the greater the likelihood of conception.

In spite of their love for one another, their understanding of the menstrual cycle and ovulation, and their ability to effectively engage in sexual intercourse, some couples are not able to conceive. There are several reasons for this, and several screening tests to determine the reason for any particular couple. Once the reason is uncovered, treatment can begin to increase the likelihood of conception.

6. *Hormone monitoring.* Several ovulation prediction kits are currently sold over the counter. These kits measure the level of luteinizing hormone (LH), the hormone causing ovulation midway through the menstrual cycle. Urine tests can also be used to measure the amount of progesterone during various phases of the cycle. Other hormones (such as prolactin, thyroid hormones, and follicle-stimulating hormone [FSH]) can be monitored as well.

7. *Cervical mucus evaluation.* The cervical mucus can be evaluated for its elasticity, its nature just before ovulation (it should be thin, watery, salty, and stretchy), and the presence of cells, debris, and proper pH level (degree of acidity or alkalinity).

8. *Ultrasonography.* High-frequency sound waves are transmitted and reflected by internal organs and structures. From the resulting pattern, detailed outlines of the reproductive system can be obtained.

9. *Hysteroscopy.* The uterus is expanded with carbon dioxide gas or liquid and is observed through a hysteroscope—a long, narrow, illuminated instrument that is inserted through the cervix into the uterus. Abnormalities such as polyps, fibroids, and adhesions can be identified in this manner.

These screening procedures determine the cause of infertility in approximately 85% of cases. (In the remaining 15% the cause of infertility is unknown.) Once the cause or causes are determined, treatment can be prescribed. Cessation of ovulation can be restarted through hormone therapy or by increasing body fat through nutritional therapy. Blocked fallopian tubes can be cleared through microsurgical techniques. Artificial insemination (projecting sperm from a male donor into the female's vagina by mechanical means) can be used when the male is not fertile. To aid women whose fallopian tubes are irreparably blocked, physicians in special clinics can unite the partner's sperm and ovum outside the woman's body. The fertilized egg is then allowed to develop in a Petri dish and is implanted in the woman's uterus to create a pregnancy. This procedure, known as *in vitro fertilization,* and artificial insemination are discussed in detail in the next section.

Assisted Reproductive Technologies

During the latter part of the 20th century, advanced reproductive technologies (ARTs) have been developed to assist infertile couples in conceiving. The first American baby conceived in vitro was born in December 1981. Since then, technologies have become increasingly sophisticated in resolving infertility. The most common ART techniques are in vitro fertilization and gamete intrafallopian transfer.

Artificial Insemination

About 20,000 babies yearly are produced by **artificial insemination**. There are two types of artificial insemination: *artificial insemination by a donor (AID)* and *artificial insemination by the husband (AIH).* Artificial insemination by the husband is generally attempted when the husband has one of a number of problems, such as a misplaced urinary meatus, impotence, or low sperm count. The semen is collected from the husband by masturbation or immediately after coitus. Either the specimen is collected by the couple and then taken to the clinic, or the man masturbates at the clinic. The sperm are then introduced into the woman's uterus by means of a syringe or by placement of the semen in a cervical cap fitted against the cervix.

artificial insemination
Introduction of semen into the uterus by noncoital means.

Artificial insemination by a donor other than the husband is done when there is no husband or in cases where the husband produces no sperm (a condition called *azoospermia*), has a sperm count too low to ensure fertilization (*oligospermia*), has sperm that are not viable enough for insemination, or has a combination of the last two conditions. The donor is screened for health factors and is matched to the husband in physical appearance and genetic background, though generally his identity is unknown to the receivers. For legal reasons, if the husband can produce even a minimal amount of sperm, some physicians mix his semen with that of the donor before inseminating the woman. Because in some states the question of legal paternity arises when AID is used, mixing sperm can help ensure the husband's status as father, because it cannot be disproved. In states that have no legal guidelines or statutes regarding paternity in such cases, lawyers encourage husbands to legally adopt children produced through AID.

Artificial insemination allows people to experience natural parenthood, even when they are unable to conceive through intercourse. And with AID, mothers at least are the biological parents of their offspring. Furthermore, many single women who are physically, emotionally, and economically capable of being mothers are unwilling to be impregnated through intercourse but are willing to be artificially inseminated. Obviously although artificial insemination offers the option of parenthood to many to whom it was barred, it also raises many questions of a moral nature—for example, whether it is fair to a child to bring it into the world with no known biological father.

In Vitro Fertilization

In vitro fertilization (IVF) has incorrectly been labeled the "test-tube baby" procedure. This is actually a highly sophisticated medical procedure, "which involves removing a ripened egg or eggs from the female's ovary, fertilizing it with semen, incubating the dividing cells in a laboratory dish, and then replacing the developing embryo in the uterus at the appropriate time" (Clapp, 1998). The woman's eggs can be used, or donor eggs can be used. The man's sperm can be used, or donor sperm can be used.

The success rate for IVF was approximately 40% in 2002 (Wright et al., 2005). Clinics are trying to improve the success rate by retrieving and fertilizing multiple eggs or transferring multiple embryos. As a result, multiple birth rates with IVF are as high as 20%. In the 1997 case of Bobbie McCaughey, seven embryos were transplanted, resulting in the birth of septuplets. In addition, women who become pregnant with more than one child through in vitro fertilization or gamete intrafallopian transfer (discussed later) have a twofold higher risk of development of preeclampsia than women who become pregnant spontaneously (Lynch et al., 2002).

IVF raises numerous ethical issues. In some cases, women find out that all the embryos have begun to develop into fetuses, and they choose to have a procedure called *selective abortion*, whereby one or more of the fetuses are aborted to give the remaining fetuses a better chance to develop. In many clinics, more eggs are harvested than needed for a single cycle and are fertilized. These embryos are then frozen so that they can be used for future IVF procedures. However, in some cases, couples have divorced before the transfer of the embryos, and so couples have fought over these embryos as part of a divorce settlement. In a few widely publicized cases, embryos have been implanted after the man has died. Is the child in that case born to a married couple, or should he or she be considered an out-of-wedlock child? And, should insurance companies and Medicaid pay for IVF? In most cases, they do not. The procedure is expensive—costing tens of thousands of dollars per cycle. Should IVF be available only to well-to-do couples?

Gamete Intrafallopian Transfer

In gamete intrafallopian transfer (GIFT), rather than transplantation of an embryo into the uterus, an ovum is transferred to one or both fallopian tubes during laparoscopy. Fertilization occurs in the tube, as it does naturally, and the embryo implants in a regular conception cycle. It is an option only for women with open fallopian tubes. One problem is that there is a higher tubal pregnancy rate for using GIFT. Consequently, less than 1% of assisted reproductive technologies involved GIFT in 2002 (Wright et al., 2005).

Exploring the
DIMENSIONS
of Human Sexuality

Our feelings, attitudes, and beliefs regarding sexuality are influenced by our internal and external environments. Go to sexuality.jbpub.com/dimensions/4e to learn more about the biological, psychological, and sociological factors that affect your sexuality.

Sociocultural Factors

- Socioeconomic status influences infant and maternal health, because poor people have less access to prenatal care than well-off people do.
- Laws restrict access to abortions during the third trimester.
- Religion, culture, and ethnic heritage influence many beliefs about pregnancy, childbirth, and parenting.
- Media and ads may influence the choice of where to have a child or whether to use the services of a midwife or a physician.
- Family, neighbors, and friends who have children can provide invaluable advice and assistance to new parents.

Biological Factors

- Hormones create gender differentiation during the second month of prenatal development.
- Physiological cycles and changes in the fetus take place at an extremely fast pace.
- Physical appearance of the mother changes (for example, clearer skin) as hormonal changes take place.
- Parents' genetic characteristics determine many attributes of their children, such as height and hair color.

Psychological Factors

- A pregnant woman's emotions can swing wildly because of hormonal shifts. The postpartum period can be associated with mild depression.
- Experience counts in pregnancy; subsequent infants go through labor faster and breastfeed more readily.
- Self-concept usually increases as a result of the responsibility of caring for another person.
- Learned attitudes and behaviors are often exhibited by pregnant couples.
- A woman's body image can suffer if she views herself as "getting fat" rather than as "carrying a child."

CASE STUDY

Pregnancy is a time of wonder and joy. For first-time parents, the world is forever changed after their infant is born. But even the degree of responsibility and emotional attachment to the child are influenced by many dimensions.

Biological age of the mother plays a factor. Teen pregnancies tend to have more medical complications for both mother and child. Risk of Down syndrome increases with age, from 1 in 885 births at age 30 years, to 1 in 109 births at age 40 years, to 1 in 32 births at age 45 years.

Socioeconomic status plays a role in the health care of children. Parents on the low end of the socioeconomic scale may lack resources for parental and infant care, as well as the education and resources for raising healthy children.

Social pressure about child rearing is exerted by grandparents as well.

When disposable diapers were introduced, Pampers advertised them as "easier." But grandparent pressure—"What was wrong with the diapers we used on you?"—caused many parents to return to cloth diapers. Pampers had to change its marketing strategy from being easier to being better for the baby.

Working parents tend to rely on a far-flung network of day care providers, friends, family, and peer parents for emotional and practical advice. Without such support, the emotional impact of raising a child can be overwhelming.

Summary

- Conception occurs in the fallopian tube. Sperm stay alive in the female reproductive tract for 24 to 72 hours. The ovum's peak fertile period is 8 to 12 hours, although an egg can be fertilized for as long as 24 hours after ovulation.

- The conceptus is known as a zygote until 8 weeks of development, when it is known as an embryo. At the beginning of the third month of development, the conceptus is known as a fetus. The embryo develops in the amniotic sac cushioned with amniotic fluid.

- Sometimes an ectopic pregnancy occurs in which the blastocyst becomes implanted in a site other than the uterus. Ectopic pregnancies are the main cause of maternal morbidity and mortality in the first trimester.

- Childbirth can occur under the supervision of a physician or a nurse–midwife. It can take place in a hospital, in a free-standing birthing center, or at home.

- Among the threats to a normal birth delivery are the use of over-the-counter drugs and alcohol, cigarettes, marijuana, cocaine, heroin and other narcotics, and birth control pills. Disease such as diabetes, HIV infection, syphilis, gonorrhea, herpes, chlamydia, and genital warts are additional threats. The pregnant woman may also experience hypertension, nausea and vomiting, hemorrhoids, and other conditions.

- Labor occurs in three stages. Stage I is the period from the onset of labor to the point at which the cervix is fully dilated. Stage II is the period from full cervical dilation through the birth of the child. Stage III is the period from the infant's birth to the delivery of the placenta, or afterbirth.

- Infertility, or the inability to reproduce, can be caused by occlusion of the fallopian tubes, blocked sperm ducts, low sperm production, or poor semen quality. Infertility can be treated by assisted reproductive technologies such as artificial insemination, in vitro fertilization, or gamete intrafallopian transfer.

Discussion Questions

1. Explain the process by which life begins, citing as much detail as possible.

2. What are the characteristics of fetal development that differentiate the three trimesters?

3. What can a pregnant woman do to increase the chance of having a healthy pregnancy and child?

4. Describe how various drugs and diseases can threaten infant health.

5. Which maternal problems may occur during pregnancy? What can be done to alleviate some of these problems?

6. Differentiate the three phases of labor and methods of reducing the pain of labor.

7. Describe the benefits of breastfeeding an infant.

8. Is sex safe during pregnancy? Explain the situations in which it is or is not.

9. Compare and contrast the prenatal undifferentiated and sex-differentiated external genitalia, including the hormones that create the sexes.

10. Explain the most common causes of infertility and the methods to treat such problems.

Application Questions

Reread the chapter-opening story and answer the following questions.

1. The Rich and Mary story underscores how the many dimensions of human sexuality play into our decision making. Although Mary believed in the social and ethical right of women to have abortions, her personal convictions and the psychological desire for another child led her to continue her pregnancy. What would you have done in Rich and Mary's situation? Which of the dimensions of human sexuality mentioned here would influence you?

2. The Rich and Mary story also underscores the fact that medical personnel often work with less than perfect information—they did not know she was carrying twins! If you had been in their situation, where could you find more information on analyzing amniocentesis test results? Would you pursue such avenues?

Critical Thinking Questions

1. A premature baby born at 24 weeks gestation (5½ months), weighing about a pound, can be saved—at a cost of more than $300,000. But that is just the start. Many "preemie" children continue to have problems in school, requiring special-education programs. Choose a side and debate for or against saving children born more premature than 35 weeks. (*Note:* This question was submitted by a parent of two premature babies to provoke discussion.)

2. Hospitals have found that birthing centers are enormously profitable ventures. In major cities, hospitals compete for patients by having birthing rooms designed to look like homes with extra amenities and "freebies" (such as a champagne breakfast the morning after). Yet

to maintain profits, patients are sent home as soon as state laws allow—usually after a 2-night stay. Do patients benefit from such an arrangement—or is it simply a business deal for the hospitals?

Critical Thinking Case

For many years, there had been concern that too many cesarean birth deliveries were being performed in the United States. In 2006, the U.S. cesarean rate of nearly 31% of all births was higher than that of other industrialized nations. Interestingly, the data indicated that the increase in the cesarean rate did not contribute to the decline in infant mortality rate. Making matters worse, maternal morbidity and mortality rates are higher in cesarean deliveries than in routine vaginal deliveries. As a result, as one of the Year 2010 national health objectives, the Department of Health and Human Services sought to decrease the rate of C-sections in women giving birth for the first time to 15% of live births, and to 63% of women giving birth who had a prior C-section.

It had previously been thought unwise and unhealthy for women who had a previous cesarean delivery to attempt a vaginal birth. The concern was for tearing of the tissue and possible infection for the baby. The standard practice was "Once a cesarean, always a cesarean." However, it was found that, barring complications, many women who had a cesarean delivery could deliver vaginally the next time without endangering their or their baby's health. Still, in 2003, only 11% of women who had previously had a C-section and delivered again had a vaginal delivery.

Are the high rates of C-sections the result of the current medicolegal climate in the United States, which causes physicians to perform C-sections more often than in the past to protect themselves against a lawsuit?

Is the fact that C-sections earn the obstetrician more money a factor in the decision to perform them?

Given the increased risk to the mother of a cesarean delivery, and the evidence that it has little effect on infant mortality rate, is the relatively high rate of cesarean deliveries ethical?

Exploring Personal Dimensions

How Much Do You Know About Pregnancy and Birth?

For each of the statements that follow, indicate whether you think the statement is true or false. The correct answers and explanations appear after the questions.

True ____ False ____ 1. Pregnant women should stop exercising as soon as they discover they are pregnant.

True ____ False ____ 2. Once a woman has had a C-section, she should have C-sections for subsequent deliveries to prevent tearing of the abdominal tissue.

True ____ False ____ 3. The use of midwives has decreased in recent years.

True ____ False ____ 4. Breastfeeding is covered by the Pregnancy Discrimination Act, which guarantees that working women may breastfeed.

True ____ False ____ 5. Teen birth rates have steadily increased and are of significant concern.

True ____ False ____ 6. In terms of a newborn baby's health, the length of time before its mother becomes pregnant again does not matter.

Answers and Explanations

Each of the statements above is false.

1. Pregnant women are encouraged to continue exercising if they exercised before becoming pregnant. Some studies have suggested that exercise during pregnancy helps make the labor and delivery easier and shorter, promotes earlier recovery after delivery, and reduces the chance of C-sections. However, women who have not maintained an exercise regimen before becoming pregnant should not begin after becoming pregnant. Rather, they should exercise by adopting a mild walking or swimming program or by consulting an expert on exercise and pregnancy for other activities that will be beneficial for them and their fetuses.

2. There is no reason why, as a matter of routine, women who have had one C-section need to have C-sections for subsequent pregnancies. C-sections need be performed only if the woman has an STI that can be transmitted during childbirth, if the baby is too large to pass through the vaginal opening, or if the stress of the delivery has the potential to cause harm to the mother.

3. Contrary to popular belief, the proportion of women who use a nurse–midwife rather than an obstetrician to deliver their babies has remained constant. One percent of births are attended by a midwife.

4. Many women have been fired or discriminated against for breastfeeding at work. However, the courts have failed to interpret the Pregnancy Discrimination Act as protecting these women. To correct this situation, legislation was passed in the U.S. House of Representatives in 1998 to encourage employers to provide support for working mothers who choose to breastfeed their infants.

5. The birth rate for teenagers increased in 2006 for the first time after 14 straight years of decline. The rate in 2006 was 41.9 births per 1,000 females aged 15–19 years, up from 40.5 births in 2005. The teen birth rate had dropped 34% from 1991 (61.8 births per 1,000) to 2005 (Martin et al., 2009). Teen birth rates are still too high and are, rightfully, of national concern.

6. Research has shown that a short interpregnancy interval is a risk factor for infant mortality. Two explanations have been offered to explain this finding. The *maternal depletion hypothesis* suggests that at least 1 year between the birth of one child and subsequent conception is essential to restore maternal nutritional resources necessary for a successful pregnancy. The postpartum stress hypothesis states that caring for an infant can be so stressful that the physical or emotional strain can interfere with the growth of the fetus. In any case, an 18-month interpregnancy interval is recommended (Conde-Agudelo, Rosas-Bermúdez, & Kafury-Goeta, 2006).

Suggested Readings

American College of Obstetricians and Gynecologists. *Your pregnancy and birth*, 4th ed. Atlanta, GA: American College of Obstetricians and Gynecologists, 2005.

Buckhanon, K. *Conception*. New York: St. Martin's Press, 2008.

Curtis, G., & Schuler, J. *Your pregnancy week by week*. Philadelphia, PA: Da Capo Press, 2004.

Jones, S., Jones, M., Westdahl, C., & Bernstein, P. S. *Great expectations: Your all-in-one resource for pregnancy and childbirth*. New York: Barnes & Noble Books, 2004.

Kitzinger, S., & May, M. (Photographer). *The complete book of pregnancy and childbirth*. New York: Knopf Publishing Group, 2003.

Murkoff, H., & Mazel, S. *What to expect when you're expecting*, 4th ed. New York: Workman, 2008.

Simkin, P. *The birth partner: A complete guide to childbirth for dads, doulas, and all other labor companions*, 3rd ed. Boston, MA: Harvard Common Press, 2007.

Stone, J., & Eddleman, K. *The pregnancy bible: Your complete guide to pregnancy and early parenthood*. Tonawanda, NY: Firefly Books, 2008.

Stoppard, M. *Conception, pregnancy and birth: The childbirth bible for today's parents*. London: DK Adult, 2008.

Web Resources

For links to the web sites below, visit *http://sexuality.jbpub.com/dimensions/4e* and click on Resource Links.

Planned Parenthood Federation of America
www.plannedparenthood.org

Includes information on how to get pregnant, decisions necessary once pregnant, options for pregnant women, and other topics pertaining to family planning issues.

Maternal and Child Health Bureau
www.mchb.hrsa.gov

A bureau of the Health Resources and Services Administration of the U.S. Department of Health and Human Services, this site provides links to information pertaining to issues of the health of mothers and their children. Included are links to programs, funding opportunities, data, and resources and publications.

National Campaign to Prevent Teen and Unplanned Pregnancy
www.teenpregnancy.org

Presents information on programs that have been successful in preventing teen pregnancy and other links to assist in this endeavor. Provides information to acquire materials to support a National Day to Prevent Teen Pregnancy.

Association of Reproductive Health Professionals
www.arhp.org

Provides information and resources pertaining to many aspects of reproduction. Among the topics about which information is provided are abortion, contraception, emergency contraception, menopause, politics and reproductive health news, international reproductive health news and issues, and patient education materials.

National Center for Fathering
www.fathers.com

Seeks to inspire and equip men to be the involved fathers, grandfathers, and father figures their children need. The center provides practical, research-based training and resources, and reaches more than 1 million dads annually through seminars, small-group training, the WATCH D.O.G.S. (Dads of Great Students) program, a daily radio program, and weekly email.

Unexpected Pregnancy Outcomes

FEATURES

Ethical Dimensions
Should Intact Dilation
and Evacuation
(D&E) Be Banned?

**Communication
Dimensions**
Debating the
Abortion Issue

Global Dimensions
A Worldwide
Preference for Boys

Gender Dimensions
Baby "Richard"

**Multicultural
Dimensions**
International
Adoptions

CHAPTER OBJECTIVES

1 Discuss abortion issues, including abortion procedures, legal history, and current attitudes toward abortion.

2 Describe the various types of adoptions and the laws surrounding them, including closed and open adoptions, agency adoptions, independent adoptions, and adoption by relatives.

sexuality.jbpub.com/dimensions/4e

Global Dimensions: A Worldwide Preference for Boys
Emotions and Abortion
Multicultural Dimensions: International Adoptions
Foster Care and Adoption

INTRODUCTION

*T*oo many pregnancies are unplanned and unwanted. The dilemma this causes for some men and women is eloquently described by the author Anna Quindlen (1988, 209–212).

It was always the look on their faces that told me first. I was the freshman dormitory counselor and they were freshmen at a women's college where everyone was smart. One of them would come into my room, a golden girl, a valedictorian, an 800 verbal score on the SATs, and her eyes would be empty, seeing only a busted future, the devastation of her life as she knew it. She had failed biology, messed up the math; she was pregnant. That was when I became prochoice.

Quindlen then describes the birth of her own son.

It was the look in his eyes that I will always remember, too. They were as black as the bottom of a well, and in them for a few minutes I thought I saw myself the way I had always wished to be—clear, simple, elemental, at peace. My child looked at me and I looked back at him in the delivery room, and I realized that out of a sea of infinite possibilities it had come down to this: a specific person, born on the hottest day of the year, conceived on a Christmas Eve, made by his father and me miraculously from scratch.

Once I believed that there was a little blob of formless protoplasm in there and a gynecologist went in there with a surgical instrument, and that was that. Then I got pregnant myself—eagerly, intentionally, by the right man, at the right time—and I began to doubt. My abdomen still flat, my stomach roiling with morning sickness, I felt not that I had protoplasm inside, but, instead, a complete human being in miniature to whom I could talk, sing, make promises. Neither of these views was accurate; instead, I think, the reality is something in the middle. And that is where I find myself now, in the middle—hating the idea of abortions, hating the idea of having them outlawed.

For I know it is the right thing in some times and places. I remember sitting in a shabby clinic far uptown with one of those freshmen, only three months after the Supreme Court had made what we were doing possible, and watching with wonder as the lovely first love she had had with a nice boy unraveled over the space of an hour as they waited for her to be called, degenerating into sniping and silences. I remember a year or two later seeing them pass on campus and not even acknowledge each other because their conjoining had caused them so much pain, and I shuddered to think of them married, with a small psyche in their unready and unwilling hands. . . .

I don't feel all one way about abortion anymore, and I don't think it serves a just cause to pretend that many of us do. For years I believed that a woman's right to choose was absolute, but now I wonder. Do I, with a stable home and marriage and sufficient stamina and money, have the freedom to choose abortion because a pregnancy is inconvenient just now? Legally I do have the right; legally I wanted always to have that right. It is the morality of exercising it under those circumstances that makes me wonder. . . .

I have taped on my VCR a public television program in which somehow, inexplicably, a film is shown of a fetus in utero *scratching its face, seemingly putting up a tiny hand to shield itself from the camera's eye. It would make a potent weapon in the arsenal of the antiabortionists. I grow sentimental about it as it floats in the salt water, part fish, part human being. It is almost living, but not quite. It has almost turned my heart around, but not quite my head.**

Many people are surprised to learn that nearly half of all pregnancies are unintended. Yet, that is the case. When an unintended pregnancy occurs, decisions are required. Should the pregnancy be terminated? If so, which method of abortion should be used? What are the legal, moral, and health implications of this decision? Should the fetus be brought to term and a baby born? If so, should the child be raised by the biological parents? Should it be placed for adoption? If placed for adoption, should adoption be arranged through an agency or through a relative? What are the legal and moral implications of this decision? This chapter explores the alternatives presented to people who experience an unintended pregnancy.

Abortion

For unplanned pregnancies, the first decision to be made is whether to continue the pregnancy. Sometimes the woman or the couple decide to allow the pregnancy to continue, but something goes wrong and the fetus stops developing. Such natural cessations of the pregnancy are called **spontaneous abortions**, or miscarriages. Abortions requiring intervention to end the pregnancy are technically called **induced abortions**.

Abortion is safest in the earliest weeks of pregnancy. If a woman thinks she is pregnant and does not want to continue the pregnancy, she should perform a home pregnancy test or go to a clinic as soon as she misses a period.

Abortion Procedures

Vacuum Aspiration

Almost all abortions in the United States are performed during the first trimester of pregnancy, using a surgical procedure called **vacuum aspiration**. It is a surgical procedure that uses suction equipment to evacuate the contents of the uterus. It can also be used in the first weeks of the second trimester. Eighty-nine percent of abortions are performed in the first 12 weeks of pregnancy (Guttmacher Institute, 2009a). Twelve percent of abortions are performed in the second trimester of pregnancy (Stubblefield, Carr-Ellis, & Borgatta, 2004).

Manual vacuum aspiration (MVA) is a variation of vacuum aspiration that can be used from the detection of pregnancy to up to 12 weeks since the last menstrual period (LMP). In contrast to traditional vacuum aspiration procedures, it uses nonelectric suction instruments. The procedure takes 5 to 15 minutes, and the woman usually leaves the clinic within 2 hours.

Medical Abortions

Medical abortions are procedures that use drugs to induce abortion, including **mifepristone** or **methotrexate** in combination with **misoprostol**. Mifepristone was discovered by a French pharmaceutical company in 1978 and was known as RU 486. (*RU* refers to Roussel Uclaf, the French pharmaceutical company.)

Mifepristone blocks the hormone progesterone, which is needed to maintain a pregnancy. A woman who is no more than 49 days LMP takes mifepristone at a clinic visit. She returns to the clinic 2 days later and takes misoprostol, a prostaglandin that causes uterine contractions. In 92% of the cases, the pregnancy is terminated (Spitz et al., 1998; World Health Organization, 2000). In the fall of 2000, mifepristone was approved by the U.S. Food and Drug Administration (FDA).

Methotrexate blocks folic acid and prevents cell division. A woman who is no more than 49 days past her last missed period receives an injection of methotrexate at a clinic and swallows misoprostol pills 2 to

spontaneous abortion (miscarriage) The natural termination of a pregnancy.

induced abortion Purposeful termination of a pregnancy.

vacuum aspiration Surgical procedure that uses a suction tube to evacuate the contents of the uterus, which can be used through the first weeks of the second trimester.

manual vacuum aspiration (MVA) A variation of vacuum aspiration that uses nonelectric suction instruments and can be used from detection of pregnancy through 12 weeks.

medical abortion A procedure that uses drugs to induce abortion.

mifepristone A drug that blocks the hormone progesterone, which is needed to maintain a pregnancy.

methotrexate A drug that blocks the hormone progesterone, which is needed to maintain a pregnancy.

misoprostol A prostaglandin that causes uterine contractions.

7 days later. This combination is 92–94% effective in terminating pregnancy (Okie, 2000).

Currently, in the United States, methotrexate medical abortions are available only on an "off-label" basis. When drugs are approved by the U.S. FDA, their safety and efficacy are judged to warrant their use for specific conditions. Often, however, physicians discover other uses for those drugs and prescribe them for these other purposes. This practice, termed *off-label use*, is perfectly legal. Methotrexate is currently approved by the FDA for use by physicians for psoriasis and for rheumatoid arthritis (Hatcher et al., 2004). Although approved for these conditions, it is used off-label by physicians for medical abortions. However, RU 486, mifepristone, was approved by the FDA for use in medical abortion on September 28, 2000.

Women who choose a medical abortion should understand that there is a 1% chance they will need to return for a surgical abortion (National Abortion Federation, 2008). Still, many women consider medical abortions as easier and more natural than a surgical procedure (Harvey, Beckman, & Satre, 2001). Ninety-six percent of women in clinical trials of mifepristone would recommend the procedure to others, 91% would choose it again, and 88% said it was very or moderately satisfactory (Winikoff et al., 1998).

Dilation and Evacuation

During the second trimester of pregnancy, **dilation and evacuation (D&E)** is the abortion procedure used. It involves dilating the cervix, scraping the walls of the uterus, and removing the endometrial lining with suction. In very rare cases (less than 1% of all abortions), a saline or prostaglandin solution is injected into the uterus to induce premature labor.

> **dilation and evacuation (D&E)**
> Surgical procedure that involves dilating the cervix, scraping the walls of the uterus, and removing the endometrial lining with suction.

The vast majority of abortions are performed early in pregnancy. Fifty-eight percent occur within the first 8 weeks, 20% between weeks 9 and 10, and 10% between weeks 11 and 12. Thus, 88% of abortions are performed during the first trimester of pregnancy (Cates, Grimes, & Schulz, 2003). Only 1.1% are performed at 21 weeks or more (Guttmacher Institute, 2009a). The procedure used during the third trimester is called an *intact D&E* and has been dubbed by opponents of legal abortion as a "partial birth abortion." This procedure is required when the fetus is too large for other abortion procedures to be performed safely and effectively (see the box on page 264).

The Law and the Debate

Because abortion is an issue debated by citizens, ruled on by the judiciary, and legislated by elected representatives—not to mention its being a major decision for people who become directly involved in unplanned pregnancies—it is a topic that needs the fullest possible study and consideration.

For more than three decades, abortion has been vehemently debated in the political sector. Although in vitro fertilization, contraception, and sterilization all have their controversial aspects, none of them generates the political, religious, and emotional heat that abortion does. Some people believe induced abortion to be murder of a baby, whereas others see it as a medical intervention into a biological process. Some people feel that the question of when life begins is central to this debate: Is it at conception, at some point when the fetus could (with help) exist outside the uterus, or at birth? But a person's view of when life begins is only one factor in shaping his or her attitudes on whether induced abortion is morally acceptable. Another central issue is whether the individual woman has the right to make a decision so basic to her own life or whether the government has that right and power. Other attitudes also enter into the debate—for instance, attitudes regarding world population, religious issues, women's "place," political power, poverty, public and private child care, and the degree of responsibility people should assume for their sexual behavior.

At this writing political groups generally typed pro-life are actively supporting candidates who are totally opposed to abortion. Their goal is to pass legislation making abortion illegal or even to pass a constitutional amendment prohibiting abortion in the United States. Groups labeled pro-choice, however, believe that women should have the right to decide for themselves what they will do with their bodies. Consequently they oppose legislative restrictions on the availability of abortion to women who choose that option, and they wish to uphold the Supreme Court decision of 1973, which established the current legal status of abortion in the United States. The Court ruled (in *Roe v. Wade*) that abortion should be available to women during the first trimester (the first 3 months) of pregnancy. The decision is made by the pregnant woman and her physician. With regard to abortion during the second trimester, the Court ruled that the states can develop the regulations they deem necessary to maintain the pregnant woman's health. In the third trimester the states can limit or prohibit abortions if the mother's health is not in jeopardy.

In 1983 the Supreme Court reaffirmed its 1973 decision and stated that the government could not interfere with abortion unless such interference was clearly justified by "accepted medical practice." In

Ethical
DIMENSIONS

Should Intact Dilation and Evacuation (D&E) Be Banned?

Intact dilation and evacuation is performed late in the second trimester when, in the judgment of the physician, it is deemed the best means of abortion—that is, the most effective and safest. Some reasons for this type of abortion are concern for the health of the pregnant woman, late determination of birth defects in the fetus, or the woman's delay in seeking abortion as a result of fear of letting others know that she is pregnant. Objections have been raised to this method of abortion because it is performed at or near viability of the fetus. Those opposed to abortion at any time in any form are understandably opposed to D&E. However, even some Americans supportive of a woman's right to abortion during the first trimester and through the second trimester until the fetus could live outside the womb are disturbed by abortions occurring so late in the pregnancy. In their desire to secure support for their position, opponents have dubbed D&E "partial birth abortion," attempting to have D&E viewed as the interference with the birth of a live baby, rather than the termination of a pregnancy.

Those opposed to placing restrictions on the type of abortion allowed argue that the most qualified person to make this decision is the physician. Therefore, they believe a ban on any type of abortion procedure would limit physicians' options at a time when performing it would be most effective and safest. Opponents to restrictions also believe that once restrictions are allowed, Right to Life supporters will use them as a wedge to introduce more restrictions, eventually eroding a woman's right to abortion.

In 1997, Congress passed a law banning D&Es. However, President Bill Clinton vetoed that law, and Congress could not muster the votes required to override the veto. The following year, Congress again passed a similar law, but it was again vetoed by President Clinton. However, this time the House overrode the veto. Once the bill arrived back in the Senate, the veto was sustained, thereby preventing the legislation from becoming law.

In June 2000, the U.S. Supreme Court ruled in *Stenberg v. Carhart* that bans on intact D&E abortion were unconstitutional. However, in 2007, the Supreme Court, in *Gonzales v. Carhart*, upheld the federal Partial-Birth Abortion Ban Act of 2003, which prohibits this type of abortion without any exemptions (that is, regardless of concerns for the woman's health). As a result, dilation and evacuation abortions are banned by the federal government. Confusion still exists, because the federal law does not provide a precise description of what is banned. Consequently, states have proposed their own laws. As of 2009, 31 states had enacted bans on "partial birth" abortions (17 of which were deemed unconstitutional because of their broad language); all of them include some sort of exemption if the woman's health is jeopardized by the pregnancy.

Do you believe D&E should be banned as an abortion procedure? Why do you believe as you do?

---

effect this ruling prohibited governmental interference even into the second trimester and invalidated state laws that required abortions during the second trimester to be performed in a hospital.

However, in 1989 a Court made more conservative by new presidential appointments revisited this issue. The justices decided in *Webster v. Reproductive Health Services* that a Minnesota law requiring physicians to test fetuses to determine whether they could survive outside the womb before performing abortions was constitutional. That opened up the possibility that other regulations of abortion would be reviewed positively by the Court. Subsequently, two other cases were taken before the Supreme Court and decided in 1990. In *Hodgson v. Minnesota*, the Court rejected a law requiring a physician to notify both parents of a minor before an abortion could be performed. The rationale for this ruling was that some minors either do not live with both parents or have abusive or otherwise uncaring parents. The Court made it clear that if this law included a judicial bypass (in which a judge could approve the abortion if the parents were not the ones most appropriately notified), this law would be considered constitutional. In fact, in *Ohio v. Akron Center for Reproductive Health*, the Court held that a similar law that required notification of one parent and that did include a judicial bypass was constitutional.

In 1992, the Supreme Court reaffirmed the constitutionality of states attaching regulations to abortions, although it also reaffirmed the right of a woman to have an abortion if she chooses. In *Planned Parenthood of Southeastern Pennsylvania v. Casey*, the Court ruled that Pennsylvania could require a woman seeking an abortion to receive counseling; to wait 24 hours before

Both sides of the abortion issue attempt to show their strength in numbers with annual marches on Washington coinciding with the anniversary of *Roe v. Wade*. The marches do not happen on the same day, to minimize conflict as well as to accommodate the huge influx of people to Washington.

an abortion could be performed; and, if a minor under 18 years old, to obtain a parent's informed consent or a judge's approval. The Court also ruled that a physician had to keep detailed records of abortions and reasons for performing late-term abortions. However, the Court refused to overturn *Roe v. Wade*, as many opposed to abortion had hoped a conservative Court would do.

In June 2000, the Supreme Court returned its most significant abortion ruling since the *Casey* case (NARAL Pro-Choice America, 2005b). In *Stenberg v. Carhart*, the Court ruled that bans on intact D&E (referred to as partial birth abortions) were unconstitutional since they did not take into account the health of the pregnant woman. Still, in 2003, the federal government passed the Partial-Birth Abortion Ban Act, which prohibited D&E abortions. In

2007, the Supreme Court upheld the constitutionality of that law.

In 1980 the Supreme Court made a decision that profoundly affected the availability of legal abortions. It ruled that the federal government could refuse to fund abortions for the poor, even though it funded other health care (Hyde Amendment). The consequence of this action has been to prohibit poor women from obtaining safe abortions—the same abortions that middle- and upper-class women can receive by paying for them—with Medicaid funds. People who oppose abortion acknowledge that an inequity exists between poor and affluent women regarding the availability of abortion, but they view this circumstance as leaving the fetuses of more wealthy women unprotected by law. Some states have taken on the financial costs of abortion for poor women who are denied federal assistance by the Hyde Amendment.

Current Laws on Abortion Services

People who oppose legalized abortion have unsuccessfully tried to outlaw abortion services completely. However, they have been successful at limiting the availability of abortion under many circumstances.

For example, in October 1998 the U.S. Congress passed a $500 billion appropriations bill, which contained many restrictions on abortion. The bill prohibited

- Abortion coverage for workers insured by the federal government

- Abortions for women in federal prisons

- Abortions in overseas military hospitals

- Federal or local funding of abortions in the District of Columbia

- Medicaid funding of abortions, which primarily affects women with disabilities and low-income women

- Abortions through the Indian Health Service

- Federally supported embryo research

Many states have also passed laws limiting abortion services (Tables IF1.1, IF1.2, IF1.3, IF1.4, IF1.5, IF1.6, IF1.7). These include laws limiting public and private funding for abortion, parental consent laws, waiting periods, and bans on certain procedures.

Who Has Abortions?

In 2005 (the latest data available at the time of this writing), 1.21 million abortions were performed in the United States, down from 1.31 million in 2000 (Jones et al., 2008). From 1995 through 2005, more

Communication
DIMENSIONS

Debating the Abortion Issue

Because of the intense emotions associated with abortion, as well as the moral and ethical implications, pro-choicers and pro-lifers tend to talk past one another. This is unnecessary, however, because there are many points on which they can agree, and others that they can understand better. In summarizing polls of Americans on the issue of abortion, *USA Today* (1996) reported wide agreement among people who make up the "great middle." Most people believe in personal choice. Fifty-nine percent opposed a constitutional amendment to ban abortion except to save the life of the mother. Eighty-eight percent believed abortion should be legal if the mother's life is endangered, 82% if the woman's physical health is endangered, 77% if the pregnancy was caused by rape or incest, and 64% during the first 3 months of the pregnancy. Still, there was agreement that there ought to be limits. Seventy-four percent favored a waiting period, 86% favored informed consent, 74% favored parental consent for minors, 70% supported spousal notification, 71% favored a partial birth abortion ban, and 82% believed abortion should be illegal during the last 3 months of pregnancy.

And yet, in arguing their positions, the two sides often take extreme positions. For example, extreme pro-lifers emphasize late-term abortions, whereas these abortions constitute only approximately 1% of all abortions. However, extreme pro-choicers oppose any restrictions on abortion through all three trimesters of pregnancy.

The result is a figurative—and too often a literal—shouting match rather than a conversation, and this form of communication can unfortunately lead to extreme actions. The National Abortion Federation reports that between 1977 and 2008, there were more than 5,924 attacks on abortion providers (National Abortion Federation, 2009).

Is this an effective way of communicating? Is this the way to resolve an ethical dilemma? How might groups such as clergy, citizens, or politicians work together to employ communication techniques that require listening as well as speaking?

than 45 million legal abortions occurred in this country. Each year, approximately 2% of women have an abortion, and, surprising to most people, 47% of them have had at least one previous abortion.

The Alan Guttmacher Institute monitors abortion laws and the characteristics of those having abortions (Guttmacher Institute, 2009a–i). It reports that about half (49%) of all pregnancies of American women are unwanted and that 40% of these are terminated by abortion. What surprises some people is that of these women 60% have had a previous birth.

Fifty percent of abortions are performed for women younger than 25 years. One-third of abortions are performed for women aged 20 to 24 years, and teenagers have 17% of all abortions.

Of the women who have abortions, 37% are African American, 34% are white, 22% are Hispanic, and 8% are other races. Because the rate of unintended pregnancy among poor women is four times that of women whose income is above 200% of the poverty level, poor women have four times the abortion rate compared to their more affluent counterparts.

Religion plays a role as well. Women who report no religious affiliation are more than four times as likely to obtain an abortion as other women. Among specific religions, 43% of women obtaining abortions identify themselves as Protestant, and 27% as Catholic (Guttmacher Institute, 2005).

Marital status is another variable associated with abortion. Seventy-nine percent of abortions are obtained by women who are not married (Strauss et al., 2004).

There are three primary reasons women give for seeking an abortion (Guttmacher Institute, 2009a). Three-quarters say that having a baby would interfere with their work, education, or other responsibilities. Approximately three-fourths say they cannot afford a child. And half say they do not want to be a single parent or are having problems with their husband or partner. In addition, some abortions are performed for health-related reasons.

The Safety of Abortion

Abortion is an extremely safe procedure. Less than 0.3% of abortion patients experience a major complication. Of these, the primary risks are pelvic infection, hemorrhaging, or unintended major surgery. For abortions performed during the first 8 weeks of pregnancy, 1 death occurs per 1 million abortions. The risk rises as the pregnancy progresses to 1 death per 29,000 during weeks 16 to 20, and 1 death per

TABLE IF1.1 **Protecting Access to Clinics**

	Specific Prohibited Actions					
State	Obstruction	Threat	Damage	Telephone Harassment	Other	Protected "Bubble Zone"
California	X	X	X			
Colorado						8-ft. zone within 100 ft. of door
District of Columbia	X	X	X	X	Noise	
Kansas	X					
Maine	X			X	Noise, odor	
Maryland	X					
Massachusetts						35-ft. zone around entrances and walkways
Michigan		X				
Minnesota	X					
Montana	X					8-ft. zone within 36 ft. of door
Nevada	X					
New York	X	X	X			
North Carolina	X	X			Weapon	
Oregon	X		X			
Washington	X	X	X	X		
Wisconsin		X				
Total	**11 + D.C.**	**6 + D.C.**	**4 + D.C.**	**2 + D.C.**	**2 + D.C.**	**3**

Source: Guttmacher Institute. *State policies in brief: Protecting access to clinics,* January 1, 2009.

11,000 after 20 weeks (Guttmacher Institute, 2009a). In comparison, the risk of death associated with childbirth is 11 times greater than that associated with abortion. Furthermore, there is no effect on subsequent pregnancies or births in women who have had the most common abortion procedure (vacuum aspiration) within the first 12 weeks.

Although there has been some concern raised about the psychological health of women as a result of experiencing an abortion, there is little evidence that women are negatively affected. In a study of more than 5,000 American women, those who had had an abortion actually had higher self-esteem and greater feelings of self-worth and capability than women who had not had an abortion (Russo & Zierk, 1992). Interestingly, women with a greater number of births or at least one unwanted birth had lower self-esteem than other women did.

Attitudes About Abortion: Changing and Unchanging

Since *Roe v. Wade*, attitudes toward abortion have been evolving, and many studies have attempted to identify Americans' attitudes. In 2003, 23% of Amer-

icans believed abortion should be legal under any circumstance, 15% under most circumstances, and 42% in only a few circumstances; 19% believed it should be *illegal* in all circumstances; and 1% had no opinion (Saad, 2003). The percentage saying abortion should be legal in all circumstances rose from 21% in 1975 to 34% in 1992, and slipped back to 25% in 1996. According to another study, 20% of Americans believe that abortion should be legal under any circumstances, 62% believe that it should be legal only under certain circumstances, and 15% believe that it should be illegal in all circumstances. These percentages have remained largely unchanged for the past 25 years (Adamson, 2000). A Gallup poll also studied this issue and found that 24% of respondents believe abortion should be legal in all circumstances, while 20% believe it should be illegal under all circumstances. Fifty-five percent believe abortion should be legal only under certain circumstances (2% had no opinion) (Gallup, 2006).

Table IF1.8 presents how Americans feel about abortion under certain circumstances and during various phases of a pregnancy. As Table IF1.8 demonstrates, abortion is considered more acceptable during the early stages of pregnancy than the later stages. In

(Text continued on p. 271)

TABLE IF1.2 State Requirements for Abortion Reporting

State	Reporting Required	Method of Payment	Complications	Reasons For Procedure					Met State Requirement for:	
				Woman's Health/Life	Rape/Incest	Fetal Abnormality	Other*	Fetus Viable	Mandated Counseling	Parental Involvement
Alabama	X†									X
Alaska	X	X				X			X	
Arizona	X			X		X	X			
Arkansas	X									X
California	▶									
Colorado	X									
Connecticut	X		X							
Delaware	X									
District of Columbia	Ω									
Florida	X†			X	X	X	X			
Georgia	X		X						X	X
Hawaii	X†		X			X				
Idaho	X		X							
Illinois	X†		X				X		X	X
Indiana	X		X					X‡		
Iowa	X									
Kansas	X							‡		
Kentucky	X									
Louisiana	X†		X	X	X	X			X	
Maine	X									
Massachusetts	X		X					‡		
Michigan	X	X	X					X		
Minnesota	X	X	X	X	X	X	X			
Mississippi	X	X	X							
Missouri	X		X					X		
Montana	X		X							
Nebraska	X		X	X	X	X	X			

State	1	2	3	4	5	6	7	8	9	10
Nevada	X†									
New Hampshire	Ω	X								
New Jersey	Ω					X				
New Mexico	X									
New York	X	X	X	X	X	X	X			
North Carolina	X		X							
North Dakota	X		X							
Ohio	X		X							
Oklahoma	X		X						X	
Oregon	X		X							
Pennsylvania	X		X					‡		
Rhode Island	X		X							
South Carolina	X		X			X			X	X
South Dakota	X	X	X	X	X	X	X		X	X
Tennessee	X†		X							
Texas	X		X					‡		
Utah	X		X	X	X	X	X	X		
Vermont	X		X			X				
Virginia	X		X			X				
Washington	X		X			X				
West Virginia	X		X	X		X			X	X
Wisconsin	X		X							
Wyoming	X		X							
Total	**46**	**7**	**26**	**9**	**6**	**14**	**8**	**4**	**8**	**8**

▶ Enforcement permanently enjoined by a court order; policy not in effect.

* States list a range of "other" reasons on their forms: elective (AZ, FL, IL, MN, SD, UT); economic (FL, MN, NE, SD); contraceptive failure or nonuse (NE); the woman's familial circumstances (NY); the woman's age (NY); "therapeutic" (UT); and the woman's being HIV positive (UT).

† Reporting form does not specifically include medication (nonsurgical) abortion.

Ω Reporting from physician to the state on abortion procedures is voluntary.

‡ State requires provider to report reasons for abortions performed after viability (IN), after 21 weeks gestation (KS), after 23 weeks gestation (MA and PA), or after the second trimester (TX); MA also asks whether the abortion resulted in a live birth.

Source: Guttmacher Institute. State policies in brief: Abortion reporting requirements, January 1, 2009.

TABLE IF1.3 Parental Involvement in Minors' Abortions

State	Consent Only	Notification and Consent	Notification Only	Judicial Bypass	Other Adult Relatives	Medical Emergency	Abuse, Assault, Incest, or Neglect
Alabama	X			X		X	
Alaska	▼						
Arizona	X			X		X	X
Arkansas	X			X		X	X
California	▼						
Colorado			X	X		X	X
Delaware		X*,†		X*,†	X†	X†	
Florida			X	X		X	
Georgia			X	X		X	
Idaho	X			X		X	X
Illinois			▼				
Indiana	X			X		X	
Iowa			X	X	X	X	X
Kansas			X	X		X	X
Kentucky	X			X		X	
Louisiana	X			X		X	
Massachusetts	X			X		X	
Michigan	X			X		X	
Minnesota			Both parents	X		X	X
Mississippi	Both parents			X		X	
Missouri	X			X			
Montana			▼				
Nebraska			X	X		X	X
Nevada			▼			X	
New Jersey			▼			X	
New Mexico	▼						
North Carolina	X			X	X	X	
North Dakota	Both parents			X		X	
Ohio	X			X			
Oklahoma		X		X		X	X
Pennsylvania	X			X		X	
Rhode Island	X			X			
South Carolina	X†			X†	X†	X†	X†
South Dakota			X	X		X	
Tennessee	X			X		X	X

Note: Except where indicated, policies require the involvement of one parent.
▼ Enforcement permanently enjoined by court order; policy not in effect.
* Allows specified health professionals to waive parental involvement in limited circumstances.
† While most states' laws apply to all minors, Delaware's law applies to women under 16 and South Carolina's law applies to women under 17.
‡ The provision only applies to parental consent requirements.
Ω The provision only applies to the parental notice requirements.
Source: Guttmacher Institute. *State policies in brief: Parental involvement in minors' abortions,* January 1, 2009.

Continued

TABLE IF1.3   **Parental Involvement in Minors' Abortions—cont'd**

State	Required Parental Involvement			Alternatives		Exceptions	
	Consent Only	Notification and Consent	Notification Only	Judicial Bypass	Other Adult Relatives	Medical Emergency	Abuse, Assault, Incest, or Neglect
Texas	X			X		X	
Utah		X		X‡		X	XΩ
Virginia	X			X	X	X	X
West Virginia			X*	X*		X	
Wisconsin	X*			X*	X	X	X
Wyoming	X			X		X	
Total	**22**	**2**	**10**	**34**	**6**	**33**	**14**

Note: Except where indicated, policies require the involvement of one parent.
▼ Enforcement permanently enjoined by court order; policy not in effect.
* Allows specified health professionals to waive parental involvement in limited circumstances.
† While most states' laws apply to all minors, Delaware's law applies to women younger than 16 and South Carolina's law applies to women younger than 17.
‡ The provision applies only to parental consent requirements.
Ω The provision applies only to the parental notice requirements.
Source: Guttmacher Institute. *State policies in brief: Parental involvement in minor's abortions,* January 1, 2009.

addition, when the women's life is endangered or the pregnancy is a result of rape or incest, a majority of Americans believe abortion ought to be an option even during the third trimester of pregnancy.

When Americans who favor U.S. funding for family planning programs and abortions in developing countries are surveyed about their beliefs, they differ significantly from those who oppose such funding. For example, over 80% of those in favor of funding these programs believe it would save women's lives, whereas only 42% of those opposed to such funding believe women's lives would be saved. Table IF1.9 depicts these differences.

The latest data indicate Americans are less supportive of abortion than in the recent past. In 2005, when asked if they favor or oppose the Supreme Court decision making abortion legal up to 3 months of pregnancy, 52% favored and 47% opposed *Roe v. Wade* (Harris Interactive, 2005). Furthermore, whereas 58% of those polled in 1992 classified themselves as pro-choice, in 2005 only 51% stated they were pro-choice; 44% were pro-life, up from 35% in 1992. In 2005, 23% of those polled favored abortion under any circumstances, 55% under some circumstances, 21% under no circumstances, and 1% were not sure. In addition, in 2005, 60% believed abortion ought to be available during the first trimester, 26% believed abortion ought to be available during the second trimester, and 12% believed abortion ought to be available during the third trimester.

Availability of Legal Abortion

It is becoming increasingly difficult for a woman to have an abortion in the United States. The number of abortion providers in the United States has fallen by 37% since 1982 (Henshaw & Finer, 2003), and 11% between 1996 and 2000 (Guttmacher Institute, 2005). Between 2000 and 2005, the number of abortion providers declined another 2% (from 1,819 to 1,787). The proportion of women who live in a county with no abortion provider increased from 28% in 1982 to 34% in 2001 (Henshaw & Finer, 2003). Eighty-seven percent of counties in the United States lacked an abortion provider in 2005 (Guttmacher Institute, 2008b). These data are not surprising considering that one study found 40% of medical schools do not offer formal education on abortion in the preclinical years, and 25% do not offer it for third-year students doing clinical rotations in obstetrics and gynecology (Espry, 2005). In another study, only 51% of residency programs in obstetrics and gynecology were found to routinely provide abortion training (although residents could opt out if they had religious or moral objections). An additional 39% of programs offered optional abortion training, and 10% did not offer abortion training at all (Eastwood et al., 2006).

Further, many abortion clinics are picketed on a regular basis. In many cities, college students volunteer as escorts at local abortion clinics in order to assure that women can use the clinic without interference.

(Text continued on p. 280)

TABLE IF1.4   Abortion Counseling and Waiting Periods

State	Length of Waiting Period (hours)	In-Person Counseling Necessitates Two Trips to Clinic	Written Materials Given or Offered	Woman Informed That Abortion Cannot Be Coerced	Description of Procedure		Fetal Development		Ability of a Fetus to Feel Pain*	Accessing Ultrasound Services
					Specific	All Common	Gestational Age of Fetus	Throughout Pregnancy		
States with Detailed Abortion-Specific Informed Consent Requirements (23 states)										
Alabama	24		Given	V,W	V	W	V	W		
Alaska			Offered		V	W	V	W	W†	
Arkansas	Prior day		Offered	V,W	V	W	V	W	V,‡ W	
Georgia	24		Offered		V	W	V	W	V,W	V^Ω
Idaho	24		Given		V	W		W		
Kansas	24		Given	W	V	W	V	W		
Kentucky	24		Offered		V		V	W		
Louisiana	24	X	Given	W	V	W	V	W	V^Ω	
Massachusetts	▶									
Michigan	24		Given		V,W	W	V,W	W		W†
Minnesota	24		Offered		V	W	V	W	V,‡ W	
Mississippi	24	X	Offered		V		V	W		
Montana	▶									
Nebraska	24		Offered		V	W	V	W		
North Dakota	24		Offered		V		V	W		
Ohio	24	X	Given		V	W	V	W		
Oklahoma	24		Offered		V	W	V	W	V,‡ W	
Pennsylvania	24		Offered	W	V	W	V	W		V,W
South Carolina	1		Offered		V	W	V	W		
South Dakota	24		Offered		V	W†	V	W	W†	
Texas	24		Offered		V	W†	V	W	W†	

Continued

Utah	24	X			V	W	V	W	W	V
Virginia	24		Given	W	V	W	V	W	W	
West Virginia	24		Offered	W†	V	W	V	W	W	
Wisconsin	24		Offered	W	V	W	V	W	W	V,W
States with Customary Informed Consent Provisions (10 states)										
California					V					
Connecticut					V		V			
Delaware		▶			V		V			
Florida					V		V			
Indiana	18	X			V		V			
Maine					V		V			
Missouri	24	X			V		V			
Nevada					V		V			
Rhode Island					V		V			
Tennessee Ψ	24	▶			V		V			
TOTAL	24	7	23	8	32	18	30	8	22	6

All states waive mandatory waiting period requirements in a medical emergency or when the woman's life or health is threatened. In Utah, the waiting period requirement is waived if the pregnancy is the result of rape or incest, the fetus has grave defects, or the patient is younger than 15. The counseling requirement is waived in cases of ectopic pregnancy or severe fetal abnormality (Alabama) and in cases of a medical emergency (Georgia and Rhode Island).

V = verbal counseling; W = written materials.

▶ Enforcement permanently enjoined by court order; policy not in effect.

* Illinois does not have a counseling and waiting period law, but it requires that a woman receiving an abortion after viability be given the option of having anesthesia provided to the fetus.

† Included in written counseling materials although not specifically mandated by state law.

‡ Information given only to women who are at 20 weeks gestation or more.

Ω The law also requires the information to be included in the written materials; however, the materials have not been updated.

Ψ Enforcement of a provision of the Tennessee law requiring that a woman be told that an abortion constitutes major surgery is enjoined.

TABLE IF1.4 Abortion Counseling and Waiting Periods—cont'd

State	Counseling on Health Risks of Abortion						Counseling on Health Risks of Pregnancy
	Future Fertility		Breast Cancer		Mental Health		
	Accurately Portrays Risk	Inaccurately Portrays Risk	Correctly Reports No Link	Inaccurately Asserts Possible Link	Correctly Reports Range of Emotional Responses	Describes Negative Emotional Responses	
States with Detailed Abortion-Specific Informed Consent Requirements (23 states)							
Alabama					W†		W
Alaska	W†			W†	W		W
Arkansas	W†				W		V,W
Georgia	W†				W		V,W
Idaho	V				W†		V,W†
Kansas	W†			W†	W†		V,W
Kentucky							V
Louisiana	W†				W†		V,W
Massachusetts							
Michigan						W	W
Minnesota	V,W†		V,W†		W		V,W
Mississippi	V,W†		V	W†			V,W†
Montana							
Nebraska	V,W†					W	V,W
North Dakota	V						V
Ohio							V
Oklahoma	W†			W†	W		V,W
Pennsylvania	W†				W		V,W

State							
South Carolina	W†						W
South Dakota	V	W†					V,W†
Texas	V	W	V	W		W†	V,W
Utah						W	V,W
Virginia					W		W
West Virginia	V			W†		W	V,W
Wisconsin	V,W				V,W		V,W
States with Customary Informed Consent Provisions (10 states)							
California							
Connecticut							
Delaware							
Florida							V
Indiana							V
Maine							V
Missouri							
Nevada					Φ		
Rhode Island							
Tennessee							V
Total	17	2	3	6	12	7	27

V = verbal counseling; W = written materials.

† Included in written counseling materials although not specified by state law.

Φ Law requires discussion of emotional impact of abortion.

Source: Guttmacher Institute. *State policies in brief: Counseling and waiting periods for abortion,* January 1, 2009.

TABLE IF1.5 Restricting Insurance Coverage of Abortion

State	Private Insurance Policies		Insurance Policies for Public Employees					
	Limited to Life Endangerment*	Limited to Life, Rape, and Incest*	Abortion Coverage Offered in Cases of:				Abortion Coverage Never Offered	Coverage in Cases of Life, Rape, and Incest Allowed By Purchase of Rider at an Additional Cost
			Life	Health	Rape/ Incest	Fetal Abnormality		
Colorado							X	
Idaho	X		X					
Illinois			X					
Kentucky	X						X	
Massachusetts			X†	X†				
Mississippi			X		X	X		
Missouri	X							
Nebraska			X‡					
North Dakota	X		X					
Ohio								X
Oklahoma		X						
Pennsylvania			X		X			
Rhode Island	▶		X		X			
South Carolina			X		X			
Virginia			X		X	X		
Total	**4**	**1**	**9**	**1**	**5**	**2**	**2**	**1**

▶ Enforcement permanently enjoined by court order; policy not in effect.
* Additional abortion coverage is available only at an additional cost.
† State specifically prohibits coverage of postviability "partial birth" abortions.
‡ The individual employee must bear the cost of abortion coverage for other circumstances.
Source: Guttmacher Institute. *State policies in brief: Restricting insurance coverage of abortion,* January 1, 2009.

TABLE IF1.6 State Funding of Abortion Under Medicaid

State	Generally Follows the Federal Standard; Funds in Cases of: Life Endangerment, Rape, and Incest	Other Exceptions	Funds All or Most Medically Necessary Abortions
Alabama	X		
Alaska			Court order
Arizona			Court order
Arkansas	X		
California			Court order
Colorado	X		
Connecticut			Court order
Delaware	X		
District of Columbia	X		
Florida	X		
Georgia	X		
Hawaii			Voluntarily
Idaho	X		
Illinois			Court order
Indiana	X	Physical health	
Iowa	X	Fetal abnormality	
Kansas	X		
Kentucky	X		
Louisiana	X		
Maine	X		
Maryland			Voluntarily
Massachusetts			Court order
Michigan	X		
Minnesota			Court order
Mississippi	X	Fetal abnormality	
Missouri	X		
Montana			Court order
Nebraska	X		
Nevada	X		
New Hampshire	X		
New Jersey			Court order
New Mexico			Court order
New York			Voluntarily
North Carolina	X		
North Dakota	X		
Ohio	X		
Oklahoma	X		
Oregon			Court order
Pennsylvania	X		
Rhode Island	X		
South Carolina	X		
South Dakota	*		

* State pays for abortions only when necessary to protect the woman's life.

Continued

TABLE IF1.6 **State Funding of Abortion Under Medicaid—cont'd**

State	Generally Follows the Federal Standard; Funds in Cases of:		Funds All or Most Medically Necessary Abortions
	Life Endangerment, Rape, and Incest	Other Exceptions	
Tennessee	X		
Texas	X		
Utah	X	Physical health/fetal abnormality	
Vermont			Court order
Virginia	X	Fetal abnormality	
Washington			Voluntarily
West Virginia			Court order
Wisconsin	X	Physical health	
Wyoming	X		
Total	**32 + D.C.**		**17**

* State pays for abortions only when necessary to protect the woman's life.
Source: Guttmacher Institute. *State policies in brief: State funding for abortion under Medicaid,* January 1, 2009.

TABLE IF1.7 **Later-Term Abortion Policies**

State	Threshold for Later-Term Abortions	Later-Term Abortion Permitted When Threat to Woman's:			When a Later-Term Abortion Is Performed a Second Physician Must:	
		Life and Health	Life and Physical Health	Life	Attend	Approve
Alabama	Viability		X			X
Arizona	Viability	X			X	
Arkansas	Viability	X*			X	
California	Viability	X				
Connecticut	Viability	X				
Delaware	▼			▼		
Florida	24 weeks	X				X
Georgia	Third trimester	X				X
Idaho	Viability			X		X
Illinois	Viability	X			X	
Indiana	Viability		X		X	
Iowa	Third trimester	X				
Kansas	Viability	X				X
Kentucky	Viability	X				
Louisiana	Viability	X			X	
Maine	Viability	X				
Maryland	Viability	X**				
Massachusetts	24 weeks	X				
Michigan	Viability			X		
Minnesota	▼	▼			▼	
Missouri	Viability	X			X	

▼ Enforcement permanently enjoined by a court order; policy not in effect.
* Also permitted in case of rape or incest.
** Also permitted in case of fetal abnormality.
† If done for mental health reasons, must have the certification of an independent psychiatrist.

Continued

TABLE IF1.7   Later-Term Abortion Policies—cont'd

State	Threshold for Later-Term Abortions	Later-Term Abortion Permitted When Threat to Woman's:			When a Later-Term Abortion Is Performed a Second Physician Must:	
		Life and Health	Life and Physical Health	Life	Attend	Approve
Montana	Viability		X			X
Nebraska	Viability	X				
Nevada	24 weeks	X				
New York	24 weeks			X	X	
North Carolina	20 weeks	X				
North Dakota	Viability	X				X
Ohio	▼		▼		▼	▼
Oklahoma	Viability	X			X	
Pennsylvania	24 weeks		X		X	X
Rhode Island	24 weeks			X		
South Carolina	Third trimester	X†				X
South Dakota	24 weeks	X				
Tennessee	Viability	X				
Texas	Third trimester	X				
Utah	▼		▼*			
Virginia	Third trimester	X				X
Washington	Viability	X				
Wisconsin	Viability	X				
Wyoming	Viability	X				
Total	**36**	**28**	**4**	**4**	**9**	**10**

▼ Enforcement permanently enjoined by a court order; policy not in effect.
* Also permitted in case of rape or incest.
** Also permitted in case of fetal abnormality.
† If done for mental health reasons, must have the certification of an independent psychiatrist.
Source: Guttmacher Institute. *State policies in brief: State policies on later-term abortions,* January 1, 2009.

TABLE IF1.8   Circumstances Under Which Abortions Should Be Legal in First and Third Trimesters

Circumstance	First Trimester	Third Trimester
When the woman's life is endangered	82%	75%
When the pregnancy was caused by rape or incest	72%	59%
When the child would be born with a life-threatening illness	60%	48%
When the child would be born mentally disabled	50%	38%
When the woman does not want the child for any reason	41%	24%

Source: Saad, L. Abortion views hold steady over past year: Public makes sharp distinction about abortion circumstances. *Gallup News Service* (June 2, 2003). Available: www.gallup.com/poll/content/default.aspx?ci=8521.

TABLE IF1.9 **Differences Among Respondents Who Favor U.S. Funding for Both Family Planning (FP) Programs and Abortion in Developing Countries, Favor Funding for Family Planning but Not Funding for Abortion, and Oppose Funding for Both**

Circumstance	Favor FP/ Favor Abortion	Favor FP/ Oppose Abortion	Oppose FP/ Oppose Abortion
Many women's lives are saved when abortion is legal, as compared to when abortion is illegal	82%	54%	42%
Too many women use abortion as a routine means of controlling birth	54%	78%	75%
Legal abortion encourages more sexual activity among teenagers and unmarried couples	38%	72%	65%
In most cases, women who have a legal abortion do so only as a last resort when their birth control fails	60%	33%	34%
Having legal contraception or birth control available encourages more sexual activity among teenagers and unmarried couples	38%	62%	65%
Percentage who favor government providing funding for abortion services for poor women in this country who want them	74%	20%	22%

Source: Adamson, D. M., Belden, N., DeVanzo, J., & Patterson, S. *How Americans view world population issues: A survey of public opinion.* Santa Monica, CA: Rand Corporation, 2000. Available: www.rand.org/publications/MR/MR1114/MR1114.html/MR1114.appd.html.

DIMENSIONS

A Worldwide Preference for Boys

Around the world, on average, there are 105 boys born for every 100 girls born. Yet in China, there are 111 boys born for every 100 girls. Why is China so different from the rest of the world? Unfortunately, it is not.

Throughout the world, especially in densely populated countries, there are many reasons that boy babies are preferred, most based on long-term gender bias. China has no social security system, leaving elders vulnerable. In a country where couples are encouraged to have only one child, boys are presumed to be more valuable, because they are able to work and support their parents as they age. Either girls are not able to earn enough money to support their parents, or they are married off and assume duties with their new families. This situation is exacerbated as China becomes a more capitalistic country requiring men to travel for business purposes, while women are expected to stay at home. Men's travel earns money and makes them still more valuable in the eyes of many Chinese parents.

So the preference is for boy babies, but what is done to ensure that more boys will be born than girls? The shocking answer is female infanticide. When a Chinese woman delivers a baby, the village midwife sometimes prepares a bucket of water in which, if it is a girl, the baby's head is submerged before she starts to breathe. In India, where boy babies are preferred to girl babies for many of the same reasons as in China, female infanticide takes on a slightly different form. Pregnant Indian women have amniocentesis to determine the gender of their fetus. If the fetus is a girl, they undergo an abortion. Although the Indian authorities attempted to outlaw the use of amniocentesis for this purpose, the populace became outraged and refused to change this practice.

Looking at the female infanticide practices from the eyes of Western culture, experts have concluded that until gender equality is achieved around the world, female infanticide will be difficult to eradicate. Along with female genital mutilation (discussed earlier in this book), female infanticide may be culturally based. Some people believe that Western culture should refrain from interfering with the practices of other cultures. Others believe that in this case interference is warranted. What do you believe?

Violence has also plagued many abortion clinics and abortion providers. Between 1977 and 2008, there were 41 bombings, 175 arsons, 96 attempted bombings and arsons, and 635 bomb threats directed at abortion providers (National Abortion Federation, 2009). Abortion providers have been murdered at the clinics where they work in Florida and Massachusetts. On October 23, 1998, an obstetrician was murdered in his home by a sniper because he provided abortions. Table IF1.10 summarizes the

TABLE IF1.10 Incidents of Violence and Disruption Against Abortion Providers in the United States and Canada

Violence	1977–1992	1993	1994	1995	1996	1997	1998	1999	2000	2001	2002	2003	2004	2005	2006	2007	2008*	Total
Murder[1]	0	1	4	0	0	0	2	0	0	0	0	0	0	0	0	0	0	7
Attempted murder	2	1	8	1	1	2	1	0	1	0	0	0	0	0	0	0	0	17
Bombing[1]	27	1	1	1	2	6	1	1	0	1	0	0	0	0	0	0	0	41
Arson[1]	101	12	11	14	3	8	4	8	2	2	1	3	2	2	0	2	0	175
Attempted bomb/arson[1]	54	7	3	1	4	2	5	1	3	2	0	0	1	6	4	2	1	96
Invasion	321	24	2	4	0	7	5	3	4	2	1	0	0	0	4	7	1	385
Vandalism	430	113	42	31	29	105	46	63	56	58	60	48	49	83	72	59	23	1,367
Trespassing	0	0	0	0	0	0	0	193	81	144	163	66	67	633	336	122	51	1,856
Butyric acid attacks	57	15	8	0	1	0	19	0	0	0	0	0	0	0	0	0	0	100
Anthrax threats	0	0	0	0	0	0	12	35	30	554	23	0	1	0	0	1	3	659
Assault and battery	79	9	7	2	1	9	4	2	7	2	1	7	8	8	11	12	2	171
Death threats	88	78	59	41	13	11	25	13	9	14	3	7	4	10	10	13	1	399
Kidnapping	2	0	0	0	0	0	1	0	0	0	0	0	0	0	1	0	0	4
Burglary	28	3	3	3	6	6	6	4	5	6	1	9	5	11	30	12	3	141
Stalking[2]	0	188	22	61	52	67	13	13	17	10	12	3	15	8	6	19	0	506
Total	1,189	452	170	159	112	223	144	336	215	795	265	143	152	761	474	249	85	5,924
Disruption																		
Hate mail/harassing calls	824	628	381	255	605	2,829	915	1,646	1,011	404	230	432	453	515	548	522	113	12,311
Email/Internet harassment	0	0	0	0	0	0	0	0	0	0	24	70	51	77	25	38	22	307
Hoax device/suspicious packages	0	0	0	0	0	0	0	0	0	0	41	13	9	16	17	23	4	123
Bomb threats	275	22	14	41	13	79	31	39	20	31	7	17	13	11	7	6	9	635
Picketing	4,082	2,279	1,407	1,356	3,932	7,518	8,402	8,727	8,478	9,969	10,241	11,348	11,640	13,415	13,505	11,113	5,129	132,541
Total	5,181	2,929	1,802	1,652	4,550	10,426	9,348	10,412	9,509	10,404	10,543	11,880	12,166	14,034	14,102	11,702	5,277	145,917
Clinic Blockades																		
Number of incidents	543	66	25	5	7	25	2	3	4	2	4	10	34	4	13	7	1	755
Number of arrests[3]	32,208	1,236	217	54	65	29	16	5	0	0	0	0	0	0	0	3	0	37,718

All numbers represent incidents reported to or obtained by NAF. Actual incidents are likely much higher. Tabulation of trespassing began in 1999 and tabulation of email harassment and hoax devices began in 2002.
1. Incidents recorded are those classified as such by the appropriate law enforcement agency. Incidents that were ruled inconclusive or accidental are not included.
2. Stalking is defined as the persistent following, threatening, and harassing of an abortion provider, staff member, or patient away from the clinic. Tabulation of stalking incidents began in 1993.
3. The "number of arrests" represents the total number of arrests, not the total number of persons arrested. Many blockaders are arrested multiple times.
Source: National Abortion Federation. NAF violence and disruption statistics, 2009. Available: www.prochoice.org/pubs_research/publications/downloads/about_abortion/violence_statistics.pdf.

Did You Know ...

incidents of abortion-related violence over the past three decades.

Thirty-five states have passed laws requiring that adolescents have parental consent or notification for abortion (Guttmacher Institute, 2009e). Twenty-four states have passed laws requiring a woman to have to make more than one visit to a clinic to have an abortion, insisting on a "waiting period."

Public and Private Funding for Abortion

The patchwork of state laws concerning public funding for abortion services is complex. As a result of the Hyde Amendment, the use of federal Medicaid funds for abortion is prohibited except in cases in which the woman's life is in danger. The amendment was expanded in 1993 to include situations in which the pregnancy resulted from rape or incest. Each state establishes its own abortion funding policy related to state revenues. In 2009, the Guttmacher Institute reported that 17 states funded abortion in their state medical assistance programs in all or most circumstances. Several states ban insurance coverage for abortion unless women pay an extra premium.

Emotions and Abortion

The emotional reactions to abortion are varied. Some women feel guilty, depressed, angry, and ashamed. Others feel none of these feelings, or feel them just to a limited extent. The same range of emotions may apply to male partners as well.

Religious and moral beliefs; reactions of the medical staff, relatives, and friends; and the strength of the relationship between the partners all affect emotional responses. In addition, the earlier the abortion is performed, the lower the emotional cost. Perhaps the lack of humanlike features of the con-

ceptus is what influences this finding. Realizing this, a film was developed by opponents of abortion and shown widely in the United States. Entitled *The Silent Scream*, this film is a 28-minute depiction of an abortion using ultrasound visualization. The viewers see a 12-week-old fetus being aborted by vacuum curettage and supposedly screaming in pain. The narrator, Dr. Bernard N. Nathanson, makes one feel that abortion is akin to infanticide because, he argues, "The unborn child is just another human being . . . all the rest of his human functions are indistinct from any of ours." Many physicians and others have taken issue with Dr. Nathanson. For example, the American College of Obstetricians and Gynecologists responded to *The Silent Scream* with a statement that there is no scientific evidence to support the assertion that a 12-week-old fetus feels pain. Others have argued the following points (Spake, 1985):

1. The cerebral cortex of a 12-week-old fetus is insufficiently developed to feel pain.

2. Fetal movements are the result of reflexive action rather than "frantic activity" away from "the abortionist's instruments."

3. Because the mouth of the fetus cannot actually be identified in the film, and because there is no air inside the fetus's lungs, the "scream" is no scream at all.

4. The fetal model used by Dr. Nathanson as he narrates is much larger than a 12-week-old fetus. In addition, many of the "fetuses" shown in the film are not fetuses but rather stillborn, premature infants.

The Silent Scream is but one example of the extreme emotion associated with the issue of abortion. Abortion facilities have been bombed, and staff and patients have been targets of harassment. Reputable abortion facilities provide counseling before the abortion to help the woman, alone or with her partner, make sure that she does indeed want an abortion performed—it is usually considered the best of several bad choices. In addition, they provide counseling after the abortion to lessen the emotional costs associated with this decision. These functions are difficult to perform well in the face of bomb threats, actual bombings, arson directed at abortion facilities, or picketing and/or harassment of patients seeking services at these facilities. Furthermore, some professionals choose not to subject themselves to this type of treatment and, therefore, refuse to work at abortion facilities. Of course, some refuse to work there because of their own moral objections as well.

For many reasons individuals or couples may choose to adopt. International adoptions are among many options available.

Adoption

Another response to an unwanted pregnancy is delivery of the baby, followed by adoption placement. Women who are unwed and choose not to raise a baby or who do not have the financial resources necessary to raise a baby often select adoption as an alternative for providing a good life for their babies.

Gender
DIMENSIONS

Baby "Richard" In June 1990, Daniella Janikova and Otakar Kirchner, both immigrants from what is now Slovakia, conceived baby "Richard" (his name has been changed to protect his identity). However, before Richard's birth, Otakar returned to his country with a former girlfriend, leaving Daniella in the United States. Before the delivery, Daniella arranged to place Richard for adoption. Daniella was then introduced to the "Warburtons," a pseudonym for a family interested in adopting Daniella's baby. Daniella signed the necessary forms to arrange for the Warburtons to adopt Richard. However, under Illinois law, the father has to agree to an adoption. When Daniella was asked for the name and address of the father, she refused to give it, falsely stating that he had abused her. Richard was born on March 16, 1991.

A few days after Richard's birth, Otakar received a call informing him that Richard had died. One month later, however, he learned that the baby was alive, and soon he returned to Daniella. Otakar then hired an attorney, who started legal proceedings for the return of his child. Subsequently, he and Daniella were married.

The Warburtons, however, contested the return of Richard, and a Cook County Circuit Court judge ruled the adoption valid, declaring Otakar unfit largely because he had not filed a petition within 30 days of the birth (as required in Illinois) and because the prior testimony of Daniella alleged that he was abusive. However, when this decision was appealed, the Illinois Supreme Court in June 1994—after Richard had been living with the Warburtons for more than 3 years—overturned the adoption, stating that Otakar was led to believe that Richard had died and, therefore, could not have been expected to pursue his parental rights in a timely fashion.

After several appeals to the United States Supreme Court proved unsuccessful, Otakar and Daniella took custody of Richard on April 30, 1995. At the time of the wrenching transfer, Richard appealed to his adoptive mother, "I'll be good. Don't make me leave. I'll be good."

This case, tragic as it was for all parties, was decided on the rights of the father to agree to adoption of his biological offspring. That right is protected even if the biological mother chooses to place the child for adoption and, apparently, even if the child has been living with adoptive parents for many years.

Myth vs Fact

Myth: Most abortions are performed late in the pregnancy.
Fact: Ninety percent of all abortions are performed during the first trimester. These abortions are usually performed by vacuum aspiration.

Myth: Abortion is a dangerous procedure.
Fact: The risk of death during childbirth is 10 times greater than it is during abortion procedures. Furthermore, fewer than 0.3% of abortion patients experience a major complication.

Myth: Late-term abortions result in partial birth of the baby.
Fact: Opponents of abortion have labeled late-term abortion "partial birth abortion." This is a political tactic rather than an accurate description of late-term abortions. The correct term for these abortions is dilation and evacuation (D&E).

Myth: Adoptions have to be coordinated through an adoption agency.
Fact: Adoptions can be arranged independently, although these adoptions require court approval. In addition, adoptions can be arranged with relatives, although, again, they require court approval.

Myth: The withholding of the names of the birth parents (confidentiality and anonymity) is guaranteed by agencies and courts that arrange adoptions.
Fact: There is a debate taking place in our society regarding the rights of the birth parents versus the rights of the child. Several states have passed or are considering legislation to unseal adoption records.

Types of Adoptions

There are two basic types of adoption. *Closed adoptions* are confidential; there is no contact between the birth parents and the adoptive parents. The identities of the birth parents and adoptive parents are kept secret. *Open adoptions* allow contact between the birth parents and the adoptive parents. In fact, the birth parents may even select the adoptive parents. Contact can occur regularly or intermittently throughout the child's upbringing.

Although there have been some highly publicized cases of birth parents' seeking to reverse them, adoptions are legally binding and irreversible after a limited period. Birth parents sign "relinquishment papers" after the baby is born, and, unless both birth parents have not signed these papers, the courts have refused to reverse adoptions.

Adoptions are arranged in three ways: agency adoption, independent adoption, and adoption by relatives (Planned Parenthood Federation, 2009). In the case of *agency adoption*, the parents relinquish their baby to an adoption agency. These agencies are licensed by the government and may offer a number of services. They provide counseling, handle legal matters, make hospital arrangements for the birth, select adoptive parents, and refer the mother to agencies if financial assistance is needed. Usually, though not always, adoptions arranged through

agencies are closed adoptions. Adoption agencies can be located through contacting most religious organizations, or by writing to the National Council for Adoption at 225 N. Washington Street, Alexandria, VA 22314-2561, phoning it at (703) 299-6633, or emailing it at *ncfa@adoptioncouncil.org*. The agency accepts collect calls from pregnant women.

In *independent adoptions*, the birth parents select the adoptive parents and relinquish the baby into their care. Independent adoptions are often arranged through a physician or a lawyer and, in some states, by independent adoption centers. Independent adoptions are usually open adoptions and, although not legal in all states, are supervised by a lawyer, who usually represents both sides. However, it is often recommended that the birth parents and the adoptive parents have separate legal representation to protect them from being exploited. Often, the adoptive parents agree to pay the medical costs associated with the pregnancy and may even agree to pay for living expenses during that time. At the birth of the baby, the adoptive parents sign a "take into care" form that allows the adoptive parents to take the baby to their home while the state investigates their ability to raise the baby. This investigation usually takes 6 to 8 weeks. At any time while this investigation is occurring, either set of parents can change their minds. At the end of the investigation, the birth parents sign "relinquishment papers." Independent adoption can be facilitated by the Independent Adoption Center at 391 Taylor Boulevard, Suite 100, Pleasant Hills, CA 94523. Its telephone number is (800) 877-6736, and its email address is *staff@adoptionhelp.org*.

Adoption by relatives is used when the birth parents want the child to stay in the family. Even so, these adoptions require the approval of the courts. As in other adoptions, the relative is investigated by the state to determine ability to provide care for the child. Once the adoption is approved, the birth parents have no more rights pertaining to the child than they would in any other form of adoption.

Contemplating Adoption

Adopting a child is a decision that requires a great deal of consideration. So does the decision to give a child up for adoption. Planned Parenthood of America suggests that anyone considering giving a child up for adoption ask these questions:

1. Can you accept your child living with someone else?

2. Will going through pregnancy and delivery change your mind?

3. Are you willing to get good prenatal care?

4. Are you choosing adoption because abortion scares you?

5. Will the child's father approve of adoption?

6. Is anyone pressuring you to choose adoption?

7. Are you confident your child will be treated well?

8. Can you not be jealous of the adoptive parents?

9. Do you care what other people will think?

10. Do you respect women who place their children for adoption?

Someone contemplating placing a child for adoption may want to discuss these questions with her partner, clergy, professional counselor, or a trusted relative or friend.

Foster Care and Adoption

For parents who are not ready to decide between placing a child for adoption and parenting, many cities and counties provide temporary residences for their children. This arrangement is termed *foster care*. To arrange for this option, the birth parents must sign a legal foster care agreement that allows another family to care for the child. Often, foster care agreements specify the frequency of visits between the child and birth parents that will be allowed, the duration of stay with the foster care family, the amount of money the birth parents will have to provide the foster care parents for caring for their child, and the number and frequency of visits to a professional counselor (usually a social worker). Although foster care arrangements and regulations vary from state to state, if the foster care agreement is violated, the birth parents can lose the child permanently.

Foster care is also provided for children who are taken from their birth parents for abuse, neglect, or other behavior that precludes them from being able to raise their children and places their children at risk. Children placed in foster care permanently are eligible for adoption, and, in fact, that is the goal of state agencies that supervise foster care arrangements.

The U.S. foster care system includes more than 496,000 children, of whom 130,000 are eligible for

Multicultural DIMENSIONS

International Adoptions

Many children from other countries are adopted by Americans. These adoptions may be the result of humanitarian concern of people who see children orphaned by war or widespread disease, or difficulty in locating the type of American child they wish to adopt. These international adoptions, though, can be very costly. The bar graph below and Table IF1.A show the number of international children adopted by Americans.

Given that there are American children waiting to be adopted, should the federal government discourage international adoptions? If so, what will happen to children orphaned by war or abused or neglected in other countries? Or should people wanting to adopt children be supported wherever those children come from?

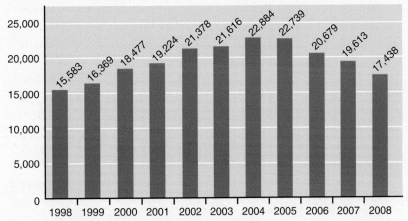

Adoptions to the United States

Source: U.S. Department of State, Office of Children's Health Issues. *Total adoptions to the United States*. 2009. Available: http://adoption.state.gov/news/total_chart.html.

Continued

Multicultural
DIMENSIONS

International Adoptions—cont'd

TABLE IF1.A   **Adoptions to the United States**

	FY 2008	FY 2007	FY 2006	FY 2005	FY 2004
1	Guatemala	China	China	China	China
	4,123	5,453	6,493	7,906	7,044
2	China	Guatemala	Guatemala	Russia	Russia
	3,909	4,728	4,135	4,639	5,865
3	Russia	Russia	Russia	Guatemala	Guatemala
	1,861	2,310	3,706	3,783	3,264
4	Ethiopia	Ethiopia	South Korea	South Korea	South Korea
	1,725	1,255	1,376	1,630	1,716
5	South Korea	South Korea	Ethiopia	Ukraine	Kazakhstan
	1,065	939	732	821	826
6	Vietnam	Vietnam	Kazakhstan	Kazakhstan	Ukraine
	751	828	587	755	723
7	Ukraine	Ukraine	Ukraine	Ethiopia	India
	457	606	460	441	406
8	Kazakhstan	Kazakhstan	Liberia	India	Haiti
	380	540	353	323	356
9	India	India	Colombia	Colombia	Ethiopia
	307	416	344	291	289
10	Colombia	Liberia	India	Philippines	Colombia
	306	314	320	271	287
11	Haiti	Colombia	Haiti	Haiti	Belarus
	302	310	309	234	202
12	Philippines	Philippines	Philippines	Liberia	Philippines
	291	265	245	183	196
13	Taiwan	Haiti	Taiwan	Taiwan	Bulgaria
	267	190	187	141	110
14	Liberia	Taiwan	Vietnam	Mexico	Poland
	249	184	163	88	102
15	Nigeria	Mexico	Mexico	Poland	Mexico
	148	89	70	73	89
16	Mexico	Poland	Poland	Thailand	Liberia
	103	84	67	72	86
17	Ghana	Thailand	Brazil	Brazil	Nepal
	101	67	66	66	73
18	Kyrgyzstan	Kyrgyzstan	Nepal	Nigeria	Nigeria
	78	61	66	65	71
19	Poland	Brazil	Nigeria	Jamaica	Brazil
	77	55	62	63	69
20	Thailand	Uganda	Thailand	Nepal	Thailand
	59	54	56	62	69

FY = fiscal year (October 1 to September 30).
Source: U.S. Department of State, Office of Children's Health Issues. *Total adoptions to the United States.* 2009. Available: http://adoption.state.gov/news/total_chart.html.

adoption (U.S. Department of Health and Human Services, 2008a). Fortunately, more and more of these children are being adopted. In 2007, 51,000 children in the foster care system were adopted. In 1997, the U.S. Congress passed the Adoption and Safe Families Act, designed to speed up adoption of children in the foster care system. That legislation provided bonuses of $4,000 to states for every child in the child protective system for whom they arranged adoption. For particularly difficult cases—such as older children or those with disabilities—states were provided $6,000 for each adoption. To further the goal of arranging for adoptions of children in foster care, in November 1998 President Clinton announced a plan to create an Internet site that would carry photographs and information about these children (Vobejda, 1998). The hope was that it would facilitate matching children eligible for adoption with parents seeking to adopt. Most states maintain web sites to facilitate adoption of children in the foster care system. Still other states provide information to private agencies that maintain such web sites.

Finding the Birth Parent

Because they seek to determine their complete history or because they are curious or have some other reason, many adults who were adopted seek to identify their birth parents. There is a good deal of disagreement as to whether and how this process should be facilitated. Some experts believe that contacting the birth parents might make them feel guilty about the adoption. Also, the birth parents might reject the adopted person, who might then have an unhealthy reaction to that rejection.

Before World War II, it was common practice for adoption records to be open. However, after the war, the combination of an increase in out-of-wedlock pregnancies and a conservative mood in the country resulted in adoption going "into the closet." Adoption records became sealed so that secrecy could be maintained. Since then, several states have passed legislation to open these records.

Residents of the state of Oregon decided this issue for themselves (Sanchez, 1998). In November 1998, Oregon voters approved a ballot initiative requiring the state to unseal confidential birth records. On request, adoptees would be given all the information about their past—in spite of the wishes of their birth parents. As you can imagine, this precipitated an outcry from opponents and supporters alike. The American Civil Liberties Union opposed the initiative, arguing that it was an invasion of the privacy earlier promised to birth parents who placed their children for adoption. Supporters argued that the question was, Who should have more rights?—a parent who gives up a child or the child who was adopted? Clearly they came down on the side of the child. Since Oregon's decision, Alabama, Alaska, Kansas, New Hampshire, and Oregon have adopted an unqualified right to view adoption records and several other states make records available if birth parents have not filed an objection (Adopting.org, 2009).

Summary

- Abortions can be spontaneous (miscarriages) or induced. Induced abortions can be performed by vacuum aspiration, manual vacuum aspiration, medical abortion, or dilation and evacuation (sometimes referred to as partial birth abortion).

- The Supreme Court legalized abortion in the *Roe v. Wade* ruling in 1973. Since then, several restrictions have been placed on abortions by the states and declared constitutional by the Supreme Court. In 2007, the Supreme Court upheld the constitutionality of the 2003 Partial-Birth Abortion Ban Act, which banned dilation and evacuation for late-term abortions.

- Forty-nine percent of pregnancies are unwanted in the United States, and approximately 40% of these pregnancies are terminated by abortion.

- Fifty percent of abortions are performed in women younger than 25, one-third in women aged 20 to 24 years of age, and 17% in teenagers. Women who report no religious affiliation are more than four times as likely to obtain an abortion as other women, and 79% of abortions are performed in unmarried women.

- Abortion is a safe procedure, with only 0.3% of abortion patients experiencing a major complication. Abortions are safest when performed during the first 8 weeks of pregnancy.

- Most Americans believe that abortions should be legal under certain circumstances (between 55% and 64% depending on the study), while 24% believe abortion ought to be legal under all circumstances and 20% believe it ought to be illegal under all circumstances.

- Adoptions can be closed—confidential with no contact between the birth parents and the adoptive parents—or open—allowing contact between birth parents and adoptive parents.

- Adoptions can be agency adoptions, in which the parents release the baby to adoption agencies; independent adoptions, in which the birth parents select the adoptive parents; or adoption by relatives.

- Although sealed in the past, adoptions records have been opened in several states. Alabama, Alaska, Kansas, New Hampshire, and Oregon have adopted an unqualified right to review adoption records, and several other states make records available if birth parents have not filed an objection.

Discussion Questions

1. What are the methods of abortion, and in which situations are they used?

2. Create a personal chart showing your own dimensions of human sexuality that relate to the abortion issue. After seeing all the issues involved, have you altered your position on abortion?

3. Explain the types of adoption available and the way each works.

Application Questions

Reread the chapter-opening story and answer the following questions.

1. The author Anna Quindlen appears to take a situational view of abortion: She thought abortion was OK for a bright college student but had second thoughts about an older and financially secure adult (herself). Does situation matter? In which situations is it acceptable to get an abortion? In which situations is it unacceptable?

2. The chapter also mentions the possibility of adoption. Should Quindlen have counseled her freshman with information about adoption? Explain why or why not.

Critical Thinking Questions

1. When the issue of abortion versus adoption is discussed, the father rarely enters into the discussion. Should the father have control over whether a woman can have an abortion or give a child up for adoption?

2. When do you believe that life begins? At conception? At a certain point in fetal development? At about 24 weeks, when the fetus can survive outside the womb (albeit with neonatal intensive care)? At about 35 weeks, when most babies can sustain life without medical intervention? Explain your answer.

3. Because many infertile couples want to adopt a child, why are there not more incentives for women to place children of unexpected pregnancies up for adoption? What could be done to motivate such a practice? Should the federal government be involved in such an effort?

Critical Thinking Case

In the late 1970s, Dr. Milfred Jefferson, an African American surgeon and chairperson of the national Right to Life organization, stated that abortion was genocide. She believed that a federally funded abortion program was aimed at eliminating the poor, African American population of the United States. Dr. Jefferson cited statistics showing that 30% of all abortions funded by Medicaid were performed on African Americans (while African Americans made up about 11% of the population). She said that "abortion is accomplishing what 200 years of slavery and 300 years of lynching didn't."

Opponents argue that the disproportionate number of Medicaid-funded abortions performed on African American women resulted from higher representation of African Americans among the poor in the United States; hence, they would have more need of financial support for abortions. Along these lines, people of lower socioeconomic status have less access to sex education, birth control information, and prescription birth control.

Abortion rates are still disproportionately high for African Americans. In 2004, the abortion rate for whites was 11 per 1,000 live births, the abortion rate for Hispanics was 28 per 1,000 live births, and the abortion rate for African Americans was 50 per 1,000 live births—more than four times the rate for whites (Henshaw & Kost, 2008).

Exploring Personal Dimensions

What is your feeling about abortion? Place an A, B, C, D, or E in the blank to the left of each of the following items, using the provided scale:

A. I *strongly agree* with the statement.

B. I *tend to agree* with the statement (some reservation).

C. I am *undecided* (uncertain about my feelings or have no feelings one way or the other).

D. I *tend to disagree* with the statement (some reservation).

E. I *strongly disagree* with the statement.

_____ 1. Abortion penalizes the unborn [child] for the mother's mistake.

_____ 2. Abortion places human life at a very low point on a scale of values.

_____ 3. A woman's desire to have an abortion should be considered sufficient reason to do so.

_____ 4. I approve of the legalization of abortion so that a woman can obtain one with proper medical attention.

_____ 5. Abortion ought to be prohibited because it is an unnatural act.

_____ 6. Having an abortion is not something to be ashamed of.

_____ 7. Abortion is a threat to our society.

_____ 8. Abortion is the destruction of one life to serve the convenience of another.

_____ 9. A woman should have no regrets if she eliminates the burden of an unwanted child with an abortion.

_____ 10. The unborn [child] should be legally protected against abortion because it cannot protect itself.

_____ 11. Abortion should be an alternative when there is contraceptive failure.

_____ 12. Abortions should be allowed because the unborn [child] is only a potential human being, not an actual human being.

_____ 13. Any person who has an abortion is probably selfish and unconcerned about others.

_____ 14. Abortion should be available as a method of improving community socio-economic conditions.

_____ 15. Many more people would favor abortion if they knew more about it.

_____ 16. A woman should have an illegitimate child rather than an abortion.

_____ 17. Liberalization of abortion laws should be viewed positively.

_____ 18. Abortion should be illegal, because the Fourteenth Amendment in the Constitution holds that no state shall "deprive any person of life, liberty, or property without due process of law."

_____ 19. The unborn child should never be aborted no matter how detrimental the possible effects on the family.

_____ 20. The social evils involved in forcing a pregnant woman to have a child are worse than any evils in destroying the unborn child.

_____ 21. Decency forbids having an abortion.

_____ 22. A pregnancy that is not wanted and not planned for should not be considered a pregnancy, but merely a condition for which there is a medical cure, abortion.

_____ 23. Abortion is the equivalent of murder.

_____ 24. Easily accessible abortions will probably cause people to become unconcerned and careless with their contraceptive practices.

_____ 25. Abortion ought to be considered a legitimate health measure.

_____ 26. The unborn child ought to have the same rights as the potential mother.

_____ 27. Any outlawing of abortion is oppressive to women.

_____ 28. Abortion should be accepted as a method of population control.

_____ 29. Abortion violates the fundamental right to life.

_____ 30. If a woman feels that a child might ruin her life, she should have an abortion.

To score this instrument, use the following point values for items 3, 4, 6, 9, 11, 12, 14, 15, 17, 20, 22, 25, 27, 28, and 30 only: A = 5, B = 4, C = 3, D = 2, E = 1.

For items 1, 2, 5, 7, 8, 10, 13, 16, 18, 19, 21, 23, 24, 26, and 29, use the following scale: A = 1, B = 2, C = 3, D = 4, E = 5.

Now add your points; the score should fall between 30 and 150. A score of 30 represents an unfavorable attitude, a score of 90 represents a neutral attitude, and a score of 150 represents a favorable attitude toward abortion.

Source: Snegroff, S. *Abortion attitude scale.* Saluda, NC: Copyright Family Life Publications. Reprinted by permission.

Suggested Readings

Beckwith, F. J. *Defending life: A moral and legal case against abortion choice.* New York: Cambridge University Press, 2007.

Hendershott, A. *The politics of abortion.* New York: Encounter Books, 2006.

Masse, S. *Her choice to heal: Finding spiritual and emotional peace after abortion.* Colorado Springs, CO: David C. Cook, 2009.

McBride, D. *Abortion in the United States: A reference handbook.* Santa Barbara, CA: ABC-CLIO, 2007.

Paris, G. *The psychology of abortion.* Putnam, CT: Spring Publications, 2007.

Shapiro, I. *Abortion: The Supreme Court decisions, 1965–2007.* Indianapolis, IN: Hackett, 2008.

Wicklund, S., & Kesselheim, A. *This common secret: My journey as an abortion doctor.* Jackson, TN: Public Affairs, 2008.

Web Resources

For links to the web sites below, visit *http://sexuality.jbpub.com/dimensions/4e* and click on Resource Links.

Alan Guttmacher Institute
www.guttmacher.org

The Alan Guttmacher Institute is a nonprofit organization focused on sexual and reproductive health research, policy analysis, and public education. The web site contains links to the Guttmacher Institute publications *Perspectives on Sexual and Reproduc-*

tive Health, International Family Planning Perspectives, The Guttmacher Report on Public Policy, and special reports on topics pertaining to sexual and reproductive health and rights. The Institute's mission is to protect the reproductive choices of women and men in the United States and throughout the world. It supports their ability to obtain the information and services needed to achieve their full human rights, safeguard their health, and exercise their individual responsibilities in regard to sexual behavior and relationships, reproduction, and family formation.

Sexuality Information and Education Council of the United States
www.siecus.org

SIECUS advocates for the right of all people to accurate information, comprehensive education about sexuality, and sexual health services. SIECUS distributes print and electronic resources to educators, advocates, parents, researchers, physicians, and others working to expand sexual health programs, policies, and understanding. SIECUS also helps individuals locate research, write accurate news articles, create sexual health curriculum, and build support for high-quality programs in their community.

National Abortion and Reproductive Rights Action League
www.naral.org

NARAL is committed to protecting the right to choose abortion and electing candidates who will promote policies to prevent unintended pregnancy. The latest laws and political issues pertaining to a woman's right to choose abortion are available on the NARAL web site, as well as related issues such as emergency contraception.

American Foster Care Resources
www.afcr.com

American Foster Care Resources, founded in 1983, is a nonprofit, tax-exempt corporation dedicated to the research, development, and production of informational and educational resources for and about family foster care. American Foster Care Resources also publishes resource materials to foster care providers, the children in care and their families, and the placing agency's staff and administration. AFCR publishes *Foster Care Journal* quarterly.

National Adoption Center
www.adopt.org

Devoted to increasing the number of children adopted, the National Adoption Center works with celebrities and corporations to advertise adoption and adoption services. Included on the web site is information on how to adopt, a resource library, and a message and chat room.

CHAPTER 9

Gender Dimensions

CHAPTER OBJECTIVES

1 Describe the biological, psychological, and sociocultural differences between males and females.

2 Explain the effects of gender identity, gender roles, and gender stereotypes on sexuality.

3 Analyze how the women's movement has affected both females and males.

sexuality.jbpub.com/dimensions/4e

Gender and Health
Global Dimensions: The Oppression of Women
Ethical Dimensions: Extreme Gender Roles—The Price of Honor
The Women's Movement

INTRODUCTION

When Mark attended college in the late 1970s, he thought all the talk about gender differences was bunk. Men and women appeared to share equal places in classrooms and in faculty positions. Women appeared to have the same opportunities as men in the outside work world. He and his classmates believed that the wage gap and glass ceiling were things that past generations dealt with. Those were the days.

But Mark still remembers one college guest speaker—a distinguished American composer. During his speech, the aging composer asserted that women were not good composers because their social upbringing left them devoid of technical skills. He told the stunned audience—among whom sat several prominent female composers—that boys take things apart and put things together, while girls play with dolls. Therefore, boys grow up with more technical abilities, which to him included the ability to orchestrate music. It seemed that everyone in attendance wrote off his comments as those of an elderly man from another era.

But as Mark joined the workforce, married, and had children, he began to witness more and more gender differences and biases. As the years passed by, the number of female friends who had experienced sexism in the workplace grew from none to all of them. It became clear that women and men did communicate differently, manage differently, work differently, play differently.

In Mark's marriage, gender roles have been reversed—because of work situations, not a deliberate decision. While his spouse works a managerial "nine-to-five job" (read, 7:00 A.M. to 6:00 P.M.), Mark writes and edits out of his home. He is responsible for raising two young children and for doing most household jobs. Because children cannot be ignored, he often has to put off work until they are in bed.

Mark has become keenly aware of the gender differences among parents. At his son's independent school, where most students' mothers do not *have a job, he is one of the few fathers who take the child to school, go to parent–teacher conferences, and volunteer for various events. This creates quite a dilemma in friendships: While playing both the mother and father roles, he really does not fit into either group. Mark also notes that teachers react differently to him: When several mothers voiced a complaint to a teacher, the teacher spoke to them directly; however, the teacher would only communicate with Mark in the presence of a senior administrator.*

Suprisingly, gender biases exist even among medical professionals. At his son's first pediatric appointment, the male doctor's first question was a stern "Where is the child's mother?" Some years later, during a hospital emergency room visit, the doctors and nurses clearly listened to every small comment his spouse made—yet brushed off Mark's input as insignificant.

As Mark's experience shows, gender plays a role in many aspects of our lives—at home, at work, and in our social activities. We develop a sexual identity, which is the outgrowth of the interaction of biology—being male or female—and social learning. Society's expectations for the behavior of men and women are conveyed to the individual by a process called socialization, which has a dominant influence on gender roles. As children model adults' behaviors, these gender roles are perpetuated, although traditional gender roles are changing as a broader range of behaviors is accepted by society.

If someone asked you whether you were a woman or a man, your first thought would probably be, What a ridiculous question! You know what gender I am. Still, that question might lead you to ask other questions about gender, such as, How did I learn to act as a man or woman? To what extent is my masculinity or femininity natural, and to what extent is it learned? Are my personal characteristics determined or influenced by my gender? In this chapter we explore some of the forces that influence our conceptions of **masculinity** *and* **femininity***.*

■ Gender Differences

When gender differences and similarities are considered, discussions often center on "nature versus nurture." Those who argue from a nature perspective attribute most characteristics to biological differences or similarities. Those who argue more for nurture believe that we become the way we are mostly as a result of social factors and learning. There are persuasive arguments on each side, and some people believe that a combination of nature and nurture makes us the way we are.

People learn attitudes and values and have their personal experiences in a "gendered world." Gender issues are dealt with differently in different societies. For example, there may be more or less gendered examples in spheres such as occupational roles, child care, clothing styles, and some social and recreational activities.

In this chapter, we discuss some gender differences related to attitude and behavior. Caution is needed when considering such differences, however,

masculinity
Those qualities characteristic of and suitable for boys and men according to the rules and expectations of a society.

femininity
Those qualities characteristic of and suitable for girls and women according to the rules and expectations of a society.

because many variations in these attitudes and behaviors exist. Overgeneralization can result in inappropriate stereotypes. At the same time, however, many argue that different genders have their own important characteristics.

Developmental Differences

There is no question that males and females differ biologically in more than their physical structure and biological function. Developmentally, girls are more advanced than boys at birth—that is, their central nervous system is more mature. Boys tend to weigh more when born, but girls have fewer physical defects and a higher survival rate. More male children are conceived, but the miscarriage rate for males is greater than for females, and more males die in the first 12 months of life. The female's two X chromosomes, compared with the XY chromosomes of the male, may be a biological advantage. The X chromosomes are larger than Ys and can supply the female with a greater variety of genetic material. Even if one of the female's X chromosomes is a carrier of genetic defects, the second one can have normal genes that offset any genetic defect.

In infancy and early childhood, growth in boys and girls is similar. The development of language, the growth of body organs and the nervous system, and perceptual and motor development proceed in sequence. The female is more developed prenatally, but the male develops more rapidly postnatally. Until age 8 years the male is heavier and taller than the female, but he reaches puberty more slowly. The onset of puberty occurs approximately 2 years earlier in the female. In the preadolescent period the female, having greater physical maturity, can perform physical and athletic tasks better than the male. With menarche, estrogen influences the increase of **adipose** (fat) tissues and enlargement of the female pelvis. Eventually the estrogen prevents growth in the skeletal long bones, and height stabilizes for girls at about age 17 years.

adipose
Pertaining to fat tissue in the body.

When the male reaches puberty, androgen increases his muscle mass and skeletal development, and thus the adolescent boy has more body mass but less fat than the girl. This androgenic effect on male development gives him more strength and more speed. Furthermore, the male's greater lung and heart capacity and greater capacity for oxygen transport to tissues, combined with his predisposition toward being taller and heavier than the female, give him more power.

Many researchers have studied the brains of males and females. Although most researchers agree

According to a 1998 study, men and women also differ in their reaction to holiday shopping. All 36 male subjects showed a dramatic increase in blood pressure when confronted with crowds and lines. But one in four females showed increased blood pressure. What physiological, psychological, and social factors would cause such a result?

that men's brains are about 10% bigger than women's, women's brains seem to have more connections between the two brain hemispheres. In some regions, the female brain is more densely packed with neurons. Women tend to use more parts of their brain to accomplish certain tasks. This might help explain why they often recover better from a stroke, because the healthy parts of the brain may more easily compensate for the injured regions. Even though men and women have different brain architectures, we really don't know yet what that might mean (Ripley, 2005).

Gender and Abilities

There are various opinions about similarities and difference in abilities between males and females. Although it is always possible to find someone who disagrees, most experts agree that until about age 11 or 12 males and females have similar verbal abilities. Around age 11 or 12, females have greater abilities in language and verbal tasks, but males perform better on visual–spatial tasks. This difference seems to persist into adulthood (see Figure 9.1). In addition, girls seem to speak sooner than boys. On average, women show more verbal skills than men.

Whether boys have better mathematical abilities than girls is still debated. Historically, math was seen as a masculine area of study in which girls were not expected or encouraged to excel. Because many females were raised thinking they should not succeed in math, their performance on math measures tended not to be high. Several decades ago, however, females'

(a) Problem-Solving Tasks Favoring Women

Women tend to perform better than men on tests of perceptual speed, in which subjects must rapidly identify matching items—for example, pairing the house on the far left with its twin:

In addition, women remember whether an object, or a series of objects, has been displaced:

On some tests of ideational fluency, such as those in which subjects must list objects that are the same color, and on tests of verbal fluency, in which participants must list words that begin with the same letter, women also outperform men:

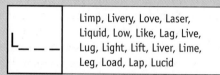

Women do better on precision manual tasks—that is, those involving fine-motor coordination—such as placing the pegs in holes on a board:

And women do better than men on mathematical calculation tests:

77	$14 \times 3 - 17 + 52$
43	$2(15 + 3) + 12 - \dfrac{15}{3}$

(b) Problem-Solving Tasks Favoring Men

Men tend to perform better than women on certain spatial tasks. They do well on tests that involve mentally rotating an object or manipulating it in some fashion, such as imagining turning this three-dimensional object:

or determining where the holes punched in a folded piece of paper will fall when the paper is unfolded:

Men also are more accurate than women in target-directed motor skills, such as guiding or intercepting projectiles:

They also do better on disembedding tests, in which they have to find a simple shape, such as the one on the left, once it is hidden within a more complex figure:

And men tend to do better than women on tests of mathematical reasoning:

1,100	If only 60% of seedlings will survive, how many must be planted to obtain 660 trees?

FIGURE 9.1 Problem-solving tasks for women and men. Research suggests that some problem-solving tasks may demonstrate gender-related performance differentiation.
Source: Kimura, D. Sex differences in the brain. *Scientific American, 267* (1992), 188–195.

perceptions of their ability to do well in math showed signs of change.

Interestingly, math scores on national tests for fourth-graders have been improving for both genders, with no statistically significant differences between boys and girls. However, girls score about 7% lower than boys on the math part of the SAT. It has been suggested that one reason for this might be that more girls than boys from lower-income families take the test (Ripley, 2005).

Looking at a different type of ability, Horgan et al. (2004) found that women more accurately recalled information concerning the appearance of other people, such as physical features, clothing, and postures. Both men and women did better at remembering the appearance of women than remembering how men looked.

Does this mean that biology is destiny when it comes to these abilities? No, because even though each gender seems to have specific abilities, there are also cultural explanations for these differences. These include teachers' assumptions and their treatment of students, parents' attitudes toward their children, the perception of society that math has been for males, each gender's self-perception and ambitions, and social pressures on adolescents—just to name some possibilities.

Boys seem to be more aggressive than most girls.

Gender and Aggression

Some experts believe that boys are more physically and verbally aggressive than girls, beginning at preschool age. Given that this seems to be true in many cultures, there may be some biological basis for this difference. Males probably remain more aggressive into their college years, but as they mature the trait diminishes. There is some evidence that boys are punished more than girls for aggression.

Intimate-partner violence continues to be a major problem in the United States. Many forms of violence have decreased in recent years, but intimate-partner violence has increased. While traditionally it was thought to be only a male-to-female activity because usually males are bigger and stronger than females, acts of violence against both women and men have increased within intimate relationships.

Tavris (2002) provided an interesting view related to female aggression. She pointed out that many authors have written about hidden and formerly secret female aggressiveness. She said that girls are not sweeter than boys, but just as bad, sexual, and aggressive—maybe even meaner, given the ruthless and sneaky ways they control one another. For example, our culture refuses girls access to open conflict, and it forces their aggression into nonphysical, indirect, and covert forms. Girls use backbiting, exclusion, rumors, name calling, and manipulation to inflict psychological pain on targeted victims. Boys, in short, resort to physical aggression; girls, to "relational" aggression.

Anger and aggression are learned behaviors and are characteristic of humans. Traditionally they have been viewed as more appropriate for males than for females. However, as we move toward humanism and less-defined parameters of what is male and what is female, we must reevaluate our cultural acceptance of these behaviors.

Gender and Health

While there is not unanimous agreement on this point, there seem to be differences in males' and females' health attitudes and behavior. Examples include women being more likely to take action to prevent health problems, men tending to rely on spouses for social support related to their health, and women being more likely to turn to friends and their children for assistance in this area. Women also seem to experience more health problems and make more extensive use of health services.

When it comes to health care, there are also some interesting comparisons between males and females. While women show a preference for a female physician in the fields of general practice and gynecology (probably due to the intimate nature of the clinical intervention), beyond that most people do not have a strong preference for a health care provider of a particular gender.

Men are more likely to avoid regular health care than are women (Galdas, Cheater, & Marshall, 2005). They often say they feel fine and do not need to consult physicians. Because of their needs related to reproductive health, women find it more difficult to avoid the health care system regardless of how well they may feel. Men and women seem to have similar experiences of daily symptoms, but women are more likely to seek medical care for these symptoms. Men also seem to have more trouble adopting the patient role than do women.

Another gender issue related to health is that some health insurance plans provide coverage for prescription drugs, but exclude coverage for prescription contraceptives. This can result in an extra financial burden on women and also make it more likely that some will use less-effective contraceptive methods—making unwanted pregnancy more likely.

Another issue related to gender and health insurance is the practice of having different rates based on gender. Some have argued that split rates are justified because younger women typically seek health care services more often than men. Some women have been paying as much as 20% more than men for the same individual coverage. Federal law prohibits employers that offer health plans from charging different rates based on gender, and in 2009 California became one of 10 states with a similar law (State Politics & Policy, 2009).

On an international level, Guptka (2001) pointed out that power imbalance increases HIV risk. For example, in many societies there is a culture of silence surrounding sexuality that dictates that "good" women are expected to be ignorant about sexual behavior and passive in sexual interactions. This makes it difficult for women to be informed about HIV risk reduction and, even if informed, to be proactive in negotiating safer sexual activity. In addition, the traditional norm of virginity for unmarried females increases young women's risk of infection, because it restricts their ability to ask for information about sexuality because of fear that they will be thought to be sexually active. In cultures in which virginity is highly valued, some young women practice alternative sexual behaviors, such as anal intercourse, to preserve their virginity. These behaviors may place them at increased risk of HIV. Accessing treatment services for STIs can be highly stigmatizing for women. Finally, using barrier methods as safer options for sexual activity can be a dilemma for women in societies in which motherhood is considered to be a feminine ideal.

Other international examples were given by Billowitz and Kukke (2004). They pointed out that gender roles can have direct implications for health outcomes. For example, in many countries female infants die at a significantly higher rate than boys because they are not as highly valued. Boys are more likely to be immunized, have better nutrition, and

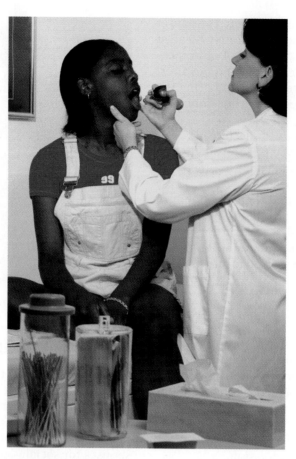

Women seem to prefer a female medical care provider in general practice and in gynecology.

receive medical care more promptly. These authors estimated that more than 1 million girls die each year from malnutrition, neglect, and abuse who would not have died had they been male. Sex-selective abortion is also still practiced in some countries where males are more highly valued.

Billowitz and Kukke (2004) also indicated other effects of gender roles. Gender norms may keep males from asking vital questions about sexuality. Men are supposed to demonstrate a bravado that makes it impossible to admit they don't know something about sexuality. In some cultures masturbation is believed to negatively affect a man's "manliness." This leads males to seek casual or commercial sexual activity when they have a desire to ejaculate, resulting in pressure to engage in frequent sexual activity with multiple partners, often without using a condom. Poor females who go to clinics may be intimidated by clinic personnel who show their attitudes about what women should do and not do. Also, in many countries economic inequities leave women few options for their livelihood, which may lead them to engage in transactional sexual activity or formal sex work, making them vulnerable to negative health consequences.

Some people think health care delivery and research benefit men at the expense of women. They believe that heart disease has been studied more in men and that women have been excluded from major national clinical studies. Others believe that women have benefited from medical research, as shown by improvements in breast cancer research as well as developments in laparoscopic surgery and ultrasound that were initially used on women's bodies (Daniel & Levine, 2001).

Kluger (2003) reported that twice as many women as men suffer from depression and twice as many men suffer from alcoholism. Similarly, women tend to be more prone to anxiety disorders, and men are more likely to have conditions stemming from impulsiveness and violence.

Multicultural DIMENSIONS

Examples of Gender Equity Promoting Programs

Nigeria

In Nigeria, girls are traditionally taught to be subservient to their male family members. The Girls' Power Initiative provides girls with information on sexuality, human rights, sexual and reproductive health and rights, leadership, self-esteem, and life skills. The girls are trained to speak out against gender inequities. There is a counterpart program that works with young men to change attitudes toward gender roles and issues.

Kenya

Maendeleo Ya Wanawake Organization, a grassroots women's organization, was the first group in Kenya to advocate for the elimination of female genital cutting (FGC). The Organization goals included raising awareness about the harmful effects of FGC, devising ways to provide a positive image of uncircumcised girls, and developing an alternative rite of passage for girls that would replace initiation by cutting. As a result, the prevalence of FGC dropped among girls ages 14 to 19, and the number of women in favor of discontinuing the practice grew substantially.

Brazil

Project H is a training project based on research into the factors necessary for young men to be "gender equitable." Activities focus on themes of sexuality and sexual/reproductive health, paternity and care, violence prevention, mental health, and HIV/

AIDS prevention and care. The project aims to reduce gender-based violence and generally improve health indicators. As a result, young men's attitudes have improved, and fewer young men are agreeing with statements such as "Men need sex more than women" and "I would be outraged if my wife asked me to use a condom." There was also a drop in STI symptoms and an increase in condom use.

India

The Better Life Options Program in India uses an empowerment approach to train low-income girls ages 12 to 20 (married and single) in family life education, literacy and vocational skills, and general and reproductive health. The project stresses leadership and social mobilization through advocacy and community involvement. Goals include building girls' self-esteem and self-confidence, as well as expanding their choices related to marriage, fertility, health, vocation, and civic participation. Girls completing the program were more likely to be literate, have completed secondary education, be employed, have learned a vocational skill, have traveled outside their village or visited the health center alone in the last 6 months, and to make autonomous decisions about going to the market, spending what they earned, and deciding when to marry.

Source: Billowitz, M., & Kukke, S. Doing gender the 'rights' way. *SIECUS Report, 32, no. 3* (Summer 2004), 5–10.

In recent decades it was found that men with a history of heart disease were two to four times more likely than females to die later of sudden cardiac death. However, now women heart attack survivors are becoming almost as likely as men to succumb to sudden cardiac death. This gender gap has narrowed a great deal (Sudden cardiac death gender gap closing in on women, 2002).

Some have pointed out a need for more gender-based medicine because of some differences between males and females (Men, women more different than thought, 2004). For example, major illnesses like heart disease and lung cancer are influenced by gender, and treatment for women may need to be slightly different from the approach used for men. Lung cancer, not breast cancer, is the number one cancer killer among women. The American Heart Association has developed heart disease prevention guidelines tailored for women. Also, heart attacks in women frequently don't involve chest pain; rather they may exhibit as more

Males report more withdrawal and physical symptoms of depression than females.

vague, flu-like symptoms. Women who do not smoke appear to be more susceptible to lung cancer than nonsmoking men. Women are less likely than men to get oral cancer, and more prone to autoimmune diseases including lupus, rheumatoid arthritis, and multiple sclerosis.

Men lead women in 12 of the 15 causes of death in the United States and die an average of 5.4 years earlier than women. In 1920 the difference was just 2 years. Although some of this gender gap may be due to biological differences, many experts now believe that much of the gap is due to inattention to men's health—from society and from men themselves. For many years there has been special attention given to women's health, but there has been no similar emphasis on men's health. There has not been a government Office of Men's Health to match the similarly named office for women. In addition, women are more likely than men to get routine preventive care; men give up on treatment plans and discontinue medications sooner than women do; men tend to see themselves as invulnerable to pain; and men's stoic attitude may further harm health by magnifying the effects of stress (Why men die younger than women, 2002).

Some people feel that men's lower life expectancies worldwide may also be because men take more risks. For example, they are more likely to work in risky occupations and more likely to engage in risky behavior such as driving carelessly. Men and boys also have higher suicide rates, and are more likely to be not only the perpetrators, but also the victims of murder.

An interesting gender twist related to nutrition has occurred. Supermarket aisles are filling up with nutrient-rich female-friendly treats (Winters, 2001). There was a nutrition bar called "Luna" decorated with silhouetted dancing girls and packed with ingredients that women are supposed to need. It quickly became the top-selling bar in natural food stores. Then there was a line of breakfast cereals from Zoe foods produced by a woman who wanted to make granola for women who were like her menopausal mother. General Mills produces Harmony cereal for women, and Quaker has a Nutrition for Women oatmeal. These foods are alike in that they are supposed to have nutrients that benefit women in particular. Manufacturers are trying to appeal as much to women's emotional needs as to their dietary ones. In reality, the basic laws of nutrition still apply to both men and women.

One final example related to gender and health focuses on college students. A survey of more than 1,400 college students in the Northeast showed that more than 83% reported having had sexual intercourse, with slightly higher rates for females (86%) than males (78%). Females (86%) were more likely than males (79%) to have had sexual intercourse without a condom. Yet, when asked if they would have sexual intercourse with a partner who refused to use

Communication
DIMENSIONS

Men Are from Mars; Women Are from Venus

John Gray, the author of the bestseller *Men Are from Mars, Women Are from Venus*, explains one reason why men and women may sometimes be frustrated in communicating with each other. He says women expand, and men contract. By this he means that women are likely to expand a topic, whereas men want them to get to the point. For example, he says that generally when a man speaks he has already silently mulled over his thought until he knows the main idea he wants to communicate. Then he speaks. A woman, in contrast (according to Gray), does not necessarily speak to make a point; speaking assists her in discovering her point. When she explores her thoughts and feelings out loud, she figures out where she wants to go.

For example, a man may want to pull away and take a little time to mull over his thoughts so he knows what he wants to say. However, a woman may find greater clarity by expanding and sharing. When she begins sharing, she is not necessarily aware of where it will take her, but she is confident it will take her where she needs to go. For her, this is a process of self-discovery.

There have been mixed feelings about Gray's book. Some feel it is inaccurate and biased, while others feel that while it may have some good points, Gray does not offer enough solutions. For example, Hamson (2004) feels that the book is completely useless as a "fix," but its popularity is invaluable for what it tells us about ourselves as a society. She points out that boys and girls/men and women share more traits than society is willing to admit. She further indicates that while we all have differences as human beings, biases and stereotypes based on gender must be understood to be not only groundless but just as divisive and nonproductive as racial prejudice.

Source: Gray, J. *Men, women and relationships.* New York: Harper Paperbacks, 1996.

a condom, significantly fewer females (8%) than males (24%) reported they would have sexual intercourse without a condom in this situation. Males (53%) were significantly more likely to report frequent condom use than females (44%) (Bontempi et al., 2009).

Gender and Dating

Some experts think there are gender issues related to dating. For example, some have indicated that females assume males will try to deceive them, but males don't seem to feel females will try to deceive them. Two issues related to sexual behavior and dating are frequency of sexual behavior and number of partners. Common sense would indicate that, on average, heterosexual men and women would have about equal numbers of sexual partners. However, males consistently report more partners than females do. Does this discrepancy arise because men are inclined to exaggerate sexual experience, and women to minimize it? Or is it because people have faulty memories? Or do women and men view sexual behavior differently?

Some think that the nature of intimacy is also a factor in male–female relationships. Many women tend to derive intimacy from talking and may be disappointed if men do not verbally share their problems, express their emotions, or listen to their feelings. In contrast, men may feel emotional closeness by working or playing side by side.

Power is fundamental to both sexuality and gender. Typically, men have been more powerful in relationships. Therefore, in sexual behavior, male pleasure often supersedes female pleasure and men have greater control than women over when, where, and how sexual behavior takes place (Gupta, 2001).

One interesting development related to dating, at least among some successful women, is the lesser boyfriend (Tan, 2001). Some women, such as Julia Roberts, Jennifer Lopez, and Ann Heche, chose less successful beaus. Today's modern woman often works and is financially independent. Some feel this is true female empowerment. Therefore, women can make a choice among men based on personality, as opposed to making a choice only within the group of men who earn as much or more. Also, in the case of celebrities, his career is not as important as hers, so when they go out, she gets all the attention. Interestingly, Jennifer Lopez changed her mind, was divorced, and later married singer Marc Anthony, another celebrity.

When the topic of "dating" is discussed with many contemporary college students, talk soon turns to "hanging out" and "hooking up." For some college students, dating is an outdated concept. Instead, they prefer to attend activities in groups or simply "hang out" with one or more people. Interestingly,

Many people seem to enjoy watching the dating practices of celebrities.

in a number of sexuality classes one of your authors has asked college students to define "hanging out" and "hooking up." In each of these conversations the conclusion was that college students do not agree on the definition of either of these terms, even though the terms are commonly used.

Other Gender Issues

Various experts have studied what males and females talk about with their friends. It is common to hear that men often discuss work issues, sports, and future goals. For women, the top three topics seem to be children, personal problems and self-doubts, and work issues. People believe that women's speech is more emotional than men's, although that stereotype has decreased in recent years (Popp et al., 2003). People also think women are more likely to show sympathy and communicate their support in problem situations (Basow & Rubenfeld, 2003). However, in a study in which men and women offered supportive communications, few differences appeared between men's and women's styles of communication (MacGeorge et al., 2004).

There are also some stereotypical things that seem to bother males and females about the other gender. Women commonly report being disturbed about men making sexual demands (making them feel sexually used or trying to force sexual behavior), making them feel inferior or stupid, and emotional constriction and

Gender
DIMENSIONS

The Social Dimensions of Sexual Behavior

Related to dating, but also to later relationships, Baumeister and Tice (2000) proposed that sexual behavior is a social exchange in which women hold the power card, and that men will do just about anything to get it. They say that the catch is if sexual activity is given too freely, men will take it and run. For women, there is a flip side: If they never have sexual activity, they then lose the value of the power they wield. When vying for attention of men, they have to walk the fine line between being a miser or a vamp.

In simple terms, according to Baumeister and Tice, women have something that men want. Whoever wants sexual activity less has a certain amount of power in a relationship. Reasons for this situation are rooted in culture. Men value women with the least number of sexual encounters, because men tend to see the value of sexual activity decreases for a woman as her sexual encounters increase. This standard does not hold for men, they say, as women gravitate toward physically robust males.

Other points made by the authors follow:
- High self-esteem enables a woman to resist the advances of men.
- Sexual possessiveness may be rooted in nature, and all cultures impose stricter penalties against wifely infidelities.
- Nature instills in people the desire for sexual activity, but culture controls that desire.
- Women prefer sexual activity with stable committed relationships rather than commitment-free sexual activity, but men like both kinds.
- Sexual fluidity affects same-gender relations, where women are more able to move from lesbian to bisexual relationships, whereas men tend to be either heterosexual or homosexual.

1. Which points made by the authors do you agree or disagree with? Why?
2. Are there any points made by the authors that are bothersome to you? If so, why?

---

excess (hiding his emotions, drinking or smoking too much). Men commonly report being disturbed about women's sexual rejection (being unresponsive to sexual advances, being a sexual tease), moodiness, and self-absorption (fussing over appearance or spending too much on clothes).

The division of household labor has long been an interest area for gender researchers because who does the various tasks reveals information about power and equity in relationships. For decades, research has indicated that even when women are employed outside the home, they still do the majority of housework and child care chores. Even though the differences are not as great today as they were in past years, women still perform about twice as much household work and child care as men do. Interestingly, gay couples seem more likely to split tasks, with each partner performing a set of chores. Lesbian couples seem more likely to alternate in sharing tasks, taking turns in performing the same chores (Sayer, 2005).

Fisher (Males, females, and evolution, 2001) has mentioned other gender differences. She says men usually want to cut straight to the point; they do not like getting distracted by side issues. Women have a more contextual view of the world and see issues as part of a larger whole. Also, young males often take many more risks than young females do. Scientists think this may be linked to differing levels of a chemical in the brain. In addition, females are more likely than males to bear grudges, sometimes for a very long time.

Peplau (2003) states that a large body of research documents four important gender differences related to sexuality. First, in many ways, men show greater sexual desire than do women. Second, compared to men, women place greater emphasis on committed relationships as a context for sexuality. Third, aggression is more strongly linked to sexuality for men than for women. Fourth, women's sexuality tends to be more malleable and capable of change over time. Obviously, not all of these differences are absolutes because men and women can vary a great deal. In general, however, these differences affect thoughts, feelings, and behavior. Also, they characterize not only heterosexuals but lesbians and gay men as well.

Gender and the Workplace

Do men and women approach things differently in the workplace? Are women being treated fairly in the workplace? Are salaries and benefits the same for males and females? These, and other interesting issues, have long provided hot topics for research and discussion.

An extensive study showed that women scored higher on orientation to production and getting results, and men scored higher on strategic planning and organizational vision. Women were seen as operating with more energy, intensity, and emotional expression; men were seen as more low-key and quiet through the control of emotional expression. Women were rated higher on people-oriented leadership skills, whereas men were rated higher on business-oriented leadership skills by bosses and peers (Do men and women lead differently?, 2000).

Eagly (2003) analyzed 45 studies of leadership styles and concluded that women in management positions were actually better leaders than men in equivalent positions. Women were more likely than men to be "transformational" leaders, or leaders who try to inspire workers and develop their skills and creativity. They serve as role models, mentor and empower workers, and encourage innovation even when the organization they lead is generally successful. Other kinds of leaders include transactional leaders, who lead by rewarding and punishing, and laissez-faire leaders, who take a hands-off approach. Previous studies indicate that transformational leaders create the most productive and satisfying work environments. Women also scored higher than men on one measure of transactional leadership—rewarding employees for good performance. One reason why women may favor transformational leadership is that such a leader operates more like an excellent teacher than a traditional boss.

Many people have assumed that women would rather work with and be supervised by other women, but some studies (Sachs, 2001) indicate that women can be each other's worst enemies on the job. According to such studies, women often betray and undermine one another; they damage other women's career aspirations; and they often fail to support other women—even actively undermining their authority and credibility. One theory is that for two women to forge a positive relationship, their self-esteem and power must be kept "dead even." When one woman gets more power, it sets off tensions and leads to hostility and sniping. One-third of the women in these studies said they would prefer a male boss.

Relatedly, Meese (2009) reported out that at least 40% of the bullies in the workplace are women. They choose other women as targets more than 70% of the time. Men seem to bully men and women pretty much equally. Reasons given for women's bullying include women believing they need to be aggressive to be promoted, women sabotaging other women because they believe helping female coworkers could

Employment opportunities for males and females have changed in recent years.

jeopardize their own careers, women withholding information such as promotional information from other women to help themselves, and other women supposedly being easier to bully than men because they are less tough than men. Many women have learned they are supposed to be nurturers and supporters, but bullying behavior is antithetical to the way they are supposed to be.

Because more than half the women with babies younger than 1 year are in the workforce, increasing numbers of them want to breastfeed their infants. In response, more companies are meeting this need by setting up a private room and a work schedule so mothers can pump their breast milk (Luscombe, 2001). Some companies provide a private room, a hospital-grade pump, a carrying case for discreet transport of the pumping paraphernalia and expressed milk, plus bottles and access to a refrigerator. One company, Cigna, in which 80% of the workforce is female, saved about $240,000 per year in health care expenses for breastfeeding mothers and their children and another $60,000 through reduced absenteeism.

Many men have assumed more responsibilty for child rearing.

This does not include the incalculable goodwill of happy new parents.

The relationship between salaries of men and salaries of women has long been of interest to some people. In 2007, more than 10.4 million men and slightly less than 3.5 million women were paid $100,000 or more. Median earnings were $59,798 for men, compared to $42,340 for women (U.S. Census Bureau, 2007). In 2009, the National Organization for Women indicated that for full-time, year-round workers, women are paid, on average, only 78% of what men are paid, and the gap is significantly wider for women of color. This gap remains despite the passage of the 1963 Equal Pay Act and a variety of legislation prohibiting employment discrimination (On Equal Pay Day NOW calls attention to persistent gender wage gap, 2009). It is difficult to interpret the meaning of these data accurately, however, without knowing more about years of experience, academic preparation, levels of responsibility, and other variables that may influence salary levels.

Differences of salaries of men and women do not necessarily indicate that wage discrimination is rampant. For example, women tend to work fewer hours than men and women tend to make educational and occupational choices that will give them flexibility if they interrupt their careers for child rearing—even though they may earn less. Women without children make about 95% as much as men with similar jobs and experience (What gender gap?, 2001).

Hilary Lips (2005) argues that there is a gender-based wage gap that exists in virtually every occupational category. She points out that this is at least partly because occupations typically associated with women are less prestigious and pay less than occupations associated with men and masculine skills. After reviewing wage trends over a number of years, she indicates there is no evidence that this wage gap is closing. She feels that employers must be convinced to re-examine assumptions that place higher value on the type of work men do than on the type of work typically done by women.

Some men say the work atmosphere turns very chilly when they seek time off to care for infants or take their kids to doctors' appointments (Grimsley, 2002). A man in Maryland was awarded $665,000 after a long legal battle to protest the state's refusal to grant him parental leave to care for his ailing wife and their infant daughter. He said he was told, "God made women to have babies," and he should not ask for leave to care for his wife and daughter.

In 2008, the Center for Women's Business Research reported that women owned 20% of U.S. businesses with revenues exceeding $1 million per year. A total of 10.1 million firms were owned by women, employing 13 million people and generating $1.9 trillion in revenues. Women business owners who exceed the $1 million revenue mark typically are "gutsy," action-oriented women; have a solutions orientation; believe that larger business provides more freedom; are energized by the "business of growing a business"; create their own rules; focus on internal business culture; and are lifelong learners (New study shows women own 20% of businesses with revenues exceeding $1 million, 2008).

An interesting study was reported by McKeen (2005). She surveyed 214 Canadian and 160 Chinese business students regarding their future spouses' employment and family roles relative to their own. Results showed that a large proportion from both countries hoped for equality between the spouses, especially in the distribution of domestic tasks. However, significant discrepancies existed between their ideal hopes and their expectations of what will actually happen. Many men and women of both countries expected that the wives would do more of the domestic work and have less prestigious jobs and lower earnings than their husbands.

Catalyst is a nonprofit organization working globally with businesses and the professions to build inclusive workplaces and expand opportunities for women and business. In 2009, several of its reports provided information on related issues. For example, in 2008 women's representation as corporate officers rose to 16.9%, an increase of 1.8% since 2006 (Jenner & Ferguson, 2009). Because men dominate executive positions, the flow of information from senior leaders tends to perpetuate gender gaps in senior leadership. In addition, gender bias inhibits the establishment of inclusive and effective talent management programs (Warren, 2009). Clearly, men have a critical role to play in inclusion and diversity efforts. Men who are more aware of gender bias are more likely to say that it is important to them to achieve gender equality. Three key barriers that undermine men's support for initiatives to end gender bias are apathy, fear, and ignorance about gender issues. Men must be helped to understand their critical role in gender initiatives (Prime & Moss-Racusin, 2009).

A Catalyst study also found that women's advancement in corporate leadership continues to stagnate, with virtually no growth seen in women's share of top positions. For example, women held 15.2% of board director positions in 2008, compared to 14.6% in 2007. They held 15.7% of corporate officer positions in 2008, compared to 15.4% in 2007 (Catalyst 2008 census of the *Fortune* 500 reveals women gained little ground, 2008). Yet another Catalyst study showed that companies with the most women in senior management had a higher return on equity.

In today's marketplace, the female management style is distinctly different, but it is essential. Women manage more cautiously than men; they focus on the long term. Men thrive on risk, especially when they are surrounded by other men. Women are less competitive, in a good way: They are consensus builders, conciliators, and collaborators (Shipman & Kay, 2009).

Although women have not held a high percentage of leadership positions in industry, in May 2009 a historical event occurred when Ursula Burns became the first African American female to head a *Fortune* 500 company (Xerox). That made her one of about 15 women leading *Fortune* 500 companies. Her ascension marked the first female-to-female transition.

Gender and Advertising

Advertising has long contributed to thinking about gender images and roles. Stereotypical examples include females with beautiful bodies often dressed in skimpy clothing being the object of another's gaze much more than their male counterparts. The authoritative male voice is still used in many commercials. It seems that through the years there

has been a change in the images of women in commercials—but not the images of men. Today women are shown more often representing managerial and professional occupations. They are shown in more diverse occupations than in the past, whereas images of men have changed little. There is probably only a small increase in images of men parenting and doing housework.

Preidt (2008) has indicated that the way men and women are portrayed in TV commercials can have a major impact on how they behave in their daily lives. Men, in particular, are influenced by commercials that more often depict them in a career setting than doing domestic chores. TV advertisements help to socially construct gender and influence how people think about their own gender as well as other genders. Most commercials featuring women focus on selling home products, such as food, cleaners, personal care items, and furniture. Men are most likely to be engaged in work behavior in commercials, whereas women are least likely to be depicted working outside the home. Only some 2% of commercials show men doing domestic chores, such as cooking, cleaning, or caring for children.

Monk-Turner et al. (2008) looked at how sexual themes are used in magazine ads. Most ads did not use a sexual theme to sell a product. If used, however, this theme was more likely to appear in an ad aimed at a male audience.

Morrison and Shaffer (2003) found that traditional participants (masculine men, feminine women) responded more favorably to traditional (i.e., gender-stereotyped) than to nontraditional advertisements. Nontraditional participants reacted more favorably to nontraditional advertisements.

Zimmerman and Dahlberg (2008) looked at attitudes of young women toward sexually objectified advertising and compared their results to findings from earlier studies. Respondents agreed that females were portrayed as sex objects in advertisements, but were less offended by these portrayals than were female respondents in 1991. Respondents also indicated that attitudes toward the advertisement have little influence on whether they intend to purchase the products. This was a significant change from the responses of the 1991 group, who indicated they were influenced by such ads.

Koernig and Granitz (2006) looked at the portrayal of women compared to men in e-commerce magazine ads. They were interested in seeing whether e-commerce ads continue to reflect negative stereotypical gender differences in relation to technology given that such portrayals may propagate harmful stereotypes to men and women. They found that, compared to past studies, ads for e-commerce products and services portray women more equitably.

Page 306

gender schema
A grouping of mental representations about male and female physical qualities, behaviors, and personality traits.

gender identity
The awareness and acceptance of one's gender.

of people change. When children learn that gender is permanent, they independently try to act the way boys or girls "should act," because of an internal need for their behaviors to be consistent with what they know.

Gender schema theory indicates that children develop a grouping of mental representations about male and female personality traits, physical qualities, and behaviors. Once they develop a gender schema, they begin to judge themselves according to traits considered relevant to their genders. By doing this, they blend their developing self-concepts with the gender schema of their culture. Many associations can be made between gender and other qualities, such as strength and affection. Traditionally, strength has been viewed as a masculine trait and affection as a feminine trait. Other gender distinctions may be viewed as important—such as men's being sexually assertive and women's being sexually passive, or men's being in leadership positions and women's being placed in lesser positions.

Gender Identity

Gender involves more than just a biological component; it also includes the biological, social, and cultural norms and something called **gender identity**. Gender identity is one's self-image as a female or a male; it is the attachment one has to one's role. Societal and cultural factors are thought to exert more influence on gender identity than the biological component. At the very least, gender identity should be considered a biopsychosocial process—it is a result of interaction of biological, psychological, and social factors.

Masculinity and femininity are not innate or instinctive. The masculinity or femininity of gender identity needs a healthy human brain in which to take root. However, the developing brain is shaped by the environment in which it grows and from which it takes its mental nourishment (Money, 1988). In this way the biological foundation is shaped by psychological and sociological influences.

Because each society defines its roles for males and females and perpetuates behaviors through gender-role socialization, boys are given reinforcement for behaving in a "masculine" way, and girls receive reinforcement for exhibiting "feminine" behaviors. Should either gender engage in cross-sex conduct, such behavior is labeled gender-role-inappropriate; when each sex behaves as the society deems normal, that behavior is labeled gender-role-appropriate and is rewarded.

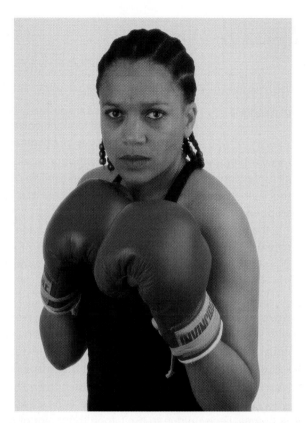

Gender roles and expectations may be defined differently by various people.

Gender roles differ markedly from society to society. Many societies discourage any deviation from the prescribed gender roles; others, such as ours, are now working toward flexibility and individualism in a wide variety of behaviors.

The expectation that people will exhibit certain characteristics and/or behaviors dictated by the customs and traditions of the society is called **stereotyping**. Expecting individuals to behave in particular ways because they are male or female is referred to as **gender-role stereotyping**. There are still many rigid, unyielding traditional attitudes about gender-role behaviors that make it difficult for people to express themselves and for society to implement change. Stereotypical images of people do not take into account individual differences. Until recently the stereotypical woman or wife in our society was passive, quiet, and concerned primarily with home, husband, and children; the stereotypical man was gruff, strong, unfeeling, and concerned mostly with work and money. The danger of such stereotypes is that people

stereotyping
The expectation that individuals will exhibit certain characteristics or behaviors.

gender-role stereotyping
Expectation that individuals will behave in certain ways because they are male or female.

The Oppression of Women

Until September 1996, Afghan women, particularly those living in cities, were highly involved in public life. They wore contemporary clothing, participated in government, and worked in all professions. In 1996, an extremist Islamic militia called the Taliban overtook two-thirds of Afghanistan and stripped females of their most basic rights.

If a woman lived in a house, the windows had to be painted black, as did all but the front windows of a car she might occupy. She could go out of the house only in the company of a close male relative.

Women could not work as doctors, nurses, or midwives and could not be treated by male doctors. Women with serious illnesses could die untreated. Women could not work outside the home, attend school, or even, for fear of terrible punishment, wear shoes that made noise when they walked. Parents could not teach their daughters to read. The Taliban did all this in the name of extremist Islamic views unique to itself; their treatment of people had nothing to do with traditional Islamic beliefs.

Mavis Leno, wife of Jay Leno, a member of the board of directors for the Feminist Majority Foundation, chaired a national campaign to demand an end to the Taliban's oppressive treatment of women.

Another example of oppression of women became public in 2001. First members of a hard-line militant group in Kashmir announced they would throw acid at women who did not wear veils and the traditional *burkah,* a long black cloak that covers a woman from head to toe. Later it was announced that women not wearing the veil would be shot. To prevent trouble, the heads of girls' schools and women's colleges asked their students to dress conservatively and to wear no makeup (Overland, 2001).

Even after American troops invaded Afghanistan, many Afghan women were still mistreated. They continued to be abused, harassed, and threatened all over Afghanistan. For example, a team of 90 women from the Ministry of Religious Affairs harassed women in Kabul's streets for "un-Islamic behavior" such as wearing makeup and, in some instances, followed them home to castigate their parents or spouses (We want to live as humans, 2002).

Source: Extreme Taliban laws oppress Afghan women, *USA Today* (October 28, 1998), 25A.

take them seriously and act on them, turning a blind eye to the qualities, capabilities, and interests of individuals—frequently denying even their own. People often believe that those who deviate from stereotypes are not as good as those who conform to them. Thus one who accepts as true the stereotypes described might look down on a woman who cared about work or a man who chose to stay home with his children. People become boxed in not only by social pressure to conform closely to the stereotype, but also by rigid customary practice (such as promoting men but not women in business and professions, hiring women but not men to nurse and teach small children, or paying men more than women, regardless of their responsibilities), as well as by law. The assumptions behind such stereotyped behavior are being challenged today, and laws are being changed as well, but popular assumptions and attitudes are slow to change and are still passed on.

Teaching Gender Roles and Stereotypes

Gender roles are taught throughout the life cycle, but parents probably have the greatest effect, especially when children are very young. Very early on, parents reinforce the behaviors deemed acceptable to their child's gender with such remarks as "What a good, sweet girl!" or "What a big, strong boy!" accompanied by smiles and nods of approval. There is no doubt that most, if not all, of the forces of socialization in our culture—parents, teachers, peers, movies, television, and books (targeted at children and adults)—encourage different behaviors in boys and girls. The resulting sets of traits are what we call *masculinity* and *femininity*. Let us look briefly at a few examples of how gender roles and stereotypes are taught.

> **gender role**
> Complex groups of ways males and females are expected to behave in a given culture.

The Influence of Schools
School personnel pass on social stereotypes in a number of ways. For example, if teachers feel that boys are naturally more aggressive or that girls are naturally more passive, how will this attitude influence the way they treat their students? If gender-role stereotyping exists in teachers' expectations, it can lead to biases in how they treat and evaluate their students.

(?) Did You Know ...

Gender differences are everywhere, even in the decision of whether to enter college or the workforce out of high school. According to a study released in June 1999 by the American Association of University Women, women were more likely than men not to attend college because of their credit-card debt or lack of scholarships and other college aid. Other bar-riers to college cited in the study were the need to care for children and lack of support from spouses. But men who go straight from high school into the workforce tend to do so be-cause they were "never that interested" in college (McQueen, 1999).

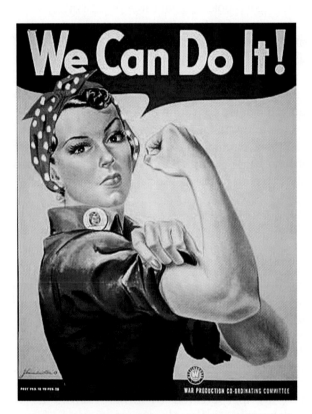

During World War II, Rosie the Riveter was part of the U.S. government's public relations campaign to get women into the workforce. Rosie shows off a strong bicep but still has a perfect manicure.

Berk (2008) mentioned a number of ways teach-ers and the school environment might contribute to gender stereotyping. For example, younger girls often gather around the teacher, following directions, while boys are attracted to other areas of the classroom where teachers are minimally involved. Consequently, boys and girls engage in different social behaviors. Teachers also use more disapproval and controlling discipline with boys. When girls misbehave, teachers tend to negotiate, coming up with a plan to improve behavior. Teachers seem to expect boys to misbehave more, a belief that seems based partly on boys' actual behavior and partly on gender stereotypes.

If teachers believe in stereotypes, they may expect one gender to excel more than the other in certain subjects, they may encourage one gender more than the other, or they may favor one gender in terms of attention and/or extra help. They may even intentionally or unintentionally pro-mote **sexism**, which is a prejudgment that because of gen-der a person will possess negative traits. In addition to these prejudgments, sexism can entail discrimina-tion against someone because of gender. For exam-ple, not hiring a man for a day care job because it is believed that males cannot nurture children would be sexism. Teachers can help promote the healthy sexual development of children if they provide equal opportunities for girls and boys, do not impose gender stereotypes, and do not use sexist language. Although young children are busy establishing their own identities, and many may exhibit stereotypical behavior, it is the role of the teacher to encourage learning and responsible behavior that does not discriminate.

> **sexism**
> The prejudgment that because of gender a person will possess negative traits.

School materials can also influence gender-role stereotyping. For example, in preschool picture books there has been a trend toward depiction of greater gender equality. At the same time, however, female characters are more likely to be shown as dependent or submissive, and males as indepen-dent and creative. Many subtle traditional expecta-tions still exist.

Some people claim bias still exists in achieve-ment tests. Language in the tests has often referred to males and their environments. Women were disproportionately shown to be homemakers, and men to be engaged in directive, leadership, achiev-ing roles. Boys were described in action terms; girls were described in helping or more passive terms. A strong bias against nontraditional behavior in both sexes has been evident in many tests.

Sadker and Zittleman (2005) point out that gender bias lives for both genders. It can be hard to detect

Multicultural DIMENSIONS

How the Economy Affects Gender Equality

Relations between men and women are influenced by race, class, and sexuality; however, the most pressing issue for men and women of color, especially those who are poor and working class, is the economy. While both the employment rates and real wages of men are down, women are working in greater numbers, and their wages are on the rise.

For working-class African Americans, Hispanics, and Native Americans, the effect of these changes has been harsh. The decline in employment for men has caused an increase in domestic violence, alcohol abuse, and other problems associated with joblessness. However, the increase in women's employment and economic resources is not enough to allow most to support a family, nor has it been accompanied by available, affordable child care.

These changes not only challenge the expectations traditionally associated with gender, but also are reshaping families along distinctive racial and class lines. For example, although families maintained by single women have become a permanent feature in all racial and class categories, this type of family is most prevalent among people of color and the poor.

Among whites, the chief cause of the increase in households headed by women is women's growing economic independence. But the growth in African American households headed by women partly reflects the employment problems of African American men.

In addition, for all immigrant groups, life in the United States leads to increased rates of single parenthood and divorce.

The economic challenges facing poor and working-class African American, Hispanic, and Native American men and women constitute the most pressing issue in relations between the sexes today. This is because racial and ethnic discrimination, combined with economic difficulties, make these groups extremely vulnerable to shifts in the economic and social climate.

Source: Dill, B. T. Economic disparity is key for all minorities, *Chronicle of Higher Education, 45, no. 6* (October 2, 1998), B7–B8.

---

because it affects boys and girls in different ways. For example, in school, the boys may be expected to "act out" and rebel at schoolwork, while the girls are expected to be docile. Both of these expectations reflect gender stereotyping, or bias. Other examples of challenges related to gender bias include:

- Boys and girls like and do well in math and science in elementary school, but girls become less positive and do less well in higher grades.

- Boys receive more math- and science-related toys than girls do.

- Girls receive higher report card grades throughout their schooling.

- Boys often regard reading and writing as "feminine" subjects, and report that reading threatens their masculinity.

- Current software products are likely to reinforce gender stereotypes and bias rather than reduce them.

- Teachers call on boys more often than girls, wait longer for boys' answers, and provide more precise feedback to boys.

- Girls are more likely to be quiet in class and praised for neatness.

Even at the college level, educators need to be sensitive to the influence of the classroom environment. It has been thought that female students participate less often and less assertively than male students in college classrooms and that the professors' discriminatory behaviors are partly responsible.

Teachers, books, and tests are powerful forces, but it is important to stress that gender stereotypes are perpetrated by other factors as well. Children take to the classroom notions of gender roles formed through the influence of parents and peers.

The Influence of Parents and Peers

In most cases, as soon as a child is born, interaction between parents and child begins—interaction that differs according to the gender of the child. Traditionally, a girl is thought to be fragile, to need protection, and to have needs that revolve around personal appearance and development. A boy is seen as tough, physically active, and unemotional. Children perceive these expectations, which tend to define their reality. Because the mother is usually the primary caregiver, the female child finds it easier to learn her appropriate gender role than does the male child. The female internalizes feminine behavior and is rewarded for her identification. The male may be in a bind. He may not have a constant

Gender DIMENSIONS

Gender Equality on the College Campus

In 1997 the New England Council of Land-Grant University Women created a document entitled *Vision 2000,* which was a call to high-level university administrators to ensure full and equitable participation by women in New England universities. The gender-equality goals in the document were intended to:

1. Foster faculty and administrative accountability for gender equality in curriculum and pedagogy
2. Implement diversity initiatives
3. Promote family-friendly policies (affordable and available child care, flex time, and parental leave policies)
4. Encourage women's academic and career development
5. Establish and support strong women's centers
6. End sexual harassment of and violence against women
7. Correct inequities in hiring, promotion, tenure, compensation, and working conditions for women employees

Critics of *Vision 2000* claim that it is a plot by women's studies faculty to stifle academic freedom—that they will determine gender-equality standards and impose them on recalcitrant faculty. They worry that feminist "indoctrination" of students will lower academic standards and destroy academic debate. Others believe that it is time to ensure gender equality in higher education. They point out that there are fewer women faculty members overall and they are concentrated in lower ranks, less well-paid career tracks, and part-time and non–tenure track positions.

Are the goals of *Vision 2000* needed at your college or university? How is your institution dealing with each of the seven areas listed? What else might have to be done on your campus?

Sources: Vision 2000, New England Council of Land-Grant University Women, February 1997. Available: http://www.umass.edu/wost/articles/vision2k/whole.htm; Ferguson, A. Gender equity on the college campus, *Boston Globe* (Feb. 23, 1997), 27.

role model because his father may not be around as much as his mother. He frequently learns from the mother's telling him that boys "don't do" certain things. Thus boys may learn to be anxious about gender-role identity.

It seems that increasing numbers of parents try to prevent teaching gender-role stereotypes to their children, but this can be hard to achieve. They may act differently toward a child, depending on the child's gender, even if they do not intend to do so. For example, if a boy is asked to participate in sports or help his father with outside chores while a girl is asked to wash dishes or clean her room, this pattern sends messages about expected gender roles.

What children observe at home in regard to sex roles also sends important messages. For example, even when both parents work outside the home in managerial or professional jobs, the redistribution of roles within the family has not yet clearly or completely occurred. American women—even those employed full time—continue to work more hours than do their husbands on household tasks, and there is little evidence that men's proportionate share of family work has changed much in recent years. Many social scientists feel parents are very influential in regard to establishing gender roles.

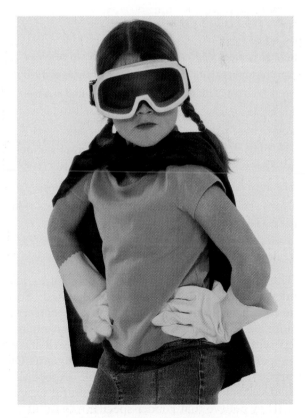

Some parents try to avoid teaching gender stereotypes.

¿? Ethical DIMENSIONS

Extreme Gender Roles—The Price of Honor

News of an interesting ethical situation related to female sexual behavior was reported in 1999 from Jordan. In 1998, Sirhan, a 35-year-old man, was proud to say that he had murdered his younger sister. She had reported to the police that she had been raped. Sirhan said, "She committed a mistake, even if it was against her will. Anyway, it's better to have one person die than to have the whole family die from shame." To Sirhan, it was more ethical to kill his sister than to suffer from the shame that would have sullied his "male honor."

For centuries, Arab men have engaged in "honor killing"—the intrafamily killing of errant females. Honor killing has its roots in the crude Arabic expression "A man's honor lies between the legs of a woman." For Arab women, virginity before marriage and fidelity afterward are considered musts. Men are expected to control their female relatives. If a woman strays, it is widely believed, the dignity of the man can be restored only by killing her.

In Jordan the 25 or so cases of honor killing documented every year make up a quarter of all homicides there.

Forbidden sexual activity is not always the issue. Marrying or divorcing against the family's wishes can also provoke murder. The law winks at honor killers. If a man catches his wife or a close female relative in the act of adultery and kills her, he is exempt from punishment.

Running away is next to impossible for women, because Arab societies are close knit, and few women have the means to live alone. "Rafa," 20 years old, was locked up in prison to protect her after her uncles and brothers vowed to murder her for having a 3-day affair with a coworker. She said, "With the mistake I made, I deserve to die."

Honor killing has started to receive media attention, and a hotline has been created by the Jordanian Women's Union for women in distress. However, honor killings are hard to combat because of the extremely strong feelings related to male and female gender roles in Jordan.

Source: Beyer, L. The price of honor, *Time, 153, no. 2* (January 18, 1999), 55.

? Did You Know...

In 2009, Barbara Millicent Roberts turned 50. In case you don't recognize that name, it is the formal name of the doll we all know as "Barbie." In 1959, Barbie debuted as a teenage fashion model—and she still is today. In 1959, 38% of women were in the workforce—today that percentage is 60%. Through the years, Barbie has been an astronaut, gone to medical school, been an Olympic athlete, served in the military, and run for president. She has had more than 108 careers and represented 50 nationalities. Some have called her the first feminist.

Others believe Barbie is not a good role model because of her emphasis on appearance. Barbie is 11.5 inches tall and weighs 7.25 ounces. This apparently translates into a woman who would be 5 feet, 9 inches tall, weighing about 110 pounds. Many have argued that this is an unrealistic and unhealthy build that promotes negative stereotypes in both males and females. Do you think Barbie has been and is a positive or negative role model?

Source: Towner, B. 50 and still a doll, *AARP Bulletin* (March 2009), 35.

The question of whether we can, or want to, raise "gender-neutral" children has been debated. Some argue that it not only is possible, but also can result in more positive self-esteem. They say that children raised with gender-neutral expectations will have a more open, positive view of the world in general. Others argue that gender and gender-role expectations are tied very closely to familial and cultural expectations. They believe that gender-specific role fulfillment is vital to certain cultures, ensuring the survival of important cultural traditions (Can we raise "gender-neutral" children?, 2003).

Sanchez-Flores (2004) pointed out that young men are exposed to many messages from different sources that inform them about what it means to be a man. Ideals such as "boys don't play with dolls," or "boys don't wear pink" may seem outdated to many adults today, but social groups still successfully transfer messages like this from generation to generation. As a result, boys live in social networks and follow norms that determine both acceptable behaviors and the consequences for not behaving that way. Another message males hear is "boys will be boys." It is most often used to dismiss actions that are challenging or seem impossible to change. This gives the impression that gender excuses behavior.

The peer group is also an important influence in learning about sex roles. Even early in life, children choose members of their own sex as playmates most of the time. This segregation by gender continues into the school years and helps contribute to sex-typing in play activities that help prepare children for adult roles.

The influence of peers becomes increasingly important by late childhood and early adolescence. Conformity can be viewed as being very important, and behaving according to traditional gender roles promotes social acceptance by peers. Those who do not behave in ways accepted by the peer group are likely to be pressured and even ridiculed.

There is no question that biology is important. There are biological factors that tilt males and females in different directions related to their interests and behavior, but numerous social factors influence the way the biological tilts can be redirected. In other words, regarding the nature versus nurture debate, biology does matter; however, the way we are treated and what we learn can drastically influence our expression of gender roles.

Gender Identity Difficulty

There are some people who experience **gender dysphoria**. They believe they are trapped in the body of the "wrong sex." They feel they are not really the gender indicated by their genitals. Sometimes the term *gender dysphoria* is used interchangeably with the term **transsexual**. Other times the term *transsexual* is used to refer to people who wish to have, or have had, their genitals surgically altered to conform to their gender identity. Therefore, an anatomically male transsexual feels that he is a female but that some quirk of fate provided him with male genitals. He wants to be socially identified as the female he believes himself to be. He does not derive sexual excitement from cross-dressing, as is the case with a transvestite, but views himself as a female. (We will discuss transvestism in In Focus: Alternative Sexual Behavior.)

Sometimes the terminology used related to gender

Danish-born Mianne Bagger, a successful amateur golfer, was barred from membership in the Australian Ladies Professional Golf Association because she was born male. Bagger's contention, like that of many transsexuals, was that she was, in fact, born female.

identity difficulty can be tricky. For example, in addition to the terms mentioned previously, in recent years the term **transgender** has become more common. According to the International Foundation for Gender Education (2005), gender is a person's innate sense of themselves as being male or female, which may differ from their biological sex. The terms "sex" and "gender" are often used interchangeably, but they are not the same. People whose sex and gender differ are known as transgender.

Transsexualism, which is a gender orientation, is not to be confused with homosexuality, a sexual orientation. Some transsexuals are homosexual, and some are heterosexual. Unless a transsexual chooses to tell another person, an observer will probably not know whether homosexual or heterosexual behavior is being practiced.

transgender
A general term used when one's identity does not match one's physical/genetic sex. It includes such diverse categories as transsexualism and transvestism.

gender dysphoria
Feeling trapped in the body of the "wrong" sex.

transsexual
A person whose gender identity does not match her or his biological sex; also a person who wishes to have, or has had, his or her gender surgically altered to conform to his or her gender identity.

According to the International Foundation for Gender Education (2003), estimates indicate that 1 in 10,000 or even 1 in 1,000 people are transsexuals. It is estimated that about half of these are female-to-male and half are male-to-female transsexuals. However, the International Foundation emphasizes that this is a very rough estimate.

Boylan (2003) wrote an interesting book on this subject entitled *She's Not There: A Life in Two Genders*. Even as a child, James Boylan felt that he was supposed to be a woman, but he thought everyone would reject him if he made the transition. So he lived as a man, married, and had children. In spite of his loving family, a successful career, and hobbies he loved, he eventually decided that he couldn't live with being a man. So he made the transition to living as a woman (Jenny Boylan). The book includes a portrait of a loving marriage—the love of James for his wife, Grace, and against all odds, the enduring love of Grace for the woman who became her "sister," Jenny. Jenny's wife, children, mother, and colleagues responded with love and acceptance. Her sister cut off contact. Boylan feels fortunate to have been given a rare gift in life—the gift of being able to see into the worlds of both men and women with clear eyes. Through it all, Boylan has been a professor of English at Colby College in Maine.

When an employee switches genders, there can be sometimes difficult issues for employers (Armour, 2005). Issues can relate to how an employee informs coworkers about switching genders, how clients might react, how others will handle a transitioning employee using the restroom, and logistical issues such as changing security badges to reflect a new gender. In many states it is legal to fire employees because they are transgender. However, in 2004 alone, more than 23 companies put policies in place to protect against discrimination of transgender employees. Major companies, such as Merrill Lynch, Chevron, BP, and Microsoft are among those with such policies.

Wilson (2005) reported on an interesting case at the University of Nebraska where, in 2005, a popular professor named Wally Bacon returned for the fall semester as a female, W. Meredith Bacon. After 29 years in the political science department, and 37 years of marriage, Ms. Bacon decided to become what she thought she was since she was a young child. In an eight-page letter, the professor explained to colleagues the decision to become a woman. Students were told that she would be happy to answer their questions if they desired. Few asked her any questions. The university administration was supportive. This had not been the case in some other situations. In one small college in New Hampshire, one man was fired after he informed the administration that he planned to become a woman. In Indiana, a professor decided to leave after his decision to disclose his sex-change plans to the college's president backfired. He says the president voiced her support, but said that he would lose his job because of the potential loss of contributions from donors who might disapprove. Ms. Bacon's wife, Lynne, remained supportive and the couple stayed together. Lynne mourned the loss of Wally, but also enjoyed counseling her spouse on her new female look.

Wilson (2005) also reported that psychiatrists estimate that 1 in 30,000 men suffer from transgendered feelings. However, groups representing transgendered people say that number of men and boys who experience "intense transsexualism" is closer to 1 in 300 to 500 with about 1 in 2,500 having undergone genital surgery. She further reported that businesses are more likely than colleges to protect employees from discrimination. According to the Human Rights Campaign, an advocacy group for gay, transgendered, and bisexual people, 73 *Fortune* 500 companies do so, compared to 37 universities.

There is no clear understanding of either the causes or the nature of transsexualism. Some theorists believe the causes relate to early parent–child relationships related to gender roles of mothers and fathers and the ways that parents treated a child. Others focus on hormonal imbalances that influenced the brain during prenatal development; however, no one knows for sure.

Gender-Reassignment Surgery

The idea of gender reassignment is controversial, and psychotherapy has not been very useful for most transsexuals. Surgery is part of gender reassignment, but, because it is irreversible, professionals usually require that the transsexual live publicly as a member of the other sex for a year before undergoing surgery. During this time it is easier for the person or the medical personnel to change their minds. Surgery is not something to be taken lightly, and it is usually done only after careful screening of the individual.

A lifetime of hormonal treatment is also necessary. Male-to-female transsexuals take estrogen. It causes fatty deposits to develop in the breasts and hips, inhibits beard growth, and softens the skin. Female-to-male transsexuals take androgens, which promote deepening of the voice, masculine hair distribution, large muscles, and loss of fatty deposits in the breasts and hips. The clitoris may also grow larger.

It is not possible to construct internal genital organs or gonads, so gender-reassignment surgery is mostly cosmetic. Male-to-female surgery is usually more successful because it is easier to construct a vagina than a working penis. The vast majority of transsexuals who undergo surgery are happy with the

Ethical
DIMENSIONS

Should Dad Dress as a Woman? Should Dad Participate in His Child's Field Trip While Dressed as a Woman?

In Saint Louis, most of the kids on a fourth-grade field trip did not notice or did not care that a classmate's father was dressed as a woman, in jeans, a sweater, and nice shoes. Most of the teachers were equally untroubled. However, one parent spotted the "cross-dressing" dad and alerted some friends. As a result, one school board member proposed a new policy that would require parent chaperones to wear "gender-appropriate" clothing for school functions.

The father described had dressed as a woman at work for years, kept his hair long, worn slacks and blouses, and used a name that could be either male or female. He had actively participated in his daughters' education and in their schools while in women's attire with no previous problems.

Some people argue that it is ethical to require parents to wear "gender-appropriate" clothing at school functions. Others argue that it is not ethical to do this because it violates the parents' rights to dress as they please—particularly because to qualify for sex-change surgery individuals must first go through a prolonged period of transition when they present themselves in public as the gender they want to become.

What do you think?

Source: Simon, S. After dad dresses as woman, field trip controversy still boils, *The Birmingham News* (January 6, 2003), 4B.

outcome. Gender-reassignment surgery is done in only a few places in the United States, is very expensive, and is usually not covered by health insurance policies. Indeed, only about 3,000 such operations have been performed in the United States since 1953. Clearly this is something to be done only with extensive counseling and medical support.

A special case of potential gender-reassignment surgery relates to the question of what should be done with intersex infants—those born with ambiguous or mixed genitalia and chromosomal structures. It is estimated that every year in the United States about 65,000 babies are born with ambiguous genitalia. Some people believe that feminizing surgery should be done at birth to ensure that the baby will be able to function later as an adult woman. Others feel that children should remain intact until they are older and decide for themselves what, if anything, to do about their ambiguous genitalia (Should parents surgically alter their intersex infants?, 2003).

Some experts point out that gender depends on more than anatomy or hormones. They feel gender is essentially hard-wired into the brain before birth. A review of 94 intersex children found that over half of the genetic males "transitioned" to become boys despite being raised as girls and undergoing female sex assignment. More doctors seem to be putting off sex-assignment surgery until later, so as to be more certain about the person's gender. The Intersex Society of North America (www.isna.org) is a good place to learn more about personal stories (Surgery may be hasty for unclear gender, 2005).

The Influence of Gender Stereotypes on Sexuality

As you can see, gender-role stereotyping limits self-expression and personal growth and development, and that limiting in turn affects sexuality. When individuals define masculinity and femininity for themselves, they express personal beliefs through gender-role behaviors. The traditional definitions are confining, emphasizing as they do conventional conformity to long-existing gender-role norms. We have referred particularly to males being socialized toward initiating, aggressive, and directive behaviors and females being socialized toward receiving, passive, and compliant behaviors. In descriptions of anatomical function, for example, the vagina has tended to be described as receiver, not for sexual pleasure but for reproduction. The penis is often described in terms of insertion based on need, dominance, and desire. Thus again, men initiate and women are passively receptive.

The pressure to conform to socialization has provoked in both sexes anxieties that we are only now beginning to discuss freely and reevaluate. The emphasis on the macho aspects of male performance tends to obliterate consideration of men as sensitive, gentle, nurturant, and intimate beings who can relate to adult partners on a variety of levels. The emphasis on the passivity of women has long neglected consideration and acknowledgment of them as full sexual beings with the same needs as men for expression and fulfillment.

Each gender needs to be able to express feelings heretofore defined as either masculine or feminine.

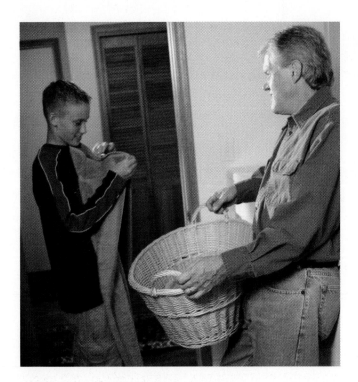

Gender roles are learned in many ways and from many different people.

Both genders need to be directive and sensitive to function effectively. Women need to make decisions in parenting, in controlling their careers, and in their sexual behavior. Men need to accept responsibility for parenting, be comfortable as receivers as well as givers, and accept that sharing intimacy and intimate acts does not mean loss of control.

Many men and women in our society still differ in their expectations for interpersonal relationships. Some women still expect assertive, in-command, successful men; some men still expect supportive, helpful, receiving women. Stereotypes of the dominant male and the submissive female continue to influence the interpersonal dynamics between the genders. Both genders have been socialized into these expectations, and socialization probably accounts for more of these distinctions than does biology.

Men have often learned to equate sexual activity with the fulfillment of their needs for support, tenderness, and the feeling of being loved. Women have often not been taught that receiving sexual pleasure has value. Mixed feelings about what they really feel and what society tells them they are supposed to feel can confuse both sexes.

Gender differences related to sexual behavior and expectations have been found among adolescents in grades 8–10. Boys initiated sexual intercourse earlier than girls, but by grade 10 the girls' rates of sexual intercourse surpassed the boys'. However, girls were less likely to intend to have sexual intercourse in the next year than were boys. Girls reported higher intention to use condoms and also felt more pressure than boys to engage in sexual intercourse (Nahom et al., 2001).

The popular press suggests that men and women may always have problems because they are so different. Examples often given are in communication (she wants more talk; he wants more action); intimacy (she needs to relax to participate in intimate sexual behavior, but he needs to participate to relax); division of household labor and child care (she says she does more; he talks about how much he does); and money and careers (she says he does not value her job as much as his; he notes that he makes more money).

Related to communication, the following are some of the ways to close the gender gap:

- **G**et honest before you get angry: Something deeper than dry cleaning or dishwashing is probably bothering you.

- **E**stablish systems for sharing chores and child care.

- **N**egotiate the division of labor and the division of love.

- **D**o not get locked into your role: Try swapping responsibilities on occasion.

- **E**xpress your emotional needs and expectations and really listen to your partner.

- **R**eview the cultural messages of your childhood to help understand the conflicts inherent in your new roles.

 Did You Know . . .

Male and female roles are often very similar.

- **G**ive each other time to change: Do not monitor or criticize.

- **A**ccept your differences and applaud each other's strengths.

- **P**rotect your intimate time together.

There is increased thinking that similarities between men and women, particularly in the human struggle for intimacy, far outweigh differences. Healthy couples appear to transcend traditional gender roles, and the roles, such as pursuer and distancer, are interchangeable. There is no one definition of an intimate, healthy relationship. Love and respect are essential in a good relationship.

In terms of human sexual expression, both partners need the freedom to be self-disclosing, intimate, and communicative. Restrictive definitions of roles serve only to repress the joy, pleasure, and emotionally fulfilling responses of sexual intimacy. And perhaps equally important is the fact that gender-role stereotyping also restricts personal fulfillment in nonsexual relationships between men and women.

The Possibilities of Androgyny

According to legend, there once were three kinds of humans—the male, the female, and the androgyne. All humans had two sets of arms and legs. The males and females had two faces and two sets of genitalia of the same gender. The androgynes each had one masculine face and one feminine face, one set of female genitalia, and one set of male genitalia. This group of humans had tremendous strength and an arrogant nature, which offended the gods.

Zeus, to punish them, split the androgynes in half and remade them as hemipeople. Thus men and women have lost their other half and seek it in other people.

The word **androgynous** originated from the story of the androgynes. An androgynous person is one who has a combination of masculine and feminine characteristics—one who exhibits some traits of both masculinity and femininity as defined by the society. Thus an androgynous male might be nurturing in addition to providing, and an androgynous female might be assertive as well as softspoken. The idea of androgyny can serve as a means of doing away with gender-role stereotyping. Many people believe that they must conform absolutely to society's notions of maleness and femaleness, especially in the ways they acknowledge and express (or repress and deny) their feelings. In conforming, they lose the opportunity to express themselves as individuals. But if, as a society, we were to view people as androgynous, then all of us might consider the expression of a variety of emotions appropriate for everyone. A significant benefit would be that people who expressed their true feelings, unswayed by the demands of gender-role stereotypes, would experience

> **androgynous**
> Exhibiting a combination of masculine and feminine traits as defined by the society.

Can you tell for sure which individuals in this picture are male and which are female?

a greater depth of sexual intimacy with their partners than would those concerned solely with how manly or womanly they appear.

The concept of androgyny has been around a long time. For example, in 1975 Sandra Bem, a noted proponent of androgyny, indicated that stereotypical gender roles were restrictive and unhealthy. She described androgynous people, by contrast, as flexible and healthy. She felt that rigidity in gender-role expectations was reflected in inflexible responses in real-life situations. To test her theory, Bem developed the Bem Sex Role Inventory. She gave a group of men and women a list of personality characteristics—some traditionally masculine (assertiveness, ambition, independence), some traditionally feminine (dependence, sensitivity, gentleness), and some neutral (friendliness, likability)—and asked the subjects to rate the accuracy of each term in describing them. Participants were then placed in situations that tested masculine and feminine behaviors such as nurturance, responsiveness to a troubled person, and conformity. Men who had described themselves as having masculine traits were not comfortable with "feminine" activities, and women who had described themselves as having feminine traits were not comfortable doing "masculine" tasks. But androgynous men and women were able to function in all situations.

It should be noted that not all studies are supportive of the androgyny concept. Yet many experts and numerous studies tend to agree that freedom from stereotypical gender roles allows for greater health and life satisfaction. People continue to do research related to androgyny. However, others criticize the concept and do not place much confidence in it.

■ The Women's Movement

In recent decades we have seen social upheaval that has changed our society in a variety of ways. Patterns of sexual behavior have been affected, for example, by contraceptive technology, abortion, and sterilization. Divorce has become more acceptable, and changes in leisure pursuits, delays in pregnancy, and the acceptance of intentional childlessness all offer women a greater diversity in lifestyle. But perhaps the single most important effect has been the women's movement. The ability of women to explore their potential has never been as great as at this time. Economic independence, control over reproduction, and choices in relationships and lifestyle have given women freedom from domination by men and the opportunity for self-direction as individuals. Statistics illustrate the increasing inroads into the labor force being made by women as they seek to achieve

Eleanor Roosevelt helped raise people's awareness about sexism.

economic independence and/or to supplement the family's income.

There were at least four groups who converged in the 1960s to help create the modern women's movement. First, there were those, such as Eleanor Roosevelt, who used John F. Kennedy's Presidential Commission on the Status of Women to reveal pervasive sexism in American society and law. Second, there were those who were from the civil rights movement, broadening the definition of equality to include women. The third group, working-class women, turned to feminism and the women's movement in their struggle for the Equal Pay Act of 1963. The fourth group was made up of white, middle-class suburban women, who found themselves stifled by gender stereotypes (Kerber, 1999).

The women's movement probably also is responsible for increased attention to victims of sexual assault and other forms of violence. A better understanding of aggressive behavior, improved services for assault victims, and greatly increased education on these topics are all evidence of this increased attention. In addition, the public discussion of sexual harassment throughout recent years must be at least partially attributed to the women's movement. There is also a growing body of literature about many issues related to gender.

With the change in the present and potential status of women, new pressures and anxieties about role

Did You Know . . .

Some people think that the women's movement started in the 1960s. There were actually many significant events prior to that time. Here is a list of selected important events related to the Women's Movement (Imbornoni, n. d.; National Women's History Project, 2005).

1769 American colonies based their laws on English common law. By marriage, husband and wife were considered one person under the law.

1777 All states passed laws taking away women's rights to vote.

1839 The first state (Mississippi) granted women the right to hold property in their own name, with their husbands' permission.

1869 The first woman suffrage law in the United States was passed in the territory of Wyoming.

1908 The first state (Wyoming) granted women the right to vote in all elections.

1916 Margaret Sanger tested New York's anticontraception law by establishing a clinic in Brooklyn. She helped establish a woman's right to control her own body.

1920 The Nineteenth Amendment to the U.S. Constitution, which states that the right to vote shall not be denied based on sex, was ratified.

1938 The Fair Labor Standards Act established a minimum wage without regard to sex.

1963 The Equal Pay Act promised equitable pay for the same work regardless of race, color, religion, national origin, or sex of the worker.

1968 Executive Order 11246 prohibited sex discrimination by government contractors and required affirmative action plans for hiring women.

1969 The Seventh Circuit Court of Appeals ruled that women meeting the physical requirements could work in many jobs that had been for men only.

California adopted the nation's first "no fault" divorce law, allowing divorce by mutual consent.

1972 Title IX prohibited sex discrimination in all aspects of education programs that receive federal support.

1973 The U.S. Supreme Court declared that the Constitution protects women's right to terminate an early pregnancy, thus making abortion legal in the United States (*Roe v. Wade*).

1974 Housing discrimination on the basis of sex and credit discrimination against women were outlawed by Congress.

1978 The Pregnancy Discrimination Act banned employment discrimination against pregnant women.

1984 Sex discrimination in membership policies of organizations such as the Jaycees, Kiwanis, and Rotary was forbidden by the Supreme Court.

1993 The U.S. Supreme Court ruled that the victim did not need to show that she suffered physical or serious psychological injury as a result of sexual harassment.

1994 Congress adopted the Gender Equity in Education Act to train teachers in gender equity, promote math and science learning for girls, counsel pregnant teens, and prevent sexual harassment.

1997 Elaborating on Title IX, the Supreme Court ruled that college athletic programs must actively involve roughly equal numbers of men and women to qualify for federal support.

1998 The Supreme Court ruled that employers are liable for sexual harassment even in instances when a supervisor's threats are not carried out. However, it also said the employer can defend itself by showing it took steps to prevent or promptly correct any sexually harassing behavior and the employee did not take advantage of available opportunities to stop the behavior or complain of the behavior.

1999 The U.S. Supreme Court ruled that a woman can sue for punitive damages for sex discrimination if the anti-discrimination law was violated with malice or indifference to the law, even if that conduct was not especially severe.

2003 The U.S. Supreme Court ruled that states can be sued in federal court for violations of the Family and Medical Leave Act.

2005 The U.S. Supreme Court ruled that Title IX, which prohibits discrimination based on sex, also inherently prohibits disciplining someone for complaining about sex-based discrimination.

2006 The U.S. Supreme Court upheld the ban on the "partial-birth" abortion procedure. It was the first ruling to ban a specific type of abortion procedure.

2009 President Obama signed the Lily Ledbetter Fair Pay Restoration Act, which allows victims of pay discrimination to file a complaint with the government against their employer within 180 days of their last paycheck. Previously, victims (mostly women) were allowed only 180 days from the date of the first unfair paycheck.

redefinition and intimate relationships have arisen. Women are more informed about their physiology and their right not only to expect sexual fulfillment and satisfaction but also to initiate or refuse sexual behavior. For many, traditional values concerning virginity, self-sacrifice for children, lifelong commitment to marriage, and the support role of women are giving way to new modes of commitment. These changes can be seen as giving both women and men a chance to explore a number of alternatives.

Some people feel true female empowerment has been shown by women (notably some movie stars) who have chosen as partners men who are less successful than they are. Because many modern women work outside the home and are financially independent, they are empowered enough to make a choice among men based on their personality, as opposed to making a choice only among men who earn as much or more. His career is less important than hers, so when they go out she gets all the attention (Tan, 2001).

The Institute for Women's Policy Research (Overview of the status of women in the states, 2001) reported that gains in education and income and an increased presence in politics helped women boost their economic and social status. Yet, even states rated highly in its report must progress for women to gain equality with men. The Institute looked at political participation, employment and earnings, economic autonomy, reproductive rights, and health and well-being in all states. Detailed results can be seen at the Institute's web site at www.iwpr.org.

In 2003 an interesting gender-equity issue arose within the sport of golf. In Virginia a 17-year-old girl won the high school boys' golf tournament. However, she won playing from tees set closer to the hole than the tees the boys used. The rules had been changed 4 years earlier to allow girls to compete with this advantage. Earlier, a woman professional golfer won a tournament to qualify to play in a men's professional tournament. She, too, had competed from tees set closer to the hole. It was later ruled that when she played in the men's professional tournament she had to play from the same tees as the men. Whether females should be required to play from the same tees as the men if they are going to compete against men remains a controversial issue. Bowen (2003) has said that once females play against males, they should play by the same rules. If a female is racing against a male in the 100-meter run, for example, she should not be able to start 20 meters ahead just because she is a female. It will be interesting to see how this issue is resolved in the coming years.

The topic of women in the military has received increasing attention in recent years. In 1990, the National Board of the National Organization of Women

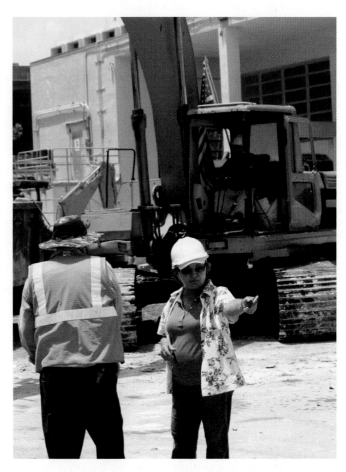

Women have had more and varied opportunities in recent years.

(NOW) adopted a policy about women in the military. It said: "NOW demands equality for women in joining the military and in training, job assignments, and benefits in the military; and NOW actively supports elimination of statutory restrictions on women in the military" (Women in the military, 1990).

Since 1995 a number of significant events have occurred related to women in the military (Chronology of significant legal and policy changes affecting women in the military: 1947–2003, 2005). For example, in 1995, the Marine Corps selected a woman for aviation training for the first time. Between 1996 and 2001, more than 15,000 American servicewomen served in Bosnia. In 1998, women aviators flew combat missions for the first time in Operation Desert Fox. In 1999, the Navy opened Coastal Mine Hunters and Mine Counter Measures ships to women. Also, women aviators participated in combat operations during the air war in Kosovo. In 2000, two women sailors were killed and several wounded in a terrorist attack on the USS *Cole*. In 2001, military women deployed to the Afghan theater as part of Operation Enduring Freedom, the war on terrorism. In 2002, the first woman

Women's sports have received increased attention in recent years.

(compared to 5% for men) between 1975 and 2001. In 2005, 200,000 more college degrees were granted to women than men. In 16 countries across the world, female graduation rates surpass male rates. In the United States, the imbalance is most prominent among blacks. In 2000, black women earned twice as many bachelor's degrees as black men (Tecson, 2005).

Not only have there been significant gains for women, but some would argue that it is becoming a woman's world. For example, in high school girls get higher grades in every subject than do boys. They have much higher reading and writing scores on national assessments. Boys still enjoy an advantage on math and science tests, but that gap is smaller and closing. Girls are more likely to be involved in the school paper or yearbook, to be elected to student government, and to be members of academic clubs (Freeman, 2005). Also, women are more likely to enroll in college. In many colleges there are now about 60 females for every 40 males. Traditionally, more men than women graduated from college. In 1985, the numbers became about even. Since 2005, about 133 women have graduated for every 100 men and the gap is expected to widen. There are two different stories here: the unprecedented success of girls and women in the education system, and the lack of comparable success for boys and men. Women receive 60% of the associate degrees, 57% of the bachelor's degrees, 59% of the master's degrees, and 45% of the doctorates. In the education system, males are less likely than females to graduate from high school, go on to college, and complete a college degree. In many ways, educational performance of males is below what it was three decades ago (Mortenson, 2005).

The National Center for Education Statistics has projected that the percentage of degrees awarded to females will slowly increase in the coming years. For example, in 2009 it was projected that females would earn 59% of the bachelor's degrees, 61% of the

Marine was killed in Afghanistan. In 2002, the Defense Authorizations Act required the Department of Defense to submit an annual report on the status of women in the services. In 2003, more than 25,400 women were deployed in support of Operation Iraqi Freedom. As of early 2009, there were more than 205,000 women on active duty, accounting for 14.2% of the total active-duty forces. In addition, 80,000 women served in the reserves (24.1% of the total) and 71,000 women were members of the National Guard (15.1% of the total) (Statistics on women in the military, 2009).

There have also been significant gains in the education of women. For example, the number of bachelor's degrees earned by women jumped by 70%

Gender DIMENSIONS

Is There Gender Equality in College Sports?

Since 1972, Title IX of the Education Amendments has forbidden sex discrimination at institutions receiving federal funds. One important, and still controversial, part of this legislation relates to college sports. After nearly 40 years of living with Title IX, there are still many viewpoints about it. Some people believe that men have been penalized for having a higher interest in athletics than women. They point to the fact that in some cases men's sports have been cut to comply with Title IX. Others believe that Title IX has not hurt men's sports, and it has greatly helped women's athletic opportunities. Efforts continue among athletic officials, college administrators, and legislators to see how to deal best with Title IX and its implications.

master's degrees, and 52% of the doctoral degrees. Small increases in these percentages are expected each year until 2017, when females will earn 60% of the bachelor's degrees, 63% of the master's degrees, and 56% of the doctoral degrees (Degrees conferred by degree-granting institutions, by level of degree and sex of student, 2009).

The Sexuality Education and Information Council of the United States (SIECUS) has issued the following position statement on gender equality and equity:

SIECUS believes that gender equality and equity are fundamental human rights. Society must recognize how gender-based stereotyping, including prejudice toward transgender, transsexual, and intersex individuals, can result in harmful consequences, such as gender-based violence and sexual, physical, and psychological abuse. Gender-based stereotyping must be eliminated, and the use of gender-inclusive language promoted. The legal system should guarantee the civil rights and protection of all people, regardless of gender, gender identity, or gender expression.

As we have pointed out throughout this chapter, some people have many different feelings about some gender issues. In 2008, the American Psychological Association (APA) adopted a policy statement related to transgender, gender identity, and gender expression nondiscrimination (American Psychological Association, 2008). Here is part of that statement:

Therefore be it resolved that APA opposes all public and private discrimination on the basis of actual or perceived gender identity and expression and urges the repeal of discriminatory laws and policies;

Therefore be it further resolved that APA supports the passage of laws and policies protecting the rights, legal benefits, and privileges of people of all gender identities and expressions;

Therefore be it further resolved that APA supports full access to employment, housing, and education regardless of gender identity and expression.

Exploring the
DIMENSIONS
of Human Sexuality

Our feelings, attitudes, and beliefs regarding sexuality are influenced by our internal and external environments. Go to sexuality.jbpub.com/dimensions/4e to learn more about the biological, psychological, and sociological factors that affect your sexuality.

Sociocultural Factors
- Gender-role orientation begins at birth. Children are treated differently according to social standards for gender.
- Family, neighbors, friends, and teachers influence our thinking about gender through their actions.
- Ethnic groups pass down gender-specific heritages and gender roles.
- Mass media are often gender-biased, portraying men and women in traditional, stereotypical roles.

Biological Factors
- Chromosomes (XX or XY) determine biological gender.
- Primitive gonadal tissues differentiate into pre-natal ovaries or testicles.
- At puberty, sex hormones cause emergence of primary and secondary sexual characteristics. Sex hormones continue to act throughout one's lifetime.
- Testosterone plays a role in aggression; estrogen has been linked to heart attack prevention.
- Most medical studies have been completed on men, and findings have been assumed to be the same for women, without taking into account gender differences in hormones and chemical makeup.

Psychological Factors
- Expressiveness and communication style differ between genders, as men withhold feelings and women express them openly.
- Women suffer more from self-esteem issues relating to body image, as they attempt to live up to the biologically impossible "Barbie" standard.
- In a society where men are presented with greater opportunities, motivation and possibility of achievement are more challenging for women.

CASE STUDY

Your gender plays a major role in how you perceive the world—and how the world perceives you. Gender plays a pervasive role in many areas that define our self-concept, including career opportunities. Men and women communicate in different styles, and they express emotions differently. Physiological differences play out in health—women do live longer, but are sick more often.

Gender roles are influenced by virtually all social and cultural aspects, including religion, ethnic heritage, family traditions, peers, and even the mass media.

In sexuality, a "double standard" still exists, as men are encouraged to be sexually aggressive and women are discouraged from being sexually active.

Summary

- Discussions about gender similarities and differences often focus on "nature versus nurture." Some attribute most of these gender-based characteristics to biological factors; others attribute them to social factors and learning.

- Gender similarities and differences usually fall into certain categories, such as developmental differences, gender and abilities, gender and aggression, gender and health, and gender and dating.

- Many gender issues have emerged related to the workplace in recent years. Issues commonly discussed include different work styles and leadership styles of men and women, rights of males and females in the workplace, and arguments about the existence of a gender-based wage gap.

- There are many feelings about gender and advertising. Some people believe numerous ads promote gender stereotypes just to sell products; others see gender-based ads as nothing very important one way or the other.

- Gender identity, roles, and stereotypes are learned in many ways. Gender roles can differ markedly from society to society.

- Gender roles and stereotypes are taught in a number of ways in society. They are strongly influenced by teachers and the school environment, and by parents and peers.

- Some people experience gender identity difficulty. A transsexual is a person whose gender identity does not match his or her biological sex. Gender-reassignment surgery is usually done only after careful screening of the individual.

- Gender-role stereotyping limits sexuality in many ways. It can limit self-expression, personal growth and development, and healthy feelings about masculinity and femininity.

- The women's movement has had many influences on gender roles as well as social and legal issues.

- Today more women than men receive bachelor's, master's, and doctoral degrees. However, many different feelings about male and female roles still exist.

Discussion Questions

1. Of the many differences between the genders, which do you believe are the most important nonbiological differences? Explain your answer. In your own college or university, are male and female students treated differently? Give specific examples.

2. Compare and contrast the feelings of males and females toward sexuality. Then discuss how the genders can bridge those differences.

3. How can women achieve sexual equality with men without becoming competitive? Does such a change need to begin with women—or with men?

Application Questions

Reread the story that opens the chapter and answer the following questions.

1. Is the writer androgynous? Explain why or why not.

2. Which conflicts has the author experienced from his "reversed" gender role?

3. Is there any merit to the composer's comment that gender play during childhood influences abilities later in life? Which other factors probably influenced the development of women composers?

4. As a student, how do you view the future of gender roles? How will life experiences affect your view of gender roles?

Critical Thinking Questions

1. Consider the expression "Candy is dandy, but liquor is quicker." Explain the gender bias of the expression. Which type of tensions might such thinking create between the genders?

2. Is there a gender bias in the United States toward the male management style? What other reasons might explain the lack of women in high-level executive positions and on boards of directors?

3. Michael Jackson was often cited as an androgynous person. Why did the popular press believe this? Was it true?

Critical Thinking Case

Because of physiological differences, men and women often have slightly different medical symptoms. The same seems true for psychological problems. For example, school-aged boys who act out in class are often considered for the *DSM-IV* diagnosis of attention-deficit/hyperactivity disorder. Boys who receive treatment can learn to do quite well in school. However, girls have been socialized not to act out in class; they tend to have different symptoms and are less often diagnosed. That difference puts those young girls at a disadvantage, leading to poor scholastic achievement and low self-esteem.

In adulthood, depression is diagnosed in women nearly twice as often as in men. Research from the 1990s suggests that when men are faced with negative emotions, they distract themselves through drinking or sports. Women, in contrast, tend to focus attention on the negative mood. If such focus intensifies the negative mood, a woman would be more prone to a diagnosis of depression.

1. Should separate diagnostic manuals for psychiatric disorders be written for men and women? Explain your answer.

2. Should psychiatrists focus their training on one gender? Or should training be generic? Explain your answer.

Exploring Personal Dimensions

Female–Male Differences and Similarities

Females and males respond in similar ways to sexual stimulation. However, in some ways they also respond dissimilarly. To assess your knowledge of these similarities and differences, determine whether each of the following statements describes a response that is similar or dissimilar for females and males. Then place a check mark to indicate your answer. The correct answers appear at the conclusion of the statements.

Similar   Dissimilar

——   ——   1. Erection occurs.

——   ——   2. When a sexual fantasy occurs, hormones are secreted.

——   ——   3. Testosterone is produced by the body.

——   ——   4. During sexual excitement, the nipples become erect.

——   ——   5. Sex flush appears during the excitement phase of the sexual response cycle.

——   ——   6. Males and females can have multiple orgasms without requiring a rest period.

Correct Answers

1. Similar. Both the penis and the clitoris become engorged with blood and become erect.

2. Similar. Hormones in both genders activate various body parts in response to sexual stimulation.

3. Similar. Testosterone is produced in the interstitial cells of the testes in men and in the ovaries of women (although in a small amount).

4. Similar. Although nipple erection is more obvious in women, it occurs in men, too.

5. Dissimilar. In men, sex flush occurs during the plateau phase; in women, it occurs during the excitement phase.

6. Dissimilar. Whereas women have the capacity to be multiorgasmic, males generally need to experience a refractory period before subsequent orgasms.

Suggested Readings

Andersen, M. *Thinking about women,* 8th ed. Boston: Allyn and Bacon, 2009.

Brannon, L. *Gender: Psychological perspectives,* 5th ed. Boston: Pearson, 2008.

Feminist Majority Foundation. Available: www.feminist.org.

Koenig, A. M. Stereotype threat in men on a test of social sensitivity. *Sex Roles: A Journal of Research 52,* no. 7–8 (April 2005), 489–496.

Lips, H. *A new psychology of women*, 3rd ed. New York: McGraw-Hill, 2006.

Lips, H. *Sex and gender*, 3rd ed. New York: McGraw-Hill, 2005.

Manning, L. *Women in the military: Where they stand*, 5th ed. Washington D.C.: Women's Research & Education Institute, 2005.

Overview of the status of women in the states. Institute for Women's Policy Research (2008). Available at: www.iwpr.org.

Rider, E. A. *Psychology of women*, 2nd ed. Indianapolis, IN: John Wiley & Sons, 2005.

Web Resources

For links to the web sites below, visit *http://sexuality.jbpub.com/dimensions/4e* and click on Resource Links.

Radford University Center for Gender Studies
http://gstudies.asp.radford.edu/sources/gsources.htm

Lists a number of Internet sites and resources relevant to studies and searches where the focus is women, men, and gender expectations. Each listing can be activated for a direct connection to that site. Beneath the tabular summary, a brief overview of each resource is provided along with a direct link to its web address.

Myths, Fallacies, Folderol and Idiotic Rumors About Military Women
http://userpages.aug.com/captbarb/myths.html

Explores reasons often given for why women should not be in military combat. The reasons are treated as myths and refuted.

National Organization for Women
www.now.org

This web site contains information about contemporary issues of particular importance to women. The content changes periodically, but issues likely to be discussed include abortion rights, breast implants, tax issues, insurance and child support, emergency contraception, and information about contraceptive options.

PATH: A Catalyst for Global Health
www.path.org

Many global health issues are discussed; however, gender-based violence is the primary topic on the web site.

WomensMedia.com—Expert Advice for Working Women
http://womensmedia.com

Emphasizes issues that might be of increased interest to women who are employed. Examples include women and investing, gender communication, male–female differences, the "old boy" network, and networking tips.

I»N»T»E»R chapter FOCUS

Body Image

FEATURES

Gender Dimensions
Dissatisfaction with
Body Parts

**Multicultural
Dimensions**
Weight and Culture

Ethical Dimensions
To Train or Not to
Train—That Is the
Question

Gender Dimensions
Why Are Eating
Disorders Mainly
Found in Women?

CHAPTER OBJECTIVES

1 Discuss body image, its role in sexuality, and the way media have created impossible body-image ideals to emulate.

2 Describe how to improve one's self-image.

3 Describe the problems that poor body image cause for females and males, including eating disorders, muscle dysmorphia, steroid use, and cosmetic surgery.

sexuality.jbpub.com/dimensions/4e

The Influence of the Media
Genetics: Building on Your Strong Points
Eating Disorders
Sports and Dieting

*I*f you had the privilege of knowing Marc Grabowski for some time, as one of your authors has, you would assume that he must have always been a confident young man. As a graduate of Boston University (class of 1999), with a double major in political science and philosophy, he worked as a trainer at a local gym while applying to law schools. Not only that: The month before he graduated, he placed fifth in the National Physique Committee's New England Body Building Competition as a heavyweight. Marc appears to be a pillar of strength and confidence.

But as with most people, Marc's confidence and bodily self-assurance have been built up over many years. In fact, Marc had very low self-esteem when he started high school. Smaller and lighter than his friends, he was picked on constantly (called "Ostrich Boy" because of his long neck). As his self-image sank, Marc decided to do something about it. He started lifting weights in his basement at age 14 years. By the time he was 16 years old, he had joined a gym. To Marc and his male friends, weight and size mattered. Their perception was that gaining any weight—fat, water weight, anything—was great.

It was not only his friends who pushed the weight issue. Marc would look at magazines like Flex and Muscle & Fitness and believe that he "could get like that": amazing abs or bulging biceps in 30 days! The articles focused on weight lifting but failed to mention nutrition, cardiovascular work, drugs (steroids), and muscle maturity. As Marc has learned, muscles take years to mature and grow dense in fibers so that they can stand out as hard as iron.

Yet those magazines continue to peddle false dreams. As Marc puts it, "They'll intentionally deceive the readers just to sell magazines." Worse than that: As many others do, Marc injured himself, rupturing the capillaries in his chest, by following the training routines in such magazines. And when the cover-boy results do not appear, that is a further blow to one's self-esteem.

Having a better body image has made Marc's social life easier. "Like it or not, the first thing people notice about you is your physical appearance. In social situations, that can be an advantage. But that is balanced against professional situations, where the negative connotations of a large size have to be overcome." Although he readily admits to "hiding behind the weight," Marc also says he enjoys life more. "It's nice to hear someone say, 'You've gotten in great shape.'"

By the time he reached Boston University, Marc set a goal to be in a bodybuilding show by the time he graduated. Although his studies always came first, Marc began the final preparations and dieting in his senior year.

The diet is what does most people in. During the off-season, Marc ate 10,000 calories or more a day. But as the contest drew nearer, he began to diet. By the last month, all Marc ate were 7 to 10 pounds of chicken and six potatoes a day! (And, of course, he drank water.) The diet takes a physical toll by depleting energy. Marc had trouble staying awake while studying for and taking exams.

The strict diet also has psychological effects. He felt "totally miserable" for the final 2 months of dieting. Marc deliberately tried to avoid social situations when he got cranky. He did not date during his final semester of college—and that, he ironically points out, somewhat defeated the original purpose of bodybuilding!

By the show, Marc was down to 206 pounds, with an incredibly low 2.7% body fat. Within 24 hours after the show, he had regained back 18 pounds (mostly water) and he gained an additional 10 pounds over the next 6 days. Marc lost the weight for a specific event but had no problem regaining it. Marc feels comfortable at an off-season weight of about 250 pounds and a body fat percentage of 10%.

As a personal trainer, Marc enjoys seeing the day-to-day growth of his clients—both in muscle and in confidence. The psychological effects of training are clear to Marc: Not only do clients have better body images, but their increased confidence is also seen in their becoming more outgoing. Clearly, a positive body image can improve your self-confidence.

As you will see in this chapter, obtaining your desired body image can be good for you both physically and psychologically. However, as Marc's story should show, it is important to keep your true goals in mind and, as you do so, respect your body and its needs.

Source: Interview with Marc T. Grabowski, June 9, 1999.

There's always a bigger fish in the water! A person in excellent shape for a young adult (bottom) can be dwarfed by a "professional" bodybuilder (top).

Body Image

Body image refers to the mental image we have of our own physical appearance. It is influenced by many factors—among them are weight, our weight distribution, our values about physical appearance, our concepts of a good physical appearance, our ethnic background, and what we see in others around us, what we hear through the media, and what we hear from others. We have previously discussed the importance of self-concept in relation to human sexuality. Self-concept is usually closely related to body image. A better body image contributes to a more confident individual; the better we feel about ourselves, the more likely we are to pursue a potential partner.

> **body image**
> The mental image we have of our own physical appearance.

Body image also affects sexual behavior. People with a positive body image are more likely to be open to sexual expression that exposes the body. Those with a poor body image might be less likely to pursue sexual expressions that cause them to reveal themselves and make them feel uncomfortable. Therefore, body image is an important part of sexual health. People who feel comfortable in their bodies are more likely to make healthy sexual decisions, such as protecting their health by using condoms. Those who feel comfortable about their sex organs are more likely to be comfortable talking openly about sexual behavior and feelings with a partner (Body image, 2009). Also, body satisfaction and, for women, the extent to which they see themselves as possessing characteristics associated with "being a sexual woman" are related to elements of subjective well-being (Donaghue, 2009).

Conversely, concerns about body image can impair sexual function and satisfaction. Sanchez and Kiefer (2007) found that body concerns negatively affect sexual pleasure and promote sexual problems for both men and women. However, Tucker and Irwin (2009) found that college students are very interested in improving their body image.

Many interesting points about body image were presented in the findings of *Psychology Today*'s 1997 body image survey (Garner, 1997). Despite the concerns of feminists and other observers, body image issues seem to be growing in importance. Body image influences much of our behavior and self-esteem. It governs whom we meet and whom we select as life partners, as well as our day-to-day interactions and our comfort level. Despite this importance, there is a growing gulf between actual and preferred shapes. As individuals, we are growing heavier, but our body preferences are growing thinner.

Results of the *Psychology Today* survey indicated that 89% of the women wanted to lose weight, and 22% of the men wanted to gain weight. Some women also reported avoiding pregnancy because of a fear of what a pregnancy would do to their bodies. Sexual experiences affect our body image, and our body image affects our sexual experiences. For example, 40% of men and 36% of women said that unpleasant sexual experiences caused negative feelings about their body. However, 70% of men and 67% of women felt that good sexual experiences contributed to satisfactory feelings about their body. In addition, 23% of women considered sexual abuse very important in negatively shaping their body image. Finally, 93% of women and 89% of men wanted models in magazines to represent the natural range of body shapes.

Women seem to be more likely than men to have poor body image. In a study with more than 3,500 participants who were university employees and bank workers, men were more likely to be overweight than

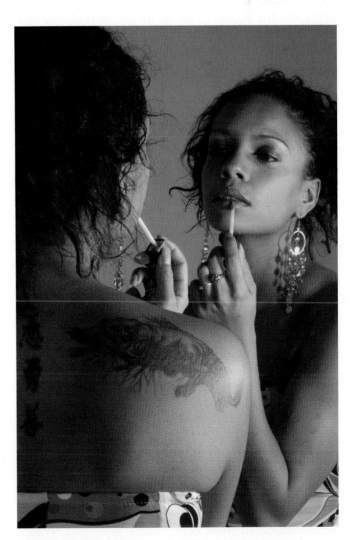

Many women feel pressure to conform to an "ideal" body image.

women. However, women were significantly more likely than men to perceive themselves as overweight, even when their weight was within the appropriate range for their height. Overall, female university employees were 3 times as likely as men, and female bank workers 10 times as likely as men, to see themselves inaccurately (Women up to 10 times more likely to have poor body image than men, 2001).

A study of women at Duke University (Lipka, 2004) found that many undergraduate women felt relentless pressure to conform to an ideal. They described a social environment that supported the expectation that a woman would be "smart, accomplished, fit, beautiful, and popular." It was also found that people at other campuses said, "It's the same way at my college." These findings stimulated discussions on campus about the extent that pressure to conform to an ideal influences women's lives.

A growing number of researchers say that many men are also suffering from body image problems—and they are often reluctant to seek help (Morgan, 2002). Some say that binge eating has become as prevalent for college men as binge drinking—about 40% of them do it. One group of researchers has named severe body-image problems in men "the Adonis complex." It can include eating disorders and a disorder called *muscle dysmorphia*, in which men perceive their bodies as perpetually puny. Some researchers argue that almost half of all college men are dissatisfied with their body.

Studies of men's body image have focused mainly on dimensions of adiposity and muscularity. Tiggemann et al. (2008), however, found that men were also dissatisfied with their head hair, body hair, height, and penis size. They were most concerned about their body weight, penis size, and height.

Research indicates that young men's body dissatisfaction increases when they see images of attractive muscular men. Those who are dissatisfied with their bodies are at risk for negative self-evaluations when exposed to idealized images, whereas those who are satisfied with their bodies seem to be protected against negative impacts from seeing such images (Blond, 2008). In addition, lower ratings of overall self-concept and higher levels of depression, anxiety, and interpersonal sensitivity are predictive of body image concerns in men (McFarland & Kaminski, 2009).

Interestingly, research has shown that gay men's body-image concerns are generally similar to those of heterosexual men (Martins, Tiggemann, & Churchett, 2008). Also, an investigation of transsexuals who had gone through sex-change operations (both male-to-female and female-to-male) showed that their body image was much improved as compared to their body image prior to the surgery (Kraemer et al., 2008).

Body image can be a unique problem for physically challenged people, such as those who have any kind of physical difficulty, including changes in body contours due to accident or disease and changes in body functioning that might relate to sexuality. People with disabilities or disease may view themselves as flawed or unattractive.

Depending on the type of physical challenge, various areas of concern need attention, including the feelings of loss of control over one's bodily functions, the inability to care for personal needs, the fear of being less of a person, and the feeling of being unacceptable. Education and counseling about body image are important and ideally should also involve the partners of challenged persons.

For many people, thinking about body image and how they would like to look implies becoming thinner. In recent years, however, there has also been a movement to acknowledge that there is a great range of beauty and attractiveness. For example, Emme became a well-known and sought-after size-16 supermodel. Also, *Mode*, a fashion magazine, was developed for women who wear average and large sizes.

For years the 11-inch-tall blonde, blue-eyed Barbie fashion doll (who celebrated her 50th birthday in 2009) represented the ideal American beauty—even though Barbie's stick-thin figure is impossible to achieve in real life. Now Barbie has some competition: the Emme doll. Based on supermodel Emme's size 14–16 figure, it is the world's first plus-size fashion doll. Emme hopes the doll will give girls the "emotional armor" to help them deal with poor body image. The doll is a vehicle for talking about health, fitness, anorexia, and obesity, she says (Mendelsohn, 2002).

There are varying opinions regarding why some people prefer certain body shapes. Research among adults has shown a preference for average weight female figures with waist-to-hip ratios of 0.7, and average weight male figures with waist-to-hip ratios of 0.9 (Connolly, Slaughter, & Mealey, 2004). In one study, more than 500 children from 6 to 17 years of age were asked to select drawings of males and females they thought looked the nicest or most attractive. The youngest children showed preferences for the underweight figures, changing to consistent preferences for the average weight figures in the teenage years.

Singh (2002) looked at cross-cultural feelings about attractiveness. He asked men and women from the Azores Islands, Guinea-Bissau, Indonesia, and the United States to judge the attractiveness of female figures differing in body weight and waist-to-hip ratio (WHR). There was a strong cross-cultural agreement for attractiveness. Figures with low WHR were judged to be more attractive than figures with high WHR within each weight category. Participants also judged attractive figures as less faithful than less-attractive

Gender DIMENSIONS

Dissatisfaction with Body Parts

It is interesting to compare the feelings of men and women about specific parts of their body. Here are the percentages of 4,000 respondents who reported feeling dissatisfied with parts of their body:

		WOMEN	MEN
1.	Overall appearance	56%	43%
2.	Weight	66%	52%
3.	Height	16%	16%
4.	Muscle tone	57%	45%
5.	Breasts/chest	34%	38%
6.	Abdomen	71%	63%
7.	Hips or upper thighs	61%	29%

Some respondents reported that body image and sexual experiences are related. For example, some said that as they feel less attractive, they have less desire for sexual activity.

Source: Garner, D. M. The 1997 Body Image Survey results, *Psychology Today, 30* (1997), 30–44.

figures. It was found that, compared to women with high WHRs, low-WHR women reported engaging in more flirting to make dates jealous, suggesting some truth to the attractiveness stereotype.

The Elusive Perfect Body

What does the perfect body look like? The answer to that question will probably depend on the purpose we have in mind. Taking a look at successful female athletes gives us some excellent examples. The best swimmers tend to be relatively tall and look like a capital *Y* from the front, with wide, flexible shoulders; long arms and hands; a narrow waist; and lightweight legs. Swimmers get by with more body fat than other athletes because it lets them ride higher in the water. Top speed skaters, in contrast, are shorter and look rather average from the waist up. Farther down, however, we see heavily muscled legs with rather short thighs. At the same time, the female gymnast probably has a lean, petite frame; a fine-boned face; small breasts; and long arms. A body that excels in one athletic context can be a hindrance in others.

Of course most of us are not training to be Olympic athletes, but there is a lesson here for all of us. The bodies closest to "perfect" are, to a large extent, born that way. We must take what we have and develop and use it as best we can. We can make the most of the genetic gifts we do have. In the end, the perfect body is the one that will allow you to do things you enjoy and allow you to live your life to the fullest—without compromising your health.

Why Models Look So Perfect

A quick glance at the covers of major fashion and sports magazines—or at the ads therein—seems to bolster the argument that "Some have it, some don't."

These models, as well as those in many movies, seem too perfect to be real. Could these people look like that all the time? The answer is, of course, no. But they may look that way only for the millisecond that the camera snaps. However, some of the images in certain magazines may be completely computer generated. They might not even be real people! Some images of models actually consist of body parts from different people.

Getting "the look" begins long before the photo shoot ever takes place. For example, months before a movie begins production, the director (and/or art director) hires a specific personal trainer who will get "the look" that the director wants. Workouts and diet are structured to transform the actor or actress.

Still in preproduction, clothes, makeup, and lighting are chosen to enhance whatever qualities have been chosen. The day of shooting starts with hours of makeup application (sometimes over the entire body), hair styling, and clothes fitting. Ever wonder how clothes can fit so skintight on some people? No problem: The clothes are literally pasted on!

Production is the time when the camera rolls (or snaps). The art director makes clear what is desired from the photographer, who in turn adjusts lighting and the camera lens to make it happen.

Then the fun begins. During postproduction, any alterations at all can be made to the pictures. You have probably heard that blemishes are covered, teeth are routinely whitened, wrinkles in clothes are deleted. But did you know that *Penthouse* routinely augments breast size? *Playboy* thinks nothing of slimming the waist and thighs of models. A knowledgeable source has told one of the authors that when photos of a playmate's rear end were not approved, the postproduction team put a new rear end on her!

To increase the sex appeal of female models, it is not uncommon for art directors to "stretch" legs

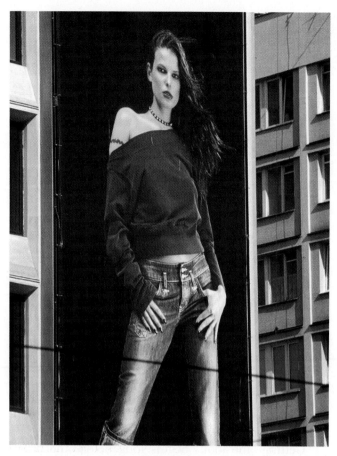

Images we see may be carefully staged and even computer generated.

to give them a longer, thinner look. Just think: You could go from being short and stocky to having the body of Cameron Diaz with a few clicks of a computer mouse!

Eventually, the picture that emerges is one that matches the art director's vision—not one that shows the person's real body. And that is not always good. To make the point that image retouching can go too far, the retouching artist Kathy Grove redid one of the most famous Depression-era photographs, Doro-

thea Lange's *Migrant Mother*. Grove's point is simple: Do not believe everything you see.

Some experts believe that the all-too-perfect models who grace magazine covers send powerful—and often negative—signals to figure-conscious adolescent girls. Mind on the Media (2009) provides some interesting related statistics: Roughly $12 billion is spent on advertising and marketing to young people every year, the average young person views more than 3,000 ads per day, the number one wish for girls ages 11–17 is to be thinner, females say the media is the most important source of pressure to be thin, and as early as age 13 approximately 53% of American girls are "unhappy with their bodies." In addition, advertisers admit that they sell more than products: They use images to affect the way we see ourselves.

The Influence of the Media

For years, some people have criticized the Barbie doll for presenting children with standards for body size and appearance that are both unrealistic and unattainable for most females. Experts also have become concerned about the impact of the "GI Joe Extreme" action figure, which has a more muscular and defined body than past GI Joe figures. At issue is whether such dolls plant the concept of the ideal body in children's minds—a concept that usually cannot be achieved without using obsessive behaviors to lose weight and gain muscle.

Relatedly, beauty pageants are another way society defines its ideal of beauty, including weight and shape. Researchers computed the body mass index (BMI) (weight divided by the square of height) of winners of the Miss America Pageant from 1922 to 1999. There was a significant decline in the BMI over that time, placing an increasing number of winners in the range of undernutrition. Pageant winners' height increased less than 2%, but body weight decreased by 12% (Rubinstein & Caballero, 2000).

 Did You Know . . .

In some places, super-skinny models have been banned. For example, in 2006, models with a body mass index (BMI) of less than 18 were not allowed to participate in Madrid, Spain, fashion shows. In 2009, the Australian Medical Association asked the government to work with the fashion industry to draw up a national code of conduct. In Milan, Italy, models with a BMI of less than 18.5 were banned from fashion shows.

BMI is the ratio of weight to the square of height. In Italy, for example, a 5 foot, 8 inch tall model weighing less than 122 pounds would be barred.

Sources: Cable News Network. Skinny models banned from catwalk. September 13, 2006. Available at: http://cnn.com/2006/WORLD/europe/09/13/spain.models/index.html; Miles, J. Call to ban skinny models. February 24, 2009. Available at: http://www.news.com.au/couriermail/story/0,23739,21324231-3102,00.html.

Even *Playboy* centerfold models have changed over time (Voracek & Fisher, 2002). A review of *Playboy* centerfold models' body measurements over a 50-year period showed that over time bust size and hip size decreased, while waist size increased. Body mass index and bust-to-hip ratio decreased, while waist-to-hip ratio, waist-to-bust ratio, and androgyny index increased. The study's authors concluded that shapely body characteristics of centerfold models have given way to more androgynous ones.

Interestingly, Bryla (2002) explored the effects of media on female image. She concluded that beyond media exposure, awareness and internalization of sociocultural ideals appear to be significant predictors of body image disturbance. In other words, looking at the effects of media on body image is not a simple matter.

Monro and Huon (2005) studied the effects of media-portrayed idealized images on female college students. They found that these images detrimentally affected the body image of the students.

There have been some attempts by advertisers to appeal to potential consumers of different sizes. One example in 2005 was the ad campaign for Dove beauty products. In the Dove ads, six women ranging from size 6 to 14 were shown wearing only bras, panties, and big smiles. The Dove marketing director said, "It is our belief that beauty comes in different shapes, sizes, and ages. Our mission is to make more women feel beautiful every day by broadening the definition of beauty" (Babwin, 2005). Dove personnel reported that responses from women of various sizes seemed to indicate that the ads helped them develop a more positive body image.

Long (2005) pointed out that in *Seventeen, Teen People, CosmoGirl!,* and *Teen Vogue,* there are bathing suit sections partially illustrated by girls with less-than-perfect figures and tips on maximizing assets and minimizing defects. More average women and fewer models are being used to reflect changing body types and to help self-conscious teens see that not everyone is perfect. In 2004, *Glamour* broke a barrier of sorts by putting the sizable Queen Latifah on the cover. *CosmoGirl!* shows five skin tones to reflect different ethnic groups. Compared

Anything is possible with photo retouching. The February 2001 issue of the U.K. edition of *GQ* magazine features a retouched image of the actress Kate Winslet. Famous for defending the appearance of fuller-figured women, Winslet has received attention not only for her acting, but also for the fluctuations in her weight. Winslet responded to the cover with shock; "I do not look like that," the actress, 27, told the *Daily Mail.* "And, more importantly, I don't desire to look like that." The controversy has highlighted how common it is for magazines to retouch photographs of models and celebrities, male and female. How do you think this practice affects the body image of young people?

Source: People (January 27, 2003).

to just a few years ago, there are now many efforts to use models of all shapes and sizes. Presenting a broader range of beauty, even under the guise of selling products, gives people more permission to believe they are attractive.

Even video games may have an influence on body image. Barlett and Harris (2008) conducted two studies to see whether playing video games that emphasized the body would increase negative body image. They found that participants in both studies had significantly lower body esteem after video game play. They concluded that video games have a negative influence on the body image of players.

Diversity and Body Image

In the past in the United States, the idea of beauty involved using the images of Barbie or Ken dolls or the like with the goal of creating some version of a white person. For example, it has been common for the winners of Latin American beauty contests to look "international": tall; not-too-dark hair; light skin; high, girlish bust; and long legs. Hispanic women often have to cope with the way the world would like to change them: if only the earrings were smaller, the makeup not so dramatic, the hair not so

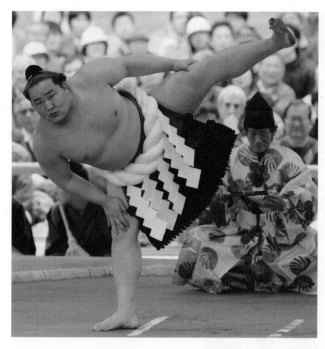

In Eastern cultures, the shape of a powerful body is that of a pyramid—with a strong base as the foundation. In Western culture the shape of a powerful body is that of an upside-down pyramid—broad shoulders and tapered waist.

wild, the walk not so sexy, the hand gestures not so expressive, the emotions not so on-the-surface, and they were thinner.

Other examples related to diversity and body image are also apparent. For example, African Amer-

ican adolescent females seem to be happier with their bodies and less likely to diet than are European American adolescent females (Wilson et al., 1996). A major problem for some African American women who seek psychological help is their skin color. For Asian American women, eye surgery is sometimes done so they will look more like whites.

However, as the result of pressure from groups interested in emphasizing the diversity of real life, products, methods, and goals relating to beauty have changed. Even plastic surgeons have learned a lot about working with people from diverse backgrounds.

■ Building a Better Self-Image

Given that none of us will be perfect, and given that we all have imperfections in our appearance, we can still look better and improve our body image. It may not always be easy, but small efforts can also make a huge difference.

When we feel good about the way we look, we are happier and likely to feel better about others. Many actions can help you improve your body image. Here are some examples:

1. Do not feel a need to apologize about every blemish you might see in your appearance. Chances are, others do not notice them anyway. None of us is perfect.

Multicultural
DIMENSIONS

Weight and Culture

The National Health and Nutrition Examination Survey (NHANES), which is conducted periodically by the U.S. Centers for Disease Control and Prevention (CDC), reported in 2007 that, after a quarter-century of increases, obesity prevalence did not measurably increase in recent years. But levels of obesity are still high—at 34% of U.S. adults aged 20 and older. Obesity means weighing at least 20% more than ideal weight. Data also suggest that the weight is not distributed evenly among ethnic and cultural groups:

• There were large race-ethnic disparities in obesity prevalence among women.
• Approximately 53% of non-Hispanic black women and 51% of Mexican American women aged 40–59 were obese, compared with 39% of non-Hispanic white women.

• Among women 60 and older, 61% of non-Hispanic black women were obese, compared with 37% of Mexican American women and 32% of non-Hispanic white women.
• Race/ethnic disparities in obesity were not observed in men.

Other researchers have also looked at cultural differences in body weight and in body image. For example, Grammas and Schwartz (2009) found that more Asian males were dissatisfied with their muscles than were Caucasian, Hispanic, or African American males. Also, Thomas et al. (2008) reported on similarities and differences in black and white women's perceptions about obesity. Black women disagreed with the ideal of being thin and family members' dissatisfaction with their weight. White women were interested in losing weight, but desired support during weight loss from other obese individuals.

2. Be careful about basing your body image on what you see and hear in advertisements. They are carefully produced to send certain messages to sell products. Few people look and act the way the people you see in the ads do.

3. Attractive people are often judged by others to be more warm, interesting, friendly, considerate, and strong than those who are less attractive. In spite of our defects, we can do things to feel more attractive. For example, clothes, styles, and personal hygiene all affect attractiveness. What can you do to feel more attractive?

4. You should be free to be yourself; however, the message you send about your appearance and the ones you receive from others may not always be the same. For example, a person might wear a certain outfit to be comfortable; another person might interpret that as a desire to be sexy. Which messages are you sending in the appearance you present?

5. The way you move your body (body language) can indicate the way you feel about yourself. Watch what others do when they are nervous, happy, or sad. Use this information to control some of your body movements so they send messages you want to send.

Here are some additional tips for a positive body image (Body image, 2009):

- Remember that health and appearance are two different things.

- Accept and value your genes—you probably inherited a lot of traits from your family members, so love those traits as you love your family.

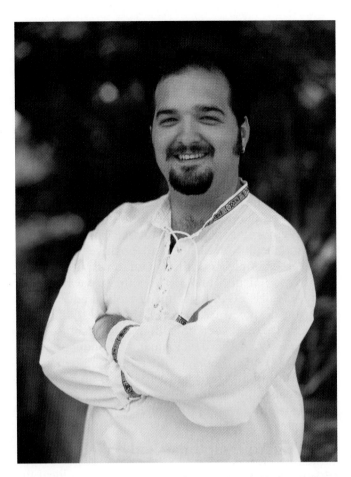

People who feel good about themselves are more attractive to others.

- Keep a list of your positive qualities that have nothing to do with your appearance.

- Surround yourself with people who are supportive and who make you feel good about yourself.

- Treat your body with respect and kindness.

Ethical DIMENSIONS

To Train or Not to Train—That Is the Question

A professionally prepared personal trainer knows how to help people develop the body to look the best it can. The trainer also knows that it is usually not possible to change the body type of a person drastically. So, what should a trainer who runs his or her own business and needs paying clients do when a person asks to look the way someone pictured in a magazine does? If the trainer agrees to help the person resemble the one in the picture, there will be false hopes created; however, you could argue that at least the person will improve his or her appearance and health—and probably body image as well. Or should the trainer tell the client that there is no way he or she can look like the picture and explain how unrealistic expectations can cause a waste of money if he or she tries to obtain objectives that cannot be reached?

Body image is important. People who feel good about themselves are more attractive to others than people who do not. Concentrate on your strengths. Do you have great hair? Eyes? Hands? Play them up. But remember your other strengths, too. Are you funny? Kind? Smart? You are more than just your looks.

There are excellent projects designed to help people improve their body image. One example is WIN Wyoming (www.uwyo.edu/winwyoming/guiding _principles.htm). It is a collaborative effort of educators and health professionals whose mission is to educate people to respect body-size diversity and to enjoy the benefits of active living, pleasurable and healthful eating, and positive self-image. Another example is Full of Ourselves: Advancing Girl Power, Health and Leadership (www.midcoast .com/~megirls/FOO.htm). It is an upbeat educational program designed to help girls improve their mental, physical, and social health and to decrease their vulnerability to the development of body preoccupation, overeating, and disordered eating behaviors. As a result of the program, girls have an improved body image, increased body satisfaction, and better body esteem.

Creating Your Optimal Body

Imagine that you are a personal trainer in a local fitness center. A center member gives you a magazine and says, "I want to look like the person in this picture, and I need you to help me do it!" What should you do?

If you are the one who wants to resemble a person in a magazine picture, it might be wise to remember that you need to optimize your own body. It does us no good to strive to be someone else. There may be qualities of other people—physical as well as others—that we want to obtain, but we cannot be exactly like another person.

Genetics: Building on Your Strong Points

A person who is 5'4" tall may strive to be an Olympic basketball player, but his or her chance of success is not good; the 6'8", 225-pound man will probably not make a good competitive gymnast. Although these examples are extreme, we need to keep them in mind when we consider what is possible and best for each of us.

Many people are not happy with the appearance of their bodies. Al Sabbah et al. (2009) surveyed adolescents in 24 countries and regions in Europe, Canada, and the United States. They found that body weight dissatisfaction was highly prev-alent but was more common in girls than boys, among overweight than non-overweight individuals, and among older adolescents than younger adolescents.

Your Body Weight

Most often when we think of body weight, we think about what the scale says when we stand on it. Although this is useful information, if you are serious about reaching your optimal body weight, it would be worthwhile to learn more about some topics beyond the scope of this book: **body mass index (BMI)** and **body composition**. Knowing about these will help you understand your body weight better and have more realistic goals.

> **body mass index (BMI)**
> Weight in kilograms divided by the square of the height in meters.
>
> **body composition**
> The percentage of fat versus lean tissue.

What the scale says is not always the complete truth, and what we see is not always what we are. For example, sometimes overweight people see themselves as heavier than they really are. When they look in a mirror, they see a bigger abdomen, rear end, and thighs than they actually have. This body image may be hard to change, even if body weight decreases.

Other overweight people may see themselves as much slimmer than they really are. They often rationalize away their need to lose weight. However, some people see themselves as they really are. Those with realistic body images tend to have the greatest success with weight control.

Diet

The diet business is big business in the United States. Despite the interest in diet products and services, few people have long-term weight control success.

To have any hope of long-term success with weight loss, our approach to diets must change. A "diet" must mean permanent changes in eating habits. Do not waste time on dieting if you are not committed to maintaining a healthy weight throughout your life. If you want to change your eating habits, you must pay close attention to the kinds and amounts of foods you eat. There is no substitute for well-balanced diets and a reduction in intake of calories—especially when combined with proper exercise habits.

Exercise

Exercise plays an important role in losing pounds and keeping them off: Researchers have compared

How can you tell if someone you love has an eating disorder? Here are possible warning signs:

1. Evidence of bulimia, such as laxatives on the dresser or vomitus in the toilet bowl.
2. Moaning about a fat behind by a person who is rail thin.
3. Hiding under baggy clothes.
4. An energy level so low that he or she sleeps much of the time.
5. The growth of baby-fine hair on arms and legs (as the shrinking body tries to keep warm).

6. Underweight by 15%.
7. Loss of menstrual cycle for 3 months.
8. Brittle nails and/or swollen joints.
9. A chronic sore throat and/or dental problems.
10. Bloating and other digestive complaints.

Source: Adapted from Gorman, C. Disappearing act, *Time, 152, no. 10* (November 2, 1998), 110.

the effects of weight loss by diet only and by exercise only. They found that the group who were only exercising lost a higher percentage of fat and had more success keeping off the weight than the group who were only dieting.

Moderate exercise suppresses appetite, rather than increasing it, as many people think. You might want to exercise just before a meal to take advantage of that effect. Another benefit of exercise is that it strengthens muscle tissue. Muscle tissue requires more calories than fat tissue does to maintain itself, so as lean muscle tissue increases, more calories are burned. This is important, because our resting metabolic rate accounts for about 70% of the calories we burn.

The ultimate goal of any weight-loss program should be the loss of body fat, not just body weight. Those who combine diet and exercise lose more fat and are more likely to keep it off. Exercise and sound eating habits result in a steady weight loss that can be maintained on a permanent basis if you maintain your exercise and dietary changes.

▇ Issues Related to Trying to Be Perfect

Although we know it is impossible to be perfect, some people are so concerned about their body image that they run into problems, such as eating disorders, obsessive muscle dysmorphia, and complications of cosmetic surgery.

Eating Disorders

In the quest to be attractive and improve one's body image, some people are willing to pay a high price. It is common to want to look as good as we can, and many people attempt to control body weight by using various diets at some time during their lives.

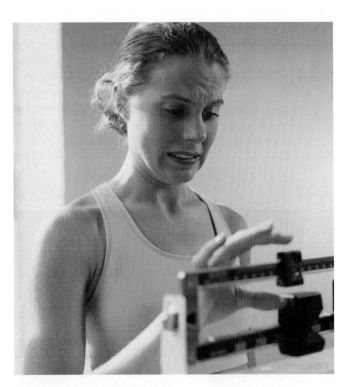

We need to pay attention to our body composition as well as our body weight.

A fear of fat seems to drive some people to extreme forms of eating behaviors. Compulsive overeating (also called *binge eating*) and compulsive dieting are the behaviors known as *eating disorders*. Striegel-Moore et al. (2008) reported that women are more likely to have eating disorders than are men. Women are significantly more likely to participate in fasting, binge eating, and vomiting. Nevertheless, a substantial minority of men have eating disorder symptoms. In addition, many college athletes show disordered eating patterns, with the greatest prevalence occurring in gymnasts and swimmers.

While they probably mean well, sometimes athletic coaches and even parents might contribute to eating disorders. They could do this by encouraging young people to diet or by demeaning their bodies by telling them they are too fat or do not have the "correct" body proportions.

The exact causes of eating disorders are not known for sure, but they seem to be triggered by life's stressors, emotional trauma, tragic events, and the media. Common health problems associated with eating disorders include intestinal problems; decayed teeth; malnutrition; dehydration; stomach ruptures; esophagus tears; serious heart, kidney, and liver damage; and death (Hughes, 2005).

Anorexia nervosa is a condition in which the individual severely limits calorie intake; it is sometimes described as self-induced starvation. The individual fears gaining weight even though he or she may already be underweight. There is also a disturbance in the way personal body weight or shape is viewed by the individual. Anorexia can be fatal. Most people with anorexia are white females

anorexia nervosa
A condition in which the individual severely limits caloric intake.

younger than 25 years of age who are focused on a goal of extreme thinness and willingly starve themselves and overexercise to reach that goal.

Over the course of a lifetime, 0.5% to 3.7% of girls and women develop anorexia nervosa. Approximately 0.5% of the female population die each year as a result of their illness, making it one of the top psychiatric illnesses leading to death (Taylor et al., 2006). Although this condition affects females 95% of the time, it may be more common than previously thought among college males. Most males with anorexia are men who depend on their thin physique for employment—such as models. Anorexia results in death in about 10% of all cases in both sexes.

Although the exact cause of anorexia is unknown, it seems to involve a combination of psychological and environmental factors. The female with anorexia might reject food in an attempt to avoid dealing with what she feels are society's demands that she become a superwoman. The severe weight loss can make the female resemble a young girl, in what some researchers feel is a conscious attempt to avoid dealing with issues related to intimacy and sexuality. People with anorexia might feel that their weight is the only factor they can control in a world where expectations of

Many female athletes turn to some form of dieting to maintain an edge in competitions. The nationally ranked gymnast Christy Henrich took her dieting too far and struggled with anorexia nervosa for several years before she died of it in 1994. Here she is seen performing in the late 1980s (left) and just before her death in 1994 (right).

others seem difficult to fulfill. One of the most difficult to understand aspects of anorexia is self-perception. Regardless of how much weight has been lost, the person with anorexia still feels too heavy (Bruess & Greenberg, 2009).

There are more than 500 web sites that deal frankly, and sometimes approvingly, with anorexia and other eating disorders. One of these web sites, ceruleanbutterfly.com, promotes the idea that an eating disorder is less a disease than a lifestyle choice—"a decision to pursue perfection" (Song, 2005). On the web site, people with eating disorders gather for support and companionship, share tips for losing weight and hiding the signs of malnutrition, and provide "thinspiration," like photos of bony fashion models. No one knows for sure how many of the estimated 11 million Americans suffering from anorexia or bulimia visit the web sites, but the developer of one of them claims to have had more than 85,000 hits in a period of about 18 months. They are often referred to as "pro-ana forums" (ana being short for anorexia). Most adolescents tend to use the web sites without their parents' knowledge, and the sites can be especially seductive. One girl said, "Now I can learn to be an anorexic from the Internet." The pro-ana sites are a world that is comforting to those with an eating disorder, and they provide a sense of belonging.

Bulimia nervosa is a condition in which the person periodically binges and purges, with an obsessive fear of becoming fat. Bulimia (insatiable appetite) has been confused with anorexia nervosa because periodic bingeing is common to both disorders; however, a number of the characteristics are different. People with bulimia are usually older than people with anorexia and may have been anorexic earlier. Whereas people with anorexia are obsessed with being thin, people with bulimia have an obsessive fear of becoming fat.

Approximately 2% to 3% of the U.S. population has bulimia. Some research indicates the rate is higher for college-age women—around 4%. The illness usually begins in late adolescence or early adult life. Only an estimated 5% to 15% of people with bulimia are male, but the incidence is increasing among males. Bulimia is often perceived to be an affliction of Caucasian girls and young women in middle and upper socioeconomic classes. However, increasing numbers of cases are being seen in men and women of all different ethnic and cultural groups. It is evident that bulimia occurs in all cultures (Schoenstadt, 2007; TieMeyer, 2007).

There is still a lot to be learned about both anorexia and bulimia. Researchers continue to discover new information about both of these eating disorders. For example, Taylor et al. (2006) found that an Internet-based intervention program may prevent some high-risk, college-age women from developing an eating disorder. In addition, Marsh et al. (2009) reported that the brain circuitry involved in regulating impulsive behavior may be less active in women suffering from bulimia. It is not clear if the brain differences are a cause or an effect of the disorder.

During their secretive eating binges, people with bulimia may consume many thousands of calories in only a few hours. Afterward, they try to purge the food through a variety of methods, including vomiting, laxatives, diuretics, and exercise. After bingeing and purging, the person with bulimia may feel discouraged about the behavior.

Binge-eating disorder (BED) is an eating disorder characterized by recurrent binge eating but not by inappropriate weight-control behaviors. Persons with BED do not regularly engage in purging, and the majority are obese. They also may be referred to as "compulsive overeaters."

Characteristics of binge eating include eating much more rapidly than normal, eating until feeling uncomfortably full, eating large amounts even though one is not hungry, eating alone because of embarrassment about eating habits, and feeling disgusted or guilty after overeating. There is usually a feeling that

> **bulimia nervosa**
> A condition in which the individual periodically binges and purges, with an obsessive fear of becoming fat.
>
> **binge-eating disorder (BED)**
> Eating disorder characterized by recurrent binge eating but not by inappropriate weight-control behaviors.

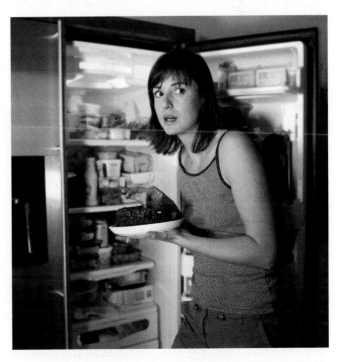

It is important to be realistic about our eating practices.

one cannot stop eating or control what or how much is being eaten.

Treating Eating Disorders

Many approaches are used in the treatment of anorexia, but the prognosis is not good. Drug therapy is used in about 25% of the cases, and behavior modification in about 45%. A combination of approaches is also used. Most specialists recommend a period of hospitalization to ensure weight gain, and families are often involved in the therapy. The prognosis for people with anorexia is worse than for people with bulimia.

Overcoming bulimia requires establishing a normal eating pattern that eliminates dieting. Although people with bulimia can hide their disorder from others, they are more likely than people with anorexia to seek treatment; however, they might expect immediate results and become frustrated with therapy. Antidepressant drugs are used in the treatment of bulimia, as is psychological therapy. Antidepressant medication and psychological treatments can also reduce binge eating of BED patients.

Muscle Dysmorphia

Body image and goals related to it may change over time. Thus, as someone makes progress with weights, or in gymnastics or figure skating, the ideal of the perfect body image may become more "perfect." A perpetual chasing of the ideal can cause people to lose perspective about their actual body image. An example of this was given in the opening story of this chapter.

One disorder that afflicts bodybuilders is essentially the opposite of anorexia nervosa. Called **muscle dysmorphia**, also known as bigorexia and reverse anorexia, it involves bodybuilders who, despite their extremely muscular bodies and tip-top shape, consider themselves to be puny (Brody, 1998). Weight lifting, for some people, can become a dangerous obsession (Bilger, 1998).

Psychiatrists have found that as many as 10% of the men and 84% of women who are bodybuilders may have this "negative anorexia." For example, men who did not think they were well built could press the equivalent of their own body weight. Even though they recognized muscularity in others, their view of themselves was very negative (Cohen, 1997). Muscle dysmorphics with body weight well above 200 pounds are sometimes so ashamed of their "undersized" bodies that they rarely leave their homes, preferring instead to follow a regimen of weight lifting in their basements, interrupted primarily for periodic protein consumption (Zorpette, 1998).

Goodale and associates (2001) used a mixed-gender sample of 323 college students to study muscle dysmorphia. She concluded that it is an increasingly common problem among athletes and nonathletes alike, that both men and women are susceptible to it, and that it has many similarities to established dieting disorders. For example, perhaps because of media glorification of lean and muscular physiques, those with muscle dysmorphia place undue emphasis on body weight and shape when judging their own worth.

Interestingly, in one study American and European college men were asked to pick a body type that they thought women would find attractive. The average pick had 20 to 30 more pounds of muscle than a normal man. When women were asked the same question, they chose the normal-sized man most of the time (Fahmy, 2004).

> **muscle dysmorphia**
> A disorder whereby a bodybuilder in top shape considers himself or herself to be puny.

Gender DIMENSIONS

Why Are Eating Disorders Mainly Found in Women?

It seems clear that physical attractiveness is more important for women than men. This is because beauty is often a central aspect of femininity (girls learn early that being pretty draws attention to them), and women's self-worth is often tied to establishing and maintaining close relationships. They can improve their feeling of self-worth based on others' opinions and approval of them.

The ideal standard of physical attractiveness has become thinner over the past few decades. This makes it even harder for women to meet the standard, so they are more likely to resort to extreme ways to control their weight—such as rigid dieting and purging.

Even when men take extreme measures to control their weight, it is usually done to improve their athletic performance (such as with jockeys and wrestlers). Their goal of losing weight is secondary to their goal of performing well. For women, however, dieting to achieve an ideal weight is related to their self-evaluation.

Source: Adapted from Wilson, G. T., et al. Eating disorders, in *Abnormal psychology: Integrating perspectives.* Needham, MA: Allyn & Bacon, 1996, 370.

A simple test for bigorexia involves questions like: (1) How often do you look at your body in the mirror? (2) Do you think your body needs to be leaner and more muscular? (3) Do you find yourself reading up on new training methods, diets, and supplements? (4) Do you eat special high-protein or low-fat diets or use food supplements to improve muscularity? (5) Do you ever wear baggy clothes to hide the body you feel is too lean—or do you avoid situations where your body might be seen? (6) Do you still train when injured because you fear losing muscle mass? (7) Do you compare yourself to other men and feel envious? (8) Do you ever think others are snickering at your puniness? (9) Would you rather spend time going to the gym than having sex, and has your libido taken a dive? (10) Have you turned down social events, taken time off from work, or skipped family responsibilities so you can work out? Typically, men who have bigorexia will say "yes" to three or more of these questions (Mind over fatter, 2005).

Muscle dysmorphia does not usually involve the serious medical complications of anorexia, but it still can have significant effects. It is certainly normal for people who go to a gym to want to improve their physique and build larger muscles. The turning point from normal goals to muscle dysmorphia occurs when the quest for "massive" size takes over one's life, destroying career, relationships, and, ironically, self-esteem.

Sports and Dieting

Eating disorders may be the gravest health problem facing female athletes, affecting gymnasts, figure skaters, swimmers, distance runners, divers, and even tennis and volleyball players. Given the importance that sport attaches to weight—and, in subjectively judged

People have various opinions about which type of physique looks attractive.

sports, to appearance—it is not surprising that eating disorders are common among athletes.

As we have mentioned, some sports, such as women's gymnastics, emphasize smallness. Vera Caslavska, who won the overall titles at the 1964 and 1968 Olympics, was a relatively normal-sized 5'3" and 121 pounds. After she was upstaged in 1968 by the pixie Olga Korbut (4'11" and 85 pounds), gymnastics was never the same (Noden, 1994). In 1976, the average woman on the U.S. Olympic team was 5'3" and 105 pounds; by 1992 she was 4'9" and 88 pounds (Noden, 1994).

But weight—and dieting—also play a major role in endurance sports. As an athlete's weight falls, his or her aerobic power increases. Put another way, it takes less energy to run if you weigh less; thus more energy can be expended on running faster. So runners and swimmers also succumb to the need to diet to win.

steroids
Synthetic versions of the male hormone testosterone that promote tissue growth.

Steroid Use

Steroids are synthetic versions of the male hormone testosterone. Steroid abuse is fast becoming a very serious problem among adolescent males, both athletes and nonathletes, who take large doses in an attempt to achieve much greater body mass quickly.

Many people look at eight-time Mr. Olympia Lee Haney only in terms of his muscles. But Haney keeps body image in perspective, placing God, family, and friends above business—and to Haney, bodybuilding was a business.

In addition to potential to halt growth and bone development, steroid use can cause testicular shrinkage, increased cholesterol levels, infertility, decreased sexual drive, prostate cancer, kidney disorders, liver malfunction, aggression and violence, suicidal tendencies, and extreme moodiness. Steroids can also be psychologically and physically addictive.

Steroid abuse is a problem among teenagers. Johnston et al. (2009) reported that there was a fairly sharp increase in the use of steroids by male teens in the late 1990s, with peak levels reached in 1999 among eighth-grade males, in 2000 among tenth-grade males, and in 2001 and 2002 among twelfth-grade males. Since those peak years, the annual prevalence rate has dropped by more than half among eighth- and tenth-grade males (to 1.2% and 1.4%, respectively), and by one-third among twelfth-grade males (to 2.5% annual prevalence in 2008). Steroid use is not limited to males, however. While the prevalence rates tend to be much lower among females, the trend toward steroid use by females is much the same as for males.

People may go to unhealthy extremes simply to look good. Goodale and coworkers (2001) reported that the most common reason male bodybuilders give for using steroids is to enhance looks.

Women in endurance sports also take steroids. Steroids help a runner in two ways: A thin runner expends less energy in running; by speeding muscle recovery, a long-distance runner is able to recover faster, train more, and thus run faster.

The adverse effects of steroids in women include lowered voice, increased body and facial hair, male-pattern baldness, enlarged clitoris, decreased breast size, and changes in or cessation of menstruation. There are not sufficient studies of female steroid users to fully understand the extent to which a woman's body may be damaged and whether the effects are permanent.

In addition to the many adverse effects of steroids listed, there is a risk of HIV transmission through shared needles. Finally, anabolic steroids are illegal in the United States; their use carries stiff fines and possible imprisonment.

Some feel that a "male body ideal" has caused increasing numbers of males to develop an "Adonis complex"—defined as a condition shared by millions of males who develop eating disorders, abuse steroids, work out compulsively, or otherwise obsess over their physical appearance. The taboo against overt male vanity inhibits men from seeking help for their disorders (Miller & Sharlet, 2000).

Makeovers and Cosmetic Surgery

If we pay attention to our favorite movie and TV stars, we see that they radically change their appearance from time to time. The makeover has become

According to the American Society of Plastic Surgeons, liposuction is the most popular cosmetic surgery procedure for men and women, after rhinoplasty. Comedian Kathy Griffin underwent liposuction in an attempt to drop from a size 4 to a size 2. Medical complications during and after the surgery, as she recounts in an article published by *Glamour* magazine, proved to be nearly fatal. Have you ever considered undergoing cosmetic surgery in pursuit of your ideal body? Do you think the benefits outweigh the risks?

a powerful draw for many stars—they feel it can renew the spirit, save a career, and even mend the heart. Indeed, Hollywood may be in the grip of a redo revolution. Some stars like to re-create themselves, increase their confidence by showing that they can wear more than one style, and avoid being linked with a look created by a past role (O'Neill, 1998).

According to the American Society of Plastic Surgeons, the number of cosmetic procedures in the United States increased to more than 10 million in 2007, a 48% increase from 2000. This increase was paralleled by a surge in reality cosmetic surgery television programming. Viewing reality cosmetic surgery shows is significantly related to more favorable cosmetic surgery attitudes, perceived pressure to have cosmetic surgery, past attainment of a cosmetic procedure, a decreased fear of surgery, and overall body dissatisfaction and disordered eating (Sperry et al., 2009).

In our quest to create the perfect look, we may see the stars radically change theirs and decide we want to do it too. People today often view their body as increasingly malleable. Sometimes, they even want to use ways that look easy, such as liposuction, implants, and plastic surgery (cosmetic surgery).

Liposuction is a technique for removing adipose (fat) tissue with a suction-pump device. A hollow suction tube, which is attached to a special vacuum, is inserted into small incisions in the skin. It is used primarily to remove and reduce areas of fat around the abdomen, breast, legs, face, and upper arms. Liposuction can be helpful for the removal of fat in particular areas, but it should not be viewed as a way to lose large amounts of fat or to change one's physique dramatically. Most people lose an average of only 3 pounds as a direct result of the procedure. According to the American Society of Aesthetic Plastic Surgery (2009), liposuction was the top cosmetic surgical procedure in 2007, with about 457,000 such procedures performed. That was 2.6 times as many procedures as were done in 1997. The cost for liposuction ranges from approximately $3,000 to $10,000 and is not usually covered by insurance.

As liposuction has become more popular, the number of inexperienced practitioners has grown. If the procedure is to be done, it must be done by a skillful, trained professional. Even in the most skilled hands, liposuction is not risk-free. A few patients are left with scarring or rippling of the skin, and some need another procedure 6 to 12 months later to fix uneven results (Graham, 1997).

As we discussed in Chapter 4, breast implants have been around for quite a few years. Silicone-gel–filled breast implants first went on the market in 1962. They were banned in 1992 by the Food and Drug Administration (FDA). The question of whether they should be used has been greatly debated. In April 2005, an FDA advisory committee voted to recommend allowing them back on the market under certain conditions—making sure women understand potential risk, having women get regular MRI exams, allowing only specially trained plastic surgeons to per-

form the insertions, and requiring continued research studies related to the implants. Women who wanted a return of the product say silicone-gel implants look and feel more natural than the saline-filled implants. The implants have been exonerated from concerns that they might cause serious or chronic illnesses such as cancer or lupus. Aside from the risk of breakage and pain, however, they can cause infection and development of painful scar tissue. About 399,000 breast enlargements and 153,000 breast reductions were performed in the United States in 2007 (FDA nears OK on silicone breast implants, 2005; American Society for Aesthetic Plastic Surgery, 2009).

Cosmetic surgery includes the procedures already mentioned, and there are also many other possibilities. Many people elect to have cosmetic surgery when a part of their body makes them self-conscious or uncomfortable. After surgery, many patients say they have a more positive self-image. Statistically, about 9% of the total number of cosmetic operations are done on men. About 89% are done on Caucasians, 9% on Hispanics, 6% on African Americans, and 5% on Asian Americans (American Society for Aesthetic Plastic Surgery, 2009).

liposuction
A technique for removing adipose tissue with a suction-pump device.

cosmetic surgery
Surgery done for the sole purpose of improving the appearance.

rhinoplasty
Surgery done to change the shape of the nose.

Another common procedure is **rhinoplasty** (surgery done to change the shape of the nose). It usually takes 1 to 2 hours and costs $2,000 to $5,000. It is not covered by insurance unless the nose structure impedes breathing. As with any surgery, there can be undesirable results. The patient may not like the aesthetic result and want a revision, the newly formed nose may make breathing difficult, or fibrous scar tissue may form. In 2007 more than 285,000 rhinoplasty procedures were performed (American Society of Plastic Surgeons, 2009).

More than 348,000 breast augmentations were performed in 2007. This was 2.6 times more than in 1997. The average cost was around $4,000 (American Society of Plastic Surgeons, 2009).

More men are turning to implants to enhance their pectoral muscles (Miller, 2002). Putting in a pair of palm-size silicone discs can cost from $4,000 to $10,000. It takes less than 2 hours and is usually performed in a doctor's office under general anesthesia. This is a relatively new procedure, but many experts feel there will be a lot more pectoral implants in coming years. In 2007, more than 1 million American men elected to have cosmetic surgery.

The top five procedures may be listed differently depending upon the source. The American Society for Aesthetic Plastic Surgery (2009) lists the top five for men as being liposuction, eyelid surgery, rhinoplasty, breast reduction to treat enlarged male breasts, and hair transplantation. For women, the top five were liposuction, breast augmentation, eyelid surgery, nose reshaping, and facelift. The grand totals were liposuction (457,000 procedures), breast augmentation (400,000), eyelid surgery (241,000), adominoplasty (tummy tuck; 185,000), and breast reduction (153,000). Men had nearly 1.1 million procedures (9% of the total), which represented a 17% increase for men since 2006.

If you watched the Austin Powers movies, you may have laughed at Austin for having a penis-enlargement pump. Men's magazines and web sites are filled with ads for pumps, pills, weights, exercises, and surgeries that are supposed to increase the length and/or the width of the penis. However, no scientific research supports the use of any nonsurgical method to enlarge the penis, and no reputable medical society endorses penis-enlargement surgery performed for purely cosmetic reasons. Many of these techniques can damage the penis and may even cause functional problems. Cosmetic surgeons have developed several enlargement techniques, but none of them are endorsed by medical organizations. Following various procedures, some men have had to undergo additional surgeries to correct deformities caused by the original procedure. Others have had scarring, shorter penises, hair on the base of the penis, low-hanging penis, loss of sensitivity, and bumps and lumps. Other complaints include loss of sexual function, urinary incompetence, and persistent pain. Surgery should only be an option for penises that have been amputated or damaged for some reason (Beware of penis-enlargement scams, 2005).

Some women want breast implants; others want to have large, heavy breasts reduced in size. The latter procedure may not necessarily be considered cosmetic surgery, depending on the intention and the situation, because it may be performed to relieve physical ailments such as back and neck pain caused by large, heavy breasts. It involves removal of fat and breast tissue and may leave noticeable scars. The procedure may also affect the ability to breastfeed. It usually takes 2 to 4 hours and costs $5,000 to $10,000, and may be covered by insurance if medical problems are associated with the size of the breasts. In 2007, approximately 153,000 breast reductions were performed on females, an increase of 3.2 times the number done in 1997 (American Society for Aesthetic Plastic Surgery, 2009).

Whereas liposuction only removes fat, the **tummy tuck** is a

tummy tuck
Extensive surgical procedure that removes excess skin and fat from the abdomen.

Young girls emulate superstars like Britney Spears, who in 1999 had breast augmentation surgery. In fact, according to the American Society of Plastic and Reconstructive Surgeons, 3,095 girls age 18 and younger had breast implants in 2002, up 19% from 2001 and up 59% from 1999. Breast augmentation surgery is the most common cosmetic surgery procedure for women, with 264,000 operations performed in 2005. Interestingly, most of the surgeries take place in California, Texas, and Florida—why do think that is the case?

more extensive surgical procedure that removes excess skin and fat from the lower abdomen and tightens the abdominal muscles. It usually requires a hip-to-hip lower-abdominal incision and takes 1 to 2 hours to complete if fat deposits are below the navel. If a more extensive procedure is needed, it can take 2 to 5 hours. It costs $5,000 to $9,000, with an average total cost of $6,400, usually not covered by insurance (American Society of Aesthetic Plastic Surgery, 2009).

Other available procedures include face lifts, upper and lower eyelid reduction, and chin implantation. In short, we can have just about any part of our body altered if we are strongly motivated and have the means to pay for it. Because it is legal in most U.S. states for any physician to advertise himself or herself as a plastic or cosmetic surgeon, candidates for surgery must select a well-trained plastic surgeon for any type of cosmetic surgery.

Several trends indicate that cosmetic surgery will continue to be a growth industry. Younger people are getting more cosmetic procedures, people who have had cosmetic procedures tend to have others, men are becoming more "vain," the number getting surgery has doubled since 1992, and the aging of the population is likely to result in more cosmetic surgery (Grant, 2001).

The top five nonsurgical cosmetic procedures in 2009 were Botox injection (2.8 million procedures); injection of hyaluronic acid (a jelly-like substance that softens facial lines and furrows; 1.45 million procedures); laser hair removal (1.41 million procedures); microdermabrasion (mechanical scraping of the top layers of the skin to soften sharp edges of surface irregularities; 830,000 procedures); and IPL (intense pulsed light) laser treatment to smooth the skin and improve the appearance (648,000 procedures). People age 35–50 had the most procedures—54 million (46% of the total). People age 19–34 had 21%, people age 51–64 had 25%, people age 65 and older had 6%, and people age 18 and younger had less than 2% of the procedures (American Society for Aesthetic Plastic Surgery, 2009).

Finally, body piercing and tattoos have been used by some people to enhance their body image. No longer a practice carried out in back rooms, body piercing and tattoos are making their way into socially acceptable studios. Although many people have questioned the motivations behind body piercing, a number of years ago Myers (1992) reported that many who use body piercing are "sane, successful people." He reported that body piercing in the United States seems to function by giving people a strong sense of self and a connection with others by marking relationship events in commitment ceremonies, by enhancing people's feelings about their body, by providing the rush of the piercing experience, and by giving people a way to rebel against mainstream society. The most common places for body piercing are the face or ears; some people pierce their tongues, nipples, abdomen, and genitals. This practice is not risk-free; it sometimes produces infection.

Summary

- Body image refers to the mental image we have of our own physical appearance. It is influenced by many factors, and in turn, influences our attitudes and behaviors.

- The media play a major role in influencing people's body images. Many media images are unattainable in real life.

- People from different cultures may view body image very differently.

- We can do a lot to build a better body image by not apologizing for all our blemishes; not basing our body image on what we see in the media; dressing and acting in ways that make us feel more attractive; and paying attention to our body language.

- Diet and exercise can play major roles related to body image.

- Some people are so concerned about their body image that they develop eating disorders such as anorexia nervosa, bulimia nervosa, and binge-eating disorder.

- Using steroids in an attempt to develop one's body is a very dangerous thing to do. Steroids cause many serious health problems.

- Cosmetic surgery has become much more popular today than it was just 10 to 12 years ago. The most common procedures include liposuction, breast augmentation, eyelid surgery, tummy tuck, and breast reduction.

Discussion Questions

1. Explain how the media have created unrealistic body images for women and men.

2. Which strategies can be used to create a more positive body image?

3. Which problems, both physical and psychological, occur when people try to make themselves more "perfect"?

Application Questions

Reread the story that opens the chapter and answer the following questions:

1. As do many teens, Marc had a poor body image. Teased by his friends ("Ostrich Boy") and haunted by the images in men's magazines, he turned to lifting weights. If you had a chance to talk to a group of 14-year-old boys, what advice would you give them on how to handle body-image issues? What about a group of 14-year-old girls?

2. One of the problems about weight lifting to improve body image is that you can "never be too big." The more muscle you gain, the more you strive for. But as goals are set higher, workouts require more time in the gym, more sleep for recovery, and more time for eating properly. How is it possible to manage the desire for continued physical improvement without becoming obsessive?

3. Consider the changes in Marc's body image as he goes to law school, gets a job, gets married, has children, and so on. How might Marc's body image change across time? If he suddenly found himself divorced and single at age 40 years, should he hit the weights again?

Critical Thinking Questions

1. Because excessive weight has been linked to many health problems, why should we all not strive to be thin? Is it more harmful to diet excessively or to be obese?

2. You are an assistant college coach. An athlete returns from summer vacation, having put on 30 pounds of muscle. He says he spent the summer "lifting his ass off." You think he may have used steroids. Would you report him to the school's athletic director? (If he were found to have taken steroids, he could be expelled from school. However, if he continued to use steroids, he could suffer serious medical problems.)

3. Would your answer to question 2 be different if a female athlete returned in the fall with an additional 15 pounds of muscle? Explain your answer.

4. The noted eating-disorder psychologist G. Terence Wilson has stated that, biologically, women cannot be thin and have large breasts. Yet many women exercise and diet until they have low body fat and then have breast implants to compensate. Role models for the thin-yet-busty type include professional bodybuilders, many of the athletes on daytime TV exercise shows, and many actresses. How do such role models affect women?

Critical Thinking Case

Before attending college, your girlfriend Amanda ran cross-country and track. But with the pressures of college studies, part-time work, and your relationship, she has little time to exercise. She has started to worry more and more about the "freshman 15," the extra weight that many college freshmen gain. She often comments on how good the cover girls on fashion magazines look. That is not all: You have noticed she rarely eats when you go out. When you mention this, she says she is trying to help save money for a vacation. When you find over-the-counter diet pills hidden under her bed, she says, "Everyone takes them." When you tell her that someone heard her throwing up in the bathroom after meals, she flatly denies it. When you tell her she is looking "rather thin," she smiles and says, "Thank you."

You have read the information in this chapter and do not believe that she has an eating disorder. However, you are concerned about Amanda's physical health and psychological well-being. How could you help her to improve her body image?

Exploring Personal Dimensions

Body Image

How do you feel about the appearance of these regions of your body?

	Quite satisfied	Somewhat satisfied	Somewhat dissatisfied	Very dissatisfied
Hair	❑	❑	❑	❑
Arms	❑	❑	❑	❑
Hands	❑	❑	❑	❑
Feet	❑	❑	❑	❑
Waist	❑	❑	❑	❑
Buttocks	❑	❑	❑	❑
Hips	❑	❑	❑	❑
Legs and ankles	❑	❑	❑	❑
Thighs	❑	❑	❑	❑
Chest/breasts	❑	❑	❑	❑
Posture	❑	❑	❑	❑
General attractiveness	❑	❑	❑	❑

1. Which of your thoughts and actions enhance your body image?
2. Which of your thoughts and actions are detrimental to your body image?
3. Which societal forces (e.g., expectations of friends and parents, advertising, celebrities and professional athletes) influence your body image most strongly?
4. What could you do to become more satisfied with your body image?

Suggested Readings

American Society of Asethetic Plastic Surgery. (2009). Available: http://surgery.org/statistics.html.

American Society of Plastic Surgeons. (2009). Available: www.plasticsurgery.org.

Anschutz, D., Engels, R. C., Becker, E. S., & van Strien, T. The bold and the beautiful: Influence of body size of televised media models on body dissatisfaction and actual food intake. *Appetite, 51, no. 3* (November 2008), 530–537.

Gerber, R. Beauty and body image in the media. Media Awareness Network (2005). Available at: www.media-awareness.ca.

Grammer, K., Renninger, L., & Fischer, B. Disco clothing, female sexual motivation, and relationship status: Is she dressed to impress? *Journal of Sex Research, 41, no. 1* (February 2004), 66–74.

Keca, J., & Cook-Cottone, C. Eating disorders: Prevention is worth every ounce. *Principal Leadership, 5, no. 8* (May 2005), 11–15.

Lin, L., & Reid, K. The relationship between media exposure and antifat attitudes: The role of dysfunctional appearance beliefs. *Body Image, 6, no. 1* (January 2009), 52–55.

Littleton, H. Body image dissatisfaction: Normative discontent? *Sex Roles, 59, no. 3–4* (August 2008), 292–293.

Swami, V., Chamorro-Premuzic, T., Bridges, S., & Furnham, A. Acceptance of cosmetic surgery: Personality and individual difference predictors. *Body Image, 6, no. 1* (January 2009), 7–13.

Web Resources

For links to the web sites below, visit *http://sexuality.jbpub.com/dimensions/4e* and click on Resource Links.

Club Drug Counselor—Male Body Issues
www.josephlafleur.com/about_Male_Body_Issues.htm

Provides information about male health issues related to body image. Includes some comparisons from different cultures.

Eating Disorder Referral and Information Center
www.pslgroup.com/dg/1d48fa.htm

Dedicated to the prevention and treatment of eating disorders. Information and treatment resources are given for all forms of eating disorders.

Media Awareness Network
www.media-awareness.ca

Deals with many issues in the media, including stereotypes about females and males. Emphasis is on female stereotypes and their effect on cultural ideas of beauty and social development. The effect of media portrayals of what masculinity means is included.

National Eating Disorder Association
www.nationaleatingdisorders.org

Provides general information about eating disorders and body-image concerns along with possible referrals for treatment, educational materials, and opportunities to help through volunteering.

Women's Issues
www.womenissues.about.com

Contains information on many women's issues including stereotypes, body image, and self-improvement.

CHAPTER 10
Sexual Orientation

CHAPTER OBJECTIVES

1 Define sexual orientation, including heterosexuality, homosexuality, situational homosexuality, and bisexuality. Discuss the validity of the Kinsey continuum.

2 Compare and contrast the theories of sexual orientation, including biological, psychological, and sociocultural theories.

3 Discuss homosexual life, including the challenges specific to homosexuality.

4 Discuss social issues that affect homosexuals.

sexuality.jbpub.com/dimensions/4e

Theories of Sexual Orientation
Homophobia
Coming Out
The Gay Rights Movement

INTRODUCTION

*B*y all appearances, Brad was an archetypal early-1970s high school male: a "good" student, a "really nice" guy with a willingness to help out with school projects and panache in fixing cars. He dated several girls. But his relationship with Peggy was extra special. They were best friends, hanging out together and attending high school parties and dances as a couple. They also engaged in a variety of sexual activities.

At first Brad could not quite understand why the idea of sexual intercourse with Peggy did not appeal to him as much as it should. Eventually Brad realized that he was gay. Peggy was hurt at first about the abrupt end of their relationship, but she cared about Brad enough to remain a close friend.

After high school, Brad attended a local college and continued to hang out with his high school friends who had accepted his sexual orientation, rather than venturing out to meet people who might not have been so accepting. Gay bashing was common, and Brad had a legitimate fear for his safety. During this time, the early 1980s, he met Brian, whom he has been with ever since.

Brad felt comfortable "coming out" to his friends, but he did not tell his elderly parents for fear of their reaction. This silence caused a bit of a problem, because his parents (and relatives) were forever introducing him to "nice girls" and wondering why nothing ever came of the dates Brad claimed he had. About the time Brad turned 30 years old, over dinner one evening, his father said to him, "You're gay, aren't you?" Although Brad's parents may have initially been hurt or confused, or may have questioned their own parenting, they continued to love and support Brad.

For Brad, as for many gays and lesbians, the AIDS crisis took a terrible toll. Many friends became sick and died. Many of Brad's friends *learned about and began practicing safer sexual activities, no longer going to bathhouses or having quick, anonymous encounters. Brad attended rallies to promote governmental funding for AIDS research.*

Brad was lucky: Both he and Brian tested negative for HIV. One thing that HIV did teach Brad, however, was that although he and Brian had been together for many years in a committed relationship, their situation was quite different from that of a legally married couple. When one of Brad's close friends died of AIDS, Brad's friend's parents, who did not want to believe their child was gay, demanded all his assets—which the deceased had intended to leave for his partner. Because the parents had the legal standing in the state in which the death occurred, the grieving partner lost everything. Even while his friend was dying, the parents were allowed to make all medical decisions and legally barred the partner from hospital visits.

In marriages, spouses automatically have each other's power of attorney, which means that if one spouse is incapacitated, the other has control over his or her affairs. A gay couple must go through lawyers to ensure that each partner has power of attorney for the other. Because Brian and Brad had purchased a home together and had made various other investments together, they realized it was imperative for them to complete the proper documentation to protect each other.

Brad's story illustrates many of the dimensions of sexual orientation. Sexual orientation takes time to develop and has an impact on many aspects of a person's life. In this chapter, we look at the ways that the many dimensions of human sexuality interact to determine sexual orientation.

Sexual Orientation

People have various feelings about sexual orientation—and even the topic of sexual orientation. The Sexuality Information and Education Council of the United States (SIECUS) position statement on sexual orientation (2009a) is as follows:

> *Sexual orientation is an essential human quality. Individuals have the right to accept, acknowledge, and live in accordance with their sexual orientation, be they bisexual, heterosexual, gay, or lesbian. The legal system should guarantee the civil rights and protection of all people, regardless of sexual orientation. Prejudice and discrimination based on sexual orientation is unconscionable.*

A person's **sexual orientation** is one's erotic, romantic, and affectional attraction to the same gen-der, to the other gender, or to both. **Sexual identity** refers to an inner sense of oneself as a sexual being, including one's identification in terms of gender and sexual orientation. **Sexual preference** is a term once used to describe sexual orientation—**bisexuality** (attracted to both genders), **heterosexuality** (attracted to members of the other

sexual orientation
One's erotic, romantic, and affectional attraction to the same gender, to the opposite gender, or to both.

sexual identity
Inner sense of oneself as a sexual being, including one's identification in terms of gender and sexual orientation.

sexual preference
Term formerly used to describe sexual orientation that is now outdated, because sexual orientation is no longer commonly considered to be a conscious individual preference or choice, but to be formed by a complicated network of factors.

bisexual
One whose erotic, romantic, and affectional attraction is toward both genders.

heterosexual
One whose primary erotic, romantic, and affectional attraction is toward members of the other gender.

homosexual
One whose primary erotic, romantic, and affectional attraction is toward members of one's own gender.

gay
Male or female homosexual. (*Gay* used alone probably refers to a male, though it is acceptable to refer to a *gay female*.)

lesbian
Female homosexual.

situational homosexuality
Homosexual behavior limited to circumstances in which members of the same gender are deprived of contact with the other gender.

gender), and **homosexuality** (attracted to members of the same gender). This term is now outdated because sexual orientation is no longer commonly considered to be one's conscious individual preference or choice; instead, it is thought to be formed by a complicated network of social, cultural, biological, economic, and political factors.

For our purposes, the terms *homosexual* and **gay** are used interchangeably to apply to either males or females. The term **lesbian**, however, applies only to a female homosexual.

The Kinsey Continuum

No clear-cut line separates homosexuality and heterosexuality; in fact, it is more accurate to think of these orientations as being on a continuum. Figure 10.1 shows a seven-point continuum of sexual orientation originally devised by Kinsey. Most of us probably experience varying degrees of sexual orientation; that is, most of us are attracted to both genders, even though we may act in only one way sexually.

The notion of a continuum of sexual orientation helps explain not only differences among people but also a phenomenon known as **situational homosexuality**—that is, sexual behavior limited to specific circumstances in which members of the same gender are generally deprived of contact with the other gender. Homosexual activity in a single-sex school or in a prison, for example, does not necessarily indicate that the individuals involved are primarily homosexual. They may never participate in homosexual activity in other situations, and their orientation may prefer sexual activity with the other gender. However, because people of the other gender are not available to them, and because they prefer sexual activity with another person to masturbation exclusively, they engage in sexual behavior with people of the same gender. You may have participated in sexual activity with someone of the same gender sometime in your life; however, unless you are sexually attracted to people of the same gender, fall in love with people of the same gender, have sexual behaviors with people of the same gender, and identify yourself as a homosexual, you are not classified as a homosexual.

The distinction we wish to make is between specific behavior and one's sexual orientation. A person's engaging in sexual activity with someone of the same gender does not indicate that person is a homosexual; someone's not engaging in sexual activity with the same gender does not indicate that person is not a homosexual. For example, a heterosexual person might engage in

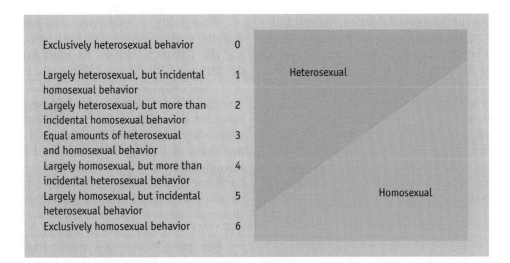

Exclusively heterosexual behavior	0
Largely heterosexual, but incidental homosexual behavior	1
Largely heterosexual, but more than incidental homosexual behavior	2
Equal amounts of heterosexual and homosexual behavior	3
Largely homosexual, but more than incidental heterosexual behavior	4
Largely homosexual, but incidental heterosexual behavior	5
Exclusively homosexual behavior	6

FIGURE 10.1 Kinsey sexual orientation continuum. The Kinsey continuum refers only to homosexual or heterosexual *behavior;* remember that it was developed in the 1950s. If such a continuum were developed today, it would likely refer to erotic, romantic, and affectional attraction, as do our definitions of sexual orientation. It would also probably recognize that a person's behavior and sexual orientation might differ. For example, a person can be heterosexually married, have sexual intercourse with a spouse, and still be a homosexual or a bisexual.

Multicultural DIMENSIONS

Race and Ethnicity and Same-Gender Sexual Behavior

Laumann and associates (1994) reported some differences in the rates of same-gender sexual behavior for people with different racial and ethnic backgrounds in the United States. For example, the proportion of people reporting same-gender sexual behavior since puberty was as follows:

> White = 7.6% of males and 4% of females
> African American = 5.8% of males and 3.5% of females
> Hispanic = 8.8% of males and 3.8% of females
> Asian = no males and 3.3% of females

The same researchers also asked people which sexual behaviors they found "very appealing." The following proportions found sexual activity with a same-gender partner "very appealing":

> White = 3.3% of males and 2.7% of females
> African American = 2.9% of males and 3.5% of females
> Hispanic = 2.9% of males and 4.4% of females
> (Sample sizes for other groups were too small to be meaningful.)

Interestingly, in most cases the proportion of people who find same-gender sexual behavior to be "very appealing" is lower than the proportion who have participated in it. We are not certain of the reason(s) for this, but perhaps some of those who participated were experimenting and learned that the behavior did not appeal to them after all.

---

sexual behavior with a person of the same gender for the purpose of experimentation, or because of a situation such as being in prison or in a single-sex school. This does not mean the person is a homosexual. Or, a homosexual might engage in sexual behavior with a person of the other gender to appear more socially acceptable and/or to hide true homosexual feelings. This does not mean that person is a heterosexual. Sexual orientation is not the same as sexual behavior.

Many of us take our sexual orientation for granted; however, about 11% of junior and senior high school students may not be sure of theirs. Uncertainty about sexual orientation declines with age, from about 26% of 12-year-old students to 5% of 17-year-old students. About 20% of gay and bisexual men surveyed on college campuses knew that they were gay or bisexual in junior high school, and 17% said they knew in grade school. Six percent of gay or bisexual women knew that they were gay or bisexual in junior high school; 11% knew in grade school (Gay, lesbian, and bisexual adolescents, 1998).

Bisexuality

If homosexuality is difficult to define accurately given the Kinsey scale, bisexuality is even more so. A bisexual person has erotic, romantic, and affectional attraction to both genders. Looking only at sexual behavior, Kinsey found that 9% of single 30-year-old women and about 16% of single 30-year-old men could be categorized as bisexual (between the numbers 2 and 4 on Kinsey's scale).

The problem with this categorization, though, is that homosexuality and heterosexuality are more than a matter of behavior, as we have discussed. Consequently, bisexuality can be considered to be a relatively equal erotic, romantic, and affectional attraction to members of both genders, even though an individual may have a favorite attraction or behavior.

Bisexuality is enjoying and engaging in sexual activity with members of both genders or recognizing the desire to do so. As with homosexuality, our definition of bisexuality allows that someone who at one time engaged in bisexual behavior may not be a bisexual, and someone who has never participated in bisexual behavior could be a bisexual. For example, someone may fantasize about sexual relations with members of both genders and find himself or herself attracted to people of both genders but may never have engaged in sexual relations with a same-gender partner. This person may nevertheless be bisexual. Bisexuals are referred to in many ways: as "switch hitters," "AC–DC," or "people who swing both ways."

For people who are really homosexual but are unwilling to acknowledge their sexual orientation even to themselves, bisexuality may be a means of coping. Many of these people eventually accept their homosexuality without the need to mask it with bisexual behavior. Others remain bisexual throughout their lives because their sexual attraction is truly to both genders.

Still others engage in bisexual behavior for a time but sooner or later revert to heterosexuality.

Bisexuals point to the variety that characterizes their sexual relationships. They are able to fully enjoy the sexual pleasures of both males and females and are open to the most erotic of activities. One of the disadvantages of bisexuality, though, is the suspicion it provokes in both the heterosexual and homosexual communities. In one sense, bisexuals are both like and unlike these groups; however, it is often the "unlikeness" that is the focus. Homosexuals view bisexuals as homosexuals who are afraid to admit to their preference. Some homosexuals reject sexual relations with bisexuals for this reason. It seems that lesbians are even more rejecting of bisexual women than are male homosexuals of bisexual men. Some lesbians want bisexual women to declare openly their lesbianism and insist there is no such thing as a true bisexual.

On some college campuses, new student organizations for bisexuals who feel shunned by gay-student support groups are emerging (Morgan, 2002). Interestingly, supporters of the new groups say many of the previous groups established for gay, lesbian, and bisexual students have exhibited the very kinds of intolerance and discrimination they were designed to fight. The name for this behavior is *biphobia*, or antipathy toward those who identify as bisexual. Supposedly, some gay students belittle bisexuality as a "cop-out" to avoid identification as gay. Others say that bisexuals are confused about their real sexual orientation.

In recent years there has been an increase in the number of research studies related to bisexuality. For example, Saewyc et al. (2009) found that bisexual adolescents had lower levels of most protective factors (family connectiveness, school connectiveness, and religious involvement) than did heterosexual adolescents. They suggested that these factors help explain the higher prevalence of risky behavior among the bisexuals.

The Ontario Consultants on Religious Tolerance (2005) summarized the following points about bisexuality:

- Bisexuality may be a difficult concept to comprehend because we are often taught to look at things as a duality: male and female, light and dark, hot and cold, etc. In this case, at least three classifications (and perhaps more) are needed to represent sexual attractions and activities.

- A bisexual is attracted to both males and females, but not necessarily to the same degree.

- Bisexuality describes how people feel, not necessarily how they act.

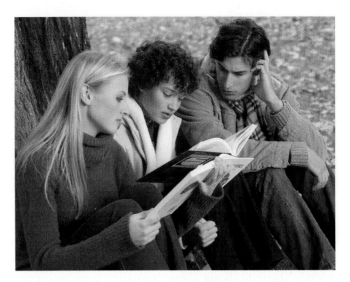

We do not know a person's sexual orientation unless they tell us what it is.

- Misinformation about bisexuality is very prevalent.

- Although it has been said that only 2% of the population is bisexual, research indicated that almost 21% of men and 18% of women admitted to same-gender sexual attraction/behavior at some time in their lives.

- Some people believe that bisexuality is just a phase. While this may be true for some people, others regard themselves bisexual throughout their lives.

- It has been said that bisexuals are only satisfied if they have sexual partners of both genders. This is not true because bisexuals do not necessarily act on their feelings of attraction.

- Some openly bisexual individuals may be subjected to prejudice from the homosexual community as well as the heterosexual community. However, this seems to be decreasing.

Asexuality

Asexuality has seldom been discussed, but more attention has been given to it in recent years. For example, the Asexual Visibility and Education Network (AVEN) was founded in 2001 with two distinct goals: creating public acceptance and discussion of asexuality, and facilitating the growth of an asexual community. It has thousands of members and can be reached at *www.asexuality.org*. According to the AVEN web site, asexual people have the same emotional needs as anyone else. Many asexual people experience attraction, but feel no need to act out that attraction sexually. Because they don't see a lack of sexual arousal as a problem to be corrected, asexual people focus their energy on enjoying other types of arousal and pleasure.

Barnes (2005) summarized some interesting points about asexuals. He indicated that asexuality isn't celibacy—the refusal to act on attraction. It is the absence of sexual attraction. Asexuals insist that theirs is a valid fourth orientation, like straight, bisexual, and gay orientations. There is nothing wrong, they say; it is simply the way they were born and they are not interested in sexual activity. Many asexuals form deep emotional bonds that they define as "romantic"—resembling those commonly understood as coupledom, except for a lack of sexual behavior. As one asexual said: "In early high school all of my friends started talking about how they were attracted to people, who they had crushes on, and I just didn't understand why sexuality was such a big deal for everyone else."

Statistically speaking, according to Barnes, there may be as many as 4.5 million Americans who are asexual. A study in Britain indicated that more than 1% of the population agreed with the statement, "I have never felt sexually attracted to anyone at all." Many experts agree that motivation to engage in sexual intimacy is a dimension that runs from zero to extremely high; thus there are probably some people at that zero end. Asexuality seems to exist in the animal world as well.

Homosexuality in the Population

It is hard to know exactly how many homosexuals live in U.S. society; most still choose to keep their sexual orientation hidden. Estimates of how many people identify as lesbian, gay, or bisexual vary widely, and there is not a lot of research on the subject. According to SIECUS (2009b), approximately 90.2% of males aged 18–44 identify as heterosexual, 2.3% identify as homosexual, 1.8% identify as bisexual, and 3.9% identify as "something else." Among females aged 18–44, 90.3% identify as heterosexual, 1.3% identify as homosexual, 2.8% identify as bisexual, and 4% identify as "something else." However, some differences arise when people are asked who they are attracted to. For example, 92.2% of males aged 18–44 report being attracted only to females, 3.9% report being attracted mostly to females, 1.7% report being attracted mostly to males, 1.5% report being attracted only to males, 1.0% report being attracted to both males and females, and 0.7% are not sure who they are attracted to. Among females aged 18–44, 85.8% report being attracted only to males, 10.2% report being attracted mostly to males, 1.9% report being attracted to both males

and females, 0.8% report being attracted mostly to females, 0.7% report being attracted only to females, and 0.8% are not sure who they are attracted to. Finally, 6% of males aged 15–44 report ever having anal or oral sexual activity with another male, and 4.5% of males ages 15–19 report having done so. Among females, 11.2% of females aged 15–44 report having sexual experience of any kind with another female. Among females aged 15–19, 10.6% report having done so. Note that the question asked of males was of more limited scope, so in this last instance the male and female numbers cannot be directly compared to each other.

In addition to the number of homosexuals who hide their orientation and the difficulty of defining exactly who is included on Kinsey's continuum, another reason for the disparity in the estimated number of homosexuals relates to political implications. For example, those lobbying for greater gay rights need to show that large numbers of people are affected by this issue. If they can demonstrate political clout—that is, a large voting bloc—they can convince politicians to support their causes. That support can translate into legislation that assures gays the rights and privileges they feel have long been denied to them. However, it is in the interest of those opposed to gay rights for these estimates to be lower, because such lower numbers would marginalize gay people. That is one reason why some gay rights organizations estimate that 10% of the population is homosexual and others use a much lower figure.

Same-gender couples head nearly 600,000 homes in the United States, according to census data considered the federal government's most thorough count yet of homosexuals (Census shows nearly 600,000 same-sex couple homes, 2001). A gay or lesbian couple heads a household

You cannot tell a person's sexual orientation just by their appearance.

in nearly every county in America. Sixteen percent of the same-gender couple homes are in California, 8% in New York, and 7% in Texas. However, such living arrangements still make up a tiny share of the nation's households—just over 0.005% of the 105.5 million U.S. homes. The results also dispel stereotypes that homosexuality is limited to large urban areas and college towns.

Heterosexuality in the Population

Regardless of the exact numbers of homosexuals and bisexuals in U.S. society, it is safe to assume that the sexual orientation of most people is heterosexual. As was seen in the statistics presented in the previous section, more than 90% of both males and females identify as being heterosexual. Because of this, some heterosexuals may have a difficult time understanding and supporting the need for equal rights and opportunities for people with different sexual orientations. Some heterosexuals may even be guilty of heterosexism, which means they think about human experience only in heterosexual terms and ignore or put down homosexual behaviors. They also may stereotype homosexuals in a negative manner and view them as dangerous to others.

While many people have wondered about the developmental process of those who do not identify themselves as heterosexuals, only in recent years have some researchers focused more on how heterosexuals develop their sexual orientation identities. For example, Worthington et al. (2002) indicated that heterosexual development encompasses the following six important dimensions to be accomplished over time:

1. Identification and awareness of one's sexual needs, as determined by sexual orientation.

2. Adoption of personal values related to sexual behavior and sexuality in general.

3. Awareness of which sexual activities are preferred.

4. Awareness of the specific characteristics that are preferred in sexual partners.

5. Awareness of preferred modes of sexual expression.

6. Recognition of one's sexual orientation and personal identification with that orientation.

People with a heterosexual orientation seem to go through some rather predictable developmental states as they integrate their sexual orientation into

their personalities. Early in life, they realize their heterosexual orientation but have not yet acted on it sexually. This stage is termed *unexplored commitment* to being heterosexual. They may then enter into an *active exploration* phase, where they intentionally try out numerous sexual ideas and fantasies, and often engage in sexual activities with members of the other gender. This helps them clarify which activities and partners they prefer. Some people experience *diffusion*, which may involve sexual exploration, but with less intentionality and goal direction than active exploration. After some exploration along with maturation, heterosexuals enter into the stage of *deepening and commitment*, which is characterized by more intimacy and loving feelings in relationships. People can move through these stages at various times, but the final status of heterosexual identity is *synthesis*, in which the various elements of identity, group membership, and attitudes toward sexual minorities have achieved congruence and meaning in the person, though this may be a difficult status to achieve. All of this helps to explain how heterosexual people gradually integrate their sexual orientation into their sense of self (Hoffman, 2004; Worthington et al., 2002).

■ Theories of Sexual Orientation

Although many studies have been done on the subject, no one knows exactly which factors shape sexual orientation. Some argue that biological factors account for a homosexual, heterosexual, or bisexual orientation. Others claim that psychological factors or learned behavior is responsible. Determining an accurate method for defining and identifying sexual orientation for the purpose of constructing representative samples of homosexuals, bisexuals, and heterosexuals is a goal of researchers. Different definitions and measures have been used to develop samples since the 1860s, when the topic of sexual orientation first attracted widespread research interest. If advances in the understanding of sexual orientations are to be made, it is critical that definitions and measures of sexual orientation be standardized.

Because the vast majority of people are heterosexuals, most theories about sexual orientation relate to homosexuality or bisexuality. It is as though heterosexuality is the "norm" and homosexuality and bisexuality are indications that something went wrong. These theories are described in the following paragraphs.

Biological Theories

Biological theories of the development of homosexuality include genetic factors and hormonal factors.

The Genetic Theory

The genetic theory of the cause of homosexuality states that something in a person's genes causes that person to be sexually attracted to members of the same sex. The most frequently cited evidence for this view is the study by Kallman (1952). Kallman studied twins (both fraternal and identical) who grew up in the same home. Fraternal twins do not share an exact genetic inheritance, whereas identical twins do share the same genetic material (they occupied the same ovum). Consequently, the environments are the same for both sets of twins, but the difference is in the genetic makeup. Kallman found identical twins had a 95% concordance rate (both twins were homosexual) compared to a 12% concordance rate for fraternal twins. He concluded that homosexuality is a function of genetic predisposition. Whitman and Diamond (1986) reported a concordance rate of 75% for identical twins and a 19% rate for fraternal twins, thereby supporting the genetic theory. However, numerous other studies over the years (Heston & Shields, 1968; Zuger, 1976) have not been able to verify Kallman's findings. Furthermore, Kallman's selection of twins for his studies was criticized. He chose twins from prisons, psychiatric settings, and charitable organizations, thereby restricting the ability to generalize his results to twins living in more typical situations.

Bailey and Pillard (1991) also studied twins. They looked at identical twins, fraternal twins, and adopted brothers, among whom one of each pair had declared himself to be a homosexual. They found that the more genetically similar each was to his gay brother, the more likely he was to be gay as well. Homosexuality was found in the remaining member of each pair in 52% of the identical twins (who developed from the

Twins have been used in research to look at theories about the cause of sexual orientation.

same ovum), 22% of the fraternal twins (who developed from different ova), and only 11% of the adopted brothers (who shared no common genetic material). The researchers estimated that between 30% and 70% of the determining factors of homosexuality are genetic. However, questions remain: Even if 70% is genetic, what accounts for the other 30%? What role do prenatal hormonal secretions play? What role does environment play once the child is born?

Several studies have supported the idea of a genetic connection to homosexuality. For example, Hamer and associates (1993) studied genetic material from 40 pairs of gay brothers and found identical pieces of the end tip of the X chromosome to a much greater degree than would have been anticipated. They concluded that there may be one or more

Gender DIMENSIONS

Gay–Straight Alliances and Gender Activism

A descriptive case study was conducted within the GSA (Gay–Straight Alliance) Network, a youth-based community organization in the San Francisco Bay Area that provides leadership and networking opportunities for youth in GSA clubs throughout California. Activism focused on sexuality identity and rights is a controversial topic. Nevertheless, an increasing number of localities are passing antidiscrimination legislation protecting youth based on sexual identity and expression. Antidiscrimination policies necessitate grounded, comprehensive educa-

tion and outreach strategies. The priority is to ensure that all youth remain safe from violence, harassment, and discrimination within schools. Many youth activists' efforts center on educating school communities toward a broader understanding of the diverse ways that all people live their gendered and sexual lives. They are focused on building a community based on difference rather than defining themselves and advocating based on a single group identity.

Source: Schindel, J. Gender 101—Beyond the binary: Gay–straight alliances and gender activism. *Sexual Research & Social Policy, 5, no. 2* (June 2008), 56–70.

Did You Know...

In *Biological Exuberance* (St. Martin's Press, 1990), the linguist and cognitive scientist Bruce Bagemihl attempts to dispel the myth that humans are the only species who practice homosexuality. In fact, he found that homosexual activity has been documented in more than 20% of the 2,000 species whose sexual activity has been observed. The following are a few examples discussed in his book:

- Male giraffes wrap their necks together until both are sexually aroused.

- Homosexual activities account for 50% of sexual activity among bonobos (chimplike apes).
- A male greylag goose may pair with another male goose for 15 years.

Source: Kluger, J. The gay side of nature, *Time, 153, no. 16* (April 26, 1999), 70.

genes that play a role in predisposing some men to homosexuality.

Many researchers feel that the most promising support for a biological reason for sexual orientation comes from genetic studies. There is a great deal of evidence that gay male and lesbian sexual orientations run in families (Bailey et al., 2000; Dawood et al., 2000; Kendler et al., 2000).

Sexuality experts do caution that a specific gene linked to homosexuality has not been identified. Also, because of the complexity of sexual orientation, it is likely that a possible genetic link is only part of the picture.

McGuire (1995) indicates that genetic analysis of behavioral differences among humans requires both careful experimental design and appropriate genetic models. He believes that all studies of the genetic basis of sexual orientation of men and women have failed to meet one or more of the criteria for such a research study—valid and precise measures, appropriate methods, randomly selected subjects, appropriate sample sizes, and appropriate genetic models.

Demir and Dickson (2005) reported on an interesting genetic study with fruit flies. They showed that a single gene in a fruit fly is sufficient to determine all aspects of the fly's sexual orientation and behavior. This means that instinctive behavior can be specified by genetic programs. However, it is not yet clear if there is a similar master gene for humans.

The Hormonal Theory

The hormonal theory of the cause of homosexuality states that homosexuality is a result of hormonal imbalances that occur before or after birth. Because it is known that prenatal hormonal treatment in animals can lead to different male and female behavior patterns (Dorner, 1968; Hutchinson, 1978; Money & Ehrhardt, 1972), some theorists have concluded that these same conditions might cause homosexuality.

Evidence for this view can be found in the work of several researchers. For instance, Dorner and associates (1975) studied the responses of homosexuals and heterosexuals to injections of the hormone estrogen and found these responses to differ. Furthermore, Gladue and colleagues (1983) found that when homosexual men were administered estrogen, their patterns of secretion of luteinizing hormone (LH) changed to be more like those of heterosexual women; in addition, their testosterone levels remained lower for a longer time than did heterosexual men's when both groups were administered estrogen. Studies have also found that a prenatal excess of androgen in females is associated with a greater incidence of lesbianism (Ehrhardt, Evers, & Money, 1968; Money & Schwartz, 1977) and that a prenatal deficiency in androgen production in males is associated with an increased incidence of male homosexuality.

One research project tentatively identified prenatal exposure to the synthetic estrogen diethylstilbestrol (DES) as predisposing female offspring to lesbianism (Ehrhardt et al., 1985). Another researcher alleges the existence of anatomical differences in the size of parts of the brains of homosexual and heterosexual men (LeVay, 1991). Yet another researcher has pointed out that there is little evidence supporting the hormonal theories and that sexual orientation is more likely determined by other personal and cultural factors (Doell, 1995).

Savic et al. (2005) reported that gay men do not respond to the smell of bodily chemicals the same way that straight men do. Previously, they had isolated bodily chemicals from both males and females. When women smelled the male chemicals, their hypothalamuses "lit up," but they had no reactions to the female chemicals. In men, the results were exactly the opposite. Then the researchers included gay men in the study. When gay men were exposed to the smell of male chemicals, their hypothalamuses lit up just like a woman's. The smell of female chemicals did nothing for them. However, this study doesn't show that sexual orientation is biologically hardwired from birth. It could also be that the brains of gay men learn to respond to the smells over time and with experience.

As is the case with the genetic theories, there are problems in research on the hormonal causation of sexual orientation. There is no convincing evidence that sexual orientation is the result of either prenatal or postnatal hormonal imbalances, or that homosexuality causes these imbalances. However, research continues in this area.

Psychological Theories

Psychological theories of the development of sexual orientation consider psychoanalytical factors and the influence of learned behavior. Although these theories were historically believed, they have not been proved valid. Today many experts do not support these theories.

The Psychoanalytical Theory

Psychoanalytical theories of the cause of sexual orientation relate to parental and family characteristics. Sigmund Freud postulated that everyone is born with the potential to be bisexual. Whether someone becomes heterosexual or homosexual is, Freud believed, a result of circumstances that affect the child's psychosexual development. For example, if a young boy is unable to resolve the Oedipal complex (an attraction for his mother) satisfactorily and becomes "fixated" at this phase of psychosexual development, he may become homosexual; or if the boy continues to fear castration ("castration complex"), he may grow up to be homosexual.

Irving Bieber and colleagues (1962) fueled this view of the influence of family background when they compared the family backgrounds of 106 homosexual men and 100 heterosexual men and found differences. Specifically, Bieber found that homosexual men more often had overprotective and dominant mothers and weak, passive, and detached fathers than did heterosexual men. Bieber hypothesized that this family upbringing made men homosexual because they were fearful of interacting with women and unable to identify with their father. The problem with Bieber's study was the manner in which he acquired his sample of homosexual men. Because there is a social stigma associated with homosexuality, thereby making many homosexuals unwilling to admit to their preference, it has often been difficult to find gay men and women to study. Consequently, homosexual samples have in the past too frequently been obtained from either psychiatric settings (patient populations), prisons, or the military. The

Some experts argue that family relationships influence sexual orientation.

ability, therefore, to generalize these results to socially functional homosexuals is suspect. Bieber's sample was obtained from patients undergoing psychoanalysis. As Clark and Epstein (1969, 575) state:

> One does not go into prisons and mental hospitals or clinics to study normal heterosexuality and then generalize to the population at large; therefore, to do so with homosexuals, as has been done so often in past research dealing with this area, is to study a sample already selectively loaded with psychopathology which may not be truly representative of the whole homosexual population.

On the one hand, evidence supporting Bieber's theory exists in the larger-than-usual population of homosexuals who have such family characteristics. On the other hand, there are many heterosexuals who grew up in similar households but never became homosexual. Clearly this theory remains just that—a theory.

The Learned Behavior Theory

Behaviorists believe that homosexuality is the result of situations experienced usually early in childhood and reinforced throughout one's life. For example, someone may experience an unsuccessful and unsatisfying heterosexual relationship that leads him or her to experiment with homosexuality, with which the person finds satisfaction. The attitude of many people is that "if they only had an effective lover, they'd never be homosexual." Others believe homosexuals are physically unattractive to the opposite sex, so their only sexual outlet is someone of the same sex. Dew (1985) found that many college students had this view. Others believe that an early

Ethical
DIMENSIONS

Research on Causes of Homosexuality

As can be seen from information presented in this chapter, many researchers are interested in what determines sexual orientation or, perhaps for some, what causes homosexuality. They would argue that it is important to know which factors determine sexual orientation because if causes are known, then sexual orientation could be influenced in whatever way might be desired.

Others argue that research into the cause(s) of homosexuality is unethical and should not be undertaken because it assumes more often than not that homosexuality is a form of mental illness or an undesirable deviance from the heterosexual norm, which should be cured (Schuklenk & Ristow, 1996).

Do you think research about the causes of sexual orientation (or homosexuality) is ethical or unethical?

childhood homosexual experience "recruits" people to homosexuality.

Studies are not supportive of these viewpoints. Homosexuals do not differ from heterosexuals in terms of their frequency of dating in high school, nor are they seduced into homosexuality as children (Bell, Weinberg, & Hammersmith, 1981), and they often report having had sexual experience with people of the opposite sex (Klach, 1974; Martin & Lyon, 1972). As with the other theories, the learned behavior theory demands further investigation before it can be supported.

Recently some researchers have argued that we have no business trying to determine the cause of homosexuality until we are able to determine what causes any form of sexual orientation. In other words, we are what we are; why we have certain sexual orientations might be scientifically interesting, but it has very little practical significance. Whether or not you accept this type of reasoning, the fact is that we still do not know why some people are homosexual and others heterosexual.

Integrated Theories

The integrated theory of the development of sexuality—homosexuality is just one form—argues that physical, psychological, and learned factors are involved. A good explanation of this view has been offered by the renowned endocrinologist John Money (1987). Money describes societies in which homosexuality is a precursor of heterosexuality. For example, in the large area in the Pacific between Sumatra through Papua New Guinea and Melanesia, homosexuality is institutionalized. Males between the ages of 9 and 19 years move out of their families' homes into the long-houses in the center of the village. There they engage regularly in homosexual activity until they reach marriage age (19 years). After marriage, homosexual activity stops or is kept

to a minimum. Likewise, the Sambian people in the eastern part of New Guinea require a boy just before puberty to give up his mother's milk for the "milk" (semen) of men. That is the only way the boy can grow and mature into a man. In fact, omission of this phase would stigmatize the man as deviant, rather than stigmatizing him as deviant for participating, as it might in American culture.

In the examples cited, homosexuality is a part of society and is learned behavior. Still, there is evidence presented by integrated theorists of the biological aspects of homosexuality. Experiments on certain animals have shown that the brain can develop in contrast to the body's form and structure. In one such study, pregnant lambs were injected with testosterone at a critical point in the pregnancy, and the resulting ewe was homosexual. That is, its brain was masculinized and it acted exactly as a ram acts in its mating and urinating behaviors. However, it possessed ovaries that secreted estrogen.

Integrationists, then, conclude that the prenatal influence on sexuality is important but that it plays out in a social context. Therefore, sexuality (heterosexuality, bisexuality, and homosexuality) is a function of the interaction of all of these factors: biology, hormones, cultural expectations, learned behavior, and psychological variables.

No single scientific theory about what causes sexual orientation has been substantiated. Studies to associate orientation exclusively with genetic, hormonal, or environmental factors have so far been inconclusive.

Effect of School Environment

Something not often considered related to sexual orientation is the environment found in educational institutions. For example, how do teachers deal with the topic of sexual orientation or with students with

Myth vs Fact

Myth: A homosexual can be easily recognized as being different from heterosexuals.
Fact: Only a small proportion of homosexuals are what can be termed "visible homosexuals." The vast majority look and act just as everyone else does and differ only in their sexual orientation.

Myth: Gay men really want to be women and lesbians really desire to be men.

Fact: Most homosexuals are perfectly happy with their gender; they just prefer relationships with someone of the same gender.

Myth: Homosexual males are effeminate and weak, and homosexual females are masculine and physically strong.
Fact: Sexual orientation has nothing to do with one's body type or style of movement, nor does body type dictate sexual orientation.

various sexual orientations? How do heterosexual peers treat gays, lesbians, and bisexuals?

Harris (1997) claimed that schools, especially junior high schools and high schools, are failing to accept gay, lesbian, and bisexual youths equally and teach acceptance to fellow students and faculty. She indicated a need for better role models in the career development of lesbian and gay youth, the importance of incorporation of the topic of homosexuality in the curriculum, and the need for open discussions about gay and lesbian issues at school.

Two men, Benjie Nycum and Mike Glatze, began traveling the country in 2001 to help promote positive self-image and a sense of belonging for gay youth. They have a web site called "Young Gay America" that they support with earnings from their day jobs. They provide safe sex information on the web site, post poems and essays from readers, and spend hours each night answering emails asking for advice. In addition, there are more than 2,000 gay–straight alliances in schools in the United States that can help create the integration that is so crucial for gay kids "feeling a sense of belonging" (Lotozo, 2003).

Although not all sexual minority youth experience difficulties, a number of issues frequently confront students who begin to perceive themselves as gay or lesbian. These include identity conflict, feelings of isolation and stigmatization, peer relationship problems, and family disruptions (Marinoble, 1998). Because awareness of a homosexual sexual orientation sometimes occurs quite early in life, it is vital that school personnel at all levels be active and informed in addressing this topic.

Fontaine (1998) pointed out that gay adolescents face the same developmental challenges as their heterosexual counterparts, with the added burden of attempting to incorporate a stigmatized sexual identity with little support from school personnel.

Teachers either avoid the topic of homosexuality or, when discussing it, frequently present it in a negative manner.

Ryan and Futterman (2001) pointed out that although the vast majority of lesbian and gay youth become well-adjusted adults who lead satisfying, productive lives, their additional developmental challenges require a range of coping skills and adaptation. Unfortunately, unlike most of their heterosexual peers, they have no built-in support system. They must learn to identify, explore, and ultimately integrate a positive adult identity despite persistent negative stereotypes of lesbian and gay people. They also must learn to protect themselves from ridicule, verbal and physical abuse, and exposure. The social and emotional isolation experienced by gay and lesbian youth is a unique stressor that increases risk for a range of health problems.

Russell (2001) added support to this idea by indicating that gay and lesbian youth have more threats of violence as well as experiences of violence, have substance use and abuse rates well above the national average, and have a higher risk of thinking about and attempting suicide. In addition, Sadowski (2001) indicates that verbal, physical, and sexual harassment of gay and lesbian students is widespread in U.S. schools and that many teachers and administrators do not deal effectively with such incidents.

Staley and coworkers (2001) indicated that the individual consequences of living as an openly gay person can be profound—rejection by family and friends, physical violence and verbal abuse, insensitive health and social services, loss of jobs or housing, and lack of protection under the law. Homosexual boys are more likely than heterosexual boys to report poor body image, binge eating, and suicide attempts.

Homosexual students face extra adjustment challenges in schools.

Frankowski (2004) and the Committee on Adolescence of the American Academy of Pediatrics pointed out that young people are recognizing their sexual orientation earlier than in the past. Nonheterosexual youth are at higher risk of dropping out of school, being kicked out of their homes, and turning to life on the streets for survival. Some of them engage in substance abuse, and they are more likely than their heterosexual peers to start using tobacco, alcohol, and illegal drugs at an earlier age. They are more likely to have had sexual intercourse, to have had more partners, and to have experienced sexual intercourse against their will. This puts them at increased risk of STIs, including HIV infection. They are also more likely to attempt suicide and be victimized. High levels of stress and lack of family support are also common.

Lesbian, gay, and bisexual (LGB) youth have a higher risk of suicidal behavior. They are nearly 1.5 to 3 times more likely to report thinking about suicide than non-LGB youth. They are nearly 1.5 to 7 times more likely to report actually attempting suicide. It is also likely that LGB youth experience higher rates of suicide deaths than their non-LGB peers, though it is difficult to know for sure because most mortality data do not include sexual orientation. Risk and protective factors do help explain suicidal behavior, however, and LGB youth generally have more risk factors and fewer protective factors than heterosexual youth. For example, LGB youth often lack important protective factors such as family support and safe schools, and more LGB young people appear to experience depression and substance abuse (Suicide Prevention Resource Center, 2008).

An additional relationship not often heard about is that LGB teens are at a higher risk of becoming pregnant or causing a pregnancy than their heterosexual peers. This is apparently because the discrimination, sexual abuse, and harassment these teens face prompt them to indulge in more sexually risky behavior, such as having sexual intercourse without using condoms, starting to have sexual intercourse before the age of 14, or having multiple sexual partners. Girls who describe themselves as lesbians or bisexuals are 2 to 2.5 times more likely to become pregnant at least once than are heterosexual girls. Males who describe themselves as bisexual or gay are 3 to 4 times more likely than heterosexual males to impregnate a girl. LGB teens may have sexual intercourse with members of the other gender for a variety of reasons. Some engage in this behavior to hide or to deflect the abuse they see inflicted on LGB teens. Others may have been told they are abnormal and wrong, so they may feel that "If I just have sexual intercourse with enough other-gender people, it will cure me" (Saewyc et al., 2008).

More and more universities are signaling to prospective students that they have gay-friendly campuses. For example, in 2003 Stanford University gave every freshman a CD highlighting the campus's gay and lesbian resources, including its community center. San Jose State University regularly features gay and lesbian people in its brochures. Several forces are driving the growing momentum to make gay students feel welcome. Students are coming out earlier and are searching for colleges where they will find social acceptance. As the gay population increases its visibility, students and scholars are demanding the same outreach efforts that ethnic groups and women fought for years ago. Also, school admissions staff are realizing that homosexual students represent an important demographic that should be reached in some way (Vo, 2003).

Lesbian, gay, and bisexual educators sometimes choose to "come out" or publicly reveal their sexual orientation. Waldo and Kemp (1997) investigated the effect of a gay instructor's coming out on his students' attitudes toward lesbians and gay men. A survey was administered to students at the beginning and the end of a semester. Midway through the semester, the gay instructor disclosed his sexual orientation to his students as part of a lesson on sexual orientation. Students in his section demonstrated improved attitudes, while students in a heterosexual professor's class showed no change in attitudes. It appears that a gay instructor's coming out may positively affect his students' attitudes toward lesbian, gay, and bisexual people. However, these efforts by individual instructors are only a small part of the more comprehensive institutional efforts needed to create a healthier climate for the appreciation of sexual diversity.

Archibald (2005) reported that a pro-gay group (Parents, Families and Friends of Lesbians and Gays) presented a workshop at the national PTA convention designed to get teachers and administrators to support gay, lesbian, bisexual, and transgender students in their identity. Presenters pointed out that these students do not feel safe in schools, and they need champions to help them. Goals of the workshop included developing support for diversity and intervening to prevent harassment of sexual-minority students. Attendees at the packed workshop largely supported the presentation, but some said, "I don't know why you need to teach this in schools."

School personnel need to be familiar with legal matters related to sexual orientation. Here are some examples (Student sexuality: How can and should schools respond?, 2004):

- Like all other students, lesbian, gay, bisexual, and transgender (LGBT) students are guaranteed equal protection under the Fourteenth Amendment to the Constitution and

Myth vs Fact

Myth: Homosexuals want to seduce children into a life of homosexuality.
Fact: Although some homosexuals seduce children, most sexual abuse of children is committed by heterosexuals. Both situations are intolerable, but to blame homosexuals alone for the sexual abuse of children is wrong.

Myth: Homosexuals should not be teachers.
Fact: It would be clearly wrong for a teacher of any sexual orientation to seduce students or to encourage them to adopt a particular sexual lifestyle, but there is no reason to expect such behavior to be more or less prevalent among homosexuals.

Myth: Homosexuals are suffering from a mental illness.
Fact: When homosexuals and heterosexuals are matched by age, IQ, and education, mental health experts cannot find differences in adjustment between the two groups.

Myth: Homosexuals are poor security risks.
Fact: There may have been some foundation for this belief in the past because homosexuals were easy targets for blackmail; however, as society grows less homophobic and as many homosexuals identify themselves publicly, the supposed risk should evaporate.

free speech and association under the First Amendment.

- The Equal Access Act requires schools to treat student clubs that address LGBT issues the same as other student groups.

- A school cannot refuse to allow a group such as a gay–straight alliance to meet because other students, teachers, administrators, parents, or community members object to the formation of the club.

- To be covered by the Equal Access Act, student clubs must be "student initiated." Outside community members may not direct, control, or regularly attend activities of student groups.

There have been attempts at helping homosexual students do better in schools by having a more positive environment for them. For example, in the San Francisco Unified School district there is a LGBTQ (lesbian, gay, bisexual, transgender, or questioning) liaison in place in every school that handles individual student concerns. The program helps to promote students' acceptance of one another. The Milwaukee high school called Alliance (started in 2005) and the Harvey Milk High School in New York City (started in 2003) are both intended specifically for LGBTQ students. Both schools were started to give these youths the chance to attend a public school populated by students like themselves and an environment in

which their differences are welcomed. These schools provide much safer environments for the students, but they also reawaken the debate about school segregation (Calefati, 2009).

It can be helpful for parents and teachers to talk about sexual orientation with school-age children. Here are some examples of important messages for young people of various ages (Why it's important to talk about sexual orientation, 2004):

Messages for young people age 5–8 include:

- Human beings can love people of the same gender and people of the other gender.
- There are men and women who are homosexual, which means they can be attracted to and fall in love with someone of the same gender.

Messages for young people age 9–12 include:

- Sexual orientation is one part of who we are.
- Gay, lesbian, or bisexual people's relationships can be as fulfilling as heterosexual people's relationships.

Messages for young people age 12–15 include:

- People do not choose their sexual orientation.
- Having discussions about sexual orientation can be difficult for some people.

Messages for young people age 15–18 include:

- The understanding and identification of one's sexual orientation may change over the course of that person's lifetime.
- Civil rights for gay, lesbian, bisexual, and transgender people are being debated in many places across the United States.

Homosexual Life

As we grow and develop, many challenges confront us regardless of our sexual orientation. Typically homosexuals are happy, well-balanced people just like anyone else. They basically enjoy the same activities as other people, have similar goals in life, and in recent years have been able to enjoy parenthood through adoption or, for some lesbians, through artificial insemination. This is not often the picture that heterosexuals get, however, because it is more commonly problematic behavior that is seen. For example, happy, healthy homosexuals do not seek psychotherapy more often than happy, healthy heterosexuals do; but we often tend to generalize about all homosexuals from those few who do seek help. If we did the same thing with heterosexuals, we would have a very skewed picture of what heterosexuals are really like.

Many homosexuals, however, are more likely to experience certain kinds of challenges than are heterosexuals. Gay, lesbian, and bisexual youth must cope with prejudiced, discriminatory, and violent behavior and messages in their families, schools, and communities. These often result in isolation, fear of stigmatization, and lack of peer or familial support (*Just the facts about sexual orientation and youth,* 2000).

An interesting case of discrimination was reported by Young (2002). A Christian group at Central College in Iowa forced one of its student leaders to give up his position as president of the InterVarsity Christian Fellowship because he would not disavow his homosexuality. The same person was also president of the student government at the college. Leaders of InterVarsity asked him to resign his leadership position because he would not agree to a statement that the only acceptable form of sexual activity is that of a man and a woman who are married. This led to a debate at the college about whether the InterVarsity Christian Fellowship should continue to be recognized on the campus.

One development on some college campuses has been the establishment of fraternities for gay students. The University of South Alabama, Kent State University, and Florida International University (FIU) are among the universities that have them. At FIU the Gamma Lambda Mu men took great pains to spell out the precise limits of their bonding. Their bylaws state that brothers may not date one another. They want to prove to their classmates that gay men can join together in the spirit of service and camaraderie and not for sexual activity. Gay and lesbian groups have gained acceptance on most college campuses, but entry into the Greek system has been much slower (DeQuine, 2003).

Alan Bell and Martin Weinberg (1978) studied the lifestyle of homosexuals and concluded that a more appropriate term than *homosexuality* would be *homosexualities.* They found that homosexual relationships could be categorized as (1) *closed couples* living together in committed, stable relationships; (2) *open couples* living together with less emotional involvement and having intercourse outside the relationship; (3) *functionals,* sexually active people uncommitted to any partner; (4) *dysfunctionals,* sexually active people with sexual problems who are dissatisfied with their sexual orientation; and (5) *asexuals,* those unhappy about being homosexual and less active sexually.

An increasing number of gays seek marriage, even though these marriages are not usually legally recognized. Some lawmakers simply ignore the issue, and others have gone out of their way to institute laws prohibiting gay marriages. Sometimes homosexuals

decide to have a marriage ceremony even though it may not be legally recognized. This can lead to other interesting issues. We will discuss more about this and other legal issues later in this chapter.

Reform Jewish rabbis have the option of presiding at gay commitment ceremonies. In approving this option, Jewish leaders said, "It is not sinful to be a gay and lesbian," and "Gay and lesbian Jews, and the committed relationships they form with their partners, deserve the recognition and respect due to people created in the image of God" (Thompson, 2000). Except that both people are of the same gender, the marriages usually resemble heterosexual ones in every way.

The Social Scene

In the United States the homosexual subculture centers on private clubs, homosexual bars, and homophile organizations. These organizations are designed to help protect homosexuals, promote their rights, promote a positive image of the gay lifestyle, and help the general public better understand homosexuality. Clubs, bars, and organizations give homosexuals opportunities to fraternize with other gays and perhaps develop social and/or intimate relationships.

Gay bars are most often cocktail lounges that cater to either male or female homosexuals, but usually not to both. They are places where dancing and socializing occur. Other than their clientele, gay bars are not very different from typical heterosexual bars.

Since the AIDS scare, gay baths attended by gay men are less popular, and many localities have actually passed legislation defining them as health hazards and outlawing them. This is because sexual activity with a stranger has been identified as a high-risk activity for HIV transmission. However, where they are legal, many gays still attend these facilities. The baths usually are dimly lit, with many rooms for dancing and socializing. The typical bath visit involves checking one's clothes on entering, being issued a towel, and finding a partner who is willing to have sexual activity in one of the private rooms or in the "orgy" room. Homosexuals seeking impersonal sexual activity can find it at the baths.

Another place where some homosexual men meet to find a sexual partner is in public restrooms. Sexual activity in public toilets, known as "tearooms," has long been a significant and controversial part of gay culture. Concern increased on many college campuses when a web site that listed popular places for sexual activity between men, including bathrooms at dozens of colleges nationwide, was discovered (Hoover, 2003). Some college police conducted undercover stings and routinely questioned men who appeared to

DIMENSIONS

Attitudes About Homosexuality in Other Countries

Significant differences exist between the homosexual behaviors of Mexican males in Mexico and those of middle-class Anglo males in the United States. Most Mexican homosexual males appear to have strong preferences for playing either the anal insertive or the anal receptive sexual role, but not both. Although they may engage in fellatio, anal intercourse provides the ultimate sexual satisfaction.

In Mexico there is a widely held belief that feminine males prefer to play the female (receptive) role. The link between effeminacy and homosexuality also results in a belief that as a result of this role preference feminine males are sexually interested only in masculine males with whom they play the passive sexual role.

One effect of homosexual role playing in Mexico is that only the feminine male is labeled as a "homosexual." The masculine self-image of Mexican males is not threatened by their homosexual behavior as long as they play the anal insertive role and also have a reputation for having sexual relations with women.

Compared to Mexican males, Anglo males are generally believed not to have a strongly developed preference for playing one sexual role over the other, and not necessarily to look on anal intercourse as the preferred or ultimate technique in homosexual sexual encounters. It seems unusual for Anglo males to adhere in the United States to a particular role, and fellatio is the most frequently practiced sexual technique.

In China, all major religions have codes that have been traditionally interpreted as being against homosexuality. At the same time, none of the major religions condemns homosexuality as a sin. Sodomy was decriminalized in 1997. Homosexuality was removed from the *Chinese Classification and Diagnostic Criteria of Mental Disorders* in 2001. Surveys show that Chinese people are becoming more tolerant toward homosexuality, and gay bashing is rare. However, some people complain that the government is indifferent and does nothing to improve the situation for homosexuals. Many cases show that gays still have to endure prejudice from the justice system and harassment from police. Same-gender marriage is still forbidden in China (Homosexuality in China, 2005).

Homosexuality has never been viewed as a sin in Japanese society and religion, and there is no specific legal prohibition. It is still true that sexual activity is not viewed in terms of morality, but rather in terms of pleasure. Gay male content is common in romantic literature, but lesbian content is much less widespread (Homosexuality in Japan, 2005).

Other examples of attitudes about homosexuality include the following (Breaking the cultural straitjacket, 2005):

- In Nigeria, homosexuality is punishable by flogging or stoning to death. Violence against sexual minorities is promoted. It is almost imperative for homosexuals to live heterosexual lives to avoid having problems.
- In India, homosexuality is prohibited. There is no climate that promotes human rights for sexual minorities. Homosexual behavior is sanctioned.
- In the Dominican Republic, homosexual behavior is considered a mental illness; homosexual activity could lead to psychological treatment including the use of drugs to "cure the disease." Gays and lesbians are a minority stigmatized and discriminated against in every field of life. Only a few people see this as a civil rights issue.

Sources: Zinn, M. B., Hondagneu-Sotelo, P., & Messner, A. *Through the prism of difference.* Boston: Allyn & Bacon, 1997; Homosexuality in China, 2005. Available: *www.absoluteastronomy.com/encyclopedia/h/ho/homosexuality_in_china.htm;* Homosexuality in Japan, 2005. Available: *www.absoluteastronomy.com/encyclopedia/h/ho/homosexuality_in_japan.htm;* Breaking the cultural straitjacket, 2005. Commission on Human Rights: Sixty-First Session, March 14–April 22, 2005. Available: *www.ngochr.org/view/index.php?basic_entity=DOCUMENT&list_ids=110.*

be loitering around bathrooms. In a twist of technology, the same web site that allowed users to post messages about their "cruising" experiences helped police determine where the activity was happening, and to gauge the success of their operations to discourage it. The tearooms have a distinct culture. Men use signals to approach each other. The sexual activity, usually fellatio, is quick. Words are rarely spoken between partners. Some people argue that colleges should not intrude upon activities that take place behind closed doors, even if the doors are those of bathroom stalls. Others feel that using a public bathroom is different from doing something in the privacy of one's own home. They consider it an issue of public decency and assert that people do not want to be solicited for sexual activity or to witness it.

The impersonal nature of the sexual activity that takes place in the stalls of the restroom is often the attraction; for others it is the only place they feel comfortable meeting sexual partners. The public has on numerous occasions been shocked to learn that a well-known figure—usually not known to be homosexual—frequents a particular public restroom to engage in homosexual acts. The restroom affords the anonymity desired while still providing a sexual outlet. These restrooms are known to harbor the tearoom trade and are subject to periodic police raids. As with the baths, however, the anonymity of the public restroom has the disadvantage of increasing the chances of contracting HIV. As such, they have become less frequently employed as a place for casual sexual activity.

Although clubs, bars, and organizations are often safe places for homosexuals, there is a fear of police harassment and of possible discovery. In addition, some homosexuals desire to have more open and intimate relationships.

Like people in general, who now use the Internet for various social reasons more than in previous years, those interested in same-gender relationships often choose this course. For example, there seems to be an association between online sexual activity seeking and risk for HIV infection among men who have sexual activity with men (MSM). Intention to go online seeking sexual activity has been found to predict more episodes of anal sexual activity. In addition, unprotected anal intercourse is a common activity with online-initiated liaisons. Therefore, MSM who go online to meet sexual partners are important targets for HIV interventions (Horvath et al., 2006).

In a permanent relationship, living together seems to be more important to lesbians than to male homosexuals. Many gays of both sexes believe that steady love relationships are quite meaningful and enjoy the warmth and understanding of such relationships.

Social Issues and Homosexuals

Additional issues related to homosexual life are being considered all the time. For example, the issue of homosexuals becoming parents has been controver-

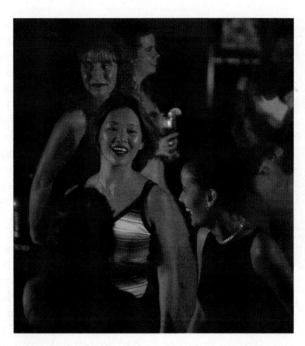

Gay bars cater to either female or male homosexuals, but usually not to both.

sial. Some people believe that homosexuals and bisexuals should have the same rights to be parents as others do. Other people believe that the inherent nature of same-gender attraction would prevent homosexuals from "properly raising" children.

Since 1994 the U.S. military has had a "Don't ask; don't tell" policy. This means that military officials are not supposed to ask about the sexual orientation of members of the military, but that they are supposed to discharge openly gay troops. Because the military is struggling to recruit and retain good people, leaders may look the other way to retain an experienced service member. At the same time, cases of antigay harassment have more than doubled (to almost 1,000 cases per year). Incidents range from verbal taunts and death threats to assaults and one murder (Stone, 2000).

Files (2005) reported that the number of men and women discharged from the military because they were discovered to be gay keeps declining. The total of such discharges was 1,227 in 2001, 885 in 2002, 770 in 2003, and 654 in 2004. This seems to show that military commanders value good service members during a time of war, whether those service members are gay or straight.

Twenty-four countries (not including the United States) allow gays and lesbians to serve openly in the military. Twenty-two of these nations are part of the coalition forces currently present in Iraq and Afghanistan. In July 2008, more than 50 retired U.S. generals and admirals released a statement calling on the U.S. Congress to repeal the ban on openly gay and lesbian soldiers serving in the military. At that time, the United States had discharged more than 11,000 service members for being gay or lesbian (Jones, 2009).

Even in professional journals there may be biases related to sexual orientation. A content analysis of 13,217 articles published in marriage and family therapy journals showed that only 77 (0.006%) focused on gay, lesbian, and/or bisexual issues or used sexual orientation as a variable (Clark & Servivich, 1997).

In 1993 the American Medical Association (AMA) banned discrimination against gay, lesbian, and bisexual doctors by adding the words *sexual orientation* to

The number of men and women discharged from the military because they are gay has declined each year.

the AMA nondiscrimination bylaws. Despite progress such as increasing support services for gay medical students, two-thirds of medical students reported hearing antigay comments from a classroom instructor, 42% said that clinical faculty had made negative remarks about homosexuality, and 7% indicated that their homosexuality had been criticized personally by an instructor. Gay and lesbian patient care needs to be integrated throughout the medical school curriculum (Wallick, 1997).

In 2004 the American Academy of Pediatrics issued a report giving guidance to clinicians in rendering pediatric care (Frankowski, 2004). The Academy reaffirmed the physician's responsibility to provide comprehensive health care and guidance in a safe and supportive environment for all adolescents, including nonheterosexual adolescents and young people struggling with issues of sexual orientation. The report outlined special needs of nonheterosexual youth as well as special considerations for them. It emphasized the importance of trying to prevent the major physical and mental health problems that may confront nonheterosexual youths in their transition to a healthy adulthood.

Evidence is accumulating that lesbians experience certain elevated health risks when compared to heterosexual women. These include increased risk of breast cancer, untreated STIs, and barriers to health care (Ellingson, 2002). The reasons for these risks are not totally clear. Reasons for increased breast cancer may include childlessness (associated with a 36% increase in the risk of development of breast cancer), higher rates of obesity and alcohol use, and less likelihood to practice breast self-examination and receive clinical breast exams. Although the prevalence of STIs is generally lower among lesbians than among heterosexual women, risk reduction behaviors also seem to

be lower. Reasons given for relatively low frequency of early detection behaviors include low perceived need, fears of and experience of homophobic care providers, and lack of insurance.

Trebay (2004) pointed out that lesbians are a powerful presence in fashion, in both predictable and unexpected ways. While old stereotypes about lesbians have not faded, they have slipped into something decidedly "cool." Although lesbians wear a variety of clothing types and styles just like anyone else, one fashion designer referred to a show where "a parade of models appeared in slashed jeans, flat shoes and mannish jackets that were hip and sexy-tough, vulnerable and imposing, just the sort of stuff one might expect a fashionable young lesbian to wear."

Gay and lesbian tourists account for more than 10% of the money Americans spend abroad in a year. However, they have felt very unwelcome close to home in the Caribbean. For example, the Cayman Islands recently turned away gay cruises. Travel agents have had to remind gay tourists to avoid public displays of affection in Barbados (where homosexuality is outlawed) or face fines and harassment. In St. Kitts, gays were thought to be a threat to national security. Partly in response to these incidents, the International Gay and Lesbian Travel Association started a campaign to boycott certain spots, encouraging gay tourists to direct their dollars only to gay-friendly destinations. A more welcoming attitude lately has been shown in St. Thomas (where they advertise gay bed-and-breakfasts and gay weddings) and in Puerto Rico (Padgett, 2005).

In 2005 MTV started a new gay cable TV channel called Logo (MTV launches new gay cable TV channel, 2005). The prospect of a television channel entirely devoted to gay programs for gay people may strike some as unnecessary and others as a sign of immoral times, but media giant Viacom thought there was money in it. A spokesperson for Concerned Women for America, which describes itself as a conservative Evangelical group, said it was "a sad day for America." She said MTV was in a powerful position to influence youth and it was "unconscionable" to present in a positive view a promiscuous lifestyle that causes "illness and diseases." The general manager of Logo cited studies saying there were some 15 million openly gay people in America, an attractive demographic for advertisers, considering that many will have no children, meaning more disposable income.

In July 2005, Oprah Winfrey devoted a show to a lifestyle called living on the "down low." This is an expression to describe men who are married or have girlfriends, but are secretly sleeping with men. The main guest on the show, J. L. King, author of *On the Down Low: A Journey into the Lives of "Straight"*

Communication DIMENSIONS

Communication About Gay and Lesbian Athletes

Being accepted and being accepting can be issues for college athletes. Traditionally there is an assumption that male athletes are heterosexually virile and desirable. Female athletes can face a very different perception—that they are all lesbians or bisexual. Straight women can go to great lengths to avoid that stereotype, leaving their homosexual teammates out in the cold. After using a series of interviews with lesbian, bisexual, and heterosexual Women's National Basketball Association (WNBA) fans, Dolance (2005) argued that the (perceived) large lesbian attendance at WNBA games enables the construction of a lesbian community by lesbian and bisexual fans in a site very different from traditional locations of lesbian community. Because the WNBA is not an explicitly lesbian space, the process of speculating about which players, coaches, and fans are lesbians is a meaningful part of being a WNBA fan for many lesbian and bisexual fans. Fantasizing a large lesbian presence enables lesbian and bisexual fans to actively and interpretively create lesbian community at the games. The women socialize and connect with other lesbian and bisexual women. WNBA games are defined as a unique space that is different from lesbian bars and other traditional "gay-only" spaces.

The highly visible men's sports of football, basketball, hockey, and baseball remain the most unaccepting of homosexual athletes. Athletes who perform individu-

ally, rather than on teams, may have an easier time being accepted (Jacobson, 2002a).

In 2002 the Rice University football coach was quoted as saying that "while he would not necessarily kick a player off the team for being gay, he probably would think hard about doing so." Immediately, the president of Rice University indicated the need for the coach to affirm his commitment to the university's nondiscrimination policy and to apologize for "the damage done by his comments." The coach did so (Jacobson, 2002b).

There are examples of communication difficulties related to homosexuality in pro sports, also. For example, in 2002 it was rumored that Mike Piazza, All-Star catcher for the New York Mets, was gay. Responding to the rumors, Piazza said that the major leagues are ready for gay players, but he is not one of them.

Also in 2002, Esera Tuaolo, who had played defensive tackle in the National Football League for 9 years, revealed that he was gay. He said that he retired from pro football in 1999 because of failing knees and shoulders, but also because of the discomfort he experienced hearing players make disparaging remarks about gays. One of his former teammates said, "Had other players known Tuaolo was gay, he would have been eaten alive" (Airing it out, 2002).

Communication related to homosexual athletes remains an important social issue.

Black Men Who Sleep with Men, said the term applies only to blacks. He also said he doesn't consider himself gay. The behavior is not a social thing. Down low is just about sexual gratification and not a relationship. According to King, down low is on college campuses, too.

In August 2005, black journalists attending a National Association of Black Journalists conference in Atlanta discussed media coverage of the black community and the down low phenomenon (Black journalists criticize media coverage of "down low" phenomenon, 2005). They hotly debated whether media coverage of the phenomenon is a public service to the black community or a "salacious distraction" from other issues affecting the black community. Many said the media coverage unfairly characterized down low as occurring only among black men and often inappropriately linked it with statistics about

the increasing number of AIDS cases in the black community. As a result, many black women went on "witch hunts" to determine whether the men in their lives were secretly gay, and people of other races wrongly assumed that this does not apply to them.

Examples of homosexual lifestyles in the media continue to grow. In 2005 a homosexual relationship was portrayed in a place that was probably unexpected—in a western film entitled *Brokeback Mountain*. The main characters, seen as very manly examples, participated in sexual encounters early in the film. Both went on to get married to females and even had children. However, after 4 years they got back together and their relationship flourished.

Another social issue is that people with disabilities who identify as LGB represent a population that has received little attention. Awareness of the unique needs and concerns of these individuals is crucial for optimizing their physical and mental well-being. This population is actually a double minority with some experiences similar to those of other minority groups (Fraley, Mona, & Theodore, 2007).

Do you think we need to make changes in society's views, or do you feel conditions are fine the way they are?

Issues Related to Religion/Morality

You are probably aware that many people have religious/moral concerns about homosexuality. The Ontario Consultants on Religious Tolerance (2005) summarized these concerns as follows:

- Same-gender activity is something that should be criminalized.

- Homosexuality is sinful and immoral, no matter what the relationship.

- Homosexuality is hated by God.

- Homosexuality is indicative of mental illness.

- Homosexuality is a choice that people make.

- Homosexuality is changeable through repentance and being saved, prayer, and/or reparative therapy.

- Homosexuality is abnormal and unnatural for everyone.

- Same-gender marriage is an extreme danger to society.

The Religious Institute on Sexual Morality, Justice, and Healing offered advice to religious foundations on securing the freedom to marry for same-gender couples (An open letter to religious leaders on marriage equality, 2004). Religious leaders within the Institute felt that there are strong civil liberties arguments for ending the exclusion of same-gender couples from the legal institution of marriage. A list of the religious foundations supporting homosexuals is available at http://religiousinstitute.org.

Many religious denominations are debating about how to deal with homosexuality in general, with homosexual religious leaders, and with same-gender marriages, among other issues. For example, in 2005 the Evangelical Lutheran Church in America retained its policy against blessing same-gender unions and ordaining gays, but suggested that sanctions could be avoided for pastors and congregations that chose to do so. Earlier, the United Methodist Church defrocked a minister in Pennsylvania who had admitted to being in a long-term lesbian relationship. She appealed the decision. The Episcopal Church USA also wrestled with how to handle homosexuality. In 2003 the Episcopal Church ordained an openly gay bishop in New Hampshire. Some Episcopal leaders called for a moratorium on ordaining bishops living in gay relationships and to halt public "rites of blessing" for same-gender unions (Banerjee, 2005).

Also in 2005, The United Church of Christ became the first mainline Christian denomination to officially support same-gender marriages (Dewan, 2005). Its ruling body passed a resolution affirming "equal marriage rights for couples regardless of gender." Symbolically, the church passed the resolution on July 4.

In "Brief Descriptions of the Sex Belief Systems," Ontario Consultants on Religious Tolerance (2009) noted that most people can be divided into one of six groups, depending on their fundamental beliefs about homosexuality. Although these six groups are stereotypical, they illustrate the typical concepts shared by many adults. Of course, some people will fit neatly into a single viewpoint, whereas others will combine the beliefs of more than one point of view. Here are the six groups:

- *Abomination:* This is the most conservative position. Based on Biblical writings, homosexual behavior is to be condemned under all circumstances.

- *Change is expected:* This viewpoint teaches that homosexuality is a product of a sinful world. Gays and lesbians can be cured and converted to heterosexuality through prayer.

- *Celibacy is expected:* This position recognizes that adult sexual orientation is fixed and homosexuals cannot change. For them, God expects a celibate lifestyle, without loving partners with whom to share their lives.

- *Marginally acceptable:* Homosexuality is a psychosexual disability that victims must try to overcome. If they are unable to change and unable to be celibate, then the least horrendous option is a monogamous, long-term, same-gender relationship.

- *Equality:* Equal status and equal rights are the goal. Homosexuals are quite capable of entering into a loving, committed same-gender relationship that is the equal of an other-gender relationship. Morality of acts is judged exactly the same way as in heterosexual relationships.

- *Liberation:* This is the most liberal position. Homosexuality is seen to be equal to heterosexuality.

Homophobia

Although society's attitudes are gradually becoming more accepting, there are still many people who have strong negative feelings about homosexuals. **Homophobia** is an irrational fear of homosexuality in others, a fear of homosexual feelings within oneself, or an unhappiness with one's own homosexuality. Homophobia probably results from ignorance, a belief in the common myths about homosexuality, or even the tendency to judge homosexuals as immoral. People with strong negative feelings often reveal their homophobia by openly insulting homosexuals and even subjecting people suspected of being homosexual to verbal or physical assault. Also, homophobics are often careful to avoid behaving in ways that could be interpreted as homosexual, for example, by shunning certain kinds of clothing or physical activities.

homophobia
An irrational fear of homosexuality.

Some people have wondered if there is a difference between males and females when it comes to homophobia. Research into this issue has not yielded clear results. However, it is interesting that Davies (2004) reported that on measures of attitudes toward homosexual behavior and homosexual persons, heterosexual men are more negative toward gay men than women are.

Homophobia is an international problem. Every 2 or 3 days a person is killed in Brazil in violence connected with his or her sexual orientation. In Mexico, the reported figure is nearly two fatalies per week. Most of the victims are men who have sexual relations with other men (UNAIDS, 2009). It has been found that gay people in the United Kingdom experience more extreme homophobia as young people than as adults. Two-thirds of young gay, lesbian, and bisexual people experienced direct bullying in British schools, 92% of young people were subject to verbal abuse, and 41% were physically assaulted. In Latin America, a gay man was killed every 2 days because of his sexual orientation (Ruscombe-King, 2009).

What can be done to tackle homophobia? Schools have an important role to play. Lesbians and gay students are more likely to feel positive about school if school personnel clearly state that homophobic behavior is against the rules. Also, it is likely that personal attitudes will become more accepting toward gay people if individuals are exposed to educational programs about homosexuality. Community-based organizations can also provide support to gay and lesbian people who might feel isolated and, at the same time, campaign for tolerance toward homosexuality. Other bodies and agencies that could positively influence the way that gay, lesbian, and bisexual peo-

On April 7, 2003, in an interview with the Associated Press, Senator Rick Santorum was quoted as comparing consensual homosexual sexual activity to bigamy, polygamy, adultery, and even incest. Sen. Santorum later admitted to having a problem "with homosexual acts" and "acts outside of traditional heterosexual relationships." While the senator's remarks sparked quite an uproar in the media, the George W. Bush administation did not immediately denounce the senator's comments. What message regarding the government's view of homosexuality did this send to the American public?

ple are treated are leaders of political parties, police forces, health services, broadcasters, and employers (Ruscombe-King, 2009).

We talked about school settings earlier; here it is appropriate again to mention teachers. A teacher can ask the following questions to create a more accepting classroom environment: (1) Do I make **heterosexist** (characterized by the belief that heterosexuality is the privileged and powerful norm) assumptions? (2) Do I ignore homophobic remarks? (3) Do I blame my audience for their own misinformation? (4) Do I use educational materials that assume that all my students are heterosexual?

heterosexist
An attitude that reinforces heterosexuality as the privileged and powerful norm.

Coming Out

The lifestyle of a gay person is greatly influenced by the extent to which he or she decides to remain in the closet—to keep his or her sexual orientation a

come out
Accept and make homosexual orientation public.

secret—or to **come out**—accepting that orientation and making it public. Each choice can be made in varying degrees.

The decision to come out involves several stages: (1) acknowledging, (2) accepting, and (3) openly expressing one's homosexuality. Some homosexuals never acknowledge their sexual orientation, even to themselves. The first step in coming out is usually to realize that one does not fit the heterosexual model. The second step is acceptance, a step that sometimes requires that the individual overcome a learned negative view of homosexuality that becomes a negative view of himself or herself.

Even when a homosexual or bisexual reaches the acceptance stage, he or she can still decide to remain in the closet. It is generally easier to pass as a heterosexual than to take the final step toward openness. However, a person who can live publicly within his or her true sexual orientation generally has a better chance of living a happier life than one who remains secretive. In some situations, however, such as being a parent, the pain of coming out may far outweigh that of staying in the closet.

Telling the family—whether parents, siblings, spouses, or children—can also be extremely difficult, and many people who would prefer an open homosexual life choose not to face this ordeal. In fact, parents are often the last to know if their son or daughter is a homosexual. D'Augelli et al. (2005) conducted an interesting study about parents' awareness of youths' sexual orientation. They found that earlier awareness and disclosure of same-gender attractions and less internalized homophobia were characteristic of youths whose parents were aware of the youths' sexual orientation. However, youths with aware parents reported more past verbal victimization on the basis of sexual orientation from parents, yet more current family support and less fear of future parental victimization on the basis of their sexual orientation.

It is no surprise that family support is an important factor when gays, lesbians, and bisexuals decide to come out. Gays, lesbians, and bisexual young adults with higher levels of family rejection during adolescence are 8.4 times more likely to attempt suicide, 5.9 times more likely to report high levels of depression, 3.4 times more likely to use illegal drugs, and 3.4 times more likely to engage in unpro-

tected sexual intercourse compared with peers from families with no or low levels of family rejection. There is a clear link between parental and caregiver rejecting behaviors and negative health problems for young lesbian, gay, and bisexual adults. Family support is crucial for reducing risk and increasing well-being for these people (Ryan et al., 2009).

For most people, the process of deciding to come out begins during their school years. As students, few homosexuals choose to disclose their sexual orientation to principals, teachers, counselors, or friends. Reasons cited for nondisclosure include fear of the consequences and not wanting others to know. Most of those who do disclose their sexual orientation receive positive feedback for doing so, but both positive and negative consequences of coming out have been reported. In one study, gay men were aware of their sexual orientation at an earlier age than lesbians and were more likely to recommend disclosure to principals and teachers. Females were more likely to disclose only to females, whereas males were likely to come out to both males and females. Both groups were cautious about coming out in the school setting (Harris, 1997).

It is not possible to predict others' response to disclosure. This move can result in a student's experiencing everything from lack of support, isolation, rejection, and ostracism to unfair discipline, taunting, harassment, verbal slurs, persistent random acts of violence, and outright vicious beatings. Students must carefully consider the pros and cons of coming

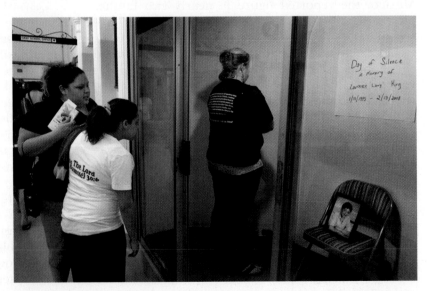

In February 2008, Lawrence "Larry" King, a gay 15-year-old student from Oxnard, California, was shot and killed by fellow student Brandon McInerney. King had reportedly asked McInerney to be his Valentine. McInerney has been charged as an adult with premeditated murder and a hate crime, and faces a maximum sentence of life in prison. The incident received nationwide attention; one news outlet described it as the most high-profile gay-bias crime since the murder of Matthew Shepard in 1998.

Communication
DIMENSIONS

Coming Out Each of us may be in a position to communicate with someone who is thinking about coming out. A few facts and a few communication suggestions may be helpful. First, the facts:

1. Coming out can be important as an affirmation of one's sexual orientation.
2. Coming out can jeopardize some relationships.
3. Coming out can promote a sense of pride in one's sexual orientation and, in the long run, actually improve relationships with both gay and straight people.
4. Coming out is usually a two-part process—first, coming out to oneself; second, coming out to others.
5. Coming out to oneself may involve gradually dealing with denial, putting matters into focus, and even dealing with personal homophobia.
6. Coming out to others probably involves stages—first involving a few very close friends or relatives, later more relatives, and then a larger public, such as employers, fellow students, and coworkers.
7. Some gays may be out only to a certain degree. For example, only families and very close friends may know about their sexual orientation.

Here are a few communication suggestions from professional counselors (Black & Underwood, 1998) that can be helpful to all of us:

1. Coming out should be postponed until the person has a reasonably high sense of self-worth and a support network.
2. The person should be secure in his or her identity before coming out to others.
3. The person should be helped to weigh the pros and cons of coming out and to examine why he or she wants to come out.
4. People who are planning to come out, or who are coming out, usually need a great deal of support and encouragement from others.
5. It is not our responsibility to "make" the person straight or gay. It is our responsibility to help provide a supportive environment.
6. It is important to be ourselves and be sincere.
7. Confidentiality must be respected.
8. Communication should be done in a helpful way but not in a forceful way.
9. Use words that do not assume that everyone is or should be heterosexual. For example, substitute terms such as *partner* or *significant other* for *boyfriend* or *girlfriend*.
10. Role playing can be used to help someone who is going to come out to be prepared to handle a variety of situations.

out and examine *why* they want to come out. In any case, coming out should be postponed until the student achieves a reasonable degree of self-esteem and a support network (Black & Underwood, 1998).

Cloud (2005) reported that the Point Foundation is one of the fastest-growing gay groups in the nation. It gives scholarships to gay students. Young people are disclosing their homosexuality with unprecedented regularly—and they are doing so at much younger ages. The average gay person comes out just before or after graduating from high school. In 1997 there were about 100 gay–straight alliances on U.S. high school campuses, but there are now more than 3,000. Nearly one in 10 high schools has one. Also, gay kids can now watch fictional and real teens who are out on shows like *Desperate Housewives*, the dating show *Next* on MTV, and *Degrassi*, a high school drama on the N network. Simon & Schuster Publishers released

over a dozen novels about gay adolescents in a recent year. Gay kids can subscribe to *YGA Magazine* (YGA stands for "young gay America"). Gay men today recall first desiring other males at an average age of 10. The average age for lesbians is 12. At many schools around the country, it is now profoundly uncool to be seen as anti-gay.

In 2005 Sheryl Swoopes, the three-time most valuable player of the Women's National Basketball Association, announced she was gay. She said she felt as if a burden had been lifted. It appeared that her announcement did not have an impact on her opportunities for endorsements or on other aspects of her career (Robbins, 2005).

Recently the Internet has played a key role in the stages of coming out. Many young men initially come out into a virtual gay community, with online observation and connection with other gay or ques-

Just a few years ago, featuring a homosexual character on a television sitcom would most likely result in a show's cancellation. Later, one of television's most popular comedies proudly and overtly addressed the topic of homosexuality. *Will & Grace,* which focused on the unique relationship between Will, who was gay, and his best friend, Grace, who was straight, won three Emmys in 2000. Through the experiences of Will and Grace and their friends Jack and Karen, the show frankly and hilariously explored the universal subjects of friendship, sex, relationships, and love, whether heterosexual or homosexual.

tioning people, well before making actual contact in the real world. This virtual coming out involves being able to watch and learn about the culture, language, and norms of gayness before actually moving into this new world. The Internet can serve as an important tool for psychological adaptation for homosexual youth, especially those who are geographically or psychologically isolated (Ross, 2007).

Unfortunately, it is difficult if not impossible to know what the reactions of people will be when a person comes out. For many reasons, the decision to come out remains difficult for most homosexuals.

The Gay Rights Movement

Gay and lesbian organizations can help gays deal with the stresses experienced as a result of their sexual orientation. There are many different organizations that can provide the social support needed to manage such stressful life situations as coming out or staying in the closet. The support of people who understand what you are experiencing and who can offer advice can be invaluable.

The gay rights movement has progressed, largely because of these homophile organizations and their ability to mobilize their membership to march, to vote, and to boycott when necessary. The movement began in earnest after a raid by the New York City police on the Stonewall gay bar in June 1969. That raid led to a 2-day riot that forever changed the tolerance level of the gay community toward societal prejudice based on sexual orientation. As a result, gays have presented a united front in voting for political candidates who are willing to sponsor their causes. In cities such as San Francisco and Washington, D.C., where there are significant numbers of homosexual citizens (voters), politicians are particularly sensitive to gay rights issues. In these cities, gays have made a difference in those elected to public office.

There is no way to know whether social activities, such as the gay rights movement, have influenced other aspects of society or whether aspects of society have influenced gay rights. There is no question that there is more openness about homosexuality in today's society. A prime example of this was Ellen DeGeneres's decision to come out on her TV show in

1998. Another example is the way that homosexual films have moved into the mainstream. In movies, homosexuals were first ignored, then scorned. By the early 1990s, with the AIDS epidemic, homosexuals began to be pitied in films. Films about them tended to be about their homosexuality and not about their overall lives. There are now more movies about homosexuals than ever, but these movies deal with overall issues and not just people's homosexuality and generally appeal to viewers of all sexual orientations (Corliss, 1998).

In 2000, a Gallup poll showed that Americans are evenly divided over the morality of homosexual relations, with 48% considering them morally acceptable and 48% saying they are morally wrong. Current attitudes are more affirming of gays than what Gallup found in 2000. Despite the divided reaction on a moral basis, the majority believes homosexual relations should be legal (55%) and accepted as an alternative lifestyle (57%). The belief that homosexuals should have equal rights in terms of job opportunities is strongly supported (89%). Giving the same legal sanction to same-gender marriage as the law does to traditional marriage is supported by 40% of Americans and opposed by 56%. During the past quarter-century, there have been important changes in public attitudes about homosexuality and gay rights. Americans have shifted from frowning on homosexuality as an alternative lifestyle and being divided over whether it should be legal, to now supporting gay rights on both fronts. Even so, support

Multicultural
DIMENSIONS

The Chinese Lawyer Who Is Out

A young Chinese lawyer named Zhou Dan started writing about being gay on Chinese web sites in 2001. He hoped his honesty would help combat prejudice. Homosexuality was, and still is, very much in the closet in China. In 2001, officials in Beijing took it off the country's official list of mental disorders. However, gay people still face discrimination and social pressures. In May 2005, Peking University authorities banned a gay-and-lesbian film festival before it was to open on campus.

Zhou's entries, signed with his own name, had an unintended consequence. Gay men from around China who had faced workplace discrimination, blackmail, and even prison time started to seek his legal counsel. Zhou helped start a hotline for sexual minorities in Shanghai in 2003. As of 2005, he was teaching China's first gradu-ate class on homosexuality and social science at Fudan University. Some claim he is China's leading voice for gay rights.

Interestingly, the first undergraduate course on gay studies ever offered at a Chinese university was also given at Fudan University in the fall of 2005 (Mooney, 2005). It drew far more applicants than the 100 available seats. The class focused on health, legal, and social issues related to homosexuality in China. The instructor said the new course's popularity stemmed from ignorance about gay issues in China. The students don't know much about homosexuality and want to learn more.

Sources: The lawyer who is out. *Time 165, no. 26* (June 27, 2005), 42–43; Mooney, P. Chinese students line up for first undergraduate gay-studies course. *Chronicle of Higher Education, Today's News.* August 23, 2005. Available: *http://chronicle.com/daily/2005/08/2005082305n.htm.*

for legalizing gay marriage lags far behind the less culturally sensitive matter of gays having equal job rights (Saad, 2008).

Legal Rights

Marriage in the United States is more than a public recognition of love. It is also a legally binding contract, providing the married couple with myriad tax and legal support benefits, from which gay relationships are usually excluded.

Gays have long argued that marriage is not a requirement for a strong family unit. In 1989, Mayor Ed Koch of New York City agreed (Koch grants benefits for domestic partners, 1989). He issued an order recognizing domestic partnerships of gays. Not merely symbolic, Koch's declaration meant that gay city employees who had live-in companions could be eligible for death benefits. It also allowed labor unions to negotiate for health benefits for such families.

Not all of New York City's politicians agreed with Koch. One argued, "I think that Koch's executive order undermines one of society's most essential institutions: marriage." Koch responded, "Over time, society changes. So must the government that serves it. Practices or policies that might have seemed unacceptable to our grandparents or unusual to our parents seem equitable, indeed necessary, to our generation. We honor the past, but we cannot be held captive to it."

Following are some of the legal benefits for married couples.

- *Income taxes*—In many instances, married couples receive a lower tax rate than would two individuals filing separately. (An exception to this, known as the "marriage penalty," occurs when both spouses earn relatively equal high incomes and consequently pay a higher rate than they would as individuals.) At any rate, any income tax benefits for married couples do not include gay couples.

- *Adoption*—Many states do not allow gay couples to adopt children. Even states that do allow it generally put married couples first in line.

- *Estate taxes*—Married couples do not have to pay any federal estate taxes (and usually only a limited amount of state estate tax) on the death of a first spouse. State laws provide (for people without wills) that property moves directly to the spouse (or spouse and children, depending on the state). Unless a gay couple has an updated will (and most people in the United States do not), the biological family of the deceased can claim all possessions.

- *Employment benefits*—Married couples share a variety of benefits from work (health, dental, and life insurance, to name some) that gay

Increasingly, gay men and lesbians are choosing in vitro fertilization or adoption to start their own families. The issue of gay and lesbian adoption was widely discussed in the media after former talk-show host Rosie O'Donnell publicly criticized President George W. Bush's opposition to gay adoption. O'Donnell, who is openly gay, has three adopted children and says that her own experiences as a mother make her certain that gay people should have the right to be parents.

partners do not. Many *Fortune* 500 companies have instituted policies in recent years to allow gay partners such rights, but there is no law requiring this. Companies like Disney and Apple offer these benefits to recruit and retain high-quality talent. Whereas many large companies can afford to do this, many smaller companies are not so inclined.

• *Social Security survivorship benefits and pensions*—At death, the law provides that the surviving spouse receive continued benefits. Not so for gays.

• *Disability decision making*—If a married person becomes seriously injured and needs medical care decisions made for him or her, the law provides that spouses can make those decisions. But in cases in which parents or siblings of a disabled gay person do not approve of his or her relationship, they can—and often do—challenge the domestic partner's decisions in court.

You can see from this list that there are many problems related to legal rights of gay couples. There is much to be done to ensure equal rights for all married couples.

In 2000 Vermont became the first state to approve same-gender unions. Although the term *marriage* was not used, this bill provided homosexual couples with essentially the same rights as heterosexual couples (Drummond, 2000). In 2004 Massachusetts began granting the first-ever marriage licenses to same-gender couples. The state's highest court had ruled that gays and lesbians had a constitutional right to marry. In 2005 Connecticut joined Vermont in approving gay civil unions (Schweitzer, 2005). Also in 2005, a federal judge struck down Nebraska's ban on same-gender marriage, saying the measure interfered not only with the rights of gay couples but also with those of foster parents, adopted children, and people in a variety of other living arrangements. The amendment to the state's constitution, which defined marriage as a union between a man and a woman, had passed overwhelmingly by voters in 2000 (Judge voids same-sex marriage ban in Nebraska, 2005).

Should same-gender couples be allowed to marry legally? Some people feel that same-gender couples should have the same human rights as others. They argue that when people work, pay taxes, enter into lifetime commitments, and raise children, there is no reason they should not be afforded the same social and legal benefits and status as heterosexual couples—including legal marriage. In opposition to this idea,

¿? Ethical DIMENSIONS

Should Gay Marriages Be Legal?

Given the many legal benefits for married couples, there seems to be increasing pressure to legalize gay marriages. Those who feel gay marriages are not proper, for whatever reasons, would argue that we should not make gay marriages legal. Those who feel we have an ethical responsibility to treat all people equally, and to recognize the rights of various groups, would argue that gay marriages should be legal.

In recent years there have been measures considered in some states to recognize the legal rights of people involved in same-gender partnerships. The question of whether it is ethical to provide or not to provide legal sanction to these partnerships fosters interesting debates.

however, an alliance of conservative groups campaigned for a 28th amendment to the U.S. Constitution that would prevent same-gender couples from getting married legally. The proposed Federal Marriage Amendment reads in part: "Marriage in the United States shall consist only of the union of a man and a woman. Neither this Constitution or the constitution of any state, nor state or federal law, shall be construed to require that marital status or the legal incidents thereof be conferred upon unmarried couples or groups" (Should same-sex couples be allowed to marry legally?, 2003).

Herdt and Kertzner (2006) argue that depriving lesbians and gays of the right to marry restricts their citizenship and hinders their health and well-being. Even though research confirms the capacity of gays and lesbians to form committed relationships and parent successfully, marriage denial continues to perpetuate an opportunity structure that disenfranchises gays and lesbians in the sociocultural, legal, economic, and political aspects of their lives. Herdt and Kertzmer point out that denial of marriage is an act of discrimination against both gays and lesbians.

In 2001 the Belgian government approved a bill to legalize same-gender weddings. It made Belgium the second country in the world to recognize gay marriages, after its northern neighbor, the Netherlands (Ames, 2001). In 2005 the Canadian government passed legislation granting same-gender couples the same legal rights as those in traditional unions between a man and a woman. According to most polls, a majority of Canadians support the right for gays and lesbians to marry in spite of the fact that the Roman Catholic Church, the predominant denomination in Canada, vigorously opposes the legislation (Duff-Bell, 2005).

Some people believe that gay marriage bans have inspired a new wave of activists. For example, in 2008 a group planned "A Day Without a Gay." The event organizers asked gay-rights supporters to avoid going to work by "calling in gay" and volunteering for the gay-rights movement instead. The burst of energy drew some comparisons to demonstrations during the early days of the AIDS crisis in the 1980s. Many activists were also motivated by the film *Milk*, which chronicled the fight by a member of the San Francisco Board of Supervisors, Harvey Milk, to beat back a 1978 ballot measure that would have barred gay teachers from California's public schools (McKinley, 2008).

As of 2009, marriage between same-gender couples was legal in seven countries. Spain was the only country that recognized same-gender marriage and other-gender marriage under the same law. In the United States, same-gender marriage was legal in Massachusetts (2004), California (2008), and Vermont (2009). However, the California law was later voted down by the people. In July 2008, New York's governor ruled that same-gender marriages performed out of state must be recognized in the state of New York. Three additional states (Connecticut, New Jersey, and New Hampshire) recognized civil unions between same-gender couples. Several other states (Oregon, Maine, Washington, and the District of Columbia) had domestic partnership laws that granted certain benefits to same-gender couples (Jones, 2009).

On the flip side, 26 states had passed constitutional amendments banning same-gender marriages, while 18 states had passed statewide laws recognizing marriage as occurring only between a man and a woman. At the same time, 13 states and the District of Columbia had enacted policies to protect against gender identity and sexual-orientation discrimination in employment. Seven other states prohibited employment discrimination based solely on sexual orientation and/or gender identity. However, in 30 states LGBT citizens could be fired on the basis of their sexual orientation and/or gender identity without any legal recourse (Jones 2009). Laws regarding same-gender marriage and relationships as well as rights can change at any time.

In 2003 the U.S. Supreme Court struck down state sodomy laws as demeaning to homosexuals, and said

People disagree about the rights of homosexual couples.

the government has no authority to regulate the sexual behavior of "consenting adults acting in private" (Murphy, 2003). Many people felt that this decision would have far-reaching implications for the popular discussion about gay rights. For example, some said that by essentially acknowledging gay relationships as legitimate, the Supreme Court justices gave the gay-rights movement a new credibility in debates about marriage, partner benefits, adoption, and parental rights.

Two interesting, but unrelated, legal rulings about homosexual rights were made in 2005. In one, the Hillsborough County Commission in Florida approved a policy directing county government to "abstain from acknowledging, promoting, or participating" in gay-pride recognition or events. It was approved after a Gay and Lesbian Pride Month display at a library upset some library patrons. Community leaders feared that the policy would damage efforts to promote the Tampa region as being multicultural and diverse (Waddell, 2005). In a second situation, the California Supreme Court ruled that country clubs must offer gay members who register as domestic partners the same discounts given to married ones. If the clubs did not do this, the court said it would be "impermissible marital status discrimination" (Leff, 2005).

Should lesbian and gay couples be allowed to adopt children? Some people start with the premise that homosexuality is wrong and believe that such a relationship is an inappropriate context in which to raise children. Because they fear that sexual orientation and behaviors can be learned, they fear that a child raised by a lesbian or gay couple would be more likely to become a lesbian or gay man. Others do not believe that sexual orientation determines one's ability to parent. They feel the most important requirements are the abilities to love, support, and care for a child. Most lesbians and gays were raised by heterosexual parents. Therefore, they believe being raised by a lesbian or gay couple will not create lesbian or gay children any more than being raised by a heterosexual married couple would guarantee heterosexuality (Should lesbian and gay couples be allowed to adopt?, 2003). Interestingly, researchers in developmental psychology have concluded that no significant differences exist between children raised by lesbians and gay men and those raised by heterosexuals (Zanghellini, 2007).

In 2005 the California Supreme Court, stepping into largely uncharted territory, ruled that both members of a lesbian couple who plan for and raise a child born to either of them should be considered the child's mothers even after their relationship ends. This meant that the law could require former members of such couples to assume parental rights and obligations. Those supporting such rights and requirements were very happy with the decision. Lawyers for groups defending what they called traditional values were troubled by the decision (Liptak, 2005).

Finally, freshmen entering college have their own ideas about legality and homosexuality. Thirty-one percent of men and 18% of women think it is important to have laws prohibiting homosexual relationships. Fifty-nine percent of men and 72% of women think same-gender couples should have the right to legal marital status (Hoover, 2009).

Exploring the
DIMENSIONS
of Human Sexuality

Our feelings, attitudes, and beliefs regarding sexuality are influenced by our internal and external environments. Go to sexuality.jbpub.com/dimensions/4e to learn more about the biological, psychological, and sociological factors that affect your sexuality.

Sociocultural Factors

- Homosexual students often feel isolated and stigmatized.
- Family life can be disrupted by disclosure of homosexuality.
- Different cultures view homosexuality in different terms.
- Some states have laws making homosexual sexual activities illegal. Further, gay marriages generally do not have legal standing for state or federal benefits. Many large corporations have begun to offer employee benefits for domestic partners.

Biological Factors

- Research into genetic factors affecting homosexuality has been inconclusive. No specific gene has been identified. Any genetic link would be only part of the picture for determining sexual orientation.
- Research into hormonal imbalances (either prenatal or postnatal) as a factor driving homosexuality has proved inconclusive. No specific hormonal factors have been identified. Any hormonal link would be only one aspect of determining sexual orientation.

Psychological Factors

- Most theories suggesting that the influence of mothers or early sexual experiences lead to changes in sexual orientation have been discounted.
- Most homosexuals lead lives as fulfilling and satisfying as those of most heterosexuals.

CASE STUDY

No single scientific theory about the biological causes of sexual orientation has been substantiated; neither have any psychological theories. It is likely that the biological, psychological, and sociocultural factors interact to influence our sexual orientation. Because the dimensions change over time, an individual's sexual orientation may change over time as well.

Culturally, not all societies view homosexuality in the same manner. In areas of the Pacific such as Papua New Guinea, boys regularly participate in homosexual activities until they reach the age of marriage (19 years). In Mexico, only a male who plays the receptive role in anal intercourse is considered homosexual.

Socially, gays and lesbians in the United States can feel stigmatized and socially isolated as a result of fear of disclosure. Those who disclose their orientation ("come out") face discrimination and possibly even violence. Further, family and friends may reject them.

Summary

- Sexual orientation can be viewed on a continuum, which Kinsey described as having seven points.

- Sexual orientations include heterosexuality, homosexuality, bisexuality, and asexuality.

- There are many theories about what determines sexual orientation, including biological, psychological, and integrated theories. None of the theories is generally agreed upon.

- Both homosexual and heterosexual youths and adolescents face the same challenges related to growth and development, but gays, lesbians, and bisexuals face additional issues related to their acceptance.

- There are many examples of discrimination against people who have a sexual orientation other than heterosexual.

- In the United States, the homosexual subculture centers on private clubs, bars, and homophile organizations. These groups are designed to protect homosexuals, promote their rights, promote a positive image of homosexual lifestyles, and help the general public better understand homosexuality.

- Social issues related to sexual orientation include military policies, discrimination based on sexual orientation, and general understanding and support for people of various sexual orientations.

- There are many points of view about sexual orientation based on religion and morality.

- The gay-rights movement has helped many people better understand homosexuals and have more positive attitudes about homosexuality in general.

- Many legal issues remain related to sexual orientation, including the legal status of same-gender relationships of various types, the right of homosexual and bisexual individuals to be parents, and legal rights concerning issues such as inheritance, health insurance coverage, income taxes, and employment benefits.

Discussion Questions

1. What defines a person's sexual orientation? Is sexual orientation constant throughout life, or can it change over time?

2. Describe the theories of the causes of sexual orientation, and indicate whether research supports their theoretical claims.

3. Compare and contrast the homosexual lifestyle with the heterosexual lifestyle.

4. What are the social issues surrounding homosexuality? How do such issues adversely affect homosexuals?

Application Questions

Reread the chapter-opening story and answer the following questions.

1. Explain why Brad was dating and engaging in sexual activities with Peggy if he thought he was gay.

2. Discuss the social and psychological effects on people who are unable to disclose their sexual orientation and introduce a lifetime partner to friends and family.

Critical Thinking Questions

1. If a genetic link were found for homosexuality, how might that affect those found to have the gene? Would society accept homosexuality as an inherited "defect"? Or would homosexuals encounter more discrimination in the workplace, in the military, and so on?

2. Assuming that studies claiming that only a small percentage of the population is gay are correct, why should efforts be made to accommodate such a small minority?

3. Consider the "Don't ask; don't tell" policy of the U.S. military. Should sexual orientation make a difference on the battlefield?

4. Given that many states ban same-gender sexual activity, is it ethical to vote admitted homosexuals into public office?

5. If homosexuality had no social stigma, would there be more or fewer people living as homosexuals? Explain your answer.

Critical Thinking Case

When the filmmaker Debra Chasnoff's son started kindergarten, she had more to worry about than the other parents. Her son thought that having two moms was great—but what would the other kids tell him?

From her own experience with school systems, Chasnoff started a film project, *It's Elementary*, which was completed in 1996. She and Helen Cohen, the film's coproducer, toured the country and filmed teachers in classrooms as they described gay and lesbian lifestyles to children. Their goal was to show that the classroom could be a place where children are taught tolerance and acceptance of lifestyles different from those of their own families.

Originally, the film was used in school systems and colleges to educate teachers about the prejudice that exists among young children regarding homosexuality. But more recently, the film has caused quite a stir on the airwaves. After PBS turned it down for national distribution, San Francisco's KQED agreed to sponsor the film.

During the early summer of 1999, 89 of 347 public stations scheduled it, 17 more were on board, and 53 were considering it. This caused some anger among the Christian Right and other conservative groups who do not believe the film should be broadcast where children might watch it without supervision, although the stations had scheduled it for nighttime airing. They also argued that the film does not take parents' rights into consideration (Ness, 1999).

What do you think? Should teachers be encouraged to educate elementary school children about the topic of homosexuality, or should this responsibility be left to parents? Should films like *It's Elementary* be broadcast on national TV if the goal is to get people talking and thinking about educational issues?

Exploring Personal Dimensions

Take a few moments to measure the strength of your feelings about homosexuality and gender identity by using this values grid.

Place in the appropriate square of the grid the *italicized* key term in the questions following that shows how you feel about the question. Note that you will be identifying the *degree* of your feelings, not whether they are positive or negative. Fill in all 16 squares, placing only one key term in any one square. (You may change your mind as you go along if you discover other key words about which you feel more or less strongly.) After you complete the grid, look it over to see how strong your feelings are. If you can find a willing partner, compare your grids and discuss your responses.

	Very Strongly	Strongly	Mildly	No Reaction
1. How would you feel if your closest *friend* told you he or she was a homosexual?	❑	❑	❑	❑
2. How do you feel about *two girls* who greet each other with a kiss after a long summer vacation?	❑	❑	❑	❑
3. How do you feel about *two boys* greeting each other with a kiss after a long summer vacation?	❑	❑	❑	❑
4. How do you feel about a person who would *beat up* a homosexual for fun?	❑	❑	❑	❑
5. How do you feel about two *girls holding hands* on the way to class?	❑	❑	❑	❑
6. How do you feel about girls wearing *boys' clothes*?	❑	❑	❑	❑

7. How do you feel about boys wearing *girls' clothes*? ❏ ❏ ❏ ❏

8. How do you feel about two *boys holding hands* on the way to class? ❏ ❏ ❏ ❏

9. How do you feel about *boys* who do not like sports? ❏ ❏ ❏ ❏

10. How do you feel about *girls* who do like sports? ❏ ❏ ❏ ❏

11. How do you feel about taking *group showers*? ❏ ❏ ❏ ❏

12. How do you feel about a man taking over the household *chores*? ❏ ❏ ❏ ❏

13. How do you feel about a male *hairdresser*? ❏ ❏ ❏ ❏

14. How do you feel about a woman who becomes a *construction worker*? ❏ ❏ ❏ ❏

15. How do you feel about going out only with persons of the *opposite sex*? ❏ ❏ ❏ ❏

16. How do you feel about going out only with persons of the *same sex*? ❏ ❏ ❏ ❏

How did you feel about these questions? Did any of them bother you for any reason? Why or why not? Do you have strong feelings about homosexuality?

Source: Bruess, C. E., & Greenberg, J. S. *Sexuality education: Theory and practice.* Sudbury, MA: Jones and Bartlett Publishers, 2004.

Suggested Readings

Barker, J. C., Herdt, G., & deVries, B. Social support in the lives of lesbians and gay men at midlife and later. *Sexuality Research and Social Policy, 3, no. 2* (June 2006), 1–23.

Bily, C. A. *Homosexuality (opposing viewpoints).* Chicago: Greenhaven Press, 2008.

Goldfarb, E. A. Lesson on homophobia and teasing. *American Journal of Sexuality Education, 1* (2006), 55–66.

Groom, C. J., & Pennebaker, J. W. The language of love, sexual orientation, and language use in online personal advertisements. *Sex Roles, 52, no. 7-8* (April 2005), 447–461.

Journal of Bisexuality. Binghamton, NY: Haworth Press. Available: www.haworthpress.com/store/product.asp?sku-j159.

Journal of Homosexuality. Binghamton, NY: Haworth Press. Available: www.haworthpress.com/store/product.asp?sku-j082.

King, J. L. *On the down low: A journey into the lives of "straight" black men who sleep with men.* New York: Broadway, 2004.

Marcus, E. *What if someone I know is gay? Answers to questions about gay and lesbian people.* Newark, NJ: Penguin Putnam, 2000.

Patterson, C. J. Children of gay and lesbian parents. *Current Directions in Psychological Science, 15, no. 5* (October 2006), 241–244.

Peters, J. A. *Keeping you a secret.* New York: Little-Brown, 2005.

Ross, M. W., Mansson, S. A., Daneback, K., & Tikkanen, R. Characteristics of men who have sex with men on the Internet, but identify as heterosexual, compared with heterosexually identified men who have sex with women. *Cyberpsychological Behavior 8, no. 2* (April, 2005), 131–139.

Walther, C. S., & Poston, D. L. Patterns of gay and lesbian partnering in the larger metropolitan areas of the United States. *Journal of Sex Research, 41, no. 2* (January 2004), 201–214.

Web Resources

For links to the web sites below, visit *http://sexuality.jbpub.com/dimensions/4e* and click on Resource Links.

American Civil Liberties Union: Lesbian Gay Bisexual Transgender Project
www.aclu.org/lgbt/index.html

Documentation of the ACLU's actions to fight discrimination and educate the public regarding LGBT rights.

American Psychological Association
www.apa.org/topics/orientation.html

Provides answers to questions about sexual orientation and homosexuality.

Hartford Institute for Religion Research: Homosexuality and Religion
http://hirr.hartsem.edu/research/homosexuality_religion.html

Articles and research on the topic of homosexuality and religion.

Lambda Legal
www.lambdalegal.org

Contains information about many legal issues including laws related to sexual orientation.

National Organization for Women: Information on Same Sex Marriages
www.now.org/issues/lgbi/marr-rep.html

Information on NOW's work on lesbian rights including support of same-gender unions.

CHAPTER 11

Sexuality in Childhood and Adolescence

FEATURES

Communication Dimensions
Tips for Discussing Sexual Messages and Scandals on TV with Children

Communication Dimensions
Resources for Becoming Askable

Ethical Dimensions
Is It Ethical to Ignore Your Child's Developing Sexuality?

Gender Dimensions
How Gender Stereotypes Affect Sexuality

Multicultural Dimensions
Racial and Ethnic Differences in Sexual Behaviors

Global Dimensions
Teenagers and Sexuality Around the World

CHAPTER OBJECTIVES

1 Explain why an infant is a sexual being; include the role that touch plays in development.

2 Explain the sexual development of children from preschool through the early elementary years.

3 Describe the differences in puberty for boys and girls.

4 Identify the three developmental stages of adolescence.

5 Compare the findings of various surveys concerning adolescent sexual behaviors and attitudes.

6 Discuss the prevalence of sexual abuse and sexual harassment of children and adolescents.

sexuality.jbpub.com/dimensions/4e

Sexual Development During Preschool and Early Elementary Years
The Media as Sexuality Educator of Children
Late Adolescence

INTRODUCTION

Shawna is a precocious five-year-old who already reads. She's been eating lunch at a nice restaurant with her mother after a morning of shopping. In the restroom before heading for home, she notices a vending machine mounted on the wall and asks, "Mama, why are they selling napkins in the bathroom when they already give them to everyone when they're eating?" Mama, visibly flustered, says, "We'll talk about it later, after we get home." Shawna feels as if she has asked something she shouldn't have mentioned and never brings it up again. Neither does her mother.

A few years later, still a precocious child, she reaches menarche just as she enters fifth grade, before she turns ten. Shawna has used the dictionary to learn all the "facts of life" she can find. She knows what is happening to her body, but is afraid to tell her mother. She privately rejoices at this sign of her physical maturity. Finally, some stained panties in the laundry disclose her secret. Then she and her mother have "the talk" about menstruation. Shawna's mother shares that when she was growing up, she was expected to announce when every period came at the breakfast table. That was very embarrassing to her, and she doesn't want Shawna to feel the same way. So she suggests, "Just let me know if there is anything you need or if something doesn't seem right." Looking back, that assurance was both positive and comforting. Shawna hopes someday she will be able to treat her own daughter with that kind of respect. But she will have "the talk" sooner and will try to answer questions candidly whenever they come up.

Now as a young mother, Shawna is in a public restroom with both her daughters, aged three and five. Her five-year-old, Samantha, asks, "Mom, how come they sell 'tampads' in here?" Remembering her own *early questions, Shawna decides to respond on the spot in front of both girls and anyone else that happens to be listening. She says, "The pads are for women or older girls who are having a menstrual period. It's a natural and healthy thing that happens every month. A period helps a girl's body to be able to have babies" (Wilson, 1991).*

As you read the chapter on Sexuality in Childhood and Adolescence, you may want to think about your own life and ask yourself, "How did I become who I am today?" "Which experiences helped promote my sexual health?" "What happened to me that I must overcome as I move into sexual adulthood?"

Learning the sexual values of parents and caregivers happens through observation and nonverbal cues, along with the "talks" that may or may not have helped move one over the speed bumps that happen as children grow up. Reflect on past experience; think about how situations might have been handled differently. Perhaps questions could have been answered more honestly. Puzzling dilemmas might have been discussed more openly.

Today, honest answers, balanced discussion, and decision-making options are more available than ever before. Reliable web sites, well-informed educators, and parental resources abound. (See suggestions in Communication Dimensions: Resources for Becoming Askable.) Yet, this open discussion leads to more sex in the media. Parents are understandably confused about how to answer their children's questions about the most recent sex scandals.

How much should they tell their children? Should they answer their children's questions directly? Should they try to shield their children from the news?

■ Sexual Development of Infants and Toddlers

Sexuality education begins in the delivery room. Of course, we are not talking about giving newborn babies facts about reproduction or sexual behaviors. But think for a minute: What is the first or second question parents ask after the birth of a child? They ask, "Is it a boy or a girl?" And sexuality education about gender roles begins.

Newborn babies develop sexually. In some ways, the first 18 months of life is one of the most important times for learning about love and touch and developing a sense of trust in the world. It is during their infancy that babies learn they are loved

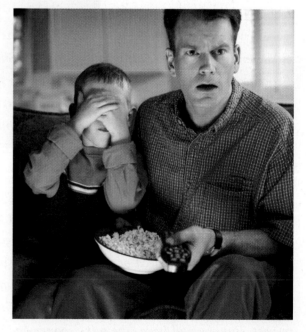

Many parents find it hard to discuss sexual relationships that are sensationalized in the media. However, it is important to realize that parents teach their children about sexuality with what they say—as well as by what they do not say. By *not* saying anything about the latest incidents in the news, parents may be inadvertently telling their children not to ask questions about sexuality.

Communication
DIMENSIONS

Tips for Discussing Sexual Messages and Scandals on TV with Children

If a sexuality scandal of a high public official or a popular entertainer makes headlines, most likely any child in school will hear about it. Many parents wonder whether they need to discuss these scandals at all. The question parents need to ask is, Who do I want to tell my children about this sad situation? Another child on the playground? An acquaintance on the school bus?

Here are some tips for discussing scandals with your children:

1. Think about values as they relate to the current situation. What are your family values about sex outside marriage, fidelity, telling the truth?

2. Find out what the children already know. Do not wait for them to ask questions. That may never happen. You can start by saying, "Tell me what you've heard about . . . ." You may be surprised how much they know.

3. Ask them to tell you what certain words mean to them. For example, a child may say that a celebrity had "oral sex" and think that means kissing.

4. Clarify the facts. Give short, age-appropriate answers. A short answer on "oral sex" for a child below the age of 10 years is, "Adults kiss, hug, or touch each other in special ways to show caring and share sexual pleasure. Oral sex is one way." Ask preteens or teenagers for their definition. Then correct any misinformation.

5. Help your children understand the larger issues surrounding sexuality scandals. These issues will affect the families of those involved, careers, and possibly the welfare of the nation.

6. You do not have to answer questions about your personal life. The answer to "Do you and Daddy do that?" is "Daddy's and my sex life is personal. When you are an adult, you will decide what sexual behaviors are comfortable for you."

Television has become a primary part of most children's sexuality education. Rather than viewing media as an adversary in efforts to educate, it can become an ally. Suit the conversation to the developmental level of the child.

Age 3–6: Focus on varied family configurations and non-normative sex roles to help little ones learn about different grown-up possibilities.

Age 7–10: Identify concerns about racial and ethnic differences, body image, clothing, and hairstyles, especially unwarranted stereotyping and advertising.

Age 11–13: Programs featuring hidden feelings and deceptions make good lessons as emotions and hormones escalate. Discuss how feelings are expressed and directed.

Age 14–17: Major adolescent concerns involve sexual behaviors and their consequences. Use viewing to discuss issues; muse aloud.

Source: Garrity, J. Tuning in to TV sex: Using television for dialogue with your children. Santa Monica, CA. Center for Media Literacy, 2002. Retrieved June 5, 2009, from http://medialit.org/reading_room/pdf/24 _TVsex_teachable.pdf.

and learn how to love when parents kiss them, hug them, and talk to them. Babies also learn whether care providers will meet their needs or whether they will have to tough it out. They learn quickly whether they can count on their care providers to respond to their basic needs.

Actually, biological sexual development begins during pregnancy. Prenatal ultrasound technology has verified that the sexual response system begins to develop in males during the middle stages of gestation. Erectile response begins to appear at around 16 weeks; respiratory function does not begin until almost 12 weeks later. And, although sexual response in female fetuses is not readily observable, it is assumed that the capacity for lubrication begins at this time as well.

During the first few months of life, **infants**, babies from birth to 1 year, begin

> **infants**
> Babies from birth to 1 year old.

to discover their bodies. By 7 or 8 months, they discover their hands and toes. About the same time, boys discover their penis. Girls, on average, seem to discover their vulva about 2 months later. Infants love to put their fingers and toes into their mouths, and they love to touch their genitals. Baby boys have erections regularly throughout the day and during sleep, as many as three or more times a night. Infant boys may become erect simply by crying, coughing, stretching, or urinating. Baby girls' vaginas are believed to lubricate about just as often, although this is not easily observable, and studies on this topic have not been done.

Psychosexual Development

Cuddling and stroking babies help them learn that their bodies feel good when they are touched and also help cement the parent–child bond. In fact, research shows that parents should hold their babies as much as possible. Touch is one of the first ways that a baby learns he or she is loved. Some psychologists theorize that a loving touch helps set the stage for adult intimacy. Touching and holding infants teach them how parents feel about them. When I am crying, will I be picked up? Can I count on you to show me that you love me? Responding to infants' needs teaches them that the world is a predictable, safe place. It boosts their self-confidence and their ability to believe that when they need help and support, they will get it. When parents and caregivers convey love and delight when they hold their infants, the infants learn they are loved.

Bonding, based on this love, begins at birth when mother and newborn are brought together. It continues during feeding, diapering, smiling, talking, and acknowledging the infant. As an active and comfortable participant in parenting, the father also bonds with the infant through touch. This fosters trust that all needs will be fulfilled and the infant is **thriving**. Developing a sense of trust in the world is an important foundation for adult mental health, including sexual health. The developmental psychologist Erik H. Erikson wrote that the first psychosocial crisis in life is to resolve "basic trust versus basic mistrust." According to Erikson, between birth and 18 months of age, children learn whether their needs will be met and whether they can trust the people and the world around them. If their needs are met, they develop the ability for intimacy and a sense of hope. Erikson wrote that feeding is the primary way that an infant resolves these issues (Erikson, 1950).

In the early 1960s, two researchers did an important experiment with rhesus monkeys. They separated some monkeys from their mothers at birth and offered them surrogate wire mothers to hold. Some of the surrogates were only wire frames; others were covered with soft fabric. The monkeys would cling to a dummy covered with soft fabric but rejected one made up just of wire, even when it had a bottle of milk attached. In other words, the baby monkeys preferred a soft touch to being fed. The baby monkeys denied touch grew up to be troubled adult monkeys. They were more likely to bite and scratch; the males did not approach females sexually; and the females were mostly infertile (Bullough & Bullough, 1994). Some psychologists believe that such studies show that a lack of touch in infancy can affect future adult sexual and intimate relationships.

Teaching Body Parts

Bath time and diaper changes are wonderful times to start teaching a child about body parts—*all* the parts of his or her body. Many parents play this game to teach body parts with their 5- or 6-month-old children: "Here is your nose, here's your tummy, here are your knees, here are your toes." In addition to teaching the names of these body parts, these parents may be inadvertently conveying an early message about their willingness to address sexual issues. These parents may be communicating to their child that many (one-third) of the body's parts have no names and that they are different from all the other parts of the body. How much more sex-positive it would be if parents could learn to say, calmly and without flinching, "Here's your nose, here's your tummy, here's your penis (or vulva), here are your knees, here are your toes." Thus all the parts of the body that the baby is exploring have names, and parents can speak about all of them.

Parents should treat all body parts equally. When parents use euphemisms only for the genitals, they give their child a message that these parts of the body are shameful or different. They may, without meaning to or realizing it, even introduce a sense of guilt about certain parts of the body. These feelings sometimes persist into adulthood, making it difficult for grown men and women to be comfortable with their bodies and sexual feelings. They may also affect a child's ability to tell about sexually abusive incidents accurately.

Infant Genital Touching

Babies begin to explore their genitals during diaper changes. This usually happens at about 7 to 10 months, a little after they discover that they have fingers and toes. And they experience for themselves that it feels good to touch all the parts of their bodies.

Many parents are uncomfortable when they see their babies touch their genitals. They wonder what, if anything, they should do. They wonder whether their child is masturbating or is becoming obsessed with this behavior. This type of genital exploration is not the same as masturbation; it is generally not purposeful and not directed at orgasm. It is about exploring and learning more about the body.

psychosexual development
The blending of sexual aspects of one's development with other psychological factors.

bonding
A process of developing a close physical and psychological relationship with one's caregiver.

thriving
Normal physical and psychological pattern of weight gain, neuromuscular development and other developmental attributes of infants.

Communication
DIMENSIONS

Resources for Becoming Askable

Here are some guidelines for becoming askable—10 healthy hints—as well as examples of questions and answers.

1. Start early, using body language and nonverbal behaviors to convey messages of approachability.
2. Giving "too much" information should not be a concern. Observe reactions to gauge how much is needed.
3. Communicate openly, even acknowledging discomfort.
4. Admit ignorance and offer to find out—together if possible.
5. Concise, simple answers are better than long lectures.
6. Too much technical information won't hurt; it allows children to sort it out and honors their ability to understand.
7. Mistakes will happen; admit them, correct them if possible and handle them as you would other mistakes.
8. Share your values about sexual matters; children want to know what you believe.
9. Encourage laughing and learning by using a sense of humor.
10. Use books as a springboard for discussion; they are lasting and can be referred to over and over (Blonna & Levitan, 2006).

Having resources at hand is helpful when talking to children about sexuality issues in the home. See the suggested reading list at the end of the chapter to begin a resource library at home.

Sex education often begins with a child's curiosity about his or her body. Let the child set the pace with his or her questions.

If your child points to a body part, simply tell him or her what it is. This is also a good time to talk about which parts of the body are private.

Expect self-stimulation. Teach your child that masturbation is a normal—but private—activity. If it happens in public, try distraction. If that fails, take your child aside for a reminder about the importance of privacy.

Curiosity about others—examining another child's sex organs—is usually normal exploration and far removed from adult sexual activity. It's harmless when only young children are involved, but as a family matter, you may want to set limits on such exploration.

Take advantage of everyday opportunities. Consider these examples:

- **How do babies get inside mommy?** You might say, "A mom and a dad make a baby by holding each other in a special way."
- **How are babies born?** It might be enough to say, "Doctors and nurses help babies who are ready to be born." If your child wants more details, you might say, "Usually a mom pushes the baby out of her vagina."
- **Why doesn't everyone have a penis?** Try a simple explanation such as, "Boys' and girls' bodies are made differently."
- **Why do you have hair down there?** Simplicity often works here, too. You might say, "Our bodies change as we get older." If your child wants more details, add, "Boys grow hair near their penises, and girls grow hair near their vaginas."

Answer specific questions using correct terminology. Even if you're uncomfortable, forge ahead. Remember—you're setting the stage for open, honest discussions in the years to come.

Source: Mayo Clinic, 2009. Retrieved June 5, 2009, from www.mayoclinic.com/health/sex-education/HQ00547.

Self-exploration lays the foundation for development of a broad range of sexual feelings and behaviors. Parental reaction also impacts development. Consider the effect of punishment—yelling, pushing the hand away, and admonishing the behavior as dirty. Conveying a strong negative message about behavior that is pleasurable creates confusion—ultimately leading to feelings of shame and fear about sex.

Some responses that encourage healthy sexual development include viewing exploratory behavior as normal learning, socializing for privacy rather than forbidding, using natural opportunities to provide basic information, and becoming more "askable."

Gender During the First Three Years

There are some innate differences between boy babies and girl babies. Studies indicate that boy babies may be more active and irritable than girl babies. On average, girl babies seem to reach such developmental

The affection displayed by parents sets an example for their children. Parents who are violent or abusive to each other around a child also set an example for the child to follow.

milestones as sitting up, reaching for objects, and talking earlier than do boy babies (Beal, 1994).

Impact of Gender Roles Before Birth

Boys and girls are also socialized differently from their earliest moments of life. In fact, parents' expectations for their children as males and females (that is, their **gender roles**) may start before birth. Mothers who know the sex of their fetus in utero even describe fetal movement differently. Pregnant mothers of boys say that the fetus's movements are strong and vigorous, whereas pregnant mothers of girls describe them as lively or moderate. When pregnant women do not know the sex of the fetus, they use words that are more gender neutral. Although studies show that male fetuses are not really more active than female fetuses, gender stereotypes affect perception even before a baby is born (Beal, 1994).

Many people prepare differently for their new baby when they know whether the child is a boy or a girl. Parents-to-be often select different wallpaper and accessories for the nursery, different-colored infant clothes, and different announcement cards. With today's frequent use of amniocentesis and ultrasound, many parents *do* know the biological sex of their child months before his or her birth. And for some parents, it is during the middle trimester of the pregnancy that they begin to think about how they want to raise that boy or girl child.

Assigned Gender from Birth Onward

Studies of parents with newborn babies show that parents often speak differently to boy infants and girl infants. In fact, many parents hold, play with, and even touch their baby girls differently than they do their baby boys. Some studies have even found that parents' views of their new babies differ by sex during the first 24 hours of life. Parents rate their new girl babies as more delicate, finer, and softer than they do their boy babies; newborn sons are rated as stronger, firmer, and hardier than newborn daughters (Beal, 1994). These differences in rearing and expectations are based on **assigned gender**.

During the first year of life, parents continue to treat their sons and daughters differently. Studies show that mothers look at their daughters more than they do their sons, hold them more, touch them more, and cuddle them more. Mothers are more emotionally expressive to daughters: They smile at them more, talk to them more, and respond to their needs more quickly. Even in the first few months of life, these behaviors encourage girls to be more social and more emotional than boys. Mothers wait longer to tend to their sons' needs, and those extra few unattended minutes perhaps give them a greater beginning sense of autonomy and independence. Fathers play with and talk to their infant sons more than they do their infant daughters, and many fathers adopt a rougher kind of horseplay with their sons than they do with their daughters (Beal, 1994).

Gender Identity Becomes Evident

During the first 18 months of life, children themselves are also beginning to learn the differences between males and females (that is, **gender identity**). Babies pick out male and female voices as early as 6 months of age. Between 1 year and 18 months, babies look longer at photographs of people of their own sex than they do of people of the other sex. Studies show that most children by the age of 3 years can identify both photographs and dolls as male

gender roles
Culturally defined behaviors that a particular society views as suitable for males and females; cultural and behavioral markers for masculinity and femininity

assigned gender
Intentional decision to raise a child as a boy or a girl, usually made at birth based on the child's genital appearance.

gender identity
Having an internal sense of self as male or female; part of one's self-image.

gender stereotypes
Beliefs about how each gender should behave, which may be over-generalized or rigidly held.

or female and can tell an adult whether they are a boy or a girl (Beal, 1994).

During the first 3 years of life, children are learning the difference between boys and girls and beginning to identify themselves as male or female. By 3 years old, they know that they will grow up to be a man or a woman, and they are absorbing a remarkable number of **gender stereotypes**.

Children learn to divide the world into "male" and "female" before they reach the age of 2 years. Depending on the behaviors they see in their homes and preschools, they identify certain behaviors as male or female. For example, in some studies, children as young as 2 years have told researchers that girls like to play with dolls and boys like to play with trucks. They say that girls like to cry and boys like to hit. They divide adult jobs into male jobs and female jobs. They even assign genders to colors: Pink and purple stuffed animals are deemed girls; black and brown stuffed animals are deemed boys. And they may even change their behaviors to fit these gender stereotypes. For example, girls and boys in the first 18 months have basically identical levels of aggressive behavior, but by the age of 2 or 3 years, girls act less aggressively than boys. Both boys and girls seem to have learned that aggression is acceptable behavior for boys but not for girls. And there is some evidence that there are, indeed, differences in male and female brains that account for some of the differences in behaviors by children of different sexes.

It is almost a cliché to say that children learn from what they observe around them. But research clearly shows that children from traditional homes are much more likely to learn these gender stereotypes. Parents often provide very different types of toys to girl and boy infants and toddlers. Girls get dolls, stuffed animals, kitchen appliances, jewelry, and dress-up clothes. Boys are given cars, trucks, balls, and sports equipment. In a study of toy catalogs, almost every catalog rigidly divided the pages into toys that were played with only by boys and toys that were played with only by girls. Girls were sometimes pictured playing "boys' games" such as ball or science projects, but no boys were pictured with dolls, kitchens, or other "playing house" toys. In every catalog, the erector set was accompanied by a picture of a boy (Haffner & Casselman, 1996). Many psychologists believe that these toy selections actually affect skills in later life: Girls learn more about nurturing and boys have more of an opportunity to develop reasoning and spatial relation skills.

◼ Sexual Development During Preschool and Early Elementary Years

During the years from age 3 years to age 5 years, children begin to develop a strong sense of gender and what that means to them and the people around them. They are finishing with toilet training, and if they are in school or a day care center, they have probably observed other children and learned for themselves that boys and girls have different body parts. At this time the child realizes that he or she will not normally change over the life span. This concept is known as **gender constancy**. Children of this age are very curious about their own and other people's bodies. This is the age when a child is first likely to ask, "Where did I come from?"

gender constancy
Recognition by a child that he or she will remain the same gender throughout life.

Preschool Genital Touching

Three- and 4-year-olds delight in their own bodies. And just as they learn it feels good when they run, jump, and cuddle, they are also discovering that it feels good when they touch their own genitals. Most professionals believe that preschool children touch their genitals as a natural part of child development. In a 1998 study of mothers of 2- to 5-year-olds, about 25% of mothers reported that their sons and 15% reported that their daughters touched their genitals in public. Sixteen percent of both preschool boys and girls had been observed masturbating with their hands (Delamater & Friedrich, 2002).

Toddlers and preschoolers touch their genitals in a much less purposeful way than older children and adolescents, and many do so without embarrassment or anxiety. In fact, it is not unusual in a preschool to have several of the boys touching their penis unconsciously throughout the day. Little girls find it pleasurable to touch their vulva and clitoris as well.

Many children appear not even to be aware that they are touching their genitals in this way. Some children do discover that this activity helps them calm down. Many children touch their genitals right before naps or bedtimes to help them fall asleep. (Just as for adults, some children never touch their genitals at all. It is normal for a preschooler to touch the genitals and it is normal for him or her not to.)

Not only do parents treat boys and girls differently, but children themselves learn gender differences in voices, levels of aggression, and even the colors of toys.

Attraction to Parents

Sigmund Freud felt that 3- to 5-year-old boys develop fantasies of possessing their mother sexually and become jealous of their father. He named it the **Oedipus complex** after the Greek tragedy in which Oedipus unknowingly kills his father and then marries his mother. According to Freud's theory, this period is accompanied by castration anxiety; boys fear that their father will retaliate against their interest in their mother by cutting off their penis. Freud also theorized that girls develop an **Electra complex**; they develop "penis envy" and want to take their father away from their mother. Girls, he said, reject their mother because they blame her for their lack of a penis. Freud named this "complex" the Electra complex after the Greek tragedy in which a princess helps kill her mother.

Most modern psychologists debunk these ideas. Feminist psychologists critique Freud's views as extremely sexist, and anthropologists point out that these "complexes" are not found in all cultures. Still, it is not uncommon for preschool children to prefer the parent of the opposite gender at this time.

Oedipus complex
Libidinal feelings of a child toward the parent of the opposite sex and hostile or jealous feelings toward the parent of the same sex.

Electra complex
Freud's theory that 3- to 5-year-old girls want to take their father away from their mother.

Preschool children love their parents intensely and may be confused about whether all love is expressed romantically. Many children try to kiss their parents romantically. Some even try to imitate adults they have seen in person or on TV or in the movies by putting their tongue into their parents' mouths.

Preschool children sometimes may even seem jealous when their parents show affection to each other. In one study, 13% of mothers of 2- to 5-year-olds reported that their children became upset when they saw adults kiss (Delamater & Friedrich, 2002).

Preschoolers and Sex Play

Many adults remember playing "doctor" or "house" with other children. Playing doctor, including undressing each other and examining each other's genitals, is quite common. As many as half of adults remember engaging in childhood sexual play (Leitenberg, Greenwald, & Tarran, 1989). Most child development experts see this type of sex play as expected and natural childhood sexual curiosity. If the children are of the same age and stage of development, experts do not believe that it is harmful. And studies of adults show that engaging in childhood sexual play does not seem to have any effect, either positive or negative, on adult sexuality.

Besides concern about childhood sex play among peers, exposure to nudity or parental sexual inter-

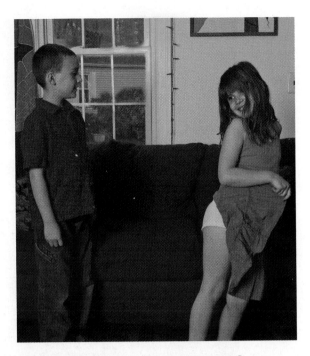

In early childhood, availability of playmates influences interaction. Games that provide opportunities for sex play and exploration such as "doctor" or "nurse" are responses to natural curiosity. According to Erickson's developmental stages (Erickson, 1950), these children need to accomplish autonomy and initiative rather than shame, doubt, or guilt.

course has been studied. The researchers concluded that such exposure is not detrimental to the mental health of children. Characterizing exposure as harmful or even a subtle form of abuse might better be conceptualized as myth (Okami et al., 1998). Another concern, that of erections among young boys as evidence of romantic interest, is also a myth. Erections come and go, rise and fall, among babies and young boys, even sleeping and waking adults, with odd timing (Schwartz & Rutter, 2000). Another study examined the impact of noncoercive sexual contact with similarly aged individuals. Researchers found that adult adjustment problems were no different from those who had no sexual abuse experience. Among those who had been abused, problems escalated according to the amount of coercion reported (Friedrich, Whiteside, & Talley, 2004).

That said, there is a big difference between normally harmless child sexual play and play that is exploitative or abusive. Children do not normally engage in painful sexual behavior, oral–genital contact, or simulated or real intercourse or penetration with fingers or objects with another child, and they do not engage in normal sexual play with children more than a few years older than they are. These behaviors may indicate a child who *may* have been sexually abused. (They could also indicate exposure to inappropriate TV or videos.) Table 11.1 provides some guidelines on distinguishing between harmless play and exploitative, inappropriate behaviors.

Questions About Reproduction

Some time between the ages of 2½ and 5 years, children ask, "Where did I come from?" Children at this age are often very curious about pregnancy and birth. According to psychologists, at around the age of 4 years, children understand that babies do not just spontaneously appear and that something must have happened for this process to begin.

The psychologist Anne C. Bernstein did research with small children about how they understand reproduction (Bernstein, 1994). She labels the preschooler asking about reproduction a "geographer." The emphasis really is on the *where*: They want to know *where* the baby comes from and *where* it was before it was born. Preschoolers can be offered a very simple answer: "You grew in a special place inside Mom called a uterus. You began from a tiny egg (the size of a pencil dot) from Mom and an even tinier sperm from Dad." This will satisfy most preschoolers. If they ask, "But how did I get into the uterus?" they can be given a very simple definition of sexual intercourse:

When two grown-ups love each other, they like to kiss and hug and touch each other in ways that feel good. Sometimes, the man and woman place the man's penis into the woman's vagina. The man's penis releases sperm into the woman and sometimes a baby begins.

TABLE 11.1 **A Quick Way to Assess Whether Childhood Sex Play Is Likely to Be Harmless or Whether Parents Should Be Concerned**

	Expected	Problematic
Age of children	Similar	More than 3 years apart
Children seem	Giggly, curious, happy	Aggressive, angry, fearful, withdrawn
Activities	Undressing, playing doctor ("You show me yours, I'll show you mine")	Oral, anal, or vaginal intercourse; penetration with fingers, objects
After parental intervention	Behavior stops	Behavior continues

Elementary School Years

The early elementary school years (kindergarten to grade 3) are years of tremendous growth and change. Naps and playtime give way to homework and tests. Preschool teacher hugs may be replaced by neutral hellos. The class of 12 now has 20 children, and individual attention is no longer the rule. Children begin to learn about sexuality issues from other children on the bus or the playground.

Freud wrote that the period from 5 to 11 years of age was the **latency period**. Although some blame Freud for mistakenly characterizing this as a period of sexual *dis*interest, Bullough describes it differently. He credits Freud with breaking the taboo on full discussions of sexuality, recognizing it as a prime factor in human development. Rather than *dis*interest, Freud expected active sexual exploration and information seeking, the prepubescent hormone surge and accompanying growth of internal and external sexual organs (Bullough, 2004).

latency period
Outdated Freudian theory that children aged 6–12 years old have no sexual feelings or interest.

Five- to 8-year-olds continue to be very interested in sexual issues; it is just that their interest is no longer as apparent to the adults in their lives as it used to be. In a 1998 study of more than 11,000 children aged 2 to 12 years, mothers reported that they had observed sexual behaviors in children at all of these ages. For example, 14% of 6- to 9-year-old boys were still touching their genitals in public, 40% did so at home, 20% tried to look at people nude, 8% wanted to watch nudity on TV, and 14% were very interested in girls. Girls this age exhibited similar sexual behaviors that were observed by their mothers (Friedrich et al., 1998).

As mentioned, 5- to 8-year-olds continue to develop as sexual persons, and they are very curious about pregnancy and birth. They develop strong friendships, and most boys and girls show a strong preference for playing with children of the same gender. They become even more aware of socially defined gender roles. They may continue to engage in sex play with children of both genders. And in private, their exploration of their genitals may become more purposeful.

Developing Empathy

Some sexologists believe that the period from age 5 years to age 8 years is critical in sexual development. They believe that the elementary school years are the most important time for people to develop as moral thinkers, and that development is important to adult sexual health. While they are preschoolers, children believe that their way of thinking is the only way possible. But in early elementary school, children begin

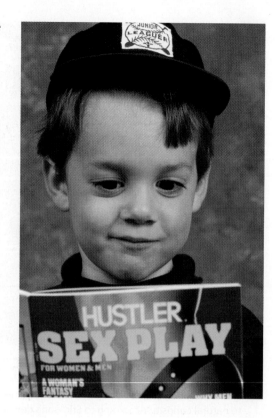

Children are naturally curious about sexuality.

to understand that there may be other points of view and ways to consider a situation. They can begin to understand the "golden rule": Treat others with the same respect you would want for yourself.

Developing an ability to empathize and make good decisions is part of the foundation for adult sexual health. A sexually healthy adult is able, for example, to make decisions about his or her sexuality that are consistent with his or her own values.

The Media as Sexuality Educator of Children

The media—television, movies, magazines, even the news—are among many children's most prominent sexuality educators. After sleeping and attending school, children aged 6 to 8 years spend more time each week watching television than they do playing, eating, doing chores, participating in sports, or attending church or synagogue. American children watch an average of 24 hours of television per week. By the time an American child graduates from high school, he or she will have spent 18,000 hours in front of a TV set, compared to only 13,000 hours in a classroom. And a child will view a staggering 20,000 commercials each year as part of that television time (Rideout & Hoff, 1996).

In addition to television, movies, music videos, video games, print, and the Internet are pervasive forms of media in today's world. According to the *Sur-*

Although it was clearly intended for preschoolers, the second largest audience for *Mister Rogers' Neighborhood* was preadolescents, who want to hear that they are special and that they are OK just as they are. What other media programs offer positive self-esteem messages to preadolescents?

geon General's Call to Action to Promote Sexual Health and Responsible Sexual Behavior (Satcher, 2001), sexual talk and behavior are increasingly explicit and frequent. Much of the content in videos and films portrays sexual eroticism, and more than half of television programming has sexual content. Thus the media do have potential for providing sexuality information and education. In a national survey, more than half the students said they learned about topics such as birth control, contraception, and preventing pregnancy from television and magazines. Yet the impact of media on actual behavior is controversial and research is indecisive (Weinstein & Rosen, 2006).

Focusing on media literacy rather than potential harm may be a way of enhancing the benefits of media as a source of useful information. More and more schools are embracing the notion that learning how information is assembled and edited will help students read, hear, and view media more critically (Goldstein, 2005). An analytical perspective can help young people entering puberty as they view media norms that present a narrow cultural definition of physical perfection. The goal is to foster an internal **locus of control** in which one's sense of identity is personally defined and not dependent on the scripts of others.

locus of control
Refers to an individual's perception of the main causes of events in life. More simply, is life's destiny controlled by the self (*internal locus*) or by external forces such as fate or other people (*external locus*)?

An example of such an educational approach for girls in grades 4–8 is called *Full of Ourselves: A Wellness Program to Advance Girl Power, Health, and Leadership* (Steiner-Adair & Sjostrom, 2006). It is a primary prevention program aimed at helping girls decrease their vulnerability to body preoccupation and eating disorders. One of the units focuses on media literacy, particularly advertising strategies. Both parents and schools are encouraged to create a supportive environment for students entering puberty.

■ Sexual Development During Puberty

Puberty, teenager, and *adolescence* are not interchangeable words. *Puberty* is the stage of maturation when a human being becomes capable of sexual reproduction. *Teenager* is defined chronologically: A teenager is a young person between the ages of 13 and 19 years. *Adolescence* is actually a relatively new concept: It is the period of development that extends from puberty (or the end of childhood) through the attainment of full adult status. Before 1900, and still today in many developing societies, children marry shortly after puberty and begin their adult responsibilities. Today, as more American young people stretch their college and graduate school education through their 20s and even 30s—and then return to live in their parents' homes—some have wondered when contemporary U.S. adolescence ends: At 30 years? When you buy your own home? Have your own children? Before your midlife crisis?

Preparing for Puberty

Young people, at some time between the ages of 8 and 16 years, go through a predictable process of biological development called *puberty*. Normal pubertal changes, indicated by the development of **secondary sexual characteristics** such as breast buds and pubic hair, may begin as early as age 8 years for girls and as early as age 9 years for boys, but some teens may not begin these changes until they are 15 or 16 years old. The median age for puberty to begin for boys is between 11 and 12 years; for girls, it is between 10 and 11 years. Still, *average* means that half of young people begin this process earlier, and half begin it later. The process of puberty from the first physical changes to obtaining a fully adult body and full reproductive potential may last 4 or 5 years. On average, boys begin and end puberty about 1 year to 2 years later than girls do.

secondary sexual characteristics
Changes occurring during adolescence—such as growth of pubic hair, breast development, and testes and penile development.

Too many young women say they are not being prepared adequately for pubertal changes. Some girls receive only minimal education in school or at a youth group meeting. In a focus group on adolescent female health (Louis Harris and Associates, 1997), one 12-year-old girl said:

> That was a big thing in the fifth grade. We had boys' education and girls' education. There was this little pamphlet we got. My friends and I were upset for the whole week.

Other girls report that they received only scant information from their mother or older siblings or friends. In the same focus group, one girl reported, "On my tenth birthday, they gave us this little package, and it was like a pad and a little booklet." Another girl reports that she really did not get the information she needed: "I think that if I knew what it was, that all girls get it, and I was told that this is going to happen to everyone, that it doesn't hurt, and that it's fine, I think it would have been all right. But in a sense, you feel such shame."

Puberty for Girls

The first noticeable sign of puberty in girls is generally the development of **breast buds**; the breast begins to elevate as a small mound. Later, the breast and the nipple get bigger. Light, sparse pubic and underarm hair begins to appear about 6 months later. Girls begin to experience a growth spurt, often growing as much as several inches in a year. Their genital and underarm areas begin to produce sweat glands, and body odor may result. Most girls begin menstrual periods about 2 years after breast budding begins, but some girls have completed breast development before their first period, and some girls' breasts continue to develop for many years after.

breast budding
First stage of breast development in females, whereby breast tissue elevates as a small mound.

Girls today are experiencing first menstruation at earlier ages than girls growing up three or four decades ago. The average age for first menstruation, **menarche** (pronounced "men-ar-key"), in the United States is now 12½ years. That means that many girls have their first period before the end of seventh grade, and many begin as early as fourth or fifth grade. It also means that many girls will at least be in the eighth grade before their first period, and some may be seniors in high school before they get a period. All of these situations are normal.

Many pediatricians use a measurement called a **Tanner scale** to rate physical sexual development in both boys and girls (see Table 11.2).

menarche
First menstruation for girls.

Tanner scale
Scale developed by Dr. John Tanner for measuring pubertal development in boys and girls.

Puberty for Boys

Puberty in boys begins on average during the sixth or seventh grade, but in some boys it begins at 9 years, and in others puberty does not begin until they are almost 14 years old. Boys experience many of the same changes as girls do. The first physical sign is usually an increase in the size of the testes; unlike breast budding in girls, this is unlikely to be observed by parents. During puberty, they too develop light, sparse pubic and underarm hair, and their sweat glands become activated. Between the ages of 12 and 14 years, their penis and scrotum begin to enlarge. At first, the testes become larger, and the skin on the scrotum reddens and coarsens. As boys mature, their penis starts to grow longer. Pubic hair slowly becomes darker, and it starts to curl. During puberty, the penis doubles in size.

By Tanner stage 3 (see Table 11.3), ejaculation has usually occurred, and there may be some production of sperm. In fact, some sexologists call this **semenarche**, to correspond to the first period of girls (menarche). Most often, a boy experiences this as nocturnal emissions, or wet dreams. By Tanner stage 4, males are fertile and able to cause a pregnancy. The average length of time for a boy to go through puberty is 3 years, but it can vary from 2 to 5 years.

Significant numbers of boys are troubled by a condition called **gynecomastia**. During puberty, they begin to develop

semenarche
First ejaculation of semen for boys.

TABLE 11.2   Tanner Scale for Girls

Tanner Stage	Pubic Hair	Breasts
1	None	None
2	Sparse	Small breast buds
3	Darker, begins to curl	Breasts and nipples enlarged
4	Coarse, less curly than adult	Continued breast development
5	Adult triangle	Mature; nipple projects

TABLE 11.3 Tanner Scale for Boys

Tanner Stage	Pubic Hair	Penis/Scrotum
1	None	Childlike
2	Sparse	Scrotum: reddened, thinner, larger; Penis childlike
3	Darker, begins to curl	Penis length increases; Scrotum continues to enlarge and darken
4	Coarse, less curly than adult	Penis increases in length and circumference
5	Adult	Adult

earlier than age 9 or 10 years. Some children even enter what is called **precocious puberty** in the first year of life. Interestingly, this seems to be largely the result of genetic coding in girls, and most often there is no underlying disease. Conversely, precocious puberty in boys is much more likely to be an indication that something is wrong. If parents observe pubertal changes in a boy younger than 7 years old, they should see a health practitioner for a medical evaluation and possible interventions.

an increase in the glandular tissue around their breasts; in fact, these boys sometimes are very worried and fearful that they are growing breasts or turning into a girl. Nearly one in five 10-year-olds will have this kind of tissue development. In rare cases, gynecomastia may be the result of diseases that are rare in young people: liver disease, **hypogonadism**, **hyperthyroidism**, or **hypothyroidism**. It could also be a sign of drug use. However, most of the time it is just a variation of male pubertal development, and it usually resolves itself within 1 year to 1½ years. It continues longer than 2 years in fewer than 1 in 10 boys.

Early and Late Developers

Although the majority of young people finish puberty a few years after the start of their teen years, some begin puberty much earlier and some go through it much later. Both early and late developers face special challenges.

Early-developing girls have special problems. Because they look more mature, adults often expect them to act more mature. A third- or fourth-grade girl with developing breasts may feel awkward and want to hide her body. She may be relentlessly teased by her male and female classmates. She may indeed feel that she is not normal. Conversely, late development in boys may be more of a problem than early development. A 15- or 16-year-old boy who is still short, has no facial hair, and has a high voice may be relentlessly teased.

Some children begin puberty much

What Is Normal?

Early, late, and average developers *all* share a common concern: *Am I normal?* Rapid body changes can be very confusing. Nine- to 12-year-olds can become obsessed with their appearance. In fact, psychologists say preteens have an **imaginary audience**: They think that everyone is looking at them. Getting dressed and preparing their hair and faces can take hours. They need adult reassurance that they are attractive, and they need to understand that it is not true that everyone is looking at them.

They are concerned about their height and breast size or penis size, and they wonder whether they are too developed or too underdeveloped. They wonder whether their feelings, which sometimes fluctuate immensely, are normal. It is important to reassure preadolescents that they are developing according to their own personal genetically predetermined clock. When they ask questions like "How come I don't have my period yet?" or "Why am I the shortest boy in the class?" the question behind the question is almost always "Am I normal?"

The reality is that during preadolescence and the years following it, conflicts with parents peak. Yet, it is important to know that only about one in six teenagers and parents experience a severe disruption in their parent–child relationship (Grunbaum et al., 2004). Preadolescents are just beginning to separate from their parents, but they are also still looking to their parents for guidance and support.

Children learn about many aspects of sexuality and relationships from their

gynecomastia
Glandular tissue development in the breasts of boys.

hypogonadism
Decreased activity of the gonads that may result in retardation of growth and sexual development.

hyperthyroidism
Excessive functional activity of the thyroid gland.

hypothyroidism
A deficiency of thyroid activity.

precocious puberty
Pubertal development before the age of 7 years.

imaginary audience
Belief in early adolescence that other people are looking at you as if you are onstage.

Development of body hair in both boys and girls and facial hair in boys results in shaving, viewed by some as a rite of passage indicating sexual maturity.

parents—much of it by astute observation rather than through discussion. Yet, the value of parental involvement and maintaining open lines of communication is well documented as a deterrent to a variety of risky behaviors. Parents can enhance their children's sense of self-worth with assurances of affection and acceptance in spite of the many changes adolescence brings (Strong et al., 2005).

Emotional Changes in Preadolescence

The rapid physical changes of puberty we have described initiate many psychosocial changes. Preadolescents are beginning to move toward independence and are often very self-conscious of their bodies. They may even be embarrassed by parents. Children at this age also need to test parental authority and sometimes the authority of teachers and other adult figures in their lives. This may include trying out values that are different from their parents'. The research literature demonstrates that most teenagers go through a period of seeming to reject their parents' values; yet, by the time they reach adulthood, almost all of them adopt values similar to their parents'.

Friends become very important during the preadolescent years. Being popular is of utmost importance. The good news is that needing to be just like friends, known by psychologists as **conformity with peers**, peaks in early adoles-

conformity with peers
Desire to be like everyone else.

cence and then starts to decline. The bad news for parents is that peer pressure can be intense during this period and usually dictates the type of clothes that are acceptable. It also can lead to experimentation with cigarettes, alcohol, and sex.

Cliques often emerge during this period. Preadolescents may for the first time feel pressure to engage in certain activities to be part of a group, and, for some young people, that means experimenting with smoking, shoplifting, or cheating on tests.

Preadolescents are also beginning to develop a sense of identity. Their ability to think abstractly has just begun. They frequently daydream and turn inward and imagine acting out different roles. Daydreaming is normal and actually quite healthy. Giving a child a diary or journal and then respecting his or her right to keep it private can be an effective way to encourage a new adolescent to think about and explore his or her feelings. Children at this age can seem very dramatic. They often feel that they are continuously onstage. They may become convinced that their problems are unique and no one understands them.

Masturbation

During puberty, many boys and girls begin to masturbate for sexual pleasure. In addition to providing relief from sexual tension, masturbation has several physical and mental health benefits (Yudt, 2004). These include relief from migraine headaches and menstrual cramps, and self-knowledge about sexual functioning that can be shared with a partner. In spite of these positive aspects, along with its relative safety—no chance of pregnancy or infection—masturbation creates anxiety. Again, questions arise about what is normal because masturbation is one of the most widely practiced forms of sexual behavior but the least discussed (Weinstein & Rosen, 2006). Data indicate that a majority of boys begin masturbating between the ages of 13 and 15, whereas the onset among girls is more gradual (Bancroft, Herbenick, & Reynolds, 2003). Frequency is also a concern, but is highly individual. Some adults masturbate every day; some, once a year. Some people never masturbate. In fact, teenagers need to know that although many preteens, teens, and adults masturbate, some never do.

■ Sexuality in Adolescence

There is public and professional consensus about what is sexually unhealthy for teenagers. Professionals, politicians, and parents across the political spectrum share a deep concern about unplanned adolescent pregnancy; out-of-wedlock childbearing; STIs, including AIDS; sexual abuse; date rape; and the potential negative emotional consequences of premature sexual behaviors.

However, there is little public, professional, or political consensus about what is sexually healthy for teenagers. The public debate about adolescent sexuality has often focused on which sexual behaviors are appropriate for adolescents and ignored the complex dimensions of sexuality.

Some groups support the "Just say no" approach to adolescent sexuality. They believe that the only healthy adolescent sexuality is abstinence from all sexual behaviors until marriage and that adults should work to eliminate teen sexual experimentation. Another approach could be described as "Just say not now." This philosophy encourages young people to abstain until they are more mature but, given the high rates of teenage sexual involvement in intercourse, recommends that it is important to provide young people with access to contraception and condoms regardless of whether adults approve of their behavior. This approach might also be labeled "If you can't say no, protect yourself!" Other adults adopt a "Don't ask; don't tell" posture and simply pretend that adolescent sexuality and sexual behavior do not exist (Grunbaum et al., 2004).

Sexuality Education

In 2004, the Sexuality Information and Education Council of the United States (SIECUS) revised the *Guidelines for Comprehensive Sexuality Education: Kindergarten–12th Grade*, third edition, compiled by the National Guidelines Task Force. The following sections are adapted with permission. "The primary

Myth vs Fact

Myth: People become sexual at puberty.
Fact: People are sexual from birth to death. Although people sexually mature at puberty and become capable of reproduction, infants and children experience sensual feelings and identify themselves as boys and girls.

Myth: Dressing boys in blue and girls in pink teaches them about their gender.
Fact: By the time they are 3 years old, almost all boys and girls identify themselves by gender. They know that they will have that gender throughout their lifetime (the concept known as gender constancy). Clothes' colors do not make a difference.

Myth: Children in elementary school go through a latency period about sexual issues.
Fact: Elementary school children remain very interested in sexuality-related issues, and many continue to be involved in sex play with friends or genital self-pleasuring. They have just learned to hide this behavior from adults.

Myth: The average age of first intercourse has plummeted in the past 5 years.
Fact: The biggest change in adolescent sexual behavior occurred in the 1970s. The average age of first intercourse has decreased by 1 year since 1971.

Myth: Most teenagers have had sexual intercourse.
Fact: Only about half of teenagers aged 15–19 years have had sexual intercourse.

Myth: Masturbating more than once a week is harmful.
Fact: There is no "standard" for frequency of masturbation. Once is too often if you do not like it. Frequency is highly individual, and it is not harmful as long as it does not interfere with school, work, or relationships.

goal of sexuality education is to promote adult sexual health. It should assist young people in developing a positive view of sexuality, provide them with information they need to take care of their sexual health, and help them acquire skills to make decisions now and in the future. Life behaviors of a sexually healthy adult are essentially outcomes of instruction. The following lists reflect the actions students will be able to take after having applied the information and skills.

Human Development Life Behaviors:
Having applied the human development subconcepts at the appropriate age, the learner will be able to:

- Appreciate one's own body.

- Seek further information about reproduction as needed.

- Affirm that human development includes sexual development, which may or may not include reproduction or sexual experience.

- Interact with all genders in respectful and appropriate ways.

Many adults become concerned when their adolescent children begin to explore their emerging sexuality. But honest communication between an adult and a child can help him or her develop into a sexually healthy adult.

- Affirm one's own sexual orientation and respect the sexual orientations of others.

- Affirm one's own gender identities and respect the gender identities of others.

Relationship Life Behaviors:

Having applied the relationships subconcepts at the appropriate age, the learner will be able to:

- Express love and intimacy in appropriate ways.

- Develop and maintain meaningful relationships.

- Avoid exploitative or manipulative relationships.

- Make informed choices about family options and relationships.

- Exhibit skills that enhance personal relationships.

Personal Skills Life Behaviors:

Having applied the personal skills subconcepts at the appropriate age, the learner will be able to:

- Identify and live according to one's own values.

- Take responsibility for one's own behavior.

- Practice effective decision making.

- Develop critical-thinking skills.

- Communicate effectively with family, peers, and romantic partners.

Sexual Behavior Life Behaviors:

Having applied the sexual behavior subconcepts at the appropriate age, the learner will be able to:

- Enjoy and express one's sexuality throughout life.

- Express one's sexuality in ways that are congruent with one's values.

- Enjoy sexual feelings without necessarily acting on them.

- Discriminate between life-enhancing sexual behaviors and those that are harmful to self and/or others.

- Express one's sexuality while respecting the rights of others.

- Seek new information to enhance one's sexuality.

- Engage in sexual relationships that are consensual, nonexploitative, honest, pleasurable, and protected.

Sexual Health Life Behaviors:

Having applied the sexual health subconcepts at the appropriate age, the learner will be able to:

- Practice health-promoting behaviors, such as regular check-ups, breast and testicular self-exam, and early identification of potential problems.

- Use contraception effectively to avoid unintended pregnancy.

- Avoid contracting or transmitting an STI, including HIV.

- Act consistently with one's own values when dealing with an unintended pregnancy.

- Seek early prenatal care.

- Help prevent sexual abuse.

Society and Culture Life Behaviors:

Having applied the society and culture subconcepts at the appropriate age, the learner will be able to:

- Demonstrate respect for people with different sexual values.

- Exercise democratic responsibility to influence legislation dealing with sexual issues.

- Assess the impact of family, cultural, media, and societal messages on one's thoughts, feelings, values, and behaviors related to sexuality.

- Critically examine the world around them for biases based on gender, sexual orientation, culture, ethnicity, and race.

¿? Ethical
DIMENSIONS

Is It Ethical to Ignore Your Child's Developing Sexuality?

One of us once attended a presentation with a group of Swedish sexuality educators who were talking about the difference in sexual mores between Sweden and the United States. One of the Swedish women told us a story about her first sexual experience. She was 17 years old and very much in love. She and her boyfriend told her parents that they were ready to have sexual intercourse, and they asked to make love in her bedroom at home. The next morning, her parents served them breakfast in bed to celebrate this passage! The American educators were stunned.

Whether parents in America would openly accommodate their teens' first experience of sexual intercourse at home or not, it *is* happening. Almost half (48%) of all high school students reported in 2007 they have had sexual intercourse, and sexual activity increased with grade level, while condom use decreased (U.S. Department of Health and Human Services, 2008). When asked the location, 68% of 16- to 18-year-olds reported their first sexual intercourse occurred in their family home (22%), their partner's family home (34%), or a friend's house (12%) (Child Trends, 2003).

The boundaries between parents and their teen children about sexuality are often difficult to negotiate and raise many moral and ethical issues. Is it ethical to ignore a teen's developing sexuality? Is it ethical to withhold information about contraception and condoms? Does talking about condoms and contraception encourage teens to experiment with sexual behaviors? Should parents help a teen obtain contraception, or is a teen who is old enough to be having intercourse old enough to go to a clinic or a drug store unassisted? And if you know your teen child is having intercourse, should you allow him or her to do so in your home? While you are out? Overnight? And what is your responsibility to the other child's parent?

How did your parents handle these issues? How do you think you will handle them when you are a parent? Which issues do you need to think about in answering these questions?

- Promote the rights of all people to accurate sexuality information.

- Avoid behaviors that exhibit prejudice and bigotry.

- Reject stereotypes about the sexuality of different populations.

- Educate others about sexuality.

The following four areas contribute to an educational experience that will encourage achievement of the life behaviors listed above.

Information: Sexuality education seeks to provide accurate information about human sexuality, including growth and development, human reproduction, anatomy, physiology, masturbation, family life, pregnancy, childbirth, parenthood, sexual response, sexual orientation, gender identity, contraception, abortion, sexual abuse, HIV/AIDS, and other STIs.

Attitudes, Values, and Insights: Sexuality education seeks to provide an opportunity for young people to question, explore, and assess their own and their community's attitudes about society, gender, and sexuality. This can help young people understand their fami-ly's values, develop their own values, improve critical thinking skills, increase self-esteem and self-efficacy, and develop insights concerning relationships with family members, individuals of all genders, sexual partners, and society at large. Sexuality education can help young people understand their obligations and responsibilities to their families and society.

Relationships and Interpersonal Skills: Sexuality education seeks to help young people develop interpersonal skills, including communication, decision making, assertiveness, and peer refusal skills, as well as the ability to create reciprocal and satisfying relationships. Sexuality education programs should prepare students to understand sexuality effectively and creatively in adult roles. This includes helping young people develop the capacity for caring, supportive, noncoercive, and mutually pleasurable intimate and sexual relationships.

Responsibility: Sexuality education seeks to help young people exercise responsibility regarding sexual relationships by addressing such issues as abstinence, how to resist pressures to become involved in unwanted early sexual intercourse, and the use of contraception and other sexual health measures" (National Guidelines Task Force, 2004).

Linking Research and Programs

While the content and goals of a comprehensive sexuality education program are presented as the ideal, the research literature identifies antecedents of risky sexual behavior and pregnancy that provide implications for program delivery. A systematic analysis of peer-reviewed research from 1994 to 2002 identified four sets of associated factors that need to be considered: race and ethnicity; socioeconomic status; social influences; and attitudes toward contraception, condoms, and pregnancy, and safer sex behavioral skills. The following is a list of eight programmatic implications drawn from research designed to reduce high-risk behaviors among adolescents.

- Programs should begin earlier and target younger adolescents.

- New program models for minority teens need to be developed.

- Risk reduction programs need to be systematically linked to other youth programs that directly address socioeconomic disadvantage.

- Programs need to understand that many youth lack the skills to practice safer sex. A variety of behavioral skills are necessary for condom use; these include communication, negotiation and refusal skills, and technical condom use skills.

- Programs need to effectively address the influence of peer groups, social norms, and pressures to have sex.

- Programs for adolescents should not assume that sexual behavior is volitional.

- Programs should not assume that sexual activity among teens is limited to vaginal sex.

- Programs cannot assume that teens are unambivalent about preventing pregnancy.

Program providers also identify impediments to program success with adolescents. These include learning disabilities and cognitive immaturity, insufficient male involvement, very early sexual activity of males (as yet largely unexplored by research), and single program opportunities due to one-time clinic visits (Kalmus et al., 2003). Another researcher, Dr. Douglas Kirby, has investigated a range of school-based sexuality and HIV education programs over many years to determine program outcomes (Kirby, 2002b). He has found that the more comprehensive programs do not increase sexual intercourse or the number of sexual partners, and some delay the onset of sexual intercourse, decrease the frequency of intercourse, and increase the use of condoms and other contraceptives. In contrast, there are methodological flaws in the evaluation of abstinence-only sexuality education programs. Therefore, Kirby concludes that evidence is lacking to support claims made for the effectiveness of these programs.

Risk and Protective Factors

Most recently, Kirby has contributed to a summary of risk and protective factors affecting teen sexual behavior, pregnancy, childbearing, and STI. More than 400 research studies were analyzed to determine which factors influence adolescents' decisions about sex and which of these factors can be altered. The likelihood that a teen will have sex, become pregnant or cause a pregnancy, or contract an STI increases as the number of risk factors in a teen's life increases and/or the number of protective factors decreases. These risk and protective factors are grouped thematically as follows: (1) individual biological factors such as age, physical maturity, and gender; (2) disadvantage, disorganization, and dysfunction in the lives of teens, including violence, substance abuse, divorce, and low levels of education; (3) sexual values, attitudes, and modeled behaviors as expressed by teens themselves and by parents, peers, and romantic partners; and (4) connection to adults and organizations that discourage sex, unprotected sex, or early childbearing, such as parents and adults in schools and places of worship (Kirby, Lepore, & Ryan, 2005).

Although more research is certainly warranted, most professionals agree that age-appropriate and targeted sexuality education is one of the best preventive means available for reducing risks and enhancing sexual health. Parents can guide, schools can inform, and other community support can be provided so that adolescents will have the knowledge and self-confidence to make informed decisions regarding their own sexual outcomes.

The Three Stages of Adolescence

Developmental psychologists and health professionals have categorized adolescence into three developmental stages: early adolescence, middle adolescence, and late adolescence. These stages are key to understanding adolescents' behavioral decisions and adolescent sexuality. Table 11.4 summarizes these stages.

While reading this section, it is important to remember that there is no such thing as an "average adolescent." Individual adolescents vary widely in the pace of their development. Adolescent sexuality emerges from cultural identities mediated by ethnicity, gender, sexual orientation, class, and physical and emotional capacity. Adolescent development is affected by parents, other family members, and other adults, as well as schools and the peer group.

Early Adolescence

The **early adolescent** (females aged 9–13 years, males aged 11–15 years) experiences body changes more rapidly than at any time since infancy—secondary sexual characteristics begin to appear; growth accelerates; and physical changes require psychological and social adjustments of the adolescent, family, and other adults. These young people are often concrete thinkers and therefore have difficulty projecting themselves into the future. This phenomenon creates problems when young people are asked to modify their behaviors and delay gratification to achieve a distant future goal. The young adolescent is beginning to separate from the family but usually values parental guidance on important issues. Peer norms, especially identification with a particular group or set of groups, assume increasing importance.

Experimenting with some sexual behaviors is common, but sexual intercourse of any kind is usually limited. Males may initiate intercourse during this stage but most often delay regular sexual activity until middle or late adolescence. Adolescent girls are much less likely to begin having sexual intercourse at this age. Of those who do, many are in relationships with much older males.

Young adolescents seek to develop a sense of identity, connection, power, and joy. For many adolescents in communities that do not support the development of personal identity in other ways, drugs and sexual experimentation may provide a way to achieve it. Early sexual involvement is one way that disadvantaged youth may meet developmental needs for power, identity, connection, and pleasure (Selverstone, 1989). Involvement in sexual behaviors may not be motivated by sexual pleasure but rather may reflect peer norms, boredom, conflicts with adults, low self-esteem, and poor ability to control impulsivity (Durban, DiClemente, & Seigel, 1993).

Middle Adolescence

Middle adolescence (females aged 13–16 years, males aged 14–17 years) is the stage that most typifies the stereotype of "teenager." The transitions in this stage are so dramatic that they seem to occur overnight. The secondary sexual characteristics become fully established, and, for girls, the growth rate decelerates. Abstract thought patterns begin to develop in significant proportions of middle adolescents.

TABLE 11.4 Highlights of Adolescent Developmental Stages

Early Adolescence

Females ages 9–13; males ages 11–15

- Puberty as hallmark
- Adjusting to pubertal changes such as secondary sexual characteristics
- Concern with body image
- Beginning of separation from family, increased parent–child conflict
- Presence of social group cliques
- Identification in reputation-based groups
- Concentration on relationships with peers
- Concrete thinking but beginning of exploration of new ability to think abstractly

Middle Adolescence

Females ages 13–16; males ages 14–17

- Increased independence from family
- Increased importance of peer group
- Experimentation with relationships and sexual behaviors
- Increased abstract thinking ability

Late Adolescence

Females ages 16 and older; males ages 17 and older

- Autonomy nearly secured
- Body image and gender-role definition nearly secured
- Empathetic relationships
- Attainment of abstract thinking
- Defining of adult roles
- Transition to adult roles
- Greater intimacy skills
- Sexual orientation nearly secured

Source: Reprinted with permission from Haffner, D. *Facing facts: Sexual health for America's adolescents.* New York: SIECUS, 1995.

early adolescence
First stage of adolescence, defined by pubertal changes—usually ages 9–13 years for females and ages 11–15 years for males.

middle adolescence
The typical "teenage years," usually ages 13–16 years for females and ages 14–17 years for males.

Middle adolescents are sometimes described as feeling omniscient, omnipotent, and invincible. These feelings provide young people with the support to develop increased autonomy but may also put them at risk. In a recent study of ninth graders, their early sexual decision-making processes highlighted active consideration of health and social risks and benefits, as well as generating options, setting boundaries and limits, and evaluating sexual experiences (Michels et al., 2005).

As adolescents continue the process of separation from the family, they cling more tightly to the peer group that they defined for themselves in early adolescence. The peer group begins to define the rules of behavior. Parents generally place more value on long-term issues such as the importance of education and career preparation than peers do. The desire to be accepted by the peer group often influences experimentation with drugs or sex. By its acceptance or rejection, the peer group influences the adolescent's self-image.

Middle adolescents often focus on themselves and assume others will, too. Many middle adolescents choose to show off their new bodies with revealing clothes. Although adults may define these styles as sexually provocative, that may not be the intent of the middle adolescent.

Middle adolescents often fall in love for the first time. Again, because they are self-centered, their love object may serve as a mirror and reflect characteristics that they admire; that is, they may not love an individual for himself or herself. Sexual experimentation is common, and many adolescents first have intercourse in middle adolescence.

Late Adolescence

Teenagers in **late adolescence** (females aged 16 years and older; males aged 17 years and older) are explicitly moving toward adult roles and responsibilities. Some are beginning full-time jobs; others are beginning families. Many are preparing for these adult roles. The late adolescent completes the process of physical maturation. Many young people at this stage achieve the ability to understand abstract concepts, and they become more aware of what their limitations are and how their past will affect their future. They understand the consequences of their actions and behaviors, and they grapple with the complexities of identity, values, and ethical principles. Within the family, they move to a more adult relationship with their parents. The peer group recedes in importance as a determinant of behavior, and sexuality may become closely tied to commitment and planning for the future.

late adolescence
Period of transition to adulthood, beginning usually at age 16 years for females and age 17 years for males.

Adolescent Developmental Tasks

Developmental psychologists have identified six key developmental tasks for adolescents. Becoming a sexually healthy adult depends on the completion of these key developmental tasks (Grunbaum et al., 2004). The six key tasks are as follows:

1. *Physical and sexual maturation:* Adolescents mature biologically into adults, a process that occurs at an earlier chronological age than it did in the past.

2. *Independence:* Adolescents develop autonomy within the structure that gave them nurture and support during their childhood. This is usually the family but may include some similar surrogate structure. The parent–child relationship is transformed during adolescence, as the young person obtains the skills to maintain satisfying relationships.

3. *Conceptual identity:* Adolescents establish and place themselves within the religious, cultural, ethnic, moral, and political constructs of their environments.

4. *Functional identity:* Adolescents begin to prepare themselves for adult roles in society. By identifying their competencies, they discover how they will support themselves and contribute to their own families and society.

5. *Cognitive development:* Children and young adolescents are concrete thinkers and focus on real objects, present actions, and immediate benefits. During adolescence they develop a greater ability to think abstractly, plan for their future, and understand the effect of their current actions on their future lives and other people.

6. *Sexual self-concept:* During adolescence, young people tend to experience their first adultlike erotic feelings, experiment with sexual behaviors, and develop a strong sense of their own gender identity and sexual orientation.

The pursuit of these developmental tasks answers three psychosocial questions that adolescents ask themselves: Am I normal? Am I competent? Am I lovable and loving? Many adolescent behaviors can be

conceptual identity
Who am I in my world?

functional identity
What adult roles will I play in the world?

cognitive development
Explains the ability to think concretely or abstractly.

sexual self-concept
Who am I as a sexual being?

attributed to the search for affirmative answers to these questions.

Physical and Sexual Maturation

As noted in the section on puberty, sexual maturation differs significantly among young men and young women. On average, young girls begin pubertal events 1 to 2 years before boys. The adolescent female completes the process of puberty in 3 to 5 years, whereas for males, the process lasts 4 to 6 years. Adjusting to the biological changes of puberty is a major task of early adolescence, and society does not adequately prepare or support young people during these changes.

Sexual cognitions of girls appear to change prior to sexual experiences such as breast fondling and genital contact. Because most research focuses on intercourse as a key marker or pivotal event, the importance of attitudes, perceptions, and sexual self-esteem may have been overlooked as an important aspect of sexual development (O'Sullivan & Brooks-Gunn, 2005). The discrepancy between maturation among young women and young men is one factor that may contribute to some young women's seeking partners older than they are. This difference in age places young women at considerable risk for sexual exploitation.

> **sexual cognitions**
> Attitudes, expectations, beliefs, and values framing one's sexual experiences

Cognitive Development

During adolescence, young people develop a range of intellectual characteristics that increase the probability that they will be able to become sexually healthy adults. Ideally, this includes developing the ability to reason abstractly, to foresee consequences of actions, and to understand the social context of behaviors. Adolescents develop an increased ability to control impulsivity, to identify the future implications of their actions, and to obtain control of their future plans.

Although the study of child development from 0 to 3 years of age has recognized the importance of brain development, study of adolescents has tended to focus more on psychological and social factors rather than on physiological ones. Recent imaging advances have allowed neuroscience—the scientific study of the biology of the brain—to demonstrate brain growth patterns. These studies in teens reveal remarkable changes during the second decade of life (Weinberger, Elvevåg, & Giedd, 2005). Of particular interest is the frontal cortex area, which governs impulse control, judgment, and decision making; that portion does not fully mature until around the age of 25. That means that teenagers, though very capable of huge intellectual and creative endeavors, are limited in strategies, organizing, and recognizing potential consequences. Conversely, the teen brain is adept at learning by example. Thus modeling behavior to be emulated could be a good tactic for both parents and teachers (Giedd, 2005).

Developmental age and general level of cognitive and emotional development may influence adolescent sexual decisions, contraceptive use, and safer sex practices. An adolescent's degree of cognitive maturity may place limits on his or her ability to plan for sexual relationships, clearly articulate personal values, negotiate with a partner, and obtain contraception and condoms. Further, the adolescent's ability to form empathetic relationships is dependent on **social cognition**: the capacity to see a situation from another person's perspective. Social cognition is one aspect of cognitive development. Understanding one's feelings and the feelings of others is central to emotional growth.

> **social cognition**
> Ability to see a situation from another person's point of view.

Adolescents express sexual cognitions, social cognitions, peer affiliations, and various aspects of gender identity such as gender role expression, behavior, and conformity as they participate in proms, graduation events, and other social activities that mark passages throughout the teen years.

Gender DIMENSIONS

How Gender Stereotypes Affect Sexuality

Gender-role stereotypes impede both young men and young women in attaining sexual health. Young women may learn that "It is better to be cute and popular than smart," "Girls have few sexual feelings," and "Girls who carry condoms are bad." Boys may learn that "Real men are always ready for sex" and that "Guys should never act like girls." In an online article for teens written by a 17-year-old male staff writer for Sex, Etc., women clearly are short-changed. He says, guys get to enjoy sex but girls are told by society they can't. Females faking orgasm is a laughing matter. Another problem is that many people, especially teens, are focused on sexual intercourse (where the "goal" is for the male to have an orgasm). Other ways of experiencing pleasure are less valued or ignored. Or, as one concerned male suggests, men are afraid they don't know how to please their partner, so they're reluctant to try. Regarding masturbation, there is silence and disdain for women but with men, it's common conversation. The suggested solution is T-A-L-K. When discussing safer sex, pleasure should be included, too. Since communication is the key to better relationships, maybe the real payoff *and* the best pleasure of all is an enhanced sexual connection (Dalal, 2005).

Although patterns of sexual involvement are increasingly similar for boys and girls, persistent gender stereotypes mean that expectations regarding sexual pleasure for young women are still quite different from those for young men.

Why do these different standards continue to exist? Will they ever change?

Sexual Self-Concept

Sexual self-concept, an individual's evaluation of his or her sexual feelings and actions, develops during adolescence. Young people develop an increasing sense of gender identity as men and women. An understanding of one's sexual orientation also develops during adolescence: Young people become more aware of their sexual attractions and love interests, and adultlike erotic feelings emerge. Sexual experimentation is common among all groups of adolescents.

Gender Identity

During adolescence, young people solidify their gender identification by observing the gender roles of their parents and other adults. Gender identification includes understanding that one is male or female, as well as understanding the roles, values, duties, and responsibilities of being a man or a woman. Most young people have a firm sense of their maleness or femaleness before adolescence, but in adolescence, clear identification with adult masculine and feminine models emerges. The markers of masculinity and femininity vary by culture and are adopted to a greater or lesser extent by adolescents. *Gender-role behavior, expression,* and *conformity* are all current terms used to describe sex-typed attributes. Differences that have been studied include peer affiliation preference, aggression, and activity level (Zucker & Bradley, 2005).

Sexual Orientation

One's erotic attraction to others is discovered as one matures sexually. Sexual orientation, whether heterosexual, homosexual, or bisexual, does not seem to be something one chooses. Gay, lesbian, and bisexual people are not seduced, recruited, or taught to become homosexual. Rather, one's sexual orientation often emerges in adolescence. In one study of students in grades 7–12, 88% of teenagers described themselves as predominantly heterosexual, 1% described themselves as bisexual or predominantly homosexual, and 11% were "unsure" of their sexual orientation. Uncertainty about sexual orientation diminished with chronological age; 26% of the 12-year-olds were "unsure" compared with only 5% of the 18-year-olds (Remafedi et al., 1992).

In retrospective studies, many gay and lesbian adults identify adolescence as a period of confusion about their sexual orientation. Although a majority of adult gay men recall feeling different as children, most did not self-identify as gay until their late teenage years.

Research to explain romantic attachments formed by gay men and heterosexual men found that sex-role nonconformity (dislike for conventionally masculine activities) and feeling different and excluded from male groups in high school predicted adult identification as a gay man. Bell believes that romantic attachments are made on the basis of heterogamy, meaning that people are drawn to those they perceive to be different from themselves. Thus it makes sense that a gay man who perceives himself as somewhat feminine or gender neutral would feel more different from men than women. Likewise, heterosexual men who perceive themselves as essentially masculine would be drawn to the difference of a feminine partner (Johnston & Bell, 1995).

Adolescent Sexual Behavior

Regardless of one's sexual orientation, almost all American adolescents engage in some type of sexual behavior (Table 11.5). Although policy debates have tended to focus on sexual intercourse and its negative consequences, young people explore dating, relationships, and intimacy from a much wider framework. *Sexual behavior is almost universal among American adolescents.*

Consider these statistics:

- About half of those aged 12 to 14 report having been on a date or having a romantic relationship in the past 18 months (Sexual behavior of young adolescents, 2003).

- Of American teenagers, 85% have had a boyfriend or girlfriend.

- Of American teenagers, 85–90% have kissed someone romantically.

- Of American teenagers, 79% have engaged in "deep kissing" (Roper Starch Worldwide, 1994).

The majority of adolescents move from kissing to other more intimate sexual behaviors during their teenage years.

- Just over half of teens (aged 15 to 19) have had oral sex, and it is now more common than sexual intercourse. About one in four teens who have *not* had sexual intercourse report they have had oral sex. Among teen boys who have not had sexual intercourse, the proportion of those who say they have had oral sex did *not* increase between 1995 and 2002, but for those who have had sexual intercourse, the proportion saying they have had oral sex increased from 82% in 1995 to 88% in 2002 (Teens and oral sex, 2005).

- Between 5% and 10% of adolescent males report having sexual experiences with someone of the same gender, compared with 6% of adolescent females (Bancoft, Herbenick, & Reynolds, 2003). These adolescents usually report their first experience was with another adolescent (DeLamater & Friedrich, 2002).

When data are collected about teen sexual behavior, the focus becomes *what, when,* and *how often,*

but rarely *with what emotional intent.* Thus it is difficult to pin down aspects of sexual experience that are nuanced. Much has been written recently about changes in relationship patterns, particularly the phenomenon of "friends with benefits" and hooking up (a euphemism for a sexual encounter, particularly oral sex, without emotional involvement). Much of the discussion is anecdotal and involves use of the Internet to post personal profiles, chat online, and arrange meetings. Whether such interaction is viewed as healthy or harmful may depend on one's age and experience. Most of the experts cited in a recent feature article in the popular press indicate that females may have less to gain than males and the ultimate risk may be increased chance of STIs. The role of commitment and dating seems to be changing, perhaps due to the expectation that marriage and romantic relationships won't happen until later in life (Denizet-Lewis, 2004).

Clearly, research is needed to measure more than numbers. Detailed studies might discover whether friends with benefits are truly a widespread and long-term change in relationship patterns or a minor blip in reaction to new technology that will be reversed when another trend appears. Some data suggest that the progression from kissing to noncoital behaviors to intercourse differs among different groups of adolescents. Many teenagers move through a progression of intimate behaviors; lower-income teenagers are less likely to follow this progression, moving more rapidly from kissing directly to sexual intercourse (Brooks-Gunn & Furstenberg, 1990).

Teenagers Who Have Intercourse

Substantial changes in adolescent sexual behavior have occurred in the past four decades. From the late 1960s until 1988 the proportion of teen women who had had sexual intercourse increased. Then the trend reversed, and from 1991 to 2001 the proportion of young women reporting having had sexual intercourse dropped from 51% to 43% (Santelli et al., 2004). However, between 2001 and 2007, the proportion of students who had ever had sexual intercourse stopped declining (Teen sexual behavior, 2008).

Contraceptive use among teens has also undergone remarkable change. In the 1970s, the most commonly used method was the birth control pill, followed by condom use and withdrawal. In the 1980s, condom use increased and the use of birth control pills declined. This trend continued into the 1990s, and now condom use among high school students has stabilized at 63% with no significant change from 2003 to 2007 (Santelli et al., 2007; Youth Risk Behavior Surveillance System, 2008).

TABLE 11.5   Trends in the Prevalence of Sexual Behaviors—National YRBS: 1991–2007

The national Youth Risk Behavior Survey (YRBS) monitors priority health risk behaviors that contribute to the leading causes of death, disability, and social problems among youth and adults in the United States. The national YRBS is conducted every 2 years during the spring semester and provides data representative of ninth- through twelfth-grade students in public and private schools throughout the United States.

	1991	1993	1995	1997	1999	2001	2003	2005	2007	Changes from 1991–2007[1]	Change from 2005–2007[2]
Ever had sexual intercourse											
	54.1 (50.5–57.8)[3]	53.0 (50.2–55.8)	53.1 (48.4–57.7)	48.4 (45.2–51.6)	49.9 (46.1–53.7)	45.6 (43.2–48.1)	46.7 (44.0–49.4)	46.8 (43.4–50.2)	47.8 (45.1–50.6)	Decreased, 1991–2007	No change
Had sexual intercourse with four or more persons during their life											
	18.7 (16.6–21.0)	18.7 (16.8–20.9)	17.8 (15.2–20.7)	16.0 (14.6–17.5)	16.2 (13.7–19.0)	14.2 (13.0–15.6)	14.4 (12.9–16.1)	14.3 (12.8–15.8)	14.9 (13.4–16.5)	Decreased, 1991–2007	No change
Currently sexually active (Had sexual intercourse with at least one person during the 3 months before the survey.)											
	37.5 (34.3–40.7)	37.5 (35.4–39.7)	37.9 (34.4–41.5)	34.8 (32.6–37.2)	36.3 (32.7–40.0)	33.4 (31.3–35.5)	34.3 (32.1–36.5)	33.9 (31.4–36.6)	35.0 (32.8–37.2)	Decreased, 1991–2007	No change
Used a condom during last sexual intercourse (Among students who were currently sexually active.)											
	46.2 (42.8–49.6)	52.8 (50.0–55.6)	54.4 (50.7–58.0)	56.8 (55.2–58.4)	58.0 (53.6–62.3)	57.9 (55.6–60.1)	63.0 (60.5–65.5)	62.8 (60.6–64.9)	61.5 (59.4–63.6)	Increased, 1991–2003 No change, 2003–2007	No change
Used birth control pills before last sexual intercourse (To prevent pregnancy, among students who were currently sexually active.)											
	20.8 (18.5–23.2)	18.4 (16.3–20.7)	17.4 (15.2–19.8)	16.6 (14.7–18.8)	16.2 (13.6–19.0)	18.2 (16.5–20.0)	17.0 (14.7–19.4)	17.6 (15.1–20.5)	16.0 (14.2–17.9)	No change, 1991–2007	No change
Drank alcohol or used drugs before last sexual intercourse (Among students who were currently sexually active.)											
	21.6 (18.7–24.8)	21.3 (19.3–23.5)	24.8 (22.1–27.8)	24.7 (22.9–26.7)	24.8 (21.8–28.0)	25.6 (23.8–27.4)	25.4 (23.2–27.8)	23.3 (21.1–25.6)	22.5 (20.7–24.5)	Increased, 1991–2001 Decreased, 2001–2007	No change
Were ever taught in school about AIDS or HIV infection											
	83.3 (80.1–86.0)	86.1 (83.4–88.4)	86.3 (79.0–91.3)	91.5 (90.3–92.5)	90.6 (89.1–91.9)	89.0 (87.6–90.3)	87.9 (85.8–89.7)	87.9 (85.8–89.7)	89.5 (88.1–90.7)	Increased, 1991–1997 Decreased, 1997–2007	No change

[1] Based on trend analyses using a logistic regression model controlling for sex, race/ethnicity, and grade.
[2] Based on *t*-test analyses, *p* < .05.
[3] 95% confidence interval.
Source: www.cdc.gov/HealthyYouth/yrbs/pdf/yrbs07_us_sexual_behaviors_trend/.pdf.

Finally, rates of teen pregnancy, including births and abortions, have changed dramatically. A record high (96 births per 1,000 teen girls aged 15–19) was reached in 1957, followed by a steady decline to the mid-1980s. Then the birth rate increased again by 24% by 1991. Since that time there has been a decrease of more than 33% in the birth rate, to a low of 41 births per 1,000 teen girls in 2004 (Santelli et al., 2004). The trend has recently changed again: After 14 years of decline, the birth rate for teens *increased* by 3% in 2006 and by 1% in 2007 (CDC, 2009). Abortion rates for teens rose in the 1970s, were mostly stable in the 1980s, and have declined steadily since 1991 (Santelli et al., 2004).

Data from the Youth Risk Behavior Surveys (YRBS) for estimates of sexual activity and contraceptive use were combined with data from National Surveys of Family Growth (NSFG) for method-specific contraceptive failure rates and from the National Vital Statistics System for pregnancy rates. These data suggest that both delayed initiation of sexual intercourse and improved contraceptive practice contributed equally to declines in the pregnancy rates among high school-aged teens during the 1990s. Specifically, decreased sexual experience accounted for 53% of the pregnancy rate decline and better contraception accounted for 47%. There was an increase in condom use from 40% to 51%, a decrease in use of withdrawal from 20% to 13%, and decline in use of no method from 17% to 13% (Santelli et al., 2004).

Although the data do not suggest a dramatic turnabout in either sexual activity or contraceptive use, they do indicate a loss of momentum when compared to the steady improvements in the 1990s. Moreover, the U.S. teen birth rate remains much higher than the rates in other developed nations. Research is lacking, but hypotheses abound, including those related to changes in the economy, attitudes, anxiety, schooling, public policy, programs and services, families, and media messages. In addition, prevention fatigue and the need for new strategies to reach teens who have not been reached by existing approaches have been suggested as critical factors (Moore, 2008).

While more teens are doing the right thing, adults debate whether the reduction in unintended pregnancies is the result of promoting abstinence or promoting better contraceptive protection. Speculation must suffice because the surveys provide little information to explain the shift in behaviors. The important point is to support teens in each decision by providing accurate information, encouragement, and validation, whether their concern is initiating sex, limiting activity or partners, or choosing to use contraception (Sonenstein, 2004).

Early Sexual Activity

- Female adolescents who first had sex prior to the age of 14 had more sexual partners than females who first had sex at age 15 or older, thus increasing their risk of STI or pregnancy.

- One in ten young women who first had sex before the age of 15 described it as nonvoluntary and many more said it was unwanted.

- Survey data indicate that younger teen girls who are sexually experienced are more likely than older teens to say they "wish they'd waited."

- Relationships between a young adolescent (aged 12–14) and an older partner (by two or more years) compared to a partner only slightly older, the same age, or younger, is more likely to include sexual intercourse.

- More than half the girls and two-thirds of the boys aged 12–14 say they used some form of contraception the most recent time they had sex. (This is a higher percentage than among 15- to 19-year-olds.)

- Approximately one in five adolescents has had sexual intercourse before his or her 15th birthday (Sexual behavior of young adolescents, 2003).

- High school boys are more likely than girls to have four or more partners (17% versus 11%). This pattern is the same across grades and racial/ethnic groups.

- Young boys (aged 12–14) are slightly more likely than older boys (aged 15–19) to think it is embarrassing to say they are virgins. Boys in general are more embarrassed than girls the same age to say they are virgins.

- Boys are slightly more likely than girls the same age to report feeling pressured to have sex (82% versus 79%). Girls say romantic partners cause pressure, while boys say pressure is most likely to come from friends (Sexual attitudes and behavior of male teens, 2003).

Table 11.6 shows teen birth rate data from 1940 to 2007. The United States has the highest rates of teen pregnancy and births in the Western industrialized world. Thirty-four percent of young women become pregnant at least once before they reach the age of 20. Eight in ten of these pregnancies are unintended. Although the teen birth rate has steadily declined since 1991, Hispanic teens have the highest

TABLE 11.6 Teen Birth Rates in the United States, 1940–2005

From 1940 to 1957, the teen birth rate increased 78% to a record high. The birth rate dropped fairly steadily from the end of the 1950s through the mid-1980s, but then increased 24% between 1986 and 1991. Between 1991 and 2005, the teen birth rate decreased 35% to a record low of 40.5% in 2005. The chart and the table reflect births per 1,000 teen girls aged 15–19 in the United States and are the most recent national data available.

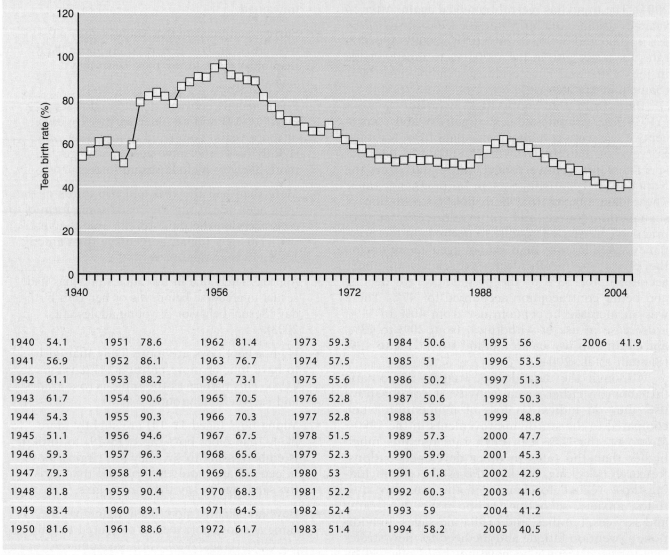

1940	54.1	1951	78.6	1962	81.4	1973	59.3	1984	50.6	1995	56	2006	41.9
1941	56.9	1952	86.1	1963	76.7	1974	57.5	1985	51	1996	53.5		
1942	61.1	1953	88.2	1964	73.1	1975	55.6	1986	50.2	1997	51.3		
1943	61.7	1954	90.6	1965	70.5	1976	52.8	1987	50.6	1998	50.3		
1944	54.3	1955	90.3	1966	70.3	1977	52.8	1988	53	1999	48.8		
1945	51.1	1956	94.6	1967	67.5	1978	51.5	1989	57.3	2000	47.7		
1946	59.3	1957	96.3	1968	65.6	1979	52.3	1990	59.9	2001	45.3		
1947	79.3	1958	91.4	1969	65.5	1980	53	1991	61.8	2002	42.9		
1948	81.8	1959	90.4	1970	68.3	1981	52.2	1992	60.3	2003	41.6		
1949	83.4	1960	89.1	1971	64.5	1982	52.4	1993	59	2004	41.2		
1950	81.6	1961	88.6	1972	61.7	1983	51.4	1994	58.2	2005	40.5		

Sources: Ventura, S. J., Mathews, T. J., & Hamilton, B. E. Births to teenagers in the United States, 1940–2000. *National Vital Statistics Reports, 49, no. 10* (2001); Hamilton, B. E., Sutton, P. D., & Ventura, S. J. Revised birth and fertility rates for the 1990s and new rates for hispanic populations, 2000 and 2001: United States. *National Vital Statistics Reports, 51, no. 12* (2003); Martin, J. A., Hamilton, B. E., Sutton, P. D., Ventura, S. J., Menacker, F., Kirmeyer, S., & Mathews, T. J. Births: Final data for 2006. *National Vital Statistics Reports, 57, no. 7* (2009).

teenage birth rate. The rate for African American teens declined the most but remains higher than other groups except Hispanic teens. Prior to 1980, most teen mothers were married, whereas today most are unmarried.

Parents are rated by most teens as trustworthy and a preferred source of birth control information. About 6 out of 10 teens find it easy to talk to their parents about relationships. Still, about 1 in 4 teens say it's difficult (National Campaign to Prevent Teen and Unplanned Pregnancy, 2007). Teens raised by two parents (biological or adoptive) from birth have a lower probability of having sex than teens growing up in any other family situation. Eight in ten girls and six in ten boys say they wish they had waited to have sex until they were older (National Campaign to Prevent Teen Pregnancy, 2005).

The self-assessment exercise at the end of this chapter raises many of the questions that a young person—indeed, an adult—needs to consider to determine his or her readiness for a sexual relationship.

◼ Sexual Abuse of Children and Adolescents

Sexual abuse occurs in all types of homes. It happens hundreds of times a day in the United States. Indeed, as many as 200,000 children are reported to be sexually abused in the United States each year. Seven percent of girls younger than 12 years old say that they have been sexually abused, and 4% of boys that age say that they have been sexually abused (Louis Harris and Associates, 1997). Girls are more likely to be sexually abused than boys, and men are more likely to be the assailants than women. However, boys are also victims of sexual abuse, and some abusers are women. And sexual abuse is every parent's nightmare.

> **sexual abuse**
> The psychological exploitation or infliction of unwanted sexual contact on one person.

Sexual Abuse of Children

Most parents teach their children not to talk to strangers, accept candy from people they do not know, or ever get into a car with a stranger. Indeed, many preschools and kindergartens offer "stranger danger programs." However, the reality is that, in 90% of the cases, the assailant was someone in the child's family or someone close to the family.

Children can also be sexually abused by other children. This is different from the sex play described earlier in this chapter. In sex play, children are usually of the same age, they are engaging in light-hearted exploration, and they appear to be enjoying themselves—at least until they realize they have been "discovered" by an adult. And, in general, once they are told by an adult that they should stop, they do.

Some children, however, engage in inappropriate behaviors and become sexually abusive to other, usually younger, children. This may include engaging in oral or genital sex with other children, with or without their consent. Many of these children have been sexually abused themselves, and many of them have inappropriately been exposed to sexually explicit materials or adult erotic behavior. In one study, all the girls who had sexually abused other children (about 25% of childhood abusers are girls) and most of the boys had been molested themselves, often years before

they committed these crimes against other children (Finkelhor, 1986).

Family and Acquaintance Sexual Abuse Using the Internet

The Internet and related technologies have transformed many aspects of communication. It is realistic to assume it will have an effect on child mistreatment as well. So far, concern has focused on online meeting crimes in which adult strangers have used the Internet to meet and develop abusive relationships with vulnerable youth. However, just as most face-to-face sexual abuse involves family members and acquaintances of the victim, so it is realistic to assume that Internet sexual abuse would also involve nonstranger sex offenders.

Internet technology provides a number of ways for this to happen. Digital photography has made online production and distribution of child pornography a more frequent component of abuse. Availability and

Myth (vs) Fact

Kiss and Tell: What Teens Say About Love, Trust, and Other Relationship Stuff

It's a relationship world. Seven in ten teens say their friends are in romantic relationships.

Relationships

The good news is that most teens (68%) say that their friends are in "healthy" romantic relationships. The proportion saying this is almost identical for teen boys and teen girls.

The not-so-good news is that one in five teens (19%) aged 15–17 say that most of their friends are in *unhealthy* relationships—those without love, trust, mutual respect, and honesty.

Trust and Honesty Rule. When it comes to relationships, teens say it's all about trust—40% of guys and 48% of gals say that *trust* is the most important part of a healthy relationship. Teens say that *honesty* is the second most important factor. Surprisingly, 10% of teen boys say that *compatibility* is most important; yet only 3% of teen girls agree. Fewer than 3% of teens say *looks* or *popularity* matters most.

Pressure

More good news is that most teens (84% of guys and 85% of gals) say they have never felt pressure to be in a romantic relationship before they were ready.

Fast Fact. Teens who are in relationships with someone who is 3 years older are far more likely to say that sex was unwanted.

Role Models

Teens in focus groups indicated that they can learn a lot about what to avoid from seeing unhealthy relationships.

Almost one in five (17%) teens say they don't know *anyone* who serves as an example of a healthy relationship.

Fast Fact. Most teens aged 15–17 say they enjoy spending time with their mother (79%) and father (76%).

Source: Kiss and tell: What teens say about love, trust, and other relationship stuff survey results. National Campaign to Prevent Teen and Unplanned Pregnancy. 2007. Retrieved June 5, 2009, from www.thenationalcampaign.org/resources/pdf/pubs/kiss_tell.pdf.

Multicultural DIMENSIONS

Racial and Ethnic Differences in Sexual Behaviors

The likelihood of having several sexual partners varies by race and ethnicity, as does condom use. Only 44% of all 15- to 19-year-old males report using a condom every time they had sex in the previous year. Consistent condom use also varies by race and ethnicity. Overall, 14% of sexually experienced males aged 15–19 reported that they had gotten a part-ner pregnant. Causing a pregnancy varies by racial/ethnic group: 22% of African American, 19% of Hispanic, and 10% of non-Hispanic white male teens reported causing a pregnancy. Since there are large disparities in sexual behavior by race and ethnicity, it is important for program leaders and educators to pay attention to these differences and target specific behaviors (Sexual attitudes and behavior of male teens, 2003).

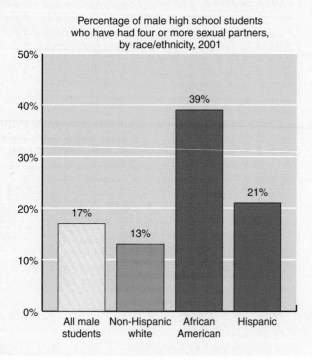

Percentage of male high school students who have had four or more sexual partners, by race/ethnicity, 2001

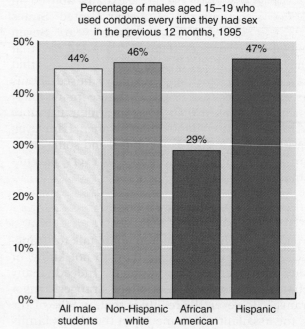

Percentage of males aged 15–19 who used condoms every time they had sex in the previous 12 months, 1995

ease of online communication may allow acquaintance and family member offenders a means of bypassing parents and other caregivers so as to develop abusive relationships with potential victims. The Internet may provide opportunities for family and acquaintance offenders to seduce children and adolescents by bringing up sexual topics and exposing potential victims to sexual images and materials.

In response to this concern, child sexual abuse researcher David Finkelhor and others designed a National Juvenile Online Victimization (N-JOV) Study. They examined information provided by law enforcement agencies on almost 800 cases of online sex crimes and found that approximately half of all the arrests involved family and acquaintance offenders. Offender demographics showed that all but 1% were male, most (87%) were over 26 years of age, and 95% were non-Hispanic whites. Almost all victims of family member abuse were female (93%) and younger than 12 (82%), whereas victims of acquaintance offenders were nearly half (49%) male and most (71%) were teenagers.

Crimes were committed in five primary ways: seduction and grooming, child pornography production, arranging meetings and other communication, rewarding victims, and advertising or selling victims. Implications from this study for law enforcement must be to expand the notion of Internet crime to include family and acquaintance offenders. For mental health professionals, Internet involvement should be an inquiry topic for victims and offenders. Both prevention messages and investigation approaches should be revised to incorporate this potential form of sexual abuse (Mitchell, Finkelhor, & Wolak, 2005).

Sexual Abuse of Adolescents

Sexual assault is not uncommon among adolescents. Six percent of boys and 15% of girls are sexually assaulted before their 16th birthday. In a study of teenage girls in foster care, 43% reported experiencing some type of sexual abuse. The most prevalent type of abuse was being touched or fondled by an adult against her wishes. One in six reported that she had been forced to have intercourse with an adult. One-third of the young women had been sexually abused before their 10th birthday (Polit, White, & Morgan, 1990). Ten thousand women younger than 18 years

DIMENSIONS

Teenagers and Sexuality Around the World

Young people around the world experiment with sexual behaviors. Young people in northern European countries and the United States have first intercourse at similar ages, but northern European teenagers have much lower pregnancy and STI rates. European countries tend to be more open about sexuality, and their official governmental policies focus on reducing unprotected intercourse rather than on eliminating sexual behaviors. There is a greater availability of sexual information and reproductive health services for teenagers.

The United States has one of the highest adolescent birth rates in the world. Teenagers in Sweden, France, Canada, Great Britain, and the United States have similar levels of sexual intercourse, but teenagers in other countries are much more successful than U.S. adolescents at preventing pregnancy and disease. For example, Sweden has one-third the U.S. rate of teenage pregnancies, despite similar levels of teenage sexual intercourse.

Reasons for these birthrate differences may include the following factors:

- Teenagers in these countries are not too immature to use contraceptives consistently and effectively.
- Teenage pregnancy rates are lower in countries where there is greater availability of confidential contraceptive services and comprehensive sexuality education.
- Social and economic well-being and equality are linked to lower teenage birthrates.
- Strong and widespread governmental support for parents and for young people's transition to adulthood may contribute to low teenage birthrates.
- Positive attitudes about sexuality and clear expectations for behavior in sexual relationships encourage responsible teenage behavior (Guttmacher Institute, 2001).

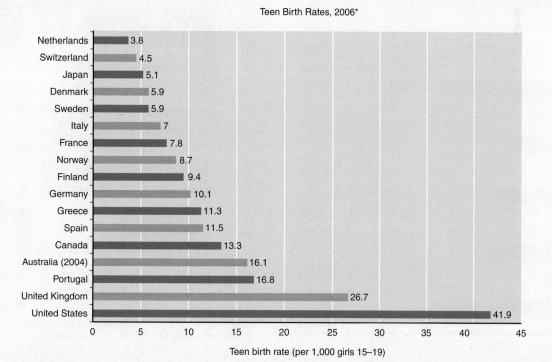

Teen Birth Rates, 2006*

Country	Teen birth rate (per 1,000 girls 15–19)
Netherlands	3.8
Switzerland	4.5
Japan	5.1
Denmark	5.9
Sweden	5.9
Italy	7
France	7.8
Norway	8.7
Finland	9.4
Germany	10.1
Greece	11.3
Spain	11.5
Canada	13.3
Australia (2004)	16.1
Portugal	16.8
United Kingdom	26.7
United States	41.9

*All birth rates are for 2006 unless otherwise noted.

Source: United Nations Statistics Divisions. *Demographic Yearbook 2006.* New York: United Nations, 2006.

Continued

Global
DIMENSIONS

**Teenagers and
Sexuality Around
the World—cont'd**

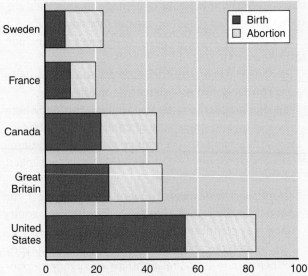

U.S. teenagers have higher pregnancy rates, birthrates, and abortion rates than adolescents in other developed countries

Birth
Abortion

Rate per 1,000 women aged 15–19

Note: Data are for mid-1990s

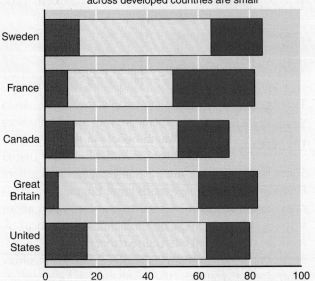

Differences in levels of teenage sexual activity across developed countries are small

Percent of women 20–24 who had sex in their teenage years

■ by age 15   □ by age 18   ■ by age 20

Note: Data are for mid-1990s.

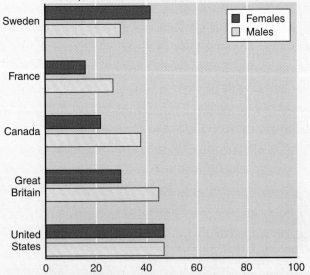

Among teenagers who had sex in the last year, those in the United States are more likely than those in other developed countries to have had two or more partners

■ Females
□ Males

Percentage of 18- to 19-year-olds who had two or more partners.
*Data are for 16- to 19-year-olds. *Note:* Data are for mid-1990s.

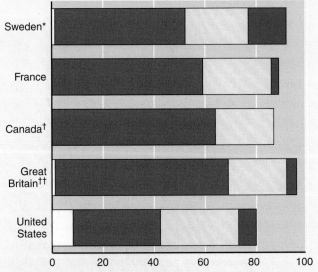

U.S. teenagers are less likely to use a contraceptive method and to use a hormonal method than teenagers in other developed countries

Percent of women 15–19 who used a contraceptive method at last intercourse

□ long-acting   ■ pill   □ condom   ■ other

*Data are for 18- to 19-year-olds. †The condom category includes all methods other than the pill, but the condom is the predominant "other method." ††Data are for 18- to 19-year-olds. *Note:* Users reporting more than one method were classified by the most effective method. Data are for early to mid-1990s.

old were raped in 1992 (Child Welfare League, 1994). In fact, one-quarter of rape victims are women 11 to 17 years of age (National Victims Center and Crime Victims Research and Treatment Center, 1992). Nearly three-quarters of young women who had intercourse before age 14 years reported having had intercourse involuntarily (Guttmacher Institute, 1994; Child Welfare League of America, 1994).

A disproportionate number of young women who become pregnant during adolescence are victims of childhood sexual abuse. In one study of teenagers who were pregnant or were parents, 70% of whites, 42% of African Americans, and 37% of Hispanics had been sexually abused as children (Boyer & Fine, 1992). In another study, 64% of parenting and pregnant teens reported that they had had at least one unwanted sexual experience (Child Welfare League of America, 1994).

Gay, lesbian, and bisexual teenagers face an additional form of abuse related to their sexuality. A study in New York City found that of lesbian, gay, and bisexual teenagers reporting an assault, almost half reported that the assault was related to their sexual orientation, and for almost two-thirds, the assault happened within their families (Hunter, 1990).

Sexual Harassment

Sexual harassment is a fact of life in most middle and high schools. *Sexual harassment in school* is defined as "unwanted and unwelcome sexual behavior that interferes with the student's life." Sexual harassment includes unwanted sexual comments, jokes, and gestures; receiving from another student sexual pictures, photographs, and notes; sexual graffiti about a specific student in the bathroom or locker room; spreading of sexual rumors; flashing or mooning; touching, grabbing, or pinching in a sexual way; brushing against another student in a sexual way; pulling clothes off; blocking another student in a sexual way; and forcing kissing and other sexual behaviors. In a study conducted by the American Association of University Women in 1993, 85% of girls and 76% of boys in grades 8 through 11 reported that they had been victims of one of these behaviors (Bryant, 1993). One-third had been harassed by the time they reached sixth grade. And almost 6 in 10 of these students report that they have engaged in these offensive behaviors themselves!

Most sexual harassment in schools occurs openly in classrooms and hallways, rather than in secluded areas. Students are usually harassed by other students, but in one in five cases, they are harassed by

> **sexual harassment**
> Unwanted sexual behavior that interferes with the student's life.

Sexual harassment in schools is common. What type of program could be instituted to help stop such harassment?

adult employees. And students report that this type of sexual harassment affects their lives. Girls in particular report that they feel less confident and more afraid to go to school after incidents of sexual harassment. This same study found that students are not likely to tell adults about these incidents. Only 7% told a teacher, and only one-quarter told a parent (Bryant, 1993).

Schools are supposed to protect students against sexual harassment. Schools need to have sexual harassment policies, with clear penalties for perpetrators, which should be communicated to students and parents. A clear procedure for handling complaints of sexual harassment should be established. A May 1999 U.S. Supreme Court decision found a school financially liable for harassment that occurred between two students (Haffner, 2001).

Recognizing a Sexually Healthy Relationship

Although sexual abuse and harassment are critical concepts to define and avoid, the components of a **sexually healthy relationship** are less often discussed. This is unfortunate because development of self-identity, particularly in personal and intimate relationships, is a key developmental task of young adults. Being skilled at recognizing a positive

> **sexually healthy relationship**
> Consensual, non-exploitative, honest, mutually pleasurable, safe and protected from unwanted pregnancy, STIs, and other harm (National Guidelines Task Force, 2004).

relationship provides protection from being exploited, misled, or victimized. Here the focus is on health rather than harm. To distinguish between potentially healthy and harmful sexual relationships, the following list provides a tool for assessing relationships by applying the defining characteristics to one's own personal relationships or those of others (Conklin & Peters, 2004).

Who is your partner? What is your relationship with this person? Sexual activity often involves many feelings and emotions that can be confusing. How will you and your partner handle these feelings if they come up? How will sex change your relationship with this person?

Do you feel safe? Consider your partner, the situation, the location . . . Do you feel safe and taken care of? Do you feel respected by your partner? Do you respect your partner? Can you talk and listen to him or her? Are you worried that someone might walk in?

Is it consensual? No one has the right to be sexual with another person without that person's explicit permission. Have you talked about which behaviors you give permission for and have permission to start? Have you talked about where you will stop? Do you feel like your partner respects your decisions? Do you respect your partner's decisions?

What is your motivation? Why are you thinking of doing this? People can have many reasons for having sex, like to become closer, to feel loved, to express love, to feel good, to satisfy curiosity, to gain popularity, to get someone to like them, to fit in, or to rebel. Let's face it, some of these aren't very good reasons for getting sexually involved with someone else. Be honest with yourself, what are your reasons?

Is it non-exploitative? Exploitation is when one person uses someone else for selfish reasons. Exploitation should not be part of sexual relationships. Partners should be interested in each other's well-being as well as their own. Are you and your partner looking out for each other?

Are you being honest? Have you talked to your partner about your feelings, what you want to do, and what you don't want to do? Were you truthful in these conversations? Being honest with yourself and your partner can help you have a better relationship.

Is it pleasurable? One reason that many people participate in various sexual activities is because these behaviors provide physical, emotional, and psychological pleasure. Does the sexual activity you are considering or engaging in feel good?

Is it protected? Most sexual behaviors carry some risk of STIs or pregnancy. It's important to protect yourself from these risks—either by avoiding behaviors and eliminating the risk or by using effective protection and reducing the risk. Do you understand the risk involved in each behavior you are considering? Do you understand the benefits of abstaining from some or all risky behaviors? Do you understand how condoms or birth control can reduce your risk? Do you know how to use condoms or birth control correctly?

What does your gut instinct say? A lot of people talk about listening to their inner voice or gut to let them know whether they are making the right decision. Whatever the decision is—if it feels wrong, it is wrong for you. And remember, you can always change your mind. You and your partner always have the right, the ability, and the responsibility to stop if either one of you changes your mind (Kemper & Rodriguez, 2005).

Exploring the DIMENSIONS of Human Sexuality

Our feelings, attitudes, and beliefs regarding sexuality are influenced by our internal and external environments. Go to sexuality.jbpub.com/dimensions/4e to learn more about the biological, psychological, and sociological factors that affect your sexuality.

Sociocultural Factors

- Socioeconomic status affects sexual behaviors. Lower-economic status youths have sexual intercourse earlier than teens who are more well off, and they experience a higher rate of STIs and births.
- Religion and ethnic heritage affect beliefs about sexuality and permissiveness.
- Many cultures' double standard expects boys to be sexually aggressive and girls to remain sexually passive.
- Media and ad information often convey information to adolescents about sexuality and sexual behavior.
- Friends often convey false information about sexual behaviors to adolescents.
- Use of the Internet can provide access to reliable sexuality information but can also lead to sexually abusive situations (Common Sense Media, 2009).

Biological Factors

- Puberty changes boys and girls into men and women.
- Genetic coding affects the onset of puberty and general overall appearance.
- Reproduction becomes possible after menarche and semenarche.
- Sexual arousal and response become important issues in an adolescent's life.
- Physical appearance changes dramatically during puberty, affecting body image.
- Growth and development, in terms of physical and mental maturity, greatly affect a person's self-concept.

CASE STUDY

Sexual maturation is a time of constant physical and psychological changes. At the same time, deeply rooted sociocultural influences, once able to provide a sense of comfort, now may cause confusion.

Many adolescents feel they have almost no control over physiological changes and the accompanying mood swings. In an attempt to preserve the child's body they once had, some girls attempt to control their food intake. But a girl with a bad self-image may develop an obsession with food intake that leads to an eating disorder.

Boys also feel out of control, experiencing erections and hormonal surges at almost any stimulus.

A cultural double standard does not help. Boys who do not want to be permissive feel out of place, as do girls who want to experience sexual behaviors. Such confusion can lead to sexual experimentation—usually in the form of unsafe sexual practices.

Psychological Factors

- Emotions are dramatically affected by hormones, which cause dramatic mood swings for adolescents.
- Early or late developers may have issues with securing their body image.
- Sexual experience used to be gained slowly, starting with kissing games, moving to petting, then intercourse. Today's teens often move directly from kissing to intercourse.
- Self-concept is influenced by social status and peers.
- Learned attitudes and behaviors are put to the test as the body goes through constant physical changes.

Summary

- Biological sexual development begins during pregnancy. Infants develop a sense of trust based on loving touch and reliable need fulfillment.

- Healthy sexual development of infants and toddlers is fostered by teaching correct names of all body parts and responding non-punitively to self-stimulation and curiosity about genitals.

- Gender is assigned at birth, usually based on genital appearance. By age 3, a child recognizes gender differences; by age 5, a child has an internal sense of being male or female (gender identity) and knows his or her gender will not change (gender constancy).

- Preschoolers develop autonomy and intiative rather than shame or guilt when curiosity-based sex play is expected as normal behavior and questions about reproduction are answered truthfully.

- Parents can use the media as an effective teaching tool, encouraging elementary-school-age children to develop empathy and to critically examine what they see and hear for sexism, gender role stereotypes, and other prejudices.

- Puberty—the predictable process of biological sexual development—usually occurs between the ages of 8 and 17; the median age is 10–11 years for girls and 11–12 years for boys. Physical changes during puberty include emergence of secondary sexual characteristics such as body and facial hair, glandular changes, growth spurt in height and weight, and reproductive maturity indicated by menarche (first menstrual period for girls) and semenarche (first ejaculation for boys).

- The goal of comprehensive sexuality education is to promote adult sexual health. Key concepts include human development, relationships, personal skills, sexual behavior, sexual health, and sexual aspects of society and culture. These concepts are learned through obtaining accurate information, exploring attitudes and values, developing interpersonal skills including communication, and exercising responsibility.

- Adolescence—the period of development from puberty to adulthood—consists of three stages during which thinking, emotions,

relationship skills, autonomy, body image, gender-role definition, and sexual self-concept become mature.

- Teen sexual behavior is often examined through the lens of risk behaviors, STIs, and teen birthrates. After 14 years of birthrate decline, attributed to decreased sexual intercourse and increased use of condoms, the birthrate among U.S. teens increased 4% from 2005 to 2007 and remains the highest in the Western industrialized world.

- Sexual abuse and harassment can occur online via the Internet—that is, electronically as well as directly.

- A sexually healthy relationship can be recognized as one that is safe, consensual, non-exploitative, honest, pleasurable, and protected.

Discussion Questions

1. Discuss how touch, including genital touching, differs for infants and toddlers versus adolescents.

2. Describe the roles that parents, peers, and the media play in teaching preschoolers and early elementary students about sexuality.

3. Compare and contrast puberty in boys and girls, both physiologically and emotionally.

4. Identify and describe the three stages of adolescence, including the development of sexual self-concept.

5. Describe how trends in sexual behaviors, attitudes, and birthrates have changed since the first YRBS was administered in 1991.

6. Distinguish between expected childhood sex play and behaviors that could be abusive.

Application Questions

Reread the chapter-opening story and answer the following questions.

1. On *Mister Rogers' Neighborhood*, Fred Rogers sings a song that says, "Boys are special on the outside/Girls are special on the inside." Is there any reason to tell a young child more than that?

2. Some parents choose to teach their young children about sexual intercourse and reproduction; many other parents do not want their children learning such information. Given that children repeat what they know, is it important to respect

the rights of those who—for religious or cultural reasons—want such information withheld from their children?

3. Given that children do hear explicit sexual references on the national news at some point, how should the mass media handle this content with adequate discretion? If you were a reporter *and* a parent, how would you balance the responsibility to report the news but protect young children?

Critical Thinking Questions

1. You are the parent of a 4-year-old and have just received a phone call from a parent who has a child the same age. It seems the two children were in the garage "examining" each other. The other parent is furious, accusing your child of initiating the "perversities." What do you say to the parent? What do you say to your child?

   You have 10 minutes before your child arrives home, time enough to check out the SIECUS web site. Which information will help you talk to your child?

2. Some pressures of adolescence are the result of society's double standard—that it is OK for men but wrong for women to be interested in engaging in sexual behaviors. Given what the chapter says about normal sexual feelings, what pressures does a double standard place on women? On men?

   Is it possible for society to eliminate the double standard and emphasize equality? If so, would society choose that both men and women have an equal right to say yes or no to sexual experiences? Explain your answer.

3. Refer to the Multicultural Dimensions feature when answering these questions. What is the influence of race and ethnicity on condom use? What might account for these differences? What is the influence of race and ethnicity on the number of sexual partners? Why might these differences exist? How might cultural differences influence partner impregnation? How can young people who choose to engage in sexual intercourse be encouraged to use condoms consistently?

Critical Thinking Case

Adolescents have a hard enough time coming to grips with their sexuality even if they receive proper information and support. But few do. In addition, some school-based sexuality education programs have a "fear-based" component. The aim of many

fear-based programs is abstinence outside marriage. There is nothing wrong with teaching abstinence; however, many fear-based programs tend to distort information and use incorrect information to make their point.

The SIECUS web site features a large section on fear-based programs, with general information and critiques of seven fear-based programs.

Choose one fear-based program and prepare a critique. What are the strong points and weak points of the program? How could it be improved? Would the fear techniques used in the program have prevented you from engaging in sexual activity?

Exploring Personal Dimensions

Readiness for a Sexual Relationship

Teenagers and young adults often wonder, "How do I know if I am ready for sex?" The following checklist may help them assess their readiness for mature sexual relationships (Winship, 1983).

This checklist may help adolescents *and* adults evaluate whether they are ready for a mature sexual relationship with a partner. Ideally, these criteria would be met *before* a young person or an adult engaged in intimate sexual behaviors, including any type of intercourse. Think about your own decisions or the decisions of people you know. Do they meet these criteria?

Are you and your partner
_____ Physically mature?
_____ Patient and understanding?
_____ Knowledgeable about sexuality and sexual response?
_____ Empathetic and able to be vulnerable?
_____ Committed to preventing unintended pregnancies?
_____ Able to handle responsibility for positive consequences?
_____ Able to handle responsibility for potential negative consequences?
_____ Honestly approving of your behavior?

Is your relationship
_____ Committed, mutually kind, and understanding?
_____ Do you trust and admire each other?
_____ Have you experimented with and found pleasure in nonpenetrative behaviors?
_____ Have you talked about sexual behaviors before they occur?
_____ Is your motivation for a sexual relationship pleasure and intimacy?
_____ Do you have a place for the sexual relationship that is safe and comfortable?

Source: Haffner, 1995.

Suggested Readings

Goldman, L. *Coming out, coming in: Nurturing the well-being and inclusion of gay youth in mainstream society.* New York: Routledge Press, 2007.

Haffner, D. W. *Beyond the big talk: A parent's guide to raising sexually healthy teens, revised and updated edition.* New York: Newmarket Press, 2008.

Haffner, D. W. *From diapers to dating: A parent's guide to raising sexually healthy children,* revised 2nd Ed. New York: Newmarket Press, 2008.

Harris, R. H., & Emberley, M. *A family library: It's not the stork! A book about girls, boys, babies, bodies, families and friends.* Cambridge, MA: Candlewick Press, 2006.

It's perfectly normal. Cambridge, MA: Candlewick Press, 2009.
It's so amazing! A book about eggs, sperm, birth, babies, and families. Cambridge, MA: Candlewick Press, 2009.

Macavinta, C., & Vander Pluym, A. *Respect: A girl's guide to getting respect and dealing when your line is crossed.* Minneapolis, MN: Free Spirit, 2005.

Parent power: What parents need to know and do to help prevent teen pregnancy. Washington, DC: National Campaign to Prevent Teen Pregnancy, 2005.

Steiner-Adair, C., & Sjostrom, L. *Full of ourselves: A wellness program to advance girl power, health, and leadership.* New York: Teachers College Press, 2006.

Web Resources

For links to the web sites below, visit *http://sexuality.jbpub.com/dimensions/4e* and click on Resource Links.

Answer/Sex, Etc.
www.sexetc.org

Sex, Etc. is part of the Teen-to-Teen Sexuality Education Project developed by Answer. Answer—part of the Center for Applied Psychology at Rutgers University—is a national organization dedicated to providing and promoting comprehensive sexuality education to young people and the adults who teach them.

Sexuality Information and Education Council of the United States
www.siecus.org

SIECUS has been a national voice for sexuality education, sexual health, and sexual rights for more than 40 years. It provides information, education, public policy, and media outreach to educators, health care providers, parents, journalists, policy makers, religious leaders, community members, and young people.

National Campaign to Prevent Teen and Unplanned Pregnancy
www.thenationalcampaign.org

Founded in 1996, this nonprofit, nonpartisan initiative is supported almost entirely by private donations. Its mission is to improve the well-being of children, youth, and families by reducing the nation's teen and unplanned pregnancy rates. It offers a host of research-based resources for teens, parents, faith leaders, researchers, and professionals.

Planned Parenthood Federation of America
www.plannedparenthood.org/teen-talk

Teen-Talk is the official teen outreach web site of Planned Parenthood. It provides honest and non-judgmental information about sexuality in language teens can understand. The goal of this site is for teens to use this knowledge to reduce their risk of unintended pregnancy and sexually transmitted infections.

CHAPTER 12

Sexuality in Adulthood

FEATURES

Multicultural Dimensions
The Jefferson–Hemings Affair

Communication Dimensions
Tempted by Digital Dalliances

Global Dimensions
Divorce in China and Sudan

Multicultural Dimensions
The Boomer Sandwich

Ethical Dimensions
Should Donor Eggs Be Used to Let Women Older Than 50 Years Produce Viable Babies?

Gender Dimensions
Coming to Terms: Masculinity and Physical Challenges

CHAPTER OBJECTIVES

1 Discuss the major theories of love and sexuality.

2 Describe the typical college relationship, including sexual activities.

3 Cite the factors that have led to the increase in the number of single people and the postponement of marriage.

4 Evaluate the advantages and disadvantages of cohabitation.

5 Describe the characteristics of a happy marriage.

6 Discuss the reasons for the high number of divorces.

7 Describe changes that occur during the aging process.

8 Discuss the sexuality challenges for the disabled and ill, as well as how to overcome them.

sexuality.jbpub.com/dimensions/4e

Cohabitation
Multicultural Dimensions: The Jefferson–Hemings Affair
Types of Marriage
Divorce

INTRODUCTION

*L*ynn and Chris first met in a small town's only junior high when they were 12 years old. By high school, they had become friends and had their first date at the homecoming dance their sophomore year. After a couple of years of dating, they lost their virginity together at age 16 years. Throughout high school, they stayed together and began planning for college and a life together.

They applied to the same colleges and entered the college where they were both accepted. The struggles of college produced many changes, but they made a conscious effort to change together. As they grew up together, they did things they perceived to be more grown-up: traveling, saving up for an apartment, and the like. During their junior year, they got an off-campus apartment in the heart of the local city.

Although they had been together for more than 5 years and were engaged, they were surprised at their parents' reactions—shock and dismay—to their living together. After all, it was the late 1970s, and both families had had other relatives who had lived together. Lynn and Chris saw living together as a "next step" toward marriage. Why, they thought, was society so backward?

Surviving college made them more determined to pursue their dream of life together, with children and good jobs. At age 24 years, they married. Four years later, a first child was born; 3 years later, a second child. With each change, they managed to adapt. But slowly—almost imperceptibly—they realized that they were not always changing in the same ways.

As they hit full stride in their careers in their mid-30s, and their children reached school age, decisions had to be made. Holding a high-level management position that requires long hours and travel also requires support at home—with children and housework. The old saying

"Behind every great man, there's a great woman" today would be phrased as "A successful person has family support."

Lynn supported the family by working from a home office and taking care of the children—schools, homework, sick days, vacation days, doctor and dentist appointments, play dates, sports, and extracurricular activities. Chris rarely returned home from work before 7:30 P.M., worked many weekends, and traveled around the world. Conflicts developed over what was important in their lives, and, because Chris made more money than Lynn, issues concerning how to spend also arose. Chris's lack of time at home increased tensions. Eventually, Lynn discovered that Chris was having an affair with a business associate.

After considering the possibility of divorce for several years, Lynn and Chris finally proceeded—after 14 years of marriage and almost 25 years together. The children stayed with Lynn, and Chris was ordered to pay child support and alimony. Both Lynn and Chris expressed a feeling of relief after the divorce was finalized.

Lynn and Chris had a great deal of positive support from friends, many of whom had been divorced themselves. It seemed that society had begun to accept divorce. But once again, they were surprised by the reaction of their parents, who felt that they should stay together and try to work out their problems. Some things never change!

In this chapter we continue our exploration of the life cycle, picking up in young adulthood. We first explore how people fall in love, then we follow the life cycle from singlehood, through cohabitation, marriage, and divorce. Finally, we take a look at sexuality and the elderly.

■ Love and Sexuality

What is love? How do you know when and whether you are in love, whether you are loved, or whether you love another person? These questions have been asked through the ages by young people just beginning to long for and seek intimacy outside their parental families. And through the ages love has never grown any easier to define. There are many types of love—love of one's parents, of a friend, of a pet. Perhaps the most difficult sort of love to describe is love of a person with whom one could potentially share a sexual relationship.

Theories About Love

Love may take a variety of forms, as Greek philosophers long ago demonstrated: *eros*, passionate and/or erotic love; *agape*, a selfless, giving love; *storge*, affectionate love, usually of the type parents have for their children; *ludus*, playful love (partners keep the relationship at a distance by keeping love at a game level); and *mania*, a love consumed by emotional extremes such as misery, possessiveness, and jealousy.

Erich Fromm presented his ideas about love in *The Art of Loving* (1956). He distinguishes brotherly

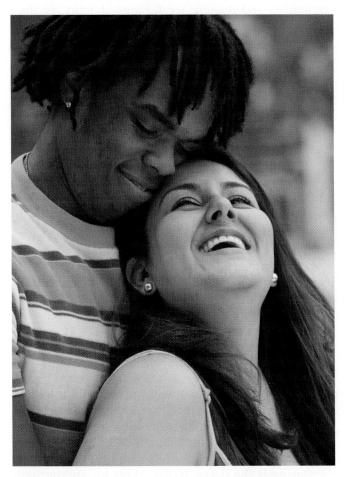

Passionate love is characterized by almost total absorption in another person.

love, motherly love, erotic love, and self-love. He believes that loving is an art—something that must be learned and practiced. Fromm indicated that immature love is characterized by a dependent relationship between two people, and mature love is characterized by care, responsibility, respect, and knowledge of the loved person. He defines erotic love as a craving for total union with another person that is exclusive and enduring.

Abraham Maslow distinguished between B-love and D-love (1968). Those who experience B-love (short for *Being* love) are unselfish in their love for another; those who experience D-love (short for *Deficiency* love) are selfish and have a strong need for love.

Rempel and Burris (2005) suggested that love is a motive based on the valuing of the other person, and is associated with the goal of preserving or promoting the other's well-being. They said that intense, powerful emotions may serve as eliciting experiences for different types of love. Benefitting the other person can be an ultimate goal for the various forms of love.

Types of Love

Love takes many forms and can be distinguished as romantic love or conscious love. Romantic love, also known as passionate love, is characterized by almost total absorption in another, with strong feelings of elation, sexual desire, anxiety, and arousal. This form of love is often accompanied by physiological reactions—perspiration, stomach churning, blushing, and increased pulse rate.

Intense, passionate love is most likely to occur early in a relationship. At this point people often overlook faults, avoid conflicts, and ignore logic and reasoned consideration. Conscious love, in contrast, is a more realistic view of another person. We see both the strengths and weaknesses of the loved one and do not depend completely on him or her to fulfill our needs and give us what we ourselves lack. The sexual activity in conscious love may be more rewarding than in romantic love because the sexual behavior communicates and expresses loving feelings. People who have an honest view of each other can enjoy giving as well as receiving. People who feel romantic (passionate) love are often intent on receiving pleasure and fulfilling their desires, rather than on giving and taking equally.

In addition to being romantic or conscious, love can take various forms—erotic, friendship, devotional, parental, or altruistic. In erotic love there is a type of biological "chemistry" that binds lovers together and leads them to form a binding relationship (Lee, 1988). Individuals experiencing erotic love are preoccupied with their love and constantly think about their partner. Erotic love becomes less intense as time goes on, but even at a lower level it can be a positive part of a relationship.

Friendship involves deep and intimate feelings, but these are not physical. The Greek term for this type of friendship or liking is *philia*. Although there are many similar attitudes and feelings among lovers as well as friends, lovers tend to differ from friends in sexual intimacy, exclusiveness, and fascination (Davis, 1985). Men and women can be friends without becoming sexually involved.

Devotional love does not involve physical contact and is a very specific kind of love. This type of love is most likely to be directed to a god, a country, an ethnic group, or other significant groups or institutions.

Parental love can be intense, but the feelings are different from other forms of love. Infants and children learn this type of love through holding and touching—even very early in life. For some people, parental love represents the most intense form of love they will ever feel.

Altruistic love is a generous giving of the self. Some say this is a special form of parental love; it is

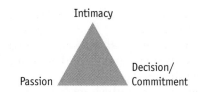

FIGURE **12.1** Sternberg's triangular theory of love.

seen in people who spend great amounts of time doing church work, volunteering in hospitals, and assisting others in a variety of ways. Some people who work in helping professions—for example, as therapists or teachers—might find they have a great capacity for altruistic love.

Sternberg (1986) has proposed a triangular theory of love suggesting that there are three components of love: intimacy, passion, and decision/commitment. These components can be visualized as points on a triangle (Figure 12.1); the triangle metaphor is used to show how a couple can be matched or mismatched in the love they have for each other. The top of the triangle is intimacy, which is the emotional component of love, according to Sternberg. Here are feelings of mutual understanding, bondedness, willingness to share, giving of emotional support, and valuing of the other person as part of your life. Passion is the motivational drive of love that includes physical attraction, sexual relations, and romance. Passion can usually differentiate romantic love from love in a friendship or of a family member. This component is usually first in a relationship but is also the first to fade. Passion and intimacy are interwoven and one may precede the other, depending on how the relationship begins. Decision/commitment is the cognitive component of the triangle, as one makes the decision to love the other person and then makes the long-term commitment to maintain the relationship.

Perfectly matched involvements of partners exist when the vertexes of the triangles are equally matched and are at the same level. Closely matched couples may be slightly off on one of the components, and this is usually not a perilous situation. Moderately mismatched partners exhibit mismatching at one or two of the vertexes and the partners are at different levels within those components. For example, they may be equally matched on the passion vertex, but one partner is slightly more

committed and has greater feelings of intimacy than the other. A severely mismatched couple is one whose partners may be equally committed but are very disparate in the passion and intimacy components.

This theory of love may help partners determine whether they are on the right track in their relationship and may help diagnose any problems.

Sternberg (1988) has outlined eight types, or phases, of love based on his triangular model. They are listed in Table 12.1.

Characteristics of Romantic Love

Because we are focusing on human relationships and sexuality in this text, it is appropriate to consider briefly the characteristics of romantic love—companionship, intimacy, caring, commitment, sexual activity, and romance. Companionship involves sharing experiences and receiving emotional support from each other. At first this characteristic might not seem as exciting as some of the others, but over time it can be enduring and very necessary.

Intimacy involves sharing thoughts and feelings with a person who is considered very special. Whereas traditionally women and not men revealed their innermost thoughts, in recent years there is a tendency for both genders to disclose highly personal feelings within a relationship (Hatfield, 1988; Pearson, 1985).

Caring is the desire to do things for another person without expecting anything in return. As in most other aspects of a relationship, balance is important. For example, it is possible to think of situations in which there is so much caring that the relationship is completely one-sided.

TABLE 12.1	**Sternberg's Types (Phases) of Love**

1. **Nonlove:** All three components of love are absent. Most personal relationships are of this type.

2. **Liking:** Intimacy is present, but passion and commitment are not.

3. **Infatuation:** There are passionate desires, but intimacy and commitment are not present. This is a kind of "love at first sight."

4. **Empty love:** Commitment exists, but passion and intimacy are missing. Relationships that once had passion and intimacy can become stagnant.

5. **Romantic love:** There is no commitment, but there is passion and intimacy.

6. **Companionate love:** A combination of intimacy and commitment exists, but passionate attraction has died down. The relationship becomes a kind of committed friendship.

7. **Fatuous love:** Passion and commitment are present, but intimacy is not. This type is associated with whirlwind romances and "quickie marriages."

8. **Consummate love:** This is the complete measure of love involving passion, intimacy, and commitment. It can be very hard to achieve this type of love, and even harder to maintain it.

Source: Sternberg, 1988.

Intimacy means sharing thoughts and feelings with someone we consider very special.

Commitment means pressing on with a relationship even during difficult times. When conflict or problems exist, commitment is needed to give other aspects of love a chance to grow.

Sexual activity sometimes seems to be the major part of romantic love; however, there are many couples who love each other but have a minimal amount of sexual activity. Sexual activity alone, even when highly pleasurable, is not enough to maintain a poor relationship (Blumstein & Schwartz, 1983). There does seem to be a connection between sexual activity and positive relationships, but a good relationship probably has a positive influence on sexual activity, rather than the converse.

The decision to participate in sexual activity can be very simple for some people, and very complicated for others. Sexual activity can have different meanings for different people. It can be a validation of deep intimacy in a relationship, it can be a way to help get to know another person, it can be done to promote reproduction, it can reduce sexual tension, it can produce excitement and risk, and for some it can be a form of recreation.

For many college students it is helpful to base decisions about sexual activity on their values. Some students may have clear guidelines based upon what they have learned from their family, their religion, or their peers; others may not have such guidelines. In either case it may be wise to consider personal values in life and relationships before getting sexually involved. This can mean thinking about the role of relationships and sexual activity in life at that time,

which norms are most highly valued and why, and what should be done for protection against unwanted pregnancy and sexually transmitted infections (STIs) if a decision is made to participate in intimate sexual activity. Communication about these decisions with a potential partner is especially important. Suggestions for such communication were provided in Chapter 3.

The nature of love typically changes as a relationship develops. For example, the passionate or romantic love of an early stage might evolve into a companionship type of love. This does not mean that passion and romance have evaporated, nor does it mean that the relationship is not as good as before. It simply means that there are common stages of relationships, and they can all be of high quality. Relationships can be thought of as having different phases of growth. At any stage there are ways to promote better relationships.

Aron et al. (2005) reported interesting research about romantic love and related changes as relationships develop. They used MRI brain scans and studied 17 college students who were intensely "in love" from 1 to 17 months. Participants alternately viewed a photograph of their beloved and a photograph of a familiar individual. The MRI detected increases or decreases of blood flow to the brain, which reflected changes in neural activity. Based on brain activity, they found that romantic love is a biological urge distinct from sexual arousal. It is close to the neural profile of drives like hunger and drug craving. In its early stages, love can be very intoxicating and the drive for romantic love can be stronger than the will to live. With time, however, the intoxication mellows and brain scans show different findings. The scans show that different parts of the brain are stimulated later in a relationship as compared to the earlier stages. The researchers indicated that, among other processes, new love involves psychologically internalizing a lover, absorbing elements of the other person's opinions, hobbies, expressions, and character, as well as sharing one's own. The expansion of the self happens very rapidly, and it is one of the most exhilarating experiences there is.

Many have traditionally believed that romantic love fades over time and evolves into warm feelings. However, Acevedo and Aron (2009) found that long-term relationships do not necessarily kill the romance. Their research indicates long-term romantic love (with intensity, sexual interest, and engagement, but without the obsessive element common in new relationships) appears to be real and is associated with marital satisfaction, mental health, and overall well-being.

The relationship between love styles and lifetime number of sexual partners has also been explored among college students. Hans (2008) found that the number of sexual partners was positively correlated with age, romantic lovers, and game-playing lovers (who typically value fun and self-indulgence over commitment and emotional involvement), and was negatively correlated with religiosity.

Hormonal and Chemical Aspects of Love

The characteristics and types of love presented so far have been mainly based upon emotional, psychological, and spiritual kinds of feelings. Some experts argue that hormonal and chemical factors are also involved in love. One reason may be related to brain chemistry. Another relates to pheromones, which are chemical substances secreted by some animals that supposedly affect the reproductive behavior of another same-species animal.

Related to brain chemistry, during the intense passion of a developing love relationship some people report a natural high, almost as though they were on drugs. Researchers (Liebowitz, 1983; Walsh, 1991) reported that this "high" results from surging levels of three brain chemicals that allow brain cells to communicate with each other. They are similar to amphetamine drugs and cause effects such as giddiness, euphoria, and elation. As with use of amphetamines, the "high" typically does not last—perhaps because the body develops a tolerance for the chemicals just as it does for amphetamines, or perhaps because the intensity of the relationship decreases.

The same researchers also point out that there are brain chemicals that help explain why some relationships develop into long-term loving relationships. These substances, called endorphins, are morphine-like chemicals that help cause a sense of security, tranquility, and peace. The researchers suggest that these chemicals help explain why abandoned lovers may feel such a loss: They are not getting their doses of feel-good chemicals.

The topic of pheromones has received greater attention in recent years. For more than a hundred years scientists have documented the effects of pheromones on mating behavior in insects and animals. The big question has been, Do pheromones have the same effects on humans?

In 1986 Dr. Winnifred Cutler began to document the effects of human pheromones (Link & Copeland, 2001). Those who believe in human pheromones claim they send signals that are picked up by organs inside the nose. We cannot smell them, but they supposedly can have a major impact on sex drive, increase in fertility, and regulation of women's menstrual cycles. Behaviors that are reported to increase as a result of pheromones include making conversation, expressing an interest in another person, being responsive to another person, paying unsolicited compliments, overtly flirting, brushing up against another person, and becoming sexually excited.

On the basis of the concept that there are natural human pheromones, entrepreneurs developed numerous products designed to mimic the alleged effects of pheromones. These include towelettes with pheromones as well as creams and oils that are supposed to help with sexual attraction. It is too early to tell whether such products are effective—and even the basic effects of pheromones are not agreed upon by experts.

The overall biology of love is still a mystery. However, many people report that biological factors and changes seem to influence their strong feelings for another person. Obvious things like increased heart rate, slight sweating, and hormonal changes do seem to occur. For example, levels of glucocorticoids and norephinephrine can increase in the bloodstream very quickly when seeing a very attractive person. These reactions, along with the potential influence of pheromones, result in biological impacts on potential love relationships (Gonzales, 2005).

At the 2009 annual meeting of the Advancing Science, Serving Society (AASA), several researchers talked about the biology of romantic love (Borenstein, 2009). Among other points, they indicated that parts of the brain respond strongly when people are around those they love romantically, brain cells make chemicals and send them to different brain regions, and love works chemically in the brain like a drug addiction.

Love Problems

With all its positive aspects, love can also create problems. Perhaps the most obvious ones are rejection, jealousy, and falling out of love. Being turned down by another person (rejection) can be difficult to experience. This can happen at various stages of a relationship, and fear of rejection is natural. Of course, as with so many other aspects of life, obtaining the many positive benefits of a relationship always entails a gamble (such as the possibility of rejection). Dealing with rejection can be difficult for some, but often it simply involves trying again. If a strong relationship already exists, it might be wise to use good communication skills and talk about the rejection with the other person. Couples counseling can help single and married couples. At any rate, rejection can also be used as a learning experience to help in future relationships.

Some jealous feelings are probably natural, but jealousy is also a bothersome feeling that can get in the way of good love relationships. It can be helpful to understand why jealous feelings occur, to use good communication skills to talk about jealousy within a relationship, and to avoid doing things that might contribute to a partner's jealous feelings. For some, effective means of coping with jealousy are thinking about one's positive qualities, selectively ignoring some activities that might be upsetting, and simply containing feelings of jealousy. It might be wise to recognize jealous feelings and accept and deal with them as part of an overall relationship.

It may be hard to deal with feelings if you are attracted to someone who is in a relationship with another person.

What Causes Attraction?

Many factors contribute to attraction and falling in love. Unlike in the fairy tale in which the prince marries the commoner, in real life we are usually attracted to someone we consider attainable. This attraction differs from adolescent crushes on movie stars, sports stars, politicians, or teachers. In adulthood, we seek intimate relationships with someone who can love us in return.

Most North Americans marry someone who has the same sociocultural dimensions, someone whose race and ethnicity, religion, age, and social class are similar to their own (Henslin, 1995). A 1994 study showed that most Americans met their spouses at school, church, or work or through friends (Laumann et al., 1994). Why do we like people who are like us? One explanation is that doing so provides us with validation for our personality characteristics and beliefs (Baron, 1998). Similarity is a very powerful determinant of attraction.

Gender also plays a role in mate selection. Researchers interviewed more than 9,000 young adults (males and females), all in their 20s, who lived in 33 countries. Subjects were given a list of 18 traits and asked to rank them in terms of most (1) to least (18) desirable in a potential mate (Buss et al., 1990). The results are listed in Table 12.2.

Buss and associates found a gender difference as well: Males in all cultures in the study placed an emphasis on youthfulness and attractiveness. Data showed that at the time of marriage, the average male was 2 to 5 years older than his partner. Women, however, placed an emphasis on mates who were somewhat older, had better prospects for financial security,

and were industrious. Buss explains the difference in terms of evolutionary needs: Males select younger, physically attractive women because such characteristics are viewed as good indicators of reproductive success. Women select older, more established males because such characteristics are viewed as good indicators of security for their offspring (Buss, 1994).

Attraction, then, can be caused by many characteristics. Features such as height, eye color and size, size of body parts, skin characteristics, musculature, and body symmetry can all play a role for some people. Related to all of this is the waist-to-hip ratio. It is determined by dividing your waist measurement by your hip measurement. For example, a ratio of 0.7 might be considered desirable for a female, while a ratio of 0.9 might be desirable for a male. The hips are measured

TABLE 12.2	Ranking of Desirable Traits in a Partner (Male and Female Combined)

1. Mutual attraction (love)
2. Dependable character
3. Emotional stability and maturity
4. Pleasing disposition
5. Good health
6. Education and intelligence
7. Sociability
8. Desire for home and children
9. Refinement, neatness
10. Good looks (ranked higher by males)
11. Ambitious and industrious
12. Good cook and housekeeper
13. Good financial prospects (ranked higher by females)
14. Similar education
15. Favorable social status or rating
16. Chastity (ranked higher by males)
17. Similar religious background
18. Similar political background

at the widest part of the buttocks, and the waist is measured at the smaller circumference of the natural waist, usually just above the belly button. Research indicates that people with "apple-shaped" bodies (with more weight around the waist) face more health risks than those with "pear-shaped" bodies who carry more weight around the hips. It has also been found that in most cultures waist-to-hip ratio is viewed as a measure of attractiveness and health for men and women (Singh, 2002).

Whatever causes attraction, it is interesting that many of us have a "love-is-blind bias" (a tendency to perceive romantic partners as more attractive than the self). For example, Swami (2009) found that both gay men and lesbians rated their partners as significantly more attractive than themselves. The author called this a "robust positive illusion in self–partner perceptions."

Sexuality During the College Years

Before the late 1960s, there were strict rules on campuses about men's and women's socializing. Older readers may remember the "one foot on the floor" rule: Women were allowed to have men in their college dorm room only with the door open and only with each person's having one foot on the floor. Curfews were common. Coed dorms were nonexistent. Today, most campuses have long given up these types of rules. Sexual activity on college campuses has increased dramatically: 12% among college men and 35% among college women during the period from 1965 to 1980 (Rubinson & Rupertis, 1991). The prevailing sexual norm on most campuses is "permissiveness with affection."

Since 2000, the American College Health Association (2008) has conducted the National College Health Assessment every fall and spring term. Some of the questions relate to sexual behavior, and more than 70,000 college students respond each term. Here are highlights from the most recent findings:

- 28.4% of respondents had ever been tested for HIV infection.

- 14.1% of sexually active women had used emergency contraception within the past school year.

- 2.3% of females and 2.5% of males who had vaginal intercourse within the past school year had become pregnant unintentionally or had gotten someone else pregnant unintentionally.

- 45.3% of students had oral sexual activity in the past 30 days.

- 49.1% of students had vaginal intercourse in the past 30 days.

- 5.2% had anal intercourse in the past 30 days.

- 31.4% had no sexual partner, 45.3% had one sexual partner, 10.1% had two sexual partners, 5.3% had three sexual partners, and 7.9% had four or more sexual partners in the past 12 months.

- Using a condom within the last 30 days (mostly or always) was reported by 49.1% of those who had vaginal intercourse and 24.7% of those who had anal intercourse. Approximately the same percentage of students used a condom the last time they had sexual intercourse of either type.

- The most common forms of birth control used by students or their partners the last time they had vaginal intercourse were condoms (35.8%), birth control pills (34.2%), and withdrawal (15.6%).

It is interesting that in general respondents thought that their college peers were participating in much more sexual activity than they actually were. This reminds us that perceptions of other people's sexual behavior are often not accurate.

While not necessarily pertaining only to students attending college, here are some interesting statistics about males and females of college age. By their late teenage years, at least 75% of all men and women have had intercourse, and more than two-thirds of all sexually experienced teens have had two or more partners. Among sexually experienced people in their 20s, 31% of men and 20% of women have had more than one sexual partner in the past year (Sexual and reproductive health, 2002).

Late high school and early college years are a time of transition to sexual activity for males. Fewer than 25% are sexually experienced by age 15, but more than 90% have intercourse before their 20th birthday. Slightly more than 20% of sexually experienced men have had only one partner by their late teens, and about 30% have had six or more (In their own right, 2002).

Types of Relationships

Most college students appear to be serially monogamous; that is, they are sexually exclusive with one partner at a time. In one study, 53% of the sexually experienced college men and 60% of the sexually experienced college women were involved in an exclusive love relationship. Still, significant percent-

Some researchers indicate that dating among college students is almost dead. Many seem to participate in random hookups or very serious relationships instead.

ages of college students have casual sexual activity. Fourteen percent of young women and 38% of young men report that they have had casual intercourse with more than one partner during their college years (Dunn, Knight, & Glascoff, 1992).

Significant proportions of college students have had several sexual partners. In one study, 38% of men and 36% of women had had vaginal intercourse with more than five partners. Although on average, these young people had been having sexual intercourse for less than 4 years, males reported an average of eight female partners and females reported an average of six male partners (Reinisch et al., 1995). In a national phone survey of college students, 36% of males and 21% of females reported that they had had nine or more partners (Survey USA, 1998).

The Institute for American Values (Mulhauser, 2001) interviewed 1,000 college women and reported that dating among college students is all but dead. Apparently, college students either participate in random hookups or are in a very serious relationship. For many, there is nothing in between. Hooking up does not have to mean having sexual intercourse. In fact, 39% of the respondents were virgins. Dating, however, was not reported to be very common. One-third of the women said they had been asked on two or fewer dates. Of the seniors interviewed, only 50% said they had been asked on six or more dates since college started. Because few people are asking for dates, what is left is an informal hookup.

Previously, noncollege singles in their 20s were almost entirely overlooked in research about sexual behavior and attitudes. Popenoe and Whitehead (2001) found that this group aspire to marriage and expect their marriage to last a lifetime. However, many are first looking to get ahead on their own. Both men and women are committed to making it on their own and getting a place of their own before marriage. The mating culture is described as "sex without strings and relationships without rings." Sexual activity is viewed as being for fun. Casual sexual activity is an expected part of the dating scene. The threat of HIV and AIDS looms large over the dating scene. However, although both men and women fear AIDS, it is mainly the women who take the initiative and responsibility for protection. Both men and women see the club scene as a place for drinking, fun, and casual sexual hookups. In seeking a high-quality relationship, these men and women say you should look for a partner through church, friends, or school. Entering a relationship usually means postponing sexual activity until you get to know each other. Before becoming seriously involved, couples often are tested for HIV and AIDS. Once a couple can prove to each other

 Did You Know . . .

Dr. Joe McIlhaney, Jr., founder of the Medical Institute for Sexual Health in Austin, Texas, feels that the pressure on college students to practice unhealthy behavior is much more intense than most adults realize. He feels that parents, university personnel, and others who care about the well-being of college students have to act. His ideas include a return to single-sex dorms and bathrooms, more abstinence and pro-marriage messages, and parent-led "inspector committees" to track high-risk health behaviors on all campuses. He is concerned that college personnel turn a blind eye to sexual behavior, while campus groups boldly advertise sex-toy sales, "fetish"

fairs, and other sexually oriented activities. Dr. McIlhaney thinks parents should be more involved on campus, while other experts do not feel this is needed.

Another expert advocates a return to dating. He says it is healthier than the casual sexual activity that comes through hookups or "friends with benefits."

How do you feel about this? Is there "sexual chaos" on college campuses?

Source: Wetzstein, C. "Sexual chaos" at college. *The Washington Times* (August 9, 2005), 9B.

that they have recently tested negative, they are less vigilant about using condoms.

Overall there has been an increase in "casual" sexual relationships among high school and college students (Surveys show change in attitudes toward sex among high school and college students, 2003). Thirteen hundred Ohio seventh- to eleventh-grade students were interviewed about dating, relationships, and sexual activity. About 55% had engaged in intercourse and one-third of those had engaged in intercourse with "someone whose attachment went no further than friendship." The study also reported a significant shift in attitudes toward oral sexual activity, noting that respondents consider it "an acceptable alternative" to intercourse and different from sexual intercourse. The proportion of young adults who have engaged in oral sexual activity has risen; one-third of 15- to 17-year-olds and two-thirds of 18- to 24-year-olds have engaged in oral sexual activity.

In more recent years, some relationships have developed over the Internet. The Internet can be a useful technology for meeting potential partners and even carrying out cyber-relationships. It can even be a unique site for sexual experimentation. However, these relationships may make it difficult to be safe when pursuing personal contact with those met via the Internet. Safety strategies include seeking reliability of a person's responses by repeated questioning, conducting Google searches on the person, setting boundaries and limits on sexual activity before the in-person meeting, and relying on intuition and gut feelings. Strategies for achieving safety during in-person encounters include meeting a person by day and in public, making safe calls during the date, using personal transportation, having a friend in the area, and carrying a cell phone. Despite all these precautions, one study showed that one-third of Internet daters had sexual activity on the first personal encounter, and nearly 80% did not use a condom or question the new partner about STIs. Perhaps this was because of "accelerated intimacy" as a result of developing the relationships via the Internet (Ross, 2007).

Safer Sexual Activities and College Students

Most studies of condom use among college students date from the early 1990s; the results then indicated that condom use was relatively rare. Studies found that between 15% and 41% of students reported that they always used condoms, and the more partners a person had, the lower the rate of condom use (Lewis et al., 1997). A 1998 telephone survey of college students was much more encouraging; 54% reported that they always or almost always use condoms, and

College students need to know about contraception and prevention of HIV and AIDS.

24% said that they sometimes did. Still, one in five respondents reported that he or she almost never used condoms (Survey USA, 1998). As a result, one in five males and nearly one in three college-age females have been infected with an STI (Reinisch et al., 1995).

Relatedly, it is interesting to note that 6 in 10 pregnancies involving teenage fathers end in a birth; 4 in 10 end in an abortion. Thirteen percent of abortions each year involve teenage men. Also, most males use a condom the first time they have intercourse, but condom use subsequently declines and reliance on female methods increases. Condom use is more common among males who are not in a union than among those who are cohabiting or married (In their own right, 2002).

In 2004 it was found that 84% of adults between the ages of 18 and 35 said they take "necessary" steps to protect themselves against STIs, but their actions did not support their claims. Although 63% of respondents said they were "well informed" about the risks associated with sexual activity, 82% said they never use protection against STIs during oral sexual activity, 64% did not use protection during anal sexual activity, and 47% did not use protection during vaginal sexual activity. In addition, although 93% said they believed their current sexual partners did not have STIs, 33% said they had never discussed the issue with their partners. About 53% said their partners had undergone screening for STIs (Survey finds gaps between safe-sex claims, behavior among U.S. adults, 2004). Sixty-eight percent of respondents said that STI tests should be part of a routine health exam, but only 51% had ever spoken to a health care provider about STIs. Also, 68% did not feel concerned about contracting an STI.

Communication is the key to an honest and protected sexual relationship. Yet, most studies indicate that college students do not talk before they have sexual activity.

Planned Parenthood (2009) indicates that these are the most important ways to practice safer sexual activities:

- Understand and be honest about the risks you take.

- Keep your blood, pre-cum, semen, or vaginal fluids out of each other's bodies.

- Always use latex male or female condoms for anal or vaginal intercourse.

- Don't have sex play when you have a sore caused by an STI.

- Find ways to make safer sex as pleasurable as possible.

In addition, be aware of your body and your partner's body. Cuts, sores, or bleeding gums may all increase the risk of spreading STIs. Lubricants can increase sexual stimulation, and they also reduce the chance that condoms or other barriers will break. Of course, abstinence is totally safe. Sexual activity with just one partner is also safe as long as neither of you is infected and neither of you ever has sexual activity or shared needles with anyone else (Safer sex guidelines, 2009).

Singlehood

For most heterosexual young adults—male and female—singlehood is a temporary status. The vast majority of people eventually marry, but they are delaying marriage longer than in the past. In 1970, the median age for first marriage was 20.6 years for women and 22.5 years for men (Renzetti & Curran, 1998); by 1997, it had reached 25 years for women and 26.8 years for men (Schmid, 1998). According to the U.S. Census Bureau, it is now about 25.3 years for women and 27.1 years for men.

Singles delay or avoid marriage for several reasons, including improved social attitudes toward being single, increased caution inspired by high divorce rates, and increased availability of effective contraceptives (Renzetti & Curran, 1998). In addition, some singles enjoy the freedom from unnecessary commitments, opportunities to meet new people and develop new relationships, room for personal growth, and the ability to have a varied sex life free of guilt (Sullivan, 1998). Further, there is less societal pressure than there used to be to marry at an early age.

But probably the most important reason why young people delay marriage are economic constraints. In the last 30 years, housing prices have increased significantly, while the number of jobs that pay a wage

Add the Internet to the places to meet singles. On singles bulletin boards, singles can read extended personal ads, complete with photos. In chat rooms, singles have the opportunity to "meet" and "talk" to prospective dates in a safe environment. But be wary—experts warn that a first encounter with someone met on the Internet should be in a public place, perhaps among other friends.

adequate for establishing an independent household has declined. Consequently, 53% of people aged 18–24 years and 12% of people aged 25–34 years live at home with their parents (Renzetti & Curran, 1998).

This group has been labeled the "twixters." They aren't kids anymore, but they're not adults either. They are a new breed of young people who won't or can't settle down (Grossman, 2005). Instead of moving from adolescence to adulthood, some experts feel there is a new, intermediate phase of development for the twixters. They are called this because they are betwixt and between. Some who study this new life phase see it as a good thing—a chance for young people to savor the pleasures of irresponsibility and search their souls for new life paths. Others are worried that twixters aren't growing up because they can't. They feel that the cultural machinery that used to turn kids into grown-ups has broken down. They fear that society no longer provides young people with the moral backbone and the financial means to take their rightful places in the adult world. They point out that growing up may be harder than it used to be.

The number of people who never marry has increased since 1970. This is true for both males and females and for every age group. Today, in the United States, approximately 28% of women and 34% of men have never married (American fact finder, 2009). In addition, 42% of U.S. residents 18 and older are unmarried, 54% of whom are women. There are 12.9 million single parents living with their children. Of those, 10.4 million are single mothers. Nine percent of households are headed by a single parent, up from 5% in 1970 (Facts for features, 2008).

Approximately 27% of all children younger than age 18 live with a single parent in the United States—up from about 9% in 1960. About 22% of white children and 58% of black children younger than age 18 live with a single parent (The social health of marriage in America, 2009). More than 78,000 of those cohabiting had partners of the same gender (Facts for features, 2008).

Of course, some people who are single would like to get married. "The majority of people still want to get married, but they see it sort of as dessert now, something that's desirable rather than necessary," said the executive director of the Albany, New York–based Alternatives to Marriage Project, which aims to fight discrimination based on marital status and to seek equality and fairness for unmarried people. He feels that people want to be sure that they don't make a marriage mistake. Also, societal pressures to marry before having children have decreased. In 2007, nearly 40% of all births were to unmarried women. That's up from 11% in 1970 (Hamilton, Martin, & Ventura, 2009).

Online dating, once viewed as a refuge for the socially inept and as a faintly disrespectable way to meet other people, is quickly becoming a fixture of single life for adults of all ages, backgrounds, and interests. Some people feel that the traditional means for getting people together are not working as well as they did previously, and that there is a need for something new. As more people choose to marry later in life, few social institutions have arisen to replace the role that local communities, families, and schools once played. The Internet is filling that need. For many, there is a disconnect between who people say they are online and what they really are like. However, many people have found success through Internet dating and feel that online dating may be making it more acceptable to openly signal what they want. But gender rules still seem to apply. Men say women rarely send the first email note. As word spreads of successful matches, the stigma of advertising for a romantic partner online rather than waiting for friends or fate to conjure one is fading (Harmon, 2003).

Online dating sites have been trying to be more like real-life matchmakers. In 2004, the fastest-growing site, *eHarmony.com*, drew 10,000 new users per day with a 436-question screen. *Match.com*, the largest of the services, added its own test as well as an advice site manned by live therapists. One in 10 web surfers uses online dating sites, which get more than 40 million hits per month (Cullen, 2004).

As of 2005, online dating was a $500 million industry. But, the old one-size-fits-all approach is outdated. New ideas related to digital romance have emerged. For example, a service called *Match.com* Mobile enables online daters to transfer their profiles to cell phones, which they then use to search for and send text messages to nearby singles. Many other variations have been provided by services with such names as *Lemondate.com*, *Truedater.com*, and *Hurrydate.com* (Date.com is so 2004, 2005).

Matchmaking has become a serious and fast-growing business. Real-life matchmakers with names like Great Expectations and It's Just Lunch are popping up around the country. The Matchmaking Institute, which offered the nation's first certification course, opened in October 2004. It describes itself as a school of matchmaking and relationship sciences and offers 22 hours of intensive training. The modern matchmaker offers much more than a dating service. It may involve acting as a pal, coach, mom, and concierge (Cullen, 2004). As an example of such a service, It's Just Lunch promises its clients low-pressure introductions on their lunch breaks or over post-work drinks. Various formats are used to help participants get to know as many other potential dating partners as possible. For $1,000 to $1,500, clients join for a year and are guaranteed a minimum of 14 dates. If a spark is ignited, they can put their memberships on hold for up to a year. Some clients indicate that a short date with no commitment set up by someone else builds self-confidence, because the whole fear of rejection is minimized (Brooks, 2004).

Cohabitation

Cohabitation is the situation in which people who live together and share a sexual relationship are not married. Just a generation or two ago people who lived together were said to be "living in sin"—a remark meant as religious scorn, not humor. Today cohabitation is not regarded as negatively as it used to be.

One reason for the increased acceptance of cohabitation is the vast increase in the number who cohabitate—from 439,000 in 1960 to more than 6.4 million in 2007. During the same time period, the number of cohabiting adult couples of the other gender living with one child or more rose from 197,000 to more than 2.5 million (The social health of marriage in America, 2009). In addition, cohabitation is particularly common among the young. About 25% of unmarried women age 25 to 39 are currently living with a partner and an additional 25% have lived with a partner at some time in the past. More than half of all first marriages

cohabitation
Situation in which people who live together and share a sexual relationship are not married.

are preceded by living together, compared to virtually none 50 years ago. Cohabitation is more common among those of lower educational and income levels as well as those who are less religious than their peers. It is also more common among those who have experienced divorce and those who have experienced parental divorce or high levels of discord during childhood. Over 40% of cohabiting couple households contain children (Popenoe & Whitehead, 2005).

Reasons for Cohabitation

Some people feel that cohabitation has become more acceptable because of the increasing numbers who cohabitate. Another reason for increased acceptance is that some major companies have extended "domestic partner benefits" to both homosexual and heterosexual cohabitors. A further reason is the availability of effective contraceptives that reduce the fear of pregnancy for those who want to live together but not start families.

Traditionally, many reasons have been given for living together. They include finding out more about the habits and character of a partner, wanting to test compatibility, avoiding the risks of being trapped in an unhappy marriage, working on personal issues before deciding to marry, and saving money.

Popenoe (2008) pointed out additional reasons why people cohabitate. He suggests that the "sexual revolution" of the 1960s gave premarital sexual activity more of a stamp of approval. Traditional norms were challenged, and relatively reliable birth control for women became available. Some men pulled back from marriage and from having children and simply lived with their sexual partners in cohabitation. Women had gained more equality in many ways and got married many years later, on average. Childbearing was also delayed, and cohabitation was a natural outcome. Also, as the number of divorces increased, people became worried about marriages going wrong. Cohabitation—rather than marriage—became increasingly popular.

Disadvantages to Cohabitation

Unmarried couples may experience discrimination in housing, insurance, taxes, child custody, and other areas. (These are some of the same issues that homosexuals face; see Chapter 10.) They may also face pressure to marry from parents and friends—who may have social and religious backgrounds different from the cohabitors'.

Some people, especially divorced people, become cohabitors because they do not want the legal and economic "entanglements" of another marriage should the relationship end. In reality, though, the legal "entanglements" of marriage can also prove to be legal "entitlements." When cohabitors break up, one partner may lose financially because of inability to prove that assets were jointly purchased. Also, if one partner dies without a will, property would pass to surviving family members—not to the intended surviving partner. For example, in Massachusetts, the property would go half to parents, half to siblings, and none to the partner. Further, if a partner is disabled or hospitalized, the cohabitor has no rights to make medical decisions and can even be legally barred from hospital visits.

After dissolution of a cohabiting relationship, formerly cohabiting men's economic standing declines moderately. However, formerly cohabiting women's economic standing declines a great deal, leaving a substantial proportion of women in poverty. This is particularly true for African American and Hispanic women (Avellar, 2005).

Are Cohabitations Successful?

Do cohabiting couples have a higher rate of success if they marry later than do married couples who did not live together first? A critical look at the body of

There is contradictory research about the effects of cohabitation.

research fails to prove whether prior cohabitors have better marriages.

It seems to be common for people to believe that cohabitation is a useful way to avoid a bad marriage. However, data do not confirm this link. In fact, evidence indicates that those who live together before marriage are more likely to break up after marriage. This evidence is controversial because it is difficult to distinguish the "selection effect" from the "experience of cohabitation." Since people who cohabit before marriage have different characteristics from those who do not, it may be these characteristics, and not the experience of cohabitation, that leads to marital instability. It can be said for certain, however, that there is no evidence that those who cohabit before marriage have stronger marriages than those who do not (Popenoe & Whitehead, 2005).

In some ways, cohabitation is replacing dating. There also seems to be an increase in "serial cohabitation," or living with one partner for a time and then another. It is interesting that women seem to perceive cohabitation as a step before marriage to that partner, whereas men tend to see cohabitation as something to do before you make a commitment. Men who live with women they eventually marry don't seem to be as committed to the union as those who didn't live with their mates before getting married (Smock et al., 2005).

There are also a growing number of older Americans living together (Census: More elderly live together, 2002). The reasons vary, but for many it is a combination of bad experiences in previous marriages, the desire to keep their finances separate, and for some, loss of benefits if they remarry. There are at least 112,000 households headed by someone 65 years or older with an unmarried partner.

Cohabitation seems to differ for older and younger adults. Older cohabitors report significantly higher levels of relationship quality and stability than younger cohabitors, although they are less likely to have plans to marry their partners. Reasons for cohabitation are similar, but assessing compatibility is a more important reason for younger cohabitors. Older cohabitors are more likely to view their relationship as an alternative to marriage, whereas younger cohabitors are more likely to view their relationship as a prelude to it (King, 2005).

A comparison of gay and lesbian cohabiting couples with heterosexual married couples showed that in many respects they do not differ. However, it seems that gay or lesbian partners function better in their relationships than heterosexual partners (Kurdek, 2004).

So, is cohabitation a positive or a negative thing? There are different opinions among different people. For example, some reports indicate that marriages of people who have cohabited and later marry are significantly more likely to end in divorce (Living together before marriage may hurt—not help—chances of successful match, 2002). Some people feel this is partly because people who choose to live together tend to be younger, to be less religious, or to have other qualities that put them at risk for divorce. Seventy percent of those who lived together for at least 5 years did eventually marry, but after 10 years 40% had broken up, as compared to 32% who did not live together first. Others argue that marriage is too great a commitment and prefer cohabitation (Should people not cohabit before getting married?, 2003). They feel that the emphasis should be on the commitment between two people and that the quality of the relationship is the most important consideration. They indicate that society discriminates against people who wish to commit themselves to another person and remain unmarried.

■ Marriage

Marriage has changed over the years, but in many respects it has remained the same. June is still the most popular time to marry, more adults marry than never marry, and marriage is still a legal entity. It involves a fee to the county, a marriage license, and a marriage ceremony—either civil or religious. Although there is no legal requirement that a wife take the husband's last name, she usually does. Most Americans spend most of their lives within a marital relationship.

Although most people marry, the marriage rate has fluctuated. The highest marriage rate (the number of marriages per 1,000 unmarried women age 15 and older) in relatively recent decades was 76.5 in 1970. It has steadily declined since then and was 39.2 per 1,000 in 2007 (The social health of marriage in America, 2009). The median age at first marriage went from 20 years for females and 23 years for males in 1960 to about 26 and 27 years, respectively, in 2005 (Popenoe, 2007).

Popenoe and Whitehead (2001) reported that although older age at first marriage seems detrimental to marriage as an institution, it may have a strongly positive effect. This is because it appears to be by far the most important factor for a leveling off of divorce rates. Nevertheless, there can be disadvantages to the trend for postponing marriage to much older ages. For example, it can result in increased exposure to the hazards of nonmarital sexual activity and childbearing, sexual exploitation, loneliness, and lack of social integration. The question of the optimal age at which to marry, then, is still open. It seems best to wait until the early 20s, but how much beyond that cannot be answered definitively.

There are many statistics available about marriage, and many articles are written about it. For example, we already mentioned that age at first marriage has been steadily increasing. Interestingly, the age at remarriage after a divorce has also been increasing. In addition, the number of interracial marriages has increased.

Although 8.6% of males and 11% of females 15 years and older in the United States were divorced as of 2007, 54.7% of males and 51.2% of females were married (The social health of marriage in America, 2008). Because it is clear that a majority of people choose to be married, it is appropriate to consider the attraction of marriage and marriage partners.

Marriage customs vary in different cultures.

The Attraction of Marriage

The attraction to marriage is the result of several factors:

1. *Marriage provides companionship.* It is nice to have someone committed to spending time with you and sharing important occasions in your life.

 Did You Know . . .

Key Findings About Cohabitation from Cross-Cultural Investigation

- Cohabitation has become a permanent part of the life-course. A great majority of people in many countries cohabit sometime during their lives.
- Cohabitation has decreased the desire of many couples to move to marriage.
- Cohabiting couples break up at a much higher rate than married couples.
- Couples who cohabit before marriage have a higher risk of divorce when they do marry.

- In most countries, cohabiting couples tend to have fewer children than married couples.
- Cohabitation has been a major contributor to the rise of unwed births and single-parent families.
- Cohabitation has negative effects on child well-being. Children in these relationships have 5 times the risk of experiencing their parents' separation and higher rates of child abuse, family violence, and lower incomes.

Source: Popenoe, D. Cohabitation, marriage and child wellbeing. National Marriage Project, 2008. Available: http://marriage.rutgers.edu/Publications/2008cohabreport.html.

2. *Marriage provides for emotional security.* The intimate nature of the marital relationship can help alleviate the anxieties, fears, and insecurities you experience in today's society.

3. *Marriage provides for a sexual outlet.* The knowledge that your sexual needs will be satisfied in a loving, caring relationship can be quite appealing.

4. *Marriage can improve your self-esteem.* Just knowing that you are worthy enough for someone else to marry can make you believe you are an attractive, appealing, valuable person.

5. *Marriage can provide financial security.* The addition of another wage earner, or someone who can earn money while you contribute to the partnership by doing chores that would cost money to pay someone else to do, can make you more financially able to live the life you desire.

6. *Marriage can legitimize reproduction.* If you want children and believe they will do best in a socially sanctioned family—a marriage—you may want to be married.

Kempner (2005) summarized the ways that marriages benefit couples. She pointed out that the benefits include legal and financial benefits ranging from family leave, health care, and parenthood to those involving taxes, property rights, and inheritance. Marriage seems to also provide a wealth-generation bonus. Married people are more likely to save money and become more economically productive. Marriage can also provide couples with an economy of scale (two can live as cheaply as one), and act as a small insurance pool against life's uncertainties such as illness or job loss. In addition, research indicates that married people are not only wealthier but happier, healthier, and having better sex lives. Married people also take fewer risks, have better health habits, and enjoy a wider social support network.

Obviously, marriage has numerous attractions that have made it the predominant family lifestyle. However, not all these attractions are present in all marriages, and, depending on the expectations before the marriage and on other important considerations—such as the personality traits of the partners and their love for each other—the resultant disappointments either are overlooked or are deemed important enough to cause divorce.

It is interesting that, in general, American women are waiting to begin families. For women who earn a 4-year college degree or better, the age at first mar-

Married people can enjoy a wide variety of activities together throughout their marriage.

riage is close to 30. After marriage, women are waiting longer before they have their first child than they did several decades ago. As a result of these trends, the years of life before children have expanded, as have the years of life after children are no longer living in the home. The years of life with children represent a shrinking share of women's life course (Whitehead & Popenoe, 2008).

Choosing a Life Partner
Interestingly, when and if you choose another person with whom to form a lifelong commitment, that person will most likely be similar to you in many ways. Most people choose others of similar religion, age, social class, race, and education (Baron, 1998). When two people join together after 20 or 30 or more years of living independently of each other, they have all the problems of adjustment you can imagine. They may have to learn to eat the same foods, wake and go to sleep at the same times, and put up with each other's myriad idiosyncrasies. In other words, they have enough problems without adding still others that occur when they have different religions, social classes, educational backgrounds, and so on. It would be unfair, however, to overlook the relationships that work in spite of the partners' dissimilarities. That elusive concept, love, can do wonders with problems. However, the odds against partners of dissimilar backgrounds are greater than those for similar partners.

A "premarital inventory" developed at the University of Minnesota could be helpful for those contemplating marriage (Zaslow, 2003). It is an example of how researchers have studied divorced couples to see which questions they wish they had asked before taking the leap. Sample items include the following: We

Multicultural
DIMENSIONS

The Jefferson–Hemings Affair

If you think some current scandals go on for a long time, consider the case of Thomas Jefferson. In 1801, the newly elected Jefferson was first accused of having children with a young black slave named Sally Hemings. But it was not until the fall of 1998 that DNA tests proved that descendants of the Hemings family were indeed related to Jefferson. Sally Hemings's youngest son, Eston, was fathered by either Thomas Jefferson or his brother.

The DNA findings do more than put to rest a question of paternity; they also lay the foundation for all the Jefferson descendants—African American and white—to join together as one openly biracial family. For the first time, descendants of Jefferson's slave were welcomed at the annual gathering of the Monticello Association (the organization of descendants of Jefferson's white daughters) at Monticello on May 15, 1999.

"It's not just our story—it resonates for the whole country," said Dr. Michelle Cooley-Quille, a Hemings descendant and a clinical psychologist at Johns Hopkins University, who attended the event. Her father was denied entry into the Monticello Association and denied burial at Monticello, a privilege accorded to all members, when he died in 1997. "It's symbolic of what we've been denied but where we belong."

Indeed, the Jefferson clan has followed the multicultural path of many Americans. The number of official interracial marriages was 1,264,000 in 1997, almost double the 651,000 in 1980. However, as the Jefferson story suggests, there have been many unrecorded interracial relationships during the history of the United States. The growing acceptance of contemporary interracial marriages—as well as the acceptance of our past—is a positive step in the direction of racial harmony.

Sources: Reed, D. Jefferson reunion adds slave's kin, AP/AOL (May 6, 1999); Edwards, T. M. Family reunion, *Time, 125, 21* (November 23, 1998); Cawthorne, N. *Sex lives of the presidents.* New York: St. Martin's, 1998; U.S. Bureau of the Census. *Statistical abstract of the United States 1998.* Washington, DC: U.S. Government Printing Office, 1998.

have some important disagreements that never seem to get resolved, and I am satisfied with the way we have decided to share household duties. It is available at *www.lifeinnovations.com* (September 2009).

Promoting a Happy Lifelong Commitment
Advice from many sources tells you how to be happy in a relationship. For example, Wallerstein (1996) lists nine "psychological tasks" that are the pillars on which good lifelong relationships rest:

1. To separate emotionally from the family of one's childhood so as to invest fully in the relationship.

2. To build togetherness based on mutual identification, shared intimacy, and an expanded conscience that includes both partners and protects each partner's autonomy.

3. To establish a rich and pleasurable sexual relationship.

4. For couples with children, while protecting their own privacy, to embrace the roles of parenthood and to absorb the effect of a baby's entrance into the marriage.

5. To confront and master the inevitable crises of life.

6. To maintain the strength of the relationship in the face of adversity. It should be a safe haven in which partners are able to express their differences, anger, and conflict.

7. To use humor and laughter to keep things in perspective.

8. To nurture and comfort each other, satisfying each partner's needs for dependency and offering continuing encouragement and support.

9. To keep alive the early romantic, idealized images of falling in love while facing the sober realities of the changes wrought by time.

Many other factors can relate to the quality of marriage. For example, Kiecolt-Glaser (2009) reported that couples whose disagreements were nastier or hostile showed large increases in stress hormones during and after an argument. Among other potential problems, it was found that women who were unhappy in their marriages had higher risks of heart and circulatory problems. This gives medical support for the need to follow the advice given previously for promoting a happy lifelong commitment.

Also, the increase in "boomerangers" can be stressful on marriages. These are people who are

It is wise to learn a lot about a potential marriage partner before getting married.

young adults or even in their 30s or 40s who move back in with their parents. This practice commonly occurs for economic reasons, and it can cause tensions for both the older and younger generations. Suggestions for dealing with this situation include talking about expectations, building in privacy for all concerned, sharing household expenses, realizing that the house is the property of the parents (grandparents?), and being realistic about expectations (Koss-Feder, 2009).

Types of Marriage

In some states heterosexual couples who have lived together for a specified period and who have represented themselves as married are recognized as legally married. These associations are called **common-law marriages**.

About 56% of children live in a **nuclear family**—a couple and their children. This is up from 51% in 1991. The portion of children living in any sort of two-parent family, including nuclear families, those living with step-parents, and those in other arrangements, is about 71% (down from 73% in 1991) (Meckler, 2001).

Peer marriages are relationships in which couples have worked out at least a 60–40 split on child rearing, housework, and control of discretionary funds and consider themselves equal. Most partners in peer marriages

common-law marriage
The recognition by some states that heterosexual couples who have lived together for a specified period and have represented themselves as married are in fact legally married.

nuclear family
A married couple and their children.

peer marriage
Relationship in which partners have equal status.

work outside the home. Partners in peer marriages require lots of honesty, a dedication to fair play, flexibility, generosity, and maturity.

In some families the fathers stay at home and the mothers work outside the home. Stay-at-home dads do the same household activities as stay-at-home moms, but they also mow the lawn, fix the dishwasher, and clean the gutters. There is not a complete role reversal when the father stays at home. Working mothers also only partially give up their traditional role. When they go home, they tend to be the "traditional mom." In a stay-at-home father family, if a child gets hurt or wakes up at night and both parents are available, the child will go to either the mother or the father. In a traditional family the child will go to the mother 80% of the time and the father 20% of the time (Working moms turn traditional when they're home, 1998).

Related to peer marriages, Orecklin (2004) pointed out that the past 30 years have seen the emergence of the working mom, the supermom, the soccer mom, and—because full-time motherhood is often considered a choice rather than a given—the stay-at-home mom. The title of "dad" has rarely been linked to a modifier. However, the majority of men today are vastly more involved in the rearing of children and maintenance of households than their fathers ever were. In straining to manage responsibilities at work and at home, many men say they don't feel an adequate sense of control in either realm. As with women of a generation ago, men are experiencing the notion of a second shift, and they are doing so in a shaky economy. They must contend with buyouts, layoffs, mergers, and a need to keep up with changing job

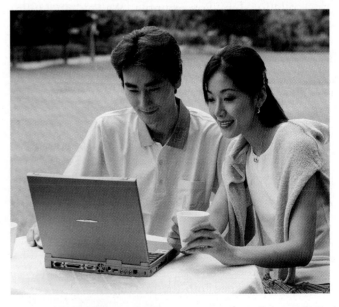

Some couples like to do online inventories and questions about relationships to learn more about themselves and each other.

Did You Know . . .

Popenoe and Whitehead (2005) listed 10 important research findings on marriage and choosing a marriage partner. While several overlap points already made, the list taken as a whole provides helpful facts for young adults and older adults about marriage. The research findings are:

1. Marrying as a teenager is the highest known risk factor for divorce.
2. The most likely way to find a future marriage partner is through an introduction by family, friends, or acquaintances.
3. The more similar people are in their values, backgrounds, and life goals, the more likely they are to have a successful marriage.
4. Women have a significantly better chance of marrying if they do not become single parents before marrying.
5. Both women and men who are college educated are more likely to marry, and less likely to divorce, than people with lower levels of education.
6. Living together before marriage has not proved useful as a "trial marriage."
7. Marriage helps people to generate income and wealth.
8. People who are married are more likely to have emotionally and physically satisfying sex lives than single people or those who just live together.
9. People who grow up in a family broken by divorce are slightly less likely to marry, and much more likely to divorce when they do marry.
10. For large segments of the population, the risk of divorce is far below 50%.

skills. There is sometimes also uncertainty in men's roles at home.

Asked how they measure success, only 3% of men said through their work, while 31% said they did so through their faith in God, 26% through being the best person possible, 22% through their network of family and friends, and 17% through maintaining a balance between home and work. Twenty-one percent said they would sacrifice family time for opportunities and higher pay at work, but 72% said they would sacrifice opportunities and higher pay at work for more time with their family. In response to a question about how they like to spend their free time, the highest response was "hanging out with family" (Orecklin, 2004).

About 16.5% of children live in a **stepfamily**, also called a *blended family*, compared to about 15% in 1991 (Meckler, 2001). Stepfamilies can be more complex than the families of first marriages, but, contrary to myth, stepfamilies have a high rate of success in raising healthy children. Stepkids seem to be very resilient. Their major source of problems is parental conflict left over from a first marriage. Stepfamilies experience most of their troubles in the first 2 years; after 5 years, stepfamilies are more stable than first-marriage families, because second marriages are generally happier than first marriages. Stepfamilies are not just make-do households limping along after loss.

stepfamily
A family with children that is formed as a result of remarriage.

Blended families come in many sizes and can look very different from each other.

All members experience real gains, notably the opportunity to thrive in a happier relationship.

One researcher indicates that there are seven basic types of relationships—three of them happy and four of them unhappy (An arrangement of marriages, 1993). The four unhappy ones make up about 75% of marriages and are labeled *devitalized, financially focused, conflicted,* and *traditional*. These relationships hinge on external elements, leisure activities, religious attitudes, financial management, children, family, and friends—and distress dominates. The three happy ones make up 25% of relationships and are labeled *balanced, harmonious,* and *vitalized.* In these relationships the partners are held together by smooth working of most or all factors intrinsic to relationships—personality compatibility, communication, conflict resolution, and sexuality.

With many new marriages in the United States destined to end in divorce, an increasing number of couples are turning to prenuptial agreements to protect their assets in the event of a marital breakup. Most such agreements simply state how assets will be divided in case of divorce or death. Some people argue that prenuptial agreements contribute to marital happiness; others believe they contribute to distrust and overemphasize personal assets.

In Louisiana and Arizona, it is legal to back up marriage laws with tougher, individually designed and legally mandated divorce standards. This is called a *covenant marriage.* In this marriage style, the option of walking out is eliminated. For example, Louisiana's covenant marriage requires premarital counseling and, for divorce, 2 years of living apart plus mandated marital counseling. The goal is to make marriage more committed (Russo, 2000).

Building a good relationship obviously takes a lot of effort. There are sources of help for couples desiring to use them. For example, the Association for Couples in Marriage Enrichment is an organization designed to preserve and strengthen relationships.

Sexual Behavior in Marriage

Nonmarital sexual behavior has received more attention than marital sexual behavior from researchers for many decades. It still does today. While the information about marital sexual behavior is comparatively limited, it is still appropriate to consider what is known.

Today's married couples have sexual intercourse more often, experience more sexual pleasure, and engage in a greater variety of sexual activities and tech-

Today's married couples experience much more sexual pleasure than those of past decades.

niques than the people surveyed in the 1950s. There is now more precoital activity and it tends to last longer than in earlier years. Oral stimulation of the breasts and manual stimulation of the genitals have increased, as has oral–genital contact (Clements, 1994; Laumann et al., 1994).

We can ascribe these changes to a loosening up of society in general and to the fact that even heterosexual sexual activity has come out of the closet. It is now permissible to talk about sexual behavior freely with one's partner and with others. Thus communication between partners has become more open and honest and certainly has had an effect on their lovemaking. Women have become more aware of their capacity for and their right to sexual satisfaction through orgasm. As a result they have been assuming an active role in lovemaking and in communicating what turns them on. When their partners have responded positively, one result has been that partners spend more time exploring each other sexually, attending to each other's bodies, and experimenting with various coital positions that may better satisfy women's needs.

Many married people also masturbate. Hunt's survey (1974) found that 72% of young married males and 68% of young married females masturbated. The frequency rates were higher for husbands (once or twice a month) than for wives (less than once a month). The reasons married people cite for masturbating vary. Some people masturbate when they are separated from their partner. Some do so as a variation on their sexual experience. Also some couples like to watch each other masturbate as part of their mutual sexual activity. Others masturbate because they do not achieve satisfaction with their partner and are unwilling to forgo it altogether.

The National Opinion Research Center (NORC) study found that frequency of sexual interactions is a factor of age, relationship duration, and marital status. In general, married couples engage in sexual activities more frequently than singles; cohabiting couples engage in sexual activities more often than married couples (Laumann et al., 1994). Nearly 40% of married couples engage in sexual activities twice a week, compared with 25% of singles (Elmer-Dewitt, 1994).

Some people wonder whether their sex life is "normal." Statistics on sexual behavior can be misleading. For example, if a couple heard that the average married couple had sexual intercourse three times a week, they may not realize that the average includes a wide range. The frequency of intercourse might range from zero for some to 15 to 20 times a week for others. So, even if their frequency of intercourse is more or less than three times a week, their behavior is within the range of normal human experience. The most important consideration isn't whether their frequency and pattern of sexual activity matches some numerical average, but whether each partner is satisfied and comfortable with the sexual relationship. There should be a feeling of overall satisfaction, relaxation, and enjoyment following sexual activity (Osborne, 2004).

As with other research, the data about frequency of marital sexual activity will vary in different research studies. However, it is generally agreed that the frequency of sexual intercourse in marriage tends to decrease the longer a couple is married. For example, for newly married couples the average rate of sexual intercourse is about three times per week. In early middle age, the average rate is about one-and-a-half to two times a week. After age 50 years the rate is about once a week or less. This does not mean that sexual activity is not important or that the marriage is no longer satisfactory. The decrease may be the result of biological aging, fatigue, and a decrease in sex drive (Call, Sprecher, & Schwartz, 1995). Higher levels of sexual satisfaction and pleasure are found in marriage than in extramarital relationships or in singlehood (Laumann et al., 1994).

The decline of marital sexual activity is explained by several factors. First, the "honeymoon effect" leads to the highest rates among the recently married, and those recently married tend to be younger. Second, biological aging reduces hormonal output, and poor health in general and sexual arousal problems increase with age. As a result, even among couples who consider their marriages to be very happy and say they are still in love, frequency of intercourse goes down with age. Third, some research indicates that the quality of sexual activity declines with marital duration and that might reduce frequency. Among married people, intercourse is more frequent among those who have happier marriages (Smith, 2003).

Are married couples generally satisfied with their sex life? According to Hunt's data, a majority of married people—60% to 66%—are satisfied. Two-thirds of the men in the sample rated their marital coitus as

Myth vs Fact

Myth: Single adults have more sexual activity than married adults.
Fact: The 1994 national survey of adults 18 to 59 years old found that married adults had more sexual activity than single adults.

Myth: Liberals enjoy sex more than conservatives.
Fact: In the same study, marriage was a great equalizer. Married couples, regardless of religious or political background or past sexual history, have roughly the same amount of sexual activity. And conservative women report more frequent orgasm than liberal women.

Myth: Almost all married couples have affairs.
Fact: Only 25% of men and 15% of women report that they have had an extramarital affair.

Myth: People lose interest in sexual activity as they get older, and, by their 60s, few people are having sexual relationships.
Fact: People can have a satisfying sexual life as they age. Sexual relationships may change as a couple ages, but many couples in their 60s, 70s, and 80s report pleasurable, exciting sexual relationships.

very pleasurable, whereas about 60% of the women said the same. Most women who said they found coitus very pleasurable were 35 to 44 years old; the men so reporting were younger. It appears, then, that as women mature and gain sexual experience, they enjoy their experiences more than at a younger age, and men experience more of their pleasure when they are young.

In general, husbands and wives closely agree on the frequency of intercourse (Smith, 2003). Married women seem to be less satisfied with sexual activity in marriage than married men. This may be because they report a lower rate of orgasm compared to that of men (Liu, 2003).

It seems that both married men and married women tend to believe that sexual activity is integral to a good marriage, and that men may be more interested in sexual activity than women. Sometimes husbands and wives experience conflict related to sexual activity and need to work emotionally to manage their own and their spouse's feelings about sexual activity (Elliott & Umberson, 2008).

One factor that can contribute to problems in marital sexual activities is timing—particularly in the years when couples are both raising children and working hard at their jobs. Married people often have sexual activities late in the evening after a long day and just before sleep. The presence of children in the family can make it hard for parents to find time to be alone. Because many people feel that a quiet and private time is necessary for sexual activities, there may be pressure to "work sex in" during the short evening.

Extramarital Relationships

Despite all the media hype over the past few years about extramarital sexual activity by government officials, the reality is that most people are faithful to their spouses. In the NORC study, a relatively large number of adults reported that they have been completely monogamous during the course of their marriage. Only 10% of women and 25% of men reported that they had had an extramarital sexual relationship (Laumann et al., 1994)—far below the 50% of men and 25% of women reported by Kinsey back in 1948 and 1953.

More recently, a NORC researcher (Smith, 2003) pointed out that there are probably more scientifically worthless "facts" on extramarital relations than on any other facet of human behavior. He said that extramarital relations are less prevalent than pop and pseudo-scientific accounts contend. The best estimates are that 3% to 4% of currently married people have a sexual partner other than their spouse in a given year. About 15% to 18% of people have had a sexual partner other than their spouse while married. It does not seem that levels have changed much in the past 20 years. The rates of extramarital relations are about twice as high among husbands as among wives. They are also more common among African Americans, those with lower incomes, those who attend church less frequently, those who have been separated or divorced, and those who are unhappy with their marriage.

Because husbands are more involved in extramarital sexual relations than wives are, presumably without their spouses' knowledge, more women may be at risk of STIs than has been thought. Research is not available on what proportion of husbands have same-gender relationships outside their marriage. However, married men and women who perceive themselves to be at no (or low) risk of STIs and HIV may, in fact, be at risk because of their partner's extramarital sexual activities (Laumann et al., 1994).

Extramarital sexual activity can take place in two different contexts: one in which the partners have no agreement (nonconsensual context) and one in which the partners agree to have sexual relations with someone else (consensual context).

Nonconsensual Extramarital Sexual Activity

Married people engage in **nonconsensual**—and therefore usually secret—extramarital relationships for many and complex reasons. On a practical level, one's spouse may be unable to have sexual intercourse because of illness, or a couple may be separated for a long period. Thus

nonconsensual
In this context, a married person's engaging in sexual intercourse without the consent of the spouse.

the person deciding on an extramarital relationship does so to have sexual relations at all. But in other situations an individual might search for someone outside the marriage simply to add excitement or variety to life. Another might feel dissatisfied sexually with his or her partner and look for a more satisfactory emotional and physical relationship while maintaining the marriage. Or a person might feel drawn to someone outside the marriage by sexual attraction alone and choose to act on that attraction.

A number of forces tend to restrain or increase extramarital sexual activity:

1. Because religiously devout people tend to have lower rates of extramarital sexual activity, rising rates can be predicted from the decline in traditional religious activity.

2. Those who participate in nonmarital sexual intercourse are more likely to participate in extramarital activity, too.

3. Because women are more aware of their right to sexual satisfaction than in years past, some females are more likely to now seek sexual pleasures outside marriage.

4. The more money a person has, the greater is the opportunity for extramarital sexual activity.

5. The changing role of women in the labor force is also a factor; women who work outside the home have a greater opportunity for extramarital activity than women who do not.

Although there are cultures in which it is expected that married people will have affairs, most people in the United States say they believe in monogamy and

Extramarital affairs are less common than the media might lead us to believe.

Global DIMENSIONS

Tempted by Digital Dalliances

Internet infidelity is a topic that would not have been mentioned too many years ago. Not all people see Internet infidelity as a real act of betrayal, but in one study the majority did see this as not only real infidelity but as also having as serious an impact on the couple as a traditional offline affair. Emotional infidelity was given as much attention as sexual infidelity was (Whitty, 2005).

The Internet's anonymity, convenience, and ready access to potential partners make it easy to participate in cyber-sex with other people. Cyber-infidelity occurs when a partner in a committed relationship uses a computer to violate agreements of sexual exclusivity. Internet affairs often go through progressive steps: non-sexually explicit flirting, sexual innuendo and explicit repartee, scheduling sex-laced chats, discussing sexual preferences and fantasies, simultaneous masturbation online, and planning or (in fewer cases) conducting face-to-face meetings and physical contact. Women are as likely to engage in cyber-affairs as men. For therapists, treating Internet affairs is no different than treating other affairs (Schnarch & Morehouse, 2002).

---

want it in their marriage. However, two of three married couples experience an affair during their marriage, and 17% of divorces are caused by infidelity. Traditionally, more men than women take part in affairs, but women are catching up. Affairs are a sign that the wandering spouse is dissatisfied in the marriage. They can be a way of expressing pain and confusion that the person cannot verbally articulate. However, an affair does not necessarily mean that he or she wants to end the marriage. An affair can be a way of expressing that there are problems that need to be resolved (Stanton, 2001).

What are the effects of extramarital sexual relationships on a marriage? Initially, many people who learn their spouse has been having affairs feel both betrayed and emotionally devastated, especially if they believe their spouse to be honest, loyal, and loving. When they learn of the affair, there is a chance that the marriage will fall apart quickly. However, if the couple can talk about the situation, taking the opportunity to improve their communication and assess their own relationship, the marriage does not necessarily dissolve.

Sometimes the type of extramarital relationship has a great effect on the eventual outcome. When a spouse has engaged in a one-night stand, the other spouse might be likely to forgive and forget. If the extramarital affair was intimate, was long-lasting, and involved a strong emotional commitment, however, the other spouse may find it difficult to get over the unfaithfulness.

Consensual Extramarital Sexual Activity

There are many types of **consensual** activities; we discuss the two major ones—open marriage and swinging. **Open marriage** became publicized with the appearance of George and Nena O'Neill's book, *Open Marriage,* in 1972. The O'Neills believed that traditional marriage was too confining and limiting for the partners and that one partner could not fulfill all the intimate needs and expectations of the other. They described an open marriage as one in which the partners allow each other to have intimate and emotional relationships—sexual or nonsexual—with others. For instance, the married couple might decide that each partner is entitled to one night a week alone to engage in another intimate relationship. The idea is that this arrangement allows the married couple to grow and contribute more to the marriage. Another aspect of the open marriage is the renewable contract. The partners formally agree that extramarital relationships are permitted in the marriage and might even foster support, loyalty, and trust between partners but that the partners may change their contract regarding extramarital activity as they continue to grow. The idea here is that the agreement is flexible and renewable so that neither partner is forced to stand by a commitment that he or she no longer feels.

Swinging is the exchange of partners among married couples. (This phenomenon used to be called *wife-swapping,* but the term lost favor with the rise of the women's movement because of its suggestion that wives were property and that men made the

consensual
In this context, a married person's engaging in extramarital sexual activity with the knowledge and permission of the spouse.

open marriage
A marriage in which partners allow each other to have intimate and emotional relationships with others.

swinging
Swapping of mates for sexual activities.

decisions.) All those involved participate willingly, and both partners in a marriage usually engage in it simultaneously.

Swingers object to calling this type of activity extramarital, because they view it as part of the marriage relationship. Most swingers do not want emotional involvements outside the marriage. Most often swingers find one another by advertising in tabloids or in special magazines devoted to swinging. People who engage in swinging are apparently very ordinary outside their sexual life.

Like other aspects of society, some for-profit ventures have developed related to extramarital sexual activity. For example, in 2002 the Ashley Madison Agency launched its web site to the public. It is designed to promote social networking. As it says on the web site, the agency deals with "risqué business." Its purpose is to cater to people who are already in relationships, but still want to date. In 3 years the agency signed up more than 500,000 members. There have been about 8.5 men for every 1.5 women who sign up on the Ashley Madison web site (Frequently asked questions, 2005).

Another related commercial venture is the Secret Lover Collection of 24 cards designed exclusively for people having affairs (Kiehl, 2005). The line was launched in May 2005. Some retailers refused to carry the cards because they did not want to alienate longtime customers. The cards have been controversial, and can be found at *www.secretlovercollection.com*.

Divorce

Today, for every two marriages there is one divorce (Marriages and divorces, 1900–2004). There are many reasons that marriages break up. Among these are greater economic independence of women, greater ease of getting a divorce, decreased stigma attached to divorce, unrealistic expectations for marriage, communication difficulties, infidelity, and feelings of incompatibility (Center for Families in Transition, 2003).

The current U.S. divorce rate (16.4 per 1,000 married women) is much higher than that of 1960 (9.2 per 1,000 married women), but has declined significantly since hitting its highest peak during the 1980s (22.6 per 1,000 married women). Two probable reasons for the decline in the divorce rate are an increase in the age at which people marry for the first time and a higher educational level of those marrying, both of which are associated with greater marital stability (Popenoe, 2007).

In 2001 the National Center for Health Statistics reported data on marriage, divorce, and remarriage (First marriage dissolution, divorce, and remarriage in the United States, 2001). The center reported that 43%

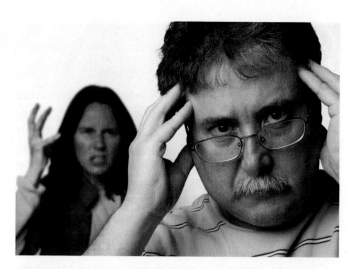

Communication difficulties are one of the major reasons for divorce.

of first marriages end in separation or divorce within 15 years. One in three first marriages ends within 10 years and one in five within 5 years. The study also showed that duration of marriage is linked to a woman's age at first marriage: The older a woman is at first marriage, the longer the marriage is likely to last. For example, 58% of marriages of brides younger than 18 years old end in separation or divorce within 15 years compared with 36% of those who married at age 20 years or older. Younger women who divorce are more likely to remarry: 82% of those divorced before age 25 years remarry within 10 years, compared with 68% of those divorced at age 25 or later.

At the same time, there has been little change in such traditionally high divorce rate differences between those who marry when they are teenagers compared to those who marry later, and the nonreligious compared to the religious. Both teenagers and the nonreligious who marry have considerably higher divorce rates (Popenoe & Whitehead, 2005).

The significant effect of divorce on family life cannot be exaggerated. The spouse who maintains custody of the children has to supervise their care, earn enough money to meet their needs, and provide, usually without help, the love and affection all children crave. In addition, the divorced parent must reestablish a social life at the same time the emotional scars from the failed marriage are healing. The children may blame themselves for the divorce and must manage without the constant contact with one parent.

Every year, more than 1 million children in the United States experience the divorce of their parents. The most important factor in how divorce affects a child's life is how parents treat each other and their children during and after the divorce (Divorce and children, 2001).

? Did You Know . . .

The Top Ten Myths of Divorce

1. **Half of all marriages end in divorce.** If today's divorce rate continues, the chance that a marriage contracted this year will end in divorce is probably a little higher than 40%.

2. **Second marriages tend to be more successful than first marriages.** The divorce rate of remarriages is higher than that of first marriages.

3. **Living together before marriage is a good way to reduce the chance of divorce.** Those who live together before marriage have a considerably *higher* chance of divorce.

4. **Problems caused for children of divorce are not long-lasting.** Many such problems are long-lasting and become worse in adulthood.

5. **Having a child will improve a marriage and prevent divorce.** The decreased risk is far less than it used to be.

6. **After divorce, the woman's standard of living plummets while the man's greatly improves.** The difference is not as great as previously thought, but the gender gap is real. A woman's loss is about 27% and a man's gain is about 10%.

7. **When parents do not get along, children are better off if their parents divorce.** Only the children in very high-conflict homes benefited from the conflict removal that divorce can effect. In lower-conflict marriages that end in divorce, the situation of the children is often much worse.

8. **Children who grow up in a home broken by divorce have as much success in their own marriages as those from intact homes.** Children of divorce have a much higher rate of divorce than those from intact families.

9. **After divorce, children involved are better off in step-families than in single-parent families.** There seems to be no difference between the two.

10. **Being very unhappy at certain points in a marriage is a good sign that the marriage will end in divorce.** Eighty-six percent of a large national sample who were unhappily married indicated 5 years later that they were happier. Three-fifths of them said they were "very happy" or "quite happy."

One additional myth: It is usually men who initiate divorce proceedings. Two-thirds of all divorces are initiated by women.

Source: Adapted from: Popenoe, D. The top ten myths of divorce. National Marriage Project, [Online]. Available: http://marriage.rutgers.edu/pubtoptenmyths.htm.

The question of whether divorce creates long-term negative effects for children has long been debated (Does divorce create long-term negative effects for children?, 2003). Some studies indicate that about twice as many children of divorced parents have emotional problems. In addition, they have greater challenges negotiating relationships once they are older, have a greater chance of choosing the "wrong" partner, and are much more likely to divorce. Critics of this research question these findings. They point out that most of the studies do not involve interviews with the children, but instead are colored by caregivers' views of how a divorce affects children. Some researchers indicate that children of divorce often have a greater sense of responsibility, independence, and maturity than their counterparts whose parents have remained together. In addition, if there has been great discord and constant fighting in the household, a divorce can provide relief to the children who have been living in that highly stressful setting.

Problems with the economy can also contribute to divorce. Money issues can drive a wedge between couples. They can lead couples to either withdraw from each other or attack each other about things that don't have anything to do with financial matters. Financial anxiety can lead spouses to alcohol or substance abuse, gambling, or extramarital affairs. At the same time, however, many couples may be motivated to make their marriages work. People are realizing it is more expensive to break up a family than it is to stay together (Johnston, 2009).

When everything is considered, your chances of divorce may be much lower than you think. While it has been said that the national divorce rate is close to 50%, for many people the actual chances of divorce are much less. If you are a reasonably well-educated person with a decent income, come from an intact family, are religious, and marry after age 25 without having a baby first, your chances of divorce are very low indeed (Popenoe, 2007).

Single-Parent Families

Families with a single parent (**single-parent families**) are becoming increasingly prevalent. According to the U.S. Census Bureau, the number of single-parent families has increased greatly, from 5% in

> **single-parent family**
> For whatever reason, only one parent who is living with a child or children.

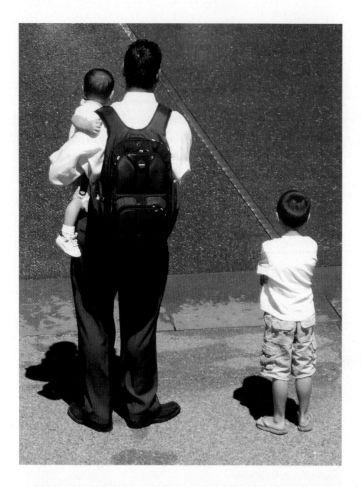

Single-parent families are becoming more common.

1970 to 9% in 2006. There were 12.9 million single parents living with their children in 2006. Single mothers accounted for 10.4 million of these parents (Facts for features, 2008).

Reasons for the increase in the number of children living with single parents include a larger proportion of births occurring to unmarried women; the delay of marriage, which means that adults were single for more years; and the growth in divorce among couples with children (Fields, 2004). Usually when we think of single-parent families, we think of them as being headed by women. However, the number of households headed by single fathers has been growing significantly.

Father-headed single-parent families often place the father in a new role. We say "often" because nowadays men in two-parent families more and more are helping with what were heretofore considered to be the wife's household chores and responsibilities. For these husbands the adjustment to heading a single-parent family will be less difficult because they are accustomed to cooking, cleaning, nurturing, and changing diapers. For the more traditional husband, the adoption of these necessary chores and responsibilities, added to

Global DIMENSIONS

Divorce in China and Sudan

Because of rapid increases in both extramarital affairs and divorces, in 1998 a "marriage and family law" was drafted in Beijing. This law resulted from 10 years of study and stipulates that husband and wife have an obligation to "mutual fidelity"; people who are unfaithful will be considered "guilty parties," and in the case of divorce the guilty party will be obliged to compensate the injured party. At the same time, living apart for 3 years will be considered grounds for divorce.

Over the last 20 years, the divorce rate in China has been steadily rising. It has risen more than 120% since 1986. In 1997 it reached one-quarter of the marriage rate.

In 1980 infidelity was the cause of divorce in only 14% of the cases, whereas by 1990 the figure reached 40%. With economic liberalization in China came a gradual increase in extramarital affairs and a corresponding increase in the number of divorces. Social change, the increasing mobility of the population, peasant migration to the cities, the arrival of foreign companies, and trends in foreign emigration have all contributed to the rising divorce rate. The divorce rate is highest in the big cities—32% in Beijing and 34% in Shanghai.

In patriarchal southern Sudan, as in much of Africa, only men have the right to file for divorce. The one legal loophole for Sudanese women is to commit adultery, a crime that is instant grounds for divorce. But even then, most husbands refuse to agree to one because they don't want to ask their relatives to return the dowry. In one case, a woman sat in prison for months, hoping to shame her husband into repaying her dowry and leaving her. She admitted breaking the law by committing adultery. This was the only way she had to try to get out of an abusive marital situation. Sudanese leaders are considering changing their laws and procedures related to divorce, but they are cautious because of the impact such changes might have on their entire society (Wax, 2005).

Source: Shuoming, J. For or against sexual liberation? *China Focus, 6, no. 10* (October 1, 1998), 1+.

the financial and emotional burdens of divorce, means that a more significant adjustment is required.

Life in a single-parent family can be stressful for the adult and the children. Members may unrealistically expect that the family can function as a two-parent family does and may feel that something is wrong if it cannot. The single parent may feel overwhelmed by the responsibility of caring for the children, maintaining a job, and keeping up with the bills and household chores. Typically, the family's finances and resources are drastically reduced by the parents' breakup.

Single-parent families deal with pressures and potential problem areas that the nuclear family does not have to face (Single parenting and today's family, 1998):

- Visitation and custody problems

- The negative effects of continuing conflict between the parents

- Fewer opportunities for parents and children to spend time together

- Negative effects of the breakup on children's school performance and peer relations

- Disruptions of extended family relationships

- Problems caused by parents' dating and entering new relationships

The demand for social services to meet the special needs of single-parent families is growing. Because single-parent families often have financial, psychological, custodial, and other needs that are more acute than those of conventional two-parent families, they need counseling and/or support groups. Many single parents have the added responsibility of providing role models for their other-sex children. Day care, a virtual necessity (as it also is for many two-parent households), solves some problems, yet it may also be a source of anxiety, or at least concern, for financial, educational, psychological, or other reasons.

Although some of these research findings might seem discouraging—or they might seem wrong to readers who come from single-parent families—it is important to remember that these findings refer to trends in groups and have no bearing on particular individuals. Children in single-parent families are often very successful. Our intention here is to suggest that single parenthood does require special care and consideration. Perhaps most of all, the special needs of single-parent families should be understood both by family members themselves and by teachers, employers, and others with whom they interact. To meet this need for understanding, a group called Parents without

Children in single-parent families can be just as successful as other children.

Partners serves as a sounding board and a source of counsel for single parents.

The need for good parenting skills remains constant regardless of the parent's marital status. However, the situation can be more demanding for both the parents and the children in single-parent households. The following are some suggested guidelines.

1. Be honest with your children about the situation that caused you to become a single parent.

2. In case of a separation or divorce, assure children that they are not responsible for the breakup of the relationship.

3. Try to maintain as much of the same routine as possible.

4. Do not try to be both mother and father to the children. Establish a family atmosphere of teamwork.

5. In the case of divorce, acknowledge that the relationship between you and your former partner is over, and do not encourage your children to hope for reconciliation.

6. Reassure children that they will continue to be loved and cared for (by both parents, if true).

7. Do not use children to gain bargaining power with a separated or divorced spouse.

8. Encourage relatives to help children maintain a sense of belonging to a continuing family.

Popenoe and Whitehead (2005) have provided helpful information to summarize this section. For example, they indicate that the percentage of children who grow up in fragile—typically fatherless—families has grown enormously over the past four decades. This is mainly due to increases in divorce, out-of-wedlock births, and unmarried cohabitation. Children in such families have negative outcomes at two to three times the rate of children in married two-parent families. In earlier times, most single mothers were divorced or widowed. Today the number of never-married single mothers is higher than that of divorced mothers. A major reason for the increase in number of never-married single mothers is that single motherhood has become a permanent status for many women.

■ Sexuality and Aging

There was a time when it was believed that sexual desire and functioning became unimportant with age. Although a gradual decline in sexual activity occurs around age 50 years and accelerates after age 70 years, sexuality remains an important part of life into old age.

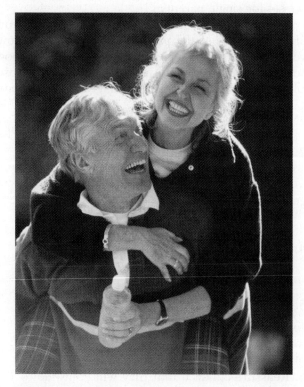

As people get older they can continue to have excellent relationships that include sexual activity.

Understanding the sexuality of elders is important because of the rapidly increasing elderly population. The population of U.S. citizens aged 65 years and older grew from 25.5 million in 1980 to 35 million in 2000. It is projected to rise to about 71 million by 2030. This will represent 20% of the total U.S. population (Healthy aging for older adults, 2009). As people live longer, it is important to understand how sexuality is affected in the later years.

Many studies have confirmed that people remain sexually active into their 70s and 80s. Bretschneider and McCoy (1988) found that 62% of the men and 30% of the women they studied engaged in intercourse. These people ranged in age from 80 to 102 years. DeBeauvoir (1973) revealed that 70% of those men older than 65 years of age who were listed in *Who's Who* had sexual intercourse on an average of four times a month. Kaplan (1974) found that women tend to want more rather than less sexual activity as they approach their middle and older years.

In 1998, the National Council on the Aging conducted a telephone survey of 1,300 Americans older than the age of 60 years. It found that nearly half engage in sexual activity at least once a month, and 4 in 10 said they would like to engage in sexual activities more frequently than they currently do. Three-quarters of the men and the women said that they are emotionally satisfied or even more satisfied with their sexual activities than they were in their 40s. Forty-three percent said that sexual relations were just as good as or better than they were in their youth, and 43% said they were less satisfying.

Older men were more than twice as likely to report wanting more sexual activity than women, and men were much more likely to be sexually active than women older than 60 years. Nearly two-thirds of senior men are currently sexually active, whereas only 37% of women are currently sexually active. This gap exists partially because women live longer and thus are much more likely to be widowed than men. However, men were much more likely to say that a medical condition prevents them from engaging in sexual activities (51% of men, 12% of women) and that medications are reducing their sexual desire (44% of men, 16% of women).

Jacoby (2005) reported the results a nationwide study conducted by the American Association of Retired People (AARP). The study focused on sexual attitudes and behavior of adults ages 45 and older. Here are some of the findings:

- The number of men who have tried treatments to improve their sexual functioning doubled from 10% in 1999 to 22% in 2005. Sixty-eight percent of those men said the treatments improved their sexual satisfaction.

Women said their own sexual satisfaction was enhanced by their partners' use of drugs and they increased their frequency of sexual activity.

- Phone sex with a spouse or intimate partner was popular among the 45 to 49 age group. Seventeen percent of the men and 18% of the women admitted to talking dirty on the phone, and 22% of men and women said they've penned erotic notes or exchanged sexy email messages.

- Slightly more than 25% of the men and 21% of women confessed to having had sexual relations in a public place, and 11% of both men and women in the 50 to 69 age group also admitted to this behavior.

- Concerning extramarital sexual activities and swinging, an overwhelming 95% said they would not do those things.

- Nearly half the women in the 45 to 49 age group reported masturbating at least once in the last six months. Twenty percent of women age 70 and older said they masturbated. A majority of all women said that self-stimulation is an important part of sexual pleasure at any age.

- About 60% of all men age 45 and older said they masturbated at least once in the last six months. More unmarried men (73%) than married men (51%) masturbated.

- While a majority of all subjects agreed that a satisfying sexual relationship is important to one's quality of life, for most it wasn't the number one priority. Good spirits, good health, close ties with friends and family, financial security, spiritual well-being, and a good relationship with a partner were all rated as more important.

- Men placed a higher value on sexual activity than did women. Sixty-six percent of men, compared to 48% of women, said that satisfying sexual activity is important to their quality of life. This gender split changes with age. In the 45 to 49 age group, men and women place almost equal importance on sexual activity. By age 60, though, 62% of men, but only 27% of women, placed a high priority on a satisfying sexual relationship.

- A majority of men and women with partners described themselves as either "extremely satisfied" or "somewhat satisfied" with their sex lives.

The Abkhasian people of Georgia (a republic of the former Soviet Union) often live to be more than 100 years old. One reason they believe they live so long is their sexual customs. The Abkhasian people believe that sexual energy should be conserved. They do not marry until about age 30 years and do not believe in premarital sexual activity. It is essential that a bride be a virgin. In marriage, sexual activity is considered a pleasure to enjoy, but for the sake of one's health it should not be overdone.

Lindau et al. (2007) reported that the prevalence of sexual activity declines with age (73% among those 57–64 years old, 53% among those 65–74 years old, and 26% among those 75–85 years old). Women were less likely than men at all ages to report sexual activity. About half of those who were sexually active reported at least one bothersome sexual problem. The most prevalent problems among women were low desire (43%), difficulty with vaginal lubrication (39%), and inability to reach climax (34%). Among men, the most prevalent sexual problems were erectile difficulties (37%). Fourteen percent of men reported using medication or supplements to improve sexual function. Men and women who rated their health as being poor were less likely to be sexually active and more likely to report sexual problems when they were sexually active.

Penhollow et al. (2009) studied a sample of older adults age 55–89 (mean age of 68). They found most of the group believed that sexual behavior is a lifelong need, that it has beneficial effects in older people, that it is a critical part of a good relationship, and that it is important to their overall quality of life. Twenty-eight percent of the men and 19% of the women were current users of sexual performance-enhancing medications.

Prevalent in our society is the performance ethic, which is concerned with the frequency of intercourse and orgasm. As we mature (age, if you will), it

Multicultural DIMENSIONS

The Boomer Sandwich

A study done by the American Association of Retired People on 45- to 55-year-olds (the sandwich generation) showed how different cultures take care of their own (The boomer sandwich, 2001). Compared with other generations, this one is better educated (38% are college graduates compared with 23% of the general population). More of them are married (67%, well above the national average). They are also more economically secure (almost a third earn more than $75,000 per year).

Who helps their aging relatives most? Forty-two percent of Asian Americans provide care for their aging relatives compared with 34% of Hispanics, 28% of African Americans, and 19% of whites. Those born outside the United States are much more likely to care for or support older family members (43%) compared with those who are born in the United States (20%). Overall, 69% do not want their children to have to look after them when they get older.

becomes apparent that other types of sexual activity become important. These include caressing, hugging, petting, kissing, and sharing of intimacies. People who experience a satisfying sexual life in their early years will most likely continue this pursuit. However, those people who are today 65 years and older lived under very different mores. Your grandparents and possibly your parents led more restricted sexual lives, especially the women. Women were not taught about masturbation, nor were they taught to ask that they be sexually satisfied.

Older people can not only be sexually satisfied by having relationships with others, but can also experience active sexual behaviors by themselves. Masturbation is a viable activity for older people, especially women. If the male loses the capacity to maintain erections, women can masturbate; or men can masturbate to orgasm even after they can no longer become erect. Mutual masturbation becomes popular, once again, as it may have been when they were younger.

Physiological changes are often attributed to changes in sexuality associated with aging. However, onset of menopause for women and declining levels of testosterone for men represent only one factor in sexuality changes. Psychological and sociocultural changes occur as well.

Some sexual dysfunction (discussed in Chapter 16) associated with aging, such as erectile disorder, can now be overcome with pharmacology. Drugs such as Viagra and Cialis can restore the physical ability to have an erection; however, it does not rekindle the psychological or social aspects that make for a loving relationship. These drugs pose special problems to a relationship: A woman may wonder whether the erection is caused by the drug or by attraction to her.

Psychological changes also occur across the aging process, such as changes in mood. For women, causes may include stress, health problems, menopause,

A new phenomena in Hollywood, both on- and off-screen, is that of a romantic involvement between a younger man and older woman. Is the pairing, such as occurred in 2003 with Demi Moore (40 years old) and Ashton Kutcher (25 years old) the start of a trend?

hormone replacement therapy, and other lifestyle changes. For men, they may include a shift in focus from career to increased focus on family, challenge to the traditional male role as leader and protector of the family, increased need for affirmation and acceptance, or irritation and anger with aging (especially the physical changes).

Social factors affecting psychological changes include the fact that socialization of people in their 70s, 80s, or 90s in regard to sexuality is substantially different from that of those in their 30s or 40s. For example, images of sexual attractiveness tend to be youth oriented and may affect the self-esteem of aging women (Sanders, 1999). Ironically, men are sometimes viewed as more attractive as they age. And Hollywood movies often capitalize on this double standard by pairing an older, experienced male actor with a young actress.

It has been common to see older men dating younger women, but a survey showed that 34% of single women ages 40 to 69 were dating younger men (Montenegro, 2003). The main reason given for women dating younger men was energy, refreshing optimism, and sexual stamina. One woman indicated that she liked dating younger guys who keep the romance stirring and their sex lives buzzing.

In addition, the acceptability of some sexual activities has changed over the past few decades. Thus, whereas younger people may engage in more oral sexual activities than their predecessors, older adults are less likely to engage in oral sexual activity (Laumann et al., 1994).

Interestingly, some long-married couples actually experience more sexual satisfaction during their older years. Once their offspring are out of the house and they are retired from working, they can devote more time to each other and have more fulfilling and rewarding lovemaking.

Finally, on a related, but different note, a growing number of older men and women are deciding to have children (Crandell, 2005). The birthrate for women 45 and older more than doubled between 1990 and 2002. Among older women having babies are celebrities like Cheryl Tiegs, Sharon Stone, Joan Lunden, and Susan Sarandon. Many older moms and dads are happy to devote what might have been leisure-filled years to the frenzy of childcare and related responsibilities. People may have to get creative to do this and use cutting-edge techniques like frozen embryos, fertility treatments and drugs, and adoption. Many older parents feel they do a better job of parenting than they would have done while they were younger.

For many years it was thought that the benefits of menopausal hormone replacement therapy might include elimination of hot flashes and vaginal dryness, protection against heart disease, and addition of calcium to the bones, thereby increasing their density and staving off osteoporosis. Other possible benefits discussed included delaying the onset of Alzheimer's disease and reducing the likelihood of developing breast cancer. Studies related to these proposed benefits have produced conflicting results, however.

Because of positive feelings about these potential benefits, for quite some time medical opinion seemed to weigh in on the side of using estrogen replacement therapy for most women. More recently, many researchers have reached the opposite conclusion. For example, starting around 2002, some studies found that women using the therapy had increased

risks of ovarian cancer, heart disease, stroke, breast cancer, colorectal cancer, and hip fracture. So, the controversy regarding the use of hormone therapy for particular women continues. Some argue that the increased risk is very small and worth the potential benefits; others argue that the risks are too great.

The National Institute on Aging suggests the following ways for women to stay healthy after menopause (Menopause, 2008):

- Don't smoke.
- Eat a healthy diet, low in fat, high in fiber, with plenty of fruits, vegetables, and whole-grain foods, as well as all the important vitamins and minerals.
- Make sure you get enough calcium and vitamin D—either in your diet or with vitamin/mineral supplements.
- Learn what your healthy weight is, and try to stay there.
- Do weight-bearing exercise, such as walking, jogging, or dancing, at least 3 days each week for healthy bones. Also try to be physically active in other ways for your general health.

Menopause

Usually between the ages of 40 and 55 years, women produce progressively less estrogen and progesterone, as an effect of aging on the ovaries. Whereas the pituitary continues to produce follicle-stimulating hormone (FSH) and luteinizing hormone (LH), the ovaries can no longer respond to these pituitary hormones as they once could. This decrease in estrogen and progesterone occurs over approximately a 5- to 10-year period and results in a cessation of menstruation. The period when these changes take place is called the **perimenopause**, or the **climacteric**; when menstruation has not occurred for a year, we call that **menopause**. Menopause is discussed in detail in Chapter 12.

Symptoms of Perimenopause and Menopause
Most perimenopausal women report mild symptoms or no symptoms at all; only about 20% report symptoms severe enough to cause them to seek medical attention. The symptoms that perimenopausal and menopausal women experience can vary

perimenopause (climacteric)
The period just before menopause when the production of estrogen and progesterone is decreasing, usually a 5- to 10-year period.

menopause
The time when a woman's menstrual cycle ceases, usually between 40 and 55 years of age.

Increased risk factors for osteoporosis include smoking, consumption of alcohol, physical inactivity, being underweight, and having a diet low in calcium.

Exercise is one way for women to prevent osteoporosis, the weakening of their bones. Thus exercise, along with proper nutrition, not smoking, and refraining from drinking alcoholic beverages, is helpful in preventing bone fractures.

from headaches, dizziness, palpitations, insomnia, anxiety, depression, and weight gain to hot flashes and vaginal dryness. **Hot flashes** (sometimes referred to as *hot flushes*) are sudden waves of heat felt throughout the body, often accompanied by reddening and sweating (National Institute on Aging, 2005). Some women experience hot flashes infrequently, whereas others may have them every few hours or so. They may last a few seconds or, in severe cases, a full 30 minutes. And some women never have hot flashes. Because hot flashes tend to occur more frequently at night, they often disturb sleep, causing the woman to awaken in a sweat. In particularly bothersome cases, they may contribute to insomnia. Hot flashes appear to be caused by hormonal fluctuations that affect the nerves governing the dilatation or constriction of the blood vessels. When the blood vessels rapidly dilate in response to hormonal secretions, a sense of warmth may result. Generally, hot flashes cease after 2 years, but in some cases they may last longer.

Vaginal dryness results from the lowered amount of estrogen in the vaginal walls, which causes shrinking and thinning and causes the vaginal mucosa to become thinner. The net result is that both the length and the width of the vagina become smaller and the

hot flashes
Intermittent sensations of heat reported by menopausal women, possibly caused by decreased estrogen production.

vagina cannot expand during penile insertion as it once could. In addition, there is diminished vaginal lubrication during perimenopause and menopause. These changes can mean painful intercourse as well as an increased risk of vaginal infection (National Institute on Aging, 2005). Over-the-counter lubricants can be helpful in these cases.

A significant symptom caused by the decrease in estrogen production is the decalcification of the bones. **Osteoporosis** is the disease that results when enough calcium is lost in the bones to make the person susceptible to bone fractures and bending (for example, curvature of the back—sometimes called "dowager's hump" because it is common among older women). Women older than 50 years of age lose about 10% of their bone mass every 10 years; the result is an increased risk of bone fractures. Women older than 60 years of age suffer many more bone fractures than do men (National Institutes of Health, 2005). It seems that osteoporosis occurs more frequently in white women who are fair skinned (especially blonds and redheads), who smoke cigarettes, who drink alcohol, who are physically inactive, who are underweight, and whose diet is low in calcium (National Institutes of Health, 2005). Osteoporosis can develop in men, too.

osteoporosis
A condition of weakened bones resulting from decalcification (loss of calcium) of bone that increases in the absence of estrogen and is of particular concern in postmenopausal women.

As if smoking weren't enough of a risk of cancer, it has been found that women who replace estrogen after menopause are at an increased risk of contracting breast cancer and ovarian cancer, not to mention the increased risk of stroke and heart disease.

Treatment for Menopause

As we have mentioned, only a minority of women have menopausal symptoms severe enough to make them seek medical attention. For those women there are several alternatives. One of the more controversial therapies considers menopause to be merely an estrogen deficiency and treats it by replacing estrogen. In fact, approximately 17 million women in the United States were taking hormones to relieve symptoms of menopause that included hot flashes, sleep disturbances, and vaginal dryness in 2002 (Redfearn, 2002). However, over the years **postmenopause hormone therapy (PHT)** (alternatively referred to as *hormone replacement therapy, or HRT*) has been controversial.

> **postmenopause hormone therapy (PHT)**
> Treatment of menopausal women who have insufficient estrogen production with synthetic estrogen supplements.

Estrogen supplements were used extensively until the 1970s, when it was found that their use increased the incidence of endometrial cancer. However, since then, progestin was added, resulting in the sloughing of the endometrial lining and the virtual elimination of endometrial cancer. Subsequently, estrogen and progestin supplements were widely prescribed (Rosenberg, 1993).

The benefits of PHT for any one woman may outweigh the small increased risk. For example, women who have osteoporosis and are at risk of hip fracture may decide, with their doctors, that the decreased risk of hip fracture associated with PHT is worth the increased risk of heart disease or breast cancer. Of course, a woman's age may also factor into this decision. It is with this reasoning that the predominant recommendation regarding PHT is that a woman and her physician consider the pros and cons, the benefits and risks, in light of the woman's particular circumstances before deciding whether to use PHT. For more information about PHT, visit the web site of the Association of Reproductive Health Professionals at *www.arhp.org*.

Other treatments for menopause disorders specific to preventing osteoporosis include sufficient physical exercise to strengthen the bones, a diet rich in calcium to slow bone decalcification, refraining from smoking of cigarettes and drinking of alcohol, and avoidance of carbonated soft drinks that contain high levels of phosphorus, which may contribute to a phosphorus–calcium imbalance associated with osteoporosis. Foods such as milk, sardines and salmon canned with bones, oysters, and dark green vegetables are recommended because they are all high in calcium.

Some physicians may also prescribe tranquilizers for women who have difficulty with the psychological aspects of menopause. It is unclear whether the depression some women report during menopause is a cause of that condition or is caused by other changes that usually occur during that stage of life (for example, children leaving home, aged parents needing more attention, or a woman's life taking a new direction).

In addition to estrogen replacement therapy, other treatments for hot flashes have been recommended. These include sleeping near an open window or fan; taking black cohosh (an ancient Native American remedy for rattlesnake bites) in capsular form; and ingesting phytoestrogens such as soy or flaxseed, vitamin E, 40 mg of red clover, combinations of bioflavanoids and vitamin C, chasteberry tea, evening primrose, and licorice (Phalen, 2001), although a study of 29 other studies (called a *meta-analysis*) found that only black cohosh relieved hot flashes (Kronenberg & Fugh-Berman, 2002).

Treatment for vaginal dryness can include the use of lubricated creams, vegetable oils, or water-soluble jellies (such as K-Y or Lubifax) and suppositories (Sexual problems overview, 2005). In addition, it appears that regular masturbation or participation in sexual intercourse helps reduce vaginal soreness.

It would be unfortunate to close this section without citing the benefits and positive aspects of menopause. Because women can no longer conceive, the fear of pregnancy is removed, and lovemaking is often more enjoyable as a result. However, a woman who has ceased to menstruate has not necessarily ceased to ovulate. So-called **change-of-life babies** have

> **change-of-life baby**
> A baby born to a menopausal woman who, in spite of not menstruating regularly, ovulated.

been known to surprise women just entering menopause who thought they could no longer conceive. Especially during perimenopause—when the menses occurs, however infrequently—caution is advised.

The anthropologist Margaret Mead talked of "postmenopausal zest" to describe the excitement, stimulation, and enjoyment that can result from menopause. If viewed in this way, the postmenopausal years can be rich with new opportunities and experiences. If its negative aspects become the focus, menopausal symptoms will probably increase, and psychological discomfort will result. It is up to a woman's friends, relatives, and colleagues at work to help her focus on the positive aspects of menopause rather than its less desirable components. In addition, many women now turn to support groups (for example, The Red Hot Mamas) or online forums to share strategies on ways to manage menopausal symptoms.

Male Climacteric

Do men have an experience analogous to menopause (termed the **male climacteric**)? The answer to this question is not clear. There is evidence that at approximately the same age at which women experience menopause, some men experience what is called a **midlife crisis**. Men wonder about the meaning of their lives thus far and worry about what the future holds for them. They may become more people oriented and less job-and-task oriented. They may grow concerned about a diminishing interest in sexual activity and a reduction of sexual potency. Some men, to reassure themselves about their sexual capabilities, begin to date younger women or initiate extramarital affairs.

The hormonal evidence usually cited for this male climacteric is a decrease in testosterone production at about age 40 to 50 years (Masters, Johnson, & Kolodny, 1985). However, the decrease in the testosterone level is believed by many experts to be minimal, too insignificant to influence male behavior. Furthermore, middle-aged women face many of the same concerns and fears about the past and the future and put themselves through similarly agonizing self-examinations. In trying to decide what accounts for the midlife crisis, researchers' difficulties in distinguishing the psychological and sociological influences from clearly identifiable physiological and hormonal changes are practically insurmountable. In women, decreased estrogen production and increased FSH production, as well as a lack of menstrual flow, serve as irrefutable evidence of menopause. No similar evidence exists for a male climacteric. Still, most observers admit that males often go through a change of life—whether hormonally, psychologically, or culturally based—that deserves recognition and attention.

male climacteric
Sometimes termed the "male menopause," which occurs at about the same age that women experience menopause, when men experience slightly decreased testosterone production and begin to question the directions in which their lives are headed.

midlife crisis
A time of life, usually between 40 and 50 years of age, during which men question the path their lives have taken and make plans for changing their goals.

Hormone Therapy

Hormone therapy is sometimes administered to men. For instance, testosterone supplements are sometimes administered to treat erectile dysfunction in older men (although testosterone levels are not low in all men who have trouble maintaining erection). Sometimes this treatment for erectile dysfunction is effective; other times it is not. The reason for this inconsistency is unclear; however, it is safe to say that the complex nature of sexuality makes it only partially responsive to hormone treatment. Testosterone supplements may not have much effect when personality, past experiences, the sexual partner, effectiveness in communication, setting, and so on, continue to have negative effects.

Other Aging-Related Physiological Changes

Direct physical changes do occur in men as they age: The testes become smaller, the scrotal skin becomes thinner and less elastic, seminal fluid may become thinner and be produced in lower quantities, and sperm become less lively. Erections occur more slowly and the plateau phase lasts longer. Another important occurrence is that older men do not feel imminent ejaculation—it is less forceful. It is common for the refractory period to become longer as men age. One possible advantage of slower response is the likelihood that middle-aged and older men can prolong sexual activity and actually be better sexual partners. It should be remembered, however, that even elderly men continue to produce sperm and can become fathers if appropriate precautions are not taken.

The capacity to enjoy sexual experiences is not lost in older men, as it is not lost in older women. Masters and Johnson (1966) maintain the importance of continued and frequent sexual experiences for aging males:

> If elevated levels of sexual activity are maintained from earlier years and neither acute nor chronic physical incapacity intervenes, aging males usually

are able to continue some form of active sexual expression into the 70- and even 80-year age groups.

Masters and Johnson further indicate that women who do not regularly participate in sexual activity tend to have difficulty accommodating a penis when they do attempt sexual intercourse. Those who can accommodate a penis and have adequate lubrication are likely to have maintained regular sexual response (once or twice a week).

If an older woman has not been sexually active for a long time, it may take a little time and patience to be able to resume sexual activity. For example, it may take longer for the vagina to swell and lubricate. Longer foreplay can be helpful, as can the use of a lubricant, such as K-Y jelly. For some women, vaginal treatment with estrogen works well. It may also take time to stretch out the vagina so it can accommodate a penis if the woman has not had sexual intercourse for a long time. Touching, cuddling, and good communication between partners help to promote sexual satisfaction (Resuming sexual activity later in life, 2004).

Influences on Sexual Activity in Later Years

Many older adults say their sex lives improve as they age. Improvements probably require more communication with partners and possible small changes both people can make. Here are a few examples (Intimacy and aging: Tips for sexual health and happiness, 2003):

- *Expand your definition of sex.* It is more than intercourse. Other options for sexual activity might be more comfortable and more fulfilling. Touching, holding, sensual massage, masturbation, and oral sexual activity are all possibilities.

- *Communicate with your partner.* Discuss changes and possible accommodations. Try different positions and activities. Ask your partner about his or her interests and needs and how you can be helpful. Communication itself can be arousing.

- *Make changes to your routine.* Change the time of day to a time when you have the most energy. Take more time to set the stage, such as a romantic dinner or an evening of dancing. Try new sexual activities.

- *Manage your expectations.* Be realistic. For example, if you didn't have much sexual

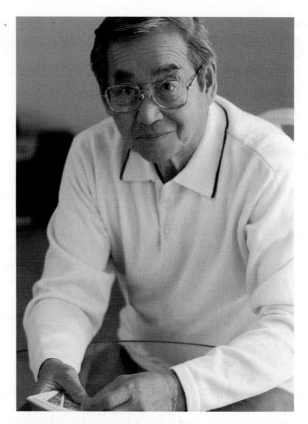

With age, men experience physiological changes that slow their sexual response.

activity when you were younger, you probably won't when you are older.

- *Take care of yourself.* Healthy living habits can help improve sexual activity at any age.

Although health problems can interfere with sexual activity for older people, they need not end all sexual activity. For example, arthritis or lower back pain might require understanding and a variety of sexual positions. Diabetes can result in diminished sexual response, but sexual pleasuring can still provide satisfaction. Stroke victims might lose some control of speech or movements but still be capable of sexual response under appropriate conditions.

Heart attacks are sometimes of particular concern in relation to sexual activity. Some people think that sexual activity may bring about a heart attack, and although in reality this is not a common problem, heart attack victims often hesitate to return to sexual activity. In general, those who have been sexually active before the heart attack will have little, if any, problem being sexually active again. Of course it makes sense to improve personal health as much as possible after a heart attack. Those who have a proper diet, exercise appropriately, and control stress responses are most likely to have satisfactory sexual activity as well.

Ethical DIMENSIONS

Should Donor Eggs Be Used to Let Women Older Than 50 Years Produce Viable Babies?

Women older than 50 years are just as likely to conceive and deliver a baby with donor eggs as younger women are. Many people argue that there is no medical reason why healthy women in their 50s should not have babies with donor eggs. They say that people in their 60s and 70s are much more active than in past years, so they have enough stamina to raise a child. Also, knowing that they can reproduce after age 50 will take the pressure off some women to reproduce when they are younger. They can concentrate more on their marriage and their careers and not worry about child rearing until later in life.

Others feel that it is wrong for a woman older than 50 years to reproduce. They feel that there is a much higher possibility of their offspring's being orphaned at a young age. Even if people are healthy and active, statistics show that many people die in their 60s and 70s. If that happens, relatively young children will be without parents for more of their lives. Also, for healthy people, raising a child takes a lot of energy and it is more likely younger parents will have that energy.

Do you think donor eggs should be used to let women older than 50 years reproduce? At what ages should women be allowed to reproduce?

Source: Rubin, R. Donor eggs can let women over 50 produce viable babies, *USA Today* (November 11, 2002), 9D.

The availability of partners for the older divorced or widowed person can present severe restrictions on intimacy. How can one have a successful relationship if there are no possible mates? Older women outnumber older men; they tend to live 7 years longer and they generally marry men a few years older than they are. Hence the older woman, who is supposed to have sexual relationships only with her spouse, is alone.

Another problem that exists for older men and women is that their sphere of friendships may be couples—that is, pairs. If one of only a few single people, the person may be omitted from social activities or may appear to be a fifth wheel, and so he or she is not very comfortable with other couples. This indeed limits sexual activity; even more importantly, it may limit intimacy and friendships in later life.

For older people living in nursing homes, there might be additional problems. For example, nursing home personnel sometimes resist sexuality programs. People may be segregated to discourage sexual activities. Medications may be prescribed without considering their effects on sexual functioning; for example, some high blood pressure or arthritis medications can lessen sexual response. Fortunately, attitudes of the staff in nursing homes as well as the families of those in the homes are changing. This is an excellent example of the need to accept people of all ages as sexual beings.

It should be noted that there are times when couples may want to sleep apart, because medication may cause a person to snore loudly, shake violently, or talk loudly, making it uncomfortable for the other partner. As well as elderly adults, some younger couples choose to sleep in separate bedrooms for similar reasons. It should be remembered that sexual activity can occur in either bedroom and at any time during the day or evening.

Aging and Safer Sexual Activity

The number of older Americans with HIV/AIDS is steadily rising. Between 2000 and 2003, about 30,000 men and women were 45 years of age or older at the time of their diagnosis of HIV. This was 23% of the total diagnoses for those years. Americans 45 or older who had been infected through heterosexual sexual activity accounted for 30% of all those diagnoses with AIDS in 2002 (Gottesman, 2005).

STI and HIV are generally thought of as diseases that the young must worry about. But the increasing number of sexually active elders has also been a factor in the increase in cases of STI and HIV. People 50 years and older account for about 13% of AIDS cases in the United States. They actually are more vulnerable to HIV infection because the linings of the vagina and anus become more fragile and more susceptible to tears during intercourse, providing a direct path into the bloodstream for the virus. The immune system also tends to grow weaker with advancing age. To make matters worse, older people are only one-fifth as likely as those in their 20s to be tested for HIV. As a consequence, the infection is typically not diagnosed until a late stage. It is important that older adults take the same safer sexual precautions as younger people (AIDS risk rising in older people,

2003; Lindau et al., 2007). As the older population continues to increase, the increase in STI and HIV is likely to continue at a corresponding rate.

One problem is that many people link pregnancy and STI risk. An elderly woman may not think to use a condom—after all, pregnancy is not possible (Broom, 1999). But condom use and safer sexual practices are still needed throughout life to prevent the transmission of STIs and HIV. And because an elderly man can impregnate a woman late into his life, safer sexual practices for men must include contraception.

Homosexuality Among the Aging

Like all sexual beings, homosexuals eventually become old and need to deal with problems caused by aging. The loss of partners and friends may be compounded for older gay men, who saw many of their friends die of AIDS during the 1980s and 1990s. For them, AIDS meant that the good-byes that would have been said as they approached old age were made not only to lifelong friends but also to younger and younger men (Swartz, 1998).

Because they grew up in such a sharply homophobic society, many gays are still cautious about coming out. Many elderly lesbians are still careful about coming out in today's somewhat more accepting society because they have become accustomed to hiding their identity. When older gay men or lesbians do not disclose their sexual identity, they prevent themselves and others from sharing in a comprehensive understanding of their lives (Altman, 1999).

Many gays may decide to keep their sexual identities secret because of fears of receiving biased or inferior services from doctors, attendants, or nursing homes. Help is available from Senior Action in a Gay Environment (SAGE), an organization concerned with gay, lesbian, bisexual, and transgender elders. It provides social services, individual and group therapy, and home visits for the homebound. It also acts as advocates on behalf of older lesbians and gays.

As people and society in general have become more open and accepting about homosexuality, changes have slowly occurred related to homosexuality and

aging as well. One germane example is the opening of retirement communities especially for homosexuals.

▪ Sexuality for the Physically and Mentally Challenged

In July 2005, the U.S. Surgeon General released a report related to disabilities. More than 54 million Americans, or one in five people, are living with at least one disability. Most Americans will experience a disability some time during the course of their lives. The Surgeon General's report emphasizes that people with disabilities can learn, get married, have a family, worship, vote, work, and live long, productive lives. There is a need to treat them as active members of society. In this spirit, the four goals of the Surgeon General's Call to Action to Improve the Health and Wellness of Persons with Disabilities are (U.S. Surgeon General issues first call to action on disability, 2005):

- Increase understanding nationwide that people with disabilities can lead long, healthy, and productive lives.

- Increase knowledge among health care professionals and provide them with tools to screen, diagnose, and treat the person with a disability with dignity.

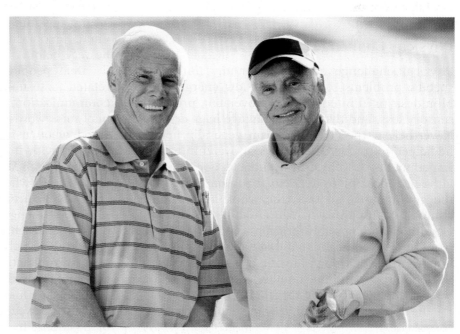

Some elderly gay and lesbian partners recall sanctions applied to homosexuals when they were younger and choose to remain "closeted," whereas others are adamant about expressing their sexuality openly in a more tolerant society.

- Increase awareness among people with disabilities regarding the steps they can take to develop and maintain a healthy lifestyle.

- Increase accessible health care and support services to promote independence for people with disabilities.

There are implications related to sexuality for each of the four goals. For example, a healthy lifestyle is important related to sexual interest and activity. It is also important for health care professionals to understand the whole person—including his or her sexuality.

Although we think of physical or mental challenges and illness as physical (biological) dimensions of sexuality, psychological and sociocultural dimensions also come into play. Mild depression is common among not only those with a chronic illness but also their caregivers and spouses, and it affects the couple's sexual activities (Pope, 1999). Further, an illness or disability may force a person to withdraw from normal social activities, thereby removing himself or herself from social support. Those who suffer from a disability also may suffer from body-image or gender-identity problems (Gerschick & Miller, 1998).

As with any sexual problem, it is not just the ill or disabled spouse who suffers. Both partners have to come to terms with changes in sexuality. Communication becomes a critical tool for acceptance of a new sexuality.

Physical Challenges

Physical challenge can result in any number of specific problems—for example, low energy levels, blindness or limited vision, movement problems, sensory loss, and the need to manage bags or tubes. Nevertheless, the challenged can generally find, or be helped to find, creative ways of overcoming such impediments to physical intimacy. For example, although most of us tend to focus on stimulating the genital area, in fact, the whole body can be stimulated and aroused. We can achieve sexual satisfaction—and possibly orgasm—without an erect penis or a well-lubricated vagina. With conscious intention and learning, anyone can use any part of the body in an infinite number of ways to achieve sexual satisfaction. For the challenged—as well as for the able-bodied—such learning can lead to a rich sexual life.

Even though sensory challenges, such as blindness and deafness, do not directly influence overall sexual responsiveness, they may affect sexuality. For

Disabilities do not have to prevent individuals from experiencing all the dimensions of human sexuality.

example, people who have been blind for most or all of their life may have difficulty in understanding a partner's anatomy. Fortunately, educational programs, including learning about sexual anatomy and intercourse positions through the use of models, can be very helpful.

Deaf people may also have special challenges related to sexuality. For example, some of the usual communication routes may be blocked. Deaf people may miss words in lipreading or may be misunderstood when using sign language if others are not familiar with it. As people without such challenges do, those with sensory challenges may feel afraid or embarrassed when attempting to communicate about sexuality. Educational programs are needed for the sensory challenged just as they are needed for people without such challenges.

Cerebral palsy usually does not preclude interest in sexual activity, fertility, or ability to experience orgasm. Depending upon the nature and extent of problems with muscle control, those with cerebral palsy may have difficulty with certain sexual activities or positions. In addition, social rejection or feelings of inadequacy may become problems. Fortunately, education and counseling to help those with cerebral palsy understand their sexuality and learn appropriate social skills can help improve body image and ability to have intimate relationships.

Sometimes challenged people have to adapt their behavior to meet new conditions. For example, a woman with severe arthritis of the hip joints may find she cannot spread her legs wide enough for intercourse in the standard frontal position or that the weight of a partner's body may produce pain. She can employ rear entry or side-by-side coital positions that reduce or eliminate discomfort.

It is important to recognize certain aspects of sexual functioning in paralyzed individuals (Woods, 1979):

1. Some components of the human sexual response cycle (such as erection) are mediated by spinal-cord reflexes. Therefore, it is not necessary to have pathways from the brain to the sex organs. For example, stimuli resulting from pressure or tension in the pelvic organs or from touch excite impulses that can cause erection.

2. The level of the spinal-cord lesion and the degree of interruption of nerve impulses influence the nature of sexual functioning. For example, the local reflexes important in female orgasm are thought to be integrated into the lumbar and sacral regions of the cord.

3. Gratification can be obtained from sexual responses other than those from the sex organs during sexual stimulation. Many physically challenged people develop other areas of stimulation to high levels.

4. Adaptation of previous sexual practices may be needed after spinal-cord injury. Sexual activity may need to take place in different positions, and sexual aids may be helpful.

5. Fertility and the ability to bear children are usually not lost by women with spinal-cord injuries.

Sexuality and Illness

The ill are another group whose sexuality has mainly been ignored. In the past both patients and medical personnel avoided any mention of sexual topics, no doubt because both were too embarrassed to discuss them. Now questions about sexual history are often asked in addition to standard questions about medical history. And physicians, patients, and partners are encouraged to discuss, when relevant, the effects of illness or other medical problems on sexual functioning.

It is important to consider the sexuality of ill people just as we consider the sexuality of all other people.

Diabetes, neurological disorders, gynecological disorders, inflammation of the male's prostate gland, castration, rectal surgery, and heart attacks usually have a direct (or assumed) effect on sexual functioning. But people with other nonrelated physical medical problems often experience sexual problems caused by psychological factors. Some of us, for example, feel guilty when we get sick and try to determine where the fault lies. Because the topic of sexuality is a leading producer of guilt, we may consciously or unconsciously avoid sexual activity. We may even allow illness to restrict our sexual life, not because restriction is necessary but because we failed to ask medical personnel whether restriction was actually required.

To reduce sexual problems associated with illness, we need to feel that sexuality is appropriate to discuss, and we need to be aware of guilt feelings. And, in all cases of illness, we need to take responsibility for finding out the earliest and safest time to resume normal sexual activity to prevent other detrimental effects on interpersonal relationships, as well as on self-concept. For example, after a heart attack it would be helpful to know the following (Sexual activity and heart disease or stroke, 2005):

1. Having heart disease, a heart attack, or undergoing heart surgery does not mean an end to a satisfying sex life.

2. Sexual activity is not really risky for the heart.

3. If a person doesn't get short of breath, have chest pain, or get tired when climbing two flights of stairs, the heart can meet the demands needed for sexual activity.

⚥ Gender DIMENSIONS

Coming to Terms: Masculinity and Physical Challenges

Men with physical challenges are marginalized and stigmatized in American society. The image and reality of men with challenges undermine cultural beliefs about men's bodies and physicality. The body is a central foundation of how men define themselves and how they are defined by others. Bodies are vehicles for determining value, which in turn translates into status and prestige. Men's bodies allow them to demonstrate the socially valuable characteristics of toughness, competitiveness, and ability . . . . Thus, one's body and relationship to it provide a way to comprehend the world and one's place in it. The bodies of men with challenges serve as a continual reminder that they are at odds with the expectations of the dominant culture. As anthropologist Robert Murphy writes of his own experiences with disability:

> *Paralytic disability constitutes emasculation of a more direct and total nature. For the male, the weakening and atrophy of the body threaten all the cultural values of masculinity: strength, activeness, speed, virility, stamina, and fortitude.*

This article seeks to sharpen our understanding of the creation, maintenance, and re-creation of gender identities by men who, by birth, accident, or illness, find themselves dealing with a physical challenge. We examine two sets of social dynamics that converge and clash in the lives of men with physical challenges. On the one side, these men must deal with the presence and pressures of hegemonic masculinity, which demands strength. On the other side, societal members perceive people with disabilities to be weak.

Recently, the literature has shifted toward understanding gender as an interactive process. Thus, it is presumed to be not only an aspect of what one *is,* but more fundamentally it is something that one *does* in interaction with others . . . . Whereas previously gender was thought to be strictly an individual phenomenon, this new understanding directs our attention to the interpersonal and institutional levels as well. The lives of men with challenges provide an instructive arena in which to study the interactional nature of gender and its effect on individual gender identities.

In *The Body Silent,* Murphy (1990) observes that men with physical challenges experience "embattled identities" because of the conflicting expectations placed on them as men and as people with disabilities. On the one side, contemporary masculinity privileges men who are strong, courageous, aggressive, independent, and self-reliant . . . . On the other side, people with challenges are perceived to be, and treated as, weak, pitiful, passive, and dependent . . . . Thus, for men with physical challenges, masculine gender identity and practice are created and maintained at the crossroads of the demands of contemporary masculinity and the stigmatization associated with disability. As such, for men with physical disabilities, being recognized as masculine by others is especially difficult, if not impossible, to accomplish. Yet not being recognized as masculine is untenable because, in our culture, everyone is expected to display an appropriate gender identity.

Source: Kimmel, M. S., & Messner, M. A. *Men's lives.* Needham, MA: Allyn & Bacon, 1998.

---

4. A person is usually able to resume sexual activity 3 to 4 weeks after a heart attack and 2 to 3 weeks after heart surgery.

5. A decrease in sexual desire after a heart attack or surgery can be expected. This is normal and should only be temporary.

The American Heart Association (2009) recommends that when people who have heart disease engage in sexual activities, they:

- Choose a time when they are rested, relaxed, and free of the stressful feelings produced by the day's schedules and responsibilities.

- Wait 1 to 3 hours after eating a full meal, so that digestion can take place.

- Select a familiar, peaceful setting that is free of interruptions.

- Take medicine before sexual relations if prescribed by a physician.

Alzheimer's disease also affects sexuality. Some Alzheimer's sufferers develop a loss of libido, whereas others develop hypersexuality—a constant desire to engage in sexual activities. However, an affected spouse may demand sexual activity but not even recognize his or her own spouse. Caregivers say that the

? Did You Know...

Persons with physical, cognitive, or emotional challenges have a right to sexuality education, sexual health care, and opportunities for socializing and for sexual expression. Family, health care workers, and other caregivers should receive training in understanding and supporting sexual development and behavior, comprehensive sexuality education, and related health care for individuals who have these challenges. The policies and procedures of social agencies and health care delivery systems should ensure that services and benefits are provided to all persons without discrimination and their caregivers have information and education about ways to minimize the risk of sexual abuse and exploitation.

Source: Position statement of Sexuality Information and Education Council of the United States, 2005.

sexual encounter may be emotionless, mechanical, or marred by inappropriate behavior, such as giggling (Pope, 1999).

We also need to realize that sexual problems can be expressed through physical symptoms; a person who asks for an examination of the genital area because of a supposed concern about cancer may actually be seeking an acceptable way to talk about a sexual difficulty. The relationship between illness and sexuality needs to be understood to help reduce the incidence of problems in medical settings and to increase our acceptance of both ourselves and others when illness is present—either in or out of the hospital.

Emotional Challenges

Throughout this text we have emphasized a comprehensive concept of human sexuality. One excellent example of this concept is the influence of emotional states upon sexual responsiveness. Many life problems, such as stress, problems at work, death of a friend or relative, or work overload, may interfere with sexual interest or response. Apprehension about intimacy, fear of pregnancy, or possibly fear of contracting an STI may influence relationships with others. Depression or poor self-esteem can also create problems related to intimate relationships.

Whatever the reason, emotional well-being has a strong influence on overall sexuality and on sexual response. It can be helpful to understand that, at times, lack of interest in sexual activity or even inability to respond can be natural and common. Fortunately, these situations are usually temporary and can be effectively handled through personal understanding or professional counseling if needed.

Sexuality of the Mentally Challenged

For many years, the sexuality of the mentally challenged was dealt with by restricting or preventing sexual behavior; indeed, the mentally challenged were sterilized to prevent any chance of pregnancy. The

Despite many factors that must be considered, including safe sex and the ability to make proper decisions regarding sexuality, the mentally challenged are certainly capable of participating in sexual relationships. With the support of education and counseling, the mentally challenged can often greatly benefit from the affection and intimacy encountered through a sexual relationship.

societal fear was that the mentally challenged would have mentally challenged children and that they would not be able to care for their children properly—thus costly medical care would be needed. A turning point in the rights of the mentally challenged occurred with the election of President John F. Kennedy in 1960. His mentally challenged sister, Rosemary, had a profound effect on him and was a major factor in his proposing of legislation to educate and help the mentally challenged (Wilson et al., 1996).

The American Association on Intellectual and Developmental Disabilities has a position statement (Sexuality, 2009) related to human sexuality. Among other points it says:

1. People with mental retardation and related developmental disabilities, like all people, have inherent sexual rights and basic needs. These rights and needs must be affirmed, defended, and respected.

2. Every person has the right to exercise choices regarding sexual expression and social relationships. The presence of mental retardation and related developmental disabilities, regardless of severity, does not, in itself, justify loss of rights related to sexuality.

3. Individuals have a right to sexual expression, information to allow informed decisions, and sexuality education including information about safe sexual practices, sexual orientation, sexual abuse, and STI.

4. Individuals have a right to sexual relationships, including marriage, with individuals of their choice.

5. Individuals have a responsibility to consider the values, rights, and feelings of others.

6. Individuals have a responsibility to seek input from families, friends, religious leaders, and others on the personal and societal values associated with sexuality.

7. Individuals have the right to choices related to birth control, deciding whether to have and raise children, and having control over their own bodies.

8. Individuals have the right to choose for themselves whether to be sterilized, regardless of the severity of their mental retardation.

Mentally challenged people who are allowed to have sexual relationships can and do build feelings of affection and tenderness that appear to contribute to their happiness and tranquility. In 1970, the United Nations passed a resolution supporting the right of mentally challenged individuals to sexuality education, cohabitation, and marriage. Although the rights of the mentally challenged are indisputable, their ability to make proper decisions regarding sexuality is often disputed.

As everyone else can, the mentally challenged can benefit from sexuality education and counseling. Because being challenged is just one more dimension of human sexuality, it needs to be factored into the decision-making process. For example, Depo-Provera or a long-term contraceptive might be selected instead of oral contraceptive pills, because contraceptive effectiveness would not depend on remembering to take a pill every day. Through factual knowledge, role playing, and personal experience, the mentally challenged are able to have fulfilling sexual lives.

Personal and Social Support

Society in general continues to deny the sexuality of the ill and the challenged. If this situation is to change, we need to remember that these people are sexual beings in the same way as everyone else. We also need to prevent public service personnel from denying the sexuality of their clientele. Attention must be paid to policy decisions influencing human services; to approaches used to serve the ill and the challenged; and to attitudes of those working with these people, as well as of society in general. Organizations that provide services to the ill and challenged need to teach classes in sexuality, not only for their patients but also for their patients' relatives and those who work with them.

Exploring the
DIMENSIONS
of Human Sexuality

Our feelings, attitudes, and beliefs regarding sexuality are influenced by our internal and external environments. Go to sexuality.jbpub.com/dimensions/4e to learn more about the biological, psychological, and sociological factors that affect your sexuality.

Sociocultural Factors

Sociocultural factors interact with biological factors to influence health.

- Laws affect what health insurers must cover. Several states in 1998 passed laws requiring Viagra to be covered as a prescription.
- Religion may affect the decision as to whether to circumcise the penis.
- The cultural bias allowing men to be sexually permissive can compromise a man's sexual health and wellness.
- Ethnic heritage influences health; for example, African American males tend to have higher levels of stress and heart disease than white men do.
- Media and ads portray the ideal man with extreme muscularity which is achievable only with tremendous work and, in many cases, illegal steroids.
- Family, neighbors, and friends often reinforce gender stereotypes.
- Behavior proscribed by society as illegal can influence health; for instance, a man can compromise his health by taking anabolic steroids.

Biological Factors

When a sperm with a Y chromosome meets an egg, a male will develop. Biological factors continue to influence development throughout life.

- Genetic coding affects physical appearance, including height; coloration of skin, hair, and eyes; muscularity; and many aspects of health.
- Physiological changes result at puberty from the hormone testosterone, which in turn affects muscle development and body size. Testosterone also increases aggression and leads to increased rates of heart attacks.
- Toward middle age, testosterone levels begin to drop, resulting in decreased muscle mass, increased fat, and a reduced sex drive.

Psychological Factors

Biological and sociocultural factors combine to influence psychological factors.

- Body image and self-concept is enhanced for many men through exercise and competitive sports.
- Men often suppress their emotions, which can result in increased levels of stress.
- Learned attitudes and behaviors about gender roles can lead to unhealthy lifestyles for men.

CASE STUDY

The life cycle of sexuality, from high school graduation through aging, offers many opportunities to see the interaction of the dimensions of human sexuality.

Consider the aging process: Biological changes, especially in levels of hormones, can bring about psychological changes, such as in mood. In addition, a psychological shift occurs in men as they shift their attention from career to family. Cultural expectations affect elderly adults' perceptions and expectations of their sexuality.

New advances in pharmacology such as the introduction of Viagra and Cialis may solve a biological problem, but the couple must then solve the psychological and social problems related to reintegrating the ability to have an erection in the relationship. Although medication can solve most erectile disorder issues, an erection is also a function of psychosocial sexual attraction—something that cannot yet be purchased.

Summary

- There are many theories about the types of love.

- It is important to understand sexual development during the college years. Many experiences and relationships with others will lay the foundation for future happiness.

- Although most people eventually marry, many are delaying marriage longer than in the past. Some people decide to remain single throughout life. In the United States, approximately 28% of women and 34% of men have never married.

- Cohabitation has drastically increased through the years. Today, some 6.5 million people live in a cohabiting relationship. There are a number of advantages and disadvantages related to cohabitation.

- Marriage is attractive to people for many reasons. More than 50% of males and females older than age 15 are married in the United States.

- There are many types of marriage—including the nuclear family, peer marriages, and stepfamilies.

- Extramarital relationships may be consensual or nonconsensual. Many worthless facts exist about extramarital relationships.

- The divorce rate has declined in the last two decades largely because of people getting married later and being better educated. Approximately 9% of males and 11% of females in the United States are divorced.

- Most older people remain interested in sexual activity and participate in various forms of sexual activity. Some health difficulties associated with aging may impede sexual activities.

- Today there is increased recognition of the sexuality of physically and mentally challenged people.

Discussion Questions

1. Compare and contrast the different theories about love. Which do you agree with? Explain why.

2. Summarize the studies about college relationships and sexual activities.

3. Discuss why increased numbers of people are remaining single.

4. Compare the advantages and disadvantages of cohabitation versus marriage.

5. Discuss why marriage is popular.

6. Discuss the reasons for divorce. What can be done to help protect children?

7. Discuss how and why the aging process affects sexuality.

Application Questions

Reread the chapter-opening story and answer the following questions.

1. The names Lynn and Chris were deliberately used as pseudonyms because they are names used by both genders. When you read the story, who did you think was the male? The female? Explain your answer. Then switch the genders of Lynn and Chris and reread the story. Does it strike you differently now? Why?

2. What advice from the chapter might have helped Lynn and Chris have a better marriage?

Critical Thinking Questions

1. Should mildly mentally challenged people be allowed to have children? Would they be any better or worse than typical parents (who have to learn from the start as well)? If mentally challenged parents are denied reproduction rights, what about those who have diagnosed psychiatric illness (such as depression)?

2. An increasing percentage of the population is remaining permanently single. Discuss whether this trend appears to be long term or just temporary. What are its implications for population growth? The future of Social Security?

3. Because of all the problems that divorce causes, should it be outlawed? What effects would such a law have on families?

4. Write a prenuptial agreement, indicating your expectations and responsibilities in marriage. Be sure to include how financial decisions, household tasks, child-rearing responsibilities, and so on, will be handled. Would such a document help or hinder a marriage?

Critical Thinking Case

Although dual-income families have become very common, equal sharing of work around the house is not as common. It is common for women to be responsible for things like shopping, cooking, and cleaning. It is common for men to more often be responsible for maintenance and repairs around the house.

The fact that many women are responsible for more of the housework has commonly been referred to as the "second shift." The first shift is the paid job outside the home, and the second shift is all the work at home. Putting the two shifts together, women put in much more work time than men.

In addition, many of women's tasks with children involve maintenance activities such as feeding, bathing, taking them to the doctor, and helping with homework. In contrast, men often help out with the more fun activities like going to the movies or playing in the park.

Consider which dimensions of human sexuality influence the continuation of this phenomenon. What could be done to break out of the stereotyped roles and create a more equal home environment? Should there be a more equal home environment?

Exploring Personal Dimensions

Are You Ready for Marriage?

The following quiz, developed by three clinical psychologists and marriage therapists, can help you decide whether marriage is right for you at this point in your life. Respond as honestly as you can to the following statements. Indicate which of the two choices more closely reflects your personal opinions and priorities by placing a check before line "a" or "b." (If you have a mate, you might each fill out the quiz separately, and then compare your answers.)

1. ____ a I wouldn't feel alive unless I were married.
   ____ b Give me liberty or give me death.
2. ____ a My "favorite things to do" are typical of married people.
   ____ b My hobbies and interests are those of a single person.
3. ____ a Being married can give me more of the security I want.
   ____ b Being single can probably give me more of the career opportunities I want.
4. ____ a I'd love to vacation alone somewhere with my spouse.
   ____ b I'd love to vacation with different people at different times.

5. ____ a Married means being sexually content.
   ____ b Single means being sexually content.
6. ____ a I prefer the stability and security of married life.
   ____ b I prefer the self-reliance and adventure of single life.
7. ____ a I want sex and affection from one reliable person.
   ____ b I want a variety of lovers.
8. ____ a Marriage is underrated.
   ____ b Marriage is overrated.
9. ____ a I'm willing to work to make my spouse happy.
   ____ b I don't want to be responsible for my mate's happiness.
10. ____ a It's morally more correct to live a married life.
    ____ b I'd like to do things when I want, without family constraints.
11. ____ a I'm ready to share my life and my credit cards.
    ____ b I'm ready to share good times, but let's not get too serious.
12. ____ a I believe that people should be married.
    ____ b I think people are happier if they are single.
13. ____ a Sex is best with one's spouse.
    ____ b Sex is too delicious to limit it to one person.
14. ____ a My career plans can tolerate or maybe even benefit from my being married.
    ____ b My career plans benefit from my being single.
15. ____ a I prefer the majority of my friends to be married.
    ____ b I prefer the majority of my friends to be single.
16. ____ a A marriage can be a beautiful experience.
    ____ b A marriage can be a trap.
17. ____ a I'd like to know whom I'll be sleeping with for the rest of my life.
    ____ b I don't want to know whom I'll be sleeping with for the rest of my life.
18. ____ a Today's smart people are getting married.
    ____ b Today's smart people are single and enjoying it.
19. ____ a The pleasures of marriage are wonderful.
    ____ b The risk of a bad marriage more than offsets any pleasure.
20. ____ a "Love" and "marriage" go together.
    ____ b "Love" and "independence" go together.

21. _____ a I don't mind sharing bank accounts and expenses.
    _____ b I'm too independent to enjoy sharing my money with a spouse.
22. _____ a I want to pour all my love into a permanent relationship.
    _____ b I'm not happy with an exclusive love relationship.
23. _____ a The economic advantages of being married are important to me.
    _____ b I like the idea of being single so I can spend my money as I wish.
24. _____ a Being married is important from a moral/religious standpoint.
    _____ b Morality and religion have little to do with marital status.
25. _____ a Lovemaking with one's spouse is certainly best.
    _____ b The many sexual opportunities of being single are a great advantage.
26. _____ a My greatest chance for personal growth is through marriage.
    _____ b My greatest chance for personal growth is through independence.
27. _____ a I'd prefer to share the risks of life with a spouse.
    _____ b My privacy is too important for me to enjoy being married.
28. _____ a I want a reliable lifetime relationship in marriage.
    _____ b I'd rather live free and easy and singly.
29. _____ a I'd be willing to make major changes, such as moving to another state, to help a spouse.
    _____ b I'm not ready to move, or make other major changes, to help a spouse.
30. _____ a Marriages are made in heaven.
    _____ b Marriages are too often made in hell.
31. _____ a My recreational interests are family oriented.
    _____ b My recreational interests are for singles.
32. _____ a I'd enjoy the security involved in being married.
    _____ b I prefer the freedom of being single.
33. _____ a I would love to have children.
    _____ b I don't want the responsibility of a family.
34. _____ a Being married offers joint tax returns and other financial benefits.
    _____ b I prefer to spend my money the way I want to.
35. _____ a I prefer sex and affection with my spouse for life.
    _____ b I prefer love affairs with many people.

36. _____ a I prefer the steady companionship of being married.
    _____ b I prefer the excitement of companionship with many lovers.
37. _____ a I'd enjoy spending leisure time with my spouse.
    _____ b I like spending my leisure time as I please.
38. _____ a If I have to choose between career advancement and marriage, I choose marriage.
    _____ b If I have to choose between career advancement and marriage, I'll take career.
39. _____ a Married people can count on sexual satisfaction from a trusted partner.
    _____ b Single people can find lovers from an endless pool of possibilities.
40. _____ a Marriage requires major compromises, and I'm willing to make them.
    _____ b Marriage requires major compromises, and I'm not yet ready to make them.

Scoring the Quiz

1. Count the number of your "a" responses and write the total here: _____
2. Compare your number of "a" responses with the following scale to determine your level.
   0–20 = Low readiness
   21–30 = Medium readiness
   31–40 = High readiness

Interpreting Your Score

Low marriage readiness: If you scored here, your values are heavily weighted toward a single lifestyle. Even if you've found a partner who shares your interests and values, the importance you attach to marriage at this time isn't enough to ensure success. Don't marry on the assumption that your values will change. They may not. And you shouldn't marry on the basis of other people's expectations or views about being married. *Yours* are the only ones that really count when it comes to marriage.

Though you may not value married life now, marriage readiness can develop rapidly. You may grow tired of the freedom and lifestyle that characterize being single, or come to appreciate more those elements associated with being married. Continue to review your marriage readiness from time to time, but do NOT marry until your values will support it.

Medium marriage readiness: Your values blend support for both single and married lifestyles, which means there's a certain level of risk if you choose to get married at this time. Probably the most important issue for you to consider is your potential mate's marriage readiness. Someone with a high readiness level can add stability to the relationship, increasing the likelihood of its success. Conversely, someone without it would dramatically reduce your already uncertain potential for a good marriage.

If he/she is less ready for marriage than you, be wary of demands for concessions. For example, he/she may say, in effect, "Do what I want or I'm getting out. I don't really want to be married as much as you do anyway." This is a destructive gambit; don't be pushed into a decision you're not ready to make.

A second major issue for you is the parity "fit" between you and your potential mate—your approximate equality in terms of personality, status, and appearance. Medium marriage readiness provides little cushion against the costs of an unequal match. High parity may lead to a successful marriage even if one or both partners possess only medium marriage readiness. But as the parity levels decrease, the greater the need for both partners to have a strong commitment to their marriage.

High marriage readiness: Your values strongly support married life, and your only challenge will be to find the right match. Be on guard, however, against projecting your own high level of marriage readiness onto a potential mate. The key for you is to realize that although you may be ready, you still need to choose your partner wisely.

Suggested Readings

Cherllin, A. J. The deinstitutionalization of American marriage. *Journal of Marriage & Family 66, no. 4* (November 2004), 848–861.

Gaboury, J. Saying "I don't." *SIECUS Report 33, no. 1* (Winter 2005), 29–33.

Geary, D. C., Vigil, J., & Bryd-Craven, J. Evolution of human mate choice. *Journal of Sex Research 41, no. 1* (February 2004), 27–29.

Menopausal symptoms and CAM. National Center for Complementary and Alternative Medicine, 2008. Available: http://nccam.nih.gov/health/menopause/menopausesymptoms.htm.

Popenoe, D., & Whitehead, B. D. The state of our unions 2007. The National Marriage Project. Rutgers, The State University of New Jersey, 2007. Available: http://marriage.rutgers.edu.

Schwartz, P., & Young, L. Sexual satisfaction in committed relationships. *Sexuality Research and Social Policy, 6, no. 1* (March 2009), 1–17.

Sexuality in later life. National Institute on Aging, 2009. Available: www.nia.nih.gov/HealthInformation/Publications/sexuality.htm.

Shildrick, M. Contested pleasures: The sociopolitical economy of disability and sexuality. *Sexuality Research and Social Policy, 4, no. 1* (March 2007), 53–66.

Stanley, S. M., Whitton, S. W., & Markman, H. J. Interpersonal commitment and premarital or nonmarital cohabitation. *Journal of Family Issues, 25, no. 4* (2004), 496–519.

Wolfson, E. Ending marriage discrimination: America in a civil rights moment. *SIECUS Report, 33, no. 1* (Winter 2005), 13–18.

Web Resources

For links to the web sites below, visit *http://sexuality.jbpub.com/dimensions/4e* and click on Resource Links.

Child Trends Data Bank
www.childtrendsdatabank.org

Information about the well-being of children, family structure, and family trends.

The National Marriage Project
http://marriage.rutgers.edu

Information about marriage, divorce, cohabitation, and some international comparisons.

U.S. Census Bureau
www.census.gov

Statistics on marriages, divorces, and various types of families and living arrangements.

Mayo Clinic.com
www.mayoclinic.com

Information on sexual health of various groups of people.

Surgeon General's Call to Action to Improve the Health and Wellness of Persons with Disabilities
www.surgeongeneral.gov/library/disabilities/index.html

Provides a copy of the full call to action along with fact sheets about parts of the call.

CHAPTER 13

Sexual Techniques and Behavior

CHAPTER OBJECTIVES

1 Identify the historical basis for present-day societal, religious, and/or cultural attitudes toward masturbation.

2 Cite the prevalence of sexual fantasy, describe its content and function, and note differences in male and female sexual fantasies.

3 Describe the role of touch, sight, smell, sound, and taste in sexual foreplay. Then list and describe various positions of sexual intercourse, including their advantages and disadvantages.

sexuality.jbpub.com/dimensions/4e

The Importance of the Senses
Global Dimensions: Global Religious Views on Sexuality

INTRODUCTION

*O*ne often hears that the 20th century's sexual revolution has led to more promiscuity and sexual freedom. The following excerpt, written before a different sort of revolution—the American Revolution—shows that many sexual techniques have not changed in a long time:

> As I kept hesitating and disconcerted under this soft distraction, Charles, with a fond impatience, took the pains to undress me; and all I can remember amidst the flutter and discomposure of my senses was some flattering exclamations of joy and admiration, more specially at the feel of my breasts now set at liberty from my stays, and which panting and rising in tumultuous throbs, swell'd upon his dear touch, and gave it the welcome pleasure of finding them well form'd, and unfail'd in firmness.

> I was soon laid in bed, and scarce languish'd an instant for the darling partner of it, before he was undress'd and got between the sheets, with his arms clasp'd round me, giving and taking, with gust inexpressible, a kiss of welcome, that my heart rising to my lips stamp'd with its warmest impression, concurring to my bliss, with that delicate and voluptuous emotion which Charles alone had the secret to excite, and which constitutes the very life, the essence of pleasure. . . .

> But as action was now a necessity to desires so much on edge as ours, Charles, after a very short prelusive dalliance, lifting up my linen and his own, laid the broad treasures of his manly chest close to my bosom, both beating with the tenderest alarms: when now, the sense of his glowing body, in naked touch with mine, took all power over my thoughts out of my own disposal, and deliver'd up every faculty of the soul to the sensiblest of joys, that affecting me infinitely more with my distinction of the person than of the sex, now brought my conscious heart deliciously into play: my heart, which eternally constant to Charles, had never taken any part in my occasional sacrifices to the calls of constitution, complaisance, or interest.

The preceding excerpt, from John Cleland's 1749 novel Fanny Hill, or Letters of a Woman of Pleasure, *shows that erotic literature has detailed sexual liaisons for centuries.*

Relatively few people actually set out to learn effective sexual arousal techniques. What learning takes place often occurs through trial and error *(with plenty of both). The results may be total pleasure, or they may be shame and embarrassment, confusion, and perhaps sexual dysfunction. Furthermore, such naivete and ignorance too often result in unwanted pregnancies. We believe that a strong foundation of sexual knowledge includes not only anatomical and physiological facts but also specific information about what people find sexually stimulating. Therefore, this chapter covers nonphysical means of arousal, as well as techniques in beginning play (foreplay), sexual intercourse, and oral–genital sexual activity.*

■ Autoerotic Sexual Behaviors

The two solitary sexual behaviors we discuss in this section are masturbation and fantasy. We should note, however, that although these are usually solitary behaviors, they can also be engaged in with a partner in the form of mutual masturbation or shared sexual fantasizing.

Masturbation

One need not have a partner to be sexually stimulated. **Masturbation** is the stimulation of one's own genitals for sexual pleasure. As Woody Allen said in the movie *Annie Hall*, masturbation is sex with the person you love most.

> **masturbation**
> Self-stimulation of the genitals.

Negative Attitudes: A Matter of History
Many of our attitudes regarding sexual activity are part of our cultural past. Masturbation is a good example of this. Ancient Hebrews believed they were partners of God in replenishing the Earth. In addition, they needed male offspring to maintain the patriarchal system and to supply needed labor. Consequently, laws were enacted to discourage nonprocreative sexual behavior. Any sexual activity that did not potentially lead to conception was devalued.

Many believe this attitude is best represented by the story of Onan in Genesis in the Old Testament. Onan was the brother of Er, whom God slayed because he was "wicked." However, Er had not yet conceived any children with his wife, Tamar. It was Judaic law that the next of kin of the husband must impregnate the widow so that the dead man had an heir. God, therefore, ordered Onan to impregnate Tamar, but Onan, not wanting to sire a child who would not be his, "wasted his seed" on the ground by withdrawing his penis just before ejaculation. The Lord killed Onan for this indiscretion, and, erroneously, masturbation came to be nicknamed *onanism*. Christian mores were influenced greatly by Jewish codes of behavior, and, consequently, masturbation was condemned by Christian law as well.

Global DIMENSIONS

Global Religious Views on Sexuality

Different religions confront sexual behaviors and sexual mores differently. For example, in Judaism, a *mikva* (ritual bath) is prescribed for women who have just finished menstruating to cleanse her physically and spiritually. Muslims and Jews perform circumcisions as part of their religious rituals, although they perform them at different times and for different reasons. Muslim circumcision of men is a rite of passage into manhood and of women is a means to prevent them from being easily sexually aroused and, therefore, potentially unfaithful to their husbands.

In Jewish practice, circumcision is performed only on young male infants 8 days old and represents a covenant with God. In Catholicism, abortion is a sin, because the religion teaches that life begins when fertilization occurs; the mother has no more status than does the unborn. In several other religions, abortion is allowed to remain a decision between the pregnant woman and her physician.

If you have a religion, what does it teach about sexuality? Perhaps you will want to interview a member of the clergy to understand better the rules, regulations, rituals, and rationale behind these teachings.

To this day our attitudes toward masturbation are colored by these ancient proscriptions. For example, although Freud believed masturbation to be a normal childhood practice, he feared that if carried into adulthood it would interfere with the formation of healthy sexual relationships. As recently as 1976 the Vatican stated in a *Declaration on Sexual Ethics* that masturbation was an "intrinsically and seriously disordered act." In 1993, Pope John Paul II reaffirmed that masturbation is an immoral act.

The Danger

No physiological harm can be attributed to masturbation. It will not cause insanity, sterility, sexual dysfunction, or any other physical affliction. Nor is there evidence that masturbation leads to an inability to establish meaningful sexual relationships. The primary danger associated with masturbation is within the individual's own mind—the guilt or shame he or she may feel about masturbating. Masturbation is so common that human sexuality experts now consider it a normal sexual act. It is normal to masturbate, and it is normal not to. As all sexual behaviors are, masturbation is a matter of personal choice. Awareness of this current thinking should go a long way toward alleviating a good deal of the guilt and shame people feel about engaging in this behavior.

Prevalence

As was discussed in Chapter 2, sexual research is fraught with limitations. Consequently we can only present data from several different studies and present a composite view about the prevalence of masturbatory behavior. The majority of studies have found that approximately 90% of adult males and slightly more than 60% of adult females report having masturbated (Arafat & Cotton, 1974; Downey, 1980; Hunt, 1974; Kinsey, Pomeroy, & Martin, 1948, 1953). These figures have remained remarkably consistent through the years (Clement, 1990). In fact, studies in the 1990s found that 60% of American men and 40% of American women had masturbated in the past year. Among couples living together, 85% of the men and 45% of the women had masturbated within the past year (Laumann et al., 1994; Michael et al., 1995). More recently, 73% of men and 37% of women reported masturbating in just the prior 4 weeks (Gerressu et al., 2008). A number of sociodemographic and behavioral factors were associated with their masturbation. Among both men and women, masturbation increased with higher levels of education and social class, and was more common among those reporting sexual func-

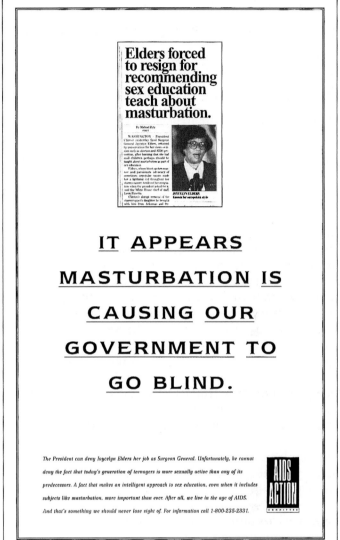

tion problems. For women, masturbation was more likely among those who had more frequent vaginal sex, who had a greater repertoire of sexual activity (such as oral and anal sex), and who had more sexual partners in the past year. In contrast, the prevalence of masturbation was lower among men reporting more frequent vaginal sex.

Techniques

Males masturbate by stroking the shaft of the penis, often stimulated by erotic literature, films, or videos. Some men use gadgets to assist them. Artificial vaginas, furlike clothes, inflatable dolls, and other devices have been reported as masturbatory aids by some men.

Women masturbate by rubbing the vulva—in particular, the clitoris—or inserting an object (a finger, a dildo, a banana, or a similarly shaped object) into the vagina. There are, of course, many variations on this theme, and the use of a vibrator to stimulate the vulva, cream to decrease friction on the area rubbed, pillows or other soft objects to rub the genitals against, and squeezing together of the thighs are all common adjuncts to the standard masturbatory techniques (see Figure 13.1).

Masturbation is a pleasurable, common, and varied sexual behavior; it is devoid of physical harm; it is more prevalent in men than women; and it continues even after marriage. The appropriateness of this and other sexual behaviors, however, relates to one's acceptance of them without guilt or shame and one's religious and moral points of view. As with other sexual behaviors, whether to masturbate is a personal choice.

The G Spot

Some women report experiencing heightened sexual arousal when an area of the interior wall of the vagina is stimulated. This area's sensitivity was first noted by the gynecologist Ernst Grafenberg; hence it is called the G spot. To stimulate the G spot, two fingers should be inserted into the vagina. The fingers should be pressed deeply into the tissue of the anterior wall of the vagina between the posterior side of the pubic bone and the cervix. Initially a woman may report a slight feeling of discomfort, a pleasurable feeling, or a sensation of needing to urinate. This latter reaction is probably due to pressure on the bladder. After a short period the tissue may swell, and unpleasant sensations may be replaced with erotic sensations. Women who experience orgasms from stimulation of the G spot often report them to be intense. Perry and Whipple (1981) describe this orgasm as resulting in a more intense uterine contraction than orgasm from stimulation of either clitoris or the vagina. Other researchers do not agree

that a "uterine orgasm" distinct from other orgasms exists (Masters, Johnson, & Kolodny, 1985).

Recently evidence has been found that might verify the existence of what appears to be a G spot in some women (Geddes, 2008; Henderson, 2008). Using vaginal ultrasound, researchers compared women who reported experiencing a vaginal orgasm with women who did not (Gravina et al., 2008). They found the tissue in the area thought to contain the G spot to be thicker in women who experienced vaginal orgasm. Still, some experts suggest this might really be a result of the size of the clitoris rather than a distinct G spot. Others wonder if the thicker vaginal wall is a result of women learning to orgasm vaginally, thereby altering their anatomy, much like exercising a muscle makes it grow. With subsequent research, perhaps the existence of the G spot will be either validated or refuted. In the meantime, the controversy continues.

Fantasy

Fantasies are thoughts and images, daydreams, and scenarios. In a sexual context, we call these **sexual fantasies**.

Prevalence of Sexual Fantasies

Sexual fantasies are quite commonplace (Halderman, Zelhart, & Jackson, 1984). One researcher surveyed middle-class women and found that only

> **sexual fantasies**
> Thoughts, images, and daydreams of a sexual nature.

FIGURE **13.1** Masturbatory techniques.

Gender DIMENSIONS

Differences Between Male and Female Sexual Fantasies

In one of the author's college classes, students are asked to write their most erotic fantasy on one side of a sheet of paper. They are then instructed to write the letter *M* or *F* on the back to indicate male or female. Of course, students can opt out of this exercise regarding what males and females find erotic, but they seldom do. The papers are collected and placed face up on a long table. Students read the fantasies, one at a time, and try to determine whether a male or a female wrote each. When all the fantasies are read, the males meet in one room and the females in another and generalize about what the opposite sex seems to find erotic. The following are typical observations:

1. In both male and female fantasies, the males were active and the females passive. In other words, males were doing "it" (whatever "it" happened to be) to the females.

2. The female fantasies involved more of a relationship between the sexual partners than did the male fantasies. For example, many females described sexual activity after a walk on the beach, dinner, or long conversation. Many female fantasies involved people with whom the writer actually had had a long-term relationship, whereas the male fantasies included more quick sex. For instance, some male fantasies involved picking up a hitchhiker and doing "it" in the back seat of the car. Others described encounters with strangers in elevators, shopping malls, or locker rooms.

3. The male fantasies were more likely to include more than one opposite-sex partner; for example, "I walked into my apartment and there were the Dallas Cowboy Cheerleaders. Boy did we get it on!" The female fantasies seldom included more than one sexual partner, but when they did, they were more likely to include both opposite-sex and same-sex partners.

4. Female fantasies included a more detailed description of the setting than did male fantasies. Females described the colors in the room, the music in the background, the candles flickering, or the bright sun-filled, leafy knoll of grass. If males described anything, it was the sexy clothing the objects of their fantasies were in the process of shedding.

The findings from our sexuality class are similar to those reported by other sexuality experts. For example, Hicks and Leitenberg (2001) studied university students and found a larger proportion of males have sexual fantasies involving someone other than their current partner than do females. They cite other studies that found "women's sexual fantasies are more likely to involve an emotional connection with a particular partner, whereas men's fantasies are more focused on explicit sexual imagery, often without romantic or emotional context" (Leitenberg & Henning, 1995, 48). Christensen (1990) puts it this way—more men than women imagine doing something to a partner, whereas more women imagine something sexual being done to them. In a review of the differences between male and female sexual fantasies, Masters, Johnson, and Kolodny (1985, 350) conclude, "Several studies have shown that the sex fantasies of women tend to be more passive than those of men (women tend to visualize their role in the fantasy as having something done to them by someone else, rather than being the active 'doer')." Obviously, there are many exceptions to these findings. Some men include romantic elements in their fantasies and some women do not. Some women include explicit, active sexual behavior by them and some men do not. However, as a generalization, it appears the findings of our students are valid.

7% had never experienced sexual daydreams or fantasies (Hariton, 1973). Earlier, Kinsey had found that 84% of men and 67% of women had sexual fantasies. Other researchers have also found sexual fantasies prevalent; for example, when studying college students, Sue (1979) found that 60% of men and women fantasized during sexual intercourse; Crepault and associates (1977) reported that 94% of their sample of women engaged in sexual fantasies; Zimmer and colleagues (1983) found that 71% of men and 72% of women fantasized about sex to become more sexually aroused; and Masters, Johnson, and Kolodny (1985) reported that 86% of the women they studied fantasized abut sex. More recently, in a study of university students and employees, 98% of men and 80% of women reported having sexual fantasies about someone other than their current partners during the past 2 months (Hicks & Leitenberg, 2001). Studies have consistently shown males have more frequent sexual fantasies than females (Leitenberg & Henning, 1995;

Hicks & Leitenberg, 2001; Ellis & Symons, 1990). Fantasies also come in many varieties. A recent study, for example, evaluated the rape fantasies of female undergraduates and found 62% of women have had a rape fantasy, which is somewhat higher than previous estimates (Bivona & Critelli, 2008).

Most people realize that it is permissible to have sexual fantasies. A *New York Times* poll (The way we live now, 2000) found that 55% of people younger than 30 years of age think it is okay to fantasize about having sex with someone other than their partners. Even many older people believed that—27% of those older than 70 thought it okay to fantasize about sex with someone other than their partners. One of the benefits of these fantasies is being able to imagine whatever one wishes unencumbered by "social convention, practical and legal barriers, or by fears of embarrassment, criticism, or rejection" (Wilson, 1997, 43). Research has demonstrated that sexual fantasizing can be healthy for both men and women (Strassberg & Lockerd, 1998; Chick & Gold, 1987–1988; Davidson, 1985; Knafo & Jaffe, 1984).

Sexual fantasies may be triggered externally, such as by a movie or by photographs. Or, they may be triggered by internal stimuli, such as thoughts of another person or a sexual situation. Alternatively, fantasies may be generated by a combination of external and internal triggers (Jones & Barlow, 1990). In addition, sexual experience appears related to sexual fantasies. For example, in two studies, women with more coital experience reported more sexual fantasies than women who were virgins or had less sexual experience (Hicks & Leitenberg, 2001; Knafo & Jaffe, 1984).

Another source of fantasy images is the Internet. Although fraught with limitations (Are students being truthful?), several studies have explored the prevalence of college students' use of the Internet to view sexually explicit material. In one study of 506 college students, 44% reported accessing sexually explicit material online (Goodson, McCormick, & Evans, 2001). In another study of 985 university students, 38% reported they used the Internet to view sexually explicit images (Rumbough, 2001).

Content of Sexual Fantasies

The content of sexual fantasies is both similar and dissimilar when gender is the variable. Interestingly, when males and females are by themselves they tend to fantasize about engaging in sexual activities with their usual partners; however, when they are engaged in sex with their usual partners, they fantasize about sex with someone else (for example, a movie star or a model) (Leitenberg & Henning, 1995). Although quite a diversity in the content of sexual fantasies exists, other prevalent fantasies

are having oral–genital sex, being found sexually irresistible by others, and having sex forced upon oneself. The most prevalent female sexual fantasies include having sex in a secluded setting, engaging in sexual activity in a different place than usual (such as a hotel), and having thoughts about an imaginary lover (Strassberg & Lockerd, 1998). Table 13.1 presents favorite male sexual fantasies. Table 13.2 lists favorite sexual fantasies of gays and lesbians. Sexual fantasies may also include group sex, sex with celebrities, voyeuristic activities (peeping or watching others engaged in sex), sadomasochism, or experimentation with other partners or other activities. In a 1995 study that reviewed more than 200 other studies of sexual fantasies, the researchers concluded that women's fantasies tended to include sex with a new male partner, sex with a celebrity, seduction of a younger man or boy, and sex with an older man. Men's favorite fantasies included seeing women nude and having sex with a new female partner, multiple sex partners, and the power to drive women wild (Leitenberg & Henning, 1995).

TABLE 13.1 Men's Favorite Sexual Fantasies

- Seeing woman nude
- Having sex with a new partner
- Having sex with multiple partners at the same time
- Having the power to drive women "wild"

Source: Leitenberg, H., & Henning, K. Sexual fantasy. *Psychological Bulletin, 117* (1995), 469–496.

TABLE 13.2 Gays' and Lesbians' Favorite Sexual Fantasies

Gays' Fantasies
- Unspecified sexual activity with another man
- Performing oral sex
- Having partner perform oral sex
- Participating in anal sexual intercourse
- Sex with another man not previously involved with

Lesbians' Fantasies
- Unspecified sexual activity with another woman
- Having partner perform oral sex
- Performing oral sex
- Anticipating sexual activity with a partner
- Being held and touched

Source: Price, J. H., & Miller, P. A. Sexual fantasies of black and white college students. *Psychological Reports, 54* (1984), 1007–1014. © *Psychological Reports* 1984, reproduced with permission.

Functions of Sexual Fantasies

Sexual fantasies serve several purposes. They are a source of pleasure, and, as such, they enhance sexual arousal. Furthermore, sexual fantasies allow people to test and rehearse various sexual activities if they are concerned about being judged by their partners. In this way the activity is tested in a nonthreatening setting and no one knows whether it works out. And sexual fantasies allow people to acknowledge sexual feelings without acting on them.

There is also research to indicate that sexual fantasies may be helpful in overcoming sexual anxiety (Coen, 1978; Leitenberg & Henning, 1995; Hicks & Leitenberg, 2001). Consequently, many sexual therapists encourage fantasies in counseling clients with sexual dysfunctions. In fact, low sexual desire in women has been found to be associated with a lack of sexual fantasizing (Nutter & Condron, 1983).

In addition, sexual fantasies allow us to be "better" than we really are—that is, better lovers, more confident, more experienced, more risky, and more desirable. They also provide us with a safe means of engaging in sexual activities in which we may never wish to participate. For example, though some women fantasize about being forced to have sex, few would actually want that fantasy to come true. It is hypothesized that the frequency with which a woman reports this forced-sex fantasy is a function of her desire to be risqué in her sexual behavior but not accountable for it, because our society generally frowns on sexually adventurous women. Another interpretation of this forced-sex fantasy is that women seek greater power rather than less, so they fantasize that they are so desirable that the man cannot resist (Leitenberg & Henning, 1995). Although Hunt (1974) found twice as many women had this fantasy as men, he did find 10% of men also had submission fantasies.

Sexual fantasies also provide us with a means of fulfilling our every desire while not hurting ourselves or those we love. It is a private and safe way of doing anything we want. It is a means of acting out our wildest dreams while never acting improperly. For example, we may wonder what sex with an animal would be like, or what the experience of sex with our lover's friend would feel like. By fantasizing about these situations we do not harm ourselves, our lovers, or our pets, yet we can experience the situation vicariously. Fantasies of this kind are safe as long as they do not become obsessive. If they do, therapy may be indicated.

There are those who argue that sexual fantasies are unhealthy. For example, Apfelbaum (1980) believes fantasizing during sex with a partner can decrease the degree of trust and intimacy in the relationship. Others have taken a similar point of view (Hollender, 1970; Shainess & Greenwald, 1971).

Maltz and Boss (2001) provide a list of nine questions to ask to determine whether, and to what extent, a sexual fantasy may be causing problems:

- Does the fantasy lead to risky or dangerous behavior?

- Does the fantasy feel out of control or compulsive?

- Is the content of the fantasy disturbing or repulsive?

- Does the fantasy hinder recovery or personal growth?

- Does the fantasy lower my self-esteem or block self-acceptance?

- Does the fantasy distance me from my real-life partner?

- Does the fantasy harm my intimate partner or anyone else?

- Does the fantasy cause sexual problems?

- Does the fantasy really belong to someone else?

The predominant view is that sexual fantasizing can enhance sexual relationships as long as it does not become obsessive and as long as there is no compulsion to act out the fantasy. Some fantasies may be acted out with the consent of the sexual partner, but if one person feels uncomfortable, problems may arise. Guilt or shame may lead to other psychological and/or sexual problems. With the willing consent of both partners, however, acting out sexual fantasies can actually enhance sexual satisfaction and improve the relationship. It appears, though, that most sexual fantasizers do not intend to act out their fantasies, and, if they do, they may be disappointed. Nancy Friday (1975) reports that most individuals who have acted out their sexual fantasies were disappointed. It seems that reality seldom matches fantasy.

■ Sexual Behavior with Others

Foreplay is the physical contact that usually precedes coitus or oral–genital sexual activity. Generally foreplay includes touching, kissing, biting, and genital fondling. The word *foreplay* is really a misnomer, because this behavior can be enjoyed for itself and need not be a prelude (*fore-*) to anything. All such activity is meant to express love, sensuousness, desire, or all these feelings.

> **foreplay**
> Physical contact preceding sexual intercourse.

Myth (vs) Fact

Myth: Sexual fantasies mean a person is fixating on sex and needs either to get professional help or to work hard to stop fantasizing.
Fact: Sexual fantasizing is prevalent and is not indicative of a sexual problem. Many males and females fantasize both before and during sexual intercourse, even if engaged in sexual intercourse with their usual partner.

Myth: Women who fantasize about being raped are "sick" and, if raped, get what they deserve.
Fact: First of all, no one "deserves" to be forced to engage in any sexual activity against his or her will. Second, having a fantasy does not indicate that someone actually wants the fantasy to come true. Rape fantasies may even indicate a woman's wish to be so desirable that men cannot resist her rather than a desire to give up control to a male.

Myth: Masturbation is normal for young people but can interfere with the healthy sexual relationship of older people, especially if they are married.
Fact: There is no evidence that masturbation is harmful either physically or psychologically. In fact, there are some times when a sexual partner is unavailable and masturbation can serve as a healthy sexual outlet. Furthermore, many married people with regular sexual intercourse still enjoy masturbating.

Myth: It is unfortunate, but people with disabilities cannot have a meaningful sex life because of the restrictions placed on them by their disabilities.
Fact: Certainly some disabilities place restrictions on sexual positions or sexual stamina. Still, there are many accommodations that can be made so that people who have heart disease, who are physically disabled, or who are ill can achieve and maintain meaningful sexual lives.

We might more appropriately term this activity *pleasuring each other*. However, foreplay does also serve to prepare the participants, both psychologically and physically, for coitus.

The importance of foreplay to sexual enjoyment has been widely acknowledged. Data (Hunt, 1974) show that unmarried people younger than 25 years of age spend an average of 15 minutes in foreplay and another 15 minutes in intercourse, whereas Kinsey's 1948 data showed that a majority of males reached orgasm just 2 minutes after penile insertion. Michael and colleagues (1994) found that for 69% of men and 71% of women, intercourse took from 15 minutes to 1 hour. Because women need more time to be vaginally lubricated sufficiently for intercourse than men do to achieve erection and be ready (Masters & Johnson, 1966), perhaps this acknowledgment represents an increased understanding of women's needs to be sexually stimulated for a longer period than men before coitus.

Interestingly, some men are fearful of foreplay. They worry about losing their erection or ejaculating before intercourse (Elder, 2009). This is unfortunate because foreplay is the perfect time for communi-

cating with your partner to find out what he or she likes (Srovny, 2009). To rush through it is to lose this opportunity.

The Importance of the Senses

Sexual stimulation in foreplay, intercourse, or any other activity involves the imagination and all of the senses: touch, sight, smell, hearing, and taste.

Touch

Sensual touching is central to sexual stimulation. Although the skin is not a sexual organ as such, stroking the skin on any part of the body can contribute to and even initiate sexual arousal. The gentle stroking of a partner's face, ear, or neck can be both exciting and effective at communicating affection. Furthermore, each manner and intensity of body contact carries its own kind of stimulation. Gentle touching, where the fingers barely make contact with the skin and perhaps focus on one part of the body, can be tantalizing. Caressing—gentle stroking or rubbing—is firmer than gentle touching and communicates affection or appreciation. Firmer touches, too, can be sexually arousing. Hugs, embraces, and squeezes are all expressions of caring. Some might consider a full-body massage the ultimate expression of the sensual touch.

So sensual touching is not necessarily focused on the genitals. But once the body and emotions are primed for sexual activity, touching in and around specific areas of the body is intensely stimulating. The breast (especially the nipple), the inner thighs, the clitoris, the penis, the neck, the ears, and the navel are particularly receptive to sensual touching because of an abundance of nerve endings. However, touching of some of the sensitive genital areas (for example, the vulva or the glans) can result in irritation unless some kind of lubricant is used. Of course, the best lubricant is that produced vaginally by the woman herself. However, any lotion, such as hydroxyethyl cellulose (K-Y jelly), that does not contain alcohol is also safe and useful for this purpose (unless you are using a condom, in which case Vaseline should not be used). Touching on all parts of the body can be of a teasing nature: moving here, then there, but not there (though almost), then back here. Genital touching should be done in a gentle manner, because rough handling (for example, of a testicle) could result in injury.

We should not overlook the use of touching for sexual self-stimulation. Masturbation is often the method by which people learn which body areas and which types of touching are most stimulating for them. Vibrators have become popular both for masturbating and for sexually stimulating partners.

Many couples masturbate each other to orgasm and find this form of sexual activity very exciting and a safe alternative to intercourse.

As with other sexual behaviors, good communication is important for guiding partners in touching each other effectively. Such phrases as "I like that," "That hurts," and "Keep doing that, but just a little more gently (or more firmly)" will help your partner use touching on the specific areas and in the particular ways most stimulating to you. If you are the toucher and do not get this feedback, ask for it.

Sight

The power of visual images is clear everywhere in modern society—for example, in advertising, in films, and in television. These images sometimes work on us without our notice, but it is possible to use sexual imagery consciously for sexual stimulation. Sexual partners sometimes use sexual imagery in books, magazines, films, and photographs to become aroused together. Clothing can also serve this purpose. Men and women often dress in a manner termed sexy, not only to attract others but to add to their partners' or their own sexual excitement. Some people are excited by the sight of hair, eyes, legs, or other body parts. Partners can learn to make use of each other's particular visual stimulants to initiate or enhance sexual arousal.

Smell

The popularity of perfumes and colognes is probably attributable to their potential for arousing sexual interest. It is no small wonder that the old-time

Smell can be sexually stimulating. Research with both animals and humans demonstrates the sexually arousing nature of certain smells. Perfume manufacturers have long recognized this fact.

bordello is associated with highly perfumed and painted women (even though these ladies might have been a far sight raunchier than their counterparts in the modern media). Animal studies have identified smell as being more important in many species than sight or sound in attracting a mate (Bhutta, 2007). Substances called **pheromones** are secreted by some female animals to attract male sexual partners. Conversely, unpleasant smells such as bad breath can interfere with sexual arousal. Attention to normal body hygiene can prevent these problems.

Although it has long been suspected that humans produce pheromones, it was only in the late 1980s that scientists verified this. Human pheromones do not actually serve as sexual attractants, but they do alter the timing of women's menstrual cycles. The Monell Chemical Studies Center and the University of Pennsylvania Medical School (Cutler et al., 1986) studied this issue for several years and found that women who experience coitus weekly are more likely to have normal menstrual cycles, fewer infertility problems, and milder menopauses than women who either are celibate or have sexual intercourse only sporadically (Rensberger, 1986). It seems that male aromatic chemicals secreted from sweat glands in the armpits, nipples, and genitalia are transmitted to their sexual partners by smell and skin absorption. Once transmitted, these chemicals affect the woman's reproductive system.

Women also produce a pheromone that affects other women's menstrual cycles. For years anecdotal reports indicated that women who live together or who work together seem to have synchronous menstrual cycles. These reports now have evidence both to support and to explain them (Preti et al., 1986).

The manner in which human pheromones work is not fully understood. The suspicion is that molecules of the substances reach receptors of the nervous and endocrine systems and act on them to stimulate signals transmitted in the brain (Keverne, 2004). These brain signals influence the endocrine system's secretion of hormones, and these hormones influence the woman's reproductive system (Lanuza et al., 2008; Spors & Sobel, 2007).

There are several potential practical applications of this knowledge regarding human pheromones. For example, nasal sprays might be developed to alleviate certain kinds of infertility problems, to regulate the menstrual cycle (for instance, to make the rhythm method of birth control more effective), or to effect the onset of menopause or minimize its effects.

> **pheromones**
> Substances that when secreted have a specific scent found to be sexually arousing.

Hearing

Have you ever heard the expression "Whisper sweet nothings in my ear"? Well, those murmurings are not just nothings! Words and sounds before and during coitus can be sexually stimulating, as can music that contributes to an erotic atmosphere. Sexual talk can take many forms. Some people are aroused by "dirty words," and others are completely turned off by them. Similarly, some people find moaning during sexual activity to be exciting, whereas others are unimpressed with such guttural goings-on. Furthermore, some people report that saying or hearing "I love you" after orgasm can be one of the most exciting and romantic experiences in the world (Haffner & Schwartz, 1998). Once again, communication between sexual partners is the key.

Taste

The use of the mouth can be quite sexually arousing. Kissing, when both partners attend to it, can be intensely stimulating, whatever the variation: open mouth, closed mouth, a nibble here, a nibble there, a tongue darting from spot to spot, and lips or teeth closing gently on a sensitive body part. Kissing with tongues touching (soul kissing, French kissing, deep kissing) can also take various forms. More on the use of the mouth, tongue, and teeth is discussed in the section on oral–genital sexual behavior. As with the other senses, taste can also be a turnoff. Obviously French kissing someone who has bad breath or licking a smelly body can be anything but arousing. Proper body hygiene and communication on such simple matters between sexual partners can go a long way toward improving sexual relations.

In the following sections, we discuss specific sexual behaviors and provide guidance for enhancing sexual satisfaction through the use of these activities.

Kissing can be a very erotic, sensual activity in and of itself.

Oral–Genital Sexual Behavior

Oral–genital sexual behavior involves contact between the mouth, lips, and tongue of one partner and the genitals of another. When a female's genitals are orally stimulated, the act is called **cunnilingus** (meaning in Latin "one who licks the vulva"). When the penis is taken into the partner's mouth, the act is called **fellatio** (from the Latin *fellare*, meaning "to suck"). As with most sexual acts, some find oral–genital sexual contact sexually arousing; others are indifferent to it or find it repulsive. It is generally agreed, however, that oral–genital activity is quite common. Hunt's (1974) study, for example, indicated that 90% of married couples younger than age 25 years had experienced oral–genital sexual stimulation. The most recent large-scale study of oral sex was conducted by Michael and associates (1994), who found that 77% of men and 68% of women reported having given oral sex *to* a partner, and 79% of men and 73% of women had received oral sex *from* a partner.

Many of the techniques described as foreplay are applicable to oral–genital sexual activity. Thus a teasing approach, gentle in nature and varied in form, involving the mouth, lips, and tongue is particularly stimulating. Some women report especially enjoying the licking or sucking of the clitoris and labia minora or a thrusting of the tongue into the vagina. Men are often aroused when their partners lick the underside of the penile shaft and the glans or lick or lightly hold a testicle in the mouth. Again, the testicles and clitoris are very sensitive and should be treated gently. And, of course, attention to personal hygiene is important to maximal—and even minimal—pleasure.

Sexual partners need to discuss whether ejaculation should occur in the mouth during fellatio. Contrary to rumor, the ejaculate is not fattening when swallowed; however, it does have a unique taste. Some like or are indifferent to the taste; others dislike it. One word of caution here, though: Because the ejaculate can contain HIV if the male is infected, unless the relationship has been monogamous for some time and both partners are known to be HIV-free, the ejaculate should not be swallowed. In any case, whether the ejaculate is swallowed does not need to diminish the pleasure of either partner.

When couples orally stimulate one another simultaneously, the act is referred to as **69** (because their bodies in position resemble

cunnilingus
The stimulation of the female genitalia by the mouth, lips, and/or tongue of the sexual partner.

fellatio
Oral contact with a male's penis.

69
Two partners' simultaneous stimulation of each other's genitalia orally. The numerals 6 and 9 visually describe the body positions.

Ethical
DIMENSIONS

Should People Who Do Not Feel Comfortable with Oral or Anal Sexual Activity Learn to Enjoy These Activities?

Some people believe that the more sexual acts one experiences, the more sexually satisfied one will be, and that to enhance our sexual lives, we need a variety of sexual expressions and sexual excitation. They feel that those who are not comfortable with oral–genital sexual activity or anal intercourse ought to be instructed in how to engage in these activities and given counseling to relieve any shame, guilt, or anxiety associated with them. People with this viewpoint argue that to ignore this discomfort is to forever accept a less satisfying sexual life than is possible; and when sexual partners have different desires related to oral and anal sexual activity, there is a threat to the relationship itself.

Others believe that sexual expression can occur in many forms and that no one person need accept all forms for himself or herself. If some sexual activities are uncomfortable, these people argue, choose other activities to include in your sexual repertoire. People should not be coerced into behaviors that they find repulsive; that is not fair. Furthermore, if one partner desires oral or anal sexual activity and the other does not, a good relationship will result if the one who does want these activities understands and accepts the other's feelings. Anything short of that and the relationship is probably not worthwhile anyhow.

What do you believe a couple who disagrees on this issue should do?

FIGURE **13.2** Simultaneous oral–genital stimulation.

the numbers 6 and 9 (Figure 13.2). Couples can perform 69 side by side or with one partner on top of the other, depending on which position they consider more comfortable and stimulating. Some couples prefer to stimulate one another simultaneously, whereas others find they cannot concentrate on their own pleasurable sensations while concentrating on pleasuring someone else.

Partners also need to discuss the need for a male to wear a condom and a female to wear a dental dam during oral–genital contact. These behaviors decrease, although they do not eliminate, the possibility of contracting HIV, as well as other STIs. That is why they are called "safer sex" behaviors. To be "safer," partners should consider agreeing to engage in these behaviors.

Anal Stimulation

Some people enjoy becoming sexually aroused anally, because there are numerous nerve endings in that area. Partners can stimulate each other by inserting a finger into the anus, stroking the anal opening, or licking the area. However, licking the anus, termed **analingus**—also commonly referred to as "rimming"—is risky to one's health. Intestinal infections, such as *Escherichia coli*, can be spread through analingus, as can hepatitis and STIs. This threat exists even though the anus may be carefully washed. In addition, minute tears that occur in the anus during **anal intercourse** provide easy entry into the body for organisms that cause STIs. This is especially likely if a condom is not used. Penile penetration of the anus is also possible, for both heterosexual and homosexual couples. **Dildos** (fake penises) can also be used for anal insertion. Because of the nature of the anus, one should take care not to tear the surrounding tissue (a lubricant should be used), and to prevent infection the penis should be thoroughly cleansed immediately after anal insertion. Because anal intercourse is one of the risk behaviors for HIV,

analingus
Licking of the anus.

anal intercourse
Insertion of the penis into the anus.

dildos
Artificial penises.

a condom should be used whenever this sexual activity is performed.

Sexual Intercourse

Variety may truly be the spice of life, at least relative to coital (penile–vaginal intercourse) positions. Although most authorities recognize four basic positions of sexual intercourse, the variations on these themes are infinite. A leg thrown over here, an arm positioned there, a hand fondling this, lips doing that can all slightly alter the sexual experience so that it differs from past experiences. Consequently this section can serve only as a guide, not the last word, on coital positions.

In addition to the desire for variety, other situations—such as pregnancy, obesity, or poor health—may dictate certain modifications. For example, it is more comfortable for a pregnant or obese woman to be on top rather than have her partner press down on her abdomen. Similarly, a man with arthritic knees may not be comfortable with his knees bent in the on-top position. In addition, some coital positions may influence the effectiveness of a condom—male or female. As an example, when the man lies on his back with the woman on top, there may be some seepage of semen from the condom, especially if it is not placed on the penis correctly. When the man is on top, this is not as likely.

1. *Man on top*. The man-on-top position (Figure 13.3) is sometimes called the "missionary position" or the male superior position. The position has a lot going for it: It allows full frontal body contact, which is usually pleasurable;

FIGURE 13.3 Man-on-top position.

(?) Did You Know . . .

Sex can be enjoyable at any age. Studies have found that the elderly engage in sex well into their 70s and 80s (Lindau et al., 2007). In a study of more than 100 white men and women aged 80 to 102 years who were living in retirement homes, there was more sex than you might imagine. Here are some of the findings:

1. The most common sexual activity was touching and caressing (82% of men and 64% of women). Masturbation was second (72% of men and 40% of women).

Sexual intercourse was third (63% of men and 30% of women).

2. Seventy percent of men and 50% of women said they often or very often fantasized or daydreamed about intimate relations with the opposite sex.

3. Only about 25% of men but almost 50% of women said they had no interest in sex.

Source: Ageless sex, *Psychology Today* (March 1989), 62.

FIGURE **13.4** Woman-on-top position.

Multicultural
DIMENSIONS

Does Level of Education Influence Sexuality?

Sexual practices vary greatly from person to person and from couple to couple. Yet, these practices seem to be influenced by education. Laumann and colleagues (1994) found that sex and education were related in the following ways.

1. Whereas 72% of men with any college education reported their last sexual encounter took between 15 minutes and 1 hour, only 61% of men with less than a high school education reported it took that long. With women, the results were comparable. Seventy-four percent of women with any college education reported their last sexual encounter took between 15 minutes and 1 hour, whereas only 60% of women with less than a high school education reported it took that long.

2. Although 81% of men and 78% of women with some college education reported having ever performed oral sex on a partner, only 59% of men and 41% of women with less than a high school education reported having ever performed oral sex on a partner. And although 84% of men and 82% of women with some college education reported ever having oral sex performed on them, only 61% of men and 50% of women with less than a high school education reported ever having oral sex performed on them.

3. In terms of anal intercourse, 28% of college educated men and 24% of college-educated women reported ever having that experience, whereas only 21% of men and 13% of women with less than a high school education reported experiencing anal intercourse.

It appears that being educated results in being less conservative sexually. Why do you think that is the case?

because the couple is lying down, their hands are free to roam; and because they are facing each other, partners can kiss, talk, and watch each other's expressions. This position is also considered the most effective for increasing the chances of pregnancy, but whether you call that an advantage depends on your circumstances. On the negative side, sexuality therapists do not recommend this position for men who have difficulty controlling ejaculation.

2. *Woman on top.* In the woman-on-top position, also called the female superior position (Figure 13.4), the woman can be either prone or on her knees. In either case this position permits more clitoral stimulation by either partner than the man-on-top position. Thus a woman who does not receive sufficient clitoral stimulation to achieve orgasm through coitus alone can reach orgasm through manual stimulation in this position while her partner's penis is inside her vagina. In this way she can experience the pleasure of orgasm around an erect penis while the man has the pleasure of feeling her orgasmic contractions on his penis. In addition, the woman is free to move rather than being pinned under her partner. This is a good position for men who are attempting to control their orgasms; the squeeze technique (described in Chapter 16) is easy to use because the penis is relatively accessible. Another advantage is that both partners' hands are free, allowing

them to caress each other. The one disadvantage of this position is that the effort by the man necessary for thrusting his penis can be tiring because the woman's weight is bearing down on his pelvis. Consequently women might do more of the movement in this position than in some others.

3. *Side-by-side.* In the side-by-side position (Figure 13.5), neither person is bearing the weight of the other. This is a relaxing position, because pelvic thrusts do not meet as much resistance as with the woman or man on top. However, because arms and legs may be pinned under other arms and legs, blood circulation can be temporarily cut off, making periodic switching or adjustment necessary for comfort. The side-by-side position also allows for kissing and face watching, and it too frees the hands for stroking and caressing. However, it is sometimes difficult to keep the penis in the vagina in this position, and even vigorous thrusting can result in little or no clitoral contact. Still, hands work well here too, as in the woman-on-top position.

4. *Rear entry.* The rear-entry position (Figure 13.6) can be performed in two ways: with both people lying down, either side-by-side or with the woman atop the man, or with the partners kneeling (called the "dog position" for reasons clear to anyone who has seen

FIGURE **13.5** The side-by-side position. Note the subtle variations that are possible.

 Did You Know . . .

In the most current comprehensive study of the sexual behavior of Americans (Michael et al., 1994), it was found that

1. The mean age of first intercourse has increased by about 6 months since the 1970s.
2. Whereas males report curiosity as the reason for having their first intercourse, females report affection for their partner as the primary reason.

3. Thirty-two percent of 18- to 24-year-olds report ever having only 1 sexual partner. However, 34% report having had 2 to 4 sexual partners, 15% 5 to 10 partners, 8% 10 to 20 partners, and 3% more than 21 partners. Males consistently have more sexual partners than do females. In fact, 17% of all males report having had more than 21 sexual partners.

FIGURE **13.6** The rear-entry position.

dogs copulating). In either case the male's hands are free to fondle his partner's breasts and stimulate her clitoris. The disadvantages of this position include the lack of face-to-face contact and the feeling of some people that they are being animal-like (others find this position sexually stimulating for this very reason). People who try the rear-entry position for the first time may be surprised by

the sound effects: Air may enter the vagina and produce noises when it leaves (some sexologists have termed this sound a "vart").

Once again we should say that the variety of coital positions is limited only by your imagination. Coitus, or any other sexual activity, can be pleasurable and exciting when the technique is pleasurable and exciting and when partners follow their inclinations. However, sexual techniques alone may not always be satisfying. The bond between sex makers that sometimes turns them into lovemakers can be as important as technique. A loving relationship of responsible people can add much to the pleasure obtained from sexual activity. Still, the very nature of sexual expression is pleasing, and it is obvious that sexual behavior can be enjoyed by people who are not in love but still care for each other. Whether such sexual behavior is moral or legal, however, is another issue, which depends on your ethics and society's—an issue discussed in Chapter 18.

Sexual Behavior of Homosexuals

With regard to the sexual activity of homosexuals, they enjoy most of the same activities as heterosexuals (Figures 13.7 and 13.8). One difference that has been noted, however (Tripp, 1976), is that intimacy and closeness seem to be more important than what is specifically done by the partners. Yet, more recently it has been reported that more gay men who have been living with a partner for 2 to 10 years have sex with someone other than their partner (79%) than do heterosexual males living with a partner 2 to 10 years (11%). In addition, gays tend to have more sexual partners than do lesbians (Peplau & Cochran, 1990; Blumstein & Schwartz, 1990). People seem to have stereotyped ideas of specific sexual acts in which homosexuals

participate (Spalding & Peplau, 1997). In contrast to these myths, both male and female homosexuals appear to take their time and make sexual activity last longer. They seem to prolong the pleasure rather than rush to orgasm (Masters & Johnson, 1979). Perhaps this is due to the fact that a person stimulating another person of the same sex can better understand what that person enjoys. Contrary to popular belief, male homosexuals do not generally have a preference to receive or insert the penis (Greenberg, 1973; Rathus, Nevid, & Fichner-Rathus, 2008, 300–301). Some people are under the misconception that one man plays the male and the other plays the female. This is not the case.

Masters and Johnson (1979), on the basis of their study of homosexuality, have reported a number of findings about the specific sexual behavior of homosexual men and women.

1. There are no major differences between the fantasy patterns of homosexuals and heterosexuals.

2. Homosexuality is learned and is definable only by overt behavior.

3. Homosexuality is a pattern of sexual interaction that a person can move into or out of at any time in life.

FIGURE **13.7** Gay men engage in varied sexual activities.

FIGURE **13.8** Oral and manual stimulation, and touching, are some of the sexual activities enjoyed by lesbians.

Communication
DIMENSIONS

Word Choice Affects Study Results

Some years ago Blumstein and Schwartz (1983) conducted a study of couples and how often they "have sex." Lesbian, male homosexual, heterosexual nonmarried couples, and heterosexual married couples participated. They reported that lesbian couples "have sex" far less frequently than any other type of couple and that lesbian couples are less "sexual" as couples and as individuals than anyone else. In their sample only about one-third of the lesbians in relationships of 2 years or longer "had sex" once a week or more; 47% of lesbians in long-term relationships "had sex" once a month or less, and among heterosexual married couples only 15% "had sex" once a month or less. They also reported that lesbians seemed to be more limited in the range of their "sexual" techniques than did other couples.

In commenting on the Blumstein and Schwartz study, Frye (1997) points out that what 85% of heterosexual married couples are doing more than once a month and what 47% of lesbian couples are doing less than once a month is not the same thing. She indicates that the comparison is not accurate because the focus has been on sexual activity whereby a penis is inserted. When the only activity that counts as "doing it" involves interactions that include some sort of penile activity, she says, it is "no wonder [lesbians] discover [themselves] to 'do it' rather less often than do pairs with one or more penises present."

Frye feels that we would get a clearer picture if we start with a wide field of passions and bodily pleasures and create meanings that weave a web across it. She says:

I suggest that we begin the creation of a vocabulary that can encode and expand our meanings by adopting a very wide and general concept of "doing it." Let it be an open, generous, commodious concept encompassing all the acts and activities by which we generate with each other pleasure and thrills, tenderness, and ecstasy, passages of passionate carnality of whatever duration or profundity. . . . Our vocabulary will arise among us as we explain and explore and define the pleasures and our preferences across this field, teaching each other what the possibilities are and how to make them real.

4. Physiologically homosexuals respond exactly as heterosexuals do to the same sexual stimuli—no sexual stimulus is unique to homosexuals.

5. Homosexuals are as amenable to treatment (with partners of their own choice) for sexual inadequacy as are heterosexuals.

6. Among established couples, homosexuals get more pleasure from lovemaking, even without intercourse, than do heterosexuals.

From a developmental standpoint, it is common for male and female homosexuals and bisexuals to have a history of sexual activity with the same and opposite genders, and to become sexually active during their early teens. No significant gender differences are found in lifetime prevalence rates or ages at initiating homosexual practices, but females tend to become sexually active at an older age than males and engage in more heterosexual activity. Sexual practices follow an initiation sequence beginning with manual sexual activity during their early teens and leading to further sexual activities during the middle and late teens (Rosario, 1996).

Lesbian Sexual Activities
In lesbian lovemaking, oral sexual activities are common, as are manual stimulation and tribadism. **Tribadism** is the rubbing of genitals against someone's body or genital area. Touching, caressing, and hugging—the emotional components of lovemaking—play a large role in lesbian lovemaking. Vaginal penetration with dildos is rare. In fact, lesbians tend to do more overall genital stimulation, rather than direct clitoral stimulation, as is often the case in heterosexual relationships (Masters & Johnson, 1979).

Gay Sexual Activities
Homosexual men engage in foreplay activities similar to those of heterosexuals, such as hugging, kissing, petting, and nipple stimulation. Anal intercourse is actually the least frequent male homosexual activity. More often, gay men participate in mutual masturbation or fellatio (oral sex). Laboratory studies by Masters and Johnson (1979) showed that gay men were likely to pay more attention to the area of the penis on the lower side than heterosexual couples.

tribadism
Rubbing genitals against someone's body or genital area.

Keeping It Going

College-age students sometimes wonder how long-term partners can maintain monogamous sexual relationships over many years. Doesn't it get stale after a while? Certainly, for some couples, it does. For many others, sex remains exciting and fulfilling. This must be the case if so many older people are still sexually active. For example, one study found that 60% of women ages 42 to 52 reported having regular sexual intercourse and 24% experienced oral sex on a regular basis (Cain et al., 2003). Another study conducted by the American Association of Retired Persons found that 19% of men 75 years of age or older have sexual intercourse at least once a week (AARP, 1999).

Although the frequency of sexual activity may decrease with age due to physical changes, such as taking longer to achieve an erection or vaginal lubrication, accommodations can be made to account for these changes. Foreplay may have to be extended, and the goal may have to be changed from achieving orgasm to intimacy and sexual pleasure.

In addition, as we've stated elsewhere in this text, variety can be vital in maintaining a satisfying sexual relationship over time. Some couples use sexual aids such as vibrators, others make use of pornographic materials to spice up their sex lives, and still others use sexual fantasy or role playing. In addition, long-term partners have learned what is sexually stimulating for each other, and the level of intimacy they develop over time goes a long way toward their still finding sex exciting.

Exploring the
DIMENSIONS
of Human Sexuality

Our feelings, attitudes, and beliefs regarding sexuality are influenced by our internal and external environments. Go to sexuality.jbpub.com/dimensions/4e to learn more about the biological, psychological, and sociological factors that affect your sexuality.

Biological Factors

- Sexual stimulation involves all five senses—touching, seeing, hearing, smelling, and tasting.
- Physical characteristics can enhance or inhibit sexual activities. For example, varying positions of intercourse offer varying degrees of comfort, depending on weight, physical stamina, or physical limitations.
- Foreplay allows for vaginal lubrication and erection before penile insertion.
- Physical disabilities may limit some sexual activities.
- Safer sexual activities decrease the risk of STI or HIV transmission.

Sociocultural Factors

- Sexual experience plays a role in what you find arousing.
- Sodomy laws prohibited certain sexual activities; however, these laws have been largely overturned.
- People who have more education tend to be less conservative sexually.
- Many religions prohibit certain sexual activities, such as premarital sex and masturbation. Pope John Paul II reaffirmed masturbation as an immoral act in 1993.
- School sexuality education programs often reflect community standards about what is perceived to be acceptable sexual behaviors. Parent and peer reactions to sexual information affect your perception of sexual activities.

Psychological Factors

- Emotional involvement with a partner plays a role in sexual pleasuring.
- Sexual fantasies are common among males and females.

CASE STUDY

Many factors influence what we find sexually arousing. Biologically, a physical disability may limit some sexual activities; however, it may also lead to other activities that are equally stimulating for a partner.

Psychologically, emotional attachment lends itself to sexual pleasuring. The greater the emotional attachment to someone we feel, often the greater the sexual pleasuring.

Schools play a broad role in developing our sense of what is acceptable or unacceptable. Community standards have an influence on what is taught, and that in turn influences student perceptions. Some fundamentalist religions ask young people to sign a public pledge to abstain from premarital sexual activity.

Communication is an important dimension. You and your partner need to be able to communicate which techniques you find sexually arousing. In addition, you must be able to communicate your love.

Family and friends influence sexual opinions as well. For example, comments by family and friends about Tiger Woods' affair may have influenced your perception of extramarital activity.

Summary

- Two autoerotic, or solitary, sexual behaviors are *masturbation* and *sexual fantasy*. These activities are considered normal with a majority of people engaging in them at one time or another. There are usually no negative physical or psychological effects of either.

- Some women report experiencing heightened sexual arousal when an area of the interior wall of the vagina is stimulated. This area is known as the *G spot,* named after Ernst Grafenberg who first discovered it. Although recent evidence has been found that might verify the presence of the G spot, experts still disagree as to its existence.

- *Foreplay* is usually the name given to the physical contact preceding coitus or oral sex. Foreplay includes touching, kissing, biting, and genital fondling. However, the term foreplay is a misnomer since it may not precede any other sexual activity but might be engaged in just for its own pleasure.

- Sexual stimulation involves all the senses: touch, sight, smell, hearing, and taste. Among these senses, the secretion of *pheromones*—substances that attract sexual partners—has long been recognized to be produced by animals. In the late 1980s, scientists verified the secretion of pheromones in humans as well.

- Oral–genital sexual behavior includes three activities. *Cunnilingus* is the oral stimulation of the female genitalia. *Fellatio* is the oral stimulation of the male genitalia. *Analingus*—commonly referred to as *rimming*—is the oral stimulation of the female or male anus.

- Sexual intercourse can include many different positions. Among the most prevalent of these are the man on top, the woman on top, side-by-side, and the rear entry positions.

- Homosexuals enjoy many of the same sexual activities as heterosexuals. Lesbian sexual activities often involve rubbing the genitals against someone's body or genital area. This is called *tribadism*.

- One of the challenges faced by long-term sexual partners is to remain monogamous over many years. Although the frequency of sexual activity may decrease with age due to physical changes, accommodations can be made to account for these changes. Foreplay may be extended, and a variety of sexual behaviors may be engaged in to spice up the relationship.

Discussion Questions

1. Discuss the many dimensions that shape current attitudes toward masturbation and fantasies. How do male and female fantasies differ?

2. Explore the role of the senses, oral–genital contact, and various intercourse positions and sexual stimulation. Describe how sexual contact with another person can be made safer.

Application Questions

Reread the chapter-opening story and answer the following questions.

1. Many people are surprised to find that such an erotic novel dates back to the mid-18th century. Given that your ancestors reproduced (if they had not, you would not be reading this text), why is it widely believed that sexuality in the 1700s was inferior to today's sexuality?

2. One major change in sexual techniques since the novel was written is the more common prevalence of oral–genital sex. What might have prompted such a change?

3. This novel, as well as *Lady Chatterly's Lover* and many others, was banned in Boston, meaning that the book was not allowed to be sold in the city. The ban was finally rendered legally useless by the mid-20th century. How do current efforts to ban or limit the distribution of sexually explicit materials differ from the efforts of our ancestors?

Critical Thinking Questions

1. If you are in a sexual relationship, is it inappropriate to masturbate? Some people believe to do so is to risk fantasizing about someone else, which is tantamount to infidelity; that it uses sexual energy that is better directed toward one's partner; and that it is an expression of dissatisfaction with one's partner, thereby insulting him or her. Others argue that masturbation has no effect on the sexual relationship; it is merely another means of sexual expression. They also believe that fantasizing about having sex with someone else is perfectly acceptable, as long as one doesn't act on that fantasy. Lastly, fantasizing can lead to uncovering new and exciting sexual activities that can be shared with one's partner. What do you think?

2. Is it better to do what is natural during sexual activity with a partner or to act according to what is learned in books such as this one?

Critical Thinking Case

The author Susan Minot, in her short story "Lust," mentions sexual technique: "I lay back with my eyes closed, luxuriating because he knew all sorts of expert angles, his hands never fumbling, going over my whole body, pressing the hair up and off the back of my head, giving an extra hip shove, as if to say *There*" (p. 15). But Minot continues the description as though the "expert" was very cold and unloving in his sexual activities.

Critics of sexuality education argue that knowing of the existence of the Grafenberg spot, erogenous zones, and the like makes sexual relationships too mechanistic. Each partner is trying so hard to recall what is stimulating and how to stimulate it that the spontaneity that makes sexual relationships so enjoyable is lost. People would be better off just "flying by the seat of their pants." Is that not the way sex has been conducted for eons? Have we not done all right with that system for generation after generation? Why add science to a nonscientific experience? Just lie back and enjoy yourself.

Others agree that sexual relationships have been adequate in the face of little knowledge of sexual arousal and response. However, they argue, adequate is not good enough. With knowledge of how the body is organized—for example, where nerve endings are accumulated—and how to achieve increased sexual excitement, sexual relationships could be enhanced. Further, there is nothing wrong with consciously, even during a highly emotional sexual encounter, thinking of how best to please your partner, because that means that your partner will be thinking of how best to please you. The result will be a more sexually satisfying relationship.

What do you think? Spontaneous sexual experiences or mechanistic ones? Thoughtless sexual experiences or thoughtful ones?

Exploring Personal Dimensions

Assessing Your Sexual Fantasies
Are your sexual fantasies similar or dissimilar to other people's sexual fantasies? In what ways are they similar? In what ways are they dissimilar? To find out, answer the following questions. A discussion follows.

1. Do you fantasize about sex? How often?
2. What do you fantasize about when you fantasize about sex?

3. Do your sexual fantasies when you are with your partner differ from those when you are alone? If so, describe the difference.
4. Do you discuss your sexual fantasies with anyone else? If so, why? If not, why not?

Discussion
In a summary of research on sexual fantasies that reviewed more than 200 studies, the *Washington Post* reported the following information. Compare your responses to the typical responses of other adults.

1. Men average seven sexual fantasies a day, five of these triggered by outside stimuli such as watching a beautiful woman and two by inner thoughts. Women average five sexual fantasies a day, three from outside stimuli and two from their internal selves.
2. Women's favorite sexual fantasies involve a new sexual partner, sex with a celebrity, and sex with either a younger man or boy or an older "gent." Men's sexual fantasies include observing women nude and having sex with a new partner, sex with multiple partners at the same time, and having the sexual prowess to "drive women wild."
3. When men and women are alone, their sexual fantasies tend to be of their usual sexual partner, if they have one. Ironically, though, when they are actually engaged in sexual activity with their usual sexual partner, they tend to fantasize about sex with someone else. Often, this fantasy involves a celebrity.
4. Because many men and women feel guilty about fantasizing about someone else while being engaged in sexual activity with their usual partner they do not discuss their sexual fantasies with their partner. A mere 26% of men and only 32% of women tell their sexual partner about their fantasies.

Well, how do you compare with the average adult female or male? Is there anything about your sexual fantasies that you will work to change?

Source: Tasker, F. X marks the fantasy, *The Washington Post* (July 27, 1995), D5.

Suggested Readings

Bakos, S. C. *The orgasm bible: The latest research and techniques for reaching more powerful climaxes more often.* Beverly, MA: Quiver, 2008.

Castleman, M. *Great sex: A man's guide to the secret principles of total-body sex.* Emmaus, PA: Rodale Press, 2004.

Davis, P. *The passion parties guide to great sex: Secrets and techniques to keep your relationship red hot.* Bel Air, CA: Broadway, 2007.

Deida, D. *The enlightened sex manual: Sexual skills for the superior lover.* Louisville, CO: Sounds True, 2007.

Foley, S. *Sex and love for grownups: A no-nonsense guide to a life of passion.* New York: Sterling, 2005.

Hooper, A. J., & Razazan, D. *Great sex games.* New York: DK Publishing, 2001.

Hutchins, D. C., & Sinclair, A. *The sensuous couple's (flip over) guide to seismic oral sex.* Philadelphia, PA: JPS, 2008.

Newman, F. *The whole lesbian sex book: A passionate guide for all of us.* San Francisco, CA: Cleis Press, 2004.

Paget, L. *The great lover playbook: 365 sexual tips and techniques to keep the fires burning all year long.* Bel Air, CA: Gotham, 2005.

Spurr, P. *Naughty tricks and sexy tips: A couple's guide to uninhibited erotic pleasure.* Berkeley, CA: Amorata Press, 2007.

Westheimer, R. K. *Sex for dummies.* New York: Wiley, John & Sons, 2001.

Web Resources

For links to the web sites below, visit *http://sexuality.jbpub.com/dimensions/4e* and click on Resource Links.

Good Vibrations
www.goodvibes.com

A web site that provides links related to sexual techniques and behaviors. Included are links to sex toys, sex education, erotic and informative books, adult DVDs, and other sexual-related materials. Products may be purchased at this web site.

Better Sex by the Sinclair Intimacy Institute
www.bettersex.com

The Sinclair Institute is a source of sexual health products for adults who want to improve the quality of intimacy and sex in their relationships. Among the products that can be acquired through this web site are adult movies, sex toys, and adult sex education materials.

About.com: Sexuality, Tips & Techniques for Better Sex
http://sexuality.about.com/od/tipstechniques/Tips_Techniques_for_Better_Sex.htm

Sexual tips and techniques from oral sex to masturbation, from female ejaculation to male multiple orgasms. Information for people of all sexual orientations, ages, and people living with disabilities. Topics include sexual intercourse positions, orgasm, masturbation, oral sex, and sexual fantasy and role play.

AllSex Guide
www.allsexguide.com

Offers links to matters pertaining to sex. Links include a guide to sex positions, learn to talk dirty, guide to having an orgasm—for women, lesbian sex, communication, erotic massage, and others.

SexualHealthConnection.com: Sex Tips and Advice
www.healthcentral.com/sexual-health/sextechniques.html

Recommendations for enhancing one's sex life. Among the topics included are speaking up for better sex, salvaging so-so sex, tantric sex, multiple orgasms, 5 steps to a healthy sex life, and 10 sexy gifts to give your partner.

chapter
I»N»T»E»R
FOCUS

Alternative Sexual Behavior

FEATURES

Communication Dimensions
Communicating Accurately

Gender Dimensions
Paraphilias and Gender Differences

Ethical Dimensions
The Ethics of Chemical Treatment for Paraphilias

CHAPTER OBJECTIVES

1 Discuss how some alternative sexual behaviors exist on a continuum of sexual activity.

2 Describe the most common paraphilias.

3 Name and define paraphilias other than the most common ones.

4 Explain what can be done to treat paraphilias.

5 Summarize what is known about sexual addiction.

sexuality.jbpub.com/dimensions/4e

The Most Common Paraphilias
Sexual Addiction

INTRODUCTION

*V*arieties of sexual behaviors have been around a long time, as have many opinions about them. Many people were surprised when a well-known sportscaster was indicted on charges of assault and sodomy. His accuser, a 41-year-old female friend whom he had known for 10 years, claimed that he viciously bit her several times on the back during an argument in his hotel room.

The woman claimed that her partner became enraged when she refused to join in a "three-way" with him and another man and that he threw her on the bed and bit her on the back 10 to 15 times. Then, according to court documents, he forced her to perform oral sexual activity. After the woman sought treatment at a local hospital, the police were notified.

To many, the charges against the sportscaster seemed very much out of character. For example, one of his producers said that on both a professional and a personal level he was a joy to be around. The executive producer of the network sports said he was "in total shock" about the charges.

As the allegations were investigated, additional stories came out about the sportscaster's sexual behavior, including his alleged fondness for wearing women's underwear and participating in threesomes. As a result, he was removed from sportscasting and taken off network shows. About three years later, he returned to broadcasting as the radio voice of a pro sports team.

Stories like this one cause people to wonder about varieties of sexual behavior and talk more about them. Although many varieties of sexual behavior are relatively uncommon, it can be important to know more about them.

Common Versus Atypical Sexual Behaviors

A few points about atypical sexual behavior in general should be noted before we consider specific behaviors. First, in many instances there are gradations of a sexual behavior existing on a continuum. For example, most people enjoy looking at other people. However, if someone spends many hours each day just looking at others, we would probably assume that person has a problem. There would be spots on the continuum between these two extremes that might be hard to judge. Is the behavior common or is it atypical? Is it acceptable or unacceptable? It is up to each individual, and society, to decide where on the continuum of sexual behavior activities become unacceptable. For instance, when is behavior obsessive (that is, the individual does not freely choose the behavior); when is it associated with emotional distress or with the inability to interact satisfactorily with other people; when is it forced on another person; when is it illegal?

Because many behaviors vary in degree, it is not surprising that many of us may recognize some degree of atypical behaviors or feelings in ourselves—perhaps only in private fantasies. In most instances, such behaviors or feelings should be accepted as natural—as long as they do not interfere with our optimal functioning or with the rights of others.

It is also common for us not to know a great deal about atypical sexual behaviors. Because in most cases such behavior is not common, and in most cases it is performed in private, it is difficult to study. Therefore, as we consider atypical sexual behaviors, many questions will be left unanswered.

It is also interesting that atypical sexual behaviors often occur in combination. For example, one well-known celebrity apparently did some cross-dressing along with participating in group sexual activity and violence.

Some people wonder about causes of paraphilias. Not a great deal is known about this topic, but theories can be grouped into psychoanalytical, behavioral, and sociobiological (Brannon & Carroll, 2008). Psychoanalytical theory centers on possible distortion of courtship phases. Some people are unable to adhere to socially acceptable norms and develop deviant or unconventional sexual practices. Behavioral theory attributes the development of certain paraphilias to the process of conditioning. For example, if nonsexual objects are frequently associated with a pleasurable sexual activity, the objects can become sexually arousing. In some cases, the constant threat of discovery may be as arousing as the act itself. Sociobiological theory includes the idea that even atypical sexual behavior relates to survival of the species. For example, different paraphilias may be responsible for enhancing society's level of sexual excitation. In turn, this increases the likelihood of people engaging in sexual acts that would ultimately lead to procreation.

Within this minichapter, we briefly discuss some of the most common atypical sexual behaviors. The more severe forms of sexual aggression (rape, incest, spousal abuse, sexual harassment, and child abuse) are discussed in Chapter 14.

The Most Common Paraphilias

Unusual or problematic sexual behaviors are scientifically known as paraphilias. **Paraphilia** means love (*philia*) beyond the usual (*para*). There are about 50 different paraphilias, and each exists in fantasy and in reality. It is generally accepted that the prevalence and variety of paraphilias are greater in males than in females, but as indicated previously, in most instances little is known about them.

Paraphilic behaviors are unconventional sexual behaviors that are obsessive and compulsive. They can interfere with love relationships and intimacy. Paraphilias are defined as recurrent, intense sexually arousing fantasies, sexual urges, or behaviors involving (1) nonhuman objects, (2) the suffering or humiliation of oneself or one's partner, or (3) chil-

> **paraphilia**
> Literally meaning "love (*philia*) beyond the usual (*para*)," this term refers to various sexual behaviors previously referred to as deviant.

 Did You Know ...

One theory suggests that paraphilias may be related to erotic target location errors (ETLEs), involving the erroneous location of erotic targets. For example, ETLEs may be responsible for people with preferred erotic targets such as children, amputees, plush animals, and real animals, to name a few.

Source: Lawrence, A. A. Erotic target location errors: An underappreciated paraphaliac dimension. *Journal of Sex Research 46, nos. 2 & 3* (March 2009), 194–215.

dren or other nonconsenting persons. Also, the behavior, urges, or fantasies cause significant stress in social, occupational, or other important areas of functioning. Some behaviors, such as sadomasochism, when they are consensual and do not impair life functioning, are not considered to be a paraphilia because they do not meet all of the diagnostic criteria (Coleman, 2005).

Paraphilias include sexual behaviors that many people view as distasteful, unusual, or abnormal and that they subsequently reject. In descending order, the most common are pedophilia (see Chapter 14), exhibitionism, voyeurism, and frotteurism. Far less common are fetishism, sexual masochism, sexual sadism, and transvestism (Paraphilias, 2005).

Exhibitionism

Exhibitionism (commonly called *flashing* or *indecent exposure*) occurs when an individual achieves sexual gratification by exhibiting the genitals to observers. The American Psychiatric Association (2005)

> **exhibitionism**
> Achievement of sexual gratification by exhibiting the genitals to observers.

has officially defined exhibitionism as "over a period of at least six months, recurrent, intense sexually arousing fantasies, sexual urges, or behaviors involving the exposure of one's genitals to an unsuspecting stranger." Though exhibitionism is a good example of a sexual behavior that is difficult to classify as one

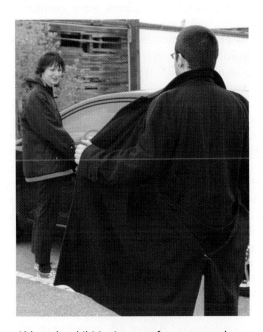

Although exhibitionists are often portrayed comically, in real life the phenomenon is quite different. Exhibitionists gain sexual pleasure from eliciting a harsh reaction to their unprovoked actions. It is best to ignore one if you are ever flashed.

that causes problems, we would probably agree that if someone's primary motivation in life is exhibitionism, that person has a problem. At what point does the behavior become abnormal?

There are three key features of true exhibitionism: (1) There is sexual arousal directly related to the shock; (2) the victim is unwilling; and (3) no further sexual contact is desired (Exhibitionism, 2005).

A few facts about exhibitionists might help to put this behavior into perspective. The exhibitionist receives sexual gratification through the victim's (observer's) response. Exhibitionists might achieve orgasm by the very act of exposure, but more likely they will masturbate either while exhibiting or later. Exhibitionists feel inadequate, they are afraid of rejection, they are shy, and commonly they have had unsatisfactory sexual relationships. They may be looking for attention or affirmation of their masculinity (most exhibitionists are male) or attempting to frighten others.

Although people often think exhibitionists are violent and aggressive, they usually are not. It is extremely rare for exhibitionists to do more than display the genitals. They do not want contact with a person. Punishment and imprisonment do not seem to prevent the recurrence of exhibitionism. Although it may be difficult, generally the best response is to ignore an exhibitionist and continue usual activities. In this way the exhibitionistic behavior is not reinforced.

Voyeurism

In a very general sense, the term **voyeurism** (or **scopophilia**, "love of viewing") means obtaining sexual pleasure from watching unsuspecting people undress or engage in sexual behavior. The American Psychiatric Association's (2000) official definition is "over a period of at least six months, recurrent, intense sexually arousing fantasies, sexual

> **voyeurism (scopophilia)**
> Obtaining pleasure from watching people who are undressing or engaging in sexual behavior.

urges, or behaviors involving the act of observing an unsuspecting person who is naked, in the process of disrobing, or engaging in sexual activity." A "peeping Tom" is a voyeur. The voyeur learns from experience where to find people to watch. His erotic excitement lies in the forbidden act of looking at the person.

The person who is being observed is nonconsenting, and not aware that he or she is being watched. The voyeur usually masturbates at the time he is watching or later while remembering the experience. Sexual contact with the person or persons observed is not sought. Because voyeurs do not hurt anyone and because they are secretive, they are rarely caught (Voyeurism, 2005). The fantasies, sexual urges, or behaviors cause clinically significant distress or impairment in social, occupational, or other important areas of functioning. Voyeurs derive sexual gratification from seeing sex organs and sexual acts (Brannon & Carroll, 2008).

Voyeurs, who are often shy and lonely and lack social skills, commonly fantasize about having sexual relations with the people they are watching and often masturbate while fantasizing. Voyeurs derive satisfaction from the fear of being caught, the anonymity of the person being watched, and the fact that the person does not know he or she is being watched. Generally voyeurs are not violent and, in fact, are fearful of any contact with the people they observe.

Some degree of voyeurism probably exists in everyone. Society even condones some forms of voyeurism; for example, some magazines are designed to satisfy peoples' voyeuristic tendencies, and the popularity of sexually explicit movies and web sites is due to voyeurism.

Obscene Communication

The most common and traditional form of obscene communication has been obscene telephone calls; through the years there have also been many exam-

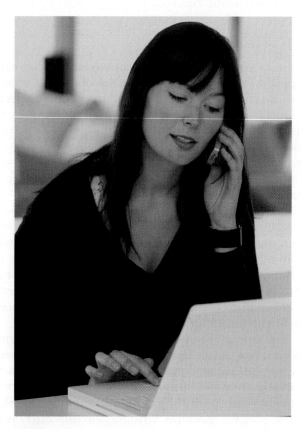

Females living in major metropolitan areas are the most likely victims of obscene communication.

ples of obscene letter writing. In more recent years obscene emails have appeared as well.

Erotic telephone calling is a form of erotic distancing. As do the exhibitionist and the voyeur, the obscene caller or writer obtains sexual pleasure from a distance and not from direct contact with another person. Telephone callers receive sexual gratification from making obscene remarks over the telephone, usually suggesting that the person meet them to have sexual relations (even though they would probably never go through with this act). The recipient may be a stranger or a consenting listener. Professional consenting listeners, trained to take part in erotic telephone fantasies, charge for playing this role.

In a national survey in Canada, Smith and Morra (1994) found that 83.2% of females had received obscene or threatening telephone calls at some time in their life. Divorced and separated females, young females, and females living in major metropolitan areas were most likely to have been victims of this harassment. The typical caller was an adult male unknown to the victim. The majority of the respondents said that the calls affected them emotionally, and the most prevalent response was fear. Katz (1994) found that in the 6 months preceding a national survey in the United States, 16% of women had received at least one call. Women younger than 65 years old and those who were neither married nor widowed were more likely to receive such a call. It appears that obscene calls occur in a pattern.

Obscene telephone callers have counterparts in those whose primary turn-on is not genital sexual activity with a partner but erotic narrations or readings. The obscene letter writer or the obscene computer message sender is hoping for sexual gratification as well.

According to the U.S. Department of Justice, "Any comment, request, suggestion, proposal, image, or other communication which is obscene or indecent, knowing that the recipient of the communication is under 18 years of age" is illegal. In addition, "any indecent communication for commercial purposes which is available to any person under 18 years of age or to any other person without that person's consent" is illegal. These offenses are punishable by a fine up to $50,000 for each violation or imprisonment of up to 6 months or both (United States Code Annotated Title 47, 2003). Note that this covers any telecommunication device, including computers.

What should someone who receives an obscene communication do? Above all, people are advised to remain calm and not reveal shock or fright: These reactions can reinforce the message sender and increase the likelihood of repeated contact. The recommended response is to say nothing and end the communication. Most people who send obscene

Communication
DIMENSIONS

Communicating Accurately

With any sexual behavior, the concept of consent is crucial. For example, if a partner wants to be tied up, that might be fine; however, prior communication about the goal is important. A student once confessed (under the influence of alcohol) to a group of people that she wanted to be tied up. Another time, though, she said that her fantasy really involved being tied down with silk ribbons to a luxurious four-poster bed. Still later she said that what she really wanted was a partner who would initiate sexual activity with her. Thus she did not always like being the aggressor, and her fantasy was really about having her lover "take charge." But in respect to her original assertions, that underlying desire would not have been known to a partner, nor would her desire for an initiating partner be fulfilled when she engaged in nonbondage activities. As always, effective communication is a must.

First, it is crucial to explain desires and intentions clearly in such situations. The student in our example was not clear, and this could have led to behavior or attempts at behavior that were not desired. This, in turn, could have caused overall relationship problems. Second, as with any form of sexual behavior, it is important to obtain consent. It is not enough to assume that you know what your partner meant or that consent is implicit because you have a good relationship. Without consent, sexual behavior is forcible. With consent, it can be enjoyable for everyone and contribute to a positive relationship.

---

messages are not dangerous, and most do not make repeat contacts with the same person. In the case of obscene phone calls, it might be helpful to get an unlisted phone number, obtain caller ID capabilities, and/or contact the police about threatening or repeated calls.

Masochism and Sadism

The American Psychiatric Association (2005) defines sexual masochism as "over a period of at least six months, recurrent, intense sexually arousing fantasies, sexual urges, or behaviors involving the act (real, not simulated) of being humiliated, beaten, bound, or otherwise made to suffer." It defines sexual sadism as "over a period of at least six months, recurrent, intense sexually arousing fantasies, sexual urges, or behaviors involving acts (real, not simulated) in which the psychological or physical suffering (including humiliation) of the victim is sexually exciting to the person."

Sexual masochism, therefore, is sexual gratification that results from experiencing pain. This might include scratching, biting, beating, and the use of various devices. The pain involved must be planned as a part of an overall experience; accidentally hitting a finger with a hammer is not the kind of experience the masochist wants. **Sexual sadism** occurs when an individual gets sexual gratification from inflicting pain on another person—the hallmark of sadism is intentional torture of the victim to sexually arouse the offender. Sadists have persistent fantasies in which sexual excitement results from inflicting psychologi-

cal or physical suffering (including humiliation and terror) on a sexual partner. At its most extreme, sadism involves illegal activities such as rape, torture, and even murder, in which case the death of the victim produces sexual excitement (Paraphilias, 2009). Sadists obviously make good partners for masochists, but sadomasochistic partner matching is difficult to achieve because it requires that the fantasies of the two people match completely. There is one sadistic scenario, however, that requires an unsuspecting partner or a stranger to be subjected to abuse. Sadism does not seem to be as common as masochism.

Domination and degradation are important to both the sadist and the masochist. Some psychiatrists feel that sadism is an expression of anger and hostility. Masochism, in contrast, is sometimes thought to result from a belief that sexual activity is dirty and evil; therefore, the activity could be viewed as just punishment for sexual sins. It is difficult to understand the true psychology of these behaviors.

Sadomasochism is a paraphilia that combines both sadistic and masochistic sexual behavior. The main characteristic is the eroticizing of pain. What appears to the outsider to be painful is experienced as somewhat painful but mostly pleasurable and very sexually arousing to the sadomasochist. Sadomasochistic sexual encounters usually occur in the context of scripted scenes that simulate interactions between master and

> **sexual masochism**
> Sexual gratification that results from experiencing pain.
>
> **sexual sadism**
> Sexual gratification that results from inflicting pain on another person.

bondage perversion
Getting sexual pleasure from being bound, tied up, or otherwise restricted.

transvestite
A person who achieves sexual satisfaction from wearing clothes usually worn by the other gender.

slave, employer and servant, and parent and child. Sadomasochists tend to alternate between masochistic and sadistic roles. In milder forms, dominance and submissive behaviors may be found in many relationships or may be an element of fantasy life (Sadomasochism, 2001).

There is more information available on masochism and sadism than on most other paraphilias, and a brief chronological review of a few studies will help to shed some light on these two behaviors. Baumeister (1997) pointed out that masochism fosters temporary escape from the stressful awareness of one's ordinary identity. Litman (1997) suggested that sexual masochism is more widespread and can be more dangerous than current literature indicates. Danger can arise from being humiliated, endangered, and enslaved and being physically bound, restrained, and rendered helpless to the degree that life is threatened. He indicates that **bondage perversion** (deriving pleasure from being bound, tied up, or otherwise restricted) can be fatal—a mix of suicide and accident.

Sexual masochism is more common in males, but the incidence in females is on the rise. Masochists often seek partners to tie up, humiliate, blindfold, or hurt. They may enjoy being whipped, beaten, shocked, or cut. Verbal abuse is common. Some masochists require pain or humiliation to function sexually (Masochism, 2001). Some sadists also require the pain or humiliation of a partner to function sexually. As long as it occurs with a consenting partner, sadism is not considered a psychological disorder. It is considered a disorder when it causes the person unhappiness or causes problems with work, social setting, or family. If the other person is not willing, sadism can be a severe and even criminal disorder. Sadism is much more common in males (Sadism, 2001). People who engage in masochism and sadism must be especially careful about diseases transmitted by body fluids, such as hepatitis and HIV.

Masochism can range from mild to extreme versions. Examples of mild versions might include bondage (being tied up for the purpose of sexual arousal), or being spanked or overpowered by physical force. The crucial point is that they are mainly symbolic enactments done under carefully controlled conditions with a trusted partner. At the opposite end of the spectrum are genuinely painful and harmful activities (Discovery Health: Paraphilia, 2005).

Sadism can also be a consensual activity in milder forms. For example, it might involve role-playing with dominant and submissive roles such as master and slave. Like masochism, however, it is important to have controlled conditions with a trusted partner to avoid unplanned injuries. Sadism is commonly found in association with other paraphilias—particularly masochism, fetishism, and transvestism (Sexual sadism, 2005).

Sadism and masochism are good examples of sexual behaviors in which we need to differentiate between fantasy and behavior. For example, many more people have reported sexual fantasies involving masochism and sadism than have actually participated in such behavior. It is possible to enjoy a sexual fantasy without needing to act it out in real life.

Transvestism

Transvestism is sometimes confused with transsexualism and homosexuality. A **transvestite** takes pleasure in wearing clothing of the other gender and is likely to achieve sexual gratification from doing so but has no interest in having a sex-change operation or in relating sexually to members of the same gender. While transvestites may be male or female, they typically are heterosexual married males (Brannon & Carroll, 2008).

Transvestism is also known as cross-dressing or dressing in drag. Some homosexual men dress in drag

Transvestites can be of many different sizes and have various appearances.

for fun. Some people with a gender identity disorder dress in clothes of the other gender to try to pass as the other gender or because they simply feel that is their proper gender. Transvestites, however, generally cross-dress for sexual arousal. Most are male and do not wish to be mistaken for women. Transvestism is considered to be a psychological disorder only when the person meets the following conditions (Transvestism, 2005). He:

- Is heterosexual, or straight.

- Has intense sexual fantasies, urges, or behaviors involving dressing in women's clothing.

- Is distressed by these fantasies, urges, or behaviors and they cause problems in his life.

Some transvestites cross-dress only periodically, and the use of female clothes (most transvestites are males) may approximate a fetish. Others may wear female clothing under their male clothes. No one knows for sure why some people are transvestites, and it is interesting to note that most transvestites have quite normal heterosexual relationships.

Most transvestites begin to experiment with cross-dressing when they are children or adolescents. Some feel guilty and uncomfortable about this preference; others do not. Many are happily married to people who understand their behaviors. Others have had relationships ruined by cross-dressing. There are numerous support groups for transvestites and their partners (Transvestism, 2001).

It is common for transvestism to be classified as a fetish. It is usually done in private, although undergarments can also be worn in public under regular street clothes. Transvestites will often masturbate while wearing female clothing and/or make-up while fondling specific items. Transvestism, by itself, is usually not associated with criminal behavior, although it could be combined with other fetishes or disorders that result in criminal behavior (Transvestic fetishism, 2005).

Fetishism

Fetishism is a paraphilia in which an inanimate object elicits sexual arousal. Articles of clothing and materials made of rubber, silk, fur, or leather are common fetishistic objects. The American Psychiatric Association (2005) defines the symptoms of fetishism as "over a period of at least six months, recurrent, intense sexually arousing fantasies, sexual urges, or behaviors involving the use of nonliving objects. The fantasies, sexual urges, or behaviors cause clinically significant distress or impairment in social, occupational, or other important areas of functioning."

The fetishist may masturbate while engaging in

Various items, articles of clothing, and materials can be fetishistic objects.

fetishistic behavior or may just enjoy stimulation from the objects. In a related paraphilia, **partialism**, people are aroused by a particular body part (breasts, muscular chests, feet, and so on). Most fetishes are practiced in private or with a willing partner.

> **fetishism**
> Paraphilia in which an inanimate object elicits sexual arousal.
>
> **partialism**
> Paraphilia in which sexual arousal is associated with a particular body part.

Generally, a person who has fetishism must have the fetish present to become sexually excited. It usually begins in childhood or adolescence and is most common among males. Although many people are aroused by undergarments or other items, this is not considered fetishism except when a person cannot perform sexually unless the partner is wearing the items (Fetishism, 2001).

The fetish may replace sexual activity with a partner or may be integrated into sexual activity with a willing partner. When the fetish becomes the sole object of sexual desire, sexual relationships often are avoided (Paraphilias, 2009). Most fetishes and partialisms are harmless. However, occasionally someone may commit burglary to obtain the fetish object.

Inanimate object fetishes can be categorized into two types: form fetishes and media fetishes. In a form fetish, it is the object and its shape that are important, such as with high-heeled shoes. In a media fetish, it is the material from which the object is made that is important, such as silk or leather. Although the list of objects that fetishists can use for sexual gratification is inexhaustible, among the more common inanimate objects are panties, bras, slips, stockings or panty hose, negligees, shoes, boots, and gloves. Common media objects include leather, rubber, silk, and fur. In most cases, the person with a fetish is no danger to others and pursues the use of the fetish objects in private, usually through masturbation. The causes of fetishism are not clearly understood. Some experts believe that it develops from early childhood experiences, in which an object was associated with a particularly powerful form of sexual arousal or gratification (Fetishism, 2005).

■ Other Paraphilias

Bestiality

Bestiality (or **zoophilia**) is sexual contact with animals. In Kinsey's research (1948, 1953), about 8% of males and 4% of females reported having had sexual experiences with animals at some time. The frequency of bestiality was higher (17% for males) for those raised in rural areas. Men most often had sexual contact with farm animals; women most often had sexual contact with household pets.

> **bestiality**
> Sexual contact with animals—also called *zoophilia*.
>
> **zoophilia**
> Sexual contact with animals—also called *bestiality*.

Human sexual relationships with animals have been an interesting topic for some people for hundreds of years. Stories of human–animal contact are found throughout ancient folklore. For example, Zeus, in the form of a swan, had sexual intercourse with Leda, the queen of Sparta. Greek and Roman mythology portrayed females having sexual relationships with bears, apes, bulls, goats, horses, wolves, snakes, and crocodiles. Historically, taboos against human–animal contact have been severe. The laws in many states treated bestiality as a felony. In eight states, the maximal penalty was life imprisonment. Many such laws remain on the books today (Bestiality, 2003).

Sexual experience with animals is usually only a transitory experience for young people who do not have acceptable sexual partners. It most likely occurs during adolescence, and most people move on to more common adult sexual relations with humans. It is generally agreed that a condition is really zoophilia only if someone prefers sexual contact with animals even if other forms of sexual activity are available.

There has been very little research on bestiality. Even though it has been present throughout history, addressing the subject often seems to evoke prejudices and emotional reactions rather than objective reflection. A large part of the information on bestiality stems from criminological reports, and this is a very limited sampling (Beetz, 2004).

Frottage

Frottage is the act of obtaining sexual pleasure from rubbing or pressing against a nonconsenting person. The American Psychiatric Association's official definition (2000) is "over a period of at least six months, recurrent, intense sexually arousing fantasies, sexual urges, or behaviors involving touching and rubbing against a nonconsenting person." It is likely to occur in crowds, on elevators, and in buses and subways. It is even possible that the frotteur will achieve orgasm. Women and girls, the usual recipients, generally find this behavior offensive. Normally no additional contact or other form of behavior follows.

Necrophilia

Necrophilia is a rather rare behavior in which a person receives sexual pleasure from viewing or having sexual relations with a dead person. Sometimes necrophiliacs (almost all of whom are men) pay women to pretend to be dead so as to provide sexual pleasure. This might even include dressing in a certain way, using white powder to look very pale, and lying very still. In this way the participants are simulated corpses.

Necrophiliacs are usually severely emotionally disturbed, sexually and socially inept, and hate and

The overcrowding of subways in Tokyo and other Japanese cities lends itself to frottage, or deriving sexual pleasure from rubbing up against a nonconsenting person. The situation is exacerbated by the male-dominated Japanese culture, which prevents police from dealing with the problem.

> **frottage**
> Obtaining of sexual pleasure from rubbing or pressing against another person.
>
> **necrophilia**
> Sexual relations with a dead person.

fear women. Although local newspapers do not report instances, law enforcement officers indicate that bodies are sometimes stolen for this purpose.

It is interesting to note that necrophilia was depicted within the range of normal expression in the television program, *Buffy the Vampire Slayer*. The sexual encounter of Buffy with Angel, two characters in the show, was presented as the natural culmination of their love for each other. The fact that Buffy was technically making love to a corpse was overlooked entirely by the audience. Over the years, a staple of the show was Buffy's relationship with vampire lovers—first Angel and then Spike. The connection between love and death and the acceptance of the undead or necrophilic lover was presented (Spaise, 2005).

Troilism

Troilism is having sexual relations with another person while a third person watches. In one respect, troilism combines elements of exhibitionism and voyeurism. In another respect, it represents an illusion of prostitution (Money, 1984) because there are elaborate ruses and pretenses of prostitution. An example might be a husband's inviting another man to have intercourse with his wife. The husband watches and is able to get an erection. He then achieves penetration and orgasm, which are not possible unless his wife plays the role of a prostitute.

Troilism clearly does not qualify as a safe sexual activity. Because multiple partners are involved, this is a high-risk activity.

Asphyxiophilia

Asphyxiophilia is the desire for a state of oxygen deficiency to enhance sexual excitement and orgasm. It has also been called *erotic* or *autorerotic suicide, sexual suicide, autoerotic strangulation, autoerotic asphyxiation, hypoxophilia,* and *autoerotic accident*. Most information about asphyxiophilia is found in reports from police or doctors of forensic medicine who examine people who have died during this behavior (Innala & Ernulf, 1989).

Self-induced oxygen deficiency is used to produce sexual euphoria, increased excitement, or heightened orgasm during masturbatory activities. Reduced supply of oxygen to the brain results in giddiness, lightheadedness, or exhilaration that is reported to enhance sexual climax (Burg, 1987).

Oxygen deficiency can be induced in many ways. Because the circumstances and features of autoerotic deaths are not commonly known, they are often misinterpreted as suicides or homicides. And death can easily result, because cutting off the flow of blood to the brain can produce unconsciousness in as little as 5 to 10 seconds. Although the person probably did not intend to die, death results when an escape mechanism fails or the person cannot recover from self-induced oxygen deprivation.

> **troilism**
> Having sexual relations with another person while a third person watches.
> **asphyxiophilia**
> Desire for a state of oxygen deficiency to enhance sexual excitement.
> **klismaphilia**
> Sexual arousal produced by the use of enemas.

Conservative estimates indicate that 500 to 1,000 autoerotic fatalities occur each year in the United States and that such deaths are steadily increasing. The majority of the victims are adolescents and young adults, almost all are male (96%) and white (94%), and most (73%) are not married (Bechtel, Westerfield, & Eddy, 1990).

Asphyxiophilia is really a subcategory of sexual masochism. Although not unheard of for it to be practiced with a partner, it is usually done as a solitary act. The practice is intended to produce sexual pleasure, but practitioners are well aware of the inherent risk element. Because of that, they use some kind of safety mechanism to prevent accidental death in the event of unconsciousness. There is no evidence that deaths from asphyxiophilia are a form of disguised suicide. Such deaths are a complete surprise to family and friends. Nearly all reported deaths have been males, and most under 40 years of age. However, the practice can begin at puberty for some. There are no known signs of predisposition to this behavior or the existence of the paraphilia. In many cases of death from asphyxiophilia, the cause of death has been attributed to suicide even though that is not what happened (Hypoxyphilia/auto-erotic asphyxia, 2005).

Klismaphilia

In **klismaphilia** sexual arousal is obtained from enema use. Klismaphiles most often prefer the receiving role, but less commonly erotic arousal may be associated with administering an enema. The background of many individuals who show klismaphilia often indicates that as infants or young children they were frequently given enemas by concerned and loving mothers. This association with loving attention, or perhaps even sexual pleasure, learned early in life may eroticize the experience for some people, so they show a need to receive an enema for sexual satisfaction as adults. Because klismaphilia involves anal contact, it is not a safe sexual activity unless latex gloves are used and there is great attention to cleanliness.

Coprophilia

In **coprophilia**, sexual pleasure is associated with feces. People who show coprophilia reach high levels of sexual excitement by watching someone defecate or by defecating on someone. The connection of feces with sexual arousal may also go back to childhood. Some children seem to enjoy holding back on a bowel movement and then carefully expelling the feces. It could also be that the connection between changing of soiled diapers and sexual stimulation during infancy eroticizes feces. Because it appears that HIV can be present in any body tissue or fluids, coprophilia is not a safe sexual activity.

Urophilia

In **urophilia**, sexual pleasure is associated with urine. Similarly to coprophilia, the person may want to urinate on someone or be urinated on. Again, as with coprophilia, there may be childhood beginnings for urophilia. For example, stimulation of the urethra during urination may become associated with pleasure, or there may have been stimulation from the changing of wet diapers. Urophilia has been referred to as "golden showers" or "water sports." Urophilia is not a

coprophilia
Sexual pleasure associated with feces.

urophilia
Sexual pleasure associated with urine.

safe sexual activity because HIV and other STIs can be transmitted through urine.

◼ Treatment for Paraphilias

A number of issues surface when one considers treatment for paraphilias. For example, people with paraphilias often do not want treatment. Also, they often feel they cannot control their urges, so they cannot accept personal responsibility for their actions. However, personal responsibility is usually a prerequisite for successful behavior change. In addition, some helping professionals think it is not their responsibility to provide treatment for paraphilias—they believe it is the responsibility of the criminal justice system. In spite of these issues, it is appropriate to consider what might be done to help those with paraphilias. Possible treatments fall into three categories: (1) psychotherapy, (2) behavior therapy, and (3) pharmacological approaches (drug therapy).

Psychotherapy

Not much information is available about successful treatment of paraphilias by psychotherapy. The purpose of psychoanalysis is to discover unconscious conflicts that are believed to originate in childhood. If conflicts can be drawn to the surface and resolved, the hope is that the particular behavior can be changed.

Gender DIMENSIONS

Paraphilias and Gender Differences

Because it is hard to find accurate statistics about the incidence of paraphilias, it is also difficult to find a great deal of information about paraphilias and gender differences. Although we know that the majority of paraphilias occur among men, here is a brief summary of what is found in the literature on this topic.

1. Janus and Janus (1993) reported that
   a. Eleven percent of both men and women have had experience with bondage.
   b. Six percent of men and 4% of women have participated in urophilia.
   c. Eleven percent of men and 6% of women have engaged in fetishistic behaviors.
   d. Six percent of men and 3% of women report cross-dressing.

2. Kinsey, Pomeroy, and Martin (1948, 1953) reported that
   a. Eight percent of men and 3% of women had experienced at least one sexual contact with animals.
   b. Twenty-two percent of males and 12% of females in their sample responded erotically to stories with sadomasochistic (SM) themes.

3. Regarding voyeurism, Person and associates (1989) reported that
   a. Among college students, 23% of women and 38% of men have watched their partners masturbate.
   b. Eleven percent of women and 18% of men have performed sexual acts in front of mirrors.
   c. Five percent of women and 4% of men have watched others engage in sexual intercourse.

Group therapy involves breaking through the denial so commonly found in people with paraphilias by surrounding them with others who share their condition. Once they begin to admit that they have a sexual divergence, the therapist begins to address individual issues such as past sexual abuse or other problems that may have led to the sexual disorder. When these issues have been identified, individual therapy may be used to help patients get past the guilt and shame that might be associated with their particular paraphilia (Brannon & Carroll, 2008).

Behavior Therapy

Behavior therapy applies learning principles to help people change their behavior. Many techniques have been used to help change paraphilic behavior. For example, in systematic desensitization the therapist tries to break the link between a sexual stimulus (such as leather for a fetishist) and the inappropriate response (sexual stimulation). The client is taught to relax muscle groups so that relaxation replaces sexual arousal in response to the stimulus.

In **aversion therapy** the undesirable behavior (such as masturbation for a voyeur) is paired repeatedly with a negative stimulus, such as a painful (but harmless) electric shock. The objective is that negative reactions to the paraphilic behavior will develop.

In **social training** the individual is helped to improve his or her social skills. It is hoped that if the person can better relate to people, he or she will be able to develop sexual relationships that would be considered more typical.

In **orgasmic reconditioning** the goal is to increase sexual arousal by socially appropriate stimuli. For example, if the person becomes sexually aroused by masturbating, as he or she approaches orgasm, "socially appropriate imagery" such as pictures of attractive people would be used. The hope is that orgasm will then be connected with these images and not the paraphilic ones.

Drug Therapy

Although no drug can eliminate paraphilic behavior, some chemicals can sometimes be helpful in reducing the intensity of sexual drives and establishing an environment for more successful treatment using one of the other approaches. For example, Prozac, which is commonly used for treating depression, has been used to help some people reduce obsessions and compulsions. Also, **antiandrogen drugs**, chemicals that reduce the sex drive by lowering the testosterone level in the bloodstream, can reduce sexual desire and erections in males. Such a drug is Depo-Provera, which must be injected weekly to be effective. However, even Depo-Provera does not change the nature of sexual stimuli for people; it only reduces the intensity of their reactions.

The International Association for the Treatment of Sexual Offenders was founded in 1998. It is

behavior therapy
Applying learning principles to help people change behavior.

aversion therapy
Pairing an undesirable sexual behavior with a painful response.

social training
Improving a person's social skills.

orgasmic reconditioning
Increasing sexual arousal to socially appropriate stimuli.

antiandrogen drugs
Chemicals that reduce the sex drive by lowering the testosterone level in the bloodstream.

Ethical DIMENSIONS

The Ethics of Chemical Treatment for Paraphilias

Is it ethical to force paraphilic sex offenders to take hormones or tranquilizers to reduce their drives for paraphilic behaviors? Although in some cases Depo-Provera reduces the paraphilic sex drive to a level that allows the person to have a more normal sex drive, in others it causes a complete elimination of the sex drive—meaning that the individual has almost no interest in any sexual behavior.

One difficulty is that some paraphilics enjoy their behavior. Therefore, they do not want treatment because they do not view their behavior as a problem.

Some experts would argue that chemical treatment for paraphilic offenders should be required to protect other people from them. Others feel that such treatments should be required only for people who have paraphilias that violate the rights of others or harm them.

When faced with the possibility of arrest or imprisonment, paraphilic sex offenders could waive their right of informed consent and sign up for treatment just to avoid legal action. It can be difficult to balance the right of society to be protected from harm against the right of a person to avoid being given chemicals that may have undesired side effects.

committed to advocate for humane, dignified, compassionate, ethical, and effective treatment of sexual offenders. It also is interested in furthering knowledge about individual and social conditions that lead to sexual offenses, and in improving treatment methods. Members of the organization are convinced that punishment is not a sufficient deterrent for sexual crimes, and that treatment will result in the reduction of sexual crimes and is a human right (Pfafflin & Eher, 2003).

Sexual Addiction

In 1998 President Clinton's sexual activity stirred up the debate over "sexual addiction." The idea that some people might have very strong, or even insatiable, sexual needs has been around a long time. The term **nymphomania** refers to an excessive, insatiable sexual drive in women. The same condition in men is referred to as **satyriasis**, or **Don Juanism**. Many professionals have argued about the appropriateness of these labels for years. They contend that the labels should not be used at all because judgments about how much sexual behavior is "normal" or "excessive" are subjective.

nymphomania
An excessive, insatiable sexual drive in women.

satyriasis
An excessive, insatiable sexual drive in men—also called *Don Juanism*.

Some experts believe that sexual addiction is mainly a male abnormality caused by childhood trauma that usually requires intense psychotherapy. Many others say this is nonsense because there is no such thing as too much sexual behavior, unless it is with the wrong partner. They say that some people who have the symptoms do not experience conflict and are not really troubled by it. Still others are concerned that use of the label *sexual addiction* may help people inappropriately excuse their behavior.

Obviously, most people engage in various forms of sexual activity without it becoming disruptive related to other behaviors. Some experts argue that some people become addicts because of changes in the chemistry of the brain. Other experts believe that this view is not correct, and the question of whether addicts experience differences in the way their brains work is still hotly debated (Bodo, 2008).

Dodge et al. (2004) found that college students who are sexually compulsive are more likely to participate in sexual behaviors that are high risk in terms of HIV and STI infections. Bancroft and Vukadinovic (2004) reported that out-of-control sexual behavior seems to result from a variety of mechanisms. They also said that sexual addicts

tend to experience increased sexual interest when they are depressed or anxious about something.

Sexual addiction can involve a wide variety of practices. They can include compulsive masturbation, multiple affairs, multiple or anonymous sexual partners and/or one-night stands, consistent use of pornography, unsafe sexual behaviors, phone or computer sex, prostitution or use of prostitutes, exhibitionism, obsessive dating through personal ads, voyeurism, sexual harassment, and molestation/rape (Sexual addiction, 2009.) Sometimes an addict has trouble with just one unwanted behavior, sometimes with many. As in other addictions, the sexual addict experiences powerlessness over a compulsive behavior. The addict may wish to stop but repeatedly fails to do so. The consequences can be loss of relationships, difficulties with work, arrests, financial troubles, a loss of interest in matters not sexual, low self-esteem, and despair (What is sexual addiction?, 2003).

Among the writings about sexual addiction have been several books by Patrick Carnes, who outlines 10 practical and useful indicators of compulsive sexual behavior.

1. A pattern of out-of-control behavior
2. Severe consequences caused by sexual behavior
3. Inability to stop despite adverse consequences
4. Persistent pursuit of self-destructive or high-risk behavior
5. Ongoing desire or effort to limit sexual behavior, usually at a partner's insistence
6. Sexual obsession and fantasy as a primary coping strategy

Cybersex addiction has become more common in recent years.

Did You Know . . .

Sexual Addiction Recovery Resources

Email Groups

Sex/Porn Addiction: *S-panon@ontos.usa.com*
Addiction research and treatment: *Addict-L@listserv.kent.edu*
Internet addiction support group: *listserv@netcom.com*
Open self-help discussion: *solution@sjuvm.stjohns.edu*

Resource and Recovery Sites

www.soberrecovery.com/
www.sexhelp.com
www.addictionresearch.com
www.gentlepath.com

National Resources

Sex Addicts Anonymous (SAA)
www.sexaa.org
(713) 869-4902
PO Box 70949
Houston, TX 77270

Sex and Love Addicts Anonymous (SLAA)
www.slaafws.org/
(210) 828-7900
1550 NE Loop 410, Suite 118
San Antonio, TX 78209

Sexual Compulsives Anonymous (SCA)
www.sca-recovery.org
(212) 606-3778
1-800-977-HEAL
PO Box 1585, Old Chelsea Station
New York, NY 10011
email: *info@sca-recovery.org*

Source: Sex Addiction Help. Available: www.sexaddicthelp.com/Links/index.htm.

7. Increasing amounts of sexual experience because the current level of activity is no longer sufficient

8. Severe mood changes related to sexual activity

9. Inordinate amounts of time spent in obtaining sexual activity, being sexual, and/or recovering from sexual experience

10. Neglect of important social, occupational, and/or recreational activities caused by behavior

The main way to identify any addictive behavior is to consider whether it is causing negative or unwelcome problems and yet the person continues it anyway. Sexual addicts are often unable to make and keep commitments to themselves and others about stopping or changing particular sexual behaviors over the long term, and most have problems with real intimacy.

In more recent years, one form of sexual addiction is cybersex addiction. There may be many symptoms of cybersex addiction; common symptoms are (1) spending increasing amounts of online time focused on sexual or romantic intrigue or involvement, (2) failed attempts to cut back on frequency of online sexual involvement, (3) online use that interferes with work and personal life, (4) secretiveness or lying about the amount of time spent on online sexual activity, and (5) a primary focus of sexual activity related to computer activity (Cybersex addiction checklist, 2001).

Most addicts live in denial of their addiction. Success in treating addiction depends on the person accepting and admitting that he or she has a problem. In many cases, like with other addictions, it takes a significant event—such as the loss of a job, the breakup of a marriage, or an arrest—to force the addict to admit his her or her problem (Sexual addiction, 2009).

Even though there is no agreement about how to deal with compulsive sexual activity—if it can be done at all—organizations have been formed to help people deal with their activities if they feel there is a problem; for example, there is a 12-step program modeled after Alcoholics Anonymous called Sex and Love Addicts Anonymous (Braanon & Carroll, 2008). Other such groups are called Sex Addicts Anonymous, Sexaholics Anonymous, and Sexual Compulsives Anonymous.

The initial process of treatment can be divided into three major stages: (1) identification of the problem, (2) behavior contracting (clearly defining specific sexual behaviors that are to be eliminated and how this will be done), and (3) relapse prevention (e.g., providing support, managing stress, improving relationships, working out financial and other problems). Recovering addicts require external sources of social reinforcement and support for changing lifelong patterns of behavior (How to approach treatment of the sexual addict, 2001).

Summary

- Because many sexual behaviors vary in degree, it is not surprising that many of us recognize some amount of atypical behaviors or feelings in ourselves.

- There is not a great deal known about atypical sexual behaviors.

- The most common paraphilias are exhibitionism, voyeurism, obscene communication, masochism and sadism, transvestism, and fetishism.

- Other paraphilias include bestiality, frottage, necrophilia, troilism, asphyxiophilia, klismaphilia, coprophilia, and urophilia.

- Possible treatments for paraphilias fall into three categories: psychotherapy, behavior therapy, and drug therapy.

- Some people have very strong, or even insatiable, sexual needs and may be sex addicts. Most treatment programs for sexual addiction resemble treatment programs for people addicted to other behaviors.

Discussion Questions

1. Describe how sexual feelings or behaviors vary from common to atypical along a continuum.

2. What are the most common forms of paraphilia? Describe the type of person who might practice them.

3. What are the less common forms of paraphilia? Discuss why someone would practice them.

4. Describe the major types of treatment programs for paraphilias, including the ways they work and their effectiveness.

5. Is "sexual addiction" a true disorder? Explain your answer.

Application Questions

Reread the chapter-opening story and answer the following questions:

1. In spite of his well-publicized sexual behavior, the sportscaster's fiancée married him. Would you have advised her to go through with the wedding? Explain your answer.

2. Discuss the issues of safer sex surrounding the sexual acts engaged in by the sportscaster.

3. In addition to causing immense embarrassment, the sportscaster's sexual habits cost him his job (and probably some friends as well). What might have caused him to take such risks? Which therapies are available to help him with his atypical behaviors?

Critical Thinking Questions

1. Look over the American Psychiatric Association's definitions for the varied paraphilias, supplied throughout the chapter. What are the common elements? On the basis of that information, how would you define "atypical sexual behavior"?

2. Given that the pornography industry takes in about $2 billion per year, are we a nation of voyeurs? What differentiates a diagnosed voyeur from someone who views porn? Explain your answers.

Critical Thinking Case

Bill and Anne, college juniors, were in a monogamous relationship for about 5 months when Bill said that he wanted to add some "variety" to their sex life. Anne's immediate reaction was to feel that she was not giving Bill enough sexual satisfaction, so she did not respond to his suggestion. As much as she loved Bill, she felt unsure about his request for variety.

After he broached the subject several more times, she finally asked him what he wanted. He said that a former girlfriend had enjoyed having another girl join them from time to time. Anne was initially aghast at the idea of including a third person, especially a girl. But a few months later, Anne and a female friend had a brief sexual encounter after drinking heavily. Anne did not enjoy it. When she told Bill what had happened, he reacted sharply: What was she doing with another sexual partner?

Why did Bill react as he did? What did Bill really want from the encounter—another girl for his girlfriend or a threesome for himself? Why was it important for him to communicate correctly what he wanted?

You want something your partner does not want. How do you approach it? How do you make sure you are comfortable?

Exploring Personal Dimensions

Respond about only your sexual activity. If you do not participate in any sexual activity, skip this assessment. Check the following items that apply to you.

_____ 1. I tell my partner what feels good.

_____ 2. I tell my partner what hurts, if anything.

——— 3. I avoid frequent sexual encounters because I do not like them.

——— 4. I let myself just go with my feelings and behave the way I want to act during sexual encounters.

——— 5. My partner and I have talked about and resolved how often to have sexual activity.

——— 6. Sexual activity is a problem for me and my partner.

——— 7. I have told my partner what I want during sexual activity.

——— 8. My partner and I enjoy holding hands, kissing, and just talking as much as we do having sexual activity.

——— 9. It is important that each time we express love or go on a date that it culminate in sexual intercourse to be a really meaningful experience.

Scoring

Give yourself the following points for the items you check, and total your score.

1.	2	4.	2	7.	2
2.	2	5.	2	8.	2
3.	−2	6.	−2	9.	−2

Interpretation

This exercise indicates whether you have healthy communication in your sexual relationship. Interpret your score as follows:

6–10 = Your communication is healthy.

0–5 = Your communication is moderately healthy.

−1–−6 = You need to improve your communication skills.

Source: Bruess, C., & Richardson, G. *Decisions for health.* Madison, WI: Brown & Benchmark, 1995.

Suggested Readings

Abracen, J. Developments in the assessment and treatment of sexual offenders: Looking backwards with a view to the future. *Journal of Interpersonal Violence, 20, no. 1* (January 2005), 12–19.

Accordina, M. P., & Hewes, R. L. Investigation of Internet use, sexual and nonconsensual sensation seeking, and sexual compulsivity among college students. *Sexual Addiction and Compulsivity: The Journal of Treatment and Prevention, 14, no. 4* (December 2007), 321–335.

Adams, K. M. Cybersex: The "crack cocaine" of sex addiction. *The National Psychologist,* 2007. Available: http://www.nationalpsychologist.com/articles/art_v17n3_3.htm.

Cloud, J. Bondage unbound. *Time, 163, no. 3* (January 19, 2004), 104–106, 109.

McBride, K. R., Reece, M., & Sanders, S. A. Using the Sexual Compulsivity Scale to predict outcomes of sexual behavior in young adults. *Sexual Addiction and Compulsivity: The Journal of Treatment and Prevention, 15, no. 2* (2008), 97–115.

Paraphilias. Sexual Conditions Health Center. *WebMD,* 2009. Available: http://www.webmd.com/sexual-conditions/paraphilias-overview.

Web Resources

For links to the web sites below, visit *http://sexuality.jbpub.com/dimensions/4e* and click on Resource Links.

BDSM Backroom
www.bcwsd.com/backroom

Contains information about bondage, dominance, sadism, and masochism for those who are curious about what BDSM is and want to learn more about it.

The Fetish Information Exchange
www.fetishexchange.org

Provides knowledge about a number of fetishes. Contains many additional sources of information including web sites about fetishes.

Society for the Scientific Study of Sexuality: What Sexual Scientists Know About Compulsive Sexual Behavior
www.sexscience.org/publications/index.php?category_id=440&subcategory_id=334

Summarizes scientific information about compulsive sexual behavior.

The Society of Janus
www.soj.org

The Society of Janus is a support and educational group for people interested in learning about BDSM. It emphasizes safe, consensual, and nonexploitative activities.

Discovery Health: Paraphilia
http://health.discovery.com/centers/sex/sexpedia/paraphilia.html

Contains information about many forms of atypical sexual behavior.

Psychology Today: Paraphilias
www.psychologytoday.com/conditions/paraphilias.html

Contains information from *Psychology Today* about various paraphilias and their treatment.

CHAPTER 14

Forcible Sexual Behaviors

CHAPTER OBJECTIVES

1 Differentiate among rape, statutory rape, stranger rape, and date (acquaintance) rape. Discuss what makes someone rape. Discuss the myths surrounding rape.

2 Discuss pedophilia, including the profile of the pedophiliac, incidence and effects of pedophilia, and prevention.

3 Describe the incidence of incest and the typical effects on incest victims.

4 Summarize important information about violence in marriage, including marital rape and domestic abuse.

5 Discuss sexual harassment in the workplace, in schools, on campus, and in the military, and indicate what can be done to prevent and deal with it.

sexuality.jbpub.com/dimensions/4e

Social Responses to Rape
Incidence of Pedophilia
Domestic Violence
Sexual Harassment

INTRODUCTION

After a discussion about forcible sexual behavior in my sexuality class, a female student who was in her late 20s asked to go to my office to talk for a few minutes. When we got there, she said that she had found the information and the discussion on forcible sexual behavior interesting and enlightening. She also said she was feeling personally troubled because it reminded her of something that had happened to her. She then told me about it.

She remembered when she was 15 years old. She said she was a typical middle-class high school girl. Although her parents and her teachers did not say a lot about sexuality, she had heard quite a bit about rape on TV and seen stories about it in magazines and newspapers. Her parents, as had many of her friends, warned her about being careful and about not trusting strangers. She dated Ed, a neighbor who lived just a block away. Ed's parents and her parents sometimes got together socially, and they had been friends for at least 10 years. Ed's parents had always been friendly to her, too, and she probably saw them at least two or three times each week.

Ed was 2 years older and a star basketball player. He was an excellent student and considered a leader and one of the most popular boys at school. She remembered that he had always seemed to be one of the best athletes as they were growing up. After a few dates, they had started to become intimate. She enjoyed the closeness with him and found him very attractive. She had some tears in her eyes when she said that on one date, after an exciting basketball game, he had intercourse with her while she was crying and asking him not to do it. Although he was a little forceful, he did not raise his voice and he did not hit her. He just paid no attention to what she was saying.

At the time she said she did not realize it was rape. She asked him why he was doing this to her, but he did not answer. Afterward she did not want to date him anymore, and her parents wondered why. Her friends thought she was crazy not to want to go out with him. She said she had not told anyone about this before, but that she just had to get it out. When we talked about forcible sexual behavior in class, all the memories rushed back to her.

Many readers of this chapter are probably survivors of forcible sexual behavior—whether it was rape, child sexual abuse, sexual harassment, or another form of forcible sexual behavior. Sometimes it can be difficult and painful to think about these topics. However, most people, such as the student in our story, find it helpful to learn more about such topics and to deal more directly with their feelings about them.

Throughout this text it has been recognized that many sexual behaviors exist and that various factors contribute to these behaviors. Most often people voluntarily choose a particular behavior, but some sexual behaviors are not voluntary. In this chapter we focus on rape and child sexual abuse because of their seriousness. By no means, however, are these the only forcible sexual behaviors. Other representative forcible sexual behaviors are also considered. A characteristic of all these behaviors is that we know very little about them because of their obvious secretive and private nature. Although knowledge about forcible sexual behavior has rapidly increased, a great need for continued study and research is evident.

■ Sexual Violence

Sexual violence is a serious problem that affects millions of people each year. The victims of sexual violence are at increased risk of being abused again. Sexual violence perpetrators are also at increased risk of perpetrating again. Statistics about sexual violence are given throughout this chapter. It is important to remember, however, that statistics about sexual violence vary due to differences in definition and how data are collected. Such data usually come from police, clinical settings, nongovernmental organizations, and survey research (Sexual violence: Fact sheet, 2005).

For more than 20 years, researchers have noted that sexual violence is a relatively common experience. For example, at least 20% of all females in the United States will be victims of sexual violence during their lives. It is a life-altering experience for many who experience sexual violence. The effects are often experienced long after the event, with many psychological, physical, and behavioral consequences such as STIs, chronic pain disorders and other physical ailments, as well as anxiety, depression, substance use, sexual problems, and interpersonal difficulties being documented in survivors of sexual violence. Even though much is known, there is a need for continued work related to research, public policy, providing treatment and prevention services, and educating the public about sexual violence. For example, it is known that childhood sexual abuse is one of the best predictors of sexual victimization in adulthood (Marx, 2005). Knowing this and other important facts will help people better understand and deal with sexual violence.

Sexual assault and abuse is any nonconsensual sexual activity, including:

- Inappropriate touching

- Vaginal, anal, or oral penetration

- Sexual intercourse after you say no

- Rape

- Attempted rape

- Child molestation

Sexual assault can be verbal, visual, or anything that forces a person to join in unwanted sexual contact or attention (What is sexual assault?, 2005).

Each year the American College Health Association surveys more than 28,000 college students about a variety of behaviors related to their health. In a recent year, 4% of males and 9% of females were sexually touched against their will. One percent of males and 4% of females said sexual penetration (vaginal, oral, or anal) was attempted against their will. One percent of males and 2% of females said they were sexually penetrated (vaginal, oral, or anal) without their consent. About 4% of each gender reported verbal threats for sexual activity against their will (American College Health Association, 2009).

As can be seen from these numbers, both males and females can be victims of sexual violence. It is true that females are victims far more often than males, and males are perpetrators of sexual violence much more often than females. Nevertheless, it is estimated that 1 out of every 6 boys will be sexually assaulted by age 16. Adult men are also victims of sexual violence. The experience of sexual assault can be very confusing for men because our society and culture often associate sexual assault with women (Porche, 2008).

◼ Rape

Rape is a forcible act. Legal definitions of rape and law enforcement procedures for handling rape cases are changing, and they differ from state to state. However, a practical definition of **rape** is "forcible sexual intercourse." This can include forced oral sexual activity, penile–vaginal sexual activity, and anal sexual activity. If a person is forced to do any of these things when he or she does not want to, that is rape.

The United States has the highest incidence of rape in the Western world—about one-half million reported cases per year. More than 90% of the victims are female, and 99% of the perpetrators are male. Almost all rapes (88%) are committed by people who

are the same race as their victims. Rapists may or may not be psychologically disturbed or have criminal records. Women are raped almost exclusively by someone they know or to whom they are related. Only 4–5% of rapes are stranger initiated (Middleton, 2002).

Within the category of rape, there are several types. For example, **statutory rape** is intercourse with a person who is younger than the age of consent (ranging from 14 to 18 years from state to state). Even with consent, statutory rape is considered to have occurred if one of the participants is not of legal age. **Stranger rape** is rape of a person by an unknown assailant. If a rape is committed by someone known to the victim, it is **acquaintance rape**, or **date rape**, both of which are discussed later in this chapter.

1 IN 4 WOMEN WILL BE RAPED IN HER LIFETIME.

WILL IT BE YOUR MOTHER, YOUR SISTER, YOUR DAUGHTER OR YOUR WIFE?

The statistics won't improve if you pretend they aren't true. Help stop the violence. Call 920-4642 for information.
The Violence Against Women Coalition

As a female, what can you do to improve your odds of preventing rape? As a male, what can you do to make sure you never are involved in forced sexual activity?

Rape Myths

In spite of the increased attention given to the topic of rape in recent years, rape myths remain prevalent (see Myth vs. Fact on pages 519–520). It is important for people to know the facts about rape to help reduce some related problems. For example, some of the more prevalent rape myths include that women lead men on and therefore deserve to be raped, women often make false accusations of rape, no woman can be raped against her will, and most rapists are strangers. *All of these statements are false!* We know that men tend to believe rape myths more than women, that those who believe rape myths are more likely to assign blame to the victim, and that those who believe rape myths are more tolerant of the rapist

rape
Forcible sexual intercourse with a person who does not give consent.

statutory rape
Intercourse with a person younger than the legal age of consent.

stranger rape
Rape of a person by an unknown person.

acquaintance rape
Rape by a friend, acquaintance, or date; also known as *date rape*.

and less tolerant of the victims (Notice to readers: Sexual Assault Awareness Month, 2005).

Society and Rape

Some people have wondered whether particular characteristics of a given society help promote rape. Even after many years of research, we don't have a definitive answer to this question. The United States has the highest rape rate among Western countries, but the reasons for this are not clear. Some people feel that the reasons may relate to the relative roles of males and females, the presence of pornography that endorses and legitimizes rape, and the fact that rape is a crime of violence in an already violent society. Others feel that these characteristics have nothing to do with the issue.

Rape is one of the most underreported crimes. This makes it difficult to accurately count the number of cases. Some researchers believe that as many as 84% of victims do not report sexual assault to the police. A primary reason given for the underreporting is cultural norms that stigmatize and blame victims for their assaults (Notice to readers: Sexual Assault Awareness Month, 2005).

Victims of rape are generally viewed more sympathetically by females than by males, and by whites more than by African Americans. However, the effect of race disappears when socioeconomic variables are controlled. Younger people and those with higher education levels are also more likely to view sexual assault victims more sympathetically (Nagel et al., 2005).

More than half (55.6%) of sexual assault victims wait years before disclosing the incident, with delays in reporting especially likely if the assault was done by a family member (42.5% of the assaults are initiated by family members). About half of the victims (51.3%) have been previously sexually assaulted, yet only 9% sought treatment. Most (69.4%) indicate they will not be filing charges against perpetrators. Psychological symptoms such as depression and anxiety are the most common reasons for eventually seeking care at a sexual assault center (Monroe et al., 2005).

Related to information already discussed about rape myths, those who score higher on a rape myth acceptance scale blame the victims of sexual assault more and are less likely to believe rape did occur (Mason & Riger, 2004). In addition, there are different responses to a marital rape scenario where the victim was dressed somberly or seductively. In one study, males rated the victim more deserving of the attack than did females. The suggestively dressed victim was rated more responsible and deserving than the somberly dressed victim. Also, those holding more traditional attitudes toward marriage assigned more victim responsibility and deservingness than those with more egalitarian attitudes (Whatley, 2005).

In Australia, the declining rate of convictions for sexual assault is attributed to the fact that juries are reluctant to convict in situations where victims know their attackers. Particularly problematic is the issue of whether there was consent. At least some of the blame for this is placed on romance novels. Traditionally, although not as common today, heroines typically rejected sexual advances, only to be overcome and later admit that they had really welcomed the advances (Philadelphoff-Puren, 2005).

Although sexual assault against women has received increasing attention over the past decades, the sexual assault of the elderly has not been well addressed. Print media and the Internet regularly report on these cases and the crises and trauma that follow for the victim and their families. Elderly victims of sexual violence represent a vulnerable and poorly understood population. They may be sexually assaulted in their homes or communities, in an assisted living facility, or in a nursing home environment. Offenders can be strangers, domestic partners, family members, nursing home residents, or caregivers. There is a need for education about sexual abuse of the elderly (Burgess & Morgenbesser, 2005).

 Did You Know . . .

Rape as a Weapon of War

Organized rape has been an integral aspect of war for a long time. In war rape, a male soldier attacks a civilian woman and does this indirectly with the aim of holding or taking a territory. The main purpose is to inflict trauma and through this to destroy family ties and group solidarity within the enemy camp. Rape is the mark of sovereignty stamped directly on the body. Through war rape, something is introduced within the woman's body (sperm or forced pregnancy), transforming her into someone who is rejected by the family, excluded by the community, and often the object of self-hate, sometimes to the point of suicide. The penetration of the woman's body works as a metaphor for the penetration of enemy lines (Diken & Laustsen, 2005).

Apparently, steps need to be taken to reduce the cultural acceptance of violence and to restructure male and female sex roles to specify equality, warmth, and supportiveness. In the past, male dominance, toughness, and violence have often been emphasized. A restructuring of the relationships between genders might reduce the high incidence of rape in American society. Steps to reduce your personal risk of sexual assault are found in Table 14.1.

The Rapist

The topics of rape and rapists are hot-button issues in American society. Some theorists argue that rape is an act of uncontrolled passion or the result of a lack of sexual partners; others suggest that it is an extreme expression of male power and violence. For others, rape is a biologically driven phenomenon whereby men forcefully try to maximize the number of women with whom they procreate.

Most rapists rape to be aggressive, to wield their power, or to degrade the victim. In most instances their motivations and satisfactions are not sexual. In fact, it is unlikely that they achieve any sexual satisfaction from the act of rape.

Many experts have developed theories about why people commit rape. For example, some believe that rape occurs to enhance the offender's sense of masculinity and power, while others believe that the rapist is angry toward women or men and wants to hurt, humiliate, or degrade someone. Still others believe that sadistic rapists may be sexually aroused in response to assault and violence, or that, for some rapists, sexual offenses may be only one component of an extensive criminal history.

It is also possible that the reasons for a rape might vary depending on the situation. For example, perhaps with separated couples, the rape might be used to punish the victim. Or, in a dating situation, the rape might occur as part of a feeling of conquest. The reason an individual commits rape can be difficult to determine in each particular instance.

According to McCabe and Wauchope (2005), there are four main types of rapists: the anger rapist, the power exploitative rapist, the power reassurance rapist, and the sadistic rapist. The anger rapist displays his anger in overt ways, such as by using a knife, using force, displaying overwhelming anger, and projecting a macho image. Even though in general rapists do not seriously harm their victims, this type can inflict serious injury, and their rage is not related to sexual satisfaction. Their anger may also be expressed as a way to humiliate victims and put them in their place.

The power exploitative rapist seems to be motivated by a desire to display hostility and power over victims by assaulting them because of his own inadequacies, particularly a sexual dysfunction or a physical deformity. The motivation seems to be domination and control of the victim sexually even though he likely has difficulties with sexual performance. This

---

TABLE 14.1 **How Can I Protect Myself from Being Sexually Assaulted?**

There are things you can do to reduce your chances of being sexually assaulted. Here are some tips from the National Crime Prevention Council (*www.ncpc.org*):

- Be aware of your surroundings—who's out there and what's going on.
- Walk with confidence. The more confident you look, the stronger you appear.
- Don't let drugs or alcohol cloud your judgment.
- Be assertive—don't let anyone violate your space.
- Trust your instincts. If you feel uncomfortable in your surroundings, leave.
- Don't prop open self-locking doors.
- Lock your doors and your windows, even if you leave for just a few minutes.
- Watch your keys. Don't lend them. Don't leave them. Don't lose them. And don't put your name and address on the key ring.
- Watch out for unwanted visitors. Know who's on the other side of the door before you open it.
- Be wary of isolated spots, like underground garages, offices after business hours, and apartment laundry rooms.
- Avoid walking or jogging alone, especially at night. Vary your route. Stay in well-traveled, well-lit areas.
- Have your key ready to use before you reach the door—home, car, or work.
- Park in well-lit areas and lock the car, even if you'll be gone only a few minutes.
- Drive on well-traveled streets, with doors and windows locked.
- Never hitchhike or pick up a hitchhiker.
- Keep your car in good shape with plenty of gas in the tank.
- In case of car trouble, call for help on your cellular phone. If you don't have a phone, put the hood up, lock the doors, and put a banner in the rear mirror that says, "Help. Call police."

Did You Know . . .

What should you do if you've been sexually assaulted? Here are tips from MedicineNet.com (*http://medicinenet.com*). Take these steps right away:

- Get away from the attacker to a safe place as fast as you can. Then call 911 or the police.
- Call a friend or family member you trust. You can also call a crisis center or hotline to talk with a counselor—for example, the National Sexual Assault Hotline at 800-656-HOPE (4673) or the National Domestic Violence Hotline at 800-799-SAFE (7233). It is important to get help from a trusted professional.
- Do not wash, comb, or clean any part of your body. Do not change clothes if possible, so the hospital staff can collect evidence. Do not touch or change anything at the scene of the assault.

- Go to the nearest hospital emergency room as soon as possible. You need to be examined, treated for any injuries, and screened for possible STIs or pregnancy.
- You or the hospital staff can call the police from the emergency room to file a report.
- Ask the hospital staff about possible support groups you can attend right away.

How can you help someone who has been sexually assaulted? Listen and offer comfort. Go with her or him to the police, the hospital, or counseling. Reinforce the message that she or he is not at fault and that it is natural to feel angry and ashamed.

Public awareness of rape and its accompanying trauma has been raised in media depiction. An early appearance of a true-to-life rape situation appeared in the sitcom *All in the Family*. During the episode, which was written and developed by rape counselors, Edith Bunker is raped in her own home. The show, plus the publicity it created, helped many real-world victims to step forward.

Most rapists rape to demonstrate power and not to obtain sexual satisfaction.

rapist gains power by targeting one of the victim's most vulnerable points. This results in dominance and control of the victim.

The behavior of the power reassurance rapist may be very similar to that of the power exploitative rapist. The main difference is that the motivation of the power reassurance is reassurance of his own status and abilities.

The sadistic rapist is motivated to assault because of sexual and aggressive fantasies. He may make excessive use of anger, force, and restraints. This rapist wants to live out personal fantasies on an unwilling victim. Except for their sadism and their greater amount of planning, these rapists can be very similar to anger rapists.

McCabe and Wauchope (2005) also point out that there is an overlap of characteristics among types of rapists, making the picture very complex.

Rapists commonly give excuses for their behavior. Some justify their actions in various ways. Others point out that sexual assault is not their fault because it is beyond their control. Some excuse their behavior because of the presence of alcohol or drugs. Still others feel their behavior was appropriate in the situation. Finally, some feel that their victims "got what they deserved."

Date Rape

Date rape, or acquaintance rape, is much more common than most people realize, although because of its nature gathering reliable data on this topic is difficult. It is suspected that some incidents of date rape might be a result of poor communication, because many people still have a difficult time talking about sexuality. At any rate, it might help those dating to realize the following: Spending money on a date does not justify expecting sexual favors; a person who participates in other forms of sexual behavior does not necessarily find intercourse acceptable; and if a date uses sexual behavior as a means of proving masculinity or femininity, it might be better to date other people.

Unfortunately, forced sexual contact has always happened between dating partners. Women often blamed themselves for "leading a date on." It was

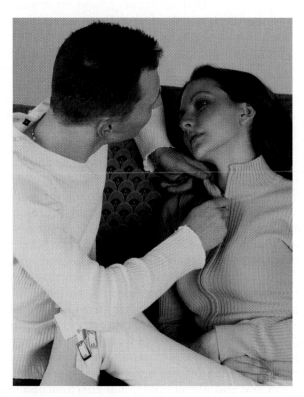

In cases of rape on college campuses, about 80% are committed by an acquaintance.

Myth vs Fact

Myth: Rape is an impulsive act of passion—meaning that men cannot control their sex drive.
Fact: Rapists themselves do not see rape as compulsive sexual behavior. The objective for rape is not usually sexual pleasure; it is to have power and to commit violence. Sexual activity is used to carry out nonsexual needs.

Myth: Women want to be raped—meaning that women have fantasies that reflect their desire to be raped.
Fact: Rape is an act of violent aggression. No healthy individual desires to be dehumanized and violated.

Myth: Women ask to be raped—meaning they tempt the man. "She should have worn a bra," "Hitchhikers get what they deserve," and "She shouldn't have been out so late at night" are examples of this thinking.
Fact: The blame and responsibility for a criminal assault are the assailant's, not the victim's.

Myth: A woman can run faster with her skirt up than a man can with his pants down—meaning a woman cannot be raped against her will.
Fact: Rape is an aggression committed under force or the threat of force on an unconsenting person. A knife, gun, or even verbal threat is often understandably stronger than a person's will.

Myth: You cannot blame a man for trying—meaning the responsibility for stopping a man is the woman's; therefore, it is her fault if matters get out of hand.
Fact: A criminal, not a victim, is responsible for criminal acts. Rape is not an impulsive act of passion. It is done for power and control.

Myth: The rapist is usually of a different race from the victim—meaning rape usually reflects ethnic or racial hatred.
Fact: In most instances the rapist and the victim are of the same race.

not until the mid-1970s that the term *date rape* was coined and women had legal rights to go after assailants they had dated.

Some statistics related to date rape are included in the periodic Youth Risk Behavior Surveillance (YRBS; Eaton et al., 2008). With regard to dating violence, during the 12 months preceding the survey, approximately 10% of students in grades 9 through 12 had been hit, slapped, or physically hurt on purpose by their boyfriend or girlfriend. Overall, the prevalence of dating violence was higher among African American students (14%) than among Hispanic (11%) and white (8%) students. Nationwide, 8% of students had ever been physically forced to have sexual intercourse when they did not want to participate. Overall, the prevalence of having been forced to have sexual intercourse was higher among female (11%) than male (5%) students, and higher among African American (11%) and Hispanic (9%) than white (7%) students.

While experts do not understand a great deal about date rape, many researchers have studied the topic. Because of the relationship of date rape to

Myth (vs) Fact

Myth: If a woman is going to be raped, she might as well relax and enjoy it—meaning it is just sexual activity.

Fact: Rape victims experience intense psychological and physical trauma. Rape is a violent, dehumanizing, and intimate invasion of a woman's privacy and integrity as a human being. The motive for rape is power; it is not sexual enjoyment. Rape is anything but enjoyable!

Myth: Most rapes are committed by strangers—meaning we are safe with people we know.

Fact: It is common for the rapist and the victim to know each other, to have been acquainted, or at least to have seen each other on the street, in the grocery store, in the student union, and so on.

Myth: It's not sexual assault if it happens after drinking or taking drugs.

Fact: A person under the influence of drugs or alcohol does not cause others to assault him or her. Many state laws say that a person who is impaired due to the influence of drugs or alcohol is not able to consent to sexual activity.

Myth: A person who has really been sexually assaulted will be hysterical.

Fact: Victims of sexual violence can show a wide variety of responses, including calm, hysteria, withdrawal, anger, apathy, denial, and shock. Reactions and the length of time needed to work through the experience vary.

Myth: Only young, attractive people are assaulted.

Fact: Sexual assault is a crime of power and control, and offenders often choose people they view as vulnerable to attack or over whom they believe they can assert power. Victims come from all walks of life and represent all ages—including males, females, and persons with disabilities.

Myth: Men can't be raped.

Fact: About 92,700 men are raped each year in the United States

Myth: I don't know anyone who's ever been raped.

Fact: Rape victims are doctors, lawyers, nurses, military personnel, cooks, accountants, or anyone. Fewer than one-third of sexual assaults are reported to the police.

---

overall dating violence, information about the two topics is often put together in research studies. From these studies we know that the vast majority of rapes on college campuses are committed by someone with whom the victim is acquainted. Many are committed on dates, and drinking alcohol and date rape often go together. Many women who are date raped do not report the assault to authorities because of feelings of self-blame and embarrassment.

Weiss (2002) studied women who experienced date rape, but did not acknowledge it to be rape. She pointed out that women often do not recognize date rape because of gendered stereotypes and classic rape scripts that preclude date rape as real rape. She found that such women tend to blame forces outside of the partner's rational control while denying that a sexually coercive incident actually occurred.

Lipman (2002) looked at women's relational and sexual functioning following date rape. She found the major themes of distrust of men, generalized disbelief, belief that intimacy is emotional, lack of pleasure in sexual activity immediately following date rape, lack of desire to participate in sexual activity immediately following date rape, feeling powerless, protection of the perpetrator, and symptoms of rape trauma syndrome. She also found the minor themes of change in the expectations of relationships, increased assertiveness about sexual wants with a current boyfriend, and change in current enjoyment of sexual activity. Immediately following date rape, victims distrusted men, blamed themselves for the rape, and continued to engage in sexual intercourse with their perpetrators even though they reported decreased sexual pleasure and desire for sexual activity. Women in the study who had pre-rape sexual experiences had positive post-rape relational and sexual experiences. However, the women who had not engaged in sexual intercourse prior to their rapes continued to report lack of pleasure and desire for sexual activity.

Putman (2002) looked at college students' perceptions of date rape. She found females and those with prior victimization indicated higher levels of victim empathy than did males and those without prior victimization. Females were more likely to report prior victimization than were males.

Howard and Wang (2003) reported that girls who were victims of dating violence were more likely to be involved in other violent behaviors. They were also more likely to report extreme sadness and suicidal actions, to use illicit substances, and to engage in risky sexual behavior. Dating violence was also associated with sad and hopeless feelings.

Kuck and Johnson (2003) presented date rape scenarios to respondents who were asked to "sentence" the convicted date rape offender. There was a lack of general consensus among the respondents and a wide range of sentences for the offender. There was little difference between male and female responses. There was a considerable amount of "blaming the victim."

Abbey et al. (2003) studied alcohol's effects on perceptions of a potential date rape. College students were randomly assigned to drink alcohol, drink a placebo beverage (a beverage they thought was alcohol, but was not), or drink a nonalcoholic beverage. All three groups read a story about a couple who had been drinking together at a party. The story ended with the woman saying "no" to sexual intercourse and the man exerting verbal pressure. Participants in the alcohol drinking group perceived the woman as being more sexually aroused and the man as behaving more appropriately than did participants in the other two groups. The researchers concluded that alcohol influences decisions related to sexual activity on dates.

Jimenez and Abreu (2003) had Hispanic and Caucasian undergraduates react to a rape vignette that manipulated victim and perpetrator race. Women reported higher perceptions of empathy than men, ascribed more credibility toward the rape victim, and were less accepting of rape myths. Compared with Hispanics, Caucasian women reported stronger positive attitudes toward rape victims and more accurate perceptions of rape when the victim was portrayed as Caucasian.

Geiger et al. (2004) studied the extent to which Israeli high school students supported date rape and victim-blaming attitudes. They found wide support for stereotypes justifying sexual coercion by time and location of the date, the victim's behavior, and the minimization of the seriousness of date rape.

Carr and VanDeusen (2004) studied risk factors for college male sexual aggression. Their results indicated that some gender attitudes, pornography use, and alcohol abuse were significant predictors of perpetration of sexual violence. Many of the males reported alcohol-related sexual coercion and held many rape-supportive attitudes and beliefs. The researchers suggested that these practices by college men contribute to pro-rape cultures found on many campuses.

McDonald and Kline (2004) had college students read several vignettes describing date rape situations. Then each participant recommended one of five punishments for the perpetrator. They found that the language used to describe the crime of date rape had a significant impact on the perceived severity of the crime. For example, using language that seemed to diffuse the responsibility for the crime between the perpetrator and the victim led to a recommendation of less punishment. However, participant gender was an even greater factor: Men tended to assign more lenient punishments than did women. The researchers pointed out that the men had more rape-tolerant attitudes.

McEwan et al. (2005) studied the relationship between date rape, ego-identity achievement, and locus of control. They found that, compared to women who had not been assaulted, date rape survivors reported lower ego-identity achievement and greater beliefs that the outcomes of their lives were controlled by luck, chance, or powerful others.

Rempala and Bernien (2005) studied the effect of target information disparity on judgments of guilt. Merely adding trivial information, such as the victim's age, college major, and city of residence, to the rape trial vignette decreased judgments of guilt for the alleged rapist. However, adding such information about the alleged rapist increased judgments of his guilt.

Lee et al. (2005) compared attitudes toward rape of Asian and Caucasian college students. Their findings suggest that Asian students are more likely than Caucasian students to believe women should be held responsible for preventing rape and to view sexual pleasure as the primary motivation for rape. Asians also had stronger beliefs than Caucasians that vic-

tims cause the rape and that most rapists are strangers and not acquaintances.

Humphreys (2007) had college students read several vignettes in which consent for sexual intercourse was ambiguous. As the degree of intimacy between the couple increased, perceptions of consent and acceptability increased. Also, men, more than women, perceived the scenarios as more consensual, acceptable, and clear regardless of relationship experience.

Marelich et al. (2008) studied the use of deception in association with sexual encounters. The three components of sexual deception used were blatant lying, self-serving lying, and avoiding confrontation. Those persons who used any of these deceptions reported more sexual partners and one-night stands. Those telling blatant lies to have sexual activity were more likely to report greater needs for sexual activity, while those using self-serving lies or having sexual intercourse to avoid confrontation experienced greater worry about partner loss. Men were more likely to use blatant lies to have sexual activity, while women were more likely to have sexual activity to avoid confrontation.

Ways to Help Prevent Acquaintance Rape

Because of the magnitude of date rape, many steps have been taken to help deal with and reduce the problem. Awareness is the first step, and materials have been developed to help college students understand date rape and how to prevent it. The American College Health Association (2008) has developed a pamphlet titled *Sexual Violence: What Everyone Should Know*, which contains suggestions for both men and women.

For example, the pamphlet indicates that alcohol and other drugs can inhibit clear thinking, make talking and listening more difficult, and make it harder to assess risk. Consenting sexual activity doesn't just happen. It requires sober, verbal communication without intimidation or threats. Many states' laws recognize that someone must be sober to give true consent. Also, being drunk or high is never an excuse for raping someone.

The pamphlet also has a section titled "What You Can Do," which indicates that you can think about how to respond to social pressures and ask yourself:

- How does sex fit into my definition of being a man or a woman?
- What role do I want sex to play in my life?
- How does alcohol affect my sexual decision-making?
- How do I learn someone's desires and limits?
- How do I express my own desires and limits?

Alcohol can play a role in acquaintance rape.

The pamphlet emphasizes the need to communicate effectively. It suggests expressing your limits clearly, listening carefully to what the other person is saying, asking rather than assuming, trusting your instincts, and remembering that effective and assertive communication may not always work. Sometimes people simply don't listen. However, no one ever *deserves* to be raped!

The Antioch College policy requiring verbal consent to sexual behavior is shown in Table 14.2. It has been the subject of many articles in which varying opinions have been expressed.

The Mentors in Violence Prevention (MVP) Program was founded at Northeastern University in 1993 and is still functioning (*www.sportinsociety.org/mvp*). It is a leadership program that motivates student-athletes and other student leaders to play a central role in helping to solve problems that have been traditionally considered "women's issues": rape, battering, and sexual harassment. The program has four main goals: (1) to raise awareness of the level of men's verbal, emotional, physical, and sexual abuse of women; (2) to challenge thinking by

countering mainstream messages about gender, sexual behavior, and violence; (3) to open a dialogue by creating a safe environment for men and women to share opinions and experiences; and (4) to inspire leadership by empowering participants with concrete options to effect change in their communities. Today the MVP program is used on a number of other campuses.

One effective, but controversial, way to prevent date rape or other rapes came from a South African inventor (South African anti-rape condom could reduce risk of pregnancy, HIV, STIs, 2005). It is called Rapex, is worn inside a woman's body like a tampon, and hooks onto a man's penis during intercourse. It is made of latex and attaches to the penis by shafts of sharp barbs. The device can be removed by surgery and is so painful that it would disable rapists immediately, allowing women to escape. It would not cause any long-term physical damage to the rapist, and could not accidentally injure the women. Some people are concerned that the device would provoke rapists and increase violence against women. They also feel that the device puts the burden on women to address the problem, instead of focusing on societal issues as motivating factors of rape. Others point out that the problem is so severe that women need protection now.

TABLE 14.2   **The Antioch College Policy Requiring Verbal Consent for Each Level of Sexual Behavior**

As part of community governance, Antioch College students developed a policy requiring students to obtain verbal consent for each level of sexual behavior. Here are the 10 reasons given to obtain verbal approval for sexual activities:

1. Because many partners find it sexy to be asked, as sexual behavior progresses, if it's okay.

2. Because sexual activity is better when each partner enjoys what is happening and no one is being forced to do something he or she doesn't want to do.

3. Because if your partner is having a good time and is not forced to do something against his or her will, he or she may be more likely to want to see you again. Mutual respect is the best basis for friendship and intimacy.

4. Because forcing sexual activity on another person can violate state and federal laws and your school's policy. In most instances, unwanted touching and fondling is sexual assault.

5. Because it prevents misunderstandings (silence is not a "yes").

6. Because you won't be accused of rape.

7. Because you won't go to jail or be expelled.

8. Because it's better to be safe than sorry.

9. Because if you want to impose your sexual will on someone, your behavior has more to do with dominating the person than with enjoying sexuality and an intimate relationship.

10. Why would you want to have sexual behavior with someone who doesn't like what you are doing?

Source: Antioch College. Ten reasons to obtain a verbal consent for sex. *About women on campus, 2* (Winter 1994).

Situational Model of Sexual Coercion

One way to comprehend better and perhaps reduce the problem of date rape is to understand a situational model of sexual coercion (Snyder & Ickes, 1985) (Figure 14.1). The model includes individual personality characteristics, situational components, cognitive processes, and behavioral effects of participants in a social situation (Craig, 1990). In other words, people introduce certain traits or dispositions to a dating situation, but they also use manipulation to express their dispositions.

In the first step of the model, the dispositions and history of the male lead him to select situations in which he can act in a particular way. Relatedly, there seems to be a common set of characteristics that distinguish between sexually coercive and noncoercive men (Craig, 1990). Coercive males tend to be more aggressive, to believe that relationships with women are basically adversarial, and to support rape myths and sex-role stereotypes. Peer approval also seems important, and sexual behavior is emphasized as a status symbol.

In the second step of the model, coercive males use selective exposure to choose situations that are likely to match their dispositions and characteristics. They tend to select certain types of women, dating situations, and relationships. For example, although there is not total agreement among researchers, it seems that women who are selected as victims by coercive males are more sexually experienced, more sexually passive, and less likely to use methods of avoidance such as running away or screaming.

Regarding the dating situation, sexual coercion seems more likely to occur when the male initiated the date, paid expenses, and drove; when there was miscommunication about sexual behavior; when an isolated location was used; when there was some consensual sexual contact; and when both persons were moderately or extremely intoxicated. In terms of the dating relationship, coercion seems more likely when there is an established relationship between the partners. Also, sexual violence seems more likely when there are differences between partners in age, intelligence, and social status.

If the factors suggested do not result in consensual sexual activity, there are additional components of the model. Through selective evaluation the male may place major importance on situational aspects that he believes encourage him to make sexual advances. For example, the female's friendliness, appearance, or behavior might cause a male's misperception of the situation.

Even after setting up a situation that increases his likelihood of engaging in sexual activity—and paying attention only to the cues that would seem to encourage sexual advances—the coercive male may still encounter resistance. He may then try to lower the woman's resistance by using alcohol or drugs or by making false statements or promises.

Cognitive restructuring is changing one's interpretations to better fit one's self-image. In relation to coercive sexual behavior, this could include use of alcohol, victim blaming (it was really her fault), and rationalization (perceiving aggressive behavior as appropriate or perceiving aggressive actions as acceptable to women).

Up to this point in the model, the goal for the male has been to make the features of the situation congruent with his self-concept. If that still has not happened, or if sexual activity still has not occurred, he may feel a need to externalize blame for his "failure."

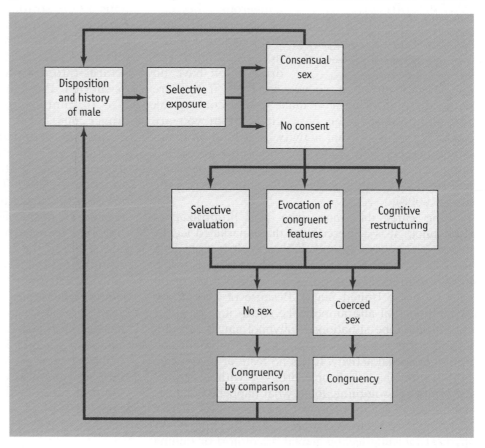

FIGURE **14.1** The situational model of coercive sexual behavior.

For example, he may indicate she was just cold or that they did not really have the opportunity.

The situational model can be helpful to understanding coercive sexual behavior in dating situations. It can also help us understand why misperceptions occur so frequently. Perhaps most importantly, it can be used in a positive way—particularly to encourage better communication at all levels of a relationship and to recognize prevention or promotion of behaviors that help prevent coercion.

Mouzon et al. (2005) studied perception of sexual coercion among African American college students. Many participants viewed verbal sexual coercion as a normative behavior often referred to as "running the game." They acknowledged the reciprocal nature of coercion as well as the fact that women use it and experience it as much as men. Poor communication skills were identified as a potential cause of sexual coercion, and a need to improve sexual communication skills was emphasized.

Date-Rape Drugs

In the early 1990s the topic of date rape was further complicated by the availability of **date-rape drugs**. These drugs are sometimes used to assist a sexual assault. They are powerful and dangerous. They can be slipped into your drink when you are not looking. The drugs often have no color, smell, or taste, so you can't tell if you are being drugged. They can make you become weak and confused—or even pass out—so that you are unable to refuse sexual activity or defend yourself. If you are drugged, you might not remember what happened while you were drugged. Date-rape drugs are used on both females and males (Date rape drugs, 2008).

One early date-rape drug was flunitrazepam (Rohypnol). It is a prescription drug marketed legally in many countries around the world. It is used as a sedative hypnotic and as a preanesthetic medication in those countries. However, it is not approved for medical use in the United States. Because of its sedative hypnotic action and amnesialike effect, it is ideal for use in date-rape situations. Rohypnol can be administered without consent to produce disinhibition and to obtain sexual activity. It has no taste or odor when mixed with alcohol. People drugged with Rohypnol may remember nothing about what happened or have only a very sketchy memory. They are often unsure that they have been raped, except that they may wake the next morning feeling genital discomfort or finding themselves undressed. Assailants typically claim the victims consented to sexual activity, and there is no way to know for sure. The effects of Rohypnol can be felt within 30 minutes and can last for several hours (Date rape drugs, 2008).

date-rape drugs
Sedative hypnotic drugs used to incapacitate victims who are then sexually molested or raped.

Date rape drugs have no taste and no odor. They are undetectable if added to a drink.

Another date-rape drug is gammahydroxybutyrate (GHB). It can be used by sexual predators to render their victims almost instantly helpless and to leave them with little or no memory of the attack. It is similar to the drug Rohypnol. GHB has no approved medical use, and it can cause depression, seizures, coma, and death. Kits can be purchased to make the drug at home for less than $100. Many argue that GHB should be an illegal substance.

A third drug being used as a date-rape drug is ketamine hydrochloride. It is used medically as an anesthetic for diagnostic and surgical purposes. It produces anesthesia within 40 seconds of intravenous administration and within 8 minutes of intramuscular administration. It is currently widely used by veterinarians. In the United States the popular method of use involves heating of the liquid until it turns into a white powder, which is then smoked or snorted. Full effects of ketamine occur in about 5 to 10 minutes and last up to 1 hour (Date rape drugs, 2008).

In 1996 President Clinton signed a bill outlawing Rohypnol and other date-rape drugs and adding 20 years to the sentence of a rapist who uses these drugs on a victim. The law also included increased penalties for illegal manufacturing, distribution, dispensing, or possession of the drugs. It was the first time that using a drug as a weapon was classified as a crime in the United States.

Although the term "date rape" is commonly used, many experts prefer the term "drug-facilitated sexual assault" when referring to these drugs. The drugs can affect a person very quickly, and the length of time that the effect lasts varies, depending on how much is taken and whether it is mixed with other substances such as alcohol. Alcohol can worsen the drug's effects. Here are some ways to protect yourself from being a victim of "drug-facilitated sexual assault" (Date rape drugs, 2005):

- Don't accept drinks from other people.
- Open containers yourself.

- Keep your drink with you at all times, even when you go into the bathroom.

- Don't share drinks.

- Don't drink from punch bowls or other large, common, open containers. They may already have drugs in them.

- Don't drink anything that tastes or smells strange. Sometimes GHB tastes salty.

- Have a nondrinking friend with you to make sure nothing happens.

- If you think you have been drugged and raped:

  - Go to the police station or hospital right away.

  - Get a urine test as soon as possible. The drugs leave your system quickly.

  - Don't urinate before getting help.

  - Don't douche, bathe, or change clothes before getting help. These actions eliminate evidence of the rape.

  - Call the National Domestic Violence Hotline at 800-799-SAFE or 800-787-3224 (TTY).

The Incidence of Sexual Assault

Because many cases are not reported, statistics on rape and sexual assault leave a lot to be desired. Estimating rates of violence, especially of sexual assault and other incidents committed by intimate offenders, continues to be a difficult task. Many factors inhibit both men and women from reporting these crimes. The private nature of the event, the perceived stigma, and the belief that no purpose would be served by reporting the crime prevent an unknown portion of the victims from talking about the attack.

Because of the difficulties of getting accurate statistics about sexual assault, numbers from different sources may vary somewhat. However, they can still give us a general picture of what is happening. For example, according to the U.S. Centers for Disease Control and Prevention (CDC), 1 in 6 women and 1 in 33 men in the United States have been victims of rape or attempted rape during their lifetimes. Eighty percent of them knew their perpetrators (Notice to readers: Sexual Assault Awareness Month, 2005).

Finkelhor et al. (2005) examined a large spectrum of crime statistics and reported that within a national representative sample of children and youth 2 to 17 years of age, 1 in 12 had experienced a sexual victimization during the study year. Campbell and Wasco (2005) reviewed reports of sexual assault and

reported that 24% of women in the San Francisco area had experienced a completed rape and 44% had experienced a completed or attempted rape. They also reported that 25% of college women in a national sample had experienced rape or attempted rape, and that 84% of them knew their attacker.

There has been substantial variation in the number of reported forcible rapes per 100,000 females through the years. For example, in 1988 there were 37.8 per 100,000. The rate slowly increased until it reached 42.8 per 100,000 in 1992. It has slowly decreased since then and was 30 per 100,000 in 2007 (Crime in the United States, 2008). Approximately 80% of rape victims are younger than 30 years old, and about half of those are younger than 18 years old. Victims younger than 12 years account for 15% of those raped, and another 29% of rape victims are between 12 and 17 years.

The amount of forcible rapes varies by region of the country. The Northeast had 12% of reported rapes, the Midwest had 25.3%, the West had 24%, and the South had the highest percentage (38.8%) (Crime in the United States, 2008).

An excellent source of sexual assault statistics is the Rape, Abuse, and Incest National Network (RAINN). It reports that someone is sexually assaulted every 2 minutes in America, and that only about 40% of rapes and other sexual assaults are reported to law enforcement personnel. Overall, RAINN indicates that, since 1993, reported cases of rape and sexual assault have fallen by more than 65%, yet there are still about 250,000 victims of rape, attempted rape, or sexual assault each year. One out of every six American women has been the victim of an attempted or completed rape in her lifetime. A total of 17.7 million women have been victims. Also, almost 3 million men have experienced an attempted or completed rape in her lifetime. In a given year, about 1 in every 10 rape

It is important to get help if sexual assault does occur.

Multicultural
DIMENSIONS

Coercive Sexual Experiences

As part of the National Health and Social Life Survey, Laumann and associates (1994) asked about coercive sexual experiences. Because of the broad nature of the question, reported incidents may not all be rape, but there are still some interesting statistics. For example, 2.8% of the men reported forcing a woman sexually, and 1.5% of the women reported forcing a man sexually. However, 1.3% of the men reported being forced by another man, and 22% of the women reported being forced by a man.

Coerced sexual activity seems to decline as people grow older. There is not a notable difference in the rate by education level. For example, 26% of women with less than a high school education reported having been coerced compared to 23% of women with a master's or advanced degree.

It is interesting to note that 31% of women with no religious affiliation reported having been coerced sexually as compared to 17% of Catholic women. This compares to an average of 23% for Protestant women.

The researchers felt that the most intriguing and unexpected pattern may be the very low rate of sexual coercion (16%) reported by women living in central cit-

ies and the relatively high rate (25%) for those living in noncity urban areas. This is not consistent with the perception of the risk of sexual assault in big cities. However, a vast majority of coerced sexual activity occurs with someone well known to the respondent, not with someone unknown, the more typical circumstance thought to predominate in large cities.

Finally, 22% of the women considered themselves to have been forced against their will to do something sexually. Asian and Hispanic women reported notably lower rates than white women, and African American women reported rates between those extremes. By race and ethnicity, the proportions who were forced were

White = 23%
African American = 19%
Hispanic = 14%
Asian = 17%

Except for offering observations about incidents in cities versus rural areas, the researchers did not provide possible explanations for the other observed differences in coercive sexual activity. We can only speculate about the reasons for the differences related to age, educational level, religious background, and race and ethnicity.

---

victims is a male. About 83.5% of the U.S. population is white, and 82.5% of rape victims are white. About 12.3% of the U.S. population is African American, and 13.3% of the victims are African American (Rape, Abuse, and Incest National Network, 2009, *www.rainn.org/statistics*).

Not only is it difficult to obtain accurate statistics about rape for reasons already mentioned, but false rape reports make it even more difficult to know for sure what is happening. For example, one study (Kanin, 1994) showed that 41% of the total reported forcible rape cases in a small Midwestern community were false rape allegations. These false rape allegations seemed to serve three major functions for the complainants: providing an alibi, seeking revenge, and obtaining sympathy and attention.

Consequences of Rape

The survivor of a rape, her friends, her family, and her husband or lover usually respond to the crime's sexual aspects, instead of the violent aspects. Rape

survivors and their loved ones need the same kinds of help to get through this difficult time as survivors of other violent acts. And beyond that, they need assistance with the specific problems that follow such a personally destructive attack.

Traumatic events, such as war, accidents, natural disasters, and sexual violence can result in serious stress and detrimental consequences for survivors and their families. Although most individuals will be able to absorb the trauma over time, many survivors will experience long-lasting problems. About 8% of survivors of traumatic events develop post-traumatic stress disorder (PTSD). PTSD symptoms include nightmares, insomnia, somatic disturbances, difficulty with intimate relationships, fear, anxiety, anger, shame, aggression, suicidal behaviors, loss of trust, and isolation (Facts about trauma, 2005).

The **rape trauma syndrome** has two phases. The acute

> **rape trauma syndrome**
> A two-phase reaction to rape. An acute phase involves intense emotional responses for several weeks. The long-term phase may last several years and involves reorganization and establishment of control.

phase can last from days to weeks, and is characterized by general stress responses such as lack of sleep, irritability, and difficulty in thinking clearly. The long-term phase can last several years and the symptoms are similar to those described for PTSD. Some experts believe that the long-term phase of the rape trauma syndrome is actually a subset of PTSD.

In addition to the psychological consequences mentioned previously, physical consequences of rape include the possibility of a pregnancy and/or an STI. Other physical consequences could be chronic pelvic pain, gastrointestinal disorders, migraines and other frequent headaches, back pain, and facial pain. Social consequences include strained family relations, less frequent contact with friends and relatives, and less emotional support from friends and family (Sexual violence: Fact sheet, 2005).

As many as 38% of women engage in more sexually risky behaviors after experiencing a sexual assault than they did before the attack, while 48% significantly reduce their risky behavior (Campbell, Sefl, & Alvon, 2004). About half of the 48% began abstaining from sexual activity after their assault. Sexually risky behavior can include sexual activity with multiple partners, without contraception, and while under the influence of alcohol or other drugs. Rape survivors who had negative interactions with police and medical professionals, and reported experiencing blame for their assault from these sources, tended to fall into the group of women who increased their sexually risky behaviors.

It is clear that individuals who are victims of sexual violence are more likely to experience depression, anxiety, and traumatic symptoms compared to nonvictims. However, the impact of sexual violence is not limited to the act itself. Instead, so-called secondary victimization may result from negative experiences within one's social group or with authorities who may hold negative attitudes toward victims of rape (Nagel et al., 2005).

Adult rape survivors experience a shattering effect on their personal stability and adjustment. Many do not wish to confide in another person and try to hold in their feelings. Some are hesitant to participate in their usual sexual relations. Personal feelings of privacy, dignity, and trust are undermined, and feelings of vulnerability are common. Many women feel they live in a world filled with threats. Anger, rage, shame, and fear profoundly influence the recovery of rape survivors. It is not unusual for this anger to be expressed toward men in general. Although some women suffer physical trauma from rape, requiring surgical repair of the perineum, vulva, or urethra, it is emotional scars that take longest to heal.

While Paul Reubens' career never quite recovered after the highly publicized charges of indecent exposure and child pornography, the same was not true for rap and R & B superstar R. Kelly, who was charged with 21 counts of child pornography stemming from a videotape that allegedly shows him having sexual activity with a 13-year-old girl. Kelly's CD in 2003 debuted at number one and the first single from the album, "Ignition," peaked at number two on the Billboard's singles chart and enjoyed consistent radio and television play, all while he faced serious charges of a sexual encounter with a minor. Does this send the message that the rap and R & B community condones such behavior?

In summary, victims of sexual assault are 3 times more likely to suffer from depression, 6 times more likely to suffer from PTSD, and 13 times more likely to abuse alcohol. In addition, they are 26 times more likely to abuse drugs, and 4 times more likely to contemplate suicide (Who are the victims?, 2009).

Many survivors of sexual assault do heal and do just fine in their lives. They probably do not forget, but they do move on. There is a great deal of hope today for such survivors.

Rape of Males

Almost all the information on rape presented so far has focused on females as victims. This is appropriate because the vast majority of survivors are females. However, in recent years there has been an increased recognition that males can be victims, too. Even the rape laws in many states now recognize the existence of male rape. Generally, male rape falls into one of three categories: male rape in prison, male rape by other males outside prison, and male rape by females.

After more than four decades of research, it is still unknown how much rape and sexually violent activity occur in prisons and jails. What is clear is that, as with rape in free society, prison rape goes largely unreported. It is very difficult to estimate the extent of the problem. The limited information available suggests that from 2% to 13% of all inmates have been raped (Prison rape, 2007). Even though research about prison rape is not conclusive, many people believe that the likelihood of being raped in prison is so great that a judge who sentences a young man to prison passes a sentence of male rape on him as surely as the prison sentence. It appears that male prison rape is an act of heterosexuals rather than homosexuals. This may sound strange at first, but in a prison situation rape is viewed as validation of masculinity and a violent act of conquest.

As one sign of concern about prison rape, in 2003 Congress passed the Prison Rape Elimination Act. This legislation calls for all correction systems to have a zero-tolerance policy regarding prison rape. It requires standards for detection, prevention, reduction, and punishment of prison rape. It standardizes collection and dissemination of information on the incidence of prison rape, and awards grants to implement the act's provisions (About the Prison Rape Elimination Act of 2003, 2007).

Even outside prison, it is probable that most rapes of males are committed by heterosexual men. This is perhaps more understandable when we consider that violence and power, rather than sexual satisfaction, are the primary motivations for rape. Statistics on the frequency of male rape are almost impossible to obtain. Perhaps this is because of the lack of research on the subject combined with the hesitation of male victims to report an attack. In addition to the reasons females hesitate to report a rape, males often feel they are supposed to be strong and "macho." To report being raped would not be consistent with this image.

A male being raped by a female is hard for many people to imagine. This is because of traditional feelings about sexuality—particularly the ideas that all males are "at the ready" for sexual activity and that males cannot be forced into submission. Although the first attitude is open to question (often based on incorrect logic), the second relates to physiological functioning. People seem to think that a male could not respond sexually while being threatened because he could not achieve a penile erection. It has been found, however, that such emotions as anger, fright, and pain can cause a sexual response, including all the usual physiological changes. This, of course, can be quite upsetting to the victim because it might be interpreted as indicating willingness. Guilt and other negative feelings can occur as well. Consequently, the responses of male rape survivors are very similar to those of female rape survivors.

Walker et al. (2005) investigated the effects of rape on a sample of 40 men recruited by media advertising. They found that most assaults had been carried out using physical or violent force, in a variety of circumstances. All victims reported some form of psychological disturbance as a result of being raped. Long-term effects included anxiety, depression, increased feelings of anger and vulnerability, loss of self-image, emotional distancing, self-blame, and self-harming behaviors.

Stermac et al. (2004) examined victim and assault characteristics among adult male victims of sexual assaults. They found that male victims presenting to an urban sexual assault care center were young, often single adults with significant vulnerabilities (living on the street or in a shelter, unemployed, and with physical disabilities). These same characteristics were not so common with female victims. Males overall were more likely to be victims of an anal and/or fellatio assault. Male stranger assailant victims were also more likely to be attacked by multiple assailants than were female victims, and more likely to be assaulted outdoors. In contrast, male acquaintance assailant victims were more likely to be assaulted in an institutional setting. Male stranger assault victims were more likely to experience assaults involving weapons. Acquaintance male assaults, however, were more likely to involve victims' alcohol use.

Most of what was discussed regarding rape trauma syndrome and post-traumatic stress disorder for female victims of sexual violence also applies to male victims. In addition, a male victim often feels that he has totally lost control over the insides of his own body, resulting in feelings of vulnerability and powerlessness. Men are often brought up to defend themselves against attack, and may consider total helplessness incompatible with masculinity. They may feel that their gender identity as a male was compromised or even demolished and reversed (Rape trauma syndrome—What everyone should know, 2005).

Prison rape is usually the act of heterosexuals rather than homosexuals.

Did You Know . . .

Myths About Male Rape

MYTH: Men can't be sexually assaulted.

FACT: Men are sexually assaulted—regardless of size, strength, appearance, or sexual orientation.

MYTH: Only gay men are sexually assaulted.

FACT: Heterosexual, gay, and bisexual men are equally likely to be sexually assaulted.

MYTH: Only gay men sexually assault other men.

FACT: Most men who sexually assault other men are heterosexuals.

MYTH: Men can't be sexually assaulted by women.

FACT: Although most perpetrators are men, women can also sexually assault men.

MYTH: Erection or ejaculation during sexual assault means you "really wanted it" or consented to it.

FACT: Erection and ejaculation are physiological responses that may result from mere physical contact or even extreme stress. These responses do not imply that you wanted or enjoyed the sexual assault.

Source: Adapted from Myths about male rape. South Eastern Centre Against Sexual Assault 2005. Available: www.secasa.com.au.

Social Responses to Rape

In many communities, sexual assault crisis centers, workshops dealing with prevention of sexual assault, and improved methods of helping survivors have become priorities. Shelters for survivors of assault have been provided so they have a place to receive help. In general, there is a better understanding of the problems in communities and the need for more support.

On many college campuses there are laudable attempts to deal with sexual assault. An effective program (1) defines and demystifies sexual assault, (2) offers educational programs, (3) empowers women to be assertive, (4) exposes the link between alcohol abuse and unwanted sexual behavior, (5) conducts institutional surveys, and (6) identifies a specific individual on campus to coordinate efforts and clinical services (Meilman, Riggs, & Turco, 1990). There is also greater recognition on college campuses of the need for more attention to the problem of sexual assault. Lighting and security on campuses have improved; courses in sexual assault prevention and self-defense are offered; and escort services are available so women need not be alone on campus, particularly after dark.

There have also been major changes in laws related to rape in the past few decades. Many of the newer rape laws (1) establish "degrees" of rape to describe types of sexual assault more accurately; (2) are gender neutral and do not apply only to attacks by men on women; (3) eliminate requirements that victims prove they resisted by "fighting back" and that corroborating evidence be presented; (4) shield victims from inquiries into past sexual experience; and (5) allow a husband to be charged with raping his wife. In fact, in many states the term *forced sex*

or *sexual assault* has replaced the word *rape*. The convicted rapist can often be sentenced to life in prison.

Changes have also been made in relation to law enforcement personnel. Training has been designed to help them become more sensitive to the problem of sexual assault. More female officers are used, and there is improved cooperation between law enforcement personnel and medical and support personnel. Guidelines for handling survivors of sexual assault have also been established.

Women who have been assaulted have begun to fight back in civil court as well. For example, a Seattle woman was awarded $300,000 from three men who raped her and a fourth who prevented her escape; a Vermont woman received $450,000 even after a defendant was acquitted of rape charges; and a Minnesota woman received $21,500 from a physician (who had been her lover) for rape.

 Did You Know . . .

Where to Find Help

The following numbers can be helpful if you want to find out more about reporting abuse or if you want more information about abuse:

Child abuse: (800) 4-A-CHILD (422-4453)

Elder abuse: (800) 677-1116

Sexual assault: (800) 656-4673

Domestic violence: (800) 799-7233

Ethical
DIMENSIONS

Should the Media Reveal the Names of Rape Survivors?

The names of rape survivors traditionally have been withheld by the news media to "protect" them. Does this special treatment do rape survivors a disservice by separating them from other survivors of violent crimes? Should the privacy of rape survivors be protected more than the privacy of survivors of other violent crimes? This issue has often been debated, and it arose again when two California teenagers were kidnapped. Their names and pictures were widely distributed to help locate them. When, after their rescue, a sheriff said they had been raped during the abduction, "What should be done now?" asked many journalists. Some media representatives stuck to their own rule and did not refer to the teenagers by name. Others called them by name, reasoning that their names had already been released.

Some people believe that the bright lights of publicity may harm the innocent in crimes of rape. They assert that rape survivors are unwillingly thrust into the limelight, their right to choose is once again removed, and their feeling of powerlessness is perpetuated. They argue that publicly identifying rape survivors without their consent compounds the trauma of rape and may discourage future survivors from reporting crimes.

Others point out that in most states it is legal to publish the names of rape survivors, and, in fact, their names should be published just as the names of people who are victims of other violent crimes are. They point out that it is discriminatory to publish the names of alleged assailants, but not the alleged survivors. They also indicate that not naming the survivors contributes to the perception that rape is a different type of crime and helps to perpetuate the notion that there is some blame or disgrace attached. It is also argued that special treatment by the news media inhibits society from treating rape as a violent crime.

Do you think it is ethical, and the best thing to do, for the media to give the names of rape survivors?

But even with the increased emphasis on prevention, a great deal must be done. Major priorities include more changes in legislation, law enforcement policies and practices, educational intervention, and media strategies. The codification of women's equality and rights is an important part of a strategy for preventing assault. Skills training, which includes avoidance strategies, appropriate resistance, and self-defense training, is also needed.

Pedophilia

The term **pedophilia** denotes feelings of adult sexual attraction to children. Even though physical force may not be used, an adult who performs a sexual act with a child is forcing himself or herself on a helpless minor in the eyes of the law. Pedophiliacs may expose their genitals to a child or fondle and even penetrate a child. There are countless ways a child might be molested; most often the term *child molestation* refers to pedophilia. For all practical purposes the terms are used interchangeably.

pedophilia
Sexual behavior in which a child is the sexual object.

The Pedophiliac

According to the American Psychiatric Association Statement on Diagnostic Criteria for Pedophilia (2003), the criteria for pedophilia are as follows:

1. Over a period of at least 6 months, recurrent, intense sexually arousing fantasies, sexual urges, or behaviors involving sexual activity with a prepubescent child or children (generally age 13 years or younger).

2. The person has acted on these sexual urges, or the sexual urges or fantasies cause marked distress or interpersonal difficulty.

3. The person is at least 16 years of age and at least 5 years older than the child or children in Criterion 1.

Pedophilia is one of the few psychiatric disorders for which the symptoms constitute a criminal act. There has not been a great deal of research on pedophilia. Child molesters are not identical to pedophiles. For example, a child molester can be anyone who has sexually molested a child. However, pedophilia involves a sexual disorder and ongoing sexual desires, urges, fantasies, and possibly, but not necessarily, behavior. Pedophilia is extremely difficult to treat and effective treatment needs to be intensive, long-term, and comprehensive, possibly with lifetime follow-up (Cohen & Galynker, 2002).

A man or a woman can be a pedophiliac, but most commonly we hear about males being the offenders. The objects of their desires may be boys, girls, or both. Their preferences with respect to practices vary from exhibition to penetration. Some have fleeting contacts with a series of children, while others look for long-term relationships, which may be sort of caring or manipulative. Many are considerate in their behavior toward children; others use force. Only a few use violent means. There are instances of consensual sexual activity between adults and children, but this raises the question: Can there ever be sexual consensus between adults and children? Also, there are many cases of nonconsensual sexual contacts between adults and children that are not traumatic for the child, although they do indeed violate the child's right of self-determination. Sexual contacts between adults and children pose a risk of lasting trauma for the latter even when they do not involve violence or the use of force (Schmidt, 2002).

Van Wijk et al. (2005) studied characteristics of sex offenders as compared to non-sex offenders. They found that juvenile sex offenders were significantly younger than other juvenile offenders at the time of their initial offense, that a larger proportion of sex offenders attended special education schools, and that violent offenders were more extraverted and impulsive and showed higher scores on lack of conscience than other offenders. Also, child molesters had significantly higher scores on neuroticism and scored worse on contact with peers. They were socially isolated because of their poorly developed social skills—and had less or no normal contact with peers.

Tardif and Van Gijseghem (2005) researched the gender identity of pedophiles. They found no differences in gender identity among pedophiles who abused male victims, pedophiles who abused female victims, or non-sexual offenders.

Most victims of child sexual abuse do not become pedophiles. However, particular experiences and patterns of childhood behavior are associated with an increased risk of victims becoming abusers in later life. These include neglect, lack of supervision, sexual abuse by a female person, being cruel to animals, and witnessing serious intrafamilial violence (Salter et al., 2003).

Although there are many biological and psychological theories, no one really knows how pedophilia develops (Pedophilia: Who are the men who "love" children in intolerable ways, 2004). The tendency may be established early in life, perhaps genetically or before birth. Hormones may be involved, but consistent hormonal abnormalities are not found in pedophiles. Some experts think that brain function may have something to do with the development of pedophilia, but no one knows for sure. Risk factors for pedophilia—and sexual offenses of all kinds—include childhood emotional abuse, family conflict, childhood behavior problems, substance abuse, and personality disorders—particularly antisocial personality. According to one theory, pedophiles compensate for feelings of powerlessness by engaging in a type of sexual activity that provides them more control than adult relationships permit. Another theory indicates that pedophilia results from a diversion of sexual development that allows immature forms of desire to persist into adulthood. Another common view is that child molestation creates pedophiles. However, as pointed out earlier in another context, most child sex abusers are not pedophiles.

Incidence of Pedophilia

As with other sexual offenses, it is difficult to know for sure how often pedophilia occurs. It is even more complicated because statistics do not differentiate between pedophilia and **child sexual abuse**. However, it is still germane to consider overall statistics regarding adult sexual contact with children.

> **child sexual abuse**
> Any sexual abuse involving fondling, erotic kissing, oral sexual activity, or genital penetration between an adult and a child, including pedophilia and incest.

According to statistics from the Rape, Abuse, and Incest National Network (Who are the victims?, 2009), approximately 44% of sexual assault and rape victims are younger than the age of 18 years. Fifteen percent are younger than age 12. Seven percent of girls in grades 5–8 and 12% of girls in grades 9–12 say they have been sexually abused. Three percent of boys in grades 5–8 and 5% of boys in grades 9–12 say they have been sexually abused. Ninety-three percent of juvenile sexual assault victims knew their attacker (34% of attackers were family members, 59% were acquaintances, and only 7% were strangers to the victim). About 75% of the sexual abuse victims are girls. Nearly 30% of child victims are between the ages of 4 and 7 years.

Overall, 7% of all victims of sexual assault reported to law enforcement agencies are younger than the age of 18; 34% of all victims are younger than age of 12 years. One out of every six victims of sexual assault reported to law enforcement agencies is younger than the age of 6 years (Sexual assault of young children as reported to law enforcement, 2005).

Regarding males, about one-sixth of men report having had unwanted sexual contact with an older person by the age of 16. On average, boys first experience sexual abuse at age 10. The age range at which

Multicultural DIMENSIONS

Sexual Contact in Various Cultures

Sexual contact between children and adults may be viewed differently in various cultures. The people following these practices are not pedophiles, but are following cultural or religious tradition. Here are some examples:

• Among the Siwans in North Africa, all men and boys engage in anal intercourse. Males are singled out as peculiar if they do not do so. Prominent Siwan men lend their sons to each other for this purpose.

• Among the Aranda in Central Australia, a man who is not yet married takes a 10- to 12-year-old boy as

his wife for several years, until the older man marries.

• In the eighteenth century in Hawaii, copulation in public between an adult male and a young girl was not considered to be indecent or improper. Sexual interactions between an adult and a child were seen as benefiting the child, rather than as gratifying the adult.

• Among the Etoro of New Guinea, from about age 10, boys would have regular oral sexual activity with older men, swallowing their semen to facilitate growth.

Source: Green, R. Is pedophilia a mental disorder? *Archives of Sexual Behavior, 31, no. 6* (December 2002), 467–471.

boys are first abused, however, is from infancy to later adolescence. Boys are most often abused by males (between 50% and 75%). However, it is hard to estimate the extent of abuse by females, because abuse by women is often covert. Also, a boy may consider it a "sexual initiation" and deny that it was abusive even though he may suffer significant trauma from the experience. A smaller proportion of sexually abused boys than sexually abused girls reports sexual abuse to authorities. While a majority of perpetrators (about 80%) were themselves abused, the vast majority of sexually abused boys (about 80%) never become adult perpetrators. Boys often feel physical sexual arousal during abuse even if they are repulsed by what is happening (Overcoming sexual victimization of boys and men, 2005).

Online Pedophilia

As the Internet has developed, so have opportunities for Internet-related crimes such as pedophilia. Children are particularly vulnerable to sexual predators, such as pedophiles, on the Internet. Pedophiles have been known to use the Internet in at least two different ways. One is a trust-based seductive model in which the pedophile tries to build up trust with the child and then attempts to plan a meeting with the child. The other is a direct sexual model in which the pedophile hopes to make contact with the child (Deirmenjian, 2002).

Wolak et al. (2004) reported on a national sample of online sex abuse cases from a national sample of law enforcement agencies. They indicated that most offenders did not deceive victims about the fact that they were adults interested in sexual relationships.

The victims, mainly 13 to 15 years of age, met and had sexual relations with the adults on more than one occasion. Half of the victims were described as being in love with or feeling close bonds with the offenders. Few offenders abducted or used force to sexually abuse their victims. Offenders targeted adolescents and not younger children. Ninety-nine percent were 13 to 17 years of age and none were younger than 12 years old. Victims and offenders had typically communicated, both online and by telephone, for more than a month prior to meeting in person.

Wolak et al. (2009) reported additional information related to online predators. There has been dramatic growth nationwide in the number of arrests of online predators who solicited law enforcement investigators posing online as juveniles. The numbers nearly quintupled from 644 in 2000 to 3,100 in 2006. While online predator arrests were increasing, overall sex offenses against children and adolescents were declining. Arrests of online predators constituted only 1% of all arrests for sex crimes committed against children and youth. These researchers also found that victims were adolescents and not younger children. Most offenders were open about their sexual motives in their online communications with youth. Few crimes (5%) involved violence.

Effects of Pedophilia

As with rape survivors, there can be a tendency to blame survivors of pedophilia. This blame can have psychological effects on the young people involved. There has been a great deal of debate about the effects of pedophilia and sexual abuse of children. Some studies connect sexual abuse to many future

Communication
DIMENSIONS

Helping Survivors of Rape and Sexual Abuse Even if you are not a trained counselor, if someone who has been raped or sexually abused talks with you about what has happened, you can be helpful by remembering the following points:

1. Listen in a supportive and nonjudgmental way, showing sympathy and concern. Ask questions and do not argue.
2. Encourage the person to express his or her feelings about the incident(s).
3. Control your own emotions. Do not react strongly and do not question the judgment of the survivor.
4. Indicate that you believe the account of what happened.
5. Let the survivor know that it was not his or her fault and that he or she is not to blame.
6. Give comfort and support.
7. Help the person focus on actions that might be needed, such as seeking medical treatment or reporting to police.
8. Try not to interrupt or ask a lot of questions.
9. Do not tell others what happened without your friend's permission.
10. The survivor must decide what to do; you cannot force him or her or make any decision you've determined.
11. Help the person find professional follow-up services—professional counseling, crisis center or domestic violence center guidance, legal assistance, medical follow-up—and accompany the person if that is appropriate and if the person desires it.
12. Survivors of rape and/or sexual abuse can respond in almost any way. They may be hysterical, amazingly calm, or anything in between. Almost any (or no) reaction is "normal."
13. Let the person know you are available to help or give support in the future.
14. Check as often as necessary to see how the person is progressing toward full recovery.

Source: Adapted from Bruess, C., & Richardson, G. *Decisions for health.* Madison, WI: Brown & Benchmark, 1995; Rape and sexual assault: Information for victims and friends. West Virginia Foundation for Rape Information and Services, 2005. Available: www.fris.org/Pages/Rape9020Info/RapeInfo.html.

---

problems, while others show little or no indication of negative effects of sexual victimization. In fact, a percentage of both men and women reported the experience as positive (McConaghy, 1998).

Researchers cannot explain the relatively large numbers of sexually abused children who have no apparent adverse psychological symptoms (Finkelhor, 1990). For those children who show symptoms, initial effects of sexual abuse include fear, anxiety, depression, anger, aggression, and sexually inappropriate behavior. The most common long-term effects are depression, self-destructive behavior, anxiety, feelings of isolation, poor self-esteem, difficulty in trusting others, substance abuse, and sexual maladjustment (Adult survivors of sex abuse in crisis, 1990; Finkelhor, 1990).

Obviously all children do not react the same way to child abuse. Some research has identified effects of child abuse that include sleeping and eating disturbances, anger, withdrawal, and guilt. Or there might be sexual preoccupation (excessive masturbation and an unusual interest in sexual organs and nudity) and a host of physical complaints such as rashes, vomiting, and headaches without medical explanation. Other common symptoms include shame, poor body image,

self-destructive behavior, nightmares, relational and/or sexual dysfunction, and compulsive behaviors like drug addiction, gambling, or overeating (Overcoming sexual victimization of boys and men, 2005).

Hillis and coworkers (2001) indicated that physical abuse and sexual abuse are related to subsequent unintended pregnancies and STI. In a study of more than 5,000 females, they found such abuse resulted in increased risk of intercourse by age 15 years and in sexual activity with multiple partners.

Exposure to childhood sexual abuse seems to be associated with increased rates of sexual risk-taking behaviors and sexual revictimization during adolescence. Young women reporting childhood sexual abuse, particularly those for whom sexual intercourse was involved, reported significantly higher rates of early-onset consensual sexual activity, teenage pregnancy, multiple sexual partners, unprotected intercourse, STIs, and sexual assault after the age of 16 years (Fergusson, Horwood, & Lynskey, 1997).

Although not a lot of information is available on the topic, the effects among homosexuals and heterosexuals seem to be very similar. For example, Arreola et al. (2008) studied the effects of forced, consensual, and no childhood sexual experiences on health

DIMENSIONS

Examples of Coercive Sexual Behaviors in Other Countries

In Japan, rape is described as having sexual intercourse with a woman through force or against her will, but there is no clear legal definition. However, the victim or her parent or legal guardian must file a complaint for the rape to be recognized as a criminal act. Fewer than 2,000 cases are reported annually throughout the country.

Protection against sexual harassment in Japan lags far behind American and European standards. The Japanese Labor Ministry has specifically forbidden sexual harassment; however, much remains to be done.

There seems to be a tolerance of violence in Japan's male-dominated society. There is a long history of violence's being condoned as a symbol of manliness. As a result, in comic books, general sexual content has been curbed but portrayals of sexual violence are common. There are even "ladies' comic books" that seem to glorify sexual violence and rape. These are not a fringe phenomenon—the leading one claims annual sales of 400,000 copies.

Late in 2005, the Supreme Court of Mexico ruled that rape within marriage is a crime. This brought Mexican laws into line with much of the world, and removed one of the many obstacles Mexican women face in reporting rape. This ended a legal battle fought since 1994 when the Supreme Court ruled that because the purpose of marriage was procreation, forced sexual relations by a spouse was not rape but "an undue exercise of conjugal rights." Many women's advocates said that there are still deep-rooted opinions that women should be subservient. They warned that entrenched attitudes still make it very difficult for women to report rape. It is thought that 9 of 10 sexual assaults go unreported in Mexico and that 18% of victims were not aware that it was a crime. Only a few countries in the world do not recognize rape within marriage as a crime. India and Malaysia are the most prominent examples.

Sources: Hatano, Y., & Shimazaki, T. Japan, in *The international encyclopedia of sexuality,* vol. 2. R. T. Francoeur, ed. New York: Continuum Publishing, 1999; Malkin, E., & Thompson, G. Mexican court says sex attack by a husband is still a rape. *The New York Times* (November 17, 2005).

---

outcomes among a sample of adult men who have sexual activity with men. They found that the forced-sex group had the highest levels of psychological distress, substance use, and HIV risk.

Often, sexual assault experiences are less traumatic for the child than for the parents. It is important that adults understand children's feelings and reactions, because a child often suffers no lasting trauma if parents can control their reactions.

Prevention

Preventing child sexual abuse demands attention. Fortunately, in recent years programs have been designed to educate children and adults to distinguish between appropriate and inappropriate touch, to say no to unwanted or uncomfortable touch, to tell a trusted adult if inappropriate touch occurs, and to identify their family and community support systems. In addition, adolescents have been encouraged to consider the risks related to certain behaviors, the selection of a mate who will not abuse their children, and ways in which they will protect children from sexual abuse.

Developing children's competence is essential, with the objective of helping children to recognize abusive situations and disclose victimization. In addi-

tion, parents can help children learn about sexual abuse in appropriate ways. They can also help children know some basic ways to help prevent sexual abuse such as (Pedophilia: Who are the men who "love" children in intolerable ways?, 2005):

- Never disclose personal information, such as your address, to strangers online.

- Never meet privately in person with anyone you have met online.

- Never get close to a car if a stranger stops and asks for directions.

- Never accept a ride from, or go anywhere alone with, an adult you don't know.

- No adult should touch you or ask you to touch him or her in any way that is confusing or frightening. If this happens, refuse and tell your parent immediately.

- No adult should ever ask you to keep a touch or a kiss secret. If this happens, tell your parent immediately.

- If any of these things happen, you will not be punished even if you have broken a rule.

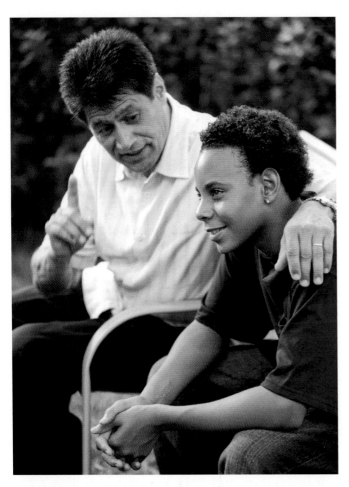

It is important to communicate about sexual abuse and how to prevent it.

A major challenge for prevention is the population of young teens who are willing to enter into voluntary sexual relationships with adults whom they meet online. People are often reluctant to confront these situations, but effective prevention requires public and private recognition of what actually happens in these cases. Teens may benefit from being told directly about why such relationships are a bad idea and made to understand that adults who care about their well-being would not propose sexual relationships or involve them in risky encounters. Efforts should be focused on the most vulnerable teens, such as those who have poor relationships with their parents, those who are lonely or depressed, or gay teens or those who are questioning their sexual orientation and turn to others on the Internet for support or information. Training is also needed for law enforcement personnel because teens may not initially see themselves as victims and may require sensitive interviewing to cooperate with investigators (Wolak et al., 2004).

Educators, parents, and other adults need to learn to recognize physical and behavioral signs of sexual abuse and pay attention to indirectly related comments made by a child. Physical signs may include irritation, pain, or injury in the genital area. Behavioral signs may include nervous, aggressive, hostile, or disruptive behavior toward adults, especially parents. It is wise to remember that one sign alone may not be a positive indication, but if a number of signs are present, the possibility of sexual abuse should be considered (*Child sexual abuse*, 1998). One should believe the child, remain calm, avoid blaming the child, avoid leading questions such as "You did that a lot?" and know where to seek help for counseling services. Adults also need to help children learn that they do not have to agree to demands for physical closeness; that touching can be good, bad, or confusing; that some secrets should not be kept; that at times adults make mistakes and do things they should not; and that there are times to ask for help and to give help when asked for help by a friend.

Another way to help prevent sexual abuse is to carefully screen professionals who work with children. For example, in many states it is necessary for teachers and other school personnel to have a background check before they can assume their responsibilities. This is usually done by requiring fingerprinting of such professionals before they are hired.

A vivid example of the need to screen individuals working with children carefully was seen in 2002

 Did You Know . . .

Law enforcement personnel are recognizing the need for special training to handle child sexual abuse cases. Without proper training, innocent people can be falsely charged, valid cases may have to be dismissed, and children and others involved may not be treated as well as possible.

Training includes the dynamics of child sexual abuse, the science of interviewing children, and approaches to verifying and corroborating allegations. Understanding the psychological needs of the victim, recognizing the sometimes vague symptoms of abuse, and knowing how to elicit sensitive information about sexual behavior from children are essential skills for law enforcement personnel.

when a Boston church scandal started a chain reaction (Kasindorf, Bayles, & Grossman, 2002). In January 2002, Boston's Cardinal Bernard Law acknowledged that he had moved a priest from parish to parish despite evidence that he had molested children. Soon afterward, church files revealed that another priest had abused children and advocated sexual activities between men and boys but still received the archdiocese's support. Before the year was over, thousands of adults filed lawsuits over abuse they said occurred when they were boys and girls—some as long as 50 years earlier. Five U.S. bishops, including Cardinal Law, resigned for reasons related to sexual abuse of children. Although he was not personally accused of abuse, Law resigned because of his failure to deal effectively with abusers who were priests. Interestingly, Law then abruptly moved to Rome and took up a series of positions in the Vatican. He was appointed archpriest of the Basilica di Santa Maria Maggiore, and also took full part in a conclave that selected the successor to Pope John Paul II (Hitchens, 2008). This certainly sent mixed signals regarding the Vatican's feelings about Law's actions.

As a result of this scandal, Roman Catholic bishops adopted a new policy for handling priests accused of sexual abuse. If a priest is found guilty by a board composed mostly of lay Catholics and at least one priest, he cannot wear a collar or give Communion, and he may be stripped of his status. In addition, most priests indicated they will tell the police about sexual abuse allegations in the future (Michaels, 2002).

In recent years, all 50 states have passed laws requiring sex offenders to alert the community to their presence. Many states run Internet sites listing such criminals. In some states judges have ordered offenders to post signs outside their homes, mandated bumper stickers, and even required temporary placards for traveling in someone else's car. Some people argue these laws are appropriate to help protect society from sex offenders; others consider it inappropriate to brand people and even punish their families. A Washington state study found that such policies did not prevent sex offenders from committing more crimes, but they did help police find and arrest repeat offenders more quickly (Thomas, 2001).

In many states there is a law requiring rapists and child molesters to register each year for inclusion in a database of sex offenders. Failure to register is usually a felony and can result in more jail time. Even so, the state of California lost track of more than 33,000 sex offenders, or 44% of the total number of registered offenders. They simply vanished after registering. Nationally, 52% of rapists are arrested for new crimes within 3 years of leaving prison, according to the U.S. Justice Department (Curtis, 2003).

In 2006, the Adam Walsh Child Protection and Safety Act was passed by the U.S. Congress. It requires all states to adopt strict standards for registering sex offenders and is meant to prevent offenders from eluding authorities, especially when they move out of state. The act made it a federal crime (a felony) to fail to reregister as a sex offender, after moving to another state and requires states to toughen their penalties for failing to register at all; currently, many states treat such failure as a misdemeanor. An estimated 100,000 sex offenders are not living where they are registered. A number of controversial points have been raised in relation to the act. State officials complain about the law's cost, may believe they have more effective laws than the federal one, and say the federal requirements violate the states' right to set their own policies. In addition, some sex offenders and civil liberties groups have argued that juvenile sex offenders should not have to be on public registries for life and note that the law does not take into account the individual circumstances of each sex offender (Goodnough & Davey, 2009).

College officials have to decide how to best deal with the Campus Sex Crimes Prevention Act, a federal law that requires sex offenders, when they register with the state, to indicate whether and where they are enrolled, employed, or volunteering on a college campus. As of October 1, 2003, college officials must tell students, faculty, and administrators where information on registered sex offenders can be obtained. Most have chosen to make the registry available for perusal in the campus police department and made its existence known either through the college's web site or by mailing of pamphlets that direct students and others to its location (Bosslett, 2003).

In many states treatment for those convicted of sexual abuse of children is required by law. It is hoped that such treatment will help prevent future sexual abuse, but much remains to be learned about effective treatment. Many treatment methods have been tried. For example, aversion therapy is used to associate a pedophilic fantasy or desire with an unpleasant sensation such as nausea or an electric shock. Behavior therapy is also used to help offenders exercise self-control by changing their beliefs and attitudes as well as their behavior. Many other psychological techniques have been tried, such as externalization where the offender learns how his or her actions look and feel to the child. A number of medications have also been tried with the hope of diminishing sexual desire. It is difficult to tell for sure just how effective various treatments have been. Research results about treatments have not been conclusive (Pedophilia: Who are the men who "love" children in intolerable ways?, 2005).

Ethical DIMENSIONS

Is It Ethical to Publicly Identify Sexual Offenders?

Named after Megan Kanka, a 7-year-old New Jersey child who was raped and murdered by a convicted sex offender who lived across the street from her, "Megan's Law" requires that authorities and the community be notified when a convicted sex offender is released or moves into their neighborhood. Variations of Megan's Law are found in a number of states. For example, Alabama's Megan's Law also forbids a convicted offender to live near a school, day care center, or past victim.

Some people want a law requiring that the identity of convicted child molesters be made known to community members. This means that if a convicted child molester moved into your community, you and all your neighbors would be informed that he or she was there and that he or she had been a child molester. Many people support such a law because they feel they have a right to protect their children.

Other people think it is a violation of individual rights and personal privacy if a convicted child molester's identity is made public. They believe that the molester, as has

any other person convicted of a crime, has paid for the crime through a prison sentence and in other possible ways, and it is not ethical to reveal his or her identity to the public. The person has a right to live privately and to start a new life if he or she desires. On the basis of these arguments, there have been legal challenges to Megan's Law in New Jersey, and similar laws have been found unconstitutional in other states.

In Virginia, state police developed a web site that lists the names of violent sex offenders. They guessed that 5,000 people would log on on the first day. In fact, in the first 12 hours, it was visited more than 45,000 times. By the second day, the site was so jammed that many people could not get through because the site can handle only six "hits" per second. Some people express the point of view that we should not be concerned about former sex offenders being harassed, because "If they don't want their names in the paper, they shouldn't commit the crime." Others question the ethics of this web site and feel it treats sex offenders unfairly.

Do you think it is ethical to require that identities of sexual offenders be made public?

Incest

Incest is sexual behavior between relatives who are too closely related to be legally married. Much of what has been said about child sexual abuse also applies to incest. However, it is helpful to consider incest separately because it is rapidly changing from a private subject to a public one.

Most contemporary research studies related to incest seem to focus on the offenders, family relationships, and possible treatments. There is not much new information about incest statistics. Because of that, much of the statistical information about incest tends to be older than might be desired. However, it still is a relatively good snapshot of the situation.

The most commonly reported form of incest is father–daughter, but in practice brother–sister incest probably happens more often (Canavan, Meyer, & Higgs, 1992). It has traditionally been estimated that about 10% of girls had a sexual experience with an adult relative, but the proportion is probably closer to 19%. In fact, when child sexual abuse by relatives out-

incest
Sexual behavior between relatives who are too closely related to be married.

side the basic family unit was included, a total of 38% of women reported at least one experience of sexual abuse before reaching the age of 18 years (Startling new study shows one in six women incestuously abused before age 18, 1986). Boys are less commonly molested by a parent or other older relative, although this also occurs.

Mother–child incest was often thought to be virtually nonexistent. This may be because of a cultural unwillingness to believe that women commit such acts or because female sex offenders have seldom been studied. Although many more males than females are guilty of incest, it is likely that the amount of sexual abuse of male and female children by women has been underestimated (Banning, 1989).

Children involved in incest are usually afraid to tell anyone about it for many of the same reasons that children do not want to tell anyone about sexual assault in general. The incest abuser may threaten the child, other family members, or friends to ensure silence. The incest abuser also says that if anyone finds out, everyone will hate and reject the child for having "participated" in this. The child, feeling violated and dirty, often believes the abuser. Guilt and shame also play a big part in a child's decision not to ask for help after incest has occurred. This is especially true if the child was raised in a home where sexual behavior is considered dirty or sinful. Also, the child may be uncertain what to think about the experience. With this uncertainty, he/she may decide it is safer not to say anything (Larsen, 2005a).

The characteristics of those involved in incest are surprising. For example, the offenders often appear to be nice guys—conventional, independent, and often very self-assured. The mothers in homes where incest occurs tend to be emotionally distant and aloof toward their children. Vulnerable family members typically view the father as the parent who loves them because he interacts more with them and provides significant caretaking, despite the incestual behavior (What families won't tell, 1986).

More than 95% of the offenders are male, and the family structure tends to be strongly patriarchal. Most families involved have lived in the same place for at least 5 years, and, contrary to popular beliefs, stepfathers are not involved more often than biological fathers. When confronted, most abusive fathers appear truly sorry for their actions, but the vast majority do not believe they have done anything particularly wrong. Incestuous fathers openly indicate they feel a right to educate their children about sex and to use their children to meet their own sexual needs. Incest is related to the father's immaturity—it is not only sex he is after but power and control. The common denominator in these men seems to be self-indulgence. Many refuse to believe that they really hurt their children. Basically, the act is so pleasurable they just do not care. It has been estimated that more than 1 million American women have been sexually abused by fathers, stepfathers, brothers, uncles, or other family members (What families won't tell, 1986).

The incest taboo is universal in human culture. It is considered by anthropologists to be the foundation of all kinship structures and even the basis of human social order (Herman, 1985). Nevertheless, incest occurs in all social classes, in all geographic areas,

Incest victims look and act like anyone else. However, they may suffer from long-term psychological consequences.

and among all ethnic and racial groups.

Compared to females who are not incest victims, female incest survivors report significantly higher anger levels in general and more anger toward their parents; anger toward mother and father is about equal. The extent of their anger is correlated with the age of the victim at the onset of incest, the duration of incest, incest involving penetration and use of force, and perceived parental responsibility for abuse (Newman & Peterson, 1996).

It is difficult, if not impossible, to separate the long-term effects of sexual abuse of children in general from those of incest, but it is important to try to understand them. The long-term consequences that affect adults in many ways include (1) post-traumatic stress disorder (including hypervigilance, intrusive thoughts, and flashbacks of the abusive experience); (2) cognitive distortions (for example, seeing the world as a dangerous place, underestimating personal self-worth, or having chronic perceptions of helplessness); (3) emotional distress; (4) impaired sense of self (relying on the reactions of others to determine their own feelings, potential to be easily manipulated by others); (5) avoidance; (6) interpersonal difficulties; and (7) health problems (Kendall-Tackett & Marshall, 1988).

The possible behavioral signs of incest are also similar to those of sexual abuse in general. They can include eating disorders or loss of appetite, extreme changes in behavioral patterns, lack of self-confidence, unexplained fear of a particular person, unusual knowledge of sexual matters, regressing to infantile behavior, poor interpersonal relationships, or attempts to run away (Larsen, 2005b). Obviously, some of the symptoms of incest can also be normal adolescent problems, but parents and teachers need to at least be aware of the possibility that incest has occurred.

Sexual abuse experts say some victims of incest use overeating to escape inner turmoil and downplay their femininity. They might gain weight so their bodies do not look so good. They might also avoid unwanted attention to their bodies by wearing baggy clothes along with gaining too much weight (McGee, 2007).

Various community organizations offer help for incest survivors and their families—for example, child-protection agencies, rape crisis centers, women's centers, and organizations that offer help for parents who are under extreme stress or are frightened about their feelings toward their children. The best strategy for preventing incest is to provide information to children as well as to parents. This means providing sexuality education at the elementary school level and above, including specific information about incest. For example, children should be taught that Uncle Charlie or Aunt Mary does not automatically have the right to touch them all over. In addition, information about pedophilia and other sexual practices should be provided at the appropriate level of understanding.

The initial focus of crisis intervention should be on stopping the sexual abuse and establishing a safe environment in the family. Once the incest is reported, it is controversial whether the child should be temporarily removed from the home. This might be destructive to the child because she may feel that she has done something wrong, that she is being punished, or that both parents are against her. It is also difficult to find an appropriate place to put the child; however, removal from the home may be the only way to ensure the child's safety.

There is also a nationwide group called Survivors of Incest Anonymous that works very much like Alcoholics Anonymous. It is a self-help group of women and men, 18 years and older, who are guided by a set of 12 Suggested Steps and 12 Traditions. The only requirement for membership is that you are a victim of child sexual abuse, and that you are not abusing any child. More information about Survivors of Incest Anonymous can be found at *www.siawso.org*.

■ Relationship Abuse

As we have seen, the topics of childhood sexual abuse and incest overlap. The same is true of various aspects of relationship abuse. For example, the abuse may take the form of forced sexual activity, use of violence without sexual activity, or both. Today it is recognized that males and females can both be victims of relationship abuse. In fact, both males and females engage in frequent minor assaults. However, females are more often the victims of severe partner assault and injury, not necessarily because males strike more often but because males strike harder (Morse, 1995). Because the number of *reported* cases of abuse of wives far exceeds the number of *reported* cases of the abuse of husbands, because physical danger to wives is usually far greater, and because most of the studies available on this topic

deal with females, most of the information here is about females as well.

Violence in relationships seems to start well before adult years. For example, in the 12 months prior to one survey, about 9% of students in grades 9 to 12 had been hit, slapped, or physically hurt on purpose by their boyfriend or girlfriend (Grunbaum et al., 2004). Overall, the prevalence of dating violence was higher among African American (13.9%) and Hispanic (9.3%) students than among white (7%) students.

Dating violence is dangerous in many ways, but one of these ways relates to the prevalence of STI, including HIV. Compared with nonabused girls, girls in grades 9 to 12 who experienced both physical and sexual dating violence were three times more likely to have been tested for STI and HIV, and 2.6 times more likely to report an STI diagnosis (Decker, Silverman, & Raj, 2005).

Marital Rape

Until the late 1970s, most states did not consider spousal rape to be a crime. In most cases, spouses were exempted from the sexual assault laws. For example, until 1993 North Carolina law stated that "a person may not be prosecuted under this article if the victim is the person's legal spouse at the time of the commission of the alleged rape or sexual offense unless the parties are living separate and apart." These laws date all the way back to the seventeenth century, when it was said that "for by their mutual matrimonial consent and contract the wife hath given up herself in this kind unto the husband which she cannot retract." In the late 1970s, feminists began efforts to change these laws. Currently, rape of a spouse is a crime in all 50 states and the District of Columbia (Spousal rape laws: 20 years later, 2004).

For obvious reasons, it is difficult to obtain accurate information on the frequency of spousal rape.

In the movie *Gone with the Wind,* the husband, Rhett Butler (played by Clark Gable), carries his wife, Scarlett O'Hara (Vivien Leigh), kicking and screaming up a staircase, implying sexual activity is to follow. Portrayed as sensual more than 60 years ago, could it be considered spousal rape by today's standards?

Based on various studies, an estimated 14% of married women report they were raped by their spouse. This percentage probably underestimates the true prevalence of marital rape. Of reporting women, 23% reported rape and sexual assault as the only abuse in the marriage. Also, 10% of all sexual assault cases reported by women involved a husband or ex-husband attacker (Marital rape, 2000).

Why spouses are raped is a question that has not been greatly explored. The few existing studies summarize common reasons as (1) entitlement to sex (thinking that the marriage contract includes the right to sexual intercourse on demand), (2) sexual jealousy, (3) rape as punishment for some "wrong" behavior, and (4) rape as a form of control (asserting of power and control) (Bergen, 1998).

A number of factors contribute to the underreporting of spousal rape and women's reluctance to discuss such experiences. They include the following:

1. Loyalty to husband/privacy of family

2. Unwillingness to accept their own victimization

3. Reluctance to label the experience as "rape"

4. Misunderstandings about a woman's role in marriage and marital responsibilities

5. Sexual inexperience and uncertainty about what constitute "normal" and "forced" sexual relations (Mahoney & Williams, 1998)

Victims of rape by a husband are different from other rape victims because they are violated by someone with whom they share their homes, lives, and maybe children. They are faced with a betrayal of trust and intimacy. Wife rape victims are more likely to be raped multiple times than stranger and acquaintance rape victims. Women who experience wife rape suffer long-lasting physical and psychological injuries that are as severe as or more severe than those of stranger rape victims (Bergen, 2009).

Why would a woman stay with a man who raped her? The answers are usually very complicated but include such reasons as the following:

1. Many women believe it is part of their "duty" to have sexual intercourse with their husband, even if it is violent and against their will.

2. Many women cannot leave because they do not have the financial resources to do so.

3. Women may fear what the offender may do to them or the children.

4. Some women may not leave because of love and loyalty to the husband, which can override their own pain and suffering (Mahoney & Williams, 1998).

It seems that women raped by a spouse are more likely to experience long-term effects than are women raped by an acquaintance or a stranger. Possible long-term effects include (1) negative feelings toward men; (2) low self-esteem; (3) fear; (4) anxiety; (5) guilt; (6) embarrassment; (7) outrage; (8) changes in behaviors, including an increase in drinking and refusal to consider remarriage; and (9) depression (Peacock, 1998).

Basile (2002a) examined national attitudes toward wife rape. She found that older, nonwhite respondents were less likely to believe wife rape occurs. Males and the less educated were less likely to believe it occurs frequently. Older and less-educated respondents were less likely to believe forced sexual scenarios between a husband and wife constitute wife rape. Among women, nonvictims were significantly less likely than current victims to believe that wife rape occurs.

Basile (2002b) looked at the amount of reported wife rape and other types of sexual coercion based upon statistics from other studies. She estimated that 34% of women were victims of some type of sexual coercion with a husband or partner in their lifetime. Of these women, 10% experienced rape by a current partner. This rate increased to 13% when only rape by a current husband was included. Other findings indicated that women had sexual activity with a current spouse or partner in return for a partner's spending money on them (24%), after the partner begged and pleaded with them (26%), and after their partner said things to bully them (9%).

Intimate-Partner Violence

Domestic violence is a significant health and social problem in the United States and many other industrialized societies. In some industrialized societies, however, it is considered to be almost nonexistent. The reasons for the variability from culture to culture have not been established. Intimate-partner violence occurs for many reasons. It can be an indication of manhood, a means of personal control, a reflection of personal animosity, and an expression of social jealousy. Women who are victims of violence are often unable or afraid to seek health care, and violence also has serious consequences for maternal mortality and child survival. Here are some related statistics about international gender-based violence (The facts on international gender-based violence, 2005):

- Intimate partners commit 40% to 70% of homicides of women worldwide.

- Around the world, 1 in 3 women have been beaten, coerced into sexual activity, and otherwise abused in their lifetime. Most often, the abuser is a family member.

- There is a strong relationship between intimate-partner violence and the spread of HIV/AIDS in the developing world. Violence and poverty force many women to remain in dangerous relationships where they are often subject to rape and HIV infection by their partners.

- Between 4% and 20% of women in developing countries experience violence during pregnancy. They then run twice the risk of miscarriage and have four times the risk of having a baby that is below average weight.

- In Nicaragua, research has shown that children of women who are abused are six times more likely to die before the age of 5 than other children.

- A study in India showed that intimate-partner violence was the cause of 16% of maternal deaths during pregnancy.

- In the United States, health care costs of intimate-partner violence against women amount to approximately $5.8 billion each year.

It is a difficult task to estimate rates of intimate-partner violence. Many factors inhibit women from reporting these crimes. The private nature of the event, the perceived stigma, and the belief that no purpose would be served by reporting the crime prevent an unknown percentage of survivors from talking about the event. Therefore, available statistics are at best estimates.

Estimates range from 960,000 incidents of violence against a current or former spouse, boyfriend, or girlfriend per year to 3 million women who are physically abused by their husband or boyfriend each year. Nearly one-third of American women report being physically or sexually abused by a husband or boyfriend at some point in their lives. Intimate-partner violence is primarily a crime against women. Women are about 85% of the victims, and men make up the remaining 15%. Women are less likely than men to be victims of crime overall; however, they are five to eight times more likely than men to be victimized by an intimate partner. Women of all races are about equally vulnerable to violence by an intimate (Prevalence of domestic violence, 2005).

In a recent year, 1,247 women were killed by an intimate partner, as were 440 men. Intimate-partner homicides account for about 33% of the murders of women, but less than 4% of the murders of men. Pregnant and recently pregnant women are more likely to be victims of homicide than to die of any other cause. Thirty-seven percent of women who sought treatment in emergency rooms for violence-related injuries were injured by a current or former spouse, boyfriend, or girlfriend (Domestic homicides, 2005).

Children are also involved in intimate-partner violence. Fifty percent of men who frequently abuse their wives also frequently abuse their children. Slightly more than half of female victims of intimate-partner violence live in households with children younger than the age of 12. Between 3.3 and 10 million children witness some form of domestic violence annually (Domestic violence and children, 2005).

Direct physical attack is the most common abuse, but a woman is also abused when she is repeatedly placed in physical danger or controlled by the use of threats to hurt her, her children, friends, family, or pets. Physical abuse can also be sexual. A marital or live-in relationship does not give a man the right to force sexual relations or practices that are unwanted, uncomfortable, or degrading. Battered women often have low self-esteem and feel humiliated and ashamed of their body. For the battering man, daily tensions seem to lead to abusive behaviors and violent explosions. Afterward, the man most likely makes excuses, apologizes, and promises it will

Back in the 1950s, the popular TV show *The Honeymooners* portrayed the blue-collar husband Ralph (Jackie Gleason) as getting mad at his wife and threatening, "One of these days, Alice … Pow … Right to the moon!" The line provoked uproarious laughter. (He never did harm her.) But there is nothing funny about intimate-partner violence. According to the National Coalition Against Domestic Abuse, 4 million U.S. women are victims of assaults by their partners each year.

not happen again. He may even make a special effort to smooth things over by trying to be nice. Because his wife wants to believe him, they often make up and she tries to forget. As time passes, tensions can build again for the abuser. Then, the violence recurs as part of a cycle of violence. This cycle has several steps. The first is "walking on eggs," where everyone is trying to be very careful within the relationship. The second step is when tensions build and violence occurs again. The third step is a time of regret and "I love you"—saying it will never happen again. Then, the cycle repeats itself.

The physical abuse associated with intimate-partner violence is probably heard about most often; such violence, however, is not limited to physical abuse. The National Resource Center on Domestic Violence (*Help end domestic violence,* n.d.) defines it as a "pattern of abusive and controlling behaviors that some individuals use against their intimate partners or former partners." In addition to physical abuse such as hitting, punching, kicking, or using weapons, it can include

- *Sexual abuse:* forcing a partner to engage in unwanted sexual behaviors.

- *Emotional abuse:* name calling and put-downs; stalking; treating a partner as inferior; using threatening looks, actions, or gestures; threatening children or pets.

- *Property/economic abuse:* stealing or destroying property and money; refusing the partner food or medical attention; or interfering with a partner's work or education.

In addition, annually in the United States, more than 503,000 women are stalked by an intimate partner. Seventy-eight percent of stalking victims are women. Eighty percent of women who are stalked by former husbands are physically assaulted by that partner, and 30% are sexually assaulted by that partner (Stalking, 2005).

Batterers often tend to absolve themselves of full responsibility, and, at the same time, they offer justifications for their abusiveness. The most common excuse is an appeal to loss of control—usually resulting either from drug or alcohol use or from a buildup of frustrations. Because awareness is impaired, there is a feeling that their impairment diminishes responsibility. The second major category of excuse is victim blaming. The men deny responsibility by claiming they were "provoked." Most often, batterers say their violence was a response to verbal aggressiveness; in some cases they say it was a response to physical aggressiveness (Ptacek, 1998).

Whereas excuses represent denial of responsibility, justifications are denials of wrongdoing by the offender.

The first category of justification is denial of injury. Offenders deny or minimize the injuries battered women suffer. The second category involves finding fault with the woman for something—perhaps not being good at cooking, not being sexually responsive, not being deferential enough to her husband, not being faithful, and so on. The assumption of entitlement, denies the wrongness of the violence. The batterer sees himself as punishing the woman for her failure to be a good wife (Ptacek, 1998).

Those who are battered may stay with a batterer for a number of reasons, including financial dependence, lack of social support (the batterer may have controlled the victim's contact with other people), fear of severe physical attack, self-blame (believing the abuse is a result of the victim's real or imagined offenses), or belief that the violence is temporary or caused by unusual circumstances. Many battered women believe the abuse will stop when "things return to normal" (Dating and domestic violence, 2009).

Intimate-partner violence doesn't stay home while its victims go to work. It also affects employees while they are at the workplace. For example, 74% of employed battered women were harassed by their partner while they were at work. On average, 1.7 million violent victimizations per year are committed against persons while at work. Homicide is the second leading cause of death on the job for women. More than 29,000 acts of rape or sexual assault are perpetrated against women at work each year. Many women report missing work as a result of stalking. In addition, 24% of women who experienced intimate-partner violence said that the abuse caused them to arrive late for work or miss days of work (The facts on the workplace and domestic violence, 2005).

There has been increased awareness of the problem of violence against women in the military. Women in the military are particularly vulnerable to abuse due to geographical isolation from family and friends, and the potential for social isolation within the military culture. The victim of intimate-partner violence in the military is mainly the female, civilian spouse of active-duty personnel. Victims normally have children and more than half have been married 2 years or less. Abused women in military communities are often fearful of reporting incidents due to the lack of confidentiality and privacy as well as limited victim services (The facts on the military and violence against women, 2005).

We have been slow to recognize the problem of intimate-partner violence. In the past, laws and common practice encouraged husbands to discipline their wives by force if they saw fit. But conditions are changing. Family violence research has made it clear that the problem of battering is too widespread

Multicultural DIMENSIONS

Examples of Female Abuse in Other Countries

Don't Talk to Strangers is a 23-part TV series that ran on Chinese networks and has been marketed abroad. The series was credited with putting the uncomfortable subject of spousal abuse in the open in China. This was surprising to many because traditional Chinese culture teaches that family problems should stay within the family. Many were surprised when the show made it past Communist Party propaganda officials, who generally frown on negative portrayals of Chinese society.

Some viewers found the show too violent, too gloomy, and too hopeless. Others consider it important to get the problem out into the open. Activists say spousal abuse occurs in one in three Chinese families compared to one in four in the United States.

In China, the marriage law of 2001 gives victims the right to protection and orders abusers punished. In divorce cases, victims of abuse can also sue for damages. However, willingness to enforce the law varies widely across the country. China's first battered women's shelters were forced to close because of lack of money or authorities' unwillingness to offer protection. Some people consider it normal for couples to fight, and it is difficult to get people to see that as violence.

In 2002, there was a well-publicized example of "honor rape" in Pakistan. Mukhtar Maj, then about 30 years old and from a lower caste, was gang-raped on the orders of the village council as a punishment because her 12-year-old brother was said to have had sexual relations with a woman from a higher caste. She did not commit suicide, as expected, but she founded two schools for children in her village and spoke out against "honor killings" and other outrages against women in her country. In 2005 she was invited to come to the United States to tell her story. The Pakistani government barred her from traveling abroad, but later lifted its travel restrictions (Pakistan lifts travel ban on raped woman, 2005).

In Kyrgyzstan, after 3 months of dating, Melis Aliyev turned to a practice that is a tradition in Kyrgyzstan, but a crime in the rest of the world. The woman he had been dating, Ainur Tairova, was kidnapped and kept in Aliyev's house for 2 days. Many friends and relatives repeatedly tried to force onto her head a white scarf signifying her acquiescence to the marriage. She eventually gave in to the man, who is still her husband 4 years later. Kidnapping to coerce a woman into marriage is on the books as a crime in Kyrgyzstan, but it is so ingrained in the country's male-dominated society that it is rarely prosecuted. In some cases, women who steadfastly refuse are raped by their captor, a crime men know likely will go unreported because filing a case with the police would brand the victim and her family with scandal (Rodriguez, 2005).

In Lagos, Nigeria, after a typical husband–wife argument, a husband followed his wife out the door. Then he beat her unconscious, and left her lying in the street near their apartment. The woman had defied her husband, and many men and women throughout sub-Saharan Africa consider that ample justification for a beating. One in three Nigerian women report having been physically abused by a male partner. In one case, a woman's husband beat her incessantly because she watched television movies. Many men feel that women are inferior and that men can do whatever they want to them. Intimate-partner violence accounts for more than 6 of 10 murder cases in court. Yet, most women remain silent about the abuse. Many men and women say that husbands have a right to beat wives who argue with them, burn the dinner, go out without the husband's permission, neglect the children, or refuse sexual activity. Nigeria's penal code specifically allows husbands to discipline their wives (LaFraniere, 2005).

Source: Bodeen, C. TV show about wife abuse grips China, *The Seattle Times* (February 3, 2003), A18.

to ignore or to explain away by blaming the victim. Many new resources are available. Battered women's shelters are particularly helpful in providing services for battered women and their children and in continuing efforts to educate people about intimate-partner violence.

Most of the research discussed so far has been about heterosexual couples. It has been only in

the last 20 years or so that literature about same-gender domestic violence started to appear. Conducting research with this population about a sensitive topic like intimate-partner violence remains difficult. However, existing studies show that the prevalence as well as the types of abuse and the dynamics of abuse are very similar between heterosexual and homosexual couples (McLennen, 2005).

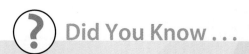
Did You Know ...

Violence by women received little attention until the mid-1970s. Now we know that women in relationships engage in violent acts as often as men. In about half of violent relationships, the violence is mutual. When there is a sole perpetrator, it is just as likely to be a female as a male. However, female use of violence, even when intended to cause harm, is mainly self-defensive.

Men tend to inflict more severe damage on women than the converse. Reasons given for this are that women tend to cease violent behaviors before causing serious injury and that men are usually physically larger and stronger than women.

The needs of battered men are somewhat different from those of battered women. Abused women have varied needs, including safety for themselves and often for their children; abused men's needs are more limited. Because they usually have the necessary resources to leave the relationship, their primary needs are legal assistance and psychological counseling.

Sources: Flynn, C. P. Relationship violence by women: Issues and implications, *Family Relations, 38, no. 2* (April 1990), 194–198; Morse, B. J. Beyond the conflict tactics scale: Assessing gender differences in partner violence, *Violence and Victims, 10, no. 4* (winter 1995), 251–272.

There are ways we can combat intimate-partner violence. Here are some possibilities (101 ways to combat domestic violence, 2003):

1. Make violence unacceptable in your life.

2. Contact your local school board and ask its members to address dating violence.

3. Contact your local media representatives and remind them that October is Domestic Violence Awareness Month. Ask them what they plan to do. Tell them about the National Domestic Violence Hotline (800-799-SAFE), and ask them to publicize it.

4. Contact community businesses and agencies, and ask them to display the number of the National Domestic Violence Hotline in prominent places.

5. Contact local schools and colleges and let students know about resources available on the Internet concerning intimate-partner violence.

6. Ask the local police department to be sure officers are trained in handling intimate-partner violence.

7. Ask your priest, pastor, rabbi, or other religious leader to have a special service devoted to intimate-partner violence.

8. Do not let jokes about violent behavior go unchallenged.

9. Work with day care centers to make information about intimate-partner violence available to their customers.

10. Learn more about policies and facilities related to intimate-partner violence in your community.

Services for survivors of intimate-partner violence have been improved through the years, but more and better services are still needed. In 1994, the Violence Against Women Act was passed by Congress; it was extended in 2000. Its purpose was to broaden the range of services and counseling available to women victims of abuse. In 2005, the act was reauthorized, and it increased funding for new rape crisis centers and increased grant money to organizations working on intimate-partner violence issues (Feminist Wire Daily Newsbriefs, 2005).

Also, the Office for Victims of Crime of the U.S. Department of Justice provided funding in 1997 to develop Sexual Assault Nurse Examiner (SANE) programs designed to improve the community response to sexual assault victims. There are now hundreds of these programs around the country, and new ones are started every month. The goal is to see that every victim receives fundamental justice and needed services (Little, 2005).

Sexual Harassment

Since the mid-1970s, courts, popular and professional periodicals, newspapers, and books have focused on **sexual harassment**. Hundreds of articles have appeared in print, increasing the national attention paid to the subject. It is not easy to define sexual harassment. Sometimes it is hard to draw the line between harassment and other behaviors, but it can include touching, verbal abuse, demanding of sexual favors, or use of threatening tones.

The U.S. Equal Employment Opportunity Commission

sexual harassment
Unwelcome verbal, physical, or sexual conduct that has the effect of creating an intimidating, hostile, or offensive environment.

(EEOC) says that sexual harassment is a form of sex discrimination that violates Title VII of the Civil Rights Act of 1964. It defines sexual harassment as unwelcome sexual advances, requests for sexual favors, and other verbal or physical conduct of a sexual nature when this conduct explicitly or implicitly affects an individual's employment, unreasonably interferes with an individual's work performance, or creates an intimidating, hostile, or offensive work environment (Sexual harassment, 2005). The EEOC also says that sexual harassment can occur in a variety of circumstances, including but not limited to the following:

- The victim as well as the harasser may be a woman or a man. The victim does not have to be of the other gender.

- The harasser can be the victim's supervisor, an agent of the employer, a supervisor in another area, a coworker, or a non-employee.

- The victim does not have to be the person harassed but could be anyone affected by the offensive conduct.

- Unlawful sexual harassment may occur without economic injury to or discharge of the victim.

- The harasser's conduct must be unwelcome.

The Commission further says that it is helpful for the victim to inform the harasser directly that the conduct is unwelcome and must stop. The victim should use any employer complaint mechanism or grievance system available.

Sexual harassment may include verbal abuse; sexist remarks regarding a person's clothing or body; patting, pinching, or brushing up against a person's body; leering or ogling; demand for sexual favors in return for hiring, promotion, or tenure; physical assault; and rape. Two categories of sexual harassment have been described. In the first, something is to be exchanged. Perhaps a boss offers a person a job opportunity in exchange for sexual favors or threatens loss of a job opportunity if the person does not comply. In the second, there is no promise or threat; however, there are sexual remarks, touching/stroking, or lewd looks.

Legally speaking, then, there are two kinds of sexual harassment. The first is quid pro quo (Latin for "something for something"): Something is to be exchanged. The second is a hostile environment, which means that speech or conduct in itself can create a hostile environment, which in turn is sexual harassment.

The EEOC has kept statistics related to sexual harassment since 1997. The number of charges filed with the EEOC each year has remained relatively con-

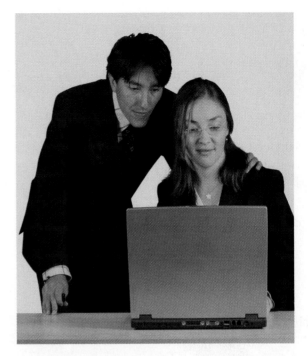

Workplace sexual harassment can include various behaviors. Coworkers need to indicate when behavior is inappropriate and unwanted.

sistent, but has decreased somewhat over the years. For example, there were almost 16,000 charges in 1997 and almost 14,000 in 2008. The percentage of charges filed by males increased from 11.6% in 2007 to about 16% in 2008 (Sexual harassment charges, 2009).

In 2009, the U.S. Supreme Court ruled that workers who cooperate with an internal investigation and report uncouth behavior by a supervisor are protected from retaliation under civil rights laws (Sexual harassment, 2009). This ruling further strengthened laws against sexual harassment in the workplace.

Efforts to end sexual harassment that rely mainly on target reporting are unlikely to be successful because most targets do not report their experiences. They tend to deny the harassment, avoid the harasser, or treat the harassment as a joke rather than confronting the harasser or reporting the behavior. It seems that the targets don't report the offenses because they want to avoid reprisal by the harasser and maintain their reputation and status in the workgroup. For this reason, some experts feel that one way for progress to be made against sexual harassment is for those who observe the harassment to be the ones who report it (Bowes-Sperry & O'Leary, 2005).

In addition to being upsetting and distracting, workplace sexual harassment can even be hazardous to health. For example, Rospenda et al. (2005) found that exposure to workplace harassment increases risk for illness, injury, or assault. Thus harassment may be hazardous not only to targets' health, but also to the

Sexual harassment lawsuits can have far-reaching effects. Anucha Browne Sanders, an executive for the New York Knicks basketball team, accused coach Isiah Thomas of sexual harassment in 2006. The lawsuit also accused team owner James Dolan of firing her in retaliation for her initial harassment complaint. The exposure in the news media led to concerns about the team's leadership and had a negative effect on the team's reputation. Browne Sanders won the lawsuit, but her job was not reinstated; it took her more than a year to find a new job. Thomas was replaced as coach in 2008. Dolan was found liable and was ordered to pay Browne Sanders $3 million, in addition to the $8.6 million ordered to be paid to her by Madison Square Garden. The total punitive damages of $11.6 million was one of the largest sexual harassment judgments in history.

bottom line of the organization in the form of costly worker's compensation claims.

One interesting multicultural aspect related to sexual harassment is that in 2005 China's parliament amended the Law on the Protection of the Rights and Interests of Women (A woman's right to sue, 2005). Amendments were then passed that made sexual harassment of women unlawful, stipulating that equality between men and women is a basic state policy. It will be interesting to see how many Chinese women take advantage of the opportunity to complain about harassment to their employers and to the "relevant department" in the government, and to bring civil suits against their tormentors.

As use of the Internet has grown, so has sexual harassment on the Internet. While it is impossible to know the extent of sexual harassment on the Internet, it seems that most victims are women (Barak, 2005).

The three general types of offline sexual harassment also exist online: (1) gender harassment—unwelcome comments that insult individuals because of their gender or that use stimuli intended to provoke negative emotions; (2) unwanted sexual attention—uninvited behaviors that communicate sexual desires or intentions toward another individual; and (3) sexual coercion—putting pressure on a person to elicit sexual cooperation. Online sexual coercion might even become actual coercion if a perpetrator uses technical knowledge to break into a person's computer and cause damage or threaten to do so. Sending frightening emails, sending viruses, and flooding an email box are just a few examples of actual sexual coercion. Sending erotic and pornographic pictures and videos are examples of gender harassment. With Internet harassment, a harasser can take advantage of being unidentifiable, anonymous, and invisible in addition to having immediate, easy-to-execute, almost untraceable escape routes.

Sexual Harassment in Schools

Initial concerns about sexual harassment focused on the workplace; however, more attention has also been given to schools and colleges. Verbal and physical sexual harassment often begin in elementary school. Four out of five girls, and almost as many boys, experience some form of sexual harassment (Sadker & Zittleman, 2005).

The American Association of University Women conducted a national survey on sexual harassment in public schools in 1993 and again in 2001 (Hostile hallways: Bullying, teasing, and sexual harassment in schools, 2001). It found that students in 2001 were much more likely to say that their schools had sexual harassment policies and distribute literature on sexual harassment. As in 1993, in 2001 80% of students experienced some form of sexual harassment at some time during their school life. There was a striking increase (from 18% to 24%) in the number of boys who often experienced sexual harassment in school. In addition, 56% of boys said they experienced sexual harassment occasionally. Girls were more likely than boys to experience sexual harassment ever (83% versus 79%). Students who experienced sexual harassment were most likely to react by avoiding the person who bothered or harassed them (40%), talking less in class (24%), wanting not to go to school (22%), changing their seat in class to get farther away from someone (21%), and finding it hard to pay attention in school (20%).

As mentioned, the number of court cases related to sexual harassment in schools is increasing. Although there have been some conflicting decisions, the Supreme Court issued a major decision in 1998 in its ruling that school districts cannot be liable for damages in a private lawsuit about teacher–student sexual harassment unless an official in a position to take corrective action knew of the harassment and was "deliberately indifferent" to it. At the same time Richard W. Riley, Secretary of Education, indicated, "Any sexual harassment of a student—particularly sexual abuse by a teacher—is a basic breach of trust between the school and the student and the family" (Walsh, 1998).

The question of whether schools should be held liable when students sexually harass their peers is extremely sensitive. Some people argue that schools should be responsible only for taking reasonable action rather than for ensuring that the behavior ends—although it can be hard to determine the definition of "reasonable." Others feel school personnel have a responsibility to take strong actions to prevent behaviors often associated with typical child growth and development—such as sexual comments, touching, and jeering. It is a real challenge to design appropriate policies and procedures related to students' sexually harassing their peers.

It is important to talk about sexual harassment with children in appropriate ways and at the appropriate level. For example, elementary school children should know that sexual harassment is unwanted and uninvited sexual attention such as teasing, touching, or taunting; sexual harassment is against the law; and they should be taught their school's sexual harassment policy. In addition, students aged 12 to 15 should know that sexual harassment can occur in a variety of settings including schools, the workplace, and extracurricular programs. They should also know where they can call for information about sexual harassment. Students aged 15 to 18 should also know that whether to report sexual harassment is a personal decision that can be hard to make, and that people who experience sexual harassment may need help and support to deal with the situation (Keeping kids sexually safe, 2004).

Sexual Harassment on Campus

Sexual harassment exists on all types of university campuses. In many cases it is unreported—and is often ignored altogether. In general, women are more likely to define behaviors as harassing and men are more likely to believe victims have contributed to their own problem. There are costs to individuals and to the institution. Victims tend to sacrifice self-confidence, academic and work opportunities, letters of recommendation, and grades. The student's professional development is hindered, and the university acquires a negative image.

Nearly two-thirds of college students experience some type of sexual harassment. Yet, less than 10%

tell a college or university employee about it, and an even smaller fraction officially report the harasser to a Title IX officer. These, and other interesting facts, are part of a major report from the American Association of University Women (Sexual harassment on campus: Drawing the line, 2005). Key research findings in the report are highlighted here:

- Sexual harassment is common on college campuses. More than one-third of college students encounter sexual harassment during their first year on campus.

- Men and women are equally likely to be harassed, but in different ways and with different responses. Females are more likely to be the target of sexual jokes, comments, gestures, or looks. Males are more likely to be called gay or a homophobic name. Females are more likely to be upset and to feel embarrassed, angry, less confident, afraid, confused, and disappointed in their college experience.

- Lesbian, gay, bisexual, and transgender students are more likely to be harassed.

- Different racial and ethnic groups experience sexual harassment in similar, but not identical ways. Generally, white, African American, and Hispanic students perceive and react to sexual harassment in similar ways.

- Men are more likely than women to harass. Both males and females are more likely to be harassed by a male.

- More than half of harassers think their actions are funny.

- Most victims don't report sexual harassment.

Bullying, teasing, and sexual harassment can be common in schools.

Gender DIMENSIONS

Same-Gender Sexual Harassment

Sexual harassment is obviously a problem for women in the workplace—and sometimes for men. Most often, the instances we hear about involve other-gender situations. However, more and more same-gender harassment cases have been filed, and lower courts have been inconsistent in their findings. One judge allowed a case to proceed only because the supervisor, accused of harassing, was admittedly gay.

The Equal Employment Opportunity Commission has for years taken the position that Title VII of the Civil Rights Act does not care which genders are involved. In 1998 the Supreme Court allowed a case to proceed in which a man working on an oil rig charged two male co-workers with making taunting comments and threatening rape.

Men and women often deal with sexual harassment differently. Whereas a woman may be more inclined to report harassing conduct, the traditional inclination of many men is just to "deal with it." This attitude has possibly led to less frequent reporting of male same-gender harassment.

Same-gender harassment cases will probably receive heavy media coverage. Treatment in the press will likely have a strong influence on whether men (or women in same-gender harassment situations) will keep harassment complaints to themselves or report them in the future.

Osman (2004) examined perceptions of sexual harassment based on a vignette in which physical or verbal harassment and the victim's facial expression were varied. She found perceptions of sexual harassment were stronger for physical harassment than verbal harassment except when the target smiled. Overall, women had stronger perceptions of harassment than did men. Also, a stronger belief that women should at least give token resistance to sex was associated with weaker perceptions of sexual harassment even when a victim verbally resisted.

Some university officials feel there should be a general statement of the university's position on sexual harassment because it is not possible to cover specific situations adequately. Others feel that the specifics should be clearly spelled out to prevent potential confusion. Some officials feel policies should prohibit even consensual sexual relationships between students and faculty members. They argue that although such relationships may appear to be consensual, they are not because of the faculty member's position of authority. Others feel that consensual relationships are not the business of the university.

As part of the emphasis on sexual harassment on campuses, many colleges and universities have developed various types of educational programs for students and faculty. It is important to understand and protect the rights of both complainants and accusers and to avoid either sensationalizing or minimizing allegations. It is also crucial for all concerned to understand the institution's policies against harassment and its procedures for handling complaints.

Sexual Harassment and the Military

In 2003 the National Organization for Women reported instances of rape and sexual harassment at the U.S. Air Force Academy. It also indicated that 78% of cadets at the Academy reported either sexual assaults or unwanted sexual advances (Military "don't tell" policy hushes up rape and sexual assault, 2003).

About the same time, Sadler et al. reported that 79% of 556 female military veterans reported experiencing sexual harassment during their military service. Thirty percent of the women reported an attempted or completed rape. They indicated their findings were consistent with research in civilian populations showing that younger women entering male-dominated work groups at lower levels of authority are those most likely to be harassed. Also, women working with superiors who made sexually demeaning comments or allowed such behavior were found to have a nearly fourfold risk of rape while in the military (Sadler et al., 2003).

Cohen (2005) reported that women in the Israeli Defense Force report hundreds of incidents of sexual harassment and rape, yet harassers usually go unpunished. Some feel that the hierarchal structure encourages males to misuse their power. Under Israeli law, those found guilty of harassment can be sentenced for up to 3 years of imprisonment. In reality, senior military officers accused of sexual harassment are rarely sent to jail.

Tyson (2005) wrote about a Department of Veterans Affairs report indicating that 60% of women and 27% of men in the military reserves and the National Guard suffered sexual assault or harassment during

Did You Know . . .

Addressing Sexual Harassment in the Military

A climate that negatively affects teamwork within a military unit impacts mission effectiveness. Consequently, the Department of Defense has specific policies and programs that support a zero-tolerance philosophy toward sexual harassment in the armed forces. Because women are essential to mission accomplishment, this is an issue that is addressed at every level of every military unit.

As gender-related incidents are investigated, they have been accompanied by a concerted effort of the Department of Defense to prevent recurrences. This has been demonstrated by the development and evaluation of programs designed to educate service members as to what constitutes sexual harassment, how to deal with it, and how to report incidents without fear of reprisal.

In an appearance before the Senate Armed Services Committee in 1997, Edwin Dorn, the Undersecretary of Defense for Personnel and Readiness, underscored the importance of military units' functioning as a team. He mentioned trust, loyalty, and self-sacrifice, issues not often relevant in large organizations. According to Dorn, a climate of discrimination and harassment will erode these elements that are essential for unit effectiveness (Dorn, 1997). Nevertheless, a policy can only be as strong as the program it supports. According to Sheila Widnall, former Secretary of the Air Force, an Equal Opportunity program to support a zero-tolerance policy on harassment must be based on the following five principles:

1. A commander's personal commitment
2. The establishment of goals, principles, and standards of performance
3. Clear, concise written policies
4. Continual training through a military member's career
5. Complaint systems that are prompt, thorough, and fair and allow for resolution, support, reprisal prevention, and sanctions (Widnell & Dorn, 1995)

The military leadership has taken the initiative for monitoring the climate within the services. Programs have been developed to improve the climate through training, prevention, and resolution. These programs have been evaluated by using instruments such as command climate surveys, sensing sessions, and other internal review processes. They have also been examined by the media, congressional inquiry, and watchdog organizations. In 2000, an assessment of four key Department of Defense human relations programs that had been fielded or modified since 1997—the Command Climate Survey, the Army Values Program, the Consideration of Others Program, and Equal Opportunity (EO) Training Programs—was conducted. The purpose of this reassessment was to determine whether the establishment or revision of these programs had improved human relations in the Army. A total of 24,000 Army leaders and soldiers were surveyed and interviewed. Among the findings were indications that although the Army provides a generally effective human relations environment, many service members do not yet consider human relations an important component of combat readiness (Johnson & Harris, 2001).

Commanders are constantly working toward achieving zero tolerance for sexual harassment; they still have a way to go. The process for reporting incidents has been improved, thus increasing the prospect of investigation and resolution. This sends a clear message that members of the various armed services must be willing to report and be vigilant, and that these behaviors are not tolerated.

Susan M. Tendy, Ed.D.
Director of Assessment, Department of Physical Education
United States Military Academy
West Point, New York

Sources: Dorn, E. DoD committed to zero tolerance of sexual harassment, *Defense Issues, 12, no. 9* (1997), 1–4. Available: http://www.defenselink.mil/speeches/1997/di1209.html. Widnall, S. E., & Dorn, E. To stop harassment, leaders must lead. *Defense Issues, 10, no. 64* (May 1995), 1–5. Available: http://www.defenselink.mil/speeches/1995/di1064.html. Johnson, E., & Harris, B. Special report 46: Human relations update 2000 executive summary (March 2001). Available: http://www.asamra.army.pentagon.mil/eo/eo_docs/human_relations.pdf.

their service. Eleven percent of women experienced rape or attempted rape, compared with 1.2% of males. More than half of the incidents took place at a military worksite and during duty hours, and in most cases military personnel were the offenders. Fewer than 19% said that they received any help for the trauma.

Boghosian (2005) indicated that the National Lawyers Guild launched a Women's Military Rights Project to challenge the long-term problem of sexual harassment and abuse within the military system through a combined program of education, legal assistance and litigation, and support for political action. This was a result of many events through the years—particularly the Navy Tailhook Association Convention in 1991, the court-martial of the most senior enlisted man in the army for sexual harassment in 1997, the accusation of the Army's most senior enlisted man in Europe of sexual harassment in 1999, the accusing of Major General Larry G. Smith of sexual harassment by the highest-ranking woman in Army history in 2000, and the Air Force Academy scandal in 2003, which erupted when 142 cadets made sexual assault charges that resulted in zero convictions. In addition, the Miles Foundation reported that from August 2002 through March 2005, there were 316 cases of sexual assault in Iraq, Afghanistan, and Kuwait. The Women's Rights Project will be involved in challenging the alleged lack of oversight of sexual abuse and harassment on the part of the U.S. military.

Reactions to Sexual Harassment

Reactions to sexual harassment are influenced by individual characteristics and the severity of the harassing behavior. Gender, attitudes toward both women and men, religiosity, and confidence all influence the way people might react to sexual harassment. Responses can range from avoidance or defusion to negotiation or confrontation. Avoidance (ignoring the harassment or doing nothing) is quite common. Defusion (which includes responses such as going along, stalling, or making a joke of it) is a more active way to minimize the impact of conflict. Negotiation is a more assertive response and involves a direct request to the harasser to stop. This shifts the focus of the interaction to the victim's needs and priorities in the relationship. Confrontation, the most assertive response on this continuum, has two components: aggressive personal responses (such as telling the harasser to stop rather than simply asking) and use of the organizational power structure (such as making a formal complaint through channels).

A person being harassed usually has several options—personal action, grievance to an employer (if applicable), union grievance (if applicable), and legal action. Each situation influences the best way to handle the harassment. There are two objectives for personal action: Attempt to stop the harassment and, if that fails, document it. If this fails and there is a grievance procedure, a complaint can be filed through prescribed channels. If none of these routes works, it may be necessary to pursue legal action.

Here are some suggestions for dealing with sexual harassment (About SSSS, 2005):

- Trust your gut. If you feel uneasy or uncomfortable, this is an important cue that something is amiss.

The sexual harasser is often a person who has authority or power over others.

- If you feel as if someone is sexually harassing you, you could either walk away or say that his or her comments or sexual attention are unwanted. Generally, the most effective response is to ask the person to stop his or her unwanted sexual behavior in a firm but cordial and non-angry way.

- Use your feelings as permission to either leave the situation or be assertive and provide the other person with good-natured feedback about how you would like to change your interaction. For example, you might say or write: "I really wanted to talk with you, and I imagine you meant well. However, your repeated touches and sexual comments felt inappropriate to me."

- Use an assertive voice and clear body language when you are telling someone else how you would like them to change their behavior. Dissuade them from thinking you are joking by looking them in the eyes and using a serious and businesslike facial expression and tone of voice.

- Try to give the person the benefit of the doubt. Treat the person who upset you as you would want to be treated. Share your concerns and negotiate how to improve future interactions with him or her personally, directly, as soon as possible.

Exploring the
DIMENSIONS
of Human Sexuality

Our feelings, attitudes, and beliefs regarding sexuality are influenced by our internal and external environments. Go to sexuality.jbpub.com/dimensions/4e to learn more about the biological, psychological, and sociological factors that affect your sexuality.

Sociocultural Factors

- Socioeconomic status plays a role in forcible sexual behaviors, as higher levels of aggression are found among lower-income populations. Pedophiles and the children they abuse are members of all socioeconomic and educational groups.
- People who believe in rape myths assign less blame to the perpetrator and more blame to the victim.
- Laws regarding sexual activity of teens vary among countries. Japanese law only prohibits sexual intercourse with someone younger than 12 years old—no other sexual activity, including child pornography, is covered.
- Deliberate interracial rape is uncommon; 88% of victims are the same race as the perpetrator.
- A cultural belief in patriarchy, whereby males have a dominant role over women, can promote abusive behavior.

Biological Factors

- Alcohol is a factor in 50% of rapes.
- Date-rape drugs produce disinhibition and an amnesia-like effect, so that victims do not remember what happened.
- Younger people commit violent acts more often than older people do.
- Although men and women attack each other at about the same rate (12%), as a result of the usually greater strength of men, women are hurt more often and live in fear of further attacks.

Psychological Factors

- Sexual abuse in childhood contributes significantly to the risk of development of mental disorders later in life. Adolescent rape survivors have more behavioral problems compared to older survivors. Women with low self-esteem tend not to end an abusive relationship.

CASE STUDY

Many positive social changes have occurred over the past few decades to help the victims of forcible sexual behaviors. Although child sexual abuse has long occurred—Freud wrote about it almost 100 years ago—it was a hushed, taboo topic. Many victims thought that they were the "only one," or that they had done something wrong. Not anymore.

The media have been a positive force for change by giving coverage to forcible sexual behavior cases. The trial of O. J. Simpson—and the surrounding coverage about battered women—gave many victims the courage to step forward. Many TV shows inform children about what to do in case someone touches them in a way that makes them feel "uncomfortable."

The legal system has made huge strides in recent years, creating and enforcing laws and helping victims of forced sexual behaviors. Police have been trained to take intimate-partner violence calls seriously, and not to let the perpetrator of violence off the hook.

Laws have been passed to help victims of sexual harassment at work or school. And, whereas in 1976 no man could be legally accused of raping his spouse, now marital rape laws have been passed in all 50 states.

Summary

- Millions of people are affected by sexual violence each year. Sexual assault and abuse include inappropriate touching; vaginal, anal, or oral penetration; sexual intercourse after a person says no; rape; attempted rape; and child molestation.

- Rape is one of the most underreported crimes. There are many myths about rape.

- Date rape, also known as acquaintance rape, is much more common than most people realize. There are many ways to help prevent acquaintance rape.

- Pedophilia entails feelings of adult sexual attraction to children. Children are particularly vulnerable to sexual predators, such as pedophiles, on the Internet.

- Preventing sexual abuse demands attention. There is a need to help children and adults distinguish between appropriate and inappropriate touch, say no to unwanted or uncomfortable touch, tell a trusted adult if inappropriate touch occurs, and identify family and community support systems.

- Incest is sexual behavior between relatives who are too closely related to be legally married. The most commonly reported form is father–daughter.

- Intimate-partner abuse is a significant health and social problem in the United States. In addition to physical abuse, it can include sexual abuse, emotional abuse, or property/economic abuse.

- Sexual harassment is unwelcome verbal, physical, or sexual conduct that has the effect of creating an intimidating, hostile, or offensive environment. It is problem in schools, colleges, and the workplace.

Discussion Questions

1. What are the different categories of rape? Who are the rapists in these categories? What are the effects on the victims?

2. What effects does child abuse have on its survivors?

3. Describe the type of person who commits incest. What drives a seemingly "normal" individual to commit incest?

4. Explain why someone in an abusive marriage stays in the relationship. Can one be absolutely sure when a spouse should leave? Or is every situation different?

5. In what ways is sexual harassment the same and different in the workplace, in schools, in colleges, and in the military? Is the intent of harassment the same in each situation?

Application Questions

Reread the chapter-opening story and answer the following questions.

1. Is date rape a form of miscommunication or a form of sexual violence? Put another way, did Ed simply misinterpret the woman's resistance, assuming that "she wanted to be convinced to have sex"? Even if that were case, did he have the right to continue sexual activity before she consented?

2. Assume for a moment that you are the woman who has just been date raped. Which actions can and should you take? What might the consequences of those actions be for both you and the rapist?

Critical Thinking Questions

1. In 1991 a Florida federal judge ruled that pictures of naked and scantily clad women displayed in a workplace qualified as sexual harassment under Title VII of the 1964 Civil Rights Act. In his written opinion, the judge said that such a "boys' club" atmosphere is "no less destructive to workplace equality than a sign declaring 'Men Only.'" At the same time, the Florida branch of the American Civil Liberties Union denounced the decision as a possible violation of free speech. Under the federal court ruling, the company involved had to institute an antiharassment policy and take down the photos. In your opinion, what was the right decision in this situation?

2. Several women in an office complained to their human resources department that a male colleague had a photo of a woman in a bikini on his desk and that the photo created a "hostile working environment." When the man was confronted by his supervisor, he stated that the photo was of his wife, and he refused to remove it. What rights does the man have to display a photo of his wife? What rights do the women in the department have to object to the photo?

3. The goal of this question/activity is to increase your awareness of relationship abuse while enabling you to reflect on your own values about what would constitute an abusive romantic or sexual relationship. Read each statement, consider how you feel about it, and discuss your feelings with others in your class to explore the various opinions that might exist in your class.

Is it abuse if . . .

1. a man and a woman are arguing when she begins to cry hysterically, and he gives her a light slap to calm her down?

2. a husband takes his wife to work every morning, meets her for lunch every day, and picks her up at the end of each afternoon?

3. a wife tells her husband that he would look better if he lost a few pounds?

4. every time a lesbian couple argues, one of the partners threatens to "out" the other to her family?

5. an 18-year-old has a sexual relationship with a 14-year-old?

6. a woman who wears tight clothing and short skirts walks down the street and men whistle and make sexual comments to her?

7. a man says he wants to have sexual intercourse, his girlfriend says she's not ready, but after talking about it, she gives in and has sexual intercourse with him, even though she doesn't really want to?

Source: Adapted from Schroeder, E. Is it abuse if . . . ? *American Journal of Sexuality Education, 1, no. 1* (2005), 141–149.

Critical Thinking Case

Paul Ingram, a deputy in the sheriff's department in Olympia, Washington, suddenly found himself accused of child abuse. His two daughters, aged 18 and 22 years, had just returned from a spiritual retreat when they suddenly recalled that their father had sexually abused them when they were children. During the retreat, a charismatic preacher had said that someone in the audience had been molested as a child—a plausible assumption in any audience given prevalence rates. The more the daughters remembered, the more their stories kept changing. The father was stunned, claiming he remembered no sexual abuse toward his daughters. But he also believed his daughters would never lie. Eventually, he confessed to abusing his daughters.

In fact, the more he remembered, the clearer his memories of the events became. A psychologist tried an experiment on Paul, in which false information about abusing his children was told to him. Within days, Paul claimed to "remember" these made-up events. When told that these events had never taken place, Paul tried to retract his other statements from the legal process. Unfortunately, he was too late. Paul was convicted and sentenced to jail for his initial recalled memories (Wilson et al., 1996).

Given this true case study of recovered memories, is it ethical to use them for treatment of a sexual abuse survivor? Is it ethical to use them to charge someone else with sexual assault or sexual abuse many years later?

Explain your answer.

Exploring Personal Dimensions

Date Rape

Directions

This exercise is for those who are single and dating. Mark all that apply to you.

_____ 1. When dating, most of the excitement is to see what degree of intimacy I will be able to reach with this person (that is, how far we will go).

_____ 2. I test how far I will go (physical intimacy) with someone by progressive fondling (holding hands, putting arm around waist, rubbing back, chest, or breast and genitals) to see at what point the person will stop me.

_____ 3. When dating, I generally go with others or go somewhere public until I know someone.

_____ 4. I ask around about someone before I go out with her or him.

_____ 5. I make it very clear what my values are about physical intimacy when dating before difficult situations arise.

_____ 6. I have tried to coerce or talk someone into having sexual activity with me.

Scoring

Give yourself the following points for the items you checked, and total your score.

1. 3
2. 3
3. −2
4. −3
5. −3
6. 5

Interpretation

3–11   You are potentially infringing on someone else's right to live within her or his value system and legal rights. You may be "date raping" or attempting date rape.

0–2   You have tendencies to infringe on someone else's right to live within her or his value system.

−1––3   You are practicing moderately healthy dating precautions to avoid date rape.

−4––8   You are practicing healthy dating precautions to avoid date rape.

Suggested Readings

Acquaintance rape. Rape, Abuse, and Incest National Network, 2009. Available: http://www.rainn.org/print/117.

Child sexual abuse. Rape, Abuse, and Incest National Network, 2009. Available: http://www.rainn.org/print/116.

Lalumiere, M. L., Harris, G. T., Quinsey, V. L., & Rice, M. E. *The causes of rape: Understanding individual differences in male propensity for sexual aggression.* Washington, DC: American Psychological Association, 2005.

Lorentzen, E., Nilsen, H., & Traeen, B. Will it ever end? The narratives of incest victims on the termination of sexual abuse. *Journal of Sex Research, 45, no. 2* (April 2008), 164–174.

Osman, S. L. Predicting perceptions of sexual harassment based on type of resistance and belief in token resistance. *Journal of Sex Research, 44, no. 4* (October 2007), 340–346.

Reed, E., Silverman, J. G., Raj, A., Rothman, E. F., Decker, M. R., Gottlieb, B. R., Molnar, B. E., & Miller, B. E. Social and environmental contexts of adolescent and young adult male perpetrators of intimate partner violence: A qualitative study. *American Journal of Men's Health, 2, no. 3* (2008), 260–271.

Walsh, W. A. Predators, pedophiles, rapists, and other sex offenders. *Violence Against Women, 11, no. 1* (January 2005), 139–142.

Wilson, R. Notoriety yields to tragedy in Iowa sexual-harassment cases. *Chronicle of Higher Education, 55, no. 24* (February 20, 2009), A1, A8–A13.

Web Resources

For links to the web sites below, visit *http://sexuality.jbpub.com/dimensions/4e* and click on Resource Links.

MaleSurvivor
www.malesurvivor.org

Provides extensive information about sexual victimization of boys and men designed to help them overcome their sexual victimization experiences.

Men Can Stop Rape
www.mencanstoprape.org

This organization works with male youth to help them be allies with women in preventing rape and other forms of men's violence. Gender equity is promoted along with men's capacity to be strong without being violent.

National Coalition Against Domestic Violence
www.ncadv.org

The mission of the National Coalition Against Domestic Violence (NCADV) is to organize for collective power to end the violence in our lives. NCADV believes violence against women and children results from the use of force or threat to achieve and maintain control over others in intimate relationships. NCADV works for major societal changes necessary to eliminate both personal and societal violence against all women and children.

National Women's Health Information Center
www.4woman.gov

The Office of Women's Health coordinates the efforts of all of the federal Health and Human Services agencies and offices involved in women's health. Its purpose is to improve the health and well-being of women and girls in the United States through education, programs, and motivating behavior change.

U.S. Department of Justice: Office on Violence Against Women
www.usdoj.gov/ovw

The Office on Violence Against Women handles legal and policy issues regarding violence against women and responds to requests for information regarding violence against women.

Rape, Abuse, and Incest National Network
www.rainn.org

The Rape, Abuse, and Incest National Network is the nation's largest anti-sexual assault organization. RAINN operates the National Sexual Assault Hotline and carries out programs to prevent sexual assault, help victims, and ensure that rapists are brought to justice.

CHAPTER 15

Sexually Transmitted Infections

CHAPTER OBJECTIVES

1 Define STIs and SRDs, describe how are they transmitted, and discuss the reasons for their prevalence.

2 Discuss the bacterially based STIs, including incidence, transmission, symptoms and complications, and diagnosis and treatment.

3 Discuss the virally based STIs, including incidence, transmission, symptoms and complications, and diagnosis and treatment.

4 Discuss the ectoparasitic infestations, including transmission, symptoms and complications, and diagnosis and treatment.

5 Describe ways that STIs and SRDs can be prevented.

sexuality.jbpub.com/dimensions/4e

Prevalence of Sexually Transmitted Infections
Bacterial Infections
Viral Infections

INTRODUCTION

J essica was enrolled in one of our human sexuality classes. One day after class, she asked whether she could stop in during office hours to discuss something "private." Over the years, we have learned that "private" can mean many things: a student just found out she is pregnant, is being abused by a romantic partner, or is concerned about a sexual disorder. In Jessica's case, though, it was a concern that she might have an STI.

Jessica went on to describe a sexual encounter with Rodney that culminated in sexual intercourse. Shortly afterward, Jessica noticed a rash on her inner thighs and became alarmed. As soon as she described her concern about having contracted an STI, I knew I would have to refer Jessica to a physician at the campus health center for testing and diagnosis. I am an educator, not a medical doctor, and I know my limitations. Still, I could not refer her immediately for fear that she would think I was uninterested and be disinclined to discuss with me other concerns she might have in the future. Consequently, we discussed the reasons for her concern—the rash appeared, Rodney had not used a condom, they had not employed any other method of birth control, she met Rodney only the week before at a party and she did not really know him well—and we explored any other symptoms she described. Although I did not feel qualified to discuss whether Jessica had an STI, I did take advantage of our private time together to talk about the wisdom of coitus without the use of a condom and/or any other method of birth control and explored with her the decision to engage in coitus with someone she had only recently met.

It turned out that all Jessica had was a rash caused by nylon underpants she wore during her weekly jog. The relief on her face said it all, and I doubt that Jessica forgot that scare the next time she was faced with a *decision regarding whether to engage in sex. That is not to say that she will refrain or become abstinent, although those are certainly possibilities and decisions others have made, but rather that she would understand better that any choice to engage in sexual activity is accompanied by both potentially pleasurable and potentially disturbing consequences. Contracting an STI, one of those disturbing consequences, is always a possibility.*

Although Jessica did not have an STI, we have encountered other students who did. Fortunately, most of those students were diagnosed early enough and treated successfully. This chapter describes the more common STIs, ways they can be prevented, and ways they are treated when they are not prevented.

What Are Sexually Transmitted Infections?

The term **sexually transmitted infections (STIs)** describes infections that can be contracted through sexual intimacy. Sexual intimacy includes oral–genital and anal sex, as well as vaginal intercourse. At least 20 STIs have been identified. There are also diseases of the sexual organs referred to as **sexually related diseases (SRDs)**, which are disorders of the reproductive tract that occur in both sexually active and sexually abstinent individuals. These can be caused by organisms that live in the healthy body but under certain conditions, such as stress, diabetes, drug use, and other health-related problems, affect the delicate chemical balance of the body and cause disease conditions of the sexual organs. Some cancers are also considered to be SRDs. A sexually related infection can sometimes be transmitted to a sexual partner, and the conditions under which this occurs are discussed in this chapter.

Whatever the sexual disease, whether contracted during sexual activity or occurring in an abstinent individual, it affects the individual's feelings about his or her sexuality. Some people feel that anyone with a disease of the sexual organs is unclean, evil, and immoral; that a sexual disease is a punishment for sexual intimacy; and that only those of low socioeconomic and low educational status contract these diseases.

sexually transmitted infections (STIs)
Infections that are primarily contracted through sexual contact.

sexually related diseases (SRDs)
Diseases of the reproductive system that can occur in either sexually active or sexually inactive individuals.

There is no truth to these beliefs. Organisms live in our bodies and can multiply when our resistance is low or, as mentioned earlier, when other conditions exist. Pathogenic organisms can sometimes adjust to their habitat, proliferate, and even change in ways that cause symptoms of disease. Not only can they affect the body of an infected individual, but they are also sometimes transferred to another individual through sexual activity.

Prevalence of Sexually Transmitted Infections

STIs have become quite common, even though we have seen a decline in the rates of some particular STIs. There are many reasons for the prevalence of STIs. For example, whereas most states require physicians to report to health departments HIV and AIDS, gonorrhea, and syphilis cases, this was not always the case. Therefore, to compare current STI rates with periods in which reporting was not required would certainly make it appear that there are more cases; in fact, there may not be. In addition, since the 1960s there has been a change in attitudes about sexual behavior. More frequent sex and earlier sex have meant an increase in the number of people subjected to STIs. Other variables include the following:

1. There is considerable social pressure for social and sexual contact, along with widespread ignorance about sexual health and disease transmission.

2. The traditional restraints on sexual behavior are weakening as families and society in general become more loosely knit. Families

Global DIMENSIONS

STIs Around the World

There are wide variations in STIs around the world. Some countries have a high incidence; others have a lower one. The reasons for these differences may at first appear obvious but on further inspection are extremely complex. For example, it is assumed that lack of education is related to STIs, and, in fact, in some countries that is the case. Better educated people have access to information about STIs, their transmission, and their prevention. Furthermore, better educated people are more likely to have better paying jobs, allowing them to act on their STI knowledge (purchase condoms, for example). Yet, this is not always the case. For example, the Joint United Nations Programme on HIV/AIDS (2004) cites sub-Saharan Africa as the region of the world most affected by HIV. In the 44 countries of this region, the majority of the infections occur among the most literate men and women.

There are several possible explanations for this surprising finding. First, more schooling may be associated with a cultural change that is also associated with behaviors that increase the risk of disease. The World Health Organization states that this may be especially true for women, who without education may be less socially mobile and be exposed to a narrow spectrum of social and sexual relations. More education also means more money to support high-risk behaviors, such as paying for prostitutes or supporting a number of sexual partners.

The reason people contract STIs varies from country to country and even within subpopulations in any one country. The keys to preventing STIs at a policy level are understanding these differences and responding to them systematically.

are more mobile; relocation can threaten the stability of family members as they move away from the support system offered by the extended family and community. Adolescents and young adults are now reared in an atmosphere favoring more personal freedom and less adult supervision. More and more families have two parents in the workforce; adolescent and young adult family members are frequently employed while attending school; and many more adolescents than in the past are unattended during certain times of the day.

3. Adolescence is a time of physical, psychological, and biochemical change and development. There is a wide range in the speed of adolescent development. Physiological maturing occurs at a faster rate than do intellectual, social, and emotional maturing. This places young people in a position of biological readiness for activities that have physical and emotional consequences for which they are not prepared. Often they face sexual decisions that affect their interests and they are not able to judge.

4. Current social values have led to widespread expectations of instant gratification. Learning, growing, and achieving goals require persistence; there seems to be a strong sense of urgency to act now, accompanied by a need for immediate satisfaction.

5. An "everybody does it" attitude undermines convictions about individual responsibility. Thus adolescents who feel stifled by external controls and are eager for independence often take actions, frequently sexual in nature, for which they are unprepared.

6. New modes of contraception have not eliminated unwanted pregnancy, but they have all but eliminated the fear of it. In the past this fear effectively inhibited sexual activity among many people of childbearing age.

One result of the combination of these factors has been an increase in sexual activity among most people—not just the young. This increase, in turn, has led to a rise in the incidence of STIs. There is no doubt that the risk of exposure is greater in people who are sexually active, especially with more than one person, because the chance of contracting an STI increases with the number of sexual contacts.

In spite of these social factors, and because of several other variables such as the fear of HIV infection, the rates of several STIs have decreased dramatically. However, accompanying this decrease in rates for some STIs is an increase in rates for others. The rates, signs, symptoms, potential complications, and means of diagnosing and treating the more prevalent STIs are presented in the following sections.

◼ Bacterial Infections

Some STIs are caused by bacteria. Among these are chlamydia, gonorrhea, nongonococcal urethritis, and syphilis. It is not uncommon for these bacterial infections to be transmitted from one partner to the other, and treatment therefore often requires refraining from sexual activity until the bacteria have been eliminated.

Chlamydia

Incidence

Chlamydial infections, caused by the intracellular parasite **Chlamydia trachomatis**, are the most common STIs in the United States today. The Centers for Disease Control and Prevention (CDC) of the Department of Health and Human Services states that because case reporting remains incomplete, estimating the total number of **chlamydia** cases is extremely difficult. However, in 2008 there were more than 1.2 million chlamydial infections reported (Centers for Disease Control and Prevention, 2009b). There are more than three times more chlamydia cases than gonorrhea cases. From 2000 through 2007, reported cases of chlamydia increased from 251 cases per 100,000 persons to 370 cases per 100,000 (see Figure 15.1). This increase reflects increased screening, recognition of the nature

> **Chlamydia trachomatis**
> An intracellular parasite that causes chlamydial infections.
>
> **chlamydia**
> A term that encompasses several major diseases caused by *Chlamydia trachomatis,* including genitourinary tract infection, a type of conjunctivitis in newborns, a type of pneumonia in infants, lymphogranuloma venereum, and trachoma.

of asymptomatic infection (especially in women), as well as actual increases in the disease.

Reported cases of chlamydia in women far exceed reported cases in men (545 cases per 100,000 to 190 per 100,000, respectively). Rates for women are highest in the 15- to 19-year-old age group (3,005 per 100,000 persons) and for 20- to 24-year-olds (2,949 per 100,000) (see Figure 15.2).

Chlamydial infection is an umbrella term that encompasses four major diseases caused by *C. trachomatis*: (1) a genitourinary tract infection in adults, (2) inclusion conjunctivitis (an acute eye infection) in newborns and chlamydial pneumonia in infants, (3) trachoma (a chronic eye infection), and (4) lymphogranuloma venereum. The two diseases of most concern in the United States are adult genitourinary tract infection and infant conjunctivitis and pneumonia.

Symptoms and Complications

Genitourinary tract chlamydial infection has been called "the silent STI." Early symptoms of this infection are often mild and therefore unrecognized. Approximately 75% of infected people are asymptomatic. Symptoms, in those who exhibit them, occur 1 to 3 weeks after exposure. In men the most common symptoms include pain or burning on urination and a white, watery discharge from the penis. Women may note painful urination, a vaginal discharge, and abdominal pain.

Diagnosis

To diagnose chlamydia, a layer of cells is scraped from the affected area. One of three tests is then used. A culture test for chlamydia is preferred by the CDC

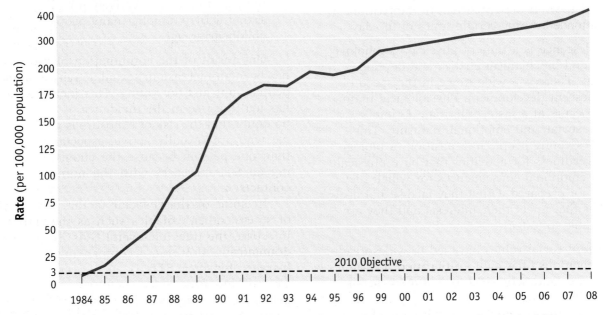

FIGURE **15.1** Chlamydia—reported rates: United States, 1984–2008. *Source:* Division of STD Prevention. *Sexually transmitted disease surveillance, 2008.* Atlanta, GA: Centers for Disease Control and Prevention, 2009, p. 88.

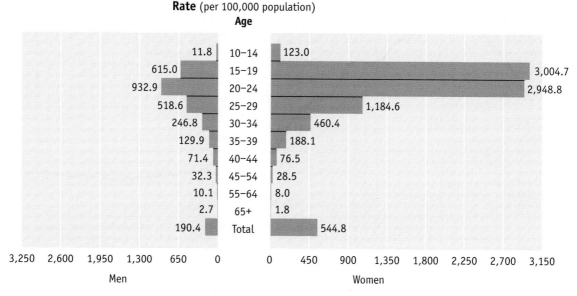

Rate (per 100,000 population)
Age

Men	Age	Women
11.8	10–14	123.0
615.0	15–19	3,004.7
932.9	20–24	2,948.8
518.6	25–29	1,184.6
246.8	30–34	460.4
129.9	35–39	188.1
71.4	40–44	76.5
32.3	45–54	28.5
10.1	55–64	8.0
2.7	65+	1.8
190.4	Total	544.8

Men: 3,250 2,600 1,950 1,300 650 0
Women: 0 450 900 1,350 1,800 2,250 2,700 3,150

FIGURE **15.2** Chlamydia—age- and gender-specific rates: United States, 2007. *Source:* Division of STD Prevention. *Sexually transmitted disease surveillance, 2007.* Atlanta, GA: Centers for Disease Control and Prevention, 2009.

because of its sensitivity and specificity. Rapid assay tests and fluorescent antibody tests are often used because results are available within 15 minutes for assays and within several hours for fluorescent tests. These tests are also less expensive than cultures.

Infants born to women with genitourinary chlamydial infections have a 70% chance of acquiring either inclusion conjunctivitis or chlamydial pneumonia during delivery (McCormack, 1984). It is estimated that in the United States more than 200,000 infants are born to chlamydia-infected mothers annually. Because of the magnitude of this health threat, the CDC recommends that all pregnant women be screened for chlamydia at their first prenatal visit, whether or not they exhibit symptoms of infection (Centers for Disease Control and Prevention, *Chlamydia,* 2005). Additionally, high-risk women should be screened again in their third trimester to prevent complications at birth. Pregnant women should not use doxycycline; erythromycin can be substituted. Because of the prevalence of chlamydia, it is recommended that primary care clinicians screen all sexually active women 25 years of age and younger for chlamydia as part of regular health care visits (Agency for Healthcare Research and Quality, 2001; Centers for Disease Control and Prevention, 2006).

Treatment
Chlamydial infections are easily treated in their early stages. The treatment of choice is a single 1-g dosage of azithromycin administered orally or 100 mg of doxycycline administered orally twice a day for 7 days. Alternatively, either erythromycin or ofloxacin may be used. To minimize the risk of reinfection, patients are

asked to refer their sexual partners for evaluation, testing, and treatment and to refrain from sexual intercourse with any partners who have not been treated. Reinfection is of prime importance. Researchers have found that nearly 20% of teenage women who have had a chlamydial infection are reinfected within 2 years (Xu et al., 2000). In fact, women aged 15 to 19 years old are four times as likely as 30- to 44-year-old women to have one repeat infection and five times as likely to be reinfected at least twice.

Unfortunately, because of the asymptomatic nature of the infection and the similarity of symptoms for chlamydia and gonorrhea, many cases of chlamydia are either improperly treated or untreated. Untreated chlamydia can lead to PID in women and to epididymitis in men. In both genders the possibility of sterility exists. Screening is therefore recommended annually for all sexually active women 25 years of age and younger (Centers for Disease Control and Prevention, 2006).

Gonorrhea

Incidence
Gonorrhea ranks high on the list of reportable communicable diseases. Only chlamydia is more prevalent. The incidence of gonorrhea decreased from 1970 to 1996. However, it increased to 132 per 100,000 population in 1999 (Centers for Disease Control and Prevention, 2001) (Figure 15.3). It decreased to 119 per 100,000 population in 2007.

> **gonorrhea**
> An STI that commonly starts with inflammation of the mucous membrane lining of the openings of the body (mouth, vagina, etc.).

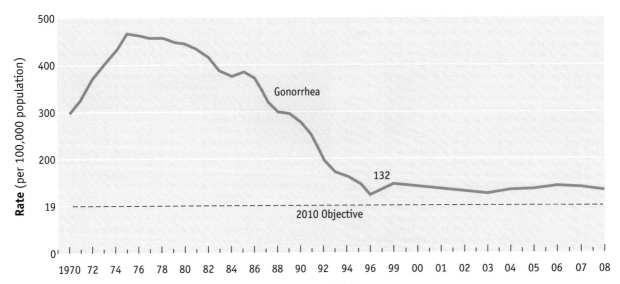

FIGURE **15.3** Gonorrhea—reported rates: United States, 1970–2003, and the *Healthy People 2010* objective. *Source:* Division of STD Prevention. *Sexually transmitted disease surveillance, 2007.* Atlanta, GA: Centers for Disease Control and Prevention, 2009.

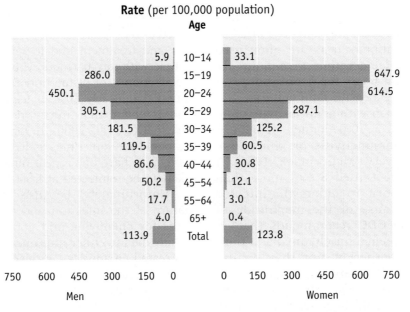

FIGURE **15.4** Gonorrhea—age- and gender-specific rates: United States, 2008. *Source:* Division of STD Prevention. *Sexually transmitted disease surveillance, 2008.* Atlanta, GA: Centers for Disease Control and Prevention, 2009.

This decrease was consistent across gender and age (see Figure 15.4). In 2007 there were 355,991 cases of gonorrhea reported in the United States. Gonorrhea rates still remain higher than the *Healthy People 2010* national health objective of 19 new cases per 100,000 persons.

When gonorrhea rates are examined by race and ethnicity, wide variations are evident (Centers for Disease Control and Prevention, 2009). In 2007, gonorrhea rates remained highest among African Americans (662.9 cases per 100,000 population). Similar to findings in recent years, the rate among African Americans was 19.1 times greater than the rate among whites (34.7 cases per 100,000 population). Gonorrhea rates were 3.1 times greater among American Indian/ Alaska Natives (107.1 cases per 100,000 population), and 2.0 times greater among Hispanics (69.2 cases per 100,000 population) than among whites in 2007. However, rates among whites were 1.8 times higher than those among Asian Pacific Islanders (18.8 cases per 100,000 population).

To put these figures into perspective, it is expected that many other cases of gonorrhea are not reported because of the social stigma still associated with STIs and the reluctance of Americans to address sexual health in an open manner. Because gonorrhea can result in pelvic inflammatory disease, sterility, ectopic pregnancy, and other serious health conditions, the number of Americans subjected to these risks, in spite of the declining rate of gonorrhea, is still disturbing.

Transmission

Gonorrhea is caused by a bacterium known as **Neisseria gonorrhoeae**, also called *gonococcus*. This bacterium grows in the mucous membrane, the moist protective coat that lines all orifices (openings) of the body. The mucous membranes lining the mouth, throat, vagina, cervix, urethra, and anal canal are all very receptive to gonococcus. When contact occurs between the site of gonococcus in one person and the moist membrane of another—as in all forms of sexual activity—bacteria are transferred. Thus oral–vaginal, oral–anal, penile–anal, oral–penile, oral–oral, and genital–genital contact can result in the transmission of the disease from an infected person to the other partner. Outside the body, however, the gonococcus dies in a few seconds, making it next to impossible to transmit the disease via toilet seats, cups, towels, or other articles used by an infected person. Interestingly enough, although bacteria travel from the mucous membrane of the infected partner to that of the uninfected partner, they sometimes die during transfer. Thus exposure does not always result in infection. It is thought that a man has about a 10% chance of contracting gonorrhea from a single exposure to a partner with the infection. A woman, however, has a greater than 40% chance of contracting the disease from a single exposure, because the mucous membrane lining of the vagina, having a large surface area, is particularly receptive to gonococcus invasion. Any small irritations in the mucous lining can allow the organism rapid entry into the woman's system. For men and women, after multiple exposures to an infected individual the attack (infection) rate increases to 80% to 90% (Fiumara, 1987). Oral–genital sexual activity can result in *gonococcal pharyngitis* (gonorrhea of the throat) in either gender.

Neisseria gonorrhoeae
The bacterium that causes gonorrhea; also known as *gonococcus*. Street names include "clap" and "drip."

Symptoms and Complications

Males are more likely than females to exhibit symptoms of gonorrhea. It is estimated that 90% to 95% of men infected with gonorrhea have symptoms (Schwebke, 1991a; Smith, Schoonover, Lauver, & Allen, 1990). The males who exhibit symptoms do so within 2 to 10 days after contact; 3 to 5 days is the most likely

Although 90–95% of males with gonorrhea experience some symptoms, almost 80% of women are asymptomatic. For males, the gonorrhea "drip" is a common symptom.

Gonorrhea lesions on the tongue.

Neisseria gonorrhoeae is the cause of gonorrhea.

interval. The primary sites in males are the urethra and the rectum. Symptoms include the sudden onset of frequent, painful urination (dysuria) and a discharge of pus from the urethra. Some males have tenderness in the groin area and noticeable swelling of lymph nodes. In anal gonorrhea, symptoms include membrane irritation, discharge, and painful defecation.

Complications in the male are seen within 2 to 3 weeks without treatment. Infection spreads up the *genitourinary tract*, the posterior urethra, the prostate, the seminal vesicles, and the epididymis. Sometimes acute inflammation of the prostate occurs, accompanied by pelvic tenderness and pain, fever, and urinary retention. Inflammation of the epididymis may occur; it can be recognized by a feeling of heaviness in the affected testicle, inflammation of the scrotal skin, and sometimes swelling in the lower part of the testicles. If the gonococcal infection spreads to the other testicle, infertility is a possible complication.

As many as 80% of the females who contract gonorrhea have no symptoms. The cervix is the primary infection site in females, and although it may be inflamed, symptoms may not be evident. Inflammation of the Bartholin's glands is possible but not common. A yellowish discharge may be present but may remain undetected. In actuality most females do not know they have a gonorrheal infection unless the infected partner tells them or they have a smear and culture done in a routine gynecological examination. This fact alone should encourage sexually active women to ask for a gonorrhea test as part of their regular checkups.

A complication of gonorrhea in women is **pelvic inflammatory disease (PID)**. In PID cases, the most common cause is gonorrhea. If the gonorrhea goes untreated in a woman, within 2 months the gonococcal organisms may cause an ascending infection into the internal reproductive organs and pelvic cavity. During menstruation and immediately after, the organisms travel rapidly. Symptoms include dyspareunia (painful intercourse), occasional nonmenstrual uterine bleeding, inflammation of the fallopian tubes with subsequent tubal infection, vaginal discharge, general abdominal pain, and fever up to 102°F. PID is a common complication in women. As the body defenses try to wall off the infection, scarring of the fallopian tubes can occur and infertility can result.

Extragenital complications of gonorrhea (those that occur in areas other than the genitals) include *gonococcal arthritis* and *gonococcal dermatitis*. These are sometimes referred to as *disseminated gonococcal infection*. Gonococcal arthritis affects the hands, wrists, ankles, knees, and elbows. Gonorrhea is the primary cause of arthritis in pregnant women and the most common cause of infectious arthritis in the United States. Gonococcal dermatitis, a rash, is most frequently seen on the hands and lower extremities. White blisters appear and eventually darken, leaving the body without scars. *Gonococcal endocarditis*, inflammation of the heart valves, is a serious but rare gonorrheal complication. Finally, *gonococcal ophthalmic infection* can occur in the newborn; that complication has been reduced by treating the eyes of all babies with silver nitrate tetracycline, or penicillin, at birth.

Diagnosis and Treatment

The most accurate method of diagnosing gonorrhea is by means of a culture of discharges taken from various body sites. In the male, the urethra is the most common site of infection, and a sample of the discharge should be taken there. Throat and rectal cultures are taken if the patient's sexual activity with an infected person involves these body areas. In the female the discharge sample is taken with a cotton-tipped applicator inserted into the cervical opening, because the environment in this area is optimal for gonococcus. Other sites from which cultures can be developed are the throat, rectum, and vagina. When gonococci are present, approximately 96% of the organism is isolated in these areas.

For many years the treatment of choice for gonorrhea was penicillin. In 1976, however, a strain of gonococcus resistant to all forms of penicillin appeared (Antibiotic-resistant strains, 1987). Called **penicillinase-producing N. gonorrhoeae (PPNG)**, this organism produces a substance that inactivates penicillin. PPNG was originally linked to foreign travel, but this is no longer the case. Today the number of reported cases of PPNG in the United States continues to rise, as infections are reported in a vast majority of the states.

Three other resistant strains of gonorrhea have also appeared. The first is known as **chromosomally mediated–resistant N. gonorrhoeae (CMRNG)**, an organism that contains intranuclear DNA capable of rendering its cell membrane impermeable to penicillin (Fiumara, 1987). The second strain is **tetracycline-resistant N. gonorrhoeae (TRNG)**. This strain of gonorrhea, similar to PPNG, produces a substance that inactivates tetracycline. The third resistant strain is **ciprofloxacin-resistant N. gonorrhoeae**. This strain, discovered in 1991, is resistant to the new drug ciprofloxacin. Approximately 6% of gonorrhea bacteria were found to be PPNG-resistant, 9% were CMRGN-resistant, 14% were TRNG-

pelvic inflammatory disease (PID)
Infection of the reproductive organs, particularly the uterus and fallopian tubes, and the pelvic cavity.

penicillinase-producing N. gonorrhoeae (PPNG)
Strain of gonococcus resistant to all forms of penicillin.

chromosomally mediated–resistant N. gonorrhoeae (CMRNG)
Strain of gonorrhea resistant to penicillin because its DNA makes its cell membrane impermeable to penicillin.

tetracycline-resistant N. gonorrhoeae (TRNG)
Strain of gonorrhea that produces a substance that inactivates tetracycline.

ciprofloxacin-resistant N. gonorrhoeae
Strain of gonorrhea resistant to the drug ciprofloxacin.

resistant, and 0.04% were resistant to ciprofloxacin. In 2007, 27% of gonorrhea cases were resistant to some antimicrobial treatment (Centers for Disease Control and Prevention, 2009a).

The current treatment of choice for gonorrhea consists of an intramuscular injection of the drug ceftriaxone or 500 mg of ciprofloxacin administered orally. Other drugs have also been used, such as cefixime, ofloxacin, and doxycycline, all of which are administered orally. Because it is suspected that more than half of those people who are infected with gonorrhea have a coexisting chlamydial infection, a dual-therapy regimen that includes a drug for the gonorrheal infection as well as doxycycline or azithromycin for the chlamydial infection has been recommended. As with all drug regimens, special populations, for example, pregnant women, require special precautions and alterations.

Nongonococcal Urethritis

Incidence
Nongonococcal urethritis (NGU) and its potential companion, *nongonococcal cervicitis* (in females), are STIs characterized by inflammation of the urethra and cervix, respectively. The signs and symptoms of NGU are similar to those of gonorrhea. If there are indications of urethritis and a laboratory test rules out gonorrhea, NGU is diagnosed.

> **nongonococcal urethritis (NGU)**
> Inflammation of the urethra caused by *Chlamydia trachomatis*, and *Ureaplasma urealyticum*, *Mycoplasma hominis*, *Trichomonas vaginalis*, herpes simplex virus, and unknown organisms.

Before the 1990s this condition was called *nonspecific urethritis* because its causes were unknown. Today researchers have been able to identify several organisms that are believed to cause NGU. Approximately 30% to 40% of NGU cases are caused by *Chlamydia trachomatis*. *Ureaplasma urealyticum, Mycoplasma hominis, Trichomonas vaginalis,* and herpes simplex virus are thought to be the causative agents in another 30% to 40% of cases. The cause of the remaining cases is still unknown (Sexually transmitted diseases treatment guidelines, 2006).

Symptoms
NGU symptoms in males include discharge from the penis and a burning sensation during urination. Women who have NGU-related infection sometimes report a mild vaginal irritation, burning, or discharge. At least 70% of infected women, however, are believed to be asymptomatic. Additionally, 10% of infected men may be asymptomatic. NGU is not a reportable communicable disease, so we have no official count of cases in the United States. It is esti-

mated that cases of NGU equal or surpass those of gonorrhea.

Treatment
Treatment consists of either 100 mg of doxycycline taken twice a day for 7 days or a single dosage of 1 g of azithromycin, both administered orally. Alternatively, erythromycin, levofloxacin, or ofloxacin may be used (Sexually transmitted diseases treatment guidelines, 2006).

Syphilis

Incidence
After falling to an all-time low in 2000, the syphilis rate in the United States rose for the seventh consecutive year in 2007 (Centers for Disease Control and Prevention, 2009). In 2007, 11,466 cases of primary and secondary syphilis were reported, a rate of 3.8 per 100,000 persons (see Figure 15.5).

Outbreaks of syphilis among gay men are believed to be largely responsible for the increasing syphilis rate. The Centers for Disease Control and Prevention estimates that 60% of all cases of primary and secondary syphilis occurred among men who have had sex with other men (Heffelfinger et al., 2004), although rates among women have also increased since 2004.

Wide disparities exist in the rates of syphilis among racial and ethnic groups. The syphilis rate for 2007 in African Americans was 7 times the rate in whites, which is substantially lower than the disparity observed in 1999, when the rate among African Americans was 29 times greater than that among whites. However, with increases in syphilis among blacks occurring since 2003 at a greater rate than those among whites, we are no longer seeing declines in this health disparity. In 2007, increases were observed among both African American men (23.2 cases per 100,000 population, up from 18.1 in 2006) and African American women (5.6 cases per 100,000 population, up from 4.9 in 2006). Smaller increases were observed among white men (3.7 cases per 100,000 population, up from 3.5 in 2006) and white women (0.4 cases per 100,000 population, up from 0.3 in 2006) (Centers for Disease Control and Prevention, 2009). Males contracted syphilis at a rate 6 times higher than females (see Figure 15.6).

Chancres of primary syphilis on penis.

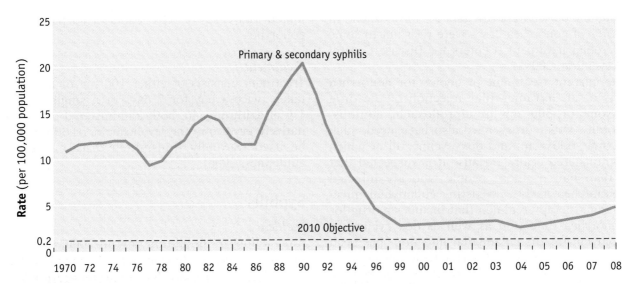

FIGURE **15.5** Primary and secondary syphilis—reported rates: United States, 1970–2008, and the *Healthy People 2010* objective. *Source:* Division of STD Prevention. *Sexually transmitted disease surveillance, 2008.* Atlanta, GA: Centers for Disease Control and Prevention, 2009.

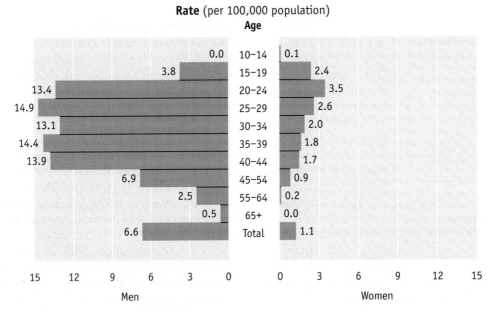

FIGURE **15.6** Primary and secondary syphilis—age- and gender-specific rates: United States, 2008. *Source:* Division of STD Prevention. *Sexually transmitted disease surveillance, 2008.* Atlanta, GA: Centers for Disease Control and Prevention, 2009.

After 14 years of decline in the United States, the rate of congenital syphilis increased 12.9% between 2006 and 2007 (from 9.3 to 10.5 cases per 100,000 live births). In 2007, 430 cases were reported, an increase from 382 cases in 2006. The increase in the rate of congenital syphilis may relate to the increase in the rate of syphilis among women that has occurred in recent years (Centers for Disease Control and Prevention, 2009).

Transmission

The cause of **syphilis** is *Treponema pallidum,* a spirochete organism that requires a warm, moist area to survive. The **spirochete** is thin and corkscrew-shaped and is transmitted from the open lesions of the infected person to the mucous membranes or cuts in the skin of the other person. The organism can be transmitted by vaginal, anal, or oral–genital contact. Only a few hours after the time of contact, the spirochete reaches the bloodstream of the newly infected person.

syphilis
An STI caused by the spirochete *Treponema pallidum.*

spirochete
A spiral-shaped bacterium, one of which, *Treponema pallidum,* causes syphilis.

? Did You Know...

In 1932, the U.S. Public Health Service began a study to determine if syphilis developed differently in African Americans than in whites. The study was conducted in Alabama under the guidance of the Tuskegee Institute, one of the foremost black universities in the United States and, therefore, became known as the Tuskegee Study. The study followed 399 black subjects, all with syphilis—and 201 control subjects who had not contracted the disease—for 40 years.

In 1951, when penicillin became available to treat syphilis, the researchers withheld treatment from the study's subjects because of concern it would interfere with their results. Even in 1966, when the morality of withholding treatment to subjects of the Tuskegee Study was raised with the director of the U.S. Public Health Service's Division of Venereal

Disease, a committee specifically organized to decide this issue voted to continue the study and continue to withhold treatment from the study's subjects. Not until a concerned researcher went public in 1972, and another committee chaired by Senator Edward Kennedy in 1973 was formed to study the issue, was a directive ordered to stop the study and treat the remaining subjects. Guidelines were subsequently developed to prevent researchers conducting studies under the aegis of the federal government to ever again behave in such an immoral manner. The remaining subjects of the Tuskegee Study sued the government and eventually settled for $10 million. However, suspicion of researchers, especially among minority populations, has still not fully recovered from the stigma of the Tuskegee Study.

A chancre is symptomatic of the primary stage of syphilis. Often, though, the chancre can appear on hidden parts of the female genital areas, making the disease asymptomatic by appearance. A woman who suspects that her partner has syphilis should request a medical exam or test.

The spirochete can also be transmitted by an infected pregnant woman through the placenta to the unborn child. Syphilis bacteria cannot cross the placenta to infect the fetus until after the fourth month of pregnancy because of protection provided by a membrane known as Langhan's layer. Therefore, if the mother is treated before the fourth month of pregnancy, the baby will be free of the disease. Women should be tested early in pregnancy, and if they suspect exposure at any time during pregnancy, they must be retested. Additionally, high-risk women should be retested in the third trimester (Sexually transmitted diseases treatment guidelines, 2006).

Symptoms and Complications

Syphilis has three stages of development: primary, secondary, and latent. *Latent* is the newer term for what used to be called the *tertiary* stage; this stage is divided into early latent and late latent, with no true delineation between the two, because the disease occurs on a continuum. Syphilis is infectious during the primary, secondary, and early latent stages.

Primary syphilis manifests itself by the appearance of a painless lesion, called a **chancre**. The chancre can appear from 10 to 90 days after exposure; on average, it appears in 21 days. Usually one lesion forms, generally on the glans penis in the male and the cervix in the female; however, the walls of the vagina and the tissues of the labia can also be sites of chancres. Because the lesions occur most frequently on hidden genital areas, they often remain undetected. Lesions can also appear on the nipples, anus, scrotum, or mouth.

Unfortunately the chancre disappears with or without treatment within 2 to 6 weeks. A person who suspects that he or she has been exposed to syphilis should have a blood test and not assume that the disappearance of the lesion means absence of the disease. During the primary stage, however, a blood test result may be negative; thus the test should be repeated. If possible, material exuding from a lesion suspected of being syphilitic should be examined under a microscope in what is called the *darkfield technique*. Sometimes this procedure, too, is repeated.

primary syphilis
The first stage of syphilis most generally manifested by the appearance of a painless lesion called a *chancre*.

chancre
A painless lesion that is symptomatic of the primary stage of syphilis and appears at the site of contact.

In the secondary stage of syphilis, a generalized rash can appear on the body 6 weeks to several months after initial exposure. Although the rash disappears within a few weeks, medical treatment should be sought for the underlying syphilis bacteria, *Treponema pallidum*.

Secondary syphilis is usually characterized by a generalized rash that appears on the body 6 weeks to several months after initial exposure. The rash does not itch, and it too subsides without treatment. Sometimes in this stage mucous patches are found in the mouth. A dull, depressed feeling; fever; and some hair loss may occur, and a blood test result is positive for the organism. In about 25% of cases of secondary syphilis, the spinal fluid also tests positive for the spirochete. This stage usually lasts from 2 to 6 weeks.

Latent syphilis has no visible symptoms, and this stage may last for years. The early latent period begins when the secondary symptoms disappear and ends 1 to 4 years later. In the late latent period, the disease may remain asymptomatic or symptoms involving the nervous system or cardiovascular system may appear. The disease can cause blindness, paralysis, crippling, brain damage, and possibly death. In the late latent period, blood tests of untreated persons yield positive findings for the spirochete, although the disease is not infectious at this stage (except to a fetus).

Diagnosis and Treatment
As noted, early diagnosis is made through a dark-field microscope examination of the material exuding from the chancre or rash, if possible, and through blood testing. The current treatment of choice is 2.4 million units of benzathine penicillin G, usually in one megadose, injected into the buttocks muscles. Because this penicillin is excreted from the body slowly, a constant level of the drug is maintained in the blood for a number of days.

◼ Viral Infections

Some STIs are caused by viruses. Among these are genital warts, herpes genitalis, and hepatitis B. Acquired immunodeficiency syndrome (AIDS) is also caused by a virus, the human immunodeficiency virus (HIV). We discuss HIV/AIDS in the next interchapter. These STIs are among the most difficult to eradicate because the viruses that cause them remain in the body even after symptoms subside. However, as we discuss, there are effective treatments for viral STIs.

Human Papillomavirus

Persistent infection with a group of viruses called **human papillomavirus (HPV)** is associated with the development of cervical cancer and/or genital warts, depending on the type of HPV. Data obtained from the National Health and Nutrition Examination Survey (NHANES) reported overall prevalence of HPV—that associated with cervical cancer and that associated with genital warts—was 26.8% (Dunne et al., 2007).

Genital Warts
In 2004, data from the National Disease and Therapeutic Index (NDTI) suggested the prevalence of genital warts was increasing. In a national study, 5.6% of sexually active 18- to 59-year-olds reported a history of genital warts (Dinh et al., 2008). However, in 2006 and 2007, prevalence rates decreased (Centers for Disease Control and Prevention, 2009). Genital warts occur in most areas of the genitals and anus. In females the warts appear on the labia, in the lower area of the vagina, on the cervix, or around the anus. In males

secondary syphilis
The second stage of syphilis, characterized by a rash.

latent syphilis
A stage of syphilis that may last for years: early latent (about 1 to 4 years in duration) and late latent (may last for years); it may be symptom free or cause degenerative complications.

human papillomavirus (HPV)
A persistent STI caused by any of a group of viruses associated with the development of cervical cancer and/or genital warts.

Communication
DIMENSIONS

Talking with a Partner About STI Prevention

Many of our students react incredulously when we suggest they speak with a potential partner about STIs before engaging in sex. "It would ruin the moment," they argue. In frustration, we sometimes respond, "Contract an STI and then let us know about ruining the moment!" If that were all we offer our students, they would be right to be angry. Instead, we also provide them with suggestions to communicate with a potential sexual partner about preventing STIs:

- Begin the conversation before matters are "hot and heavy." Once people are sexually excited, it is more difficult for them to make sensible decisions or to participate in meaningful conversation.
- Make inspecting genitalia part of sexual play. Laughter, soft touch, and expressions of admiration can make the moment enjoyable rather than clinical.
- Suggest that your partner examine you for signs of disease first. This will make it less threatening when it is your partner's turn to be examined.

- Discuss your prior sexual history, as it relates to STI risk, with your partner before asking your partner to share his or her history. Engage in this discussion by disclosing as much detail as you feel comfortable discussing. If expressed in an erotic manner, this discussion can be sexually stimulating as it concurrently accomplishes the purpose of preventing exposure to disease-causing organisms.
- Demonstrate effective communication skills. Lean forward, nod your head, and look your partner in the eyes to communicate interest. Periodically paraphrase what your partner has said and what you guess he or she is feeling to demonstrate you have been listening. Do not interrupt, raise your voice, or frown in a way that interferes with your partner's communication.

There are ways to make communicating about STIs less embarrassing, less confrontational, and more effective. Discussing STIs with sexual partners is important. Your very health, maybe even your life, may depend on it!

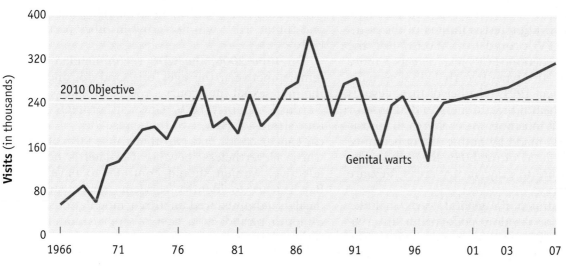

FIGURE **15.7** Human papillomavirus (genital warts)—initial visits to physicians' offices: United States, 1966–2007, and the *Healthy People 2010* objective. *Source:* Division of STD Prevention. *Sexually transmitted disease surveillance, 2007*. Atlanta, GA: Centers for Disease Control and Prevention, 2009.

they appear on the glans, foreskin, and shaft of the penis; on the scrotum; and in the anal area as well. It is estimated that there are more than 20 million women with genital warts in the United States, and three-fourths of their sexual partners are infected (see Figure 15.7). The incubation period ranges from 3 weeks to 3 months after contact with an infected person. Some lesions are moist and some are dry; the moist lesions respond well to treatment. Most genital wart infections are subclinical, meaning that they are not readily apparent to the infected individual and may often be overlooked by a physician during an

examination. A study at the University of California at Berkeley found that almost half of the 467 young women who consulted the university health service for a routine gynecological exam were infected with HPV (Bauer et al., 1991). Of the women examined, only 1% had genital warts visible at the time of examination, and only 9% had a history of genital warts. The rest of the women who had a positive test result for HPV had subclinical infection that would generally be undetected. Bauer and her colleagues believe that their results are applicable to other young college women.

It is estimated that more than 20 million women and 15 million men have genital warts. Most people have a subclinical condition; in other words, the warts are not readily visible. Although the condition is treatable, it is not curable.

Diagnosis and Treatment

Because it is difficult to diagnose subclinical cases of HPV infection, many cases are undetected. Several tissue biopsy tests are used by HPV researchers. The dot blot hybridization test is limited in the number of strains of HPV it can detect. Another test, the polymerase chain reaction (PCR) test, detects a more broad spectrum of HPV types (Nearly half of sexually active college women, 1991). Neither of these tests is routinely used by health practitioners to diagnose or detect cases of HPV infection. Most often a diagnosis of HPV infection is made by noting the appearance of warts. In moist areas of the body, they tend to be white, pink, or white to gray; in dry areas they are hard and yellow-gray.

The usual treatment for genital warts includes either cryotherapy or the drug podophyllin. In cryotherapy the warts are frozen with liquid nitrogen. The tissue then dies and is replaced with healthy normal tissue. The drug podophyllin is an irritant that causes the outer skin containing the virus to be sloughed off. Neither of these techniques kills the virus; both remove the infected tissue. Podophyllin should not be used during pregnancy because it may cause birth defects. Surgery may be necessary to remove especially large warts (Krilov, 1991). Regardless of the method used to treat genital warts, the recurrence rate is high.

Patient-applied treatments are also available. These include podofilox solution or gel that is applied with a cotton swab or the finger to the infected area twice a day for 3 days, followed by 4 days of no treatment.

This cycle can be repeated for up to 4 weeks. Imiquimod cream may also be applied at bedtime three times a week for as long as 16 weeks.

Cervical Cancer and HPV

HPV causes approximately 95% of the cervical cancer cases in the United States (Janicek & Averette, 2001). According to the American Cancer Society, between 50% and 75% of people who have ever had sexual intercourse will contract HPV, although the immune system usually clears out 70% of the virus within 1 year and 90% within 2 years (American Cancer Society, 2009). Risk factors associated with cervical cancer include initiation of sexual intercourse as a teenager and sexual intercourse with multiple partners. HPV is attracted to and able to live only in squamous epithelial cells in the body. Squamous epithelial cells are thin, flat cells that are found on the surface of the skin, cervix, vagina, anus, vulva, head of the penis, mouth, and throat. HPV will not grow in other parts of the body.

In June 2006, the CDC recommended that all females between the ages of 9 and 16, and before the first sexual intercourse, receive a new vaccine—Gardasil—against HPV. Gardasil protects against four strains of HPV: two that cause 70% of all cervical cancer cases, and two that cause 90% of genital warts. Nevertheless, because Gardasil is not 100% effective, women should continue to have annual Pap smears to identify cervical cancer early. Gardasil is administered in three inoculations over a 6-month period, at a cost of approximately $360. Although it is too soon to state conclusions confidently, it appears that the vaccine remains effective for at least 5 years. Because HPV causes genital warts in men, studies are under way to determine if young men should also be vaccinated. At present, the vaccination recommendation pertains only to young females.

Whereas health advocates welcome and support the CDC's recommendation that all females, especially those between ages 9 and 16, be inoculated, this support is not universal. Some individuals and groups argue that inoculating young girls encourages sexual behavior, whereas others question the wisdom of undertaking widespread inoculation before the vaccine has been studied over a longer period of time. No federal law requires inoculation; these are state matters. Some states have passed legislation requiring HPV inoculation for entry to school, whereas others merely recommend inoculation.

Herpes Genitalis

Incidence

The cause of **genital herpes** is a virus called **herpes simplex virus (HSV)**, which belongs to a family of more than 70 herpesviruses. Humans play host to four herpesviruses:

1. Herpes simplex virus, the agent for fever blisters and genital herpes

2. Cytomegalovirus, a virus that can cause death or retardation if acquired by a fetus

3. Varicella-zoster virus, the agent that causes chickenpox and shingles

4. Epstein-Barr virus, the agent of Burkitt's lymphoma in humans

In 1961, it was found that two types of HSV exist. Type 1 (HSV-1) is seen more frequently in areas of the body above the waist; type 2 (HSV-2) is seen more frequently below the waist. Although most cases of recurrent genital herpes (70%) are caused by type 2, 5% to 30% are caused by type 1. In addition, genital herpes can appear above the waist. For example, when HSV is transmitted through oral–genital sex, a sore may appear on the mouth.

Most patients who experience a first episode of HSV-2 infection experience recurrent episodes of genital lesions. However, clinical recurrences are much less frequent for HSV-1 infection than for HSV-2 infection. Therefore, identifying the causative agent has implications for treatment and counseling. For patients who have frequent recurrences of lesions (six or more recurrences a year), daily oral administration of acyclovir (400 mg twice a day) can decrease the rate of recurrence by 75% or greater.

Genital herpes had been diagnosed by 2003 in 45 million Americans (Division of STD Prevention, 2004); many other cases remain undiagnosed (Figure 15.8). In 2007, 317,000 new cases of genital herpes were reported (Centers for Disease Control and Pre-

> **genital herpes**
> An STI characterized by tiny fluid-filled blisters that appear on the genitals and in the genital tract.
>
> **herpes simplex virus (HSV)**
> The virus that causes oral and genital herpes infections.

Herpes simplex type 1 can manifest itself as a cold sore.

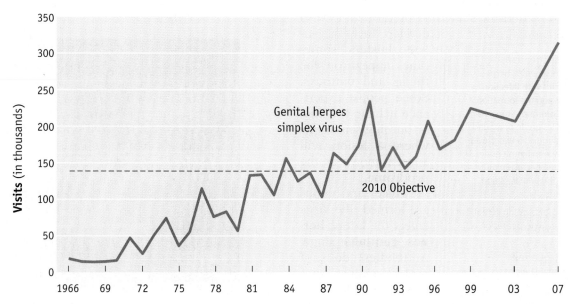

FIGURE 15.8 Genital herpes simplex virus infections—initial visits to physicians' offices: United States, 1996–2007, and the *Healthy People 2010* objective. *Source:* Division of STD Prevention. *Sexually transmitted disease surveillance, 2007.* Atlanta, GA: Centers for Disease Control and Prevention, 2009.

vention, 2009b). The *Healthy People 2010* national health objectives set a goal of reducing the incidence of genital herpes from 17% of the population to 14%. It is believed that 50% of pregnant women have antibodies to herpes that have developed as a result of a past contact with a herpesvirus and pass the antibodies to their unborn child through the placenta. Possibly as many as 70% of children 10 to 14 years of age have herpes antibodies, and by 50 years of age about 90% of people have such antibodies, which indicate that they have had some contact with a herpesvirus.

Symptoms and Complications

A herpes infection may be categorized into four stages (Fiumara, 1986b). **Primary herpes genitalis** corresponds with the time of actual infection by the herpesvirus and the formation of antibodies. A primary (first occurrence) herpes infection can be very painful but can also be completely symptom free. Fewer than 40% of those infected experience noticeable signs and symptoms. The other infected individuals become carriers of the herpesvirus and are unaware of their infection (Johnson et al., 1989). The time between exposure and development of the primary infection is 2 to 20 days, with an average of 6 days (Smith et al., 1990). In women the cervix is the main site of infection, although the vagina and vulva may also be involved. Symptoms include painful lesions, a sluggish feeling, and fever, along with possible lymph-node enlargement. Tiny blisters form, filled with a clear fluid in which the virus thrives. The area may become reddened and infected, and when blisters appear the site is in its most infectious state. The open lesions crust over as healing begins. In men, blisters and ulcers appear on the glans penis and the shaft, and urethritis may also develop. In both genders blisters sometimes appear on the thighs and buttocks. Some people experience itching, tingling, or burning sensations where a lesion will appear, known as the **prodrome**.

Once antibodies are formed, the virus enters the **latent herpes genitalis** stage. Antibodies do not protect against reinfection, but they do tend to make any recurrent infection less severe. During the latent stage the herpesvirus travels up the afferent nerve to the sacral ganglion, where it remains inactive (Figure 15.9). At this point in the infection there are no signs and symptoms.

The virus can become reactivated in the sacral ganglion without producing clinical signs. This occurrence is termed **shedding herpes genitalis**. During this stage, the virus is excreted from the body even though the infected individual is experiencing no symptoms. HSV is readily transmitted when blisters or ulcers are present. However, the infection is more commonly transmitted through asymptomatic viral shedding (virus shedding without detectable lesions). Asymptomatic HSV shedding is common (Australian Herpes Management Forum, 2007).

Patients with recurrent genital herpes can be treated with antiviral drugs that can be used intermittently (to treat each episode) or continuously (to prevent episodes) (Cowan, 1994). Intermittent drug treatment will decrease viral shedding during the treatment period. However, it will affect asymptomatic viral shedding only during the time of treatment. Continuous drug treatment is effective in suppressing recurrences and reducing symptomatic and asymptomatic shedding of HSV (Wald, et al., 1997).

primary herpes genitalis
The first stage of a genital herpes infection; it begins with infection by the herpesvirus and the formation of antibodies. Common symptoms include painful lesions in or around the genital area, a sluggish feeling, fever, and possibly swollen lymph nodes. Up to 75% of infected persons may be asymptomatic in the primary stage.

prodrome
Itching, tingling, or burning sensations that occur where a herpes lesion will appear.

latent herpes genitalis
The stage of genital herpes characterized by inactivity of the herpesvirus, during which an infected individual is asymptomatic and transmission of the virus is rare.

shedding herpes genitalis
The third stage of a genital herpes infection, during which virus is excreted from the body even though an infected individual experiences no signs or symptoms.

recurrent herpes genitalis
The fourth stage of a genital herpes infection, which is characterized by a reactivation of the virus and the appearance of blisters on the skin. Not all people with herpes have recurrences.

Symptoms of primary herpes genitalis include painful lesions, a sluggish feeling, and fever, along with lymph node enlargement.

To brain

Spinal cord
(cross section)

Ganglion

Herpesvirus
hides here

To lower body

Bundle
of nerve fibers

Virus travels
up nerve

Sensory
nerves

Skin cells

Herpesvirus enters
mucous membrane, eye,
or cut in skin and
reproduces

FIGURE **15.9** An initial herpes infection takes place when the virus (dots) enters cells of the mucous membranes, eyes, or skin. It reproduces and travels up (arrows) the sensory nerves until it reaches a ganglion (cluster of nerve cell bodies). There it hides, protected from attack by the body's immune system, which overcomes the infection at the place of entry. Though the entry wound soon heals, when conditions allow, the virus may later travel back down the nerve pathway to reinfect skin cells.

or which factors trigger recurrence. It has been suggested that stress, menstruation, or illness may bring on a recurrence; however, more research is needed to clarify the mechanisms at work in the recurrence stage of genital herpes.

The recurrence stage of herpes causes special problems for those infected. Recurrences are not always apparent as blisters may appear inside the genital tract where they cannot be seen, or symptoms may be so mild they are unnoticed. Psychological stress increases for many herpes sufferers because they are constantly in fear that symptoms will reappear. They are faced with the difficult decision of whether to tell new partners that they have had herpes. They feel vulnerable to rejection and therefore unwilling to share the information, yet they feel guilty if they are not honest. A variety of local groups across the country help herpes sufferers express their feelings about the disease and work through emotional problems.

The fourth stage of a herpes infection is termed **recurrent herpes genitalis**, characterized by reactivation of the virus with clinical manifestations. During this stage the virus travels down the nerve root to the skin, often causing new herpes blisters to erupt. Many individuals experience prodrome symptoms before a recurrence. Symptoms of recurrent infections are usually milder than those of the primary herpes infection and are of shorter duration, lasting from 2 to 10 days. The lesions are infectious for about 5 days. The frequency of outbreaks also varies, ranging from one or two recurrences in a lifetime to several outbreaks a month. Researchers have not been able to determine who experiences recurrences

Diagnosis and Treatment

Most diagnoses of herpes are made from the clinical signs: The patient has the vesicle-type lesions and the herpesvirus is isolated by tissue culture (the current preferred diagnostic procedure) or by blood test or Pap test (which is less accurate than a tissue culture). Cultures are taken from saliva, semen, and the cervix. The virus is known to grow slowly at times, so a culture result is not concluded to be negative for 2 weeks. Even with this procedure, conclusive diagnosis cannot always be made.

Herpes simplex on penis.

The best treatment for genital herpes is prevention. Some recommended preventive treatment procedures are as follows:

1. Many cases of genital herpes are transmitted by persons who are unaware that they have the infection or are asymptomatic when transmission occurs. In light of this realization, and because of the possibility of asymptomatic shedding of the virus between recurrences, it is recommended that condoms and spermicides always be used during sexual intercourse.

2. Persons with genital herpes should refrain from sexual activity when lesions or symptoms (prodrome) are present and inform their sexual partners that they have herpes. Prodromal symptoms precede herpes recurrences and include itching and burning and a "pins and needles" sensation at the site of infection.

3. Because there is a risk of transmitting herpes to a fetus neonatally, childbearing-aged women who have genital herpes should inform their health care providers, especially those who care for them during a pregnancy, about the infection.

4. Those experiencing a first episode of genital herpes should be advised to seek episodic therapy with antiviral medications and to minimize or prevent recurring symptoms with suppressive antiviral therapy.

5. Sexual partners should be evaluated for genital herpes and counseled regarding the disease regardless of the results of that evaluation.

6. Patients should be informed that the presence of lesions makes them more susceptible to HIV infection. Therefore, special precautions to refrain from HIV high-risk behaviors should be taken.

7. Because stress can induce recurrences, it is advisable for persons with genital herpes to learn stress management techniques and employ them on a regular basis. These include relaxation techniques, such as yoga, meditation autogenics, and progressive relaxation, as means of perceiving events as less stressful (Greenberg, 2009).

8. To help prevent secondary infections and thereby prolong the recurrent episode, persons with genital herpes should be advised to wash the affected area with warm water and soap several times a day. Dry the area by patting it with a soft towel, sprinkle cornstarch or baby powder on the area to keep it dry, and wear loose-fitting cotton underwear to allow moisture to evaporate from the area (nylon traps moisture).

Although there is no cure for genital herpes, there is effective treatment that can manage the symptoms and minimize or prevent recurrences. Treatment includes oral prescription antiviral medications, including acyclovir (Zovirax), famciclovir (Famvir), and valacyclovir (Valtrex), to help heal the sores sooner and reduce the frequency of relapses. If taken daily, these medications may also reduce the chance of transmission of the herpes virus (Mayo Clinic Staff,

 Did You Know...

Individuals infected with an STI are at a higher risk for becoming infected with HIV, the virus that causes AIDS. Researchers believe that the genital lesions characteristic of STIs provide HIV with an easy entry point to the body. Thus individuals who engage in unsafe sexual practices while an open lesion exists on the genitals lose an important line of defense against infection—unbroken skin.

2008a; WebMD, 2007). Treatment also may include a daily regimen to reduce the frequency of genital herpes recurrences. These treatments, called *suppressive therapy,* can reduce recurrence by as much as 75% among patients who have frequent recurrences (six or more a year).

The most important adverse effects of genital herpes are the long-term problems; everyone—infected or not—needs to be aware of these. One serious implication is the association between the virus and cervical cancer, although this relationship is neither absolute nor conclusive. Epidemiological studies have suggested a fivefold increase in risk for cervical cancer in women with herpes virus type 2 infection (Sexuality update, 1987). Therefore it is generally recommended that women with genital herpes have a Pap smear every 6 to 12 months (Centers for Disease Control and Prevention, 2005).

One serious effect of genital herpes is that it can lead to potentially fatal infections in babies. It is important that women avoid contracting herpes during pregnancy because a newly acquired infection during late pregnancy poses a greater risk of transmission to the baby (Centers for Disease Control and Prevention, 2008b). As already noted, the contagious virus is contained within the lesions. If vaginal lesions leak fluid during childbirth, the virus is transmitted to the infant and can result in encephalitis, brain damage, or both. Though less common, HSV can also be transmitted to a fetus through the placenta, thus causing infection before birth.

At this time it is not considered practical or feasible to test all women for herpes during their pregnancies, but women with a history of herpes definitely should be examined weekly from 32 weeks of gestation until delivery to see whether lesions recur. Any primary genital herpes lesions are likely to be detected in the frequent routine prenatal visits. If genital herpes is present at the time of delivery, the infant should be delivered by cesarean section. If laboratory examinations for active herpesvirus yield negative findings at delivery, the infant can be delivered vaginally with little risk of infection.

Hepatitis B

Incidence

Anywhere from 80,000 to 1.4 million people in the United States are infected with the virus that attacks the liver and causes hepatitis B. In fact, it is estimated that 1 in 20 people in the United States is infected by hepatitis B virus (HBV) at some time in life. HBV is transmitted through blood or blood products, semen, vaginal secretions, and saliva. The following populations are at increased risk of becoming

Photomicrograph of cells infected with the herpes simplex virus.

infected with HBV (Centers for Disease Control and Prevention, 2008a):

- Infants born to infected mothers

- Sexual partners of infected persons

- Sexually active persons who are not in a long-term, mutually monogamous relationship (e.g., more than one sexual partner during the previous 6 months)

- Men who have sex with men

- Injection drug users

- Household contacts of persons with chronic HBV infection

- Health care and public safety workers at risk for occupational exposure to blood or blood-contaminated body fluids

- Hemodialysis patients

- Residents and staff of facilities for developmentally disabled persons

- Travelers to countries with intermediate or high prevalence of HBV infection

Symptoms and Complications

Approximately 30% of those infected with HBV are asymptomatic. In those cases, only a blood test can reveal the disease. In other instances, in those infected the eyes or the skin turns yellow (jaundice); the appetite suffers; nausea, vomiting, fever, or stomach or joint pain may occur; and the person may feel extremely tired and unable to work for weeks or months. Although the mortality rate is lower than that of other forms of hepatitis, 2,000 to 4,000 people die each year of untreated hepatitis B.

Diagnosis and Treatment

Hepatitis B is diagnosed by a blood test for hepatitis antibodies or antigens. At the time of this writing, there is no cure for hepatitis B. That is why prevention is so important. Once hepatitis B is diagnosed, treatment consists of bed rest and ingestion of adequate amounts of fluid to prevent dehydration. Usually feelings of fatigue subside in a few weeks, although they may not subside for several months in severe cases. For patients in whom liver disease develops, alpha interferon and lamivudine are two drugs that have proved to be effective in approximately 40% of patients.

As with all of the STIs, prevention is the first avenue of protection from infection by HBV. Of course, limiting the number of sexual partners and having no sexual activity with someone who is infected is good advice. In addition, refraining from handling blood or blood products, semen, vaginal secretions, and saliva is an effective preventive measure. And, of course, injecting no drugs, being tattooed or having body piercing from an artist who practices good health practices, and sharing no personal care items such as razors or toothbrushes are also good preventive practices. There is a vaccination to prevent HBV infection that has been available since 1982. The CDC recommends that the following persons be vaccinated against hepatitis B:

- All infants, beginning at birth

- All children younger than 19 years of age who have not been vaccinated previously

- Susceptible sex partners of HBV-positive persons

- Sexually active persons who are not in a long-term, mutually monogamous relationship (e.g., more than one sex partner during the previous 6 months)

- Persons seeking evaluation or treatment for an STI

- Men who have sex with men

- Injection drug users

- Susceptible household contacts of HBV-positive persons

- Health care and public safety workers at risk for exposure to blood or blood-contaminated body fluids

- Persons with end-stage renal disease and home dialysis patients

- Residents and staff of facilities for developmentally disabled persons

- Travelers to regions with intermediate or high rates of endemic HBV infection

- Persons with chronic liver disease

Hepatitis B is diagnosed by a blood test that looks for antibodies or antigens that are present when exposed to the hepatitis B virus.

- Persons with HIV infection

- All other persons seeking protection from HBV infection—acknowledgment of a specific risk factor is not a requirement for vaccination

The vaccination consists of three doses administered over several months.

■ Vaginal Infections

One category of infection, vaginitises or vaginal infections, occurs in response to changes in an individual's own body and has, therefore, been referred to as a *sexually related disease* (SRD). Two of these vaginitises, trichomoniasis and candidiasis, can also be transmitted from partner to partner and are considered relatively common in women (see Figure 15.10).

Trichomoniasis

Trichomonas vaginalis is a one-celled organism that burrows under the vaginal mucosa to cause **trichomoniasis**, or **trick**. According to the National Institute for Allergy and Infectious Diseases, the estimated annual incidence is approximately 3.7 million cases. The common mode of transmission is through sexual intercourse, but tricho-

> **trichomoniasis (trick)**
> A type of vaginitis that can be an STI or an SRD. Symptoms include a foul-smelling, foamy white or yellow-green discharge that irritates the vagina and vulva. Urethritis may also be present.

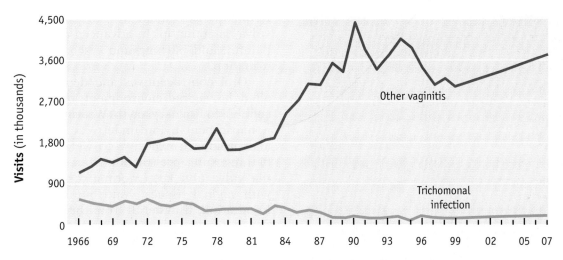

FIGURE **15.10** Trichomonal and other vaginal infections—initial visits to physicians' offices: United States, 1966–2007. *Source:* Division of STD Prevention. *Sexually transmitted disease surveillance, 2007.* Atlanta, GA: Centers for Disease Control and Prevention, 2009.

Micrograph of vaginal discharge revealing the presence of *Trichomoniasis vaginalis,* a common vaginal infection. Prolonged, untreated, or inadequately treated trichomoniasis can result in an increased risk of cancer.

moniasis can be contracted by prolonged exposure to moisture (for example, wet bathing suits, towels, or other clothing). Women who are pregnant or who use an oral contraceptive may be more prone to trichomoniasis infections. These women have high levels of progesterone, which increase the alkalinity in the vagina, creating a hospitable environment for the *Trichomonas* organism. The main symptom of trichomoniasis is an odorous, foamy, white or yellow-green discharge that irritates the vagina and vulva. Frequently trichomoniasis is accompanied by urethritis. A microscopic examination of a sample of the discharge can reveal what caused the condition.

Because the infection can be passed back and forth between partners (the Ping-Pong effect), both partners should be treated when trichomoniasis is confirmed in a woman. The man may harbor the disease organism but be asymptomatic. Metronidazole (trade name Flagyl) is the drug of choice, although tinidazole has also been used as a treatment. Topical agents are also sometimes prescribed. Both partners follow the regimen, which is one megadose administered in 1 day. Consumer advocates have suggested, however, that metronidazole is linked with cancer, because cancer appeared in laboratory animals given massive doses of the drug. Others argue that much greater doses than those used in treating trichomoniasis were administered to these laboratory animals and that it poses no danger to humans. Nevertheless, an increased risk of cancer of the cervix does exist in women with a history of trichomoniasis infections. The white blood cell count lowers with the intake of Flagyl, but it returns to normal in a short time. If a second round of the drug is necessary, a white blood cell test is recommended. Prolonged, untreated, or inadequately treated trichomoniasis may result in a greater risk of cancer than does use of the recommended dosage of Flagyl.

Flagyl should not be taken during the first 3 months of pregnancy; a pregnancy test should always precede prescription of this drug. Also, both partners taking metronidazole are advised against drinking alcoholic beverages because of undesirable side effects, such as headache and nausea.

Candidiasis

The second most common form of vaginitis, **candidiasis**, also called *moniliasis, Monilia,* or *yeast infection,* is caused by the fungus *Candida albicans.* This fungus normally lives and grows in the vagina.

candidiasis
A common form of vaginitis, sometimes called a yeast infection, which is caused by the fungus *Candida albicans.*

The second most common form of vaginitis is candidiasis, or yeast infection. It can result in white and curdy discharge, as shown here.

frequently associated with a rash or redness of the vulva, is common. In advanced cases intercourse is painful, and burning and discomfort occur during urination.

Oral contraceptives and deodorant sprays also alter the vaginal environment, making it more susceptible to fungus growth. Wearing of tight jeans and nonabsorbent nylon underwear and outer clothing and prolonged exposure to wet, synthetic material bathing suits prevent air from circulating around the vulva and keep normal discharges in contact with vaginal tissues, contributing to yeast growth. In addition, if material from the bowel is carried to the vagina, the person becomes more susceptible to moniliasis, because the bowel harbors the *Candida* fungus.

Clothes should serve as a means for absorbing normal discharges. Good hygiene and wearing of cotton or cotton-crotch underclothing go far in offering protection. For women with confirmed yeast infections, mycostatin tablets inserted high into the vagina twice a day for a few weeks is the standard treatment, although vaginal suppositories or creams can also be used. Alternative remedies include tea tree oil, yogurt (which contains the antifungal *Lactobacillus acidophilus*), garlic (taken orally), echinacea (taken orally), gentian violet, and oregano oil, though there is little evidence that these are effective (Mayo Clinic Staff, 2008b).

■ Ectoparasitic Infestations

There are two common STIs that are not diseases as such, but rather infestations of parasites. These are pubic lice and scabies. Parasites are found among all socioeconomic classes and are spread by close physical contact.

Pubic Lice

Pubic lice, commonly referred to as crabs, are parasites. Actually there are three different kinds of lice, known as **pediculosis lice**, and each seems to prefer its own habitat. *Pediculus corporis* is a body louse; *Pediculus capitus* is a head louse; and *Pediculus pubis* is the louse of the pubic area. Pubic lice are usually transmitted from person to person by sexual contact. The organism grips the pubic hair and feeds on tiny blood vessels of the skin.

Female crabs live 1 to 2 months and

lactobacilli
Bacteria in the vagina that aid in keeping it healthy; also called *Doderlein bacilli.*

It is also known to be present in the mouth and intestine of many men and women. On occasion when the **lactobacilli**, or *Doderlein bacilli*, that are necessary for a healthy vaginal condition are reduced in number, the yeast multiply and outgrow other vaginal organisms. Women normally have these lactobacilli in the vagina, where they are necessary to maintain a healthy environment. They protect against a variety of infections, particularly those caused by bacteria in the urinary tract and the colon. The protective lactobacilli can be reduced by general poor health or lowered resistance, by too frequent douching, and by use of antibiotics (which can kill the lactobacilli as well as the bacteria causing the disease for which the antibiotic is prescribed). When the normally acid environment is changed, the yeast multiply and outgrow other vaginal organisms, resulting in a white and curdy discharge. Examination reveals a whitish plaque around the vagina and on its walls. Itching,

pubic lice
A parasite, commonly referred to as crabs, a louse that grips the pubic hair and feeds on tiny blood vessels of the skin.

pediculosis lice
Also known as crabs, of three common types: *Pediculus corporis*, a body louse; *Pediculus capitis*, a head louse; and *Pediculus pubis*, a pubic louse.

Multicultural
DIMENSIONS

STIs and Minorities Surveillance data show high rates of STIs for some minority racial or ethnic groups compared with rates for whites. Race and ethnicity in the United States are risk markers that correlate with other more fundamental determinants of health status such as poverty, access to high-quality health care, health-care-seeking behavior, illicit drug use, and residence in communities with high prevalence of STIs.

- In 2007, 48% of all chlamydia cases occurred among African Americans. Overall, the chlamydia rate among African Americans was more than 8 times that among whites. The chlamydia rate among African American women was more than 7 times higher than the rate among white women. The chlamydia rate among African American men was more than 11 times higher than the rate among white men.
- In 2007, the chlamydia rate among Hispanics was nearly 3 times higher than the rate among whites. The chlamydia rate among American Indians/Alaska Natives was more than 5 times higher than the rate among whites.
- In 2007, approximately 70% of the total number of reported cases of gonorrhea occurred among African Americans. Overall, the rate of gonorrhea among African Americans in the United States was 19 times greater than that among whites. This disparity was higher for African American men (26.1 times higher) than for African American women (14.9 times higher). Among those aged 20 to 24 years, the gonorrhea rate among African Americans was 16.5 times greater than that among whites (2,618.3 versus 158.8 cases per 100,000 population).

- In 2007, the gonorrhea rate among American Indians/Alaska Natives was 107.1 cases per 100,000 population, which was 3.1 times higher than the rate among whites. The gonorrhea rate among Asians/Pacific Islanders was lower than the rate among whites, and the rate among Hispanics was higher than the rate among whites.
- In 2007, 46.0% of all cases of primary and secondary syphilis occurred in African Americans. Compared to whites, the overall 2007 rate of primary and secondary syphilis among African Americans was 7 times higher.
- Compared to whites, the 2007 primary and secondary syphilis rate among American Indians/Alaska Natives was 1.7 times higher, and the rate among Hispanics was 2.2 times higher.

Reducing the prevalence of many of these STIs in minority populations will require a combination of strategies. Of course, education about prevention is important. Still, education will not have a significant effect in minority populations if it is not combined with strategies to reduce poverty, increase access to good-quality health care, decrease drug abuse and the sharing of drug "works," and create comprehensive sexuality education programs that start in schools at early ages and continue through community agencies into the adult years.

Source: Division of STI Prevention. *Sexually transmitted disease surveillance, 2007.* U.S. Department of Health and Human Services, Public Health Service. Atlanta: Centers for Disease Control and Prevention, 2009.

lay up to 10 eggs a day. As they feed on the human skin and blood, they irritate the skin, causing itching and occasionally swelling of glands in the groin. The nits, or eggs, stick to the pubic hair with a thick substance. Aided by body warmth, the eggs hatch and the new lice perpetuate the cycle of feeding on the human before dropping off. They can live for about 1 day off the body and are visible to the naked eye on clothing and bedsheets. Two different preparations are effective: A-200 Pyrinate, an over-the-counter preparation, and gamma benzene (Kwell), available only by prescription. Either one is applied to the pubic hair. Directions should be carefully followed. One dose is usually curative, but sometimes the nits, though inactive, adhere to the pubic hair for

Pubic lice, commonly called "crabs," are usually transmitted from person to person by sexual contact. Direct treatment, plus cleaning of clothes and bedding, eliminate the lice.

weeks after treatment unless removed. A fine-toothed comb dipped first into vinegar, then into water, and combed through the pubic hair dissolves them. And, of course, clothing and bed linen used before treatment should be washed.

Scabies

Scabies is caused by a tiny mite that can barely be seen. The organism generally lives for up to 2 months. The female burrows under the skin at night, probably for the warmth of the human host, and the results are intense itching and the formation of pus. There is a characteristic distribution pattern of scabies. It is seen most commonly on the wrists, in the spaces between the fingers, under the breasts, and on the buttocks. Nodular scabies (raised lesions) can last up to 1 year. The mites lay two to three eggs a day, and in 2 or 3 weeks a new cycle begins. Because the incubation period is 4 to 8 weeks, one individual can transmit scabies to another before being aware of its existence. Close contact that is usually (but not exclusively) sexual can transmit the mites. Scabies is rarely contracted from clothing, bedding, or toilet seats.

To diagnose scabies, a physician scrapes a burrow and puts the scraping on a slide, often with mineral oil to make the swimming mite more readily visible (Centers for Disease Control and Prevention, *Scabies—CDC fact sheet*, 2005). Lindane (Kwell) is the medication used to treat scabies, as well as crabs. It must be applied very judiciously, because it can be toxic to some people. In particular there is concern about the safety of pregnant women using lindane. Consequently, pregnant women are advised to wear gloves when applying this medication (National Library of Medicine, 2008).

> **scabies**
> Skin irritation caused by a tiny mite that is transferred from one person to another by close contact, sexual or otherwise.

Scabies lesions can last for up to a year and can be transmitted before being aware of its existence.

▮ Prevention

On the one hand, STIs are often like other diseases in that, for many, there are effective treatments that result in elimination of the disease. On the other hand, for some STIs, even though there are effective treatments, there are no cures (for example, herpes genitalis). Still other STIs have only recently had potentially effective treatments developed to treat them and, until then, inevitably led to incapacity and death (for example, syphilis). Even when cured, people who have contracted some STIs can be affected for their entire lives—for example, when the disease results in infertility. STIs, therefore, are serious conditions that we would be best advised to prevent. Fortunately, there are actions we can take to prevent contracting an STI or at least minimize the likelihood of contracting one.

Abstinence

The most certain way to avoid contracting an STI is to abstain from sexual activity, meaning not just coitus. As we have learned, STIs can be contracted through oral sex and anal sex, as well as skin-to-skin contact.

For some people, abstinence is a viable choice. However, it is clear that for many others, abstinence

Did You Know . . .

Although it is impossible to determine the exact number of STIs each year, it is agreed that the cost of these diseases is extensive. One estimate is that STI expenditures on direct medical care and related services, as well as the indirect costs associated with the loss of productivity, totaled $15.9 billion in 2008 (Centers for Disease Control and Prevention, 2009b). This estimate excludes costs attributed to HIV and AIDS.

¿? Ethical DIMENSIONS

Notifying Partners About STIs

There are many reasons why people with STIs choose not to notify their sexual partner(s) about their infection. They may be embarrassed to do so, they may be married and have contracted the STI during extramarital sex or homosexual contact, or they may not want anyone to know about their infection for fear they will not be able to get dates or other sexual partners.

Similarly, there are many reasons people with STIs choose to notify their sexual partners. They may believe that all sexual partners, past and present, should be notified of a sexual partner's STI status. In this way, they can get tested and retested if they are infected. And they can prevent the spread of the infection by refraining from sex with other people until they are disease free.

On the one hand, some people argue that *absent any signs or symptoms,* notifying a sexual partner might do more harm than good. For example, if the disease was contracted during an extramarital affair, notification might result in divorce. If contracted during homosexual activity, notification might mean the loss of a job or other discriminatory actions. Furthermore, notification might unduly frighten the unsuspecting partner, causing potentially unhealthy consequences associated with stress.

On the other hand, some people argue that to disclose an STI is consistent with the ethical principles of honesty and nonmaleficence (do no harm). Even if the result of the sexual behavior is accompanied by sanctions (such as divorce or the loss of one's job), they believe it further compounds the violation of trust to withhold information that a loved one can use to protect his or her health.

What do you think is the ethical thing to do?

---

is not acceptable. This may be for many reasons. They may have an interest in sex and find it so pleasurable that they are not willing to forgo it. They may be older and not married and intend never to marry. They may be homosexual with legal marriage unavailable to them. For those not willing to remain abstinent, other strategies for preventing contraction of an STI are available.

Monogamy

If a sexual partner is STI free, and he or she is the only person with whom you engage in sexual activity, then you will not contract an STI. Monogamy with an uninfected partner, though, can be problematic. How are you to be sure your partner is uninfected? If the relationship is a long-term one, there probably is a greater reason to assume your partner is uninfected if he or she tells you so. However, unless you see the results of medical tests for STIs, you can never really be sure. Furthermore, even if the results are negative for HIV, for instance, sufficient antibodies may not have been formed to allow the test to detect them. This usually takes months. Even if you assume a partner is monogamous, some seemingly trustworthy sexual partners have been shown to be anything but. For these reasons, relying on monogamy with an uninfected partner as protection against contracting an STI can be risky.

If sexually active, the best way to prevent contracting an STI is by maintaining a monogamous relationship in which both partners are STI free.

Myth (vs) Fact

Myth: If you get syphilis, you will know it because a rash will break out.
Fact: A rash may not appear until secondary syphilis has occurred. Furthermore, although a chancre (a sore) may develop early in the course of the disease, it may not be visible or may be dismissed as inconsequential. Also, in women, the early signs of syphilis may not be readily visible on the genitalia.

Myth: Gonorrhea is no more serious than the common cold and can be cured easily.
Fact: Gonorrhea can cause infertility, arthritis, or endocarditis (inflammation of the heart valves). In addition, certain antibiotic-resistant strains of gonorrhea raise concern about the ability to continue to treat this STI with present medications.

Myth: If you get an STI once, you acquire an immunity to it and cannot contract it a second time.
Fact: You do not have immunity to STIs and can contract them anew each time you have contact with the disease-causing organisms.

Myth: STIs occur only in or on the genital organs.
Fact: You can acquire an STI through oral–genital contact, in which case the signs of the disease would occur in the mouth and on the face. Or, you can have contact with an STI-causing organism by touching an infected area with your fingers, in which case the signs of the disease would appear on your fingers and hands.

Reduce the Number of Sexual Partners

If a person is unwilling or unable to maintain a monogamous relationship, decreasing the number of sexual partners lessens his or her odds of contracting an STI. The greater number of sexual partners, the greater the likelihood that one of them will be infected.

Refrain from the Use of Alcohol and Other Drugs

Decisions regarding important aspects of your life deserve thoughtful consideration. What more important decision is there than that concerning whether you will engage in an activity that has the potential of causing serious, sometimes life-threatening illness? Alcohol and other drugs can interfere with decision making by decreasing inhibitions and affecting judgment. Therefore, protection against STIs should include abstention from the use of mind-altering drugs.

Discuss STI Concerns with Potential Sexual Partners

Any new sexual partners should discuss concern about STIs before engaging in sexual activity. Whether they know they are infected, the high-risk behaviors they have engaged in and the results of any medical screenings they have had should be shared. This kind of a conversation can lead to concern about a potential sexual partner and a decision to refrain from sex altogether—or at least until a new medical screening can be obtained. Such a conversation will also make it easier to engage in the inspection of external signs of STIs described in the following section.

Examine Yourself and Your Partner

Although it may be embarrassing for some people, inspecting yourself and your sexual partner for signs of STIs can help prevent their spread. However, if this activity is done as sexual play, the embarrassment can be minimized.

Examine the skin of the genitals for lesions, blisters, and infected sores. Genital warts, chancres, and signs of herpes can be detected in this way. Note any foul-smelling odors. For males, the penis should be checked for any discharge by "milking" the urethra. This can be done by holding the penis and squeezing it gently but firmly. For females, the vulva should be examined for any external signs of infection. In addition, evidence of any vaginal discharge should be sought by inserting a finger into the vagina.

Because you are not a medical expert, do not rely on your own inclinations or interpretations of any unusual signs you notice. If any doubt is raised by your inspection, refrain from sexual activity until a medical screening has been arranged. That does not mean you have to abandon your relationship with a partner who has signs of an STI or that you have to be abandoned if you have these signs. All it means is that you need to protect yourself and a sexual partner from a disease that can be prevented with a little caution and patience. Recognizing an STI is disturbing and sometimes scary. However, until the results of medical screening are obtained, and afterward if the results indicate an STI, partners should express caring and concern.

Use Latex Condoms

The pores of a latex condom are too small for some organisms that cause STIs to penetrate. Therefore, the use of a latex condom during coitus and fellatio is effective in reducing the risk of contracting an STI. The National Institutes for Health formed a panel of experts to study the effectiveness of condoms in preventing STIs and HIV and AIDS. The panel concluded that condoms are effective in preventing HIV and AIDS and gonorrhea acquired by men from women (American Public Health Association, 2001). It also concluded that there was not conclusive

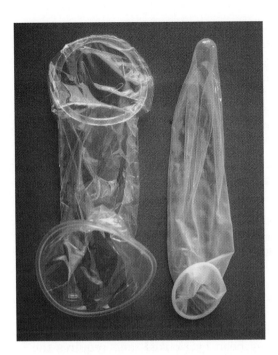

The male and female condoms prevent STIs by establishing a barrier between the disease-causing organism and the body. This barrier prevents the organism from finding a pathway into the body.

epidemiological evidence that condoms prevented the transmission of chlamydia, syphilis, chancroid, trichomoniasis, genital herpes, and human papillomavirus infection. These findings have, unfortunately, been misinterpreted in too many media reports. The panel did not state that condoms did not prevent these STIs. Rather, it stated only that there was no convincing epidemiological evidence that they do. It also stated that more studies were needed to warrant such a statement. Experts still recommend the use of condoms to reduce the risk of HIV and AIDS and STIs, awaiting the supportive evidence they expect to have soon.

It should be noted that condoms can only decrease the risk of contracting an STI, not eliminate it. Condoms will not offer protection against STIs that are transmitted by contact with other parts of the body—diseases such as herpes, warts, or ectoparasitic infections.

Avoid High-Risk Behaviors

Because organisms that cause STIs are present in semen and vaginal secretions, the goal is to prevent them from being transmitted from an infected person to a person not infected. Coitus without the use of a condom can result in the depositing of semen that includes disease-causing organisms within a partner's body. So can fellatio without a condom and cunnilingus without a dental dam. Anal sex is a par-

ticularly high-risk behavior because the friction creates fissures (tears in the lining) in the anus, allowing easy entrance to disease-causing organisms into the bloodstream. Furthermore, because organisms that cause STIs reside in the blood, using needles or other products that may contain drops of blood from another person puts one at high risk for disease. Sharing needles is one of the more common ways of contracting HIV in the United States.

Other Protective Measures

Still other behaviors can lessen the likelihood of contracting an STI or increase the likelihood of detecting one at an early stage:

- Wash the genitals before and after sex.
- Obtain regular medical checkups.
- Inspect the genitalia regularly.
- Do not share razors, hypodermic needles, or scissors.
- Do not handle towels, wet bedding, or undergarments immediately after these have been in contact with another person.
- For women, using a diaphragm, spermicide, or other barrier method of contraception may offer protection against some STIs.

If you suspect you have been exposed to an STI, see a physician or visit a health clinic in your community or on your campus. It is unwise to try to diagnose and treat the condition yourself. It is also extremely important to comply with the treatment regimen, which includes taking all the medication prescribed at the appropriate times and returning for any follow-up visits. Also, if you have an STI, notify your partner(s). Failing to tell a partner of the possibility of infection could result in the spread of the disease, not just to a single individual but possibly to many (see Figure 15.11).

Sexuality Education and STIs

Alarmed at what it called the "hidden epidemic," the Institute of Medicine (IOM) convened a 15-member expert panel in 1994 to strategize ways to address the STI problem. The IOM concluded that society's unwillingness to confront sexual issues is the main barrier to responding to STIs (Eng & Butler, 1996). The IOM report went on to explain that this attitude hinders the dissemination of accurate, straightforward information about STIs in educational programs for adolescents and interferes with communication between parents and their children and

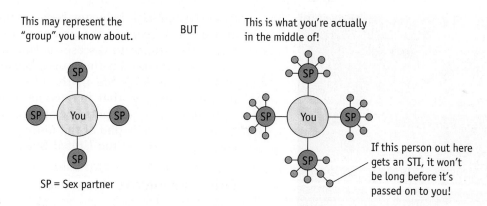

This may represent the "group" you know about.

BUT

This is what you're actually in the middle of!

SP = Sex partner

If this person out here gets an STI, it won't be long before it's passed on to you!

FIGURE 15.11 STIs: a fact of life for the sexually active. By "sexually active," we do not mean having a lot of sex. Instead we are using the term to mean having sex with different people. In general, the fact of life is that, sooner or later, sexually active people will either be exposed to an STI or contract one.

between sexual partners. Furthermore, this attitude compromises health care professionals' ability to counsel patients, impedes research on sexual behavior, and leads to unbalanced messages being sent via the media. The members of the expert panel noted several studies that found that almost two-thirds of respondents knew little or nothing about STIs other than HIV and AIDS and that most people seriously underestimate their risk of acquiring an STI, as well as its consequences. Not much has changed in the intervening years.

The need for education about STIs is evident, has long been overlooked, and requires the involvement of many different segments of our society, working together to prevent their occurrence and to develop more effective treatments if and when they do occur.

Exploring the
DIMENSIONS
of Human Sexuality

Our feelings, attitudes, and beliefs regarding sexuality are influenced by our internal and external environments. Go to sexuality.jbpub.com/dimensions/4e to learn more about the biological, psychological, and sociological factors that affect your sexuality.

Biological Factors

- STIs are contracted primarily through sexual contact.
- SRDs are diseases of the reproductive system that can occur in either sexually active or sexually inactive individuals. For example, cervical cancer has been linked to herpes type 2.
- Individuals with an STI have a higher risk of becoming infected with HIV, possibly because the genital lesions characteristic of STIs give HIV access to the body.
- STIs can be passed to a baby both before and during birth.

Sociocultural Factors

- Society's unwillingness to confront sexual issues is a major barrier in responding to STIs.
- Some ethnic groups have higher rates of STIs than others. Southern states have higher rates of syphilis than the national average.
- Economically, the cost of treating STIs—and the associated lost productivity—exceeds $15 billion per year.

Psychological Factors

Biological and sociocultural factors combine to influence psychological factors.

- Having an STD affects an individual's feelings about his or her sexuality.
- Learning later in life that you became sterile due to an undiagnosed STD can have a devastating psychological effect.
- Psychological stress increases for genital herpes sufferers because they are constantly in fear that symptoms will reappear. They must decide whether to tell new partners of their condition, which can lead to rejection.

Sexually transmitted infections are quite prevalent, especially among young people. Some STIs and SRDs are curable; some are treatable but chronic. Because many cases are asymptomatic or early symptoms are ignored, treatment does not always occur. The STI can then be transmitted further.

Having a curable STI is, at a minimum, embarrassing. Yet having a chronic STI such as genital herpes or genital warts can have a profound psychological impact on a person's life. The STI will affect the individual's sexual activities for an entire lifetime. The fear of rejection after informing a potential sexual partner might cause the individual to say nothing. Self-esteem can diminish.

Socially, race and ethnicity correlate with fundamental determinants of health status such as poverty, access to health care, health-care-seeking behavior, and residence in areas with a high prevalence of STIs. Thus a higher prevalence of gonorrhea or syphilis among African Americans has social—not biological—underpinnings.

Prevent STIs through abstinence, monogamy, reduction in the number of sexual partners, abstinence from alcohol or other drugs, communication with partners, examination of yourself and your partner, use of latex condoms, and avoidance of high-risk behaviors.

Summary

- Sexually transmitted infections (STIs) are infections contracted through sexual activities. There are also diseases of the sexual organs referred to as sexually related diseases (SRDs), which can occur in both sexually active and sexually abstinent individuals.

- Chlamydia is the most prevalent STI. More than 1.1 million cases were reported in 2007, more than three times the number of gonorrhea cases reported. Symptoms are often asymptomatic, although men may notice pain or burning during urination and women may notice a vaginal discharge and abdominal pain.

- Gonorrhea is the second most prevalent STI. In 2007, almost 356,000 cases were reported. Males are more likely to experience symptoms from gonorrhea infection than are females. Males may experience frequent and painful urination and a discharge of pus from the urethra. Females are usually asymptomatic, although some may notice a yellowish discharge.

- Syphilis rates have been rising since 2000. Initial symptoms include the development of a lesion (chancre), which disappears in 2 to 4 weeks. Soon afterward, a rash, fever, and some hair loss can occur. If syphilis goes untreated, blindness, paralysis, brain damage, and death are possible.

- Among viral causes of STIs are human papillomavirus (HPV), which is associated with the development of genital warts and cervical cancer. A vaccine, Gardasil, is now available that can prevent as much as 70% of cervical cancers and 90% of genital warts caused by HPV. Other viral causes of STIs include herpes simplex virus (HSV), which is associated with the development of genital herpes, and hepatitis B virus (HBV), which is associated with the development of hepatitis B.

- Sexually related diseases include vaginal infections (such as trichomoniasis and candidiasis) and ectoparasitic infections (such as pubic lice and scabies).

- Among the means of preventing or minimizing the risk of developing an STI are sexual abstinence, maintaining a monogamous sexual relationship, reducing the number of sexual partners, refraining from the use of alcohol or other drugs, examining yourself and your sexual partner, and using latex condoms.

Discussion Questions

1. What are STIs, how are they transmitted, and what are the reasons for their prevalence?

2. What are the bacterially based STIs? Include their incidence, transmission, symptoms and complications, and diagnosis and treatment in your answer.

3. What are the virally based STIs? Include their incidence, transmission, symptoms and complications, and diagnosis and treatment in your answer.

4. What are the ectoparasitic infestations? Include their incidence, transmission, symptoms and complications, and diagnosis and treatment in your answer.

5. List the key ways to prevent STIs, evaluating the theoretical and user effectiveness of each in the real world.

Application Questions

Reread the chapter-opening story and answer the following questions.

1. Jessica chose to ask her human sexuality professor about her potential STI. Why didn't she go to the student health clinic or her primary care physician?

2. The author describes several of the "private" conversations students wish to have with human sexuality professors, concerning pregnancy, abuse, sexual disorders, and STIs. Where on your campus (or in your community) could you go for help for each of these problems? Be specific, creating a list with phone numbers.

3. Should professors discuss personal sexuality issues with students? Explain why or why not.

Critical Thinking Questions

1. Applications for marriage licenses in many states require a blood test for syphilis but not for the other STIs. Because many STIs are asymptomatic, should marriage tests require testing for all the major STIs? What difficulties would implementing such a program involve? (Hint: Consider how each disease is diagnosed.)

2. How can undetected STIs affect fetuses and newborns?

3. Criminal laws generally provide that someone who deliberately inflicts harm on another person should be punished. Civil laws allow the victim to seek compensation for harm done. Should people who know they are infected with STIs but who have unprotected sex with others and infect them be prosecuted? Should the people they infect be able to sue for physical and psychological damages?

Critical Thinking Case

Most of us believe that STIs afflict young people. But STIs strike people of all ages—including senior citizens. People who are widowed or divorced do not become asexual; rather, they usually begin dating new people. In fact, 90% of postmenopausal women remain sexually active.

Dr. Peter Leone, medical director of the Wake County, North Carolina, STI Clinic, says: "Women who are past menopause often think they can't get an STI. People link pregnancy and STI risk. But methods to prevent pregnancy aren't the best ones for preventing STIs. On the other hand, some people think, 'Why should I use a condom? I can't get pregnant.' "

Although the STI incidence rates per 100,000 people has remained low for senior citizens, the number of seniors is growing dramatically. So, even if rates remain low, the number will continue to increase. Consequently, in 2006, people 50 years old and older accounted for 18% of the total AIDS cases reported in the United States.

Consider your parents or your parents' friends who are divorced or widowed. How could you, as a student in this class, give them information about taking responsibility for their sexual behavior?

Ironically, it seems that senior citizens share the attitude of young people regarding sexual behavior: It cannot happen to me. Explain this attitude. Do young people and seniors have different reasons for their beliefs?

Exploring Personal Dimensions

Can You Be Assertive When You Need to Be?

To take the necessary actions to prevent contracting an STI, you will have to be assertive: That is, you will need to resist pressure to engage in sexual activity if you choose not to, and you will need to insist on the use of a condom and other safer sex precautions if you decide to engage in sex. Do you have assertiveness skills? To find out, write an assertive response to each of the situations described.

1. You are on a date and your partner insists on engaging in a sexual activity that you decide is not for you at that time. You say:

_____

_____

_____

2. Your partner argues that condoms diminish the sensation. You respond by saying:

_____

_____

_____

3. Your partner states that she or he has been tested for STIs and the test result was negative. Therefore, there are no reasons for using safer sex techniques. You respond by saying:

_____

_____

_____

To be assertive, you need to:

1. Specify the behavior or situation to which the statement refers.

2. Relate your feelings about that situation.

3. Suggest a remedy or what your preference is.

4. Identify the consequences of the change: what will happen if it occurs and what will happen if it does not occur.

Now check your responses and revise them to be consistent with these assertiveness principles.

Suggested Readings

Handsfield, H. H., Hook, E. W. J., Lipshutz, J. A., & Aral, S. O. *Behavioral interventions for prevention and control of sexually transmitted diseases.* New York: Springer, 2008.

Holmes, K., Sparling, P., Stamm, W., Piot, P., Wasserheit, J., Corey, L., & Cohen, M. *Sexually transmitted diseases.* New York: McGraw-Hill, 2007.

Klausner, J., & Hook, E. *Current diagnosis and treatment of sexually transmitted diseases.* New York: McGraw-Hill, 2007.

Marr, L. *Sexually transmitted diseases: A physician tells you what you need to know.* Baltimore, MD: Johns Hopkins University Press, 2007.

Moore, E. A., & Moore, L. M. *Encyclopedia of sexually transmitted diseases.* Jefferson, NC: McFarland, 2008.

Naff, C. F. *Sexually transmitted diseases: Perspectives on diseases and disorders.* Chicago, IL: Greenhaven Press, 2008.

Zenilman, J. *Sexually transmitted diseases and reproductive health.* Philadelphia, PA: W. B. Saunders, 2009.

Web Resources

For links to the web sites below, visit *http://sexuality.jbpub.com/dimensions/4e* and click on Resource Links.

Centers for Disease Control and Prevention
www.cdc.gov

An agency of the federal government, CDC provides links to information about STIs including HIV/AIDS, resources available, prevention, and treatments available.

Department of Health and Human Services
www.hhs.gov

An agency of the federal government, DHHS provides links to various diseases and infections including STIs and HIV/AIDS, policies and guidelines, laws and regulations, statistics, and faith-based programs.

National Center for Infectious Diseases
www.healthfinder.gov/orgs/hr2611.htm

This site offers information about disease surveillance systems operating within or collaborating with the National Center for Infectious Diseases (NCID); among these is information about STIs and HIV/AIDS. The site also maintains links to disease reports, data, and publications that these systems publish.

Division of STD Prevention
www.cdc.gov/std

This site provides statistics and reports pertaining to STIs. Among the links are those pertaining to bacterial vaginosis, chlamydia, genital herpes, gonorrhea, hepatitis (viral), HIV/AIDS, human papillomavirus infection, pelvic inflammatory disease, pregnancy and STIs, syphilis, trichomoniasis, and general information about STIs.

American Social Health Association
www.ashastd.org

The American Social Health Association develops and delivers accurate, medically reliable information about STIs. ASHA publishes educational pamphlets and books for clients and students. It helps community-based organizations communicate about risk, transmission, prevention, testing and treatment of STIs. Links to statistics, prevention tips, and information about particular STIs are included on this web site.

I»N»T»E»R chapter FOCUS

HIV and AIDS

CHAPTER OBJECTIVES

1 Describe acquired immunodeficiency syndrome (AIDS), the opportunistic diseases associated with it, and the way in which the human immunodeficiency virus (HIV) invades the body and causes AIDS.

2 Discuss different treatments for HIV infection and AIDS, including how the mortality rate has declined as a result of these treatments.

3 Cite ways in which HIV infection can be prevented.

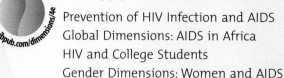

sexuality.jbpub.com/dimensions/4e

Prevention of HIV Infection and AIDS
Global Dimensions: AIDS in Africa
HIV and College Students
Gender Dimensions: Women and AIDS

INTRODUCTION

*T*om applied for a graduate assistantship in our department and, because of his impressive academic record and the nature of his experiences, was awarded one. He was a pleasure to have around, always smiling and willing to help in whatever way he could. Because of his personality and his conscientiousness Tom's graduate assistantship was extended into the next year and several years thereafter.

It was during his fourth year with us that Tom began losing weight and missing some days at school. Attributing it to the flu or a similar condition, no one seemed to take much notice—that is, until Tom started missing even more days and looking emaciated. Before long, the rumor spread that Tom had AIDS and did not have long to live. Unfortunately, the rumor was true and before many more months, Tom died.

With today's new medications and combination of medications, Tom might be alive today. Or at least he would have lived longer with HIV than he did. Of course, that troubles those of us who knew and cared for Tom. However, other issues are also troubling. Until he told us, we did not even know Tom was gay. He contracted HIV through unprotected sex. Why did he feel the need to hide his identity, and how much torment did that hiding create? More to the point, what did we (the department, the faculty, the university, and the society at large) convey to Tom that led him to conclude we would reject him if we knew his secrets? And how many others are in a situation similar to Tom's and are in torment as he was?

We hope that this chapter, by presenting information about HIV and AIDS, will help us all become more understanding of those who are wrestling with not only the physical and psychological effects of HIV infection but also the social consequences.

■ Acquired Immune Deficiency Syndrome (AIDS)

Acquired immune deficiency syndrome (AIDS), so named because it attacks and slowly destroys the body's immune system, was first identified by American physicians in mid-1981. At that time, physicians noted the unusual occurrence of five cases of *Pneumocystis carinii* pneumonia among previously healthy homosexual men in Los Angeles. Soon thereafter, reports surfaced of a rare form of cancer, Kaposi's sarcoma, also among young homosexual men in New York and California. These observations led to the recognition of AIDS, a disease characterized by **opportunistic diseases** in an immune-compromised individual. Diseases such as *P. carinii* pneumonia and Kaposi's sarcoma are labeled opportunistic because they rarely occur in young healthy individuals, instead relying on the opportunity presented by a depressed immune system. AIDS is considered a syndrome because it is characterized by a range of opportunistic diseases, rather than one particular disease (Table IF4.1).

Research conducted by Robert Gallo at the National Institutes of Health and by Luc Montagnier and colleagues at the Pasteur Institute in Paris led to the discovery of a new virus believed to cause AIDS. Gallo named the virus human T-lymphotropic virus type III (HTLV-III); Montagnier identified it by the name lymphadenopathy-associated virus (LAV). In May 1986 the International Committee on Taxonomy of Viruses announced its recommendation that the virus be consistently identified by the name **human immunodeficiency virus (HIV)** (AIDS virus gets new name amid feuding, 1986). Today we know that HIV is the cause of AIDS.

acquired immune deficiency syndrome (AIDS)
A syndrome caused by the human immunodeficiency virus (HIV), characterized by a depressed immune system and the presence of one or more opportunistic diseases.

opportunistic diseases
A major manifestation of AIDS, diseases that occur in the presence of a suppressed immune system.

human immunodeficiency virus (HIV)
A retrovirus that causes AIDS.

HIV belongs to a special class of viruses called **retroviruses**. Retroviruses consist of a protein shell surrounding the genetic material ribonucleic acid (RNA) (Figure IF4.1). For HIV to attack a human cell, it must first attach itself to a special receptor on the cell's surface. In humans HIV attaches to T4 lymphocytes, a type of white blood cell that plays an important role in the immune response to disease. Once attached to the T4 cell, HIV enters the cell and releases its RNA. The RNA is then converted into DNA by an enzyme (reverse transcriptase) also carried by HIV. This HIV DNA combines with the cell's DNA, causing the cell to reproduce HIV (Figure IF4.2). In essence, HIV converts the cells it attacks into factories producing HIV, which then go on to infect other T4 cells. As this process progresses, T4 cells are destroyed and the body becomes unable

retroviruses
A group of viruses consisting of ribonucleic acid (RNA) surrounded by a protein coat that can convert their RNA into deoxyribonucleic acid (DNA) once they have invaded a living cell, allowing them to take over the cell and reproduce themselves.

TABLE IF4.1 Common Opportunistic Diseases

Cancers

Kaposi's sarcoma

Primary lymphoma of the brain

Protozoal and Helminthic

Cryptosporidiosis, intestinal (causing diarrhea for more than 1 month)

Pneumocystis carinii pneumonia

Strongyloidiasis (pneumonia, central nervous system [CNS] infection, or disseminated infection)

Toxoplasmosis (pneumonia or CNS infection)

Fungal Infections

Aspergillosis (CNS or disseminated infection)

Candidiasis (esophagitis)

Cryptococcosis (pulmonary, CNS, or disseminated infection)

Histoplasmosis (disseminated)

Bacterial Infection

Atypical *Mycobacterium* species other than *M. tuberculosis* or *M. leprae* (disseminated infection)

Viral Infection

Cytomegalovirus (pulmonary, gastrointestinal tract, or CNS infection)

Herpes simplex virus

   Chronic mucocutaneous ulcers persisting longer than 1 month

   Pulmonary, gastrointestinal tract, or disseminated infection

Progressive multifocal leukoencephalopathy (presumed papovavirus)

Source: Allen, J. R. Definitions: Surveillance definition of AIDS, in *AIDS: A basic guide for clinicians,* Ebbeson, P., et al., eds. Philadelphia: W. B. Saunders, 1985, 233–234.

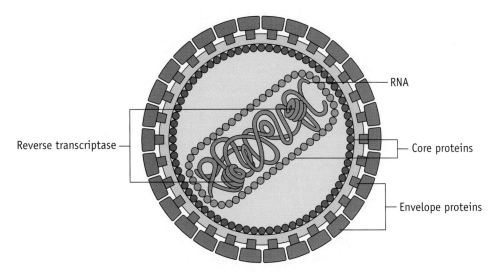

FIGURE IF4.1 HIV consists of an outer shell, or protein envelope, that surrounds a protein core that protects the ribonucleic acid (RNA) and the enzyme reverse transcriptase. *Source: FDA Consumer* (October 1987), 10.

FIGURE IF4.2 HIV infection and replication in a human cell. The virus enters the cell and releases RNA, its genetic material. Using the enzyme reverse transcriptase (RT), the virus converts its RNA into deoxyribonucleic acid (DNA), which enters the cell nucleus and combines with the cell DNA. The cell's altered genetic material then produces messenger RNA (mRNA), which codes for new virus. *Source: FDA Consumer* (October 1987), 10.

to defend itself against organisms that would normally be no threat to health. Thus the opportunistic diseases that characterize AIDS infect the individual, usually leading to death.

Incidence of HIV and AIDS

As noted in Table IF4.2, through December 2006, more than 983,343 adults and adolescents had acquired AIDS. HIV infection is the seventh leading cause of death among African Americans in the United States. Between 1985 and 2003, almost 377,000 white Americans, 368,000 African Americans, and 173,000 Hispanics contracted AIDS. Almost 4½ times as many American males as females contracted AIDS between those years.

HIV affects different age groups at different rates. Whereas in 2003 HIV infection was the tenth leading cause of death among 15- to 24-year-olds, it ranked sixth among 25- to 44-year-olds. What these rankings indicate is that HIV is contracted when people are teenagers and in their early 20s and is manifested after several years when they are older.

Although the death rate from HIV infection increased steadily from 6 per 100,000 in 1987 to 17 per 100,000 in 1995, it dropped for the first time to 11.1 per 100,000 in 1996. It has continued to decline ever since (see Figure IF4.3). This drop was primarily a result of new treatments, although education campaigns may have played a part. It is in no small part related to the increased funding for HIV and AIDS research, which increased dramatically over the years.

TABLE IF4.2 Reported AIDS Cases, by Age Category, Transmission Category, and Sex, 2006 and Cumulative—United States and Dependent Areas

Adult or Adolescent Transmission Category	Males 2006 Number	%	Males Cumulative Number	%	Females 2006 Number	%	Females Cumulative Number	%	Total 2006 Number	%	Total Cumulative Number	%
Male-to-male sexual contact	13,775	49	429,897	54	0	0	0	0	13,775	35	429,897	44
Injection drug use	3,413	12	163,070	21	1,826	17	67,693	35	5,239	13	230,763	23
Male-to-male sexual contact and injection drug use	1,603	6	65,524	8	0	0	0	0	1,603	4	65,524	7
Hemophilia/coagulation disorder	43	0	5,176	1	11	0	348	0	54	0	5,524	1
High-risk heterosexual contact	2,997	11	49,610	6	4,839	46	85,186	44	7,836	20	134,796	14
Receipt of blood transfusion, blood components, or tissue	63	0	5,213	1	68	1	4,176	2	131	0	9,389	1
Other/risk factor not reported or identified	6,484	23	73,136	9	3,793	36	34,311	18	10,278	26	107,450	11
Total	28,378	100	791,626	100	10,537	100	191,714	100	38,916	100	983,343	100

Source: Centers for Disease Control and Prevention. *Cases of HIV infection and AIDS in the United States and dependent areas, 2006.* Atlanta, GA: Author, 2008.

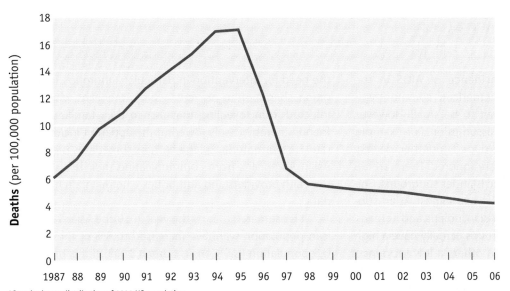

FIGURE IF4.3 Trends in annual age-adjusted* rate of death due to HIV disease, United States, 1987–2006.

*Standard: age distribution of 2000 US population
Note: For comparison with data for 1999 and later years, data for 1987–1998 were modified to account for *ICD-10* rules instead of *ICD-9* rules.
Source: Centers for Disease Control and Prevention, *HIV Mortality (Through 2005)*. Available: http://www.cdc.gov/hiv/topics/surveillance/resources/slides/mortality.

The United Nations reports that there were some 33 million HIV infections in 2007 (Joint United Nations Programme on HIV/AIDS, 2008). Most of these appeared in sub-Saharan Africa (between 21 and 24 million), another 4 million in South and Southeast Asia, 1.6 million in Latin America, and 230,000 in the Caribbean. In North America, there were 1.3 million infections in 2007. In contrast to the incidence in the United States, where most cases of HIV are the result of homosexual contact, the majority of HIV infections in those other regions of the world are transmitted by heterosexual contact.

Transmission

HIV is found in large concentrations in two human body fluids: semen and blood. This is related to the large number of white blood cells present in these body fluids. It appears that a concentration of HIV is probably necessary for the transmission of HIV from one individual to another. Thus the most common modes of transmission are those that involve the exchange of semen or blood between individuals. Unprotected sexual intercourse with an infected individual is the most common way that infected semen is transmitted; however, cases of AIDS related to artificial insemination have been reported (Confirmation of transmission, 1986). The majority of AIDS cases in the United States, more than 50%, have involved men who had sex with men (Table IF4.2). The prevalence of anal intercourse among homosexual and bisexual men and their often large

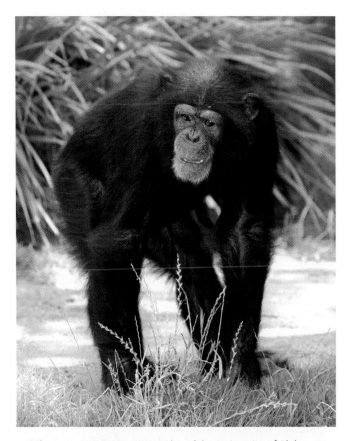

In February 1999, Dr. Beatrice Hahn of the University of Alabama at Birmingham announced that she had tracked HIV's ancestor to a virus that has long infected *Pan troglodytes,* a subspecies of African chimpanzees. In an effort to help human HIV patients, researchers are looking into why the monkeys do not appear to become sick from the virus.

Multicultural DIMENSIONS

AIDS Among Asian Americans

The incidence of AIDS in the Asian American community is assumed to be small. However, there are problems with this assumption. For example, when Asian Americans are grouped together, diverse ethnic and racial subgroups are ignored. There are 28 Asian subgroups and 20 Pacific Islander subgroups. Chinese and Filipinos make up the two largest Asian subgroups, followed by Japanese, Asian Indians, and Koreans. The result is that certain subgroups actually have a high incidence of HIV infection and others a low incidence. For example, in 2002, 16% of Asian Americans with AIDS were born in the Philippines and 7% in Vietnam, whereas only 2% were born in Cambodia and South Korea, and fewer yet (1%) were born in Laos (Zaidi et al., 2005). Grouping Asian American subgroups together conceals the need for intervention in particular subgroups. In addition, shame often prevents Asian Americans who are infected from revealing that fact to their families and friends, thereby falsely lowering the apparent incidence rate. Furthermore, language barriers sometimes prevent Asian Americans from communicating their HIV status to health providers and authorities who maintain health data.

It is estimated that by the year 2050, the Asian American population will have increased to 8% of the total U.S. population (U.S. Census Bureau, 2008). If this projection is accurate, there will be more than 34 million Asian Americans in the United States by the year 2050. It is time that HIV and AIDS in the Asian American community be studied more systematically and interventions adopted as necessary.

number of sexual partners have been cited as reasons for this large percentage of cases.

Of the total reported adult/adolescent AIDS cases in 2006, approximately 20% appear to be related to heterosexual transmission (Centers for Disease Control and Prevention, 2008c). In the United States, this transmission category includes individuals who reported heterosexual contact with a person considered to be at risk for AIDS and of individuals born in a country where heterosexual transmission is believed to be the major mode of transmission. Heterosexual transmission is of particular concern to women—for them, 46% of reported cases are thought to have been transmitted by heterosexual contact, compared to only 11% of male reported cases. Many women who become infected with HIV through heterosexual contact have partners who are injecting drug users. Women in this category are not necessarily injecting drug users themselves; they become infected through sexual intercourse with partners who are.

The transmission of HIV related to injecting drug use is also of concern. Through December 2006, injecting drug use was associated with HIV transmission in 18% of all reported AIDS cases. Infection occurs through the sharing of needles contaminated with HIV. Additionally, these injecting drug users can transmit the virus to their sexual partners through intercourse, and, in the case of female injecting drug users, to their infants prenatally or postnatally. Injecting drug use is currently thought to constitute the major threat of HIV transmission to the heterosexual population. This mode of transmission disproportionately affects the urban poor and minority populations, especially African Americans and Hispanics. It is estimated that 22% of African Americans and 19% of Hispanic men with AIDS are injecting drug users. The number of injecting drug users among minority women with AIDS is 23% of the reported cases of AIDS in African American women and Hispanic women (Centers for Disease Control and Prevention, 2004).

Between 1979 and mid-1985, HIV transmission through blood transfusions was of great concern to health professionals and the public. In the spring

Did You Know ...

Do mosquitoes transmit HIV? Scientific experiments have shown that HIV does not multiply in insects such as biting flies, mosquitoes, and bedbugs (Centers for Disease Control and Prevention, 2006). Additionally, it has been noted that the mouths of such insects cannot hold enough blood of one person to be capable of infecting another person. Epidemiological evidence also supports the hypothesis that transmission by insects does not occur.

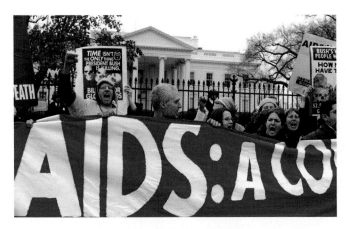

The efforts of the gay community to garner media attention for the HIV and AIDS crisis brought it to the forefront of the U.S. medical agenda during the 1980s. Because of these efforts, HIV and AIDS research and medical funding garnered a far greater percentage of government spending than it would otherwise have, which resulted in a significant reduction of HIV incidence in the mainstream gay community. Unfortunately, within the gay community, gay men are currently experiencing a resurgence of the HIV and AIDS epidemic. In actuality, we have little more today in the way of prevention than we had two decades ago. Despite the efforts of both the gay and mainstream communities and tremendous scientific advances in treatments for the virus, this crisis is far from averted.

of 1985 an HIV antibody test was approved by the FDA for the purpose of screening blood donations. **Antibody** tests do an excellent job of protecting the U.S. blood supply from contamination with HIV. There is, however, still a slight risk that the test will miss HIV antibodies (resulting in a false negative test result). Additionally, the test may not detect HIV-infected blood because a person who is infected with HIV may not produce a detectable level of antibodies for up to 3 months after infection. It must be emphasized that this risk is very small. The CDC and the American Red Cross reported that the risk of contracting AIDS through blood transfusions was only 1 in 28,000 way back in 1987 (Blood supply grows safer, 1990). Additionally, they reported that the chance that HIV-infected blood will not be detected through the blood screening process was decreasing by more than 30% per year. There is no risk of becoming infected with HIV through donation of blood.

> **antibodies**
> A class of proteins secreted by the immune system that bonds with antigens. Antibodies fight off disease-causing organisms.

AIDS and the Gay Community

Originally, AIDS was discovered in gay men. Of course, it was soon realized that risky behavior is associated with HIV infection, not one's sexual identity or one's

country of origin. (Haitians were targeted with discriminatory immigration regulations because of the relatively high incidence of AIDS in Haiti.) However, given the high incidence of HIV infection in the gay community, much effort has been made to educate gays about safer sex practices. This effort had been quite successful: Gay men had been engaging in sex with fewer partners (Seigel & Raveis, 1993), using condoms more frequently during sex, and somewhat decreasing anal sexual intercourse behavior. Unfortunately, the number of HIV/AIDS cases among men who have sex with men has been increasing since 2003. In 2003, 15,409 cases were reported, whereas in 2006 there were 17,465 new cases (Centers for Disease Control and Prevention, 2008d). Some gay men who are infected tend to discontinue their sexual activities, for many reasons: They may not feel up to it physically, they may not be able to acquire a willing sexual partner, they may perceive themselves as less attractive as the disease progresses, they may become depressed, and they may be concerned about infecting another person. It is for these reasons that many gay men choose a sexual partner who is also HIV positive (Hoff et al., 1992).

Not to be overlooked is the effect of the lobbying efforts by the gay community—males and females—for increased funding for AIDS research and more rapid approval of drugs with the potential for treating HIV infection and AIDS. As more and more people, including celebrities (for example, Rock Hudson, Keith Haring, Freddy Mercury, and Greg Louganis) contracted HIV, the alarm was sounded throughout the gay community and beyond. That alarm led the way to successful local and national lobbying efforts. When compared to that for other diseases, funding for AIDS research far exceeds its ranking in terms of deaths or incidence, a direct result of the gay community's involvement. Imagine what the status of treatment for HIV and AIDS would be today—not to mention the advancements on the horizon—without the gay community's efforts.

Stages of HIV Infection

Once an individual is infected with HIV, the natural course of the infection progresses in three stages. The first stage is **silent infection**. This stage is an asymptomatic period during which the only evidence of infection is the presence of HIV antibodies. The development of antibodies takes at least 2 weeks, and it is often 6 to 8 weeks before antibody levels are high enough to be detected by current tests.

> **silent infection**
> A stage of HIV infection characterized by no symptoms other than the presence of HIV antibodies.

FIGURE IF4.4 Estimated rates (per 100,000 population) for adults and adolescents living with HIV infection (not AIDS) or with AIDS, 2006—United States and dependent areas. *Source:* Centers for Disease Control and Prevention. *Cases of HIV infection and AIDS in the United States and dependent areas, 2006.* Atlanta, GA: Author, 2008.

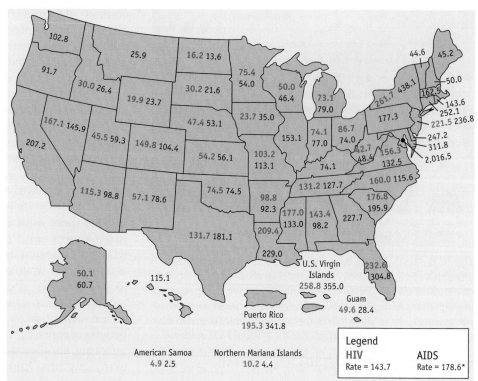

*Includes persons whose area of residence is unknown.

Some infected individuals (it is not known how many) progress to the second stage of infection—**symptomatic infection**. This stage consists of several general signs and symptoms, the most prominent of which is persistent swelling of the lymph glands, especially in the neck, armpits, and back of the mouth. Other common signs include fatigue, unexplained weight loss, night sweats, persistent fever, and diarrhea. It is currently believed that most, if not all, individuals who have symptomatic HIV infection will progress to the third and final stage—AIDS.

In the latest reporting period at the time of this writing, in the year 2006 there were 38,916 new cases of AIDS reported in the United States and its territories (Figure IF4.4). People who have AIDS have all the general signs and symptoms of infection described, but they also have one or more of the opportunistic diseases such as *Pneumocystis carinii* pneumonia or Kaposi's sarcoma. HIV can cross the blood–brain barrier and cause personality changes, deterioration of memory and judgment, dementia, and brain tumors (Redfield & Burke, 1989).

Although AIDS is classified as a terminal disease, people now live with AIDS for a long time. Newer medication regimens, accompanied by an enthusiastic research agenda, lead some to conclude that AIDS will be considered a chronic disease (like hypertension and diabetes) that can be controlled, if not eradicated.

Testing for HIV

There are several HIV tests. The initial one performed is called the *enzyme-linked immunosorbent assay (ELISA)* test. The ELISA test identifies the presence of HIV antibodies. If antibodies are present, the person is said to be **seropositive**. If no antibodies are present, the person is said to be **seronegative**. However, even though the test results show that HIV antibodies are present, they may be "false positive." Therefore, once the ELISA finding is positive, a more sensitive, and more expensive, test is administered, the Western blot. If the Western blot result confirms the presence of HIV antibodies, the person can be assured that he or she is infected. It should be noted that both of these tests do not directly test for the presence of HIV. Rather, they test for the presence of antibodies produced in response to HIV infection. Thus it is possible that the infection has not yet produced sufficient antibodies to be measured even though the person being tested is infected with HIV. If it is too early for the antibodies to be present in sufficient numbers to be measured, the person can transmit the virus nevertheless.

One test that looks for HIV itself is known as the *polymerase chain reaction (PCR)*. The PCR is more costly and more labor-intensive than the other tests and, therefore, is not used routinely.

The OraQuick Rapid HIV-1 antibody test is another test, which was approved

symptomatic infection
The second stage of HIV infection, characterized by HIV antibodies as well as general signs and symptoms such as swollen lymph glands, fatigue, unexplained weight loss, night sweats, persistent fever, and diarrhea.

seropositive
The result of a blood test for antibodies to HIV that indicates that such antibodies have been found in the blood.

seronegative
The result of a blood test for antibodies to HIV that indicates no presence of such antibodies.

Total number of new individuals named at each stage of investigation

FIGURE IF4.5 Partner notification programs can be highly productive, as illustrated by results of a South Carolina investigation that began with one HIV-positive man. Of the 19 sexual contacts he named, all but one were tested, and three were seropositive. Those three then named 20 sexual contacts not already identified, leading to the discovery of two more HIV-positive men, who in turn named 24 other previously unidentified contacts, and so forth. When the investigation reached its end point of no new HIV-positive contacts, it had identified a total of 90 persons at risk, tested 68 of them, and found 12 who either were seropositive or seroconverted 6 months after initial testing.

by the FDA in 2002. It uses a finger stick and provides results in 20 minutes.

Until 1996, the only way to get tested for HIV was to be tested under a doctor's supervision. However, in 1996 the FDA approved the first home-collection HIV testing systems. At this time, only one HIV home-collection test system is approved by FDA and legally sold in the United States. This test system, sold as either "The Home Access HIV-1 Test System," or "The Home Access Express HIV-1 Test System," is manufactured by Home Access Health Corporation and allows blood samples to be taken at home, which people then send to a laboratory for testing. This test system may be purchased on the Internet.

An oral HIV test is also available. In 1997, the Whitman-Walker Clinic in Washington, D.C., became the first major AIDS clinic in the United States to administer this oral test. The oral test, OraSure, requires a person to place a flat inch-long cotton swab, attached to a stick, between the gum and cheek for 2 minutes. The swab draws fluid from the mucous membrane, which contains HIV antibodies if the person is infected. This test is ideal for persons who are afraid of needles.

An individual who receives a positive HIV test finding should be given medical and psychological counseling as well as education intended to prevent HIV transmission to others. Additionally, it is important at this time to initiate the process of *partner notification*. The CDC recommends that "persons who are HIV-antibody positive should be instructed in how to notify their partners and to refer them for counseling and testing. If they are unwilling to notify their partners, or if it cannot be assured that their partners will seek counseling, physicians or health department personnel should use confidential procedures to assure that the partners are notified" (Partner notification, 1988).

The notification of partners is an important step in stopping the spread of HIV (Figure IF4.5). However, an HIV-positive person may not feel capable of contacting sexual or needle-sharing partners for a variety of reasons, including fear of discrimination or legal action (Judson, 1990). In one study, Marks and associates (1991) found that 52% of sexually active HIV-positive persons did not inform their partners of their HIV antibody status. In such instances, when an HIV-infected person does not feel able to disclose HIV antibody test results, a representative from the health department should notify and counsel the partner(s) of that person. The name of the HIV-positive individual is not revealed, nor is the alleged HIV exposure date. Thus confidentiality is maintained for HIV-infected individuals while knowledge of exposure to HIV is provided to partners.

■ Treatment of HIV and AIDS

In 1987 the FDA approved **zidovudine** (brand name Retrovir; formerly azidothymidine [AZT]) as the first drug licensed in the United States for the

zidovudine
The first drug (brand name Retrovir; also known as AZT) approved by the FDA for the treatment of AIDS. This antiviral drug slows the replication of the AIDS virus, thus slowing the course of the syndrome.

treatment of AIDS patients. Zidovudine is an antiviral drug that slows the replication of HIV in human cells. Originally, zidovudine was approved for use by AIDS patients who had not developed Kaposi's sarcoma or opportunistic infections other than *Pneumocystis carinii* pneumonia. The FDA has approved the use of zidovudine for people infected with HIV who do not yet have AIDS, for children as young as 6 months who have AIDS (Use of AZT expanded, 1990; Zidovudine for children, 1990), and for pregnant women who are HIV positive. Studies indicate that zidovudine not only slows the progression of HIV infection when given in early stages, but also prolongs survival and decreases the incidence and severity of opportunistic infections in people living with AIDS. It should be emphasized that zidovudine is not a cure for AIDS. Additionally, the drug is not without risks; zidovudine has been shown to depress essential white and red blood cell production in some individuals (Fast-tracking the first AIDS drug, 1987).

Research on AIDS treatment and prevention continues to receive top priority. The results of this research have been the development of several possible vaccines now being tested and of a new generation of drugs to treat HIV infection.

The Vaccine

In 1998, after an experimental AIDS vaccine had been tested on animals, 5,000 volunteers began receiving injections. The volunteers consisted of people at high risk for HIV infection, such as gay men and women whose sexual partners were infected. Manufactured by VaxGen, Inc., the vaccine AIDSvax, was made of dead virus and therefore could not cause HIV infection. It was hoped that it would produce antibodies in sufficient number to provide protection against HIV. However, it was found in 2003 that the vaccine did not work. Researchers continue to look for an effective vaccine.

Ethical DIMENSIONS

Should HIV Testing Be Mandatory for Pregnant Women?

If pregnant women are infected with HIV, they can pass on that infection to their babies in utero. Yet, there is a simple way to prevent many of these babies from being born infected—that is, by administering to pregnant women a regimen of the AIDS drug AZT. In fact, the likelihood of HIV transmission to babies of HIV-positive pregnant women drops from approximately 26% to 8% when AZT is administered. For this reason, many physicians and legislators advocate that pregnant women be required to be tested for HIV as part of their routine prenatal care. In that way, the danger to the fetus is identified, and treatment can be administered to the women whose fetuses are at risk.

However, this issue is more complicated than it appears at first glance. For example, if women are required to be HIV tested during prenatal care, many may forgo prenatal care to avoid the test and its possible repercussions. These repercussions may include losing one's job, one's housing, or one's partner. In addition, a woman who lives in a rural area may not be able to find a physician willing to manage her pregnancy and help in the delivery of her child. Avoiding prenatal care places the fetus at risk of being born at low birth weight and/or with a variety of birth defects. Opponents of mandatory testing point out that no other segment of society is required to be HIV tested. Therefore, to require this of pregnant women is to discriminate against these women. There is no disagreement that pregnant women ought to be counseled about the risks and benefits of being tested and that there is a treatment to help prevent their babies from being born infected with HIV even if the mother is infected. But, the choice to be tested for HIV should be the woman's.

Proponents of mandatory HIV testing for pregnant women argue that counseling alone will not persuade enough women to be tested. Too many would choose to avoid testing, and the result would be that too many babies would be born with HIV. To protect the babies, they maintain, women should be required to be tested and their HIV status determined. Only then can pregnant women infected with HIV be administered effective medication, thereby indirectly treating their fetuses. In addition, women who test positive for HIV can be educated about the risk of breastfeeding, another means through which HIV can be transmitted to their babies.

Should the privacy of the mother be protected, or is her privacy less important than the benefits to the fetus? This is not only a policy issue, but also an ethical issue. On which side of this argument do you find yourself?

Triple-Drug Therapy

The new generation of drugs has produced the most dramatic advancement in the fight against AIDS to date. There are now six classes of antiretroviral drug therapies (U.S. Department of Health and Human Services, 2008):

1. *Nucleoside reverse transcriptase inhibitors* (zidovudine, didanosine, stavudine, and so on): These drugs block the action of reverse transcriptase, thereby preventing HIV RNA from reproducing.

2. *Protease inhibitors* (such as indinavir, nelfinavir, ritonavir, and saquinavir mesylate): These drugs shut down HIV replication by preventing the viral enzyme protease from cutting other viral protein into shorter pieces needed by HIV to make new viral copies for infecting new T4 cells.

3. *Nonnucleoside reverse transcriptase inhibitors* (such as delavirdine and nevirapine): These drugs block the reverse transcriptase directly.

4. *Entry/fusion inhibitors* (such as enfuvirtide and maraviroc): These drugs block the entry of HIV into the cells.

5. *Integrase inhibitors* (raltegravir): These drugs disable integrase, a protein the HIV uses to insert its viral genetic material into the generic material of an infected cell.

6. *Fixed-dose combination* (such as abacavir, lamivudine, and zidovudine): This regimen consists of a combination of two or more anti-HIV drugs from one or more classes of drugs.

These medications are administered together in what is called *combination therapy*, or the *AIDS cocktail*. Combination therapy makes sense because it attacks the virus at different steps in the life cycle rather than at one step. Studies have reported that combination therapy delays the progression of HIV infection to AIDS and reduces mortality rate (Hammer et al., 1996; Katzenstein et al., 1996). However, combination therapy is expensive. In 2003, it was estimated that the average annual cost of treating someone with HIV was between $10,000 and $15,000; for AIDS the annual cost was between $15,000 and $22,000. The effect of these astronomical costs is that some people with AIDS, such as the poor or unemployed, cannot afford the most effective treatments available to them; the government has to decide how much financial support to provide for the treatment of AIDS (an economic issue with tax implications). The most effective treatments were originally withheld from developing countries where HIV and AIDS are prevalent (both a financial issue and an ethical issue). In 2000, drug companies started discounting drugs to developing countries so more people with HIV and AIDS could be treated. And recognition of the financial costs—not to mention all the other costs of contracting HIV to the person and the person's friends and family—leads many experts to conclude that the best way to prevent HIV and AIDS is by educational campaigns.

■ Prevention of HIV Infection and AIDS

Until a cure for AIDS or a vaccine is discovered, efforts to prevent HIV infection and AIDS will be critical to controlling this epidemic. Currently there are two major emphases: (1) preventing the initiation of behaviors or conditions that will put an individual at risk of infection and (2) changing behaviors to reduce the chances that an individual will become infected if exposed to HIV.

The best method available to prevent infection with HIV is abstinence: abstaining from sexual activity with an HIV-infected partner and abstaining from injecting drug use. This is an important message of HIV and AIDS education efforts—especially for adolescents and young adults who are in a developmental stage at which sexual and drug experimentation

People with HIV must cope not only with the knowledge of their illness but also with society's fear of HIV. Support groups offer emotional support and firsthand advice on coping with the illness.

In November 1991, the basketball star Magic Johnson announced that he had acquired HIV infection through unprotected sexual intercourse with an unknown infected woman. Johnson provides living proof of the effectiveness of the AIDS cocktail: The level of HIV in his body has been reduced to an undetectable level.

is common. Today such experimentation carries a deadly risk of HIV and AIDS.

Abstaining from sexual activity throughout one's life is impractical and undesirable for most people. For those who are uninfected and sexually active, maintaining a mutually faithful monogamous relationship with an uninfected partner prevents the sexual transmission of HIV. Each partner would also need to abstain from injecting drug use, another high-risk behavior for HIV transmission.

Many people have previously engaged in behaviors that put them "at high risk" of being infected with HIV. People should be considered at risk if they have shared needles or syringes to inject drugs or steroids; are male and have had anal sex (even once) with another male; have had sex with someone they believe may have been infected with HIV; have had another STI; received blood transfusions or blood products between 1978 and 1985; or have had sex with someone who has any of these risk characteristics. In addition, the more sexual partners a person has had, the greater the chances that person will have had contact with an HIV-infected person. The former basketball player Magic Johnson brought this point home to many people when he announced to the world that he was infected with HIV from unprotected sexual intercourse with a woman he could not identify because of his numerous sexual partners over the years. It is important to remember, however, that unprotected sexual intercourse with just one person is risky if that person is infected with HIV.

If an individual decides to engage in sexual activity with a person who is at risk for or is infected with HIV, public health authorities recommend that a condom be used during sexual intercourse (vaginal or anal). Latex condoms have been shown to be an effective barrier to HIV (Tests confirm condoms block AIDS virus, 1986). Although condoms are not 100% effective in preventing HIV transmission, they are considered to be among the most important components of safer sex.

Yet, even with all the educational efforts and mass attention directed at the issue of condoms and safer sex, studies indicate that most people do not consistently use condoms. In a study of almost 6,500 women between the ages of 20 and 44, the women reported that they were frequently sexually active. Among the single women in the study, 22% had two or more sexual partners in the past year (26% of women 20 to 29 years of age had two or more partners in the past year). Yet only 19% reported always using condoms, 54% used condoms sometimes, and 27% never used condoms (Linberg & Singh, 2008). In another large-scale study conducted by the Centers for Disease Control and Prevention as part of the Behavioral Risk Factor Surveillance System, males

 Did You Know...

The World Health Organization, in collaboration with UNAIDS, released the *AIDS Epidemic Update* in 2007, which estimated that 2.5 million new infections with HIV occurred in 2007. Of those new infections, 420,000 occurred in children younger than 15 years of age. Furthermore, in 2007, 2.1 million deaths occurred worldwide as a result of AIDS, 330,000 of whom were children younger than 15 years of age.

who had two or more sexual partners used condoms only 63% of the time, and females only 45% of the time (Centers for Disease Control and Prevention, 2002). Even gay and bisexual men, who are generally at increased risk of HIV, do not use condoms as they should. In a study of gay and bisexual men, only 53% used a condom every time or almost every time during anal sex, whereas 39% never used a condom during anal sex. In addition, only 1% used a condom during oral sex, whereas 87% never did (Gullette & Turner, 2003).

In 1990, the CDC surveyed a representative sample of 11,631 U.S. high school students about their sexual behavior (Sexual behavior among high school students, 1992). A majority of the students surveyed (54.2%) reported that they had engaged in sexual intercourse; 39.4% reported having had sexual intercourse within the past 3 months. Of those latter students, only 44.9% indicated that they had used a condom during their last act of intercourse. In a study of adolescent use of condoms (Ford, Woosung, & Lepkowski, 2001), researchers found that condoms were used in 59% of relationships, although not necessarily during every sexual intercourse encounter. White adolescents were more likely to use condoms than either African American or Hispanic adolescents; adolescents whose partners were of a different race or ethnicity were more likely to use condoms; and the longer the relationship, the more likely it was condoms were used. Further research is needed to identify educational programs that successfully increase condom use in people at risk for HIV infection. In 2002, only 24% of women ages 15 to 44 who used some form of contraception used a condom (National Center for Health Statistics, 2006).

Other safer sex strategies are also recommended. If an individual or a sexual partner is at risk for HIV infection, he or she should avoid mouth contact with the penis, vagina, or rectum. Sex with prostitutes should also be avoided, because both male and female prostitutes are often injecting drug users. The possibility of prostitutes having sexual intercourse with high-risk individuals is also great.

Because the current antibody tests for HIV are not 100% accurate, those who are at high risk of HIV infection and those who are known to be infected are asked not to donate blood. Women infected with HIV should prevent pregnancy, as HIV can be transmitted to the unborn child (see the Ethical Dimensions box on page 600).

Screening tests for HIV are an important preventive tool. It is currently recommended that those who have engaged in any of the risk behaviors described take an HIV antibody test. There are many public and private testing sites that provide confidential or

HIV infection is determined by a blood test that looks for antibodies produced in response to HIV. Testing is accompanied by counseling and education to interpret the results and to discuss ways to prevent infection, or to seek treatment if the test is positive.

anonymous HIV testing. HIV testing should always be accompanied by counseling and education as well. Even for those who test negative, the time of finding out their results can be an important "teachable moment."

Of course, among the ways to prevent the spread of HIV are for those who are infected to let their sexual partners know of their HIV status and to take all the necessary precautions to prevent its transmission. Many people do disclose their HIV status to their partners. Still, in a review of several studies of this issue, the American Public Health Association found that only 60% of those who knew they were infected with HIV disclosed this information to all their partners (Many people, 1998). Of the 40% who did not share this information, half of those did not tell their primary partner. To make matters worse, only 42% used condoms all of the time during sexual intercourse. Given that disclosure can lead to stigmatization and other consequences that have been described previously in this chapter, it is understandable, though not acceptable, that some people who are HIV positive refrain from informing others. In the end, however, this is selfish and dangerous.

HIV and AIDS and Young Adults

HIV and AIDS are of particular concern for young adults who have a lot of years left to live. Unfortunately, the HIV and AIDS rate for young adults is a growing problem. In 2006, 9,680 children and adults younger than age 25 years were living with AIDS. The

The remarkable AIDS quilt is made up of 44,000 panels, each representing a life lost to AIDS. It was created both as a living memorial for those who died and as a brilliant way to help the public visualize the growing toll that AIDS was taking.

reasons for the large number of AIDS cases among young adults include the following:

- Young adults tend to have more sexual partners, thereby increasing their risk of encountering one who is HIV positive.

- Young people tend to consider themselves invulnerable and are therefore more likely to engage in sexual intercourse without using a condom.

- Young people may feel self-conscious about purchasing condoms and therefore not have them available when they decide to engage in coitus.

- For some of the reasons given, young people become infected with STIs more often than older people; that incidence in turn makes them more susceptible to contracting HIV.

- Young adults tend to use mood-altering drugs that diminish their capacity to make healthy decisions when they are sexually aroused.

However, in recent years young people have tended to change some high-risk behaviors. For instance, the proportion of youths in grades 9–12 who engaged in coitus declined between 1993 and 2003 (from 50% to 45% among women and from 56% to 48% among men) (Kaiser Family Foundation, 2005). In 2007, 48% of all high school students reported having experienced sexual intercourse (National Campaign to Prevent Teen and Unplanned Pregnancy, 2008). The *Healthy People 2010* National Health Objectives goal is

that 75% of males and females ages 15 to 17 years will have never engaged in sexual intercourse. The *Healthy People 2010* objective is to increase further the number of sexually active African American women who use condoms, recognizing that African American women have a high incidence of HIV. The Guttmacher Institute (2008a) reports that 45% of teenage women using contraceptives choose a condom, either alone (19%) or with another method (25%). There are other signs of progress as well. Among women ages 15 to 44 who have ever had sexual intercourse, the percentage who had a male partner use a condom increased from 52% in 1982 to 90% in 2002 (Mosher et al., 2004).

HIV and College Students

In the absence of a cure for AIDS and the prevalence of STIs, preventive measures will continue to be the primary method of responding to the threat of these diseases. Because young adults, such as college students, tend to have more sexual partners than those older or younger, they are particularly at risk for these diseases. That is why HIV and AIDS and STI educational campaigns have targeted this population. The results of these educational efforts have been heartening at times and disturbing at others.

The American College Health Association (2006) found that 71% of college students reported having had sexual intercourse during the past year. Many had had multiple partners. Eleven percent of male college students and 6% of female college students reported having had four or more sexual partners in the past year. Forty-five percent reported having engaged in

DIMENSIONS

AIDS in Africa Imagine! In some areas of Africa, 35% of the population is infected with HIV. The United Nations reported that in 2004, throughout the world, more than 39 million people were infected with HIV (Joint United Nations Programme on HIV/AIDS, 2004). An estimated 25 million people are living with HIV in sub-Saharan Africa alone. Sub-Saharan Africa is home to slightly more than 10% of the world's population, and almost two-thirds of all people living with HIV. In 2003, an estimated 3 million people became infected and 2.2 million died (75% of the 3 million AIDS deaths globally that year).

However, in six African countries, adult HIV prevalence is less than 2%. In six other countries in the region, it exceeds 20%. In southern Africa all seven countries have prevalence rates greater than 17%, with Botswana and Swaziland having prevalence greater than 35%. In West Africa, HIV prevalence is much lower, with no country having a prevalence greater than 10% and most having prevalence between 1% and 5%. Adult prevalence in countries in Central and East Africa falls somewhere between these two groups, ranging from 4% to 13%. African women are at greater risk, becoming infected at an earlier age than men. Today there are on average 13 infected women for every 10 infected men in sub-Saharan Africa, up from a ratio of 12:10 in 2002.

Sub-Saharan Africa has the world's highest prevalence of AIDS and faces the greatest demographic impact. In the worst-affected countries of eastern and southern Africa, if current infection rates continue and there is no large-scale treatment program, as many as 60% of today's 15-year-olds will not reach their 60th birthday.

The stark differences in access to antiretroviral treatment are reflected in mortality rates. In low- and middle-income African countries, mortality rates among 15- to 49-year-olds are now up to 20 times greater than death rates for people living with HIV in industrialized countries. In seven African countries where HIV prevalence is more than 20%, the average life expectancy of a person born between 1995 and 2000 is 49 years. That is 13 years less than in the absence of AIDS. In Swaziland, Zambia, and Zimbabwe, which lack antiretroviral programs, the average life expectancy is predicted to drop to less than 35 years.

The African situation is even more perilous when one considers these countries' inability to afford costly drugs shown to be effective in treating HIV infection and AIDS. The triple-drug treatment, which has become routine in the United States, for example, was long unheard of in many parts of Africa and other developing countries. In a humanitarian gesture, drug companies have begun discounting the drugs to these countries.

---

oral sex one or more times, and 5% reported having anal sex one or more times, during the past 30 days. When asked if they used a condom during the last time they engaged in sexual activity, 52% did so during sexual intercourse, 4% during oral sex, and 28% during anal sex.

As evidenced by these statistics, too many males and females still engage in unhealthy sexual practices that place them at risk of contracting an STI or becoming infected with HIV. Are college students, who are the most educated people in our society, ready to engage in safer sex? A study of 376 university students concluded that they are not (Dahl, Gorn, & Weinberg, 1997). With the rationale that carrying condoms is the one way to ensure that a condom is available when needed, researchers surveyed college students regarding their likelihood of carrying a condom in different situations (a bar, a concert, a party, and a first date). Part of the study involved the researchers interviewing 346 students (137 females

and 209 males) at a university bar known for "fun, cheap beer and . . . sex." They offered a five-dollar food coupon for every condom each student possessed. Only 16 students were carrying a condom (less than 5%). What do you think the results of this study would be if conducted today at a bar near your campus?

Why do students not use condoms during sexual activities? A partial answer was provided by students themselves in a study that asked them that very question (Bradford & Beck, 1991). Among the most frequently cited reasons for not using a condom were the belief that condoms reduced pleasure and that their partners would not approve of condom use. In another study, college students who did not to use condoms had high perceptions of invulnerability and low perception of risk associated with their sexual behavior (Thompson et al., 2006). These students also believed they had the ability to identify a partner's HIV status. Other reasons for college

Bill and Melinda Gates have established a foundation that has donated millions of dollars to combat HIV infection and AIDS, especially on the African continent

Gender
DIMENSIONS

Women and AIDS AIDS was originally identified as a disease affecting gay men. However, the face of AIDS has changed. Certainly, gay men are still the largest category of those infected with HIV in the United States. In 1993, 45% of new adult HIV infections occurred in women. By 2004 almost half of new HIV infections were in women (UNAIDS, Uniting the world against AIDS: Women, 2006. Available:www.unaids.org/en/getstarted/women.asp).In the United States, new cases among women are increasing at a greater rate than among men, although men still have a greater number of cases (Centers for Disease Control and Prevention, 2007b).

Although HIV infection is affecting women to a greater extent than before, it is especially affecting women of color. AIDS is the leading cause of death among African American women. Furthermore, 64% of women living with AIDS are African American (Centers for Disease Control and Prevention, 2008d).High-risk heterosexual contact was the source of 80% of newly diag-

nosed cases of HIV infection. More alarming is that new cases of HIV/AIDS occur more often in women aged 15 to 39 than in other age groups. Given that these are the childbearing years, often these women's babies are born infected.

Poor women and women of color are more likely to contract HIV from a male sexual partner who is infected (most likely from intravenous drug use) than other women. They are also more likely to use drugs themselves, share needles, and/or engage in sex for drugs with other drug users who may be infected. Furthermore, poor women often lack access to education about AIDS and safer sex techniques, to medical care, and to economic and social support systems.

Instituting needle-exchange programs and community educational campaigns, putting health providers in the community through health clinics and walking of the neighborhoods, and using community health workers to encourage women to seek treatment are ways we can respond to the problem of women and AIDS.

students not using condoms during sexual activities include past failure or lack of experience with condoms, embarrassment in purchasing or using condoms, interference of the effects of alcohol with the use of condoms, hesitation to offend partners, belief that condom use decreases sexual pleasure, loss of spontaneity, loss of erection, lack of a condom when sexual intercourse was desired, low comfort level in communicating feelings about condom use with a partner, and fear of rejection if insisting on the use of a condom.

With so much at stake in terms of life and death, why do the factors cited seem so insurmountable to many college students and young adults?

Summary

- Acquired immune deficiency syndrome (AIDS) attacks and slowly destroys the immune system, resulting in the development of opportunistic infections such as pneumonia and cancer.

- AIDS is caused by the human immunodeficiency virus (HIV), which is transmitted through the transfer of bodily fluids such as semen, vaginal secretions, and blood. HIV infection is contracted primarily through sexual contact such as coitus, oral sex, or anal sex.

- Although AIDS is still considered a terminal illness, the death rate from this cause has steadily declined since 1996. This decline is predominantly due to new medications that seek to transform AIDS into a manageable chronic illness.

- Most AIDS cases occur among men who have sex with men, although the number of women developing AIDS has increased in recent years. Eighty percent of women who contract HIV infection do so through sexual activity with men.

- There are several tests available to diagnose HIV infection and the eventual development of AIDS. Some screening tests employ blood analysis, whereas others test saliva samples. One home testing kit has been approved by the FDA for the diagnosis of HIV infection.

- AIDS is treated with one of six classes of antiviral medications: nucleoside reverse transcriptase inhibitors, protease inhibitors, nonnucleoside reverse transcriptase inhibitors, entry/fusion inhibitors, integrase inhibitors, and fixed-dose combination. Each works on a different aspect of HIV infection, such as preventing HIV from reproducing or preventing HIV from invading the cells.

- Among the safer-sex behaviors to prevent HIV infection are remaining sexually abstinent, being in a sexually monogamous relationship, using a condom or dental dam, and avoiding high-risk behaviors such as anal intercourse.

- College students are particularly vulnerable to HIV infection owing to their relatively frequent sexual activity, their feelings of invulnerability, and the fact that they frequently engage in sexual activities without using a condom.

Discussion Questions

1. Explain the ways HIV is transmitted, the stages of infection, the tests for infection, and how opportunistic diseases occur as a result of AIDS.

2. Which treatments are available for HIV infection? What limits their worldwide availability?

3. List the safer-sex practices that reduce the risk of HIV transmission.

Application Questions

Reread the chapter-opening story and answer the following questions.

1. On June 25, 1998, the Supreme Court ruled that HIV-infected people are protected by a federal ban on discrimination against the disabled—even if they suffer no symptoms of AIDS. If that ruling had been made when Tim was diagnosed with HIV, do you think he might have been more willing to disclose his condition? Why or why not?

2. Regardless of the law, if you were a professor considering granting a graduate assistantship to a student (or an employer making a hiring decision), would the knowledge that the candidate was infected with HIV make a difference? How about if the person were being treated for cancer? Or heart disease? Why should such information make a difference?

3. How would you feel if you knew a fellow classmate or employee were HIV infected?

Critical Thinking Questions

1. Is it fair that the federal government spends a disproportionate share of medical research money on HIV research? Put another way, should federal research money be spent in proportion to the number of people who contract an illness and die of it (such as cancer or heart disease)? Or should the potential threat of a disease becoming more widespread take precedence?

2. You may remember this gender-related issue from another chapter: Men who carry condoms are considered to be "responsible," but women who carry condoms are considered "sluts." Given the need for more condom use to prevent the spread of STIs and HIV, how can this double standard be overcome?

Critical Thinking Cases

Deciding whether to disclose HIV infection is clearly a troubling decision for anyone to make. But do people have an obligation to disclose that information to protect others?

Consider the case of the two-time double–Olympic diving gold medalist Greg Louganis, who was HIV positive during his second Olympics. Louganis did not disclose his HIV status to Olympic officials. During one dive, Louganis hit the diving board with the back of his head and received a wound that bled. A doctor treated him without knowing of the HIV condition—and thus did not take extra precautions. Also, Olympic competitors are required to supply urine samples to test for illegal substances (such as steroids). Because urine would contain HIV, anyone handling Louganis's sample would have also been at risk unless proper precautions were taken.

Should Louganis have been required to disclose his status before the Olympics? What discrimination may result against an athlete who discloses his or her HIV-infected status? (You may reflect on the problems Magic Johnson faced when he disclosed his status.)

What about typical recreational athletes—people who work out in gyms, play basketball in leagues, fence (saber, epee, or foil), or participate in any recreational activity in which they can be injured accidentally? When do HIV-infected people need to disclose their status?

Exploring Personal Dimensions

Could You Negotiate Safer Sex?

The following items ask you to agree (A) or disagree (D) with the statements presented. Indicate the items about which you are unsure (U) of your response. Compare your responses to those of a friend. Discuss each item about which you said you were unsure of your response. Are there items about which you and a friend disagree? Which changes or adaptations would you or your friend have to make to take on a safer orientation toward sex with a partner?

I believe that . . .

_____ I could use a condom effectively.

_____ I could buy condoms without embarrassment.

_____ If my partner did not want to use a condom during sexual intercourse, I could convince him or her to do otherwise.

_____ Consumption of alcohol or use of other recreational drugs would in no way affect my determination to use a condom or to convince my partner to respect my wishes.

_____ Having to remember to buy, carry, and use condoms would interfere with sexual spontaneity.

_____ If I suggested using a condom, my partner would think that I must have had many previous sexual partners.

_____ I would feel comfortable insisting on using a condom with a new sexual partner.

_____ I would not feel self-conscious about putting a condom on myself (or on my partner).

_____ I would be able to discuss use of condoms with a partner even before we had any physical intimacy such as touching, caressing, or kissing.

_____ If I suggested using a condom, my partner would think I did not trust him or her.

_____ Using a condom during sexual intercourse would interfere with sexual pleasure or sexual functioning.

_____ Using condoms is an activity primarily for people who have many sexual partners.

_____ Having to use a condom might subsequently prove to be embarrassing to me or my partner if the mechanics of using one resulted in loss of erection.

_____ I could tactfully remove and dispose of a condom after sexual intercourse.

_____ I could convince my partner that use of a condom can be a stimulating part of sexual foreplay.

Suggested Readings

Bartlett, J. G., & Finkbeiner, A. K. *The guide to living with HIV infection: Developed at the Johns Hopkins AIDS Clinic*. Baltimore, MD: Johns Hopkins Press, 2006.

Bauer, H. M. *The origin, persistence and failings of HIV/AIDS theory*. Jefferson, NC: McFarland & Company, 2007.

Chalmers, J. *Legal responses to HIV and AIDS*. Oxford, UK: Hart, 2008.

Dube, M. W. *The HIV and AIDS bible: Selected essays*. Scranton, PA: University of Scranton Press, 2008.

Gallant, J. *100 questions and answers about HIV and AIDS*. Sudbury, MA: Jones and Bartlett, 2007.

Grodeck, B., & Berger, D. S. *The first year: HIV: An essential guide for the newly diagnosed*. Cambridge, MA: Da Capo Press, 2007.

Hunter, S. *AIDS in America*. New York: Palgrave Macmillan, 2006.

Sanford, J. P., Gilbert, D. N., Robert C., Jr. Moellering, R. C., & Eliopoulos, G. M. *The Sanford guide to HIV/AIDS therapy 2009*. Hyde Park, VT: Antimicrobial Therapy, 2008.

Stine, G. *AIDS update 2008*. New York: McGraw-Hill/Dushkin, 2008.

Web Resources

For links to the web sites below, visit *http://sexuality.jbpub.com/dimensions/4e* and click on Resource Links.

Maternal HIV Consumer Information Project
www.cms.hhs.gov/HIVAIDSRes

This web site is managed by the U.S. Department of Health and Human Services. Its index page links you to information about the Centers for Medicare and Medicaid Services (CMS). Each link represents a topic. Topic links are grouped by category, such as HIV or AIDS.

Henry J. Kaiser Family Foundation: Kaiser Daily U.S. HIV/AIDS Report
http://dailyreports.kff.org/Daily-Report.aspx

This web site provides a daily report with information pertaining to HIV and AIDS. Medical information and political issues are presented. Both global and issues specific to the United States are discussed.

National Institute of Allergy and Infectious Diseases
http://www3.niaid.nih.gov

Managed by the federal government, this web site presents information pertaining to HIV and AIDS. Links include health and science, research, news and events, the latest news, and research funding.

National AIDS Control Organisation
www.nacoonline.org

Provides links relative to HIV/AIDS pertaining to news, facts and figures, glossary/abbreviations, resources, partnerships and collaborations, photo gallery, programs, publications, and state AIDS control societies.

National AIDS Research Institute
www.nari-icmr.res.in

Managed by the government of India, this web site is devoted to presenting research findings pertaining to HIV and AIDS, publishing research findings and reports, answering frequently asked questions about HIV/AIDS, and providing links to other organizations concerned with HIV/AIDS issues.

CHAPTER 16

Sexual Dysfunction and Therapy

FEATURES

Gender Dimensions
Sexual Issues for Older Men and Women

Communication Dimensions
Discussing Sexual Dysfunction

Multicultural Dimensions
Sexual Dysfunction and Latino Populations

Global Dimensions
Sexual Disorders Around the World

Ethical Dimensions
Should Surrogates Be Used in Sexual Therapy?

CHAPTER OBJECTIVES

1 Describe the major male and female sexual dysfunctions, including the desire dysfunctions. Evaluate what makes the inability to perform sexually a clinical dysfunction.

2 Identify the multidimensional causes of sexual dysfunction, including the physical, psychological, and sociocultural aspects.

3 Compare and contrast the varied approaches to treating sexual dysfunctions. Explain why many different models of therapy exist.

sexuality.jbpub.com/dimensions/4e
Male Sexual Dysfunction
Female Sexual Dysfunction
Treating Sexual Dysfunction

INTRODUCTION

After he was diagnosed with prostate cancer in 1991, Senator Bob Dole underwent treatment, including surgery. He has since avidly promoted the importance of early detection and encouraged men to speak frankly with their doctors about prostate-related problems.

But it was in May 1998 that Dole made his biggest disclosure: He said on Larry King's talk show that he had been among the men who took part in the trials for the drug Viagra (sildenafil citrate). Viagra is a drug to treat men who have difficulty achieving an erection (erectile dysfunction). In effect, Bob Dole was admitting that he, as do millions of other men, had a sexual dysfunction—specifically, erectile disorder. The next day, Elizabeth Dole, his wife, was asked about the drug during a public appearance. She laughed and said with a beaming smile, "It's a great drug!"

Such public disclosures by celebrities and politicians make taboo topics—such as sexual dysfunctions—the subject of discussion among friends, colleagues, classmates, and even couples. Dole's 1998 public announcement, followed by commercials in March 1999, offered frank and genuine advice: If you have a problem, see a doctor. In the case of erectile disorder, about 80% of problems are physical and can be solved with a prescription or a medical procedure. Other disorders, though, have psychological or sociocultural dimensions at their root.

The Viagra story also touches on the socioeconomic and political dimensions of sexuality. As recently as the 1970s, insurers would not have covered treatments for erectile disorder, because the condition was believed to be psychological. Insurers began coverage as research proved there were physical causes as well. Coverage for Viagra is limited generally to 12 pills per month—the recommended dosage.

When the FDA approved Viagra on March 27, 1998, it was not covered under Medicaid. Thus it was unavailable to those in lower economic brackets. But the political ramifications of denying this wonder drug to the poor caused an uproar. Politicians know that older citizens are more likely to vote. Consequently, many states required Medicaid coverage for Viagra. However, under a law signed by President George W. Bush, as of January 2006, Medicaid no longer covers erectile dysfunction medications, and Medicare stopped coverage as of January 2007.

Sources: Why is Mrs. Dole smiling? *Washington Post* (May 9, 1998); Postmarketing safety of sildenafil citrate (Viagra), www.fda.gov/cder/consumerinfo/viagra/viagraupdate721.htm; Stark, K. Will insurers pay? Clamor for Viagra could cinch it, *Philadelphia Inquirer* (April 24, 1998).

■ Sexual Dysfunction

Are you perfect? What seems a silly question has great importance for sexual functioning. Of course, none of us is perfect. And yet, the occasional inability to function sexually (for example, to achieve and maintain an erection or to secrete adequate vaginal lubrication) leads many of us to conclude that something is drastically wrong with us.

This lack of response may be caused by a number of factors that have no bearing at all on your sexual functioning. For example, the ingestion of alcoholic beverages can interfere with sexual response, as can use of drugs such as hypertension medication, narcotics, and barbiturates. In addition, some people have partners with whom it is difficult to respond sexually. For example, your partner may have poor hygiene; he may know so little about sexual physiology that he attempts penile insertion before sufficient vaginal lubrication; or she may touch the scrotum and handle the testicles in a way that causes pain and discomfort. And yet, if the individuals with these sexual partners do not respond as one would expect under more conducive circumstances, they themselves are sometimes accused of having an "abnormality." It might be more accurate to suggest that those who are sexually responsive to dirty, smelly, clumsy sexual partners are the ones experiencing some abnormality.

The media also help to establish unrealistic sexual expectations that, when not met, may lead people to think of themselves as dysfunctional. For example, when movies portray gorgeous specimens of men and women in romantic settings, who seem to have nothing else on their minds but sex, and who are willing and able to engage in any sexual activity that comes to mind, we and our lovers may not measure up. We might conclude something is wrong with us or

our love life, although in reality something is wrong with this portrayal. We will discuss the commercialism of sex in detail in Chapter 17. Suffice it to say here that soap operas, movies, plays, and advertisements sometimes lead people to decide they are not as sexually adequate as those they see "performing" on satin sheets with unblemished bodies glistening under flattering spotlights.

However, there are people who experience difficulty responding sexually and who wish their sexual responses could be healthier and more sexually satisfying. They may find it difficult to achieve and/or maintain an erection or to relax enough to allow penile penetration. They may ejaculate too soon, or they may experience disturbing pain during coitus. They may wonder why they do not feel sexually aroused enough or do not experience orgasm. Men and women, heterosexuals and homosexuals, experience these concerns. They may be young or old, African American or white, well educated or lacking in schooling, and from any socioeconomic group. The one characteristic they have in common, though, is dissatisfaction with their sexual life, and this dissatisfaction often affects other aspects of their relationships.

This chapter explores some of these matters. We discuss which kinds of sexual problems people experience, what causes these problems, and how they can be treated. Notice the difficulty in diagnosing particular sexual dysfunctions (even the experts do not always agree about whether a dysfunction exists) and the varied approaches to treating them once they are identified. This, too, is discussed and its implications explored. We begin with a definition of sexual dysfunction.

Sexual dysfunction is a chronic inability to respond sexually in a way

sexual dysfunction
A specific, chronic disorder involving sexual performance.

that one finds satisfying. We do not use the term to describe those situations, common to many people, in which they are temporarily uninterested in sexual activity or unable to respond sexually because of exhaustion, excessive use of alcohol, anger, and so on. The key word in our definition is *chronic*—that is, a consistent long-term inability to respond. It applies both to people who have never had satisfactory sexual relations—primary dysfunctions—and to people who have had successful sexual relations at some time but are now having chronic difficulty—secondary dysfunction.

The amount of sexual dysfunction prevalent in society is difficult, if not impossible, to determine. As evidence of this difficulty, it has been estimated that at some time in their marriage, about half of all married couples experience sexual difficulties (Ende, Rockwell, & Glasgow, 1984; McCarthy, Ryan, & Johnson, 1975; Nathan, 1986) that can be classified as (chronic) sexual dysfunctions. Yet, a more recent study concluded only 22% of married women experience a sexual dysfunction (Lauman, Paik, & Rosen, 1999). Obviously it is impossible to determine the number of people who do not satisfactorily respond sexually but who never seek treatment. But the number of people seeking treatment has increased in recent years (Leiblum, 2003). Table 16.1 lists the percentages of men and women who experience various sexual dysfunctions. Although several years old, these data are still the most current and most extensive information we have regarding the prevalence of sexual dysfunctions.

There are several possible explanations for this increase. First, the increasing amount of information on the subject has made admitting sexual dysfunctions less embarrassing. Second, more effective therapy is now available and people are more willing to take advantage of it. Third, as the physiological fea-

People who experience chronic sexual dysfunction often feel shameful and inadequate. Yet, there are successful treatments for most sexual dysfunctions, whether they are caused by physical or psychological factors.

tures of sexual response are understood by more people, more nonorgasmic women and men with erectile problems realize they are not permanently unresponsive but have sexual dysfunctions that can be treated effectively. Fourth, the amount of sexual dysfunction might actually be increasing among men because as women become aware of their right to sexual satisfaction, more men may find themselves overanxious about meeting their partners' expectations.

The underlying cause of any sexual dysfunction may be either physical or psychological, but most experts agree that psychological causes, broadly defined, are much more prevalent, causing anywhere from 40% to 90% of sexual dysfunctions. Masters and Johnson's 1970 conclusion, which is probably still relevant, was that "sociocultural deprivation and ignorance of sexual physiology, rather than psychiatric or medical illness," were at the source of most sexual dysfunction. We would add that although poor communication about sex may not actually cause a dysfunction, it can certainly allow conditions to worsen

TABLE 16.1	Percent of Men and Women Who Experienced a Sexual Dysfunction for Several Months During the Past Year	
Type of Dysfunction	**Men (%)**	**Women (%)**
Pain experienced during sex	3.0	14.4
Sex not pleasurable	8.1	21.2
Unable to experience an orgasm	8.3	24.1
Lack of interest in sex	15.8	33.4
Anxiety about sexual performance	17.0	11.5
Reaching climax too quickly	28.5	10.3
Unable to maintain an erection	10.4	—
Trouble lubricating	—	18.8

Source: Lauman, E. O., Gagnon, J. H., Michael, R. T., & Michaels, S. *The social organization of sexuality: Sexual practices in the United States.* Chicago, IL: University of Chicago Press, 1994.

♂♀ Gender DIMENSIONS

Sexual Issues for Older Men and Women

Contrary to common belief, older people remain sexually active. Still, as with younger men and women, older men engage in sexual activity more often than do older women. In a large scale study[1] of the sexual behavior and health of older Americans, it was found that 84% of men and 62% of women between ages 57 and 64 participated in a sexual activity with a partner at least once during the previous year. Furthermore, although sexual activity declined as respondents got older, 39% of men and 17% of women between ages 75 and 85 still reported engaging in sexual activity with a partner at least once during the previous year.

Older men and women also differed in the sexual problems they experienced. The most prevalent sexual problems experienced by older women were low sexual desire (43%), insufficient vaginal lubrication (39%), and an inability to achieve an orgasm (34%). The most common sexual problems experienced by older men were erectile dysfunction (37%), lack of interest in sex (28%), premature ejaculation (28%), and performance anxiety (27%).

[1]Lindau, S. T., Schumm, L. P., Lauman, E. O., Levinson, W., Muircheartaigh, C. A., & Waite, L. J. A study of sexuality and health among older adults in the United States. *New England Journal of Medicine, 357, no. 8* (2007), 762–774.

rather than improve and can contribute to making otherwise temporary troubles chronic. Likewise, most problems are best solved through the cooperation of partners (Wylie, 2002).

We now turn our attention to the types of dysfuctions people experience, and we begin with those experienced by men.

Male Sexual Dysfunctions

Sexual dysfunction in males can be traumatic. In our society, men are expected to be experienced and talented in matters of sex. They are supposed to be the leaders with their sexual partners, serving as a guide to sexual bliss. When men cannot perform in this manner, they may consider themselves less manly and, as a result, experience a range of other psychological problems.

In addition to the effect sexual dysfunctions can have on a man's psychological health, his relationships can be devastated. A man would most likely not want to initiate or participate in sexual activity when the results might be failure and a demonstration of ineptness. Only a masochist would allow himself to be placed in such a situation continually and, consequently, his sexual activity would become sporadic. The partner then might wonder why she was not good enough or appealing enough and the total relationship would be at risk.

Sexual dysfunctions need not be viewed as exclusively negative. There is a positive side to this situation. Researchers report that people who engage in sexual therapy often become less anxious, commu-

nicate better (Zilbergeld & Kilmann, 1984), become more assertive with their sexual partners (Tullman et al., 1981), and feel more positive about their sexual selves (Cotton-Houston & Wheeler, 1983). You might not choose to have a sexual problem even if you could acquire these benefits of sexual therapy, but the fact that this potential exists is often a welcome surprise.

Men experience four main types of sexual dysfunctions: erectile dysfunction, premature ejaculation, ejaculatory incompetence, and dyspareunia.

Erectile Dysfunction

A man's difficulty in achieving and maintaining an erection is popularly known as **impotence**. This term is Latin and means "without power." The word *impotence* is used to connote that a man has lost power—is no longer "manly"—when he cannot achieve or maintain an erection. Furthermore, he has lost power as a lover and has lost his reproductive capacity. The more understanding, more professional, more sensitive, and more accurate term is **erectile dysfunction**. To imply that a man with a sexual dysfunction is generally without power is untrue and unfair and only exacerbates the situation. Men who are unable to achieve or maintain erections may be satisfying lovers nevertheless; they may be very effective at cunnilingus or manual masturba-

impotence
Difficulty in achieving and maintaining an erection.

erectile dysfunction
The inability of a man to maintain an erection long enough to have sexual intercourse; commonly known as *impotence*.

tion. Furthermore, they may be in "powerful" positions (such as a corporate executive) or be adequate in all other aspects of their lives.

The best estimate is that one in three men suffer from erectile dysfunction (Jarrow & Amawalt, 2006). Approximately 6% of men experience erectile dysfunction (Saigal, Wessells, & Wilt, 2006). As men age, they are more prone to experience erection problems. Whereas 2% of men aged 20 to 29 report erectile dysfunction, 17% of men aged 60 to 69, 22% of men aged 70 to 74, and 48% of men aged 75 and older report erection problems. Besides men included in these data, it is not unusual for men not classified as having erectile dysfunction to experience occasional difficulty in achieving an erection. For example, alcohol can interfere with developing penile erection. If a sexual partner is unclean or disliked, this too can interfere with male sexual arousal. Men who have never had an erection sufficient to have sexual intercourse are said to have **primary erectile dysfunction**. Men who have previously been able to maintain an erection long enough to have intercourse but subsequently have an erection problem are said to have **secondary erectile dysfunction**. Secondary erectile dysfunction is approximately 10 times more prevalent than primary erectile dysfunction (Kaplan, 1974; Kolodny, Masters, & Johnson, 1979). Some men achieve an erection only to lose it on vaginal insertion. Others achieve and maintain an erection long enough during masturbation to have an orgasm but cannot be coitally connected and maintain that erection. These, too, are examples of erectile dysfunction.

Making a precise diagnosis of erectile dysfunction is not as easy as it might appear. Many men are at times unable to have an erection or lose it before vaginal penetration. They may be uninterested in their partners, they may have ingested too much alcohol, or they may be using certain medications that interfere with the erectile reflex. How often does this have to occur before the condition is classified as erectile dysfunction? Masters and Johnson (1970) classified men who, in at least 25% of their sexual encounters, are unable to maintain an erection long enough for penile insertion as having secondary erectile dysfunction. Crooks and Baur (2002) believe it inappropriate to specify a cutoff point (for example, 25%). They prefer to ask the couple whether they believe a problem exists; if they say it does, then erectile dysfunction is diagnosed.

primary erectile dysfunction
A condition in which an adult male has never had an erection sufficient to engage in sexual intercourse.

secondary erectile dysfunction
A condition in which an adult male has previously had an erection sufficient to engage in sexual intercourse but no longer has.

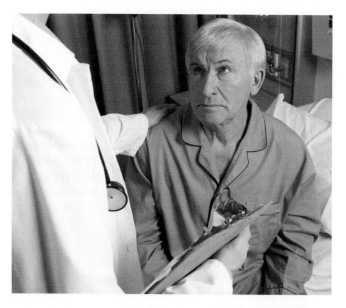

It used to be thought that erectile dysfunction was the result of psychological factors. It is now known that most erectile dysfunctions are the results of physical maladies such as clogged penile arteries.

Erectile dysfunction is caused by myriad factors. Whereas it was previously believed that most erectile dysfunctions were caused by psychological factors, the latest thinking is that 70% are at least partially the result of physiological factors (National Kidney and Urologic Diseases Information Clearinghouse, 2003). Among these factors are diabetes (National Kidney and Urologic Diseases Information Clearinghouse, 2003). Between 35% and 50% of men with diabetes experience erectile dysfunction (National Institute of Diabetes and Digestive and Kidney Disorders, 2005). Other causes include damage to nerves, arteries, and smooth muscle that are a result of kidney disease, chronic alcoholism, multiple sclerosis, and neurological diseases. Heart disease and its risk factors—smoking, being overweight, and a lack of exercise—can also contribute to the development of erectile dysfunction, as can surgery for prostate or bladder cancer. Lastly, some common medications such as blood pressure drugs, antihistamines, antidepressants, tranquilizers, and appetite suppressants can produce erectile dysfunction as a side effect. Even riding a bicycle more than 100 miles per week (obviously among serious bikers) can cause erection problems (Schrader, Breitenstein, & Lowe, 2008).

There is some convincing evidence implicating lifestyle behavior risk factors with the development of erectile dysfunction. These risk factors include obesity, a sedentary lifestyle, hypertension, hypercholesterolemia, and a high body mass index (Feldman et al., 2000; Fung, Bettencourt, & Barrett-Conner,

2004). These are all recognizable as coronary heart disease risk factors. Just as coronary blood vessels can become blocked when these risk factors are present, so can penile arteries. In an 8-year study, those men who were more active and less obese developed erectile dysfunction to a lesser degree than those who were less active and more obese (Derby et al., 2000). Other researchers have also concluded that healthy lifestyle factors are associated with the maintenance of erectile function (Bacon et al., 2003). These findings have led some experts to suggest that before medications are prescribed, men who are having difficulty achieving an erection should participate in lifestyle programs designed to decrease weight and increase physical activity. Such a program was developed for obese men and was found to reduce the risk of erectile dysfunction by 70% (Esposito et al., 2004). However, whereas pharmaceuticals for erectile dysfunction is big business, as one cynical researcher stated, "this study provides evidence of efficacy for what perhaps should be the first-line treatment for obese patients with ED. . . . Unfortunately, however, this is one treatment for ED that will not be accompanied by free pens, free notepads, and its own Super Bowl commercial" (Saigal, 2004).

Among the nonorganic causes are fear of sexual performance—"Will I be an adequate sexual partner or show my ineptitude?" This fear can result in a self-fulfilling prophecy; that is, the fear may make the man so anxious that he is unable to achieve and maintain an erection. The result could be lowered self-esteem, which itself feeds into the original fear. Thus a cycle of erectile dysfunction develops. In addition, guilt or shame about sexual activity can interfere with an erection.

All men are capable of having difficulty in achieving an erection at one time or other, even college-age men. Perhaps they have just ingested alcohol, which is a central nervous system depressant; or they find their partner unappealing; or the surroundings are not conducive to sexual stimulation. In any case, infrequent erectile difficulties are not cause for alarm. However, if they persist, professional help should be sought.

Some novel ways to diagnose the causes of erectile dysfunction exist. For example, knowing men normally have erections during their sleep, physicians sometimes place electronic devices around the flaccid penises of men with erection problems while they sleep to determine the presence and frequency of erections (Spark, 2008). If a problem exists during sleep, the cause is organic. A man who is concerned about an erection problem but who does not yet want to consult a physician or counselor can place a ring of postage stamps around his penis before going to sleep. If the stamps are placed snugly around the flac-

cid penis and an erection occurs, the ring of stamps will be broken in the morning. To determine further whether erectile dysfunction is a result of physiological causes, the man is questioned about how abruptly the problem presented itself. If it is a psychological problem, it usually develops gradually; if it is physiological, it usually develops abruptly (Stipp, 1987).

It is an unfortunate fact that erectile dysfunction can permeate an entire relationship. This is true not only because sexual activity is a significant part of a total relationship, and consequently has an effect on other aspects of the relationship, but also because the woman or man may blame herself or himself for the partner's erectile problems—"Am I not attractive enough?" "Am I not skilled enough?" "What am I doing wrong?" Also, the sexual partner may assume that the problem stems from the man engaging in sexual activity with someone else. In any case, the effect may place such strain and pressure on the relationship that counseling should include these considerations among its foci (American Urological Association, 2005a).

Premature Ejaculation

Premature ejaculation, or rapid ejaculation, is the most common sexual dysfunction in men. It is estimated that 30% of men worldwide experience premature ejaculation (Carson & Gunn, 2006). However, as with some of the other dysfunctions, this condition is not easily defined. Years ago, *premature ejaculation* meant the man could not maintain penile insertion without ejaculating within a minimal amount of time (for example, 2 minutes) or could not perform a minimal number of penile thrusts before ejaculating. Masters and Johnson (1970) even proposed a definition that classified the ejaculate as premature if the man's partner was not satisfied in at least 50% of their coital episodes. Helen Singer Kaplan (1974) defined *premature ejaculation* as the man's inability to control his ejaculate voluntarily.

The problems with these definitions were several. The couples in these studies differed in their perception of what was premature. Some couples were perfectly happy for coitus to last a short period, whereas other couples were dissatisfied with only 2 minutes of insertion or a minimal number of penile thrusts. In addition, Masters and Johnson's definition overlooked the fact that some women do not experience orgasms during coitus and would not achieve orgasm, regardless of the timing of their partner's ejaculation. Kaplan's definition neglected to recognize that men, as a rule, do not possess total voluntary control over ejaculation;

premature ejaculation
The inability of a man to control ejaculation for a sufficient length of time during coitus.

Communication
DIMENSIONS

Discussing Sexual Dysfunction

Two people who love and care for each other can deal with sexual dysfunction together. The key to the resolution of this situation, however, lies in the total relationship, not just the sexual part. Sexual communication is just one form of communication. If the relationship is characterized by ineffective communication in general, assuming that communicating about sex will be different is unrealistic. So, the first step in resolving sexual problems is to develop a relationship of caring, concern, mutual respect, and understanding. For this reason, some sex therapists work with clients to improve their interaction in general and concurrently help them respond to their sexual concerns.

Assuming that the relationship is minimally communicative, the first step is to provide support for each other and the promise of hope: "That's okay, honey; we'll get help and work it out." "It's not that I care any less for you, sweetheart, but something's interfering with my sex-making right now." This form of communication can reduce partners' anxieties that may be interfering with sexual function. Imagine the embarrassment of experiencing a sexual

dysfunction and the resulting pressure during each subsequent sexual encounter. The fear of "failure" and the anticipation of disappointing one's partner can be so frustrating that they can feed on themselves, contributing to, and exacerbating, the sexual problem. Communicating that it is okay, that help can be obtained, that the problem will be faced together, and that there is a commitment to work to make matters better can go a long way in intervening between dysfunctional feelings and resulting dysfunctional sex.

Once counseling starts, the couple needs to continue communicating with each other but now must also begin communicating with the counselor. To be effective, communication with the counselor must be candid. Without candor, the source of the problems may never be uncovered, or at least it will take longer to discover. A commitment is then required to adhere conscientiously to the treatment regimen and remain with it until the problem is resolved.

Certainly, sexual dysfunction puts a strain on both people involved, but caring, supportive lovers can become even closer through facing this problem and overcoming it.

this definition would classify most men as sexually dysfunctional.

Newer research considers the desires of the couple in the definition of premature ejaculation. For example, one definition divides premature ejaculation into a continuum ranging from ejaculation before penile insertion to ejaculation 7 minutes after insertion (Schover et al., 1982). The ejaculate is not classified as premature, however, unless either the man or the woman considers it to be so. We define premature ejaculation as a condition in which the man cannot maintain vaginal insertion long enough—long enough as judged by the man himself and his partner—without ejaculating. This requires that either the man or his partner must be dissatisfied with the timing of the ejaculate for a problem to exist. This definition is consistent with that in the American Psychiatric Association's *Diagnostic and Statistical Manual (DSM-IV)*, which states that premature ejaculation is "the persistent or recurrent ejaculation with minimal sexual stimulation, or, before, upon, or shortly after penetration and before the person wishes it." However, because this definition leaves open the questions of what is "minimal sexual

stimulation" and what does "shortly" mean, we prefer our definition, which requires that either one or both partners perceive there to be a problem.

The effects of ejaculating prematurely can be harmful to the relationship and to the psychological health of the man. Men may feel less than manly and may have a lowered self-esteem. Not wanting to disclose their problem, these men may refrain from sexual intercourse, thereby disappointing their partners and/or making them wonder about the viability of the relationship. Because premature ejaculation is estimated to affect approximately 20% of American men at least moderately (American Urological Association, 2005b; Laumann & Rosen, 1999), the number of people affected—men and women—is significant.

Several self-help techniques for overcoming rapid ejaculation have been proposed (Mayo Clinic Staff, 2007c). The use of a condom seems to help because the glans penis is not stimulated directly. Some men drink an alcoholic beverage to decrease the rapidity of their sexual response. Others allow themselves a rapid orgasm, or a small orgasm, knowing that the next one will take longer to arrive. Waiting for sufficient vaginal lubrication may also help prolong ejaculation. The glans penis may experience too much friction if the vagina is insufficiently lubricated, causing increased sensitivity and rapid ejaculation. Relaxing or switching positions to decrease muscle tension is another technique recommended, because rapid ejaculation is encouraged by too much muscular tension. Finally, creams designed to decrease sensitivity can be placed on the glans penis. Whether the benefit of controlling the ejaculate is worth the price of deadened sensations during coitus is a decision that only the man and his partner can make.

Ejaculatory Incompetence

For some men, the problem is not ejaculating too soon, but rather being unable to ejaculate in the vagina at all. This condition is known as **ejaculatory incompetence**, sometimes referred to as **retarded ejaculation**. Ejaculatory incompetence has a relatively low prevalence—approximately 3% (Perelmen & Rowland, 2006). When a man has never ejaculated in the vagina and is incapable of doing so, he is classified as having primary ejaculatory incompetence. When he has previously been able to ejaculate in the vagina but can no longer do so, he is classified as having secondary ejaculatory incompetence. These men may still be able to maintain an erection and/or stay sexually aroused. Or they may be able to ejaculate through masturbation or oral–genital stimulation. Sometimes, though rarely, this condition can be specific to only one partner or to specific situations (Munjack & Kanno, 1979).

We use the term *ejaculatory incompetence* with some hesitation. It is unfair and inaccurate to suggest that men who have difficulty with ejaculating are incompetent. But because the professional literature refers to this condition as *ejaculatory incompetence*, we do so as well.

Another form of retarded ejaculation is called **partial ejaculatory incompetence**. This condition results in a "half" orgasm—that is, a seepage of semen without true orgasmic sensations. Kaplan (1974) writes of men who, when fatigued or in conflict, "come without realizing they have." Originally thought to be rare, this form of ejaculatory incompetence seems relatively common among men.

Ejaculatory incompetence is a dis-

Men who experience pain during sexual intercourse may be experiencing dyspareunia. Pain may be caused by infection of the sexual organs or by allergic reactions to spermicidal creams or foams used by their partner.

order that may have interesting side effects. For example, the ability to maintain penile insertion for long periods without ejaculating may be valued by many men and appreciated by their sexual partners. However, the extreme of being unable to ejaculate in the vagina at all can result in the partner's questioning her own sexual abilities. In this case, the benefit of prolonged insertion quickly dissipates, and frustration and doubt set in. Another side effect is that when the man fakes orgasm to prevent his partner from feeling inadequate, not only does he remain sexually unsatisfied, but deceit, rather than trust and openness, can begin to characterize the relationship as a whole. As with many of the other sexual dysfunctions, treatment must be directed at the relationship as well as at the specific disorder.

Dyspareunia

Painful sexual intercourse is called **dyspareunia**. During sexual intercourse, men may feel pain in the penis, testes, or some other part of the body. Pain during coitus can be caused by both organic and nonorganic factors. For example, infections of the penis, foreskin, testes, urethra, or prostate can cause such pain, as can allergic reactions to a spermicidal cream or foam used as a contraceptive. Some men report irritation of the glans penis caused by an intrauterine device (IUD) string, which extends out of the uterus into the vagina.

ejaculatory incompetence
A condition in which a male is unable to ejaculate in the vagina; sometimes referred to as retarded ejaculation.

retarded ejaculation
A condition in which penile erection occurs during sexual intercourse but ejaculation does not; sometimes termed ejaculatory incompetence.

partial ejaculatory incompetence
A condition in which, during ejaculation, only a seepage of semen occurs, and orgasm lacks pleasurable sensations.

dyspareunia
Pain in the genital area during sexual intercourse.

Other causes of dyspareunia in men include a foreskin that is too tight and causes pain when an erection develops; smegma (a cheeselike substance secreted by the glans penis) that has not been washed away from the glans penis and causes an infection and/or irritates the glans; and Peyronie's disease, in which fibrous tissue and calcium deposits develop in the area around the cavernous bodies of the penis and may cause pain.

Female Sexual Dysfunctions

It wasn't too long ago that females were first allowed to express their sexual needs and to be viewed as entitled to sexual satisfaction at the same level as men. However, a double standard is still alive and well. Some men consider women suspect if they initiate sexual activity or are vocal in appreciating it. They are still supposed to be coy, letting the man take the lead, for fear of what might be thought of them if they act too assertively. Given this situation, too many women have adopted a passive attitude toward sexual activity and sometimes have developed shame, guilt, or embarrassment about their sexual behavior. For some women, this has progressed into an inability to function in a sexually healthy and satisfying way. In particular, the sexual dysfunctions women sometimes experience are sexual unresponsiveness, orgasmic dysfunction, vaginismus, and dyspareunia.

Sexual Unresponsiveness

Popularly known as **frigidity**, the condition in which a woman "is uninterested in sex" (Haas & Haas, 1990) or receives no erotic pleasure from sexually oriented stimulation is more appropriately termed **sexual unresponsiveness** or, technically speaking, female sexual arousal disorder. The word *frigidity* connotes a cold feeling or a lack of emotion. On the contrary, the opposite might be true; that is, a woman may be a caring and sensitive person who is just unable to respond to sexual stimulation. The physiological manifestations of sexual unresponsiveness include lack of vaginal lubrication, lack of vasocongestion, and lack of change in the size of the vagina during sexual stimulation. One study found 27% of premenopausal women and 52% of menopausal women experienced hypoactive sexual desire disorder (West et al., 2008).

One out of three women report lack of interest in sex, 10% report lubrication difficulties, and 20% find the sex not to be pleasurable (Gladu, 2002). Furthermore, women experiencing sexual

sexual unresponsiveness
Commonly referred to as *frigidity* or female sexual arousal disorder, a sexual dysfunction that causes a woman to experience little or no erotic pleasure through sexual stimulation.

arousal disorder have fewer sexual fantasies than do other women (Brotto, Heiman, & Tolman, 2009). However, sexual arousal disorder is more complicated than it appears initially. Experts have recommended considering the sexual partner and environmental conditions when diagnosing sexual arousal disorder (Brotto, Bitzer, Laan, Leiblum, & Luria, 2010).

Sexual unresponsiveness can be caused by nonpsychogenic factors (such as low estrogen levels or medications for hypertension or depression), shame, fear, guilt, or embarrassment about sexual activity or one's body. Before treatment can begin, the cause(s) must be identified. Obviously, if the causes are psychogenic in nature, treatment will differ from treatment for organic causes.

Orgasmic Dysfunction

Some women have difficulty experiencing orgasm; this condition is known as **orgasmic dysfunction**. (Table 16.4). Women who have never had an orgasm are said to have *primary orgasmic dysfunction*, or *primary anorgasmia* (some term this *inorgasmia*). Those who have at one time experienced orgasm but do not now are said to have *secondary orgasmic dysfunction*, or *secondary anorgasmia*. Some women have orgasms under certain circumstances but not others—for example, while masturbating but not when stimulated by a partner. This condition is referred to as *situational orgasmic dysfunction*, or *situational anorgasmia*. If the inability to experience an orgasm is limited to coital episodes, that is known as *coital sexual dysfunction*, or *coital anorgasmia*.

orgasmic dysfunction
The consistent or frequent inability of a woman to achieve an orgasm.

The data regarding the incidence of orgasmic dysfunction have been remarkably consistent over the years. Earlier studies that found that approximately 10% of women were coitally anorgasmic (Female orgasmic disorder, 2005; Kinsey, Pomeroy, & Martin, 1953; Levin & Levin, 1975) have been supported by more recent research (Hayes et al., 2008; Spector & Carey, 1990). However, Laumann et al. (1999) reported that 24% of women they studied were unable to reach orgasm for several months over the past year. Furthermore, 33% to 50% of women report they are dissatisfied with how often they reach orgasm (National Library of Medicine, 2009a). Many women reach orgasm through clitoral stimulation but not by sexual intercourse alone. These statistics have generated some controversy as to whether coital anorgasmia should be considered a problem. Remember our discussion of premature ejaculation, in which we stated the need for one or both of the sexual partners to feel a problem

Some women experience pain during intercourse. Possible causes include disorders of the reproductive organs, vaginal infections, or irritation due to the use of some contraceptive products.

exists. Similarly, experts argue that if women achieve orgasm through direct clitoral stimulation or through oral–genital sex only, and they and their partners are satisfied with this situation, the condition should not be considered dysfunctional. It is further argued that coital orgasms are an inappropriate "goal" of sexual activity—a goal imposed by men, who are only rarely anorgasmic, on women. The argument continues that because women's sexual response cycles have greater variability than men's, women are more content to enjoy sex—even coitus—without orgasm. Furthermore, most women can have regular orgasms, but not through intercourse alone. They require clitoral stimulation. If women do not experience orgasm through intercourse, they should not be considered dysfunctional.

An opposing view is presented by Masters, Johnson, and Kolodny (1985). They argue that accepting coital anorgasmia because it affects so many women is akin to accepting premature ejaculation as within normal limits, because both conditions affect approximately the same number of people. They continue that because many women who are coitally anorgasmic can be taught, through therapy, to achieve orgasms during coitus, why discourage these women from doing something about their coitally anorgasmic condition by describing it as normal? Finally, they argue there is no evidence that a large percentage of women are incapable of orgasm. Consequently, those who are incapable of orgasm should be offered help to rectify their situation.

Only about 5% of the cases of orgasmic dysfunction are the result of organic causes (Masters, Johnson, & Kolodny, 1985). Organic causes are usually such chronic illnesses as diabetes, alcoholism, hor-

mone deficiencies, or pelvic infections. The other 95% are the result of psychogenic factors such as shame and guilt associated with sexual activity. Depression is also a major contributor (Female orgasmic disorder, 2005; Orgasmic dysfunction, 2009). These states of mind interfere with the woman's ability to relax and allow the natural body processes to occur. Each episode then feeds on the last, until coitus is anticipated with fear and embarrassment. It is no wonder that orgasms do not occur under these circumstances.

Vaginismus
Some women cannot relax the muscles around the entrance to the vagina enough to allow for penetration of the penis or even a narrower object—for example, a finger. The recurrent or persistent involuntary spasm of the outer third of the vagina that interferes with sexual intercourse is known as **vaginismus** (Simons & Carey, 2001). *Primary vaginismus* occurs when a woman has never been able to achieve vaginal penetration. *Secondary vaginismus* occurs when a woman has previously been able to achieve pain-free vaginal penetration but subsequently cannot (Cordell, 2008). In less severe cases, spasms occur only when coitus is attempted. In even less severe cases, coitus is possible but is accompanied by discomfort. Figure 16.1 depicts the normal vagina opening as well as the contractions of the vaginal muscles during vaginismus.

vaginismus
The involuntary contraction of the muscles surrounding the vaginal entrance so that entry of the penis is prevented.

It is estimated that 0.5% to 1% of women experience vaginismus (Greziottin, 2004; Laumann, Paik, & Rosen, 1999). Interestingly, most of these women do not have a problem with sexual arousal. They experience vaginal lubrication normally, then enjoy foreplay, and they can be orgasmic (Kolodny, Masters, & Johnson, 1979). The causes of vaginismus are usually psychogenic (National Library of Medicine, 2009b)—that is, shame, fear, or embarrassment, the most common cause of which is childhood sexual abuse (Perry, 1992). In addition, dyspareunia can lead to vaginismus. It is not difficult to imagine how a woman who experiences pain during sexual intercourse could tense up in fear of pain when penile insertion is imminent. In this case, when the dyspareunia is eliminated, the vaginismus usually disappears.

Vaginismus is also associated with erectile dysfunction in a woman's male partner, strong religious teachings about sexuality, homosexual feelings, and negative or hostile feelings about one's partner (Lewis et al., 2004).

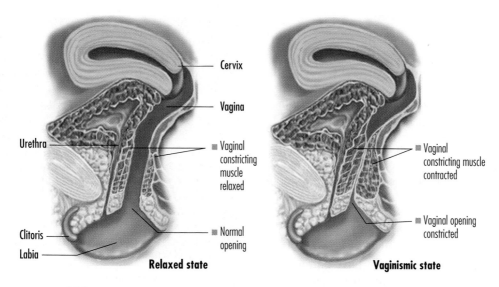

Cervix

Vagina

Urethra

Vaginal constricting muscle relaxed

Normal opening

Clitoris

Labia

Relaxed state

Vaginal constricting muscle contracted

Vaginal opening constricted

Vaginismic state

FIGURE **16.1** Vaginismus is the involuntary contraction of the muscles in the outer third of the vagina.

Dyspareunia

Some women experience pain during sexual intercourse. Recurrent or persistent genital pain associated with sexual intercourse is known as *dyspareunia* (Dyspareunia, 2009). Although all women may experience some pain during some particular coital episode, dyspareunia is a chronic condition. Often this pain manifests itself as a burning feeling or cramping and may occur externally, in the vagina, or elsewhere in the pelvis. It is estimated that 7% of women experience dyspareunia regularly (Jamieson & Steege, 2003).

Dyspareunia may be caused by disorders of the introitus, vagina, uterus, fallopian tubes, and/or ovaries (Dyspareunia, 2003). It may be a result of vaginal infections: yeast, bacterial, or trichomoniasis. Some contraceptive foams, creams, or gels or some condoms or diaphragms may irritate the vagina, resulting in pain during sexual intercourse. Even an intact hymen or scar tissue from a ruptured hymen can cause pain during penile insertion. More rarely, smegma—oily glandular secretions—accumulates under the clitoral hood and, when moved during coitus, may cause irritation and pain. Other pain may result when internal organs (such as the ovaries or uterus) are jarred during sexual intercourse (this may be remedied by the woman's being on top during coitus so she can control the depth of the penile thrusts).

One of the concerns regarding dyspareunia is its potential to lead to other sexual dysfunctions. For example, if a woman anticipates pain during coitus, she may tense her vaginal muscles, resulting in vaginismus; she may not be sexually responsive; or she may be anorgasmic. Treatment must identify any secondary dysfunctions and respond to those as well.

 Did You Know . . .

Testosterone has been used to increase the sex drives of women. In several well-conducted, randomized trials, testosterone delivered in various ways (for example, injections, implants, and patches) resulted in an increase in women's sexual desire, sexual responsiveness, and frequency of sexual intercourse (Heiman, 2006). Yet, as with all medications, there are potential side effects of testosterone use for low sexual desire. Among these side effects are unwanted hair growth and the unanswered question regarding the relationship between testosterone administration and the development of breast cancer (Davis et al., 2008). Despite these concerns, the North American Menopause Society (2005) supports the use of testosterone "in appropriate post-menopausal women . . . administered at the lowest doses for the shortest time that meets treatment goals." It also recommends counseling women about the risks and benefits of testosterone use.

Sexual Desire Dysfunctions

In addition to the sexual dysfunctions described, both men and women sometimes experience problems with their interest in sexual activity. These dysfunctions include *inhibited sexual desire, dissatisfaction with sexual activity frequency,* and *sexual aversion.*

Inhibited Sexual Desire

Kaplan (1979, 1989) described **inhibited sexual desire (ISD)**, sometimes referred to as *hypoactive sexual desire disorder (HSDD)*, as a lack of sexual appetite (Berney, 2009). It is characterized by a lack of interest in various types of sexual activity—for example, coitus, oral–genital sex, and even sexual fantasizing. ISD is the most common reason people seek sexual therapy. People with ISD do not necessarily have some other sexual dysfunction as well. For instance, a man with ISD may not be interested in sexual activity initially but may be able to achieve an erection and have an orgasm once encouraged to participate; or a woman with a lack of interest in sexual activity may be orgasmic once convinced to participate.

As with many sexual dysfunctions, the prevalence of HSDD is difficult to determine. One study found 27% of premenopausal women and 52% of menopausal women experienced HSDD (West et al., 2008). Another reported 10% to 51% of women surveyed worldwide have HSDD (Basson, 2006). In a large-scale study of women's health across the United States, 40% of participants reported that they never or infrequently felt sexual desire (Avis et al., 2005). Men also experience HSDD. One expert reports between 4% and 25% of men experience HSDD (Grant & Potenza, 2006) and another study found 15% do (Rosen, 2000).

Primary ISD is a rare condition in which a person was not interested in sexual activity even as a child to the extent that he or she did not masturbate or fantasize about sexual matters. As adults, these people remain uninterested in sexual activity even if they are in a close relationship and/or married. More prevalent is **secondary ISD**, in which a lack of interest in sexual activity develops after a time of interest. With secondary ISD, lack of interest may be limited to a particular sexual partner or a specific situation. For example, the person may lack interest in sexual activity with the spouse but not with another lover, or in coitus but not in masturbation.

Although people differ in their interest in sexual activity, when one partner experiences inhibited sexual desire, the other partner may become frustrated and even angry. Understanding and seeking treatment is necessary at this point.

Defining ISD is as difficult as defining other sexual dysfunctions. Because each person's interest in sexual activity varies, when is too little interest really too little? When the lack of interest is specific to a sexual partner, is it the partner's fault? As we have stated, sexual interest in a smelly and dirty partner may be a dysfunction. One definition of ISD looks at the number of orgasms experienced in a certain period. Schover and associates (1982) diagnose ISD when the person experiences less than one orgasm every 2 weeks from masturbation or sexual activity with a partner. This definition ignores the fact that some women may be interested in sexual activity but are anorgasmic. In spite of this oversight, and as with several other dysfunctions discussed in this chapter, if the person or the couple does not perceive a sexual problem to exist, perhaps one does not. If the degree of interest between two people in a relationship is similar, and the relationship is otherwise healthy, should therapists advise the couple that they have a problem? Should they attempt to change the couple's degree of interest in sexual activity? Should one person accommodate his or her partner's lack of interest or adopt sexual behaviors to meet the interested person's needs? For example, should an uninterested person engage in oral–genital activity to satisfy the interest of the partner? Does this situation need correcting? These are not easy questions to answer.

The causes of ISD include organic and psychogenic factors. Approximately 10% to 20% of men with ISD have pituitary tumors that cause too much of the hormone prolactin to be produced. Excessive prolactin level reduces the level of testosterone produced and can lead to ISD or erectile dysfunction (Schwartz &

inhibited sexual desire (ISD)
A lack of interest in sexual activity of various sorts; also called *hypoactive sexual disorder (HSD)*.

primary ISD
A condition in which a person has always been uninterested in sexual activity.

secondary ISD
A condition in which a person was at one time interested in sexual activity but is no longer interested.

Multicultural
DIMENSIONS

Sexual Dysfunction and Latino Populations

The Hispanic community, as do all subgroups within the United States, has some unique features that need to be considered regarding sexual dysfunction. Many of these features preclude Latinos from seeking professional help for sexual dysfunction. One of these is the language barrier. Not speaking English, or not speaking it well, means that if a sexual dysfunction arises, the person's ability to communicate the condition may prevent him or her from seeking help.

Hispanics also view the family as an extended one, not distinguishing between the nuclear family and the extended family. Cousins, aunts, uncles, and other family members are assumed to be part of the family, and advice is traditionally sought from family members as opposed to people outside the family, such as health professionals. However, matters of sexual function are considered inappropriate for a family discussion and, therefore, often are ignored.

Hispanics also maintain a sense of fatalism. Expressions such as *que sea lo que Dios quiera* ("it's in God's hands") and *esta enfermedad es una prueba de Dios* ("this illness is a test of God") are examples of this view

of health-related problems. Therefore, a sexual dysfunction might be considered a matter for God, not for a sex therapist.

In addition, Latino communities tend to be male dominated, and that condition may interfere with admitting to a sexual dysfunction. In a project to enroll more children in government-sponsored health insurance programs, one of us found that what works for Anglo families does not work for Hispanic families. In Anglo families, it is the mother who is targeted for improving the health of the family's children. In Hispanic families we found it necessary to influence the fathers first. This is because of the concept of *machismo* (in which males are projected as strong, virile, powerful, and in control), which manifests itself in male-dominated families. Given the need to maintain this sense of machismo, Hispanic males are reluctant to admit a "weakness," especially a sexual dysfunction.

Culturally sensitive approaches are needed in all matters, particularly sexual ones. Sexual dysfunction is no exception.

Source: Perez, M. A., Pinzón, H. L., & Garza, R. D. Latino families: Partners for success in school settings, *Journal of School Health, 67* (1997), 182–184.

Bauman, 1981). However, the majority of ISD cases are the result of such factors as poor self-esteem, a bad relationship, embarrassment regarding one's body, or a history of sexual abuse (Basson, 2006; Empower Health Corporation, 1998). ISD can also develop in response to another sexual dysfunction. For example, a man who has erectile dysfunction may develop ISD. When the thought of or opportunity for sexual activity is present, this man, rather than becoming excited, may envision only a threat to his self-image and, quite naturally, lack interest.

Dissatisfaction with Sexual Activity Frequency

Not everyone is as interested in sex as his or her partner. As we earlier described, a guest speaker in one of our classes characterized this disharmony as only a matter of the mind. To illustrate his point he referred to the way he responds to his spouse's occasional "Leave me alone, I've got a headache" when he is "ready and primed to go." Whereas some men would argue or pout, he usually says, "Where does your head ache?" and proceeds to massage her head and temples, cheeks and neck gently. After a while

he moves to her shoulders and asks, "Does this feel good?" One full body massage later, his spouse's lack of interest has been transformed. Men and women alike can learn to tune into the temporary inhibition, exhaustion, anxiety, or preoccupation that may diminish a partner's sexual interest and learn how that person likes to be treated in such circumstances.

Regardless of the cause, study after study finds men more interested in sexual activity than women (Brecher, 1984; Hicks & Leitenberg, 2001; Leitenberg & Henning, 1995; Mancini & Orthner, 1978; McCarthy, 1989), but that should not lead us to assume that all men or all women are alike. This difference can have a negative effect on other aspects of a relationship. When this disparity in sexual interest is illuminated—that is, when one person feels he or she is pressuring the other or the other feels pressured—the potential for disagreement is evident. The result may be that both partners feel unloved and guilty. Accommodations are possible, however, as when a less interested partner helps his or her lover experience orgasm by oral–genital sexual activity or masturbation. To remedy this problem the couple must

Studies show that males are usually more interested in sexual activity than are women. To resolve these differences, communication is vital for satisfying, long-term sexual relationships to develop.

maintain effective communication rather than avoid it. In some cases, the assistance of a sex therapist may be warranted.

Sexual Aversion

Some people have an irrational fear—a phobia—of sexual activity that leads them to avoid it. That condition is termed **sexual aversion** (Association of Reproductive Health Specialists, 2005). When sexual activity is even imagined, these people may experience a stress reaction: increased heart rate, muscle tension, perspiration, and nausea or diarrhea. Sexual aversion is usually caused by severe negative attitudes toward sexual activity expressed by parents, a history of sexual trauma such as rape or incest (Association of Reproductive Health Professionals, 2005), the constant pressuring by a long-term partner, and/or gender identity confusion in men. Both men and women experience sexual aversion, and the therapy success rate is high for both (Moelker, 2003; Psychiatric Disorders.com, 2008).

sexual aversion
An irrational fear of sexual activity.

Sexual Dysfunction and Self-Esteem

Some of us would like to think that sexual functioning is similar to other physical functioning—or that at least it ought to be considered so. If self-worth does not diminish when our digestive functioning goes haywire, why should we think less of ourselves if our sexual

functioning is problematic? Well, no matter what we would like to think, sexual functioning is more closely connected to self-esteem than are other body processes. Men and women with sexual dysfunctions often feel less masculine or less feminine because they do not function sexually as they want to. Aside from their desire to function sexually for their own satisfaction, the sexually dysfunctional feel they are depriving their partners of satisfaction. Furthermore, they may fear that their partners will seek other sexual partners and/or leave them, fears that further diminish self-esteem. Not surprisingly, the partners of the sexually dysfunctional may also lose some self-esteem. They may feel that the dysfunction is due to their own lack of attractiveness, skill, or attention or that the partner no longer cares for them.

Therapists and counselors have become increasingly sensitive to the matter of self-esteem, of both the person experiencing sexual dysfunction and his or her partner.

■ Causes of Sexual Dysfunction

Sexual dysfunctions can have physical causes, psychological causes, and social causes. To prevent and treat sexual problems, these factors need to be understood.

Physical (Organic) Causes

It was previously believed that approximately 10% to 20% of male sexual dysfunctions were organic. Now we know that, at least for erectile dysfunction, 80% to 90% are the result of organic problems (National Institute of Diabetes and Digestive and Kidney Disorders, 2005). Furthermore, many diseases and a number of drugs can alter sexual response. Erectile dysfunction can result from heart, kidney, and lung disease; from liver disease such as hepatitis, cirrhosis, and mononucleosis; from circulatory and blood vessel problems in which the penile veins allow blood to leak out of the erectile tissue; and from a number of endocrine disorders such as hypothyroidism, Addison's disease, and diabetes. Erectile dysfunction can also result from infections of the urethra or prostate, tuberculosis, mumps, malnutrition, spina bifida, multiple sclerosis, leukemia, sickle-cell disorders, and thrombosis of the veins or arteries of the penis. Ejaculatory disturbances can result from some surgical procedures, such as those for cancer of the prostate. Drugs known to decrease sexual responsiveness include alcohol and barbiturates, which, except in small amounts, are system depressants (Endocrinology Society, 1998). Certain antidepressants cause premature ejaculation. Medications that lower blood pressure also interfere with normal sexual functioning in males. Frequent masturbation does not seem to cause premature ejaculation (Rowland et al., 2000).

Other than interviewing patients and obtaining a medical history, sex therapists have developed some unique ways to determine whether a sexual dysfunction is a result of physiological factors or is predominantly psychological. For example, a therapist who knows that a man with erectile dysfunction caused primarily by psychogenic factors has erections while he sleeps or when he arises in the morning may instruct the client to place a device (plethysmograph) around the penis that measures penile erection. This device graphs erections that occur during sleep (Tower Urology Group, 1998).

A previous sexual trauma, such as child sexual abuse or a rape, can lead to a sexual dysfunction as this event is recalled during sex.

Although sexual dysfunctions in women are most likely the result of nonorganic factors, many of them have physiological causes. For example, sexual unresponsiveness can result from disorders of major organs such as the heart or kidneys; orgasmic dysfunction may be caused by damage to the spine; vaginismus may be a consequence of anatomical or mechanical interference resulting from accident, surgery, or radiation for cervical cancer; and dyspareunia can result from infection of the vagina or allergic reactions. Given the many physical conditions that can cause sexual dysfunction, most sex therapists require that a client have a complete medical examination at the beginning of therapy.

Psychological Causes

Many sexual dysfunctions have no known physiological cause, but rather a psychological basis. Anxiety related to meeting a partner's expectations, guilt about sexual relations or masturbatory behavior, shame about sexual behavior or about one's body, feelings of inferiority, and unconscious fear of castration or injury can all cause sexual dysfunctions. Decreased sexual desire, for example, can be caused by traumatic experiences, such as child sexual abuse, and by depression. Although erectile dysfunction is primarily caused by physiological factors, psychological causes are also at work. Among these are having a domi-

nant, overcontrolling parent who may have caused low self-esteem; having conflicted homosexual feelings; and experiencing stress. Stress leads to an increase in the hormone epinephrine in the blood, which in turn can interfere with erection (of the penis or the clitoris). One researcher of sexual dysfunctions believes this could explain "the effects of performance anxiety" (Buvat et al., 1990).

Snegroff (1986) studied stressors associated with nonmarital sexual intercourse and found that males differed in some of these stressors and not in others. For males, the following were of most concern:

1. Can I satisfy her?
2. Is my penis the right size?
3. Will I achieve and/or maintain an erection?
4. Will she want a commitment?
5. Will I perform well?

For females, the following were of most concern:

1. Can I satisfy him?
2. Will he like my body?
3. Will he respect me afterward?
4. Does he love/care for me?
5. Will I have an orgasm?
6. Are my breasts large enough?

A previous embarrassing sexual encounter in which the inability to be fully functional led to feelings of inadequacy can also lead to sexual dysfunction. Furthermore, orgasmic disorders also have psychological causes. Emotional reactions to one's partner can lead to resentment, shame, jealousy, boredom, or even disgust, which can cause an orgasmic disorder. These may be temporary feelings or, if the relationship experiences long-term disharmony, become permanent.

It is quite understandable that psychological factors can cause someone difficulty in functioning in an effective manner sexually. Is it any wonder that someone who is self-conscious about his or her

Global DIMENSIONS

Sexual Disorders Around the World

The various perspectives and cultural mores of different countries may contribute to the development of sexual disorders, or at least to a diagnosis of a sexual dysfunction. For example, in China and other countries in which homosexuality is considered immoral, homosexuals, thinking every time they engage in sex they are doing something "dirty" and opposed by their society's expectations, might develop a sexual dysfunction. In Islamic countries in which female genital mutilation is customary, women may have hypoactive sexual disorder. On the island of Inis Beag, off the coast of Ireland, it is considered abnormal for women to experience orgasm. Therefore, women on the island engage in sex but prevent orgasm. Are they then experiencing orgasmic dysfunction? When men of Inis Beag attempt to ejaculate quickly so as to make sure their partners do not experience orgasm, are they then to be diagnosed with premature ejaculation?

In contrast, countries that have more relaxed sexual mores and accept a wider array of sexual behavior as "normal" tend to cultivate a sexually healthier population. For example, Sweden and Denmark have low rates of sexual dysfunction and teenage pregnancy. In Polynesian countries, known for encouraging sexual exploration at young ages, embarrassment and anxiety associated with sex are almost nonexistent.

Where you grew up and where you live now can have a tremendous effect on your sexual health. What influenced your sexual health? How?

body might not function well sexually? Imagine just waiting for a partner to laugh or cringe! Anxiety, guilt, and shame are hardly conducive to healthy sexual functioning.

Cultural Causes

Society also influences sexual functioning. For example, the double standard that judges women as less than moral if they actively seek sexual satisfaction can create shame and guilt that, in turn, interfere with normal sexual functioning. Furthermore, if the double standard is interpreted to mean that the male initiates sex and is more expert at it than a female partner, the pressure to behave in this manner can block the male's normal function. However, if females are taught to expect sexual satisfaction in their relationships comparable to that expected by their male partners, they might unintentionally put the onus for their fulfillment on their partners rather than assume that responsibility for themselves. With the onus placed on them, males may succumb to pressure and be unable to function as usual.

The way we perceive sex is also dependent on what our culture has taught us. Someone once said that sex is so "dirty" it should be saved for someone you love. Thinking of sex as dirty can create negative feelings such as embarrassment and guilt, which can result in sexual dysfunction.

Education, such as that to prevent HIV and AIDS, can also affect sexual function. For example, some people believe that premature ejaculation can be a function of men's not using condoms, because intercourse without a condom allows direct skin-to-skin stimulation, leading to premature ejaculation. Thus, with the advent of condom use as a means of preventing HIV and AIDS, it might be expected that fewer cases of premature ejaculation might occur.

Others (Mayo Clinic Staff, 2007c) believe premature ejaculation results from boys' learning by their early teenage years to masturbate. Associated with their masturbatory behavior is guilt that causes them to speed up their orgasm. Having learned to ejaculate rapidly, they have difficulty controlling their ejaculation when they get older.

Religion is also related to sexual function. As one author states: "Rigid adherence to orthodox religious beliefs and practices is a common factor in the backgrounds of men and women with different forms of sexual dysfunction. Strict religious teaching—regardless of the particular religion—often results in negative attitudes toward sexuality. Individuals come to believe that sex is sinful" (Wilson et al., 1996, 241). Of course, not all people who hold such religious beliefs develop a sexual problem, and these beliefs often influence behaviors in a healthy manner. Still, Masters and Johnson (1970) and other sex therapists have concluded that, in fact, strong religious beliefs increase the likelihood that a person who has those beliefs will experience sexual dysfunction.

Another significant cause of sexual dysfunction is related to a lack of information about sexual functioning—for example, not knowing or forgetting that foreplay is necessary to lubricate the vagina before penile entry. Other possible causes are nonsexual problems between sexual partners, ineffective communication (about sex and other matters), and traumatic past sexual experiences (for example, rape). Thus sexual unresponsiveness might, for instance, be caused by an inexperienced, inept, hasty, or insensitive lover; by situational factors, such as thoughts of a sick relative or deep-seated career concerns; or by sexual relations with impotent men.

Sexual Dysfunction and Aging

Elders have given up sex and have debilitating sexual dysfunctions—at least that is the prevailing myth. What is the truth?

In a survey commissioned by the National Council on the Aging (1998), 1,300 Americans 60 years of age and older were asked about their sex lives. The results go a long way toward eliminating the stereotype that elders have put sex aside to care for back pain, financial portfolios, or life in a nursing home. Here are the results:

- Nearly half of the elders surveyed reported engaging in sexual activity at least once a month.

- As people aged they engaged in sex less frequently; still, 57% of men and 30% of women in their 70s reported being sexually active.

- Of those questioned, 74% of male respondents and 70% of female respondents said they were as satisfied or more satisfied with their sex life now than when they were in their 40s.

A more recent study verified that sex continues well into people's advanced years (Lindau et al., 2007). Table 16.5 highlights the findings from this study.

In summarizing the results of the National Council on the Aging survey, James Firman, president and chief executive officer of the group, stated: "Our study debunks the prevailing myth about sexuality in older years. For many Americans, sex remains an important and vital part of their lives."

An alternative, and more humorous, way of looking at these results is the comment an elder made to a sexuality expert: "Look, everything we do may be slower, but we have more time."

■ Treating Sexual Dysfunction

In the past few decades many highly effective therapeutic approaches to sexual dysfunction have emerged (although love and concern

Although the elderly are often perceived as asexual, that is far from the truth. Almost half of adults 60 years of age and older report engaging in sexual activity at least once a month.

between partners are still important). Because the effectiveness of the various therapeutic approaches is well publicized, not only do more sufferers seek treatment—a positive step—but more people want to become sex therapists. As might be expected in a field that is emerging, charlatans and quacks, in

TABLE 16.2 **Percentage of Older Adults Engaging in Sexual Activity in the Previous 12 Months**

Sexual Activity	Age		
	57–64	65–74	75–85
Sexual Activity with a Partner			
Men	84	67	39
Women	62	40	17
Vaginal Intercourse (Usually or Always)			
Men	91	79	84
Women	87	85	74
Oral Sex			
Men	62	48	28
Women	53	47	35
Masturbation			
Men	63	53	28
Women	32	22	16

Source: Lindau, S. T., Schumm, L. P., Laumann, E. O., Levinson, W., O'Muircheartaigh, C. A., & Waite, L. J. A study of sexuality and health among older adults in the United States. *New England Journal of Medicine, 357* (2007), 762–774.

addition to well-trained professionals, have set up practice. Therefore, anyone experiencing sexual problems would be well advised to investigate the training and experience of a sex therapist carefully before seeking that person's services. To help people select a professional therapist, the American Association of Sex Educators, Counselors, and Therapists (AASECT) has made public its requirements for certifying individuals as sex counselors or sex therapists. AASECT has also published a code of ethics. This code provides guidance for sex counselors and sex therapists, as well as for patients. Counselors and therapists whose behavior is inconsistent with this code may be incompetent and/or unethical.

Generally, sexual therapy for both men and women entails three components, regardless of the number and type of therapists involved: (1) an initial period of abstinence from coitus to reduce anxiety and facilitate communication; (2) the use of systematic tactile stimulation and exploration to focus on the giving and receiving of pleasure, rather than on the exclusive goal of orgasm; and (3) specific technical suggestions and direction, including sequences and variations on those techniques that facilitate and reinforce success.

Usually the couple is first seen together by the therapist or therapists. Then they are interviewed separately so they will feel free to discuss matters with the therapist that they might not yet feel comfortable discussing with their partner. Once

the nature of the problem is identified, instruction and/or counseling can begin, following the sequence outlined earlier. Usually the couple is at first instructed to abstain from sexual intercourse and to learn how to experience pleasure in non-genital touching. Then genital fondling is allowed, and eventually coitus. The touching and coitus are private, away from the therapist's office, without the therapist present or in a room with one-way mirrors. Although it is rare, sometimes a *surrogate,* or substitute, partner is used to provide instruction, practice, and feedback for someone with a sexual problem. The use of sexual surrogates is highly controversial, both within the profession and among the public.

Approaches to Sexual Therapy

Several models of sexual therapy have been proposed. Perhaps a good place to begin a discussion of these models is first to consider a stepwise approach to sexual therapy.

The PLISSIT Model
Jack Annon (1976) suggested that relatively minor treatment may be effective for some sexual dysfunctions, whereas more intensive treatment may be required for others. Annon's model of sexual therapy is known as the **PLISSIT** model (an acronym of *P*ermission, *L*imited

Ethical DIMENSIONS

Should Surrogates Be Used in Sexual Therapy?

Early on, some therapists believed that the use of a substitute sexual partner was a vital and necessary component of sexual therapy. This substitute, or surrogate, was an experienced and trained sexual partner who could teach the sexually dysfunctional client effective sexual arousal techniques. Further, the surrogate let the client practice these techniques in a nonthreatening situation, because the surrogate was not a person with whom the client had a relationship or whom the client would ever see again. Advocates of the use of surrogates believed the therapy to be more effective if the client practiced on and received feedback from a real person.

Those opposed to surrogates usually based their arguments on one of two premises—either that sexual activity between people not married to each other is im-

moral or that the knowledge, skills, and attitudes learned with a surrogate are not readily transferred to one's usual sexual partner. A client's ability to function well with a surrogate does not ensure ability to function well with the usual sexual partner. Those arguing this position believed that sexual dysfunction is a problem between sexual partners and, therefore, needs to be worked out by both partners. Because the couple would have to practice sexually arousing techniques anyhow, why not practice them together from the outset of the therapy? And, finally, some people believed a surrogate was akin to a prostitute. Those employing such a method, therefore, should be subject to criminal prosecution.

Do you think surrogates should be used in sexual therapy? Why or why not?

PLISSIT
A model of sexual therapy that consists of moving through the stages of giving permission, limited information, specific suggestion, and, if that does not work, intensive therapy.

*I*nformation, *S*pecific *S*uggestion, and *I*ntensive *T*herapy). This model extends from the simplest to the more advanced levels of treatment.

During the permission stage the therapist helps people accept their fantasies and desires and, where appropriate, even gives them permission *not* to engage in sexual intercourse until they are ready to do so. The therapist helps couples not to compare themselves with other couples or with an idealized sexual relationship.

During the limited information stage the therapist provides the factual information that may help the person become more functional sexually. For example, a person may not realize it is natural to fantasize about sexual activity or perceive it as a natural part of one's life. Information can give clients a more realistic perception, thereby removing an impediment to their sexual functioning. Other kinds of information, such as information about penis size and its limited effect on sexual satisfaction, clitoral sensitivity, or proper hygiene, may be all that is needed to help people overcome their sexual dysfunctions.

Specific suggestion is the level of therapy at which the therapist actually recommends activities for the clients. For example, self-stimulation, sensate focus, and the squeeze technique may be suggested. Many of these techniques were developed by Masters and Johnson (1970) but have since been modified by other sexual therapists. These techniques can help the person reduce sexual anxiety, improve communication between partners, or enhance arousal.

Intensive therapy may be required when permission, limited information, and specific suggestion are not successful in resolving a sexual problem. Intensive therapy entails a longer-term therapeutic treatment that identifies the deep-seated reasons that interfere with sexual functioning. This therapy has been called *psychosexual therapy* (Kaplan, 1974). Some therapists believe sexual dysfunction is caused by guilt or shame about sex, which leads to sexual anxiety, and the best treatment is intensive therapy to uncover the causes of these feelings.

The Masters and Johnson Model

William Masters and Virginia Johnson present a model of sexual therapy with several unique components. First, they believe that sexual problems are relationship problems, and, therefore, therapy works only with couples. Even seemingly healthy partners can learn how to respond and contribute better to their partner's response through sexual

Myth (vs) Fact

Myth: Sexual dysfunctions occur because someone either has been sexually abused or raped or has masturbated too often.
Fact: It is true that sexual abuse, such as rape and child abuse, can contribute to the development of a sexual dysfunction. Yet, there are many people who experience those traumatic events and never develop a sexual dysfunction. Regarding masturbation, there is no evidence that the frequency of masturbation is in any way related to the subsequent development of a sexual dysfunction.

Myth: Guys who "can't get it up" are not real men.
Fact: Most cases of erectile dysfunction are caused by physiological problems. To classify these men as less than real men is analogous to characterizing any man who has any physical illness as not a real man. The inability to achieve and maintain an erection is in no way related to manliness.

Myth: Women are not naturally interested in sex, so a woman who cannot be sexually aroused is quite normal.
Fact: Males and females have a natural interest in and capacity for sex. When they do not, they are exhibiting a sexual dysfunction termed *inhibited sexual desire* and should seek professional help to treat this condition.

therapy. Second, they believe if couples are to be treated, the therapy team should be a couple—that is, a male and a female therapist. They believe that such a team can best appreciate the perspectives and best represent the couple in therapy. In addition, Masters and Johnson feel that clients can better identify with the therapist of the same gender, who may understand them better. Third, clients are medically screened for any potential organic causes of their dysfunction and given a complete psychological evaluation. Finally, treatment at the Masters and Johnson Institute is intensive; couples are seen every day for a 2-week period. This means that the couple must live near the institute, and there is significant expense. Masters and Johnson argue that this intensive interaction between the therapists and the clients is necessary initially to reduce anxiety and help the couple concentrate on overcoming the sexual problem.

Kaplan's Model

Kaplan (1974, 1979, 1983) employs many of the specific techniques of sexual therapy recommended by Masters and Johnson. However, Kaplan believes more intensive therapy is required to uncover the reasons for the sexual anxiety that interferes with normal sexual functioning. Kaplan's triphasic model consists of desire, arousal, and orgasm phases. Desire phase problems are the most difficult to treat because of their association with deep-seated psychological difficulties.

Myth (vs) Fact

Myth: Treatment for sexual dysfunctions must entail counseling over the long term to be successful.

Fact: Treatments for sexual dysfunctions vary, depending on the nature of the particular dysfunction and the people involved. In many cases, the cause is a physical one, and medications can successfully treat it. In other cases, all that is needed is to educate the couple about effective techniques of sexual arousal. In relatively few cases is long-term counseling necessary.

Myth: Any couple who are not engaging in sexual activities frequently enough, with enough variety, and with orgasm have a sexual dysfunction for which they should seek sexual counseling.

Fact: Some experts believe that, for a sexual dysfunction to exist, one or both of the sexual partners must be dissatisfied with the sexual relationship. If both partners are satisfied, regardless of the nature of their sexual relationship, no sexual dysfunction exists.

Consequently, Kaplan recommends a longer period of sexual therapy to uncover the unconscious rationale for behavior and thought. Kaplan believes that sexual dysfunctions have their roots in multiple causes, some readily accessible and others requiring more intensive therapy to determine them. In addition, Kaplan treats premature ejaculation with the stop–start technique developed by James Semans (1956) rather than the squeeze technique developed by Masters and Johnson. Both the squeeze and the stop–start technique are described later in this chapter.

Other Approaches to Sexual Therapy

There are many other ways in which therapists treat sexual dysfunctions. For example, some behaviorists (LoPiccolo, 1977; Leiblum & Pervin, 1980) believe most sexual problems are learned and can be unlearned. Behaviorists use positive and negative reinforcement to encourage healthy behaviors and use gradual approaches to problematic sexual behavior. This latter approach is based on the early work of Joseph Wolpe (1958), who argued that one could not be anxious and relaxed at the same time. Consequently, Wolpe taught his clients deep muscle relaxation (for example, meditation) and gradually, over time, introduced more and more components of the anxiety-producing behavior. The sensate focus activity described later in this chapter is an example of Wolpe's desensitization technique.

Barbach (1980, 2000, 2001) organized groups of women to treat sexual dysfunction, in particular, orgasmic dysfunction and sexual unresponsiveness. Barbach's methods include exercises for the woman to do for herself. These exercises are also described later in the chapter.

Ellis and Harper (1975, 1979) developed a therapy model called *rational emotive therapy*. This model is based on the assumption that much of our behavior is a result of our thoughts and interpretations. Sexual problems arise from (irrational) thoughts and interpretations, and these problems can be treated by helping people recognize their irrationality and change these thoughts and interpretations into more rational ones.

Barry McCarthy believes that in the great majority of cases the sexual problem stems from a lack of knowledge, from communication problems, or from psychological difficulties. Consequently he views psychologists, social workers, marriage counselors, and ministers as better suited to working with such patients than physicians. In McCarthy et al.'s (1975) model of sexual therapy, a single therapist sees both sexual partners once a week, sometimes together, sometimes apart. This therapist is not a physician. Because a physical examination is a prerequisite to acceptance in the program, McCarthy considers a physician's skills unnecessary during therapy.

Treating Erectile Dysfunction

There are many effective ways to treat problems related to achieving and maintaining an erection. Because approximately 80% to 90% of cases of erectile dysfunction are caused by physical problems, medical scientists have successfully researched ways to counteract these physical limitations. These remedies include several different medications. A British researcher found a novel way to demonstrate the effectiveness of one of them. At a conference of urologists in Las Vegas in 1983, he presented a paper on the effectiveness of one of the medications and, in the middle of his presentation, stood up to show off his own erection, which he had induced with this drug. Urologists who began using the drug with their patients found it highly effective.

Some of these medications are injected into the penis and so are called *injection therapy* (men report only minimal pain). Until recently, the most commonly used injectable drugs were papaverine (brand name Pavabid or Cerespan) and phentolamine (brand name Regitine). Recently, however, another drug, alprostadil (brand name Caverject or Edex) has been used in injection therapy for erectile dysfunction and found to be even more effective (NIDUS Information Service, 1998). Alprostadil is usually sold in a six-dose kit that costs between $110 and $140. Erection occurs within 20 minutes of injection and lasts approximately an hour. An alternative way of administering alprostadil is by inserting a tube into the urethral opening and pressing a button that releases a pellet containing the drug.

One need not go through such an ordeal, however. Oral medications have been found to be effec-

The former Senator Bob Dole decided in 1999 to do what he called a "public service announcement" sponsored by Pfizer, makers of Viagra. The ad addressed the subject of erectile dysfunction but did not directly endorse Viagra. Dole struggled with the decision to make the ad until he "thought about the 30 million men who live with this problem and are afraid to talk about it, and [then] it was easy for me to make up my mind."

tive in treating erectile dysfunction. Although limited to men with hypogonadism (in which the testes do not produce sufficient amounts of testosterone), testosterone therapy has been used. More common has been the use of the drug yohimbine, which seems to improve blood flow to the penis.

Since 1997, excitement and a great deal of publicity have been focused on another drug, Viagra (sildenafil citrate). Viagra increases the level of cyclic guanosine monophosphate (GMP), a chemical that is produced in the penis during sexual activity and whose function is to increase blood flow. Viagra is highly effective against erectile dysfunction, up to 70% to 97%, depending on the study, and when it is taken as prescribed, it is very safe (Nagao et al., 2004; Natali et al., 2009; Toshiyasu et al., 2009). Although a few deaths of men who have used Viagra were reported, they were predominantly men who had cardiac disorders and used nitrate heart medications. Viagra is taken orally approximately an hour before sex but not more than once daily (National Library of Medicine, 2005a). It is not effective for men who experience inhibited sexual desire or no desire for their partners; desire must be present for Viagra to work.

Although it was suspected that Viagra would help women who experienced sexual dysfunction as it helped men (Women, too, may benefit from Viagra, 2000), that hope has not been realized for large numbers of women. However, the profit made from Viagra, Cialis, and Levitra has spurred research into medications that may help women who experience sexual dysfunction. Viagra-like drugs work by increasing blood flow to the penis; they are for men whose erectile dysfunction is a direct result of a physical problem. These medications can work for the 20% of women reported to have difficulties with vaginal lubrication, but are of little help for those women with other sexual dysfunctions (Gearon, 2005).

An interesting "side effect" of Viagra may benefit women in an unforeseen way. Because Viagra is covered by some insurance companies and considered a medical treatment for a valid medical condition, health insurance companies were lobbied to treat women in the same manner by including contraceptive services as a covered benefit. Such prestigious organizations as the American Medical Association and the American College of Gynecologists and Obstetricians organized efforts to influence legislation that would require health insurance companies to include contraceptive pills as a covered benefit, as they do with other prescription drugs. As of 2002, 89% of insurance plans covered contraception (Sonfield et al., 2004).

Since the success of Viagra, two other medications for erectile dysfunction have been developed and approved as competitors. Cialis (tadalafil), for example, increases blood flow to the penis. Cialis pills are ingested prior to intercourse, and effects can last up to 36 hours (National Library of Medicine, 2005b). Levitra (vardenafil) is the other drug developed that competes with Viagra (National Library of Medicine, 2005c). It is taken 1 hour before sexual intercourse.

As with all medications, side effects are possible, as are interactions with other medications. Consequently, consultation with a physician is required before these medications are taken. Recently, the Food and Drug Administration reported 43 cases of sudden blindness (non-arteritic anterior ischemic optic neuropathy) in men using erectile dysfunction medications (Kaufman, 2005). As a result, the FDA issued an alert for Viagra, Cialis, and Levitra users and their prescribing physicians to be on the lookout for this condition. The FDA identified men at greater risk of sudden blindness to be older than 50 years of age who use tobacco products and have high blood pressure, high blood cholesterol, or heart disease.

Another approach to organically caused erectile dysfunction is *bypass surgery*. When blood vessels that usually route blood to fill the cavernous bodies in the penis are blocked, surgeons can graft a blood vessel from another part of the body to bypass the blocked vessel, thereby allowing blood to flow into the cavernous bodies and make erection possible. However, very few men are candidates for this procedure, which is still considered experimental and has a high failure rate.

Sometimes the problem is not blood flowing into the cavernous bodies but blood leaking out (venous leakage). In this case, *venous ligation,* a surgical procedure that repairs the veins, can be employed. The problem with venous ligation, however, is that it is usually only a temporary remedy, and subsequent surgery is often required within a few years.

When erectile dysfunctions have irreversible physical causes, it is possible to treat them by implanting *penile prostheses,* commonly called *penile implants.* Approximately 200,000 of these devices were implanted in American men between 1982 and 1989 (NIDUS Information Services, 1998). Despite the continuing development of other therapies to treat erectile dysfunction, the number of penile prostheses implanted has actually increased each year (Mulcahy, 2008). There are three types of penile prostheses: semirigid rods, multicomponent inflatable implants, and self-contained inflatable implants. *Semirigid rods* contain stainless steel wires or plastic joints held together by a cable and coated with silicone. Two bendable rods are implanted in the corpus cavernosum, with the result that the penis is always erect (but it can be bent down).

Multicomponent inflatable implants involve placing an inflatable cylinder in the corpora, a fluid reservoir in the abdomen, and a pump in the scrotum. In preparation for intercourse, the male merely squeezes the pump, thereby moving fluid from the reservoir to the cylinders, causing the penis to become erect. When intercourse is completed, the male squeezes the pump release valve to move the fluid from the cylinder back to the reservoir.

Self-contained inflatable implants consist of two cylinders implanted in the penis, each containing a pump, fluid, and a release valve. When planning for intercourse, the male squeezes the penis glans, forcing fluid to move to the forward chamber, resulting in erection. At completion of coitus, the penis is slightly bent, causing the return of fluid to the storage area and a loss of erection.

Vacuum devices have also been successfully employed to treat erectile dysfunction. When the penis is placed in a plastic cylinder and a vacuum is created, causing blood to flow into the penis, an erection occurs. Once erection appears, a band is placed snugly around the base of the penis to maintain the erection. Although this seems "unnatural," it is very effective when the psychological barriers are overcome. One note of caution: To prevent injury to the penis, only a medically approved device should be used, not one sold in sexual paraphernalia catalogues or magazines.

Many erectile dysfunctions do not have physical causes. These conditions are treated with counseling and several techniques described later in this section.

Treating Premature Ejaculation

Two techniques are used to help men control premature ejaculation. The first is the **squeeze technique**, developed by Masters and Johnson (Figure 16.2), which entails a gentle squeezing of the penis while the man is experiencing full erection. When the man begins to feel the urge to ejaculate, the partner grasps the penis with the thumb on the underside where the shaft ends and the head begins and two fingers on the opposite side. The partner then squeezes for 3 to 4 seconds, after which the urge to ejaculate will have passed. After 15 to 30 seconds, stimulation is provided to full erection once more and the procedure is repeated as necessary. Eventually the man learns to control his ejaculation without his partner's help.

The second technique for learning ejaculatory control is called the **Semans stop–start method**, named for its developer, James Semans. The man lies on his back and concentrates on his feelings and sensations as his partner stimulates his penis manually (Figure 16.3). When he feels ejaculation approaching, he tells his partner to stop stimulating him. The couple repeats the procedure until the man learns ejaculatory control.

However, other remedies also exist. For example, changing the tempo of thrusting may result in decreased stimulation. Also, changing the angle or depth of penetration may help. Shifting one's thoughts to other events, talking to oneself ("self-talk"), and focusing on the nongenital aspects of the experience can all be of help in control-

squeeze technique
A method of helping men control premature ejaculation whereby the penis is gently squeezed when the man senses ejaculation is imminent.

Semans stop–start method
A method of controlling premature ejaculation (developed by James Semans) in which the man tells his partner to stop stimulating him when he feels ejaculation approaching.

FIGURE **16.2** The squeeze technique. The man signals his partner to squeeze when ejaculation is approaching.

FIGURE **16.3** The Semans procedure. The man signals his partner to stop stimulation when he senses that ejaculation is close.

ling ejaculation. Finally, some antidepressant medications, such as Prozac and Anafranil, have been found to control premature ejaculation (Mayo Clinic Staff, 2007; University of Toronto Sexual Education Centre, 1998).

Treating Retarded Ejaculation

The therapy for retarded ejaculation includes the technique known as sensate focus (described in the next paragraph), which helps the man focus on his sensual feelings and learn to derive pleasure from sexual behavior. Included in this treatment, in a stepwise fashion, is learning to ejaculate by masturbating alone, by masturbating with his sexual partner present, by asking the partner to masturbate him to ejaculation, and by asking the partner to masturbate him to the point just short of ejaculation and then inserting the penis into the vagina to ejaculate.

Sensate Focus

Sexual therapists treat sexual unresponsiveness in both men and women by teaching the couple a technique termed **sensate focus**. The idea behind this method is to encourage the man and woman to experience erotic feelings short of intercourse

> **sensate focus**
> A method of alleviating sexual unresponsiveness by procedures designed to encourage erotic feelings and sexual pleasuring.

so that they will learn to accept sexual pleasuring (both giving and receiving) as part of their lives. The therapist gives the unresponsive partner permission and encouragement to feel nonthreatening sexual feelings, on the assumption that the client has withheld permission from himself or herself (for whatever individual subconscious reason). Eventually the therapy incorporates coitus into the sensate focus program. Figure 16.4 illustrates one of the sensate-focusing positions taught to couples.

FIGURE **16.4** Sensate focus allows for nondemanding stimulation.

Barbach's Technique

Barbach's technique, effective in treating both sexual unresponsiveness and orgasmic dysfunction in women, has been widely disseminated to the general public through Lonnie Barbach's book *For Yourself: The Fulfillment of Female Sexuality* (2000). A woman begins the program by setting aside an hour a day for exploring her body visually (with a mirror) and manually (using body lotion or powder), all the time focusing upon feelings and sensations. Next she is led to do a vulva self-examination and vulva self-stimulation with a body lotion or oil. It is important at this stage that orgasm *not* be the goal of the self-stimulation. Rather the woman is encouraged to become aware of and focus on pleasurable sensations. Eventually the program leads the woman to seek orgasm by using the touching technique she found to be most pleasurable during the self-stimulation stage. The use of a vibrator is recommended for women who still find orgasm elusive after manual stimulation. However, after the woman experiences orgasm with a vibrator, she is encouraged to practice manual stimulation. This transfer is important in helping her to have orgasm with a sexual partner.

> **Barbach's technique**
> A method of treating orgasmic dysfunction and sexual unresponsiveness developed by Lonnie Barbach that focuses on awareness of feelings and sensations through self-exploration and stimulation.

Combating Vaginismus and Dyspareunia

Vaginismus and dyspareunia are treated by a combination of education and practice. The education component entails instruction about the anatomy and physiology of the human sexual response and reproductive systems. Once it is understood that the problem stems from contraction of the muscles of the vagina that prevents penile penetration, training to control these muscles can begin. The best manner in which to carry out this training appears to be teaching the woman to contract and relax the muscles, becoming conscious of the sensations that accompany both contracted and relaxed vaginal muscles. Next slender rods—first a very narrow one and eventually wider ones—are inserted by the woman into the vagina with relaxed muscles. Once this is mastered (about 1 week), the next step is coitus, when the woman controls inserting the penis.

Dyspareunia, when not caused by physical problems, tends to stem from insufficient vaginal lubrication. In such cases the treatment is similar to that described for sexual unresponsiveness (that is, sensate focus).

Behavior Therapy Model

As stated previously, Joseph Wolpe developed a manner of treating anxiety as the cause of sexual dysfunction. Termed **systematic desensitization**, this model can be applied to people who are anxious about sex. Wolpe reasoned that if people were muscularly relaxed, they could not be anxious at the same time. Consequently, he taught people deep muscle relaxation techniques and then instructed them to think of the anxiety-provoking stimulus. For example, sexually dysfunctional patients might imagine their arms and legs are heavy, warm, and tingly (a relaxation technique called *autogenic training*). Once relaxed, they could imagine the sexual activity about which they feel anxious.

> **systematic desensitization**
> A means of overcoming anxiety by approaching the anxiety-provoking stimulus in small steps.

Systematic desensitization also assumes that the gradual introduction of anxiety-provoking stimuli will not produce anxious feelings. Thus this technique involves a fear hierarchy: The initial stimuli are not anxiety provoking, but very gradually more anxiety-provoking stimuli are introduced. For example, the following might be the fear hierarchy of a married woman (Ted's wife) who experiences vaginismus:

1. I go out to a movie with Ted.
2. Ted and I return home and are alone.
3. Ted places his arm around me.
4. Ted nuzzles my neck.
5. Ted fondles my breast.
6. Ted takes my clothes off.
7. Ted removes his clothing.
8. Ted stimulates my clitoris and vagina.
9. Ted inserts his finger into my vagina.
10. Ted inserts his penis into my vagina.

The woman is then asked to imagine the first event in the fear hierarchy without feeling anxious—that is, without an increasing heart rate and rapid, shallow breathing. If she can imagine that event for 30 seconds without feeling anxious, she does deep muscle relaxation for 30 seconds. Then she moves to the next event of the hierarchy. The idea is to take very small steps from something that does not make her anxious to the point at which she is involved in the activity that was the problem (in the example, allowing penile insertion) (Greenberg, 2009).

Behaviorists are concerned with the behavior in question, not the underlying reasons for that behavior. They do not spend a great deal of time analyzing why someone feels or thinks as he or she does. Rather, they begin to manipulate the behavior so it is transformed into the desired behavior. To do this, therapists sometimes employ a technique called *shaping*. Shaping involves rewarding small behaviors along the way to developing the behavior that is the goal of the therapy. For example, if a person becomes anxious on dates and, therefore, refuses to accept a date, the therapist might have the person begin by just speaking to a love interest on the telephone. For doing that, he or she would receive a reward (for example, maybe a pass to a movie theater). To receive a reward the next week, however, the patient needs to spend a few minutes in face-to-face contact with that other person—and so on, until the patient goes out on a date without anxiety.

Self-Care Model

Several of the models and techniques of sexual therapy can be self-administered. For example, couples can employ the stop–start technique or the squeeze technique, and individuals can try systematic desensitization or shaping by themselves. They will thereby save some money and whatever inconvenience is associated with attending therapy. A good first step to solving problems associated with sexual functioning, given that any medical cause has been ruled out, is to employ these self-care techniques. If they are not successful, the person should consider seeking the help of a trained sex counselor or therapist. Often the trained eye can observe something that the untrained cannot.

Other Kinds of Therapy

There are other kinds of therapy that treat sexual dysfunction. However, forms of therapy and counseling that are not focused particularly on sexual response can also help people with sexual dysfunctions, especially when conditions are rooted in a more generalized lack of self-acceptance and self-esteem. Also beneficial in some cases is counseling or therapy directed toward improving communication in the nonsexual aspects of a relationship—for example, marriage counseling, family counseling, or crisis counseling for couples.

If you experience any of the sexual dysfunctions described in this chapter, you may want to ask your instructor or student-health service personnel for a referral to a qualified sex therapist. Paying attention to your sexual responsiveness is part of maintaining total well-being. A dysfunction in the sexual aspect of your life requires the same concern and treatment as any other chronic ailment. We are fortunate to live in a time when effective sexual therapy based on sound scientific research is generally available.

Choosing a Sex Therapist

For sex therapy to be effective, the therapist must be qualified. How can you determine this? Someone who claims to be a sex therapist is not necessarily competent in that particular area of expertise. To enhance your chances of choosing a qualified sex therapist, consider the following points:

1. *Does this person have a degree in a recognized profession related to counseling and therapy?* Psychology, marriage and family counseling, pastoral counseling, and social work are examples.

2. *Does this person hold a license or a certification related to counseling and therapy?* Some professions are licensed by the state (psychologists), whereas others are certified by professional organizations (for example, marriage counselors).

3. *Is this person certified by the American Association of Sex Educators, Counselors, and Therapists (AASECT)?* Certification by this professional organization attests to the training specific to sexuality issues the person has had.

4. *Do you know other people who have been helped by this therapist?* Sometimes the best referral is that of someone who has experienced therapy and benefited from it.

To begin choosing a sex therapist, consult local resources. A local hospital might be a good beginning. Perhaps the local medical association can make a referral. The psychology, counseling, social work, or health education department at your university might be able to help, as might your campus health center. Alternatively, you could contact AASECT for a referral in your area.

When first meeting the therapist, or talking with office personnel on the telephone, do not hesitate to inquire about the fee, the therapist's background and qualifications, the licenses and/or certifications the therapist holds, and the usual course of therapy provided for situations such as yours (length of treatment, type of treatment, and so on). Any therapist who objects to your asking these questions should be considered suspect. Reputable therapists should be glad that you are taking such an active interest in obtaining effective treatment. That sort of motivation is critical for a successful outcome.

Exploring the
DIMENSIONS
of Human Sexuality

Our feelings, attitudes, and beliefs regarding sexuality are influenced by our internal and external environments. Go to sexuality.jbpub.com/dimensions/4e to learn more about the biological, psychological, and sociological factors that affect your sexuality.

Biological Factors

- Some sexual dysfunctions, including 80% to 90% of erectile disorder cases, are of a physiological nature. Age is sometimes a factor, as normal changes in the human body affect sexual desire and arousal.
- Alcohol, drug abuse, and certain medications (e.g., for hypertension) can interfere with sexual response.

Sociocultural Factors

- The sexual double standard suggests that men be experienced and talented in sexual matters, leading their partners to sexual bliss. Failure to live up to such expectations can lead to psychological problems.
- Mass media create unrealistic sexual expectations that no real person can meet.
- Relationship problems can lead to some disorders.
- Rigid religious convictions that certain sexual activities are immoral may lead to negative attitudes toward sexuality.
- Masters and Johnson asserted that "sociocultural deprivation and ignorance of sexual physiology, rather than psychiatric or medical illness," were the source of most sexual dysfunction.

Psychological Factors

- Sexual functioning is closely connected to self-esteem. Men and women with sexual dysfunctions often feel less masculine or feminine because they do not function as well sexually as they wish. Low self-esteem, guilt, or depression can lead to some sexual disorders.
- Gays seeking treatment for disorders must also confront society's negative attitudes about homosexuality.
- Failure to perform as expected can be devastating psychologically. In turn, such perceived failure would likely lead to isolation from sexual activities, which would cause further embarrassment. Fear of future sexual inadequacy can create a self-fulfilling prophecy that can result in lowered self-esteem.

CASE STUDY

Many of the sexual disorders are multidimensional. In fact, at different times, there can be different causes. Consider an otherwise healthy male who, after getting too little sleep during the week and ingesting too much alcohol, is unable to achieve and maintain an erection through intercourse. The dysfunction here is likely physiological. If he understands that alcohol and lack of sleep are to blame, he will probably be fine. However, if he perceives that he "failed" sexually, he may suffer from performance anxiety during his next sexual encounter.

Partners, too, may blame themselves for sexual dysfunction. When partners call into question their attractiveness or sexual ability, their self-esteem may suffer. Further, they may isolate themselves from sexual situations so as not to "cause" failure again.

Both sexuality education and communication can help couples avoid sexual anxiety. The former would help both partners realize why the initial dysfunction occurred. And communication could help both partners' self-esteem, by letting the other person know that he or she is desired.

Summary

- An individual's sexual desire is not constant; it varies according to situational, emotional, and physical factors. Sexual dysfunction is a *chronic* inability to respond sexually in a way one finds satisfying.

- Primary sexual dysfunctions are those in which the person has never been functional in a sexual activity. Secondary sexual dysfunctions are those in which the person was functional at one time but no longer is.

- Male sexual dysfunctions include erectile dysfunction (inability to achieve an erection), premature ejaculation (not maintaining penile insertion long enough before ejaculating), ejaculatory incompetence (inability to ejaculate in the vagina), and dyspareunia (genital pain during coitus).

- Female sexual dysfunctions include sexual unresponsiveness (not experiencing erotic pleasure from sexual stimulation), orgasmic dysfunction (inability to have an orgasm during sexual activities), and vaginismus (the involuntary contraction of the outer walls of the vagina, preventing penetration).

- Both males and females may experience sexual desire dysfunctions in which they have a lack of interest in sexual activities. Among sexual desire dysfunctions are inhibited sexual desire, referred to as hypoactive sexual desire disorder (HSDD). HSDD includes a lack of appetite for various types of sexual activities, dissatisfaction with sexual frequency, and sexual aversion (an irrational fear of sexual activity that leads to avoiding these activities).

- Sexual dysfunctions can have physical causes such as diseases, malnutrition, medications, or blocked blood vessels. They may also be caused by psychological factors such as low self-esteem, guilt and shame, past sexual abuse, or performance anxiety.

- Generally, sexual therapy entails three components: (1) an initial period of abstinence from coitus to reduce anxiety and facilitate communication, (2) the use of systematic tactile stimulation and exploration to focus on the giving and receiving of pleasure, and (3) specific technical suggestions and directions that facilitate and reinforce success.

- Among the approaches to treat sexual dysfunctions are the PLISSIT model, teams of cotherapists, the squeeze technique, the stop–start method, sensate focus, surgery, and medication.

Discussion Questions

1. Review the major male and female sexual dysfunctions, including features of diagnosis. What determines what a typical person might consider a sexual problem and what a sexual therapist diagnoses as a sexual dysfunction?

2. List the specific physical, psychological, and sociocultural dimensions that can affect sexual performance. Explain how each could have an effect. (Be specific: Religion is a factor, but state the specific religion. Would it affect all members of that religion or only specific people with a high degree of religious fervor?)

3. Examine the many types of sexual therapy available. Then evaluate which you think would work best for erectile disorder, vaginismus, and inhibited sexual desire dysfunction. Explain your answer.

Application Questions

Reread the chapter-opening story and answer the following questions.

1. Explain why when a celebrity or a politician discloses a personal problem, it seems easier for the general public to talk about the issue involved. Contrast that with how you might react if a classmate announced in class that he or she had a sexual dysfunction.

2. We know that Elizabeth Dole smiled when asked about Viagra. But if she had been asked about her sex life with Bob before his disclosure, how might she have reacted? Would she have revealed his "dysfunction" (related to prostate-cancer surgery)? If Viagra had not been developed, would either Bob or Elizabeth have realized that there was a dysfunction?

Critical Thinking Questions

1. Masters and Johnson claimed that male and female cotherapists were needed to treat a couple. They reasoned that only a person of the same gender as the client could really understand a sexual problem or dysfunction. Do you agree with Masters and Johnson, or could a couple be successfully treated by one therapist (of either gender)? Explain your answer.

2. The success of the drug Viagra was unprecedented: 36,000 prescriptions in the first week, 3.6 million prescriptions in the first 4 months. Although it is clear that many of the patients had erectile disorders, there is strong anecdotal information to suggest that some men were experimenting with Viagra to improve their sex life. Consider the physical, psychological, and sociocultural dimensions of such experimentation (for example, belief you cannot perform without the pill, the ethics of getting a doctor to write a prescription). Would you take a drug that could possibly improve your sex life, even if it had associated risks?

Critical Thinking Case

Before the 1960s hardly anyone had heard of sexual dysfunction. However, soon after Masters and Johnson's book *Human Sexual Response* was published in 1966, the prevalence of sexual dysfunctions seemed to skyrocket. Some have argued that there are more sexual problems than in previous years because of the greater emphasis people place on sex today. We can now rent X-rated movies for home viewing or even order them into our homes via cable TV, we can purchase erotic print media at the local bookstore or listen to sexually charged music and lyrics on CDs and the radio, and we can even observe simulated sex during daytime hours on TV soap operas or on the Internet. This emphasis on sex, the argument continues, has created unrealistic expectations for people, and when they cannot "perform" as they observe others can, they become dysfunctional.

There is another view, however. Perhaps there was as much sexual dysfunction before 1966 as there is today; however, sex was not a topic for conversation, so problems remained undisclosed. The result was that people were unable to achieve sexual satisfaction.

What is your view? Is there more sexual dysfunction now, or has disclosure of sexual problems increased? Is the situation better today, or was it better before 1966? Is there too much pressure for people to "perform" sexually today?

Exploring Personal Dimensions

What Constitutes Sexual Dysfunction?

Perspectives on what constitutes a sexual dysfunction vary. One important consideration is that if you and your partner are satisfied with your sexual relationship, you probably do not have a disorder. If you do not participate in any sexual activity, skip this assessment. With that in mind, answer the following statements with one of the following responses:

a. Rarely or never   b. Sometimes
c. Often   d. All or most of the time

1. I fantasize about sex.
2. I think about sex.
3. I am able to become aroused.
4. I remain aroused during sexual activities.
5. I enjoy having sex with my partner.
6. I engage in masturbation more than I feel is normal.
7. I worry about my sexual performance.
8. I feel worried about having sexual relations.

Male:

9. I experience pain when I have an erection or ejaculate.
10. I am able to achieve an erection.

Female:

9. I experience pain during intercourse.
10. I have difficulty reaching an orgasm.

This self-assessment is not meant to be scored. Rather, it is intended as a tool to allow you to think critically about sexual performance and dysfunction.

After you have given initial responses to these questions, go back and review them two more times. The first time, consider whether you are satisfied with your initial response. In other words, think about whether you are happy with a particular aspect of your sexuality. Then consider whether your partner may be satisfied with your initial response.

For example, a man with a spinal-cord injury may not be able to achieve an erection. That situation may still be acceptable to both him and his partner, if they have found other satisfying sexual activities in which to engage.

Suggested Readings

Alterowitz, R., & Alterowitz, R. J. *Intimacy with impotence: The couple's guide to better sex after prostate disease.* Philadelphia, PA: Da Capo Press, 2004.

Broderick, G. A. *Oral drug therapy of sexual dysfunction: A guide to clinical management.* Totowa, NJ: Humana Press, 2005.

Fagan, P. J., & McHugh, P. R. *Sexual disorders: Perspectives on diagnosis and treatment.* Baltimore, MD: Johns Hopkins University Press, 2003.

Goldstein, S. W., & Arleque, L. *When sex isn't good: Stories and solutions of women with sexual dysfunction.* Lincoln, NE: iUniverse, 2007.

Kloner, R. A. *Heart disease and erectile dysfunction.* Totowa, NJ: Humana Press, 2004.

Metz, M. E., & McCarthy, B. *Coping with erectile dysfunction: How to regain confidence and enjoy great sex.* Oakland, CA: New Harbinger Publications, 2004.

Wincze, J. *Enhancing sexuality: A problem-solving approach to treating dysfunction therapist guide (treatments that work).* New York: Oxford University Press, 2009.

Web Resources

For links to the web sites below, visit *http://sexuality.jbpub.com/dimensions/4e* and click on Resource Links.

MayoClinic.com
www.mayoclinic.com/health/female-sexual -dysfunction/DS00701

This resource presents discussion of female sexual response issues with definitions, causes of female sexual dysfunctions, treatments, and the relationship between the mind and the body as it relates to sexual response. In addition, related links to other web sites are provided.

MedlinePlus: Female Sexual Dysfunction
www.nlm.nih.gov/medlineplus/ femalesexualdysfunction.html

Managed by the National Library of Medicine, this web site provides links to an overview of female sexual dysfunctions, diagnosis, symptoms, treatment, prevention and screening, coping, management, clinical trials, and others.

Healthcommunities.com
www.urologychannel.com/fsd/index.shtml

This web site presents an overview of female sexual dysfunctions, incidence and prevalence information, and information about the female sexual response cycle.

Sexual Dysfunction Association
www.sda.uk.net

Managed by Pfizer Pharmaceuticals, this web site provides information about male and female sexual dysfunctions with links to news and articles and frequently asked questions. It also provides an online survey pertaining to erectile dysfunction.

Society for Sex Therapy and Research
www.sstarnet.org

The Society for Sex Therapy and Research (SSTAR) is composed of a broad range of professionals who have clinical or research interests in human sexual concerns. SSTAR's goals are to facilitate communications among clinicians who treat problems of sexual function, sexual identity, and reproductive life, and to provide a forum for exchange of ideas between those interested in research in human sexuality and those whose primary activities are patient care.

CHAPTER 17

Sexual Consumerism

CHAPTER OBJECTIVES

1 Describe the ways in which sexuality is used in the mass media, including advertising, TV, movies, literature, popular music, and on the Internet.

2 Discuss what constitutes sexually explicit materials, the results of research on their effects, and efforts to control their distribution.

3 Describe the different types of sex workers and the economic factors associated with sex work.

sexuality.jbpub.com/dimensions/4e
Advertising
Literature
The Control of Sexually Explicit Materials

INTRODUCTION

*N*ot long ago, in a human sexuality class, the conversation turned to the relationship between sexuality and money. Some students were surprised when others became very interested in the topic. They seemed to feel that there was nothing to be gained by continuing the conversation because they did not see a relationship between sexuality and money.

The students interested in the topic persisted. One of the communication majors pointed out that in his classes he learned that messages and products related to sexuality are big business. The saying "You've come a long way, baby" definitely applies to this topic for better or worse, he pointed out. He went on to say that we are all bombarded with sexual themes daily; that you cannot turn on TV, pick up a magazine, or see a billboard without being confronted with sexual topics and themes. This use of sexual content, he indicated, is designed to sell even products that have no relation to sexuality.

Some other students warmed up to the discussion. One student, a psychology major, mentioned that commercialism related to sexuality has taken another form as well. Products specifically related to sexuality are available in large numbers and in great variety. Whether you want to put it in, dangle it about, or place it on, there is a store where you can get whatever "it" is.

Several students started arguing about whether the use of sexual themes to influence consumers is good or bad. One health education major argued that the use of sexual themes to sell products unrelated to sexuality is sexploitation, with the potential for sexism. He said this situation could prompt people to view others as sex objects, and it could interfere with personal relationships and sexual satisfaction as well—because when one compares one's partner against the commercialized ideal seen in the media, one is likely to be disappointed. This could lead to frustration and a mean-spiritedness that might translate into poor communication, sexual and otherwise.

Another student, a business major, jumped into the fray and added that the pressure to be like people in the ads—sexy, gorgeous, hunky—may cause people to feel inferior and ashamed of their body. Feelings of inferiority and shame, as we learned earlier (Chapter 16), can progress to sexual dysfunction.

Still another student pointed out that appearance may not be the only concern. She expressed concern that as the result of observing the sexual prowess of television and movie stars on-screen, we assume that all of us should be able to affect our partners the same way. If they do not swoon at the very thought of a caress from us, if they do not get light-headed when we place an arm around them, if they do not lick their lips when they see us in a state of semiundress, we may believe that we are ineffective lovers. Thus, because of unrealistic depictions of sexual behavior in the movies and TV, ordinary people like us may fear losing our lovers because we cannot sexually satisfy them.

A nursing major argued that some people value sexual commercialization. Whether because idealized views of sexual activity are exciting, because they have potential for improving sexual relationships by indicating new ways to relate, or because they help to desensitize people to an emotionally charged topic (namely, sexuality), these views are considered a positive trend by many people, he said.

The students' discussion was useful in that it covered most of the points that the instructor wanted to raise before starting the chapter on sexuality and commercial activities. Regardless of our points of view, sexual commercialization is probably here to stay. This chapter considers how sexuality is used in a commercial sense and will help you become a better sexual consumer.

■ Mass Media and the Arts

Advertising

Advertisements in magazines and newspapers that use sexual themes to sell products are abundant. One need only turn at random to any page and more than likely an ad or an article that has some relationship to sex or sexual attractiveness will be evident. In the 1990s, there was a controversy related to ads for con-

doms. Because of increasing incidence of HIV/AIDS, many people argued that condom ads were needed to help prevent further spread of disease. Many others argued that there should not be condom ads because they feared such ads would encourage more sexual activity—particularly among adolescents and other unmarried people. Little by little, ads for condoms have become more common, and there have not been increases in sexual activity. In fact, in other countries, where condoms have been openly advertised for years, there are lower rates of STIs, lower rates of unwanted pregnancies, and fewer abortions.

After so much controversy about condom ads, it has been interesting to observe the response to ads for Viagra, Cialis, Levitra, and other products with the sole purpose of enhancing sexual pleasure. These ads are found in newspapers, magazines, on the Internet, and on TV. For some reason, there has not been much controversy about these ads. In some cases, well-known celebrities have talked about how well the products work and how they have helped with their relationships. The presence of these ads seems to have made it more acceptable to talk about sexual behavior in general—even for people in older age groups. This is an excellent example of the impact that advertising can have in certain circumstances.

Most advertising with sexual themes is pretty obvious if you give it a moment's thought, but in the 1970s a book called *Subliminal Seduction*—about subliminal sexual selling—created a furor (Key, 1973). The main premise of the author, Wilson Key, was that many advertisers who used sexual imagery to sell their products intended it to work on the viewer's subconscious, not conscious, awareness. To support his premise Key cited the following kinds of imagery he had found in enlarged photographs taken from magazine ads:

1. Images of people engaged in sexual activity, hidden in the shading of ice cubes in liquor advertisements

2. The word *fuck* or *sex*, written in very small letters, hidden in the ads

3. Pictures that appeared innocent on one side of a magazine page but that made sexual suggestion when held up to the light—for example, a picture of a woman standing on the front of a blank sheet, backed by a picture of a projectile (such as an airplane or cigar) aimed at her vagina

4. Pictures composed to suggest genitals—for instance, of liquor bottles with small round objects on each side (such as oranges or apples) suggesting a penis and two testicles

Some critics have argued that Key went too far and that looking for sexual connotations in ice cubes is in itself perverse. In fact, many feel that Key had no evidence or research to support his ideas. Some marketers today believe that subliminal advertising is a farce. However, research is still done on subliminal exposure. For example, Gillath et al. (2007) looked at the effects of subliminal exposure to sexual

---

Myth (vs) Fact

Myth: In recent years, there has been an increased and about equal use of male and female body exposure in advertisements.
Fact: There has been an increase in breast and total female body exposure, but female body exposure is about four times more common than male body exposure.

Myth: Women appear more often than men in television beer commercials.
Fact: Men appear twice as often as women in television beer commercials.

Myth: Television is the main source of information about sexuality for teenagers.
Fact: Friends are the main source of information about sexuality for teenagers.

Myth: Fraudulent sexual aids are not among the top sources of health fraud in the United States.
Fact: According to the Food and Drug Administration, fraudulent sexual aids are among the top 10 sources of health fraud in the United States.

---

stimuli on men and women. They found that some subliminal exposure to sexual stimuli did not affect the sexual arousal of men, but caused women to have lower sexual arousal. Other subliminal exposure led to more sex-related thoughts in both men and women. So, we are still not certain about the overall influence of subliminal advertising.

Ads crafted to appeal to basic needs are apparently highly effective, even without the kinds of things Key described. For example, some would argue that Paris Hilton washing a car while eating a hamburger is a more recent example of advertising that might be called subliminal advertising and that it appeals to basic needs.

As we shall see in this chapter, we buy many products without fully understanding why. Those selling us these products, though, know that one of the hidden motivations behind our buying habits relates to sexuality. We want to appear sexy, appeal to a potential sex mate, and feel attractive; knowing this, salespeople use these needs to persuade us to buy products, even though we think we are buying them for reasons totally divorced from sexuality.

Advertisers seem to have made a study of sexual motivation. Some research from as long ago as 1973 suggested that since oral–genital activity had become relatively acceptable and widely practiced (Hunt, 1974), it found its way into product advertising. What better way to sell cigarettes to women, for example, than to associate cigarettes with penises? For years cigarettes have been used as phallic symbols. Beginning in the 1930s, cigarette ads featured only men offering cigarettes to women, employing phallic symbolism. We remember cigarette ads with words such as *longer, firmer, rounder, more satisfying,*

Myth (vs) Fact

Myth: There are special exercises and/or creams that are helpful in increasing the size of a female's breasts.

Fact: Breast size and shape are the result of glandular influences and cannot be altered by exercise or by application of anything to the breast.

Myth: Prostitution is illegal in most countries around the world.

Fact: In many countries there are no laws against prostitution. In fact, the United Nations adopted a resolution in favor of decriminalization of prostitution.

Myth: It is illegal to release the names of those accused of using prostitutes or the prostitutes themselves publicly until they have been shown to be guilty in a court of law.

Fact: Although some civil liberties groups object, in some states the identities of prostitutes and their customers are made public as soon as they are arrested— before any court action occurs.

better tasting, and *more pleasing* (not to mention *more fully packed*).

Automobile advertisements make obvious use of sexual appeals, along with appeals to such other needs as recognition and esteem. When cars were long and well adorned, they were presented as phallic symbols. *Real* men, the ads suggested, wanted long cars. The tips of automobiles were even ornamented. Today, although car companies sell smaller cars as a rule, their ads still associate the product with sexuality, sometimes by posing pretty, well-endowed, scantily clad, and perfectly proportioned females beside cars. At automobile shows, held in coliseums and arenas throughout the United States, companies employ young female models (again scantily clad) to adorn their displays.

Liquor ads are particularly notable for link-

Victoria's Secret became a multibillion-dollar company by redefining the market for underwear. Here a model shows off the "Angels" line of lingerie at a fashion show. After a single TV ad shown during the 1999 Super Bowl, more than 1 million people inundated the Victoria's Secret web site, hoping for a glimpse of more "fashion."

ing sexual imagery to our aspirations for living well. The people depicted as liquor drinkers are handsome, well dressed, sophisticated, flirtatious, and the object of someone else's unconcealed attention. Readers are supposed to envy the exciting life these attractive people live and, through their choice of liquor purchases, to emulate them.

Whether intended for this purpose or not, advertisements can send sexual messages as well as messages related to gender bias. For example, over a 10-year period there was a significant increase in breast exposure and total female body exposure even though fashion trends did not account for this change. In addition, female body exposure was about four times more common than male body exposure, in part because women were displayed in underwear and bikini swimsuits more often than were men (Plous & Neptune, 1997).

The use of sexual themes to sell products has expanded in some interesting ways. For example, in 2001 Abercrombie & Fitch said its summer catalog was sexy in a wholesome sort of way. Critics called it soft porn and joined forces to boycott the trendy youth-oriented retailer. The catalog featured young unclad male and female models to woo younger customers and use sexual themes to popularize the image of the company (Crary, 2001).

Interestingly, in 2005 Abercrombie and Fitch had another related difficulty with its products. The Women & Girls Foundation of Southwest Pennsylvania promoted a national "girlcott" of a new line of Abercrombie and Fitch T-shirts that had "sexist" slogans such as "Who needs brains when you have these," "Blondes are adored, brunettes are ignored," "Give me something to scream about," and "Available for parties." The retailer issued a statement acknowledging that the shirts that were meant to be humorous might be troubling to some. It agreed to stop selling the shirts.

In Europe, Durex, the world's number one condom maker, started a TV and print advertising campaign using humor. In one TV ad a young man walking down the street to meet his date is followed by a boisterous and excited crowd of men dressed in white sperm costumes. The sperm are suddenly trapped, squirming, in a huge condom in the middle of the street. The ad has the tagline "Durex: For a Hundred Million Reasons" (Durex condom maker using "humor" ads to sell condoms in Europe, 2001).

In 2005 another controversy erupted over another type of advertising—store mannequins. Local residents in McLean, Virginia, and Wauwatosa, Wisconsin, were upset about Victoria's Secret scantily clad and provocatively posed mannequins. There were female mannequins on all fours, others intertwined on a bed, and still others in "garters and whatnot, and the only thing missing is a whip," said one resident. Some residents of these communities were very upset, while others failed to see what the fuss was about. A spokesman for Victoria's Secret said: "All we're trying to do is market what we sell. You see bras and underwear. That's lingerie. That's what we sell." In other examples, Diesel's ad campaign celebrated "the world of individual hedonistic pleasure pursuits." One shot featured women with whips. Hipster chain American Apparel had softcore-styled ads including a tight focus on barely covered backsides of women (Barker, 2005).

A different type of controversy arose in 2009 related to Bayer's advertising campaign for its contraceptive Yaz, the most popular birth control pill in the United States. In an agreement with the U.S. Food and Drug Administration (FDA), Bayer launched a $20 million ad campaign to correct previous misleading marketing of Yaz. The FDA believed that Bayer ads had overstated Yaz's ability to treat acne and improve women's moods, while downplaying its health risks. Bayer had to run commercials to set the record straight. In the new ads, an actress said, "You may have seen some Yaz commercials recently that were not clear. The FDA wants us to correct a few points in those ads" ("Unusual" FDA order requiring corrections to Yaz ad campaign, 2009).

Television Advertising and Programming

Kuriansky (1996) provided an interesting historical overview of sexuality and television advertising. Here are some of the highlights:

1. Beer led the way for using sexual themes to sell. One TV ad in the 1950s showed a tired husband growing perky after drinking a beer. He then chased his wife around the room while disrobing.

2. Car spots also pioneered the sexy sell by using sexy models draped over the hood or stroking the wheel suggestively.

Many sexual themes are used as part of advertising on TV.

3. In 1980 then-15-year-old Brooke Shields panted that nothing came between her and her Calvins. Though some versions of the ad were banned, jeans sales doubled.

4. In the early 1990s a group of female employees sued Stroh's brewery for sexual harassment and named the company's "Swedish Bikini Team" campaign (featuring buxom, blonde, bikini-clad women) as contributing to a "hostile work environment."

5. In 1995 the FBI investigated a Calvin Klein ad featuring an underage teen stripping for a photographer. Many pairs of jeans were sold.

6. Candies hiking boots received more free exposure than paid air time when a furor erupted over the censorship of scenes of a nude couple straddling a chair.

7. What is acceptable on U.S. TV is often tame compared to that in other parts of the world where full frontal nudity is used to sell every-

 Did You Know . . .

Personal ads in newspapers have been around for many years but are much more prevalent now. They can be found on the Internet, in newspapers, in magazines, and on the radio. A radio station that has a phone-dating service will hook you up with people of a similar demographic and music-taste level. Even legitimate regional magazines, like *Boston* magazine,

carry personal ads. Your choice of whom you want may be partially influenced by where he or she advertises. For example, advertising in *Boston* magazine is much more expensive than advertising in the local newspapers, so such ads may attract a more upscale clientele.

thing from shock absorbers to sardines. In a Danish TV spot, a newspaper is draped over a man's erect penis as he spies on ladies in the steam room.

8. Cloaking sexuality in romance is one way to prevent controversy. The Taster's Choice soap-opera-like spots follow a handsome neighbor invited in for coffee and whatever else.

9. Humor also relieves the anxiety of sexual suggestion. In another ad, the actress Annie Potts is lifted into a hulk's arms while extolling the virtues of large popcorn kernels.

10. It seems that sexual themes will always sell. The Candies CEO said: "In 30 to 60 seconds, to keep people from going to the refrigerator, you have to astound them. And sex does."

Relatedly, dating shows have become to the 21st century what sleazy talk and courtroom shows were to the late 1990s (Poniewozik, 2002). The popularity of shows such as *Blind Date, Temptation Island, The Bachelor, The Dating Experiment, Love Shack, Who Wants to Marry a Millionaire,* and *The Bachelorette* has shown that people want to observe others in their sexual relationships. In 2005 and 2006 new shows called *Wife Swap* and *Trading Spouses* were added to the mix of TV shows. While not specifically about dating, these shows also dealt with personal relationships. All of these shows can make love and romance look phony at best, vicious at worst. But large numbers of people seem to enjoy these shows.

The Kaiser Family Foundation reported that the number of sexual scenes on TV nearly doubled from 1998 to 2005. Approximately 70% of all shows include some sexual content, and these shows average 5 sexual scenes per hour. This compares to 56% and 3.2 scenes per hour in 1998 and 64% and 4.4 scenes per hour in 2002. About 14% of shows with sexual content include reference to sexual risks and responsibilities (such as waiting to have sexual intercourse, using protection, or possible consequences of unprotected sexual activity). This rate is up from 9% in 1998 and about the same as the rate in 2002 (TV sexual scenes nearly double since 1998, 2005).

The Parents' Television Council reported that children watching TV during the first hour of prime time are assaulted by violence, profanity, or sexual content once every 3.5 minutes of noncommercial time. Incidence of sexual content increased by 22.1% from 2002 to 2007. Broadcasters also greatly increased the prevalence of harsh language obscured by bleeps or partial editing such as "f-words" or "s-words" (PTC study: Broadcast TV family hour fare filthier than ever, 2007).

Television is a major source of information about sexuality for people of all ages.

Many people have protested the television industry's portrayal of sexual themes in everyday life. Although objections to the portrayal of explicit sexual activities and the use of sexual language have been raised for some time, today people are beginning to object to the nature and quality of the sexual relationships enacted—stereotypical roles, sexual violence and hostility, incessant teasing, and more physical than emotional display—and to be concerned about the effects of these views of sexuality on socialization of the young.

A television rating system was adopted in 1997. The ratings system includes age-based symbols like those for movies, such as TV-G, TV-PG, TV-14, and TV-MA, as well as the codes V, S, L, and D to indicate violence, sexual themes, "adult" language, and suggestive dialogue.

Television can be an excellent way to educate people about healthy sexual practices. For instance, the Surgeon General of the United States warned that the spread of HIV and AIDS could be slowed only by sexual abstinence or the use of condoms during coitus. Fortunately, in recent years we have seen an increase in condom ads on television.

Some broadcasters worry that the public disapproves of condom ads, and some worry they would lose sponsors that do not want their ads run alongside condom ads. However, 71% of Americans favor allowing condom ads on TV: 37% support the ads running at any time and 34% support the ads running at certain times, such as after 10 P.M. Even more support exists among adults younger than 50 years of age, of whom 82% say that condom ads should be allowed (Pardun & Forde, 2002/2003).

On cable TV, the fastest-growing segment is adult programming that portrays explicit sexual behavior. As cable availability expands to a potential 500 channels, even more such programming is expected.

Many television programs have been devoted to educating the public about HIV and AIDS, and other programs have focused on such topics as sexual orientation and extramarital sexual activities. Many of these programs follow a talk-show format or are presented as documentaries; however, some sexual topics and issues are dramatized with the intent of entertaining and educating at the same time. For example, one situation comedy depicted a teenager being instructed to use a condom with his girlfriend, and another weekly comedy show depicted an unmarried couple living together and the problems they encountered.

Addressing the media in general, a position statement of the Sexuality Information and Education Council of the United States (SIECUS, 2005) indicates that

> . . . the media have a powerful influence on all aspects of society. With this power goes a major responsibility to present the complexities of human sexuality at all stages of the life cycle in a manner that is accurate, sensitive to diversity, and free of exploitation, gratuitous sexual violence, and dehumanizing sexual portrayals.

Recommendations for realistic, accurate images concerning sexuality in the media include the following (Edwards, 1996):

1. Dialogue that shows true communication among children, their parents, and trusted adults

2. Situations that show planned mature relationships as opposed to spur-of-the-moment responses to passion

3. Situations in which unprotected sexual encounters have negative repercussions

4. Articulate responsible characters with whom teenagers can identify

Interestingly, teens 15 to 17 years old believe that sexual content on TV influences the behavior of their peers, but not their own. They also report some positive aspects of sexual content on TV. They say they had learned how to say no in an uncomfortable sexual situation, that they had learned how to communicate with a partner about safer sex, and that they had talked with their parents about a sexuality-related issue because of something they saw on TV (Notes from the research, 2002).

In 2004, Collins et al. conducted a national longitudinal survey of 1792 adolescents between 12 and 17 years of age. They found that watching sexual themes on TV predicts and may hasten adolescent sexual initiation. They also reported that reducing the amount of sexual content on TV, reducing adolescent expo-

Communication
DIMENSIONS

Feelings About Sexual Themes

In Chapter 3 we outlined a basic communication model. We also talked about common communication problems, including (1) frame of reference, (2) emotional interference, and (3) physical distractions. Talk with two or three of your classmates about difficulties two people in an intimate relationship might have in these three areas when they are discussing the following topics:

1. Which characters do you think are the sexiest in current television shows? Why?

2. Which ads on TV or in magazines do you find most offensive? Why?

3. What does it take for materials to be considered obscene?

4. Which TV shows and/or movies do you think are most sexually stimulating? Why?

5. If you were a writer for a television series, how would you use sexual themes?

For example, in a discussion about sexy television shows, there could be a difference in which language is considered acceptable or in what might be considered sexy. This could cause emotional interference. Or perhaps one person could not relate to why something is sexually stimulating to another person. Thus one person's frame of reference could cause a problem. Go through each of the five questions with at least two or three other people and see which other possible barriers you can identify. Why do you think these barriers exist? What might be done about them to improve communication?

sure to the content, or increasing references to and depictions of possible negative consequences of sexual activity could appreciably delay the initiation of coital and noncoital activities. Alternatively, parents may be able to reduce the effects of sexual content by watching TV with their children and discussing their own beliefs about sexuality and the behaviors portrayed.

Escobar-Chaves et al. (2005) studied the impact of the media on adolescent sexual attitudes and behaviors. In their discussion and in their findings they made many germane points. Among them are:

- Few studies have examined the effects of mass media on adolescent sexual attitudes and behavior.

- Young people report that media messages are an important influence in their lives.

- Two-thirds of youth aged 8 to 18 report having a TV in their bedroom, and more than one-third have their own VCR.

- American adolescents spend an average of 6 to 7 hours per day with some form of media, including TV, videotapes, movies, radio, print media, computers, the Internet, and video games.

- The average teenager spends about 3 hours per day watching TV.

- Much daily TV viewing occurs alone.

- Few parents establish rules about when or what their children may view on TV.

- The overall proportion of programming with sexual content continues to increase.

- Of programs popular with teens, 83% have sexual content, and 20% contain explicit or implicit sexual intercourse. On average, each hour of programs popular with teens contains 6.7 scenes that include sexual topics.

- Most sexual behavior on TV (79%) occurs between people who are not married to each other.

- Negative consequences of sexual activity are rarely portrayed. Very few programs have a primary emphasis on sexual risk and responsibility.

- Watching TV with sexual content has the effect of artificially aging children. Those who watch more than average behave sexually as though they were 9 to 17 months older. The 12-year-olds who watch the most have the sexual behaviors of the 14- and 15-year-olds who watch the least.

- Sexually experienced students are more likely to seek out sexual content on TV than non-sexually experienced youth.

- Adolescents who have just watched an hour of MTV are more likely to report approval of premarital sexual activity than those who have not.

Although a number of researchers have tried, it is difficult to definitively establish the relationship between sexual attitudes and behavior and TV viewing. In various studies it has been reported that those persons who watch more TV initiate sexual intercourse earlier, girls view more sexual content on TV than do boys, younger adolescents view more sexual content on TV than do older adolescents, those who watch more romantic programming are more likely to endorse traditional gender-role beliefs, and college students who are shown sexual TV content and perceive it as realistic are more likely to endorse permissive sexual attitudes and to estimate that more of their female peers are sexually active (Rich, 2008).

Chandra et al. (2008) indicated that teens exposed to high levels of television sexual content are twice as likely to experience a pregnancy in the subsequent 3 years as compared with those with lower levels of exposure. Conversely, Schroeder (2008) pointed out that "We should all raise a skeptical eyebrow whenever any research claims that there's a direct cause–effect relationship between one thing, such as TV viewing, and something as complex as teenage pregnancy." In other words, maybe the same people who are more likely to become pregnant as teenagers are also the same people who want to watch more sexual content on TV—maybe one doesn't cause the other at all.

On a related note, in 1997 MTV partnered with the Kaiser Family Foundation to launch a campaign to inform young people about HIV/AIDS, other STIs, and related issues. The partnership included targeted public service announcements, documentary and entertainment programming, news segments, and a comprehensive web site (*www.mtv.com/thinkmtv/sexual_health/*). In 2005 the campaign was branded under MTV's prosocial initiative called "Think: Sexual Health." It included free resources, such as a booklet entitled *It's Your (Sex) Life (www.think.mtv.com)* and information on decision making, communication, and other related issues.

Sexuality and the Movies

Any cursory glance at the entertainment section of your local newspaper will show that movies are often marketed to the public by means of sexual themes—and have been for some time. In *The Blue Angel*, a

1930 film starring Marlene Dietrich (1930 was a time when women's bathing suits were much more than three small patches of flimsy cloth precariously held together by string), images of Marlene's bare thighs in a cabaret outfit made men's heads whirl. In *She Done Him Wrong*, when Mae West invited Cary Grant to "come up and see me some time," men's knees knocked. When Clark Gable (Rhett Butler) carried Vivian Leigh (Scarlett O'Hara) up a flight of stairs to her bedroom in *Gone with the Wind*, women swooned; when Marlon Brando appeared in his ripped undershirt in *A Streetcar Named Desire*, they panted. People's imaginations and perceptions, rather than nudity or sexual activity on film, were integral components of cinematic sexuality during the 1930s, 1940s, and 1950s.

By the 1960s and the 1970s, sexual permissiveness and experimentation had permeated the movies, as well as other segments of society. Movies previously shown as stag films and often called blue movies were elevated to respectable status. With the showing of *I Am Curious (Yellow)*, *Deep Throat*, *Beyond the Valley of the Dolls*, *Vixen*, *The Lickerish Quartet*, and *Behind the Green Door* in movie theaters (in spite of attempts by local communities to ban them), people seemed to be less shocked. Although well-known movie stars had sometimes appeared nude in films in earlier years, a new era began when Marlon Brando appeared in the X-rated *Last Tango in Paris* in the early 1970s. The films of the past 25 years leave little to the imagination and appeal more to the voyeur in us.

To help parents and others make decisions about the appropriateness of a particular movie for themselves or their children, a rating system was developed by the Motion Picture Association of America:

G—Appropriate for the general audience

PG—Appropriate for the general audience; however, parental guidance is advised. There may be brief nudity or some brief moments of sexually explicit language.

PG-13—Parents are advised that some of the material may be inappropriate for younger children.

R—Restricted to people at least 17 years of age or those accompanied by an adult due to sexual content, sexually explicit language, or violence

NC-17—No one under 17 years of age admitted. Extremely sexual in nature, and/or containing explicit sexual language, or extremely violent (but not necessarily pornographic).

In 2004, after parents complained that they wanted to let their kids see R-rated movies but didn't want to sit through the films themselves, a number of theaters in the Midwest started using a parent-

Linda Lovelace, former porn star, now openly campaigns against sexually explicit movies. Lovelace was threatened into starring in *Deep Throat* by a physically abusive husband/manager. As were countless other young actresses, Lovelace was led to believe that appearing in adult films would open the door to legitimate film work. Yet only one well-known porn star, "Traci Lords," has ever made that transition.

approved pass card. To get the card, parents had to accompany their adolescent to the movie theater and sign for the photo ID R-card. Then, the student could get into R-rated films without the parent being present. This started a debate over convenience versus parental responsibility (Dennis, 2004).

Gunasekera et al. (2005) analyzed the portrayal of sexual themes in the most popular movies of the previous 20 years. Sexual activity, STI prevention, and birth control measures discussed or depicted were recorded. They reviewed 87 movies and found only one suggestion of condom use, which was the only reference to any form of birth control. There were no depictions of important consequences of unprotected sexual behavior such as unwanted pregnancies, HIV, or other STIs. Sexual depictions in popular movies lacked safe sex messages.

Corliss (2005) reported that European films are showing more sexual behavior. It is not pretend sexual behavior, but the real thing. For example, the film *9 Songs* explicitly gives the details of a summer affair.

Corliss suggested that the film might better be called *9 Sex Acts.*

As with television and advertising, some people believe that the sexual explicitness of movies is detrimental to society, and others see this trend as positive. The opponents cite the weak commitments of sexual partners as partly responsible for the soaring adultery and divorce rates by setting poor examples of the meaning of intimate relationships. Those in favor of sexual explicitness in movies see this as just one sign of our increased openness about sexuality and the pleasures inherent in sexual behavior. We must make our own decisions about the appropriateness of this trend.

There have been a number of examples of the U.S. federal government's escalating war on indecency (Woellert, 2005). The George W. Bush administration launched a broad assault on sexual content that targeted the entertainment industry from Hollywood production to hotels. The offensive included creation of a Justice Department Obscenity Prosecution Task Force, an FBI anti-porn squad, a crackdown on indecent programming by the Federal Communications Commission, and a wave of indecency legislation. Many in Congress wanted to give regulators more power. However, business has been fighting back. Those selling cell phones, video iPods, and X-rated products could stand to lose a lot of money if the federal government's war on indecency succeeds.

Videotapes, DVDs, and Video Games

The videotape and DVD rental business has grown by leaps and bounds. In almost any community, video rental shops are found. These stores stock popular movies soon after they are shown in neighborhood theaters. In addition to these popular movies, often a separate area houses the X-rated video library, usually out of view so customers are not offended by the movies' enticing packages and children are not exposed to them. Shelves and shelves of the most sexually explicit films are available to rent and to view in the privacy of one's home.

The availability of sexually explicit material has alarmed some people. They consider these X-rated movies to be pure trash with the potential to instigate sexual violence and to stereotype females as sex objects. They argue that these materials are obscene and pornographic and, as such, should be prohibited. However, others view the openness toward sexual expression of various kinds to be healthy. They argue that a couple's sexual relationship can be enhanced by viewing sexually explicit films, learning about new sexual activities, or being implicitly given permission to act out sexual fantasies. The courts have ruled that people have the right to rent sexually explicit videos

and rental shop owners have the right to make such videos available. However, pressure from local groups in some communities has convinced shop owners voluntarily to remove the X-rated videos from their stock. In one view, this expression of community standards is considered healthy and the epitome of the democratic process at work. In another view, it is described as the "uptight" majority's dictating sexual mores to the more sexually comfortable minority. As we learned previously, one's view of sexual morality relates to the valuing of one's ethical principles; this is an example of that process at work.

In 1994 the Entertainment Software Rating Board was formed under heat from Congress to crack down on violent video games. It is a self-regulating video game industry group. It uses the following rating system:

- EC (Early Childhood—ages 3+) contains no material parents would find inappropriate.

- E (Everyone—ages 6+) contains minimal cartoon, fantasy, or mild violence and/or infrequent use of mild language.

- E10+ (Everyone—ages 10+) contains more cartoon, fantasy, or mild violence, mild profanity, and/or minimally suggestive themes.

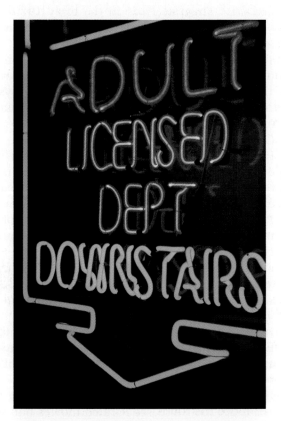

People have various opinions about the legality and availability of sexually explicit materials.

- T (Teen—13+) contains violence, suggestive themes, crude humor, minimal blood, and/or infrequent use of strong language.

- M (Mature—17+) contains mature sexual themes, more intense violence, and/or strong language.

- AO (Adults Only—18+) contains graphic depictions of sex and/or violence.

An interesting controversy arose in 2005 related to the series of *Grand Theft Auto* games (Lohr, 2005). In the M-rated game (the top seller one year), the main character seeks bloody vengeance on gang-filled streets, firing automatic weapons and picking up scantily clad women. Family-oriented media watchdog groups became very upset when the PC version had additional scenes in which nude "girlfriends" join in explicit sex acts. The scenes become "playable" with the help of a freely available download. However, had such sexually explicit content been clearly a part of the retail version, it would have likely earned the game an "adults-only" rating that would have cost millions in lost sales. In an attempt to protect children from "nasty" video games, the Illinois legislature passed a bill making it a crime to sell violent or sexually explicit games to kids under 18. Then-Senator Hillary Clinton worked on a similar bill at the national level.

Evidence suggests that about 70% of adult videos are rented by women. They are rented most frequently on weekend nights and used by married couples after the kids have gone to bed. Four common themes have been noted in sexually explicit videos: high levels of sexual desire, diverse sexual activity, many sexual partners readily available, and pleasure as the purpose of sexual activity (Brosius, Weaver, & Staab, 1993). Video rentals and sales represent multibillions of dollars in sales each year. They are a substantial part of the home-video industry's revenue. Some videos have been produced for use by couples in their homes. Sexologists have made videos that provide explicit graphic instruction to help improve sexual relationships.

In 2009, Benedetti observed that video game makers used sexual themes mainly as a means of shocking players and as a means to sell their products. She pointed that in early 2009 *Afro Samurai* had lots of swordplay, including a scene where players got to slice and dice four topless ninja strippers. In another game, the curvaceous Ayumi, a sword-swinging relic hunter, was dressed in a bumbaring thong and a bikini top. In addition, in a version of *Grand Theft Auto IV*, a man receiving a massage dropped his towel and revealed his flaccid penis for all to see. In these, and many more instances, flesh is used as a tool to sell games.

Ross (2007) pointed out that what is really different about the Internet is that it provides people with the capacity for anonymity in carrying out private cybersex activities. It can serve as a unique site for sexual experimentation. It can also serve as a very important tool for psychological adaptation for gay and lesbian youth.

Literature

As with the content of movies, TV programs, and videos, the public has become desensitized to sexually explicit material in books. However, it was not always this way. For example, in 1928 D. H. Lawrence's *Lady Chatterly's Lover* was published. Because of its sexual explicitness, it was banned in the United States until 1959. James Joyce's *Ulysses,* published in 1934, deals with masturbation, prostitution, adultery, and voyeurism. It was not allowed into the United States for years but is now considered to be a masterpiece.

In the last few decades thousands of books of varying literary quality that openly treat sexual topics have been published. Sometimes they weave themes related to sexuality into a meaningful story, but other times their authors seem to be gratuitously writing about sexual thoughts and activity as much as possible. Many earlier works appear tame compared to what is now available. What was previously considered risque, if not actually immoral or illegal, has now come to be expected in a bestseller.

Sexually arousing material, of course, has existed for centuries. The ancient *Kamasutra* and *The Perfumed Garden,* Chaucer's *Canterbury Tales* and Boccaccio's *Decameron* (both 14th-century works), Li Yu's *Flesh Prayer Mat,* and the *Memoirs of Casanova* are examples of early erotic literature. However, more and more of our popular literature that is not

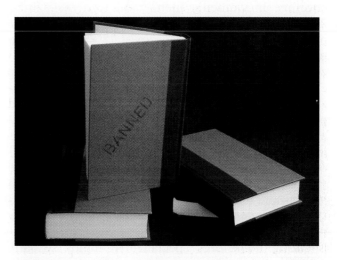

Sexually arousing books and other materials have been available for centuries.

primarily erotic is at least partly concerned with its characters' sexual activities. For example, romance literature relies on fantasy rather than sexual explicitness; its purpose is to tantalize and to nourish sexual fantasies, rather than to tell a good story. About 46% of all mass-market paperbacks are romance novels, read by both women and men (Bartley, 1994).

Magazines have made their mark as well. *Esquire: The Magazine for Men* appeared in 1933. Twenty years later *Playboy* appeared on the newsstands. It offered information about sexuality, an open philosophy toward sexuality, and photographs of nude women along with some stimulating stories. Its approach was followed by many other magazines. In the late 1960s other magazines, such as *Penthouse, Oui,* and *Hustler,* published pictures of nude males and females as well as people engaged in assorted sexual activities. Some even had a classified section allowing people to advertise their sexual services or request sexual partners.

As women asked for a more balanced view, magazines such as *Cosmopolitan* and *Playgirl* began printing photos of nude men and stories with appeal for women. Traditionally, women's magazines have focused on two broad topics: what a woman should do to get a man (*Cosmopolitan*) and what a woman should do once she has the man and his children (*Redbook*). Other magazines have attempted to include other aspects of women's lives. For example, *Working Woman* and *Savvy* are aimed at women who work outside the home. *Ms.* magazine, the only women's magazine explicitly dedicated to feminism and the facts about women's sexuality, struggled for 20 years to attract enough advertising. The magazine finally gave up on advertising and now relies on a hefty subscription price for revenue. Consequently, circulation of around 500,000 dropped to 179,000 (Brown & Steele, 1996).

Magazines collectively play a role as communicators on a range of sexual health topics (Sexual health coverage in women's, men's, and teen magazines, 2000). The Kaiser Family Foundation found that 34% of articles in women's magazines, 28% of articles in men's magazines, and 42% of articles in teen magazines focused on sexual health issues. However, the emphasis is different. For example, women's magazines emphasize pregnancy, and especially planned pregnancy, contraception, and abortion. Men's magazines mainly address concerns such as STIs, including HIV and AIDS, and the few male-controlled methods of contraception. Teen magazines focus on the potential adverse outcomes of sexual activity, such as STIs and unintended pregnancy. They also address the difficult decisions many teens face about whether to become sexually active.

Adult bookstores specialize in highly sexually arousing books. These stores are adult in the sense that a person must be of legal age to enter. Such establishments also sell sex-illustrated magazines, newspapers, postcards, decks of playing cards, and videotapes. Many communities have attempted to outlaw adult bookstores (through the courts and local government statute) or to limit their location to one part of the community. Nevertheless, all major cities have them, as do many smaller cities and towns. Furthermore, many conventional bookstores, recognizing a market for sexually explicit literature, maintain sections devoted to such books and magazines. As with sexuality in the movies, the cost and benefit of adult bookstores versus the risks of censorship is a topic of heated debate.

In addition to sexually explicit fiction, a how-to publishing business has developed to help people reach their sexual potential. Thus we now have countless books about such topics as using sexual techniques, expressing gay and lesbian sexuality, helping ourselves and our partners to be sensuous women or men, improving our overall sexual relationships, and using sexual aids for pleasure.

Popular Music

The mass phenomenon that may affect more young people than any other is popular music. And in this arena, as in most others, blatant sexuality has become a style. Lyrics (words and grunts), performance (movement and costume), and provocative photos on album covers use sexual suggestion and appeal to our sexual fantasies to sell the music and the entertainer.

Perhaps the epitome of sex in music was Elvis ("The Pelvis") Presley, with his gyrating hips. Aside from his hips, however, Elvis's songs were by today's standards tame. "Heartbreak Hotel," "Love Me Tender," and "Let Me Be Your Teddy Bear," all recorded in the late 1950s, were sexually appealing mainly because of Presley's soft, sultry voice and innuendo, rather than direct sexual language—a far cry from today's popular music and music videos that contain frequent references to relationships, romance, and sexual behavior. Lyrics about sexuality are mixed with lyrics about love, violence, rejection, and loneliness.

Music videos, available on many cable networks, may be influential sources of sexual information for adolescents because they combine visuals of their favorite musicians with music. Many of the visual elements are sexual. Rap music is particularly explicit about both sexuality and violence.

Groups of citizens have attempted to ban some of this music from local radio stations and have sometimes been successful. Whether sexually explicit music is harmful (in particular, it is argued, to youths in developmental states) is debatable and depends somewhat on our values.

it deems objectionable. Wal-Mart stores will not carry anything with a parental advisory on it. Blockbuster and K-Mart have joined Wal-Mart in this practice (Rolfe, 2005).

Online Material

Advertising, newspapers, books, magazines, television, movies, videos, and music have been around for a long time; a newer entrant on the sexual consumerism scene is online material. An increasing number of people of all ages have access to computers and the Internet and, therefore, to countless materials related to sexuality. There are at least five reasons that account for the explosion in the amount of sexual materials available via computer networks (Rimm, 1998):

1. Consumers enjoy considerable privacy on computer networks and can easily avoid the embarrassment of acquiring sexual materials elsewhere.

2. Consumers have the ability to download only those images they find most sexually arousing.

3. Easy, discrete storage of sexually explicit images on a computer enables customers to conceal them from family members and others.

4. The prevalence and fear of HIV and AIDS and STIs have helped pornographers successfully market modem sex and autoeroticism as safe and viable alternatives to the dangers of real sex.

5. New and highly advanced computer technologies are quickly being absorbed into the mainstream, permitting an ever-expanding audience to gain access to digitized pornography available on the information superhighway.

Pornography has even become a relatively big thing in the workplace. For example, 25% of employees who use the Internet visit porn sites during the workday. Hits are higher during office hours than at any other time of day. Some believe that the people who engage in this activity are looking for an escape, and think their bosses are too busy to notice. Another factor is that there is an evolving sense—not universally shared—that porn is no big deal. A number of employees have been fired for viewing porn sites frequently while on the job. The threat to companies isn't just the lost hours of work and the risk of sexual-harassment lawsuits; rather porn sites expose computers to viruses, adware, and spyware. In one case

Many entertainers use sexual themes to sell themselves and their products.

In 1985 the Recording Industry Association of America (RIAA) reached an agreement with the National Parent-Teacher Association and the Parents Music Resource Center. The agreement specified that music releases containing explicit lyrics, including explicit depictions of violence and sex, be identified so parents can make intelligent listening choices for their children. The Parental Advisory Label on music releases has become a notice to consumers that recordings with the label may contain strong language or depictions of violence, sex, or substance abuse. Parental discretion is then advised. The label is a nonremovable logo that record companies voluntarily place on products to better inform consumers and retailers while also protecting the rights of artists. The decision to label a particular sound recording is made by each record company in conjunction with the artist. The industry as a whole and its individual companies take this program seriously. In 1996 the RIAA strengthened the program by revising the logo to apply to both audio and video products (Parental Advisory, 2003).

Wal-Mart, the nation's leading seller of pop music, has refused to stock music with lyrics or artwork that

¿? Ethical
DIMENSIONS

Controlling
Cyberspace

In 1995 the U. S. Senate Commerce Committee proposed banning sexually explicit materials in cyberspace and considered the Communications Decency Act (CDA), which would have made the transmission of "obscene, lewd, lascivious, filthy or indecent" images, e-mail, text files, or other on-line communications punishable by up to $100,000 in fines and 2 years in prison. It was passed by Congress in 1996. In 1997, the Supreme Court held in a unanimous opinion that this kind of censorship could not be tolerated under the First Amendment of the U.S. Constitution.

Many people believe that attempts to ban sexually explicit materials on the Internet are, in addition to being unconstitutional, unethical. They believe that laws governing obscenity and child pornography already exist and apply to cases involving the Internet. Child pornography is not protected by free speech, so they argue that further control is not needed. In fact, they point out that such control would also deny people of all ages access to needed information about sexuality. Besides, if people want to protect children from certain information, they can do so with Internet blocking software.

Clearly, the CDA would not have been proposed if some people did not consider it ethical to ban sexually explicit materials in cyberspace. They believe such materials should not be available for viewing by anyone of any age. They also fear that even with Internet-blocking software and well-intended parents, young people will have contact with sexually explicit materials that will be harmful to them. Therefore, it is ethical to ban such materials.

Is it ethical to establish laws to ban sexually explicit materials in cyberspace? Is it ethical to transmit sexually explicit materials in cyberspace? How can the potential need for regulation be balanced with constitutional rights?

Source: Adapted from Portelli, C. J., & Meade, C. W. Censorship and the Internet: No easy answers, *SIECUS Report, 27, no. 1* (October–November 1998), 4–8.

it was learned that an executive spent many hours a day on adult sites—a fact discovered because his computer was always crashing (Kuchment & Springen, 2008).

Computer technology has influenced laws as well as behavior. For example, in 1996 federal legislation banning computer-generated depictions of children engaging in sexual conduct was passed. The act outlawed "any visual depiction" that "appears to be of a minor engaging in sexually explicit conduct." This could include scenes from a movie in which an adult portraying a minor is engaged in sexual activity (Thought police recruited in new child porn law, 1998). Although the law was challenged by sex film distributors and the ACLU, a federal judge upheld it in 1997 (New federal law upheld despite vagueness concerns, 1998).

For some people, X-rated email can be a problem. Unsolicited email messages that, with a click of a hot-linked universal resource locator (URL), can deliver pornographic web sites to your computer screen have become relatively common intrusions online. Some have telltale IDs like "Sue2nite" or "4HotTime," but others are more deceptive. For example, in one instance an innocuous-looking message said that clicking on its hot link would provide information on how to fix a computer problem. One

click of the hot link revealed a sample of sexually explicit pictures. This is probably not illegal, but it can be very annoying. The FTC encourages all consumers to forward any unsolicited, unfair, or deceptive spams to its special spam mailbox where investigators keep a database of possibly illegal email solicitations.

On the Internet, people can carry on sensual conversations, play X-rated computer games with each other (for example, they can create the appearance of their characters and engage in a variety of behaviors with characters controlled by other subscribers), obtain recent information on a variety of sexual topics, leave sexual messages for other people on bulletin boards, and obtain and use software designed to help with sexual dysfunction and other problems. Computer bulletin boards and forums exist for just about all sexual interests and fetishes.

In 2005 one of the first studies investigating the characteristics of those who participate in cybersex was reported (Daneback et al., 2005). Cybersex was defined as when two or more people engage in simulated sex talk while online for the purposes of sexual pleasure. It was found that men and women participate in cybersex to a similar extent. Women between 35 and 49 years of age had significantly more experience with cybersex than men of the same age. Men's interest in cybersex seemed to decrease with age, while women's interest stayed almost the same. Women's main reasons for engaging in cybersex were interaction with others and "education" around sexual matters. Homosexual men were more than four times more likely to have cybersex than were heterosexual men. Cybersex was found not to be primarily a "singles" activity. The amount was about the same for singles as for married people. Married people who participated did not seem to view cybersex as infidelity. Those who engage in cybersex were more likely to be sexually active offline as well—having had a greater number of sex partners during the past year as compared with those without cybersex experience.

Internet chat rooms related to sexuality are also becoming more common. For example, a person can "sit" with other people or "soak" in a hot tub and discuss sexual fantasies or participate in Internet sexual activities. Flirting and discussion about sexual relationships and desires are everyday occurrences in such chat rooms.

Computers can also be used to create virtual reality (VR) sexual activity. Soon, cable TV subscribers will be able to use VR equipment, such as gloves, goggles, and body sensors, to create their own VR sexual activity.

There can be big money involved with Internet and web site activities, as Beth Mansfield discovered (Small operators can make big killings on the web, 1997). In 1995 she was a struggling accountant wondering how she and her husband would ever put their two young children through college. She decided to try her hand at creating a web site with adult content. Within

Web sites like "Persian Kitty's" provide links to free pornographic material and generate a fortune from advertisers for their operators. However, the relative ease of obtaining sexually explicit material that such a site offers raises ethical issues. Should such sites be required to provide age verification? If not, should "Persian Kitty's" be held liable if minors follow the links to sexually explicit material?

5 months people were clamoring to buy advertising on "Persian Kitty's," a directory of sexually oriented sites she named for her three cats, and soon she grossed more than $900,000 per year.

One of the web's most successful adult-oriented sites is operated by Danni Ashe. It is called "Danni's Hard Drive." According to information at the web site, Danni Ashe is a former model and stripper who created and launched her own site in 1995. The site's initial 70,000 hits per day have grown to 5 million, gross revenue has grown by more than 2,000% and her original staff of one part-time assistant has grown to 15 full-time employees. Monthly fees of $9.95 give members access to a library of nude photos and interviews with nude models.

In 2001 the *Guinness Book of World Records* awarded Danni Ashe an award as the "most downloaded woman." At that time she had already been downloaded 7 million times into the computers of others. It is estimated that 1 in 5 hits on the web is sex-related and that sexual themes are the web's top moneymaker (Pastor's column hits the growth of porn, 2001).

Danni Ashe is more popular on the Internet than many well-known stars. For example, her web site receives more hits than the web sites for Martha Stewart, Oprah Winfrey, Britney Spears, Cindy Margolis, and Cindy Crawford (How popular is Danni Ashe compared to other stars?, 2003).

Of the 1,000 most visited sites on the Internet, 10% are adult sex oriented. In addition, portrayals of violent sexual scenes have increased. Web sites offer both still photographs and X-rated videos of every level of visual (and auditory) explicitness (Escobar-Chaves et al., 2005).

Some people feel that the Internet has been a major factor in unleashing women's interest in all things sexual. Women account for more than a quarter of all visitors to sites with adult content, with more than 10 million women logging on in a recent month (Navarro, 2004).

In 2005, a red-light district tentatively was cleared for construction on the Internet. The need for such a site was at least partially justified by the fact that 2 in 5 Internet users visited an adult site in a given month. It was billed by backers as a chance for the $12 billion online porn industry to clean up its act. The Internet's key oversight body, the Internet Corporation for Assigned Names and Numbers, voted to proceed with a .xxx designation for porn. One argument for this was that it would allow software filters to block all .xxx names and, therefore, help with limiting access to these sites by minors. Skeptics argued that porn sites were likely to also keep their .com storefronts, which would reduce the effectiveness of filters (Jesdanun, 2005).

Another development related to sexuality and the Internet has been podcasting—a blanket term used to describe a collection of technologies for automatically distributing audio and video programs over the Internet via a publish-and-subscribe model. At *podcast.net* the second most searched-for term is "porn." Six of the top 20 shows are adult oriented. Other sites also report that sexually explicit shows are growing quickly in popularity. Many parents are not pleased about this trend because filtering software is useless against this technology (Summers, 2005). Now even cell phones can be used as a lucrative way for the pornography industry to distribute sexually explicit audio and video programs.

Traditionally, some people were worried about pornography being transmitted into the home. However, web camera technology potentially inverts this relationship by transmitting activities in the home to outside viewers. One high-profile case occurred when teenagers used their home computers, web cameras, and other web-based commercial establishments such as PayPal to establish and conduct their own home-based, interactive pornography businesses (Soderlund, 2008).

On a related note, "Sex and Tech" (2008) reported that 20% of teens (ages 13–19) and 33% of young adults (ages 20–26) have electronically sent, or posted online, nude or semi-nude pictures or videos of themselves. Sexually suggestive messages were even more common (sent by 39% of teens and 59% of young adults). The term "sexting" has been used to refer to these practices.

Another use of the Internet related to sexuality was seen in 2005 when a chess grandmaster wanted to raise the profile of the game and give chess some glamour (McClain, 2005). He started a web site called the World Chess Beauty Contest (*www.1wcbc.com*) to rank the most beautiful women in the game. One of the female players also sells her bikini-clad image through her own web site. Such efforts to spice up the game of chess emanated from Eastern Europe, where players have long dominated the game of chess, and where "cheesecake displays" are less likely to draw complaints about the exploitation and objectification of women.

Of course, the Internet also has the potential for abuse with respect to sexuality. Some people have claimed they have been sexually harassed by anonymous participants in computer bulletin boards. Others have been concerned about the transmission of sexual photos of children. There is also concern about uncontrolled access to sexual materials by underage people.

In addition, it is estimated that one in five young people aged 10–17 years who use the Internet at least once a month receives unwanted sexual solicitations. Only 10% were reported to police, school officials, or Internet service providers. Solicitations involve requests to talk on the telephone, communicate by mail, and meet strangers who have established contact online (Wong, 2001).

Authorities estimate that, at any given moment, there are about 20,000 sexual predators online trying to lure unsuspecting young teenagers. FBI agents often pose as teens to help snare these predators. The FBI turned to teenage girls to help the agents convincingly pass and communicate as a young teen. Several girls helped train 500 undercover FBI agents from around the country. They tested them on the latest music, movies, teenage preferences, and lingo—especially online chat abbreviations. During the time the girls were teaching, the FBI secured 2,600 convictions. The FBI had to hire new teenage teachers when the girls became too old for the job—at age 16 (Teen girls help FBI nab cyber stalkers, 2005).

Some people have used the Internet to meet others through online ads. Padgett (2007) surveyed 740 women who had met in person with a man who answered their online personal ads. She found that women used email prior to a face-to-face meeting to negotiate such issues as safety, boundaries, sexual preferences, history of STIs, and condom use. Thirty percent of respondents engaged in sexual activity on their first encounter. Seventy-seven percent did not use condoms for their first sexual encounter. The large amount of email communication prior to meeting seemed to accelerate the intimacy for people involved and may have affected women's decisions to engage in risky sexual behaviors.

What seems to be a very positive use of the Internet for sexuality education occurred late in 2001 (Goodwill ambassador, 2001). Geri Halliwell, a former Spice Girl, launched a sexuality education web site in Britain. Titled "Like It Is," the interactive site is geared toward school-aged children and teens and offers information on reproductive health and services, including teen pregnancy, birth control, and emergency contraception. Halliwell said, "This site gives frank information, but in a way that is appropriate and safe for young people." The site can be viewed at *www.likeitis.org.uk*.

Another example of positive use of the Internet related to sexuality occurred in 2009, when the New York City Health Department launched a Facebook page to promote condom use. In just one afternoon, 1,500 Facebook messages, called e-condoms, were sent through the Web site. One more example occurred in 2009 when the U.S. Department of Justice unveiled new public-service announcements to educate people about potential dangers that children face online and, for the first time, warned potential online predators that exploiting a child online is a serious federal offense.

Sex toys are just one part of the commercialization of sexuality. It is estimated that the U.S. sex industry generates $9 billion in annual sales. With so much money at stake, do you think it would be difficult to control and regulate such an industry?

Sexual Aids

Another aspect of the commercialization of sexuality is selling the promise (and sometimes the reality) of more satisfying sexual activity through the use of sexual devices and other aids. There is a big business in the manufacture and sale of sexual aids and enhancers. Some, such as penile implants and vibrators, are used in treating sexual dysfunctions. Films on techniques for achieving orgasm and enhancing the sexual experience are often used by sex therapists as an adjunct to their treatment programs.

Previously we discussed some of the uses of vibrators. They come in a variety of colors and shapes and can be electrically or battery operated. They can be used by either sex for solitary masturbation or as a part of heterosexual or homosexual encounters. Many are sold in ordinary retail outlets for massage purposes.

One vibratorlike device, called the Eroscillator, even has its own web page. It points out that the Eroscillator is *not* a vibrator. "It provides a totally unique, gentle 'oscillating' motion which moves naturally and softly from side to side rather than up and down like a vibrator." If you believe the ad, the Eroscillator has three different levels of intensity, is completely safe, is specifically designed to meet your needs, and has no risk of irritation.

Magazines and newspapers are full of ads claiming that women may add extra inches to their breasts with only a few minutes of specific exercise daily or by using creams, massage, or worthless gadgets—all for a price. Just as the Eroscillator does, a breast cream called Enhancia has its own web page. One woman claims she noticed a difference in about 2 weeks: an increase of almost 1 inch around her bust.

In fact, breast size and shape are the result of glandular influences that cannot be altered by applying anything to the breast. It is also impossible to increase breast size through exercise. The effect of exercise is to enlarge muscle tissue. Because there is no muscle tissue in the breast, exercise cannot enhance the breast. Only injections or implants can enlarge the breast. As discussed in In Focus: Body Image, these procedures are controversial and expensive, and they can have dangerous long-term effects.

Underclothing that particularly emphasizes the genitals is manufactured to satisfy a range of tastes. It is sold by mail-order businesses, by email, and by expensive boutiques. Other sexual products are more exotic. A few examples of these products will demonstrate their nature:

1. Some manufacturers have gone beyond the standard type of vibrator that therapists recommend to enhance sexual pleasure. For example, one manufacturer advertises the Sensual Encounter, a 7-inch vibrator with

various attachments: natural veined penis, French tickler, fuzzy tongue, and others. This same ad describes the Anal Intruder vibrator for the novice analist.

2. A variety of aphrodisiacs and lotions are available: Motion Lotion, Joy Jelly, Korean Ginseng capsules, Man Power capsules, Spanish Fly Sugar powder, Jungle Love Sugar powder, or Wild Passion Ginseng capsules. They are unlikely to be effective.

3. A man dissatisfied with the size of his penis may be persuaded to buy a "penis enlarger vacuum," and a female dissatisfied with the size of her breasts can buy a "breast enlarger."

4. Penis extenders are used by those who want to give their partner the sensation of penetration by a larger penis. They are worn at the tip of the penis and are held in place by a condom or straps. Penis erectors vary in design, but many are like splints designed to support a nonerect penis. Another variety is a "cock ring," which fits around the base of the penis after erection and maintains the erection while it is in place. Also available is an artificial penis attached to a motor that moves the penis in a thrusting manner.

5. Artificial vaginas are available for males for masturbatory purposes; artificial penises (dildos) can be used by either males or females for insertion into the vagina or anus.

6. Another product advertises by asking men whether they have ever experienced fellatio while driving a car. If they have and enjoyed the sensation, or would like such an experience, they are invited to buy the Auto Suck Vagina. The product resembles an automobile vacuum and thus, the ad reassuringly advises, keeps its user out of trouble with the highway police should he be stopped "at the moment of climax."

Sexual aids used to be sold almost exclusively out of "porno-sleaze" shops in such places as New York's Times Square, but they have become such big business that they are now sold in women's sex-toy boutiques. Many of these boutiques run a very profitable catalogue business. An example of this type of organization is the Xandria Collection located in San Francisco. Through its catalogue one can purchase dildos, vibrators that fit over the penis for self-stimulation, prosthetic penis aids, penis extensions, clitoral stimulators, penis rings, and Ben-Wa balls (small balls to insert into the vagina that move

around, thereby stimulating the woman), not to mention the various lotions and potions and underwear with holes in just the right places. In addition, the Xandria Collection sells sex manuals: *Sexual Adventures in Marriage, Yesterday's Porno, Sexual Pleasures from A to Z,* and *Sex Comic Classics.*

Another means of selling sexual aids has as its model the famous Tupperware parties. Here is how it works: Someone volunteers the use of her house for the party and invites a group of friends, and a saleswoman shows all sorts of sexual aids, ranging from soft leather to French ticklers (penis sleeves with ribs to stimulate the vagina). Thousands of women are supplementing incomes and sometimes even becoming wealthy by selling sex products at home demonstrations. Passion Parties is one of the largest such companies, with 3,200 saleswomen. Sales grew more than 50% each year over a 3-year period to more than $20 million annually. Eleven Passion Parties saleswomen each sold more than $1 million worth of products in a recent year (Navarro, 2004). Good Vibrations (*www.goodvibes.com*) is an example of a company that advertises numerous sexual toys. Its representatives will come to private homes to host parties and sell sex products. As an example of the company's advertising on the Good Vibrations web site it indicates you can "make it a birthday party or bridal shower they'll never forget."

As you can see, the use of sex to sell products, combined with the manufacture and sale of sexual aids, is significant. You can hardly open a magazine or newspaper, read a book, watch television, attend the theater, or listen to popular music without encountering sexual themes; sexual explicitness (and implicitness) is part of our everyday existence. We need to be aware of its presence so that we can better control its effect on our behavior and attitudes. By way of example, knowing that the scantily clad model has no relation to our need to own a new car, we might be better able to ignore the sexual appeal of the ads and purchase a car that is suited to our needs and financial constraints.

Being aware of the uses of sexuality in the marketplace can make you a better consumer, a more enlightened citizen, and a healthier person sexually.

■ Sexually Explicit Materials

Terminology is critical, but somewhat confusing, in relation to sexually explicit materials. You may hear different people use the same terms to describe different things, so it is important to establish definitions. **Pornography** is visual and written material

> **pornography**
> Visual and written materials used for the purpose of sexual arousal.

Sexually explicit materials are easily available to people of all ages.

that is used for purposes of sexual arousal. It has been said that pornography, as is beauty, is in the eye of the beholder. Opinions about what it is, its possible uses, and its legal status are extremely varied.

Definitions

The legal definition of *obscenity*, established by the Supreme Court in 1973, is that for something to be obscene it must meet all three of the following conditions:

1. The average person, applying contemporary community standards, would find that the work, taken as a whole, appeals to **prurient** interest.

2. The work depicts or describes, in a patently offensive way, sexual conduct specifically defined by the applicable state (or federal) law.

3. The work, taken as a whole, lacks serious literary, artistic, political, or scientific value.

Therefore, although sexually explicit materials are legal in the United States, obscenity is not. Taking the three Supreme Court criteria just listed together, a reasonable definition of **obscenity** is a personal or soci-

prurient
Characterized by lustful thoughts or wishes.

obscenity
Personal or societal judgment that something is offensive.

etal judgment that something is offensive. Therefore, one person may consider obscene something that another does not.

erotica
Sexually oriented material that may be artistically produced or motivated.

Another important term is **erotica**, which usually describes sexually oriented material that can be evaluated positively, in contrast to obscenity, which is offensive. Erotica consists of "depictions of sexuality which display mutuality, respect, affection, and a balance of power" (Stock, 1985). Some people will differentiate between pornography and erotica by indicating that pornography provides a degrading or demeaning portrayal of human beings. In contrast, erotica is not degrading or demeaning anyone. Therefore, a person may find pornography to be unacceptable and erotica to be acceptable based upon this differentiation.

Effects of Sexually Explicit Materials

Traditionally many people have been opposed to sexually explicit materials. Perhaps this is because they feared that the materials had many undesirable effects, such as causing people to participate in sexual activity they might not otherwise have engaged in, increasing the number of sexual offenses, and corrupting the minds of children. It is difficult to do research in an area where there are so many personal and social variables, but a brief look at research findings about the effects of sexually explicit materials may be helpful.

The report of the Commission on Obscenity and Pornography (1970), sponsored by the federal government, and a review of this report by two researchers at Johns Hopkins University (Money & Athanasiou, 1973) give us some information about the effects of pornography. According to these sources, the following appear to be true:

1. There is little, if any, difference in males' and females' sexual responses to sexually explicit materials.

2. People are stimulated only by portrayals of sexual ideas or acts that turn them on. In other words, sexually explicit materials do not seem to plant in people's minds ideas or desires that they do not already have.

3. Exposure to sexually explicit materials does not seem to alter a person's sexual behavior patterns in the long run.

4. Continued exposure to sexually explicit materials tends to lead to indifference and boredom. John Money (1973) believes that stimuli in

Gender
DIMENSIONS

Male and Female Use of Autoerotic Materials

As part of the National Health and Social Life Survey, Laumann and associates (1994) reported on the number of men and women who had used autoerotic materials in the past year. The main activities indicated by the subjects were viewing X-rated movies or videos (23% of the males and 11% of the females), going to a club that has nude or seminude dancers (22% of the males and 4% of the females), and using sexually explicit books or magazines (16% of the males and 4% of the females). Vibrators or dildos were used by 2% of the males and 2% of the females, and other sex toys were used by 1% of the males and 2% of the females. Forty-one percent of the men and 16% of the women reported using autoerotic materials during the past year.

Interestingly, thinking about sex frequently (defined as "every day" or "several times a day") was reported by 54% of the males and 19% of the females. Thinking about sex infrequently (defined as "a few times a month" to "a few times a week") was reported by 43% of the males and 67% of the females. Thinking about sex never or rarely (defined as "less than once a month") was reported by 4% of the males and 16% of the females.

Source: Laumann, E. O., Gagnon, J. H., Michael, R. T., & Michaels, S. *The social organization of sexuality.* Chicago: University of Chicago Press, 1994.

---

sexually explicit materials are effective for 2 to 4 hours. After this time a person becomes either more selective or indifferent to the stimuli.

5. Filling out questionnaires on responses to sexually explicit material may be more stimulating than the material itself. (Perhaps this is best explained by human beings' great capacity to fantasize.)

6. Convicted sex offenders have been exposed to fewer sexually explicit and sexuality education materials during their life than nonoffenders. This fact contradicts the common belief that exposure to sexually explicit materials causes people to commit sexual offenses.

The Society for the Scientific Study of Sexuality (What scientists know about pornography, 2007) provides the following summary regarding effects of exposure to sexually explicit material:

- In general, when exposed to nonviolent erotica, men and women show small, short-term increases in the sexual behaviors they already are used to engaging in, but generally they do not add anything new to their sexual repertoire.

- Both men and women are sexually aroused by erotic material, but women report more negative emotional reactions than men, and women seem to be less likely to access sexually explicit materials.

- Findings on the effects of exposure to violent pornography are more mixed. Some researchers have found that exposure to sexually violent materials increases the acceptance of rape myths (beliefs that ascribe responsibility to women who are the victims) and increases men's self-reported likelihood of raping a woman. Other studies have found just the opposite. Still others have found no association between use of sexually explicit media and negative attitudes toward women.

Rich (2008) summarized research related to the effects of relatively violent pornography on adolescents. Male adolescents were more likely to believe women enjoy forced sexual activity after seeing an excerpt in which a woman was shown as aroused by nonconsenting intercourse. Males who watched films that portrayed violence against females as justifiable and with positive consequences showed increased belief in rape myths and acceptance of violence against women as compared with males who saw films with no sexual violence. Females had the opposite reaction to the same films. Both male and female viewers reported they were more sexually aroused by nonaggressive rather than aggressive sexually explicit materials.

Kingston et al. (2009) looked at pornography's influence on sexually aggressive behavior. They found that pornography use can be a risk factor for sexually aggressive outcomes, principally for men who rate high on other risk factors and who use pornography frequently.

Albright (2008) surveyed more than 15,000 men and women related to pornography. Seventy-five percent of men and 41% of women had intentionally viewed pornography. Women reported more negative consequences, including lowered body image, their partner being critical of their body, increased pressure to perform acts seen in pornographic films, and less actual sexual behavior. Men reported being more critical of their partners' body and less interested in actual sexual behavior.

For years some people have suggested that sexually explicit materials might be stimulating to men, but not to women. Today we know that such materials can be stimulating to both genders, but that there are individual differences in responses. We also know that in most cases exposure to pornography does not influence long-term behaviors or change interests in most sexual behaviors one way or the other.

For many people it was surprising that evidence from the President's Commission (1973) showed that sexually explicit materials might have some educational benefit. For example, if the information is factual, it can enlighten the ignorant. It also seems to foster less inhibited attitudes toward sexuality: "Well timed in its use and supported by good moral principles, visual erotica can become a positive and constructive aid in the service of developing sexual normalcy" (Money, 1973, 143). Although there is no strong evidence, it could also be argued that sexually explicit materials can provide variety and add spice to the life of some people. Given the emphasis on safer sex alternatives today, sexually explicit materials can be helpful in providing sexual stimulation and pleasure without potential exposure to HIV.

Child Pornography

So far we have considered sexually explicit materials about adults for adults. There is increasing concern about the use of children in pornographic materials and, more recently, about continued eroticization of young children in the print media and on television.

The use of minors in sexually explicit media—**child pornography**—is now prohibited. In the past, many magazine publishers and film producers used their own children in sexually explicit materials they developed. Others advertised in magazines catering to readers of pornography. Still, in spite of the law, magazines and films that depict children in sexually erotic conditions are produced and sold. Given the current societal concern for child abuse (sexual and otherwise) and for missing children, law enforcement agencies have organized to crack down on the kiddie porn industry.

child pornography
Use of minors in sexually explicit media.

People who might support the availability of sexually explicit materials for adults usually do not condone child pornography.

In 1984, the National Center for Missing and Exploited Children was established by the federal government. In 1997, an Exploited Child Unit was established within this agency to deal with child pornography and other crimes. In 1998, the CyberTipline was launched to have a means of reporting incidents of child sexual exploitation including the possession, manufacture, or distribution of child pornography; online enticement; child prostitution; child sex tourism; extrafamilial child sexual molestation; unsolicited obscene material sent to a child; and misleading domain names, words, or digital images. The CyberTipline (*www.cybertipline.com*) is staffed 24 hours a day, 7 days a week. It received its 200,000th report in 2004, and by April 2009 it had received almost 600,000 reports. In 2002, a Child Victim Identification Program was established to identify victims of child pornography.

In 2006, the Sex Offender Registration and Notification Act was passed. It was passed for two reasons: (1) to establish a national database that tracks the location and movements of people convicted of a criminal offense against a victim who is a minor, have been convicted of a sexually violent offense, or are sexually violent predators, and (2) to register and verify the addresses of sex offenders who reside in

Ethical DIMENSIONS

Should Kids Be Sexualized?

In 2005 there was a great deal of discussion related to whether to control the routines of high school bands, cheerleaders, and dancers. A Texas legislator sponsored a bill to ban "sexually suggestive" cheerleading in the public schools. A school superintendent in Alabama told bands to clean up their acts. These actions prompted a variety of responses.

On the one hand, one Alabama parent said, "As long as they're not taking any clothes off, I don't see anything wrong with it." A PTA president said, "If we're going to limit our children doing their routines, then take the Dallas Cowgirls off TV."

On the other hand, one band director said, "It is a family show, and high school girls shouldn't be doing college-girl dance routines." A school superintendent said, "It would be much more appealing to have fine sounds produced by the bands than vulgar routines."

Is it ethical for high school bands, cheerleaders, and dancers to be allowed to do suggestive routines? Is it right to have legislation, such as that in Texas, designed to ban "sexually suggestive" cheerleading? Who should decide what is right or wrong related to the possibility of sexualizing students in public schools?

Technological advances have made controlling access to sexually explicit materials very difficult. Debates continue about whether or not it should be controlled at all.

states without a "minimally sufficient" sex offender registry program. (Today all 50 states have minimally sufficient programs.) Guidelines for this act can be seen at *www.ojp.usdoj.gov/smart/pdfs/fr_2008_07_02.pdf*.

Under federal legislation, child pornography is defined as any visual depiction where a minor is used to engage in sexually explicit conduct, or a technological image is used that is indistinguishable from that of a minor, or it appears that a minor is engaging in sexually explicit conduct. It is a federal crime to knowingly produce, distribute, receive, or possess with intent to distribute, a visual depiction of any kind, including a drawing, cartoon, sculpture, or painting that meets these criteria. A minor is defined as a person younger than the age of 18.

Child pornography exists in multiple formats, including print media, videotape, film, CD-ROM, and DVD. It is transmitted on various platforms within the Internet.

The Control of Sexually Explicit Materials

Should sexually explicit materials be censored and controlled? There are varying opinions. In an attempt to keep sexually explicit materials on the Internet away from the 16 million users younger than 17 years old in the United States, Congress passed the Child Online Protection Act, which forced web sites to require a credit card number or some other adult ID. The law made it a crime to knowingly communicate to a minor "for commercial purposes" any online material that is "harmful to minors." Penalties included fines up to $50,000 per day for each violation and up to 6 months in prison. At best, however, the law would make sexually explicit material a bit more difficult for minors to reach. It does not touch areas not on the web, such as email or Usenet newsgroups. It also does not affect noncommercial sites or operations based outside the United States (Child Online Protection Act of 1998, 2003). On February 1, 1999, U.S. District Judge Lowell Reed extended indefinitely a preliminary injunction against the act, ruling it violates free speech (*ACLU v. Reno II*). This law has been controversial. Some people believe that it is in society's best interest to protect children from sexually explicit materials. Free speech advocates, in contrast, challenge the law on constitutional grounds, arguing it would affect everybody on the web.

In 2004 the Supreme Court kept in place the 1999 order blocking enforcement of the Child Online Protection Act. The court said that the government must show why the voluntary use of filters to screen out material unsuitable for children would not work as well as the law's criminal penalties (Greenhouse, 2004).

In 2009, the long legal drive to shield children from sexually explicit material on the web ended. The Supreme Court struck down the law on free-speech grounds. Judges said parents can protect their children in their own way by installing software filters on their computers.

The Child Pornography and Protection Act was passed in 1996 (High court to hear arguments on child porn amendment, 2001). Since then supporters have claimed that the act was an essential tool to prevent pedophiles from preying on children. Those who disagree have argued that it is so vaguely worded that there is no way to know what is over the line and what is not. Through the years court challenges related to the act have had inconsistent outcomes. For example, one federal district court judge found the law constitutional, and one U.S. court of appeals struck it down. The debate continues.

A major related event occurred in June 2003 when the U.S. Supreme Court upheld a federal law requiring public library personnel to install pornography filters on all computers providing Internet access, as a condition of continuing to receive federal subsidies and grants (Greenhouse, 2003). The law, enacted in 2001, had been blocked by a lower court and never taken effect. Under the law, filters are required for all library users, not just children. The law authorizes, but does not require, librarians to unblock Internet sites at the request of adult users. Many opinions exist about the wisdom of this law and how it relates to First Amendment rights to free speech.

Certain segments of the public are very concerned about the increased availability of sexually explicit materials and have organized to combat this trend. They point out that many X-rated movies, CDs, and DVDs are purchased and rented. They

Myth vs Fact

Myth: There is no difference between obscenity and pornography.
Fact: Yes, there is. Obscenity is not protected by the Constitution. It follows the Supreme Court definition, but pornography is material designed to arouse and has no legal or consistent definition.

Myth: Sexually explicit material causes violence against women.
Fact: No reputable research in the United States, Europe, or Asia finds a causal link between pornography and violence.

Myth: Men watch pornography and imitate it or force women to do what they see.
Fact: Violence and intimidation existed for thousands of years before commercial pornography. People do not mimic what they read or view in knee-jerk fashion.

Men do not learn coercion from sexual pictures.

Myth: Pornography degrades women.
Fact: Sexism, not sexual behavior, degrades women. Opponents of sexual speech do not understand that it is in everyone's interest to allow a variety of pleasurable materials that enhance well-being and sexual fulfillment.

Myth: Pornography is only for men.
Fact: Half the adult videos in the United States are bought or rented by women alone or women in couples. AIDS and other STIs have made it a public health necessity to encourage sexual fantasy material that offers women and men safe alternatives to unhealthy sexual contact.

talk about the popularity of cable television channels, such as the Playboy Channel, that specialize in sexual broadcasts; they also emphasize the success of such sexually explicit magazines as *Penthouse* and *Playboy*.

The interesting aspect of the organized opposition to sexually explicit materials is that it has united diverse groups. National conservative groups as well as some national feminist groups have joined a loose network of local groups to fight the "Porn War." Among the conservative organizations are the National Federation for Decency, the Citizens for Decency through Law, Morality in Media, the Moral Majority, and the Citizens for Legislation Against Decadence. Among the feminist groups are Women Against Pornography, Feminists Against Pornography, the Pornography Resource Center, and Women Against Violence Against Women.

The objections of these groups to sexually explicit materials are several. Some consider an explicit description or image of sexual acts immoral and irreligious. Others object to women being portrayed as sex objects and believe this view of women will be generalized to "real life." Still others perceive that women in sexually explicit materials are treated violently and fear that this type of portrayal

Myth vs Fact

Myth: Women in pornography are exploited or victimized.
Fact: Women are exploited and harassed in all fields, including pornography. Exploitation will stop when it is vigorously prosecuted everywhere it occurs. Some women in pornography say their work gives them independence and a sense of accomplishment; banning it would worsen their lives.

Myth: As an aid to masturbation, pornography is action that is not protected by the First Amendment.
Fact: Pornography may lead to masturbation much as a novel or film may lead to tears or laughter.

Feminists for Free Expression does not believe policing masturbation is the proper business of government or well-meaning committees.

Myth: Banning sexual material will protect or help women.
Fact: Historically, censorship has hurt women. It has prevented them from getting information about sexuality and reproduction. The best protection for women's ideas is the constitutional protection of free speech. The answer to bad pornography is good pornography, not no pornography.

might cause more violence toward women. For example, Women Against Pornography (WAP) has demanded that sexually explicit materials be prohibited from depicting rape, whipping, or bondage. WAP believes that such depictions lead men to feel superior to women and extend that idea of superiority to nonsexual relationships (such as those in the workplace). Women Against Violence Against Women concentrates predominantly on music and advertising, asserting that commercial degradation of women fosters sexism.

Many groups of women are most vocal in their opinions. However, though not organized, men also suffer from sexploitation. When men are shown performing violent acts on women, they are being taught to be powerful and dominant over the other sex. They are learning that sexual relationships require a measure of forcefulness that in actuality interferes with sexual arousal rather than enhances it. When men learn to treat women as sexual objects, their relationships suffer. Depictions of men and women sharing equally in sexual and love relationships would teach both sexes that sexual fulfillment is a mutual responsibility; the results would be a decrease of pressure on men to know what to do and how to do it and fewer sexually frustrated women.

The ACLU says that it is no accident that freedom of speech is the first freedom mentioned in the First Amendment. It is not limited to "pure speech"—books, newspapers, leaflets, and rallies. It also protects "symbolic speech"—nonverbal expression whose purpose it is to communicate ideas. It exists precisely to protect the most offensive and controversial speech from government suppression. The best means to counter obnoxious speech is speech. Persuasion, not coercion, is the solution. The ACLU also indicates that the innovation and citizen empowerment inspired by online communications will be lost if civil liberties do not also apply in cyberspace. Furthermore, there are three reasons freedom of expression is essential to a free society: (1) The right to express one's thoughts and to communicate freely with others is the foundation of self-fulfillment. (2) It is vital to the attainment and advancement of knowledge and the search for the truth. (3) It is necessary to our system of self-government and gives the American people a "checking function" against government excess and corruption.

Feminists for Free Expression (FFE) is a leading voice opposing state and national legislation that threatens free speech. This organization defends the right of free expression in court cases, supports the rights of activists whose works have been suppressed or censored, and provides expert speakers. On the topic of sexually explicit materials, FFE published *Feminism and Free Speech: Pornography* to aid in the understanding of pornography, its uses and benefits, and its relation to violence. An overview of its scientific and cross-cultural research is provided in the Myth vs Fact box about pornography on this page. Relatedly, there is more erotica being developed that is not sexist but feminist and gender friendly. It is designed to portray equitable relationships.

In October 2002 the Museum of Sex opened in New York City. The purpose of the museum is to preserve and present the history, evolution, and cultural significance of human sexuality. Not everyone approves of it. William Donohue, president of the Catholic League for Religions and Civil Rights, denounced the museum for celebrating "smut as sex." He accused the museum of championing or associating with racists, pornographers, and individuals who "exhibit pathological characteristics." On the other side, June Reinisch, a historian adviser to the museum and director emeritus of the Kinsey Institute, characterized it as a serious endeavor, in the sense that it wants to inform and educate as well as to entertain. "Sexuality is a very important part of individual life and to culture," she said. "To not understand it is to be handicapped in your understanding of human relations and culture" (James, 2002). It will be interesting to see how the Museum of Sex is regarded as time goes by.

Finally, the position of the Sexuality Information and Education Council of the United States on sexually explicit materials is as follows:

> When sensitively used in a manner appropriate to the viewer's age and developmental level, sexually explicit visual, printed, or online materials can be valuable educational or personal aids, helping to reduce ignorance and confusion and contributing to a wholesome concept of sexuality. However, the use of violence, exploitation, or degradation, or the portrayal of children in sexually explicit materials is reprehensible. Minors should be legally protected from all forms of sexual exploitation.
>
> Adults should have the right of access to sexually explicit materials for personal use. Legislative and judicial efforts to prevent the production and distribution of sexually explicit materials endanger constitutionally guaranteed freedoms of speech and press and could be employed to restrict the appropriate professional use of such materials by sexuality educators, therapists, and researchers.

Sex Workers

An important consideration in the study of sexual commercial enterprises is the topic of sex work, or prostitution. The term **prostitution** refers to any situation in

prostitution
Participating in sexual activity for pay or profit.

which one person pays another for sexual gratification. Sex workers may be males as well as females, but primarily sex workers have been and are females. Women do sex work mainly to make money, but other factors can also motivate them. For example, the lack of education of most sex workers limits their job opportunities. In addition, some women think sex work will be exciting and glamorous, whereas others are motivated to become sex workers because they do not like the discipline and boredom of regular jobs. Some women who are drug addicts turn to sex work to support the habit. The background of many sex workers has included emotional deprivation and sexual abuse—even within the family. Some sex workers therefore feel that by providing sexual pleasure they can gain intimacy and attention.

Types of Sex Workers

It is difficult to estimate the number of persons who currently work or have ever worked as sex workers because there are various definitions of prostitution and because sex work is usually illegal. There are many types of sex workers; the major types are call girls, house prostitutes, streetwalkers, massage parlor prostitutes, and bar girls and strippers.

Heidi Fleiss, the so-called Hollywood Madam, ran a high-priced call girl ring in Beverly Hills. She was arrested and convicted on several charges ranging from pandering to tax evasion. However, the case raised ethical questions, because all the call girls were granted immunity and none of the clients was charged. Should prosecutors use government resources to pursue prostitutes' customers?

Call Girls
Call girls are at the top of the profession. They do not solicit; rather, their "dates" are arranged by personal referral or by another person. They have regular clients who pay high fees and also pay their bills.

House Prostitutes
House (brothel) prostitutes work in more structured conditions in brothels (houses in which prostitutes work) and serve more men at cheaper rates than call girls would charge. Brothels are legal in some counties of Nevada but are illegal in all other areas of the United States.

Streetwalkers
Streetwalkers are more independent than house prostitutes but lack the contacts or ability to become call girls. They stand or stroll on streets and approach passing males. Because of their visibility, streetwalkers are the most frequently arrested sex workers.

The ratio of on-street prostitution to off-street prostitution in cities varies with local law, police, and custom. Whereas street prostitution accounts for 10% to 20% of the prostitution in larger cities, in some smaller cities with limited indoor venues street prostitution may

call girls
Highly paid female sex workers who work by appointment only.

house (brothel) prostitutes
Sex workers who work in brothels.

streetwalkers
Sex workers who work on the streets.

constitute about 50% (Prostitution in the United States—the statistics, 1998).

Many women who engage in street sex work experience pregnancies and become mothers. They report that being pregnant or parenting while regularly working the street caused them to feel ashamed of themselves and their work and anxious for their own and their children's safety. Pregnancies and parenting responsibilities also altered their working productivity and practices (Sloss & Harper, 2004).

Massage Parlor Sex Workers

Certainly many **massage parlors** offer only massages, but at others a client can find many "extras." The environment offers an indoor place to work that is safer than the streets, and massage parlor workers may be motivated to earn extra money by providing sexual favors. Fellatio is popular among both customers and masseuses. Many men claim they cannot get their regular partners to participate in fellatio. The masseuses appreciate it because it is efficient: They are trying to earn as much money as they can, so it is useful to be able to service a number of men in a short period.

Bar Girls and Strippers

Many times **bar girls** and strippers are supposed to act available so men will buy them drinks. This helps the establishment make more on the sale of liquor. Sometimes, however, paid sexual activity is also offered.

Examples of this type of activity can be found in many countries. For example, an increasing number of Cambodian "beer girls," who sell international beers, wines, and liquors at outdoor eateries and in bars, are also selling sex. If the women refuse a client's offer of sex for money, they may lose a beer sale. Because they depend heavily on commis-

sions, they feel they have to do something to convince the client to buy. To make matters worse, beer girls are less likely than brothel workers to use condoms, and surveys show that as many as one-fifth of them are HIV positive (Increasing number of Cambodian "beer girls" selling sex, 2003).

Japan's sex trade, estimated at $13 billion per year, is one of the nation's fastest-growing industries. Record unemployment has forced many women to work at brothels euphemistically known as fashion, health, soapland, pink salons, or telephone clubs. Only 6% to 25% of sex workers and the public use condoms. HIV has not been widespread in Japan, but the prevalence rate is highest among female sex workers, close to 3%. Because of the lack of HIV and AIDS education, the very low rate of condom use, and the relatively rapid increase in rates of HIV among sex workers, it is feared that HIV and AIDS could become a significant problem in Japan (Kakuchi, 2003).

Kershaw (2004) reported that stripping can be a springboard either to something better or to an abyss of drugs, alcohol, abuse, and prostitution. Sometimes stripping is just a living—the rent. Many dancers say they love what they do, if not for the money then for the attention, or for the power they wield over men who are "stupid enough to pay to see you naked." Most dancers seem to aspire to something else—being an actress, a model, a good mother, or a successful career person. Some make more than $2,000 to $3,000 per week.

There has been greater female attendance at strip clubs in recent years. Some dancers have incorporated female patrons into a sexualized space traditionally designed for men. They have tailored their lap dances for a female patron. In this way, the strip club becomes a potential space for engaging in same-gender eroticism that includes elements of play (Wosick-Correa & Joseph, 2008).

Male Sex Workers

Whereas the majority of sex workers are women, some men also sell sexual services to women or to other men. **Gigolos** provide escort and sexual ser-

---

massage parlors
Places where sex workers can be hired to perform sexual acts under the guise of giving a massage.

bar girls
Sex workers who are supposed to act available so customers will buy them drinks.

gigolo
A man who is paid to provide escort and sexual services, usually for wealthy, middle-aged women.

hustler
A male sex worker who performs homosexual acts for pay.

pimps
Individuals who set up female sex workers with clients.

vices for women, and **hustlers** are male sex workers who perform homosexual acts for pay. Male sex workers may be classified as female sex workers are, but the differences are often not obvious.

Percentages of male and female sex workers vary from city to city. Estimates in some larger cities suggest that 20% to 30% of sex workers are male. In San Francisco, it has been estimated that 25% of the female sex workers are transgendered (Prostitution in the United States—the statistics, 1998).

In Bangkok, Thailand, a nonprofit group called Swing provides services—including education about condom use—to male sex workers (*Bangkok Post* profiles group providing services for male commercial sex workers, 2005). It is the first organization to focus on Thailand's approximately 4,000 male sex workers. Swing offers English classes, Internet access, and places to nap and shower. The group plans to offer exercise equipment and medical assistance. Although Thai society has become "more tolerant" of female sex workers, it is "less accepting" of male sex workers. People look down on them because they think they are lazy and terrible people. Male sex workers also have experienced stigma in doctors' offices and sometimes avoid being treated for STIs if a doctor or nurse makes them feel uncomfortable. Swing establishes relationships with doctors to make "appropriate referrals" for its clients, and the group plans to have its own in-house physician.

In 2005 Heidi Fleiss, the former "Hollywood Madam," decided to open the "Heidi Stud Farm" in Nevada (Hollywood madam caters for ladies, 2005). She was sure her new service for women would be a hit. She said, "Women make more money these days, they're calling the shots, they're more powerful. And let's face it, it's hard to meet someone."

Pimps

The people who set up sex workers with clients are called **pimps**. Sex workers give the money they earn to their pimps in exchange for affection, concern, and love. Pimps recruit newcomers into sex work, they manage the sex workers' business and provide them counsel, bail them out of jail when necessary, and regulate the streetwalking prostitution enterprise (without a pimp, streetwalking sex workers might be in danger in certain neighborhoods).

Although most sex workers are women, it is thought that as many as 20% to 30% of sex workers are men.

Pitts et al. (2004) sought to answer the question, "Who pays for sex and why?" As compared to those who had not been clients, they found that male clients of sex workers were significantly older, less likely to have been educated beyond high school, less likely to report having a regular partner in the past 6 months, and more likely to report that their most recent sexual encounter was with a casual partner. Clients said their major reasons for paying for sexual activity were to satisfy their sexual needs (44%), followed by the belief that paying for sexual activity was less trouble (36%), and that it would be entertaining (36%).

Little is known about the magnitude of prostitution or changes in its incidence. Because prostitution is an illegal (except in rural Nevada) and socially stigmatized profession in the United States, the amount of reliable information is very limited. Smith (2003) summarized existing studies indicating that between 1.6% to 2% of U.S. women had ever had sexual activity in exchange for money or drugs. He also indicated that 0.6% of U.S. men had a prostitute for a sex partner during the last year, 5.9% within the past 5 years, and 16.3% at some point in the past. Sexual activity with prostitutes does not consistently vary by education or age. It is higher among those living in metropolitan areas, African Americans, those with lower incomes, veterans (probably when in military service), those who attend church less frequently, and those who have gone through a divorce.

Phone Sex Workers

Female employees of a phone sex company were interviewed to find out who they are and why they work at a job they often can't mention publicly (Rich, 2004). The women ranged in age from 21 to 45 and came from a variety of educational backgrounds. Many felt they held an important social role. While some lost respect for men as a result of their job, others believed that by taking callers with rape fantasies, they kept potentially violent men from enacting real-life crimes. Because some callers claim to be virgins, some employees reported that they were educating men about female sexuality. Some workers cited that they liked the casual environment, or the chance to have fun before settling down in a more serious career. The main reason they took their jobs was money. They made more than most felt they could earn elsewhere. They said the income came at a price, however, because they could not be honest with people about what they do to make money.

Public Health Perspective

The issue of commercial sex work causes a lot of debate among public health professionals (Kempner, 2005). Historically, public health professionals focused on sex workers as disease vectors—those who could spread STIs to the wider population. Interventions, therefore, focused not on the health of the sex workers but rather on their role in shaping the health of society. More recently, the World Health Organization indicated that interventions can have a positive impact on both the spread of disease and the lives of those involved in sex work. Paying more attention to the health of sex workers involves adopting a nonjudgmental attitude, respecting sex workers' human rights, involving sex workers in program development, and recognizing that sex workers are part of the solution. This kind of model can be controversial because it seeks to improve conditions and health without necessarily eliminating potentially harmful behavior or behavior that some people would feel is wrong or immoral.

Sexual Slavery

Various types of forced labor are increasing worldwide. One researcher concluded there were 27 million people around the world trapped in virtual prisons on farms, in sweatshops, or in brothels. Many women and girls are forced into prostitution, moved from country to country each year by criminals who

sell them into virtual slavery or demand they work to pay off exorbitant "debts" (Memmott, 2001).

From the former Soviet Union alone, an estimated 50,000 women are trafficked abroad each year and forced into sexual slavery. The women are told they will be given jobs as waitresses, nannies, or dancers in foreign countries. However, once they arrive at their destination, they are told they owe hundreds of dollars in job placement fees and airfare. They are threatened with beating and rape and told their family members will be hurt if they do not comply. To ensure compliance by the women, traffickers usually confiscate passports, then beat, rape, and drug them. Profits from trafficking in women reach $7 to $12 billion per year (Dolgov, 2001).

Sex trafficking has become one of the world's growth industries (Kristof, 2005). In Cambodia, for example, it is like an aquarium. Beyond a glass wall are dozens of teenage girls in skimpy white outfits, each with a number. The customer orders a girl by number, and the manager delivers her a moment later to a private room. The U.S. State Department estimates that 600,000 to 800,000 people are trafficked across international borders each year, mostly girls and most of them for the sex industry. Many more are trafficked within a country. As it becomes a global industry, sex trafficking is increasingly controlled by organized crime.

Girls are lured from other countries to the United States. They are promised restaurant jobs, modeling jobs, and other opportunities. But then people who traffic in sex slaves seize their passports. They tell the girls that they owe a large sum of money to pay for their trip and other expenses. Of course, the girls don't have the money so they are forced to work in brothels. Some of the girls are baited by promises of legitimate jobs and a better life in America, many are abducted, and others have been bought from or abandoned by their impoverished families. Some women are sold four or five times to different people like a piece of property (Vitagliano, 2004).

In 2005, *48 Hours*, a CBS News presentation, did a special on sex slavery (Rescued from sex slavery, 2005). Reporters traveled to Romania with hidden cameras to find out if it were really possible to purchase a sex slave. In a very short time, they learned about girls who were for sale as slaves. One contact told them that, "You can buy 10 girls in one night if you want to." The contact helped them meet with a sex trafficker. The woman brought out a young girl who was for sale. She had the girl undress to show that she didn't have any marks or skin disease. After some haggling, Peter Van Sant, the CBS newsman, bought the girl for $1,800. Later, the girl told the newsman it was the first time she had been outside for over a year. She said her owners brutally beat

Did You Know...

Even obtaining the services of a sex worker has changed with the advent of the Internet. For example, you can search under "prostitutes" and "[name of city]" and get a listing of the best spots to find a sex worker. Local police monitor such sites as well. Also, you can link up with an "escort" service via the Internet, ordering online.

her, and that she was fed like a dog. She had become a sex slave after her mother abandoned her in an orphanage. The *48 Hours* crew brought the girl to a shelter where she started a new life. They had demonstrated how easy it was to buy a sex slave.

The Trafficking Victims Protection Act of 2000 and its reauthorizations in 2003, 2005, and 2008 define a human trafficking victim as a person induced to perform labor or a commercial sex act through force, fraud, or coercion. The act was put in place to combat international trafficking in persons, to combat trafficking in persons in the United States, and to provide funding to assist with these efforts. In its first 21 months of operation (January 2007 to September 2008), the Human Trafficking Reporting System recorded information on more than 1,200 alleged incidents of human trafficking in the United States. Most (83%) of the incidents involved sex trafficking. About one-third of the 1,200 incidents involved children (More than 1,200 alleged incidents of human trafficking reported in the U.S., 2009).

Even though the Trafficking Victims Protection Act enables the federal government to distribute funding for victims of severe forms of trafficking, there has been controversy about use of the money. In 2009, the ACLU filed a lawsuit against the U.S. Department of Health and Human Services alleging that the agency was allowing a Roman Catholic organization to limit grant money to organizations that do not provide access to contraception and abortion services for human trafficking victims. The ACLU said the restrictions present serious health risks because sex trafficking victims have a higher incidence of HIV and other STIs. It further said that the organization was misusing taxpayer money and attempting to impose its religious beliefs on trafficking victims (ACLU sues HHS over religious restrictions on funds for programs serving sex trafficking victims, 2009).

The U.S. Department of State has an Office to Monitor and Combat Trafficking in Persons. Annually, it publishes a *Trafficking in Persons Report* that is available at *www.state.gov/g/tip*. Organizations that work on the issue of sex slavery include the International Justice Mission (*www.ijm.org*) and Free the Slaves (*http://freetheslaves.net*).

Opinions About Sex Work

The subject of sex workers produces strong emotional reactions in many people. For example, some people believe sex workers should have the right to do their work. Others believe that this practice maintains a world where women are subordinate and sex workers reinforce broad patterns of discrimination. From an economic perspective, it has been argued that sex work helps many women escape poverty and hunger. They get paid much more than they could earn by doing anything else, so they can better help their families. Also, legalizing sex work would make it easier for sex workers to organize into unions as other workers have, which could help improve their working conditions, raise the status of their profession, and promote respect for their human rights.

Of course many people would argue against sex work on moral grounds. Perhaps they feel that sexual activity should be restricted to marital relations or that it is immoral for sex workers to participate in sexual activity with many different people.

In contrast to those who organize against sex work, the North American Task Force on Prostitution (NTFP) was founded in 1979 to act as an umbrella organization for prostitutes and prostitutes' rights organizations. It is a network of sex workers and their supporters that advocates for the rights of sex workers to organize on their own behalf, work safely and without legal repression, travel without legal restrictions, have families and raise children, and enjoy the same rights, responsibilities, and privileges as other people. The goals of the NTFP are to (1) repeal the existing prostitution laws; (2) ensure the right of prostitutes and other sex workers to bargain with their employers, when they work for third parties, to improve their working conditions; (3) inform the public about a wide range of issues related to prostitution and other forms of sex work; (4) promote the development of support services for sex workers, including HIV, AIDS, and STIs and violence-prevention projects, as well as health and social support services for sex workers (including supportive programs to deal with STIs, violence, and substance abuse), legal assistance projects, and job retraining and other programs to assist prostitutes who wish to change

Multicultural
DIMENSIONS

"Values" of Prostitution in Other Countries?

In Russia, tens of thousands of female college students work as prostitutes or carry on exclusive relationships with so-called sponsors to pay for college. The Russian Internet is replete with web sites that offer free search engines that match potential clients with students. Most sites provide the woman's age, body measurements, types of sex she practices, corresponding costs, and even reviews by former clients. One girl used to work as an elementary teacher earning the equivalent of $60 per month. Now she works as a prostitute and earns the equivalent of $200 to $300 for a night of sexual activities. Of course, the women have expenses such as paying for a madam (agent) and use of an apartment or other appropriate facility. When asked how her parents feel about her work, one student said, "We tell them we work as waitresses. They don't ask any questions" (MacWilliams, 2002).

In some situations, prostitutes are very concerned about their rights. For example, in Paris hundreds of prostitutes wearing white masks with tears painted on them rallied in front of the French Senate to protest a high-profile government crackdown on their livelihood (French prostitutes protest crackdown, 2002).

their occupation; and (5) end the public stigma associated with sex work.

There are other examples of giving a louder voice to a business that has thrived in silence (Navarro, 2004). In Huntsville, Alabama, a chapter of the Sex Workers Outreach Project was formed. It is part of a national movement to demand greater acceptance and protection for sex workers. In San Francisco there is a Center for Sex and Culture where prostitutes met to plot their next political move after losing a ballot initiative that would have eased police enforcement of prostitution laws. In New York there is a magazine for people in the sex industry. On the Internet, prostitutes have found ways to find one another, form online communities, and connect with groups in other communities. The ultimate goal for some in the movement is decriminalization of prostitution. They say there are safe ways to work—that sex work is only a risk when it is illegal. They also argue that prostitution is a viable source of income for many people, and that sexual activity between adults for money should be treated as any other form of legal labor. However, some former prostitutes oppose this movement because they see the business as inherently exploitative and degrading.

In 2005 the United Kingdom Royal College of Nursing called on the British government to decriminalize prostitution in an attempt to limit associated negative health consequences (Prostitutes are people too, 2005). It was pointed out that prostitutes face many occupational hazards such as STIs, physical violence, psychological disorders, and a lifestyle associated with substance abuse. Compounding the situation is a propensity for them to be excluded from routine preventive and therapeutic health care. It was further indicated that prostitutes, be they men or women, are real people and suffer real illness and experience real pain from circumstances forced on them. They need medical care and treatment with the same respect afforded to other members of the community. The conclusion was that decriminalization of prostitution would be a fundamental step to help these often vulnerable people.

Controlling Sex Work

Some officials have tried various ways to manage sex work. For example, San Francisco took a laissez-faire approach. As a result, sex work is highly visible in tourist sections in the form of massage parlors, escort services, bar sex workers, hotel sex workers, and call girls (or boys). The major benefit of this approach has been to restrict sex work to nonresidential parts of the city. The control model—whereby certain neighborhoods strictly enforce laws against sex work—has been employed in North Dallas; the results have been reductions in crime and in visibility of sex workers. The regulation model—whereby sex work is legalized and subject to certain regulations—has been tried in rural Nevada, where it has resulted in a minimal amount of crime and where, for the most part, sex work is limited to controlled brothels. Finally, there is the zoning model—whereby sex work is tolerated but not legal only in certain parts of the city. With this model, sex workers are supposedly visible only in a certain part of the city, and crime associated with sex work is limited to that area. None of these approaches has been totally successful, and each has advantages and disadvantages.

Another method of trying to control sex work has been making public the identities of sex workers and their customers. For example, in 1997

Multicultural
DIMENSIONS

Organizations for Sex Workers

One organization for sex workers is Call Off Your Tired Ethics (COYOTE), which was founded in 1973. It works for the rights of all sex workers of all genders and persuasions. COYOTE supports programs to assist sex workers if they choose to change their occupation, works to prevent the scapegoating of sex workers for AIDS and other STIs, and educates sex workers, their clients, and the general public about safer sex.

Prostitutes of New York (PONY) is a support and advocacy group for all people in the sex industry. PONY advocates the decriminalization of prostitution and calls for an end to illegal police activity in the enforcement of existing laws. It provides legal and health referrals to sex workers and encourages members to recommend doctors, therapists, and other professionals who provide high-quality service to sex workers. PONY encourages all people who sell sex or profit from sex to learn about the diversity of their industry, to promote professional standards in their sector, and to learn more about the history of the world's oldest profession (and its allied industries).

There are similar groups in other countries. One example is the Prostitutes Collective of Victoria (PCV) (Australia), which is a community-based organization developed to include and represent sex-industry workers' concerns about the issue of prostitution as a part of a worldwide prostitutes' rights movement. It works for basic human rights and occupational health and safety rights for all prostitution workers.

The Network of Sex Work Projects (NSWP) was formed in 1991. It consists of sex workers and organizations that provide services to sex workers in more than 40 countries. The NSWP focuses on issues similar to those of interest to the other groups and aims to facilitate opportunities for the voices of sex workers to be heard in relevant international forums.

"John TV" started in Kansas City. Every Wednesday morning viewers of the local government cable TV channel saw the names, photographs, dates of birth, and addresses of people—mostly men—who were arrested for visiting sex workers. Above each picture was this disclaimer: "This person is innocent until found guilty by a court." The ACLU objected to this practice because it targeted people before they were convicted of a crime and used a government-controlled medium to deliver its message of humiliation.

"John TV" has been used in other places as well. In Oklahoma, its goals include to expose and identify those who have preyed upon women lost to drug addiction and street prostitution, use those caught and published as an example to dissuade others, and to forward the ideology of decriminalization of 100% private, consensual and nonorganized prostitution so that the community's limited resources can be focused on street, forced, and organized prostitution and trafficking. More detail is available about John TV at *http://johntv.com*.

Another method of controlling sex workers involves organizations that provide help and support for sex workers who desire to change their life and stop being sex workers. One such organization is the Council for Prostitution Alternatives in Portland, Oregon. Its goal is to help women who want to leave the sex industry find alternatives to lives in prostitution. A number of services are provided, including education, health care, referrals to services when needed, legal assistance, mentoring, and hospitality. More information can be found at *www.prostitutionalternatives.org*. Children of the Night is a similar organization located in San Francisco.

A different approach to controlling sex work came about in 1996 when the Lusty Lady Theater in San Francisco became the first women-managed strip club in the United States to unionize. This resulted in elimination of racist hiring practices and the practice of customers being allowed to videotape dancers without their consent via one-way mirrors. It also resulted in having consistent disciplinary policies, better health benefits, and better job security (Brooks, 2005).

The federal government has tried another way to control sex work. Since 2003 all foreign nongovernmental organizations seeking U.S. global HIV/AIDS funds have been required to pledge their opposition to prostitution and sex trafficking to be eligible to partner with the U.S. government in combating HIV/AIDS in the developing world. In 2005 the rule was extended to American organizations as well (U.S. requirement that AIDS groups sign pledge against commercial sex work "harms" AIDS work, 2005).

Ditmore (2005) pointed out that many agencies are severely restricted by the policy. For example, some projects advocate the empowerment of sex workers to help them develop better lives. Other projects assist trafficked persons and sex workers in

Global DIMENSIONS

Sex Work in Other Countries

Sex work occurs all over the world. There has been a recent demand for Russian women (Pope, 1997). Young, pretty women have been told they have modeling jobs but are later forced into the sex industry. They are given false papers, assumed identities, and phony marriage partners so they can work abroad.

Israel is said to have a $450 million per year sex work ring. Young women describe hostagelike conditions, severe beatings, and rape as punishment by their captors (Pope, 1997).

Here is a sampling of facts about sex work in other countries (Caron, 1998):

- Sex work is legal in Australia, but sex workers must be at least 18 years old. There are laws against pimping. Condoms are compulsory in sexual relationships with sex workers.
- Sex work is legal in Brazil. There are street sex workers and women working out of bars, hotels, massage parlors, saunas, and escort services. Child sex work is an expanding market in Brazil.

- Sex work is legal in Canada, but pimping and solicitation in public are not.
- In 1991 sex work was prohibited in China. Forced reeducation is punishment that includes legal and moral education and manual labor in a specified camp for 6 months to 2 years, for both sex workers and johns.
- In Denmark sex work is not a criminal offense, and the legal age of consent for sexual activity is 15 years old.
- In Finland prostitution is neither illegal nor regulated. Pimping and promoting sex work are forbidden.

In India, the Hindustan Latex company started selling female condoms in 2005 to help curb the spread of HIV. They cost about $2.30 each, but the government subsidized the product to bring the cost to 12 cents per condom for commercial sex workers. Since about 15% of India's 5.1 million HIV-positive people are sex workers, officials want to give a woman a choice so she is not dependent upon a man's decision (India-based company to begin selling female condoms, 2005).

---

various ways. Some help sex workers to obtain high school diplomas so they can get other employment. As one project administrator said: "How can we ask prostitutes to take a position against themselves?" As a result of the governmental policy, those in a number of worthwhile projects decided to turn down the money. This meant they could not help as many people.

The Law and Prostitution

Should prostitution be legal? This question has been argued for many years. Some people believe there are potential benefits of legalizing prostitution, such as increased human rights protection and health precautions. They argue that prostitution always has been and always will be. Legalization would increase condom use and, in turn, lead to a reduction of HIV and AIDS and other STIs. They feel prostitutes have the right to choose the way they earn their income; therefore, how can society stand in the way of someone's earning a good living?

Opponents of prostitution argue that most prostitutes are forced into sexual slavery. They suggest that legalization would give rise to a black market

that would be frightening and abusive. For some opponents to prostitution, the issue is a moral one because prostitution gives rise to dehumanizing, unsafe, illegal activities. It is morally reprehensible, they say, for prostitutes to be treated as too many are treated. They conclude that the abuses and potential threat for ongoing abuse far outweigh any potential benefits of legalization. And the argument continues (Should prostitution be legal?, 2003).

Agustin (2008) has pointed out that a large number of those who would be governed by legislation on commercial sexual activity don't identify with such legislation or consider it useful to their lives. Even in those places in the world where sex workers can legally register and operate within the law, many do not bother to do so because they fail to see any benefit. Few sex workers join trade unions or interest groups where they exist.

Child Prostitution

A particularly disturbing feature of sex work is the presence of minors selling sexual activity. Child prostitution has become more common in recent years. In some instances, children are forced by adults to per-

To survive on the streets, adolescents who have run away from home often sell drugs or their bodies.

form sexual acts. In other instances, the minors may appear to be selling sexual activity by choice—though many would argue that it is not really voluntary.

Cultures exist around the world in which children, as belongings, are property to be bought and sold. Tens of millions of children are repeatedly raped, tortured, and shamed for the sexual gratification of adults. Worldwide there are perhaps as many as 100 million child prostitutes. In the United States there are about 2.4 million (Joseph, 1995).

In some developing countries, boys outnumber girls on the streets because girls are often put into brothels. These children are prostituted, or even sold, to prevent themselves and their families from starving. The customers who purchase the children or their services are adults who are commonly pedophiles or sadists.

In some instances there can be links between child prostitution and child pornography. For example, costumed children might act out a customer's fantasy in special surroundings while filming is done. The acting might be done as part of a story, such as an abduction of a virgin or a "schoolgirl tease," or the action might simply be rape and torture. There is money to be made from the prostitution activities and the selling of films or videos (Joseph, 1995).

In the United States a large number of adolescent sex workers are runaways who are looking for companionship, friendship, love, and approval, as well as a way of supporting themselves financially. Unfortunately, many of them are ideal targets for gangs, drug pushers, and pimps. To survive on the streets, runaways often sell drugs or their bodies, and a large number turn to other types of crime to support themselves.

It is estimated that between 300,000 and 400,000 girls and boys, aged 9–17 years, trade their bodies to pay for food, shelter, clothing, and other basic needs to survive on America's streets (Uhlman, 2001). Some U.S. children engage in commercial sexual activity while living at home and generally find customers among their peers. Those children at highest risk for commercial sexual exploitation are those who run away or are thrown out by their relatives. Fewer than 25% are members of impoverished families. A significant number of their customers are married men, many with children of their own. Other children at higher risk to become victims of commercial sexual activity include female gang members who get involved to raise money for the gang; foreign children; and teenagers living along the Canadian or Mexican borders who cross into those countries specifically to solicit sexual activity.

The fact that runaways make up a significant percentage of adolescent sex workers creates a particularly difficult problem for law enforcement personnel. When they arrest a child sex worker, it does little good to send the child back to a poor home environment. In fact, there have been reports of children setting up their own prostitution rings, while living at home, to earn spending money.

In response to childhood sex work, law enforcement personnel have attempted to crack down on pimps of adolescent sex workers and at the same time better coordinate with other law enforcement agencies to recognize and help runaways when possible. Service programs for runaways have incorporated a medical component to treat the physical and mental health needs of runaways who have turned to sex work (and of other runaways, too). Runaway shelters provide services to help reduce the need for runaways to turn to sex work. Such services include medical services, crisis intervention services, individual and group counseling, vocational training and job placement, legal services, independent living skills training, and support and friendship. The hope is that the many shelters and service centers around the United States will help convince young people that they need not turn to pimps and sex work to meet their needs.

Thousands of British university students have turned to sex work to cover their college expenses. They work as strippers, lap dancers, escorts, and pornographic movie actors. One student said she cannot find another job that fits in with her academic obligations. Another said that taking his clothes off is easier than waiting on tables and he makes 10 times more. In Leeds, 60% of the city's sex workers are university students. One madam opened a brothel close to the University of Leeds to make it easier for students to commute to work (Birchard, 2001).

Research about all forms of sex work has changed more in recent years than at any time in the past. We now know more about the extent of sex work and its changing nature worldwide, but particularly in the West. We also have a better grasp of the reasons why some people enter the sex industry. With the growth of sex-worker organizations, there is greater access to research subjects. The existence of a pool of volunteers willing to contribute to both their own research projects and those of others has the potential of adding greatly to our knowledge about this area of human sexual behavior.

Exploring the DIMENSIONS of Human Sexuality

Our feelings, attitudes, and beliefs regarding sexuality are influenced by our internal and external environments. Go to sexuality.jbpub.com/dimensions/4e to learn more about the biological, psychological, and sociological factors that affect your sexuality.

Biological Factors

- Prostitutes in general have a much higher rate of HIV infection. About one-third of New York City streetwalkers are infected with HIV.
- No externally used products can enlarge the penis or breasts.

Sociocultural Factors

- Fraudulent sexual aids are among the top 10 sources of health fraud in the United States.
- Prostitution is outlawed in every U.S. state except Nevada (and even there it is legal in only a few counties).
- Many countries allow prostitution. South Korea issues identification cards to prostitutes that serve as hotel passes. South Korea and Thailand consider prostitution of young girls to be a tourist attraction.
- Some countries, such as Iran and China, have attempted to ban distribution of sexually explicit materials. Laws govern distribution and possession of sexually explicit photos of children.
- Media often fail to depict safer sexual practices in books, articles, TV shows, and movies.
- Sexually explicit materials helped create and expand the market for home VCRs and the Internet.

Psychological Factors

- Media images may negatively impact body image and self-esteem.
- Many ads use sexual imagery to attract attention and stimulate senses.

CASE STUDY

Marketing of sexual products and use of sexual imagery to market nonsexual products are multibillion-dollar businesses. The alluring imagery may draw attention to the product but does not necessarily result in a sale unless the product is sexually related, such as a product to enhance one's appearance.

As marketers attempt to target certain groups (typically younger populations) with sexual imagery, they need to be aware that other people may find their ads offensive.

Marketing of sexually explicit materials to consumers in conditions of privacy (i.e., at home) has driven the markets for the VCR, the DVD, and the Internet.

But marketers also face legal challenges to distributing sexually explicit material. Because "community standards" are used to judge whether material is obscene, a web site operator in one state can be charged with obscenity under the community standards of a person in another state who downloads the materials.

Marketing of any sexually explicit material involving children is prosecuted harshly. Even just downloading such material is a violation of the law.

677

Summary

- There are countless advertisements in magazines, in newspapers, and on TV that use sexual themes to sell products. Advertisers seem to have made a careful study of sexual motivation.

- The sexual content of TV programs has increased immensely in the past few decades. TV can be an excellent way to educate people about healthy sexual practices, but it is rarely used that way.

- The sexuality content of movies has also increased greatly in the past few decades. Some people believe the sexual explicitness is detrimental to society, whereas others see this trend as positive.

- The availability of sexual material in videotapes, DVDs, and video games continues to increase. Businesses related to these products have grown by leaps and bounds.

- The mass phenomenon that may affect more young people than any other is popular music. Blatant sexual themes in music are very common today.

- Sexual content available on the Internet has raised many interesting issues. Among them is whether and how to apply censorship, whether and how to control access to the Internet for children, and how to deal with sexual predators on the Internet.

- Sexually explicit materials have been around for centuries and have often spawned controversy. Some people believe it is necessary to strictly control such materials, but others feel they are not harmful if used by adults. Most agree that child pornography should be prohibited.

- There are many types of sex workers, including call girls, house prostitutes, streetwalkers, massage parlor sex workers, bar girls, gigolos, hustlers, and pimps. In addition, in more recent years new types have emerged—phone and Internet sex workers, sex shop operators, and owners of stores that sell toys and devices related to sexuality.

- Sexual slavery has become a huge international problem. Millions of people around the world are trapped in virtual prisons on farms, in sweatshops, or in brothels.

Discussion Questions

1. Analyze the value of sexuality in selling products. Discuss sexually oriented ads, including the ways sex helps sell products (bikini-clad calendars, sexually explicit rap music, "dirty" classic literature, and so on).

2. Create a legal standard for distributing sexually explicit materials. Include in the standard what constitutes art, child pornography, literature, and the like.

3. Compare and contrast the varied types of sex workers. Then describe efforts to control sex work.

Application Questions

Reread the chapter-opening story and answer the following questions.

1. Of the students who had opinions about sexual consumerism, with whom do you agree? Explain your answer, citing contemporary examples.

2. In what ways do actor portrayals of sexuality—or models with "perfect" bodies—make us feel inferior? (You may want to review In Focus: Body Image when answering this question.) Could those same images be said to promote erotic feelings and thus have value?

3. Does the use of naked flesh make ads sexier? Or have ads from the past, albeit with less flesh, been just as sexually oriented?

Critical Thinking Questions

1. When planning an ad campaign, a marketer needs to think about all audiences who will view the ad. Consider the anecdotal story that has appeared in various advertising publications about the former first lady Nancy Reagan and her daughter, Patty Davis: During the early 1990s, the two women were waiting in a hotel lobby when the conversation turned to sexual consumerism. Mrs. Reagan, showing her daugh-

ter a perfume ad in a magazine, said that she did not like having to look at a nearly naked man in the ad. Her daughter replied, "Well, I sure do!" They both laughed.

Clearly, the marketer was targeting the demographics of Reagan's daughter. But should a marketer have to be concerned about offending people in other demographics—older and more conservative people as well as minors? Describe the steps a marketer should have to take before placing ads.

2. Although it is billed as the "world's oldest profession," prostitution is not legal in the United States except in a few counties in Nevada. Should prostitution be legalized? Consider the social, legal (including tax ramifications), health, moral, and other dimensions of sexuality of both clients and prostitutes in your answer.

3. Former stars of sexually explicit films, such as Linda Lovelace and Traci Lords, have described the world of porn films as one of physical abuse (actual and threatened) and drugs. If an actress participated in explicit sexual activity under such coercion, does that constitute rape? Should distribution of such movies be illegal?

4. Distribution of photos of naked minors is illegal. But prominent "art" photographers often take photos of naked minors, and such photos are distributed in photo anthologies through major bookstore chains. How is it possible to differentiate between art and child pornography?

5. China, Iran, and other countries limit Internet access for their citizens. Two major concerns are antigovernment rhetoric and sexually explicit material. Given the ease with which minors can access sexually explicit material, should the U.S. government restrict the Internet access of U.S. citizens? Should the Internet be regulated?

Critical Thinking Case

In parts of Japan, December 24 is the "hottest" night of the year. Societal pressure is strong for every unmarried person to have a date on Christmas Eve and for that date to include an overnight stay. In this respect December 24 is not dissimilar to prom night here in America. Just about every major hotel in Tokyo is sold out for that night months in advance. The Japanese describe Christmas Eve as a night to make love and refer to it as "H-Day" (for "hormone," the Japanese euphemism for sex).

This evening is quite expensive for young Japanese, as the cost typically exceeds $1,000. Men are expected to buy their date a present ($215), take her to Tokyo Disneyland ($100), provide dinner at a fancy restaurant ($385), take a room at a nice hotel (between $350 and $650), have breakfast the next morning ($35), and rent a limousine ($150)—all of this in a country less than 1% Christian and where December 25 is a normal working day.

1. Discuss H-Day in terms of the dimensions of sexuality. Include safer-sex practices, the psychological implications of engaging in sexual activity with someone because of societal pressure, religion, culture, and other factors.

2. Which cultural factors would prevent H-Day from being accepted in the United States? (Assume that the date would be changed from December 24.)

Exploring Personal Dimensions

Are You a Good Sexual Consumer?
Answer the following statements with one of the following responses. When you are finished, total your points and find out how good a sexual consumer you are.
1. Rarely or never
2. Sometimes
3. Often
4. All or most of the time

_____ 1. I make sure the date on any product (such as condoms or oral contraceptives) has not expired.

_____ 2. I am not influenced by sexually alluring images to purchase products.

_____ 3. I am aware of whether any sexually explicit material I view involves minors.

_____ 4. I make sure that any sexually explicit material I view is kept away from minors.

_____ 5. I understand that sharing sexual aids (or toys) with others is a high-risk activity, capable of transmitting STIs and AIDS.

_____ 6. I am aware that sexual contact with sex workers or former sex workers is a high-risk activity because of the potential for STI and/or HIV transmission.

_____ 7. I believe that aphrodisiacs offer no sexual help physiologically, and I consider their side effects before using them.

_____ 8. I evaluate "research" claims made by marketers before buying a product.

_____ 9. I consider the source of sexual health information before purchasing any product.

_____10. I have sought recommendations from friends for whom to consult in case of sexually related health care needs.

_____11. I have regular exams by a physician.

_____12. I understand that certain prescription drugs (such as antibiotics) can affect the effectiveness of oral contraceptives.

_____13. I read labels of health products and follow directions.

_____14. I do a monthly breast or testicular self-exam.

_____15. When friends state a sexual myth as though it were a fact, I use knowledge from this course to correct them tactfully.

Scoring

0–15   Your sexual consumer skills are weak.
16–30   Your sexual consumer skills are below what they should be.
31–45   Your sexual consumer skills are good but can stand improvement.

Suggested Readings

Brennan, B. Competing claims of victimhood? Foreign and domestic victims of trafficking in the United States. *Sexuality Research & Social Policy, 5, no. 4* (December 2008), 45–61.

Herbenick, D., & Reece, M. Sex education in adult retail stores: Positioning consumers' questions as teachable moments. *American Journal of Sexuality Education, 2, no. 1* (2006), 57–75.

Johansson, T., & Hammaren, N. Hegemonic masculinity and pornography: Young people's attitudes toward and relations to pornography. *Journal of Men's Studies, 15, no. 1* (January 2007), 57–70.

O'Neil, R. O. What limits should campus networks place on pornography? *Chronicle of Higher Education, 49, no. 28* (March 21, 2003), B20.

Sex on TV4. The Kaiser Family Foundation, 2005. Available: *www.kff.org.*

Soderlund, G., Journalist or panderer? Framing underage webcam sites. *Sexuality Research & Social Policy, 5, no. 4* (December 2008), 62–72.

Stachowiak, J. A., Sherman, S., Konakova, A., Krushkova, I., & Beyrer, C. Health risks and power among female sex workers in Moscow. *SIECUS Report 33, no. 2* (Spring 2005), 18–25.

Teens talk About TV, sex, and real life. Available: www.hawaii.edu/hivandaids/Teens%20Talk%20 About%20TV,%20Sex%20and%20Real%20Life .pdf.

Web Resources

For links to the web sites below, visit *http://sexuality.jbpub.com/dimensions/4e* and click on Resource Links.

The Dove Foundation
www.dove.org

The Dove Foundation supports efforts to move Hollywood in a more family-friendly direction. It provides film reviews for consideration by consumers.

The Free Speech Museum
www.spectacle.org/musm.html

The Free Speech Museum is intended to serve as a permanent Internet resource on the freedom of speech. It is very concerned that many current efforts are designed to cut down or eliminate free speech.

Good Vibrations
www.goodvibes.com

Good Vibrations considers itself the place to go for sex toys, sex education, erotic and informative books, adult DVDs, and more.

National Coalition for the Protection of Children and Families
www.nationalcoalition.org

The Coalition's mission is to move the people of God to embrace, live out, preserve, and advance the biblical truth of sexuality. It wants to educate the Christian community on sexual ethics according to a biblical worldview, encourage and challenge Christians to live sexually pure lives, engage Christians in public policy relative to sexual ethics, and embrace those harmed by pornography and help restore them to sexual wholeness.

Prostitution Research and Education
www.prostitutionresearch.com

The purpose of Prostitution Research and Education is to abolish prostitution and advocate for alternatives to prostitution—including emotional and physical health care for women in prostitution. PRE seeks to give voice to those who are among the world's most disenfranchised groups: prostituted/trafficked women and children. Its goal is to empower this constituency by documenting their perspectives through research, public education, and arts projects.

Veronica's Voice
www.veronicasvoice.org

This organization encourages prostitutes to choose lifestyle changes that lead to recovery of their minds, bodies, and spirits. It is targeted to help women make the choice to leave prostitution, drug addiction, and a life of violence, transitioning into new lives free from abuse. Survivors of the sex industry direct the program.

CHAPTER 18

Sexual Ethics, Morality, and the Law

FEATURES

Ethical Dimensions
Extramarital Sex

Gender Dimensions
The "Umbrelly"
(A Little Humor)

Global Dimensions
Marital Age Around
the World

Communication Dimensions
The Morality of
Requesting a Variety
of Sexual Behaviors

CHAPTER OBJECTIVES

1 Define *ethics, morals, ethical principles, ethical dilemmas, values,* and the five ethical principles that serve as a basis for deciding whether a decision is moral.

2 State the ethical considerations of such sexually related topics as sexually transmitted infections, sexual activity between unmarried partners, sodomy, contraception, abortion, amniocentesis, fetal tissue implantation, prostitution, in vitro fertilization, genetic engineering, and sexual responsibility to a partner.

3 Identify the rationale for laws pertaining to homosexuality, obscenity and pornography, rape, statutory rape, adultery, and divorce.

sexuality.jbpub.com/dimensions/4e

Commonly Accepted Ethical Principles
Genetic Engineering

INTRODUCTION

Wendy Weaver was a well-respected high school philosophy teacher and girls' volleyball coach in the Nebo, Utah, school district (Associated Press, 1998). Concerned about her student athletes, in the summer of 1997 she telephoned each one to ask about her summer camp schedule. That is when it happened. A student asked, "Are you gay?" Weaver answered that she was, eliciting a response from the student that she would not play on Weaver's volleyball team in the fall. When school district officials heard what Wendy Weaver disclosed to the student, they immediately fired her from her coaching responsibilities and instructed her not to speak of her sexual orientation to either students or school staff, in or outside school.

The Nebo school district officials believed they were right to protect young people in their school from what they perceived to be disclosure of immoral behavior. They believed that homosexuality was wrong and that it was sinful.

Wendy Weaver, however, believed that she had a moral right to express her sexuality in any way she sought, as long as she did not impose it on her students. After all, she argued, heterosexual teachers are not forbidden to disclose their sexual orientation. Therefore, she asserted that it was wrong—immoral—to forbid her to do so.

Eventually a judge determined the legal issues involved in this case. In November 1997, U.S. District Court Judge Bruce Jenkins ruled that Wendy Weaver's rights of free speech, equal protection under the law, and due process were violated. He ordered that the gag order be lifted and that Wendy Weaver be reinstated as coach of the girls' volleyball team. In his ruling Judge Jenkins stated, "Although the Constitution cannot control prejudices, neither this court nor any other court should, directly or indirectly, legitimize them."

This case includes issues of morality, ethics, and law. The school officials believed that they were acting morally by protecting young people from a teacher they thought might inappropriately affect their sexual orientation. Wendy believed she was acting morally when she answered the team member honestly and when she asserted her constitutional rights. And the judge believed he was acting morally when he applied a law designed to prevent prejudice from depriving a person of her rights in a democratic society. Certainly everyone could not be right; nor could everyone be wrong. Certainly, everyone was not purposefully acting immorally. We shall see in this chapter how complex issues of morality really are and how a systematic approach can manage some of this complexity when these issues relate to matters of sexuality. Furthermore, we shall see how the law is used to codify societal consensus about morality and how it is applied to express societal mores.

Many ethical dilemmas relate to sexuality. For example, whether women should use intrauterine devices (IUDs) as a means of contraception that may prevent fertilized ova from successfully implanting on the uterus's endometrial lining involves the moral question of when life begins. Whether fetal tissue or stem cells—that is, from aborted fetuses—should be made available as a treatment for such conditions as Parkinson's disease concerns the moral issue of the sanctity of the human body.

These and other questions of sexual morality are pervasive. They affect every one of us, if not directly and daily, then certainly as members of a society wrestling with their resolutions. They are also emotionally charged. This point should not go unnoticed. When issues evoke emotional reactions—as sexual issues tend to do—these emotions too often interfere with a rational investigation. Consequently, people argue their own viewpoints while ignoring other perspectives, and that method of argument is not conducive to learning.

Before this discussion begins, however, we must prevent any possible confusion. The topics we consider in this chapter are all discussed elsewhere in this text in detail, and the various implications, ramifications, and idiosyncrasies associated with them are presented. The discussion of these topics here, however, serves to explore the morality and ethics of particular sexually related behaviors or decisions in a unified, systematic manner. In addition, it highlights the importance of considering the ethics and morality of all sexual matters.

The story of Wendy Weaver illustrates the multidimensional facets of ethics, morality, and the law.

Talking about sexual morality is not easy. Whose morality should we focus on? Which morals, if any, should we advocate? How can we prevent offending people whose morals differ from ours? It would be arrogant for us to insist that everyone adopt a single set of sexual morals, and it would be particularly impertinent to suggest that our own morals be the ones adopted. Therefore, in this chapter, rather than advocating a particular set of morals or ethical principles, we describe the process of moral reasoning. We sketch our society's moral stance on STIs, contraception, in vitro fertilization, rape, prostitution, and so on, and describe the background and enforcement of some laws. Along the way we acknowledge some of the religious, philosophical, cultural, family-related, and experiential reasons for the differences in sexual morality among individuals and among societies.

Ethics: The Basis for Making Decisions

To begin investigating sexual morality, we need to distinguish between the terms *ethics* and *moral*. **Ethics** refers to a *system* by which we determine whether some action is moral or immoral. An action is **moral** if it is judged to be *good* or *right;* it is **immoral** if it is judged to be *bad* or *wrong*. To guide the decision of whether an action is moral or immoral, the system of ethics employs **ethical principles**. These ethical principles provide answers to abstract questions—they are general guidelines, not meant for individual cases. With regard to abortion, for example, ethicists would be more concerned with the general question of when life begins or with a woman's right to control her own reproductive capacity than with whether abortion is appropriate in a particular case. Decisions about what is moral are determined by many different experiences and influences. Religious beliefs and values, social mores, humanistic views, education, culture, and friends and family are but a few of these influences.

When a set of ethical principles is available and accepted by a society, the people of that society know how they are expected to behave. Professional societies attempt to develop guiding principles—or *codes of ethics*—to govern their members' behaviors. The code of ethics developed by the American Association of Sex Educators, Counselors, and Therapists, for example, sets guidelines for its members.

Ethical Principles

Table 18.1 introduces five examples of ethical principles that can be used to make moral decisions. As will be discussed, though, these kinds of principles may be in opposition to one another in any given situation.

ethics
A system that uses ethical principles to make decisions about morality.

moral
What is judged to be right according to a system of ethics.

immoral
What is judged to be wrong according to a system of ethics.

ethical principles
Guides by which we can judge an action or decision as moral or immoral.

TABLE 18.1 **Selected Ethical Principles**

1. Nonmaleficence	Whatever else, do no harm. This includes preventing harm, not inflicting harm, and removing harm when it is present.
2. Beneficence	Not only should one not do harm, but one is also obligated to do good.
3. Autonomy/liberty	People should be free to decide their own course of action as long as they do not harm others.
4. Justice/fairness	Each person should be treated fairly.
5. Social utility	The greatest good for the greatest number should be considered. What is best for society may outweigh what is best for the individual.

Ethical DIMENSIONS

Extramarital Sex   Actually making a decision regarding sexual morality may help you comprehend the rather abstract material to come. Therefore, we quote here an argument that adultery, or extramarital relationships, can be moral and ask you to react to it. (Bear in mind that although this argument describes only men, women have extramarital affairs.)

Albert Ellis, a prominent psychologist, wrote that there is a healthy adulterer. Although Ellis's argument was presented a number of years ago, it is as applicable today as it was then. Ellis wrote (1977, 374–375):

1. The healthy adulterer is nondemanding and noncompulsive. He prefers but he does not need extramarital affairs. He believes that he can live better with than without them, and therefore he tries to have them from time to time. But he is also able to have a happy general and marital life if no such affairs are practicable.

2. The undisturbed adulterer usually manages to carry on his extramarital affairs without unduly disturbing his marriage and family relationships nor his general existence. He is sufficiently discreet about his adultery, on the one hand, and appropriately frank and honest about it with his close associates, on the other hand, so that most people he intimately knows are able to tolerate his affairs and not get too upset about them.

3. He fully accepts his own extramarital desires and acts and never condemns himself or punishes himself because of them, even though he may sometimes decide that they are unwise and may make specific attempts to bring them to a halt.

4. He faces his specific problems with his wife and family as well as his general life difficulties and does not use his adulterous relationships as a means of avoiding any of his serious problems.

5. He is usually tolerant of himself when he acts poorly or makes errors; he is minimally hostile when his wife and family members behave in a less than desirable manner; and he fully accepts the fact that the world is rough and life is often grim, but that there is no reason why it must be otherwise and that he can live happily even when conditions around him are not great. Consequently, he does not drive himself to adultery because of self-deprecation, self-pity, or hostility to others.

6. He is sexually adequate with his spouse as well as with others and therefore has extramarital affairs out of sex interest rather than for sex therapy.

Although the adulterer who lives up to these criteria may have still other emotional disturbances and may be having extramarital affairs for various neurotic reasons, Ellis argues that there is also a good chance that this is not true.

Nonmaleficence

Is it moral to convince someone else to engage in sexual intercourse in spite of his or her reluctance? One ethical principle that speaks to this issue is maleficence—the act of committing harm or evil. The principle of *nonmaleficence* is that whatever is moral—right or good—can be determined by asking whether it does any harm. If it does harm, it is not moral. Does coercing someone to engage in sex do physical, psychological, or spiritual harm? If so, that behavior is immoral.

Beneficence

For some ethicists, doing no harm is not enough. For an action to be moral, it has to do good. That is what is meant by the ethical principle of *beneficence*. School officials who banned Wendy Weaver from coaching volleyball thought they were doing good for the students in that school. Therefore, they thought they were acting morally. Those who opposed the ban believed they were doing good by upholding the right of people to acknowledge their sexuality in an appropriate and honest manner, regardless of their particular sexual orientation. Therefore, they thought they were acting morally. We will soon discuss how these contradictions can be resolved.

Autonomy/Liberty

The ethical principle of *autonomy* or *liberty* requires people be free to decide an issue for themselves before that decision can qualify as moral. That does not mean that every decision made freely is a moral one, only that any decision made under coercion is immoral. Was the decision to bar Wendy Weaver made freely by school officials, or was it coerced by a small group of vocal parents? Was Weaver allowed to decide freely whether she would discuss her sexual orientation, as could heterosexuals teaching in that school, or was she being coerced by school officials? The way you answer these questions will help you determine which actions you think were moral in this case.

Justice/Fairness

Some ethicists believe that for an action to be moral, it must treat people fairly. They term this ethical principle *justice* or *fairness*. That does not mean that people must be treated equally. For example, our culture has determined that homosexuals and heterosexuals may be treated differently by different segments of society. That is, in private clubs or homes, or in certain churches or synagogues, gays may be excluded. However, our society has determined that excluding gays from public facilities is not just or fair—it is immoral—and has codified that decision by making a law defining that behavior illegal/unconstitutional.

Social Utility

Sometimes there is a clash between individual rights and the rights of a large group of people. In these instances, some ethicists use the ethical principle of *social utility* to determine the morality of various actions being contemplated. Social utility defines the moral decision as the one that is best for society (or the large group) rather than what is best for the individual (or the small group). School officials in Nebo, Utah, determined that removing Wendy Weaver from coaching was the greater good for the greater number of people (the students). Whether they were aware of it or not, they were using social utility to justify their decision. Of course, others might argue that the greater number of people in this instance ought to have been the gay community throughout the United States whose rights have been violated for far too long.

Ethical Dilemmas

We often experience situations in which one ethical principle clashes with another. We call these clashes **ethical dilemmas**. For example, consider again the question of adultery. Suppose you held the following ethical principles: Marriage should be a sexually monogamous relationship and people have a right to a satisfying, fulfilling sexual life. Obviously if you were in a marriage in which you were sexually unfulfilled for some reason, these two ethical

ethical dilemma
When two or more ethical principles work in opposing fashion in a particular situation, resulting in bewilderment regarding what is moral and what is immoral.

principles would conflict. In such a situation which principle would be operative? Which one would take precedence over the other? Sometimes religion or culture provides answers to ethical dilemmas. For instance, in Islamic countries adultery is opposed by tradition and the law; such a society has resolved our ethical dilemma—at least officially—by placing the higher value on fidelity within marriage. Where there are no such prohibitions, individuals must rank their own values to make a choice.

rule ethics
Guiding principles used in all situations to arrive at moral decisions, which are considered applicable to all situations.

situation ethics
A belief that no one set of rules can apply to all situations and each specific situation must be analyzed to determine which ethical principles are applicable.

The existence of such dilemmas has led to the development of situation ethics, in contrast to rule ethics. **Rule ethics** are exhaustive principles intended to guide people in their moral decision making in all situations. These principles are explicit, specific, and all-encompassing. People who hold to the letter of the law and proponents of religious dogmas are rule ethicists. **Situation ethics**, in contrast, are based on the premise that all situations are unique, and therefore no one set of rules is applicable in all cases. Consequently a situation ethicist faced with a moral decision carefully reviews, analyzes, and evaluates each specific situation to determine which principles are applicable; a rule ethicist applies a given principle, regardless of the specific circumstances. As an example, a rule ethicist believes abortion is wrong in all cases. A situation ethicist may also believe abortion is wrong but may also believe it is moral in the case of a 12-year-old rape victim who becomes pregnant.

Trying to decide which viewpoint—rule ethics or situation ethics—is correct is itself an ethical dilemma. When we narrow our focus to sexual behavior, we can see that the rule/situation dichotomy has relevance. Are there general rules to guide sexual behavior, or does each situation require its own set of rules? Which rules, if any, will guide your behavior? Given your intuitive responses to the questions we raise in this chapter, see whether you consider yourself a rule or situation ethicist.

■ Moral Decision Making and Sexual Behavior

What influences the decisions we make about sexuality? Such factors as our knowledge or lack of knowledge; our sense of who we are; our ideals regarding fidelity and responsibility; our desire to express affection, passion, and delight; the emotional excitement

Deciding whether a rule should be applied to a particular ethical issue, or whether the situation is unique and requires a unique decision, is a dilemma faced by ethicists.

we experience while facing the decision; and external cultural influences such as the double standard are all involved. The questions one asks in making moral decisions about sexuality or any other area of life are, What is *right*? What is *good*? What is *wrong*? What is *bad*? If it is right or good, it is moral! If it is wrong or bad, it is immoral! Thus morals relate to concrete decisions in particular situations.

To determine whether an action or decision is moral or immoral, we use our system of ethics. This system of ethics involves our ethical principles, which are guides by which we can judge an action or decision as moral or immoral. If the decision is inconsistent with our ethical principles, it is immoral; if it is consistent with them, it is moral.

Ethical principles specific to sexual matters include the following:

1. Sexual behavior should not be forced on anyone.

2. Sexual behavior between consenting adults is acceptable.

3. Fidelity (faithfulness) in marriage is a must.

4. Marriage partners and loved ones must be responsive to each other's needs (Bruess & Greenberg, 2009).

Unfortunately, most situations are not so cut and dried. Applying ethical principles is often a complex matter because they provide only guidance, not ready-made answers. If our principles are in conflict, we must examine our personal values to rank conflicting ethical principles in order of importance. By personal *values* we mean the worth or importance we assign to our ethical principles. If we personally value our commitment to a monogamous relationship more than we value sexual fulfillment, for example, then we resolve a conflict between the two by choosing not to have extramarital relationships. If we value sexual fulfillment more highly, then we resolve the same conflict differently.

To summarize, then, we decide the morality of an action or decision after identifying and ranking ethi-

cal principles in order of our personal values. Most people learn that the many moral decisions they make about sexual behavior are ultimately based on their personal values.

Our intention is to help you explore your own values and ethical principles so you may apply them in specific situations, and thereby act morally.

Commonly Accepted Ethical Principles

This discussion is not intended to convey the notion that *anything goes*. Although we value and recognize the need for diversity, as a society we have reached agreement on a set of ethical principles. For example, we have societal consensus that caring, respect, honesty, responsibility, and trust ought to guide our decisions regarding morality. In fact, a whole educational movement that seeks to convey these principles to school-aged children and youth has sprouted. That movement is called *Character Education*. Its objectives are consistent with the societal consensus regarding ethical principles described: respect for the rights of all people regardless of their race, religion, gender, age, and sexual orientation; understanding, sympathy, concern, and compassion for others; and personal integrity and honesty. These are principles to which all citizens should adhere, and to emphasize their importance, society has passed laws specifying sanctions for acting contrary to them. For example, we have laws against discrimination by gender, race, and ethnicity, and in many states, sexual orientation. And we have laws punishing those who sexually abuse others. If someone lies to a sexual partner about his or her HIV status and infects that partner, we have laws to punish that behavior. If someone takes advantage of someone else by engaging in coitus with that person while he or she is incapable of deciding freely to participate (for example, if intoxicated or mentally impaired), we have laws punishing that behavior. And if someone fires someone else from a job solely because of that person's sexual orientation, we have

Although people may value ethical principles differently, there is agreement on a set of common principles such as caring, respect, and honesty.

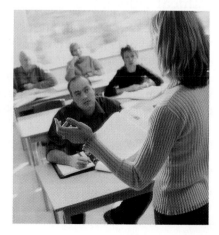

laws to punish that behavior (as the school officials who fired Wendy Weaver found out).

In matters of sexuality and sexual morality, it is important to keep these consensually agreed-on ethical principles in the forefront. Certainly we, as the writers of this textbook, value diversity and recognize the influence of different experiences and values as they play out in various ethical dilemmas. Still, these consensually accepted ethical principles are ones to which we are committed. The problem arises when behaving consistently with one or more of these principles means violating one or more of the others. This is what we earlier described as an ethical dilemma. Ethical dilemmas apply to human sexuality, as we shall now see.

Government Control and Regulation

As will be evident in the rest of this chapter, each sexual ethical issue can be controlled or regulated by government. The broader issue, then, is how much control should we expect the government to exert through regulation, and how much should individuals be allowed to decide these issues for themselves. Laws are a reflection of moral judgments. For example, we judge stealing from another to be immoral so we pass laws penalizing those who steal. Because many sexual ethical issues are controversial, passing regulations or laws to control sexual behavior can be problematic. Whose morals should be the basis for law? How will the minority view of morality be protected? These are important, but not easily answered, questions. The government has an obligation to pass laws to regulate behaviors believed to be harmful— that is, to protect the health of Americans. Where should the line between individual freedoms and governmental protections be drawn?

To resolve many of these sexual ethical issues raised by government regulations, as manifested in laws, these laws are juxtaposed against constitutional protections. The U.S. Constitution is the arbiter of issues that divide the populace. It offers guidance to lawmakers and others to help them protect the public without infringing on their rights. As you will soon see, it is not unusual for the government to pass laws pertaining to sexual behavior (for example, sodomy) or other sexually related issues (such as abortion), only to have these laws challenged, and sometimes overturned, by the U.S. Supreme Court.

Sexually Transmitted Infections

To treat sexually transmitted infections (STIs) effectively on a large scale, health care workers often ask their patients to identify their sexual contacts. The purpose is to inform these contacts that they have been exposed to a disease and encourage them to seek treatment. Generally the carrier is inclined, at least fleetingly, to protect the anonymity of his or her sexual contacts (and perhaps his or her own identity and reputation). One of the ethical principles commonly underlying such a reaction is probably, *One should not discuss other people's private sexual behavior.* However, a competing ethical principle might be, *People should not intentionally harm the health of others.* Most individuals would probably value the second principle over the first and would therefore identify their sexual contacts. Observers who also value health over confidentiality would judge this decision to be moral. If the infected person is married and has contracted the disease through nonconsensual extramarital activity, the principle of not harming others becomes harder to apply. In this situation the patient would have to decide whether the health of the marriage partner was more valuable than potential damage to the marital relationship and the family and whether the couple had an agreement regarding fidelity that had been breached.

As we discussed in In Focus: HIV and AIDS, an important ethical issue raised by the HIV and AIDS epidemic is whether to require pregnant women to be tested for HIV. With modern medications and medical regimens, approximately two-thirds of HIV and AIDS can be prevented in babies born to infected mothers. Consequently, using the ethical principle of beneficence, some medical experts argue that all pregnant women should be required to be tested for HIV, thereby identifying mothers who ought to be treated before their babies' births and newborns who ought to be treated as soon after birth as possible. However, others argue that requiring all pregnant women to be tested would actually harm newborns (maleficence). They believe that if pregnant women are required to be tested they will refrain from identifying themselves as pregnant, thereby depriving their babies of the prenatal care that can prevent all kinds of health problems, not just HIV and AIDS. This would, in turn, increase the infant mortality rate, which is already too high, especially in low-socioeconomic-status populations. Therefore, opponents of mandatory pregnancy testing for HIV believe testing ought to be voluntary (autonomy/liberty) with educational campaigns to communicate the advantages of being tested.

There are other ethical issues related to HIV and AIDS. For example, should research funds be used for treating AIDS patients or for finding a cure or for developing a vaccine? What is the appropriate balance in this funding? Are funds best used for education about HIV and AIDS to prevent the greatest possible number of cases?

These questions are more than issues for academic consideration: Decisions are being made on a regular basis by research institutes, the government, and insurance companies. Are these decisions being made ethically? Are they moral decisions? Your answers to these questions depend on the way you value your ethical principles. Although no one answer will meet with everyone's approval, society adopts a consensus view of morality as a matter of necessity. That is, *something* must be decided, even if the decision is to ignore the situation. Further, because we are citizens in a society that allows for our input, we are contributing to this ethical exercise by our votes, letters, and attitudes (as determined by opinion polls).

One ethical dilemma is whether sexual intercourse between unmarried partners is moral. Should the age of the partners matter? Should the quality of the relationship matter? What other factors do you think need to be considered when deciding on the morality of coitus between unmarried partners?

Sexual Activity Between Unmarried Partners

Whether to participate in sexual activity without being married is another common moral decision. Those who decide that such behavior is immoral might value the following ethical principle: *Marriage is a unique relationship blessed by God and allowing for a total expression of love.* Those who consider sexual intercourse to be moral in any circumstance, unless one participant is harmed in some way, might value another principle more, such as *You should experience life fully.* However, decisions regarding premarital or nonmarital sexual behavior are usually more complicated than a choice between two principles. Situation ethicists pondering the morality of premarital sex in a given situation might ask the following questions:

1. How old are the people involved? Seventeen? Forty-five?

2. What do the people feel for each other?

3. Is their intention to marry or enter into a union? Soon?

4. What are their religious beliefs?

5. In which society (country, culture) do they live?

In your own situation, which special considerations are or were relevant to your decisions about the morality of your sexual behavior?

Sodomy

It is impossible to define the term **sodomy** because states lump together those sexual activities they consider immoral and codify their views by passing laws that make these sexual behaviors illegal. Usually sodomy laws refer to such sexual activities as anal intercourse, oral–genital sexual behavior, homosexual activities, and any sexual behavior with animals. In earlier years, some states defined *sodomy* as any sexual activity of anyone other than a married couple. In fact, as late as 1990, a bill was proposed by a Washington state legislator that would allow the state to prosecute anyone younger than 18 years old who was "necking" or "petting." The proposed penalty was a maximal sentence of 90 days in jail and a $5,000 fine.

> **sodomy**
> A term that specifically refers to anal intercourse, but is often used to refer to almost any sexual behavior someone might not consider normal.

Most sodomy laws were applied primarily against homosexuals. The penalties varied from state to state, ranging from a $200 fine to 20 years of imprisonment. Violators of sodomy laws have been imprisoned, lost their jobs and homes, lost custody of their children, and even been beaten and killed. One test of the constitutionality of sodomy laws occurred in 1986. In the *Bowers v. Hardwick* case, an Atlanta man was arrested after police officers entered his home at the request of his roommate regarding another matter and found him in bed with another man. When this case finally reached the U.S. Supreme Court, the Court upheld Georgia's sodomy law in spite of recognizing that the Constitution creates "zones of privacy." Dissenting from this decision was Justice Harry A. Blackmun, who wrote that the Court mistakenly refused to recognize "the fundamental interest all individuals have in controlling the nature of their intimate associations with others." However, on June 26, 2003, in a landmark ruling on sexuality and privacy, the U.S. Supreme Court overturned *Bowers v.*

Hardwick. In *Lawrence v. Texas*, the Court found that *Bowers* "was not correct when it was decided, is not correct today, and is hereby overruled." Further, the *Lawrence* decision states, "When homosexual conduct is made criminal by the law of the State, that declaration in and of itself is an invitation to subject homosexual persons to discrimination both in the public and private spheres. . . Its continuance as precedent demeans the lives of homosexual persons."

Contraception

People who oppose so-called artificial methods of contraception for religious reasons are usually guided by the ethic, *All life is sacred*. They argue that prevention of a conception that would occur without interference is interference with God's creation of life. Proponents of modern birth control, in contrast, are often guided by the ethic, *Every child deserves to be wanted and loved*. They argue that when unwanted children are born, the quality of life diminishes for the parents and the society, and the children themselves often have difficult lives as well.

In 1914 Margaret Sanger began publishing her newspaper, *The Woman Rebel*, in which she argued that women should be free to choose whether to bear children. Sanger had witnessed the death of a young woman who tried to perform an abortion on herself and cited this incident as her motivation for working for a woman's right to control her fertility.

For some people, certain types of fertility-control methods are acceptable and others are not. For example, methods that prevent a fertilized egg from implanting on the endometrial lining of the uterus might be unacceptable to people who believe life begins at conception. For others, any action taken before birth is acceptable because they believe that birth is when human life begins.

Then there is the issue pertaining to who should be responsible for contraception. Some people wonder why most methods of contraception are designed to be used by women. Accompanying these methods of contraception are potential side effects that can have significant health implications. Why aren't men subjected to the same risks, some wonder (see Gender Dimensions). Is it moral to subject women to

Gender DIMENSIONS

The "Umbrelly" (A Little Humor)

Critics of research on contraceptive technology argue that research is immoral—that is, sexist. It focuses on female techniques, largely ignoring male methods of contraception. Others argue it is the characteristics and complexities of the male reproductive system that make the development of effective male contraception difficult. In an attempt to have males develop a greater appreciation for how the critics view the morality of contraceptive research, the following facetious description of a new male contraceptive was written:

The newest development in male contraception was unveiled recently at the American Women's Surgical Symposium held at the Ann Arbor Medical Center. Dr. Sophia Merkin, of the Merkin Clinic, announced the preliminary findings of a study conducted on 763 unsuspecting male grad students at a large Midwest university. In her report Dr. Merkin stated that the new contraceptive—the IPD—was a breakthrough in male contraception. It will be marketed under the trade name "Umbrelly."

The IPD (intrapenal device) resembles a tiny folded umbrella that is inserted through the head of the penis and pushed into the scrotum with a plunger-like instrument. Occasionally there is perforation of the scrotum but this is disregarded, since it is known that the male has few nerve

endings in this area of his body. The underside of the umbrella contains a spermicidal jelly, hence "Umbrelly."

Experiments on a thousand white whales from the Continental Shelf (whose sexual apparatus is said to be closest to man's) proved the Umbrelly to be 100% effective in preventing production of sperm and eminently satisfactory to the female whale, since it doesn't interfere with her rutting pleasure.

Dr. Merkin declared the Umbrelly to be statistically safe for the human male. She reported that of the 763 grad students tested with the device, only two died of scrotal infection, only 20 experienced swelling of the tissues, three developed cancer of the testicles, and 13 were too depressed to have an erection. She stated that common complaints ranged from cramping and bleeding to acute abdominal pain. She emphasized that these symptoms were merely indications that the man's body had not yet adjusted to the device. Hopefully the symptoms would disappear within a year.

One complication caused by the IPD and briefly mentioned by Dr. Merkin was the incidence of massive scrotal infection necessitating the surgical removal of the testicles. "But this is a rare case," said Merkin, "too rare to be statistically important." She and the other distinguished members of the Women's College of Surgeons agreed that the benefits far outweighed the risk to any individual man.

Source: Unknown.

health risks disproportionate to the risk expected of men so as to prevent conception?

Lastly, different cultural groups view the morality of contraception differently. Some countries' health insurance plans will not reimburse its subscribers for contraceptive devices or pills. In other countries, contraceptive services are part of reimbursable expenses. Countries with large Hispanic populations, such as in Latin America, with a strong belief in Catholicism, may not be as accepting of contraception as non-Catholics. Once again, morality is influenced by many variables and, therefore, what one person determines to be moral, another may determine to be immoral.

Emergency Contraception

A more recent contraceptive development pertains to *emergency contraception*. This is the use of oral contraceptives after unprotected sexual intercourse has occurred and there is a fear of pregnancy. For example, emergency contraception can be used in the case of rape or condom failure to prevent conception. The oral contraceptives must be taken within 72 hours of intercourse. A more detailed discussion of emergency contraception appears in Chapter 7. Here we limit the discussion to the ethical issues surrounding its use and availability.

One of the issues debated was whether to allow women access to emergency contraception without a physician's prescription. An expert Food and Drug Administration (FDA) panel recommended the FDA approve emergency contraception to be disbursed by pharmacists. The FDA asked the panel to gather more information and did not follow through on its recommendation. Some accused the FDA of bowing to political pressure from social conservatives (Kaufman, 2005). They argued that making emergency contraception available through pharmacists would make emergency contraception more effective. Their reasoning was that since it has to be used within 72 hours of coitus, why jeopardize that time frame by requiring a physician be contacted and a prescription be written. Further, they argued, studies have shown emergency contraception to be safe and effective.

Others, though, considered emergency contraception to be an abortion pill. That is, it prevents a fertilized egg from developing into a fetus and, eventually, a baby. They were opposed to any action that interfered with a pregnancy. They also believed that with emergency contraception available as a backup, people (in particular, youth) might engage in riskier sexual behavior. Studies, however, have found this fear to be unfounded (Kaufman, 2005). Whether and how emergency contraception should be available elicits more debate. As a responsible citizen, you should keep abreast of this debate and let your elected representatives know your views.

Abortion

Is induced, or voluntary, abortion simply a method of fertility control and as such the right of every woman, or is it taking of life that has a right to exist? Can it be both? If so, how can the dilemma be resolved? Some people seek to solve the problem by looking for evidence—or a definition—of when life begins. Does it begin at conception or does it begin when a fetus is capable of living outside the mother (at birth, or shortly before)? Others seek to solve it by asking who controls a woman's reproductive capacity. One must decide whether preserving the life and quality of life of the living is more or less important than maintaining the existence or viability of the unborn. This ethical dilemma is one of the most divisive issues in modern society. Laws are no sooner made than they are challenged. The morality of abortion is a subject of ongoing debate in many arenas of modern life—from the purely personal to the political.

Amniocentesis

Amniocentesis involves withdrawing, via a needle inserted into the uterus through the abdominal wall, a small amount of amniotic fluid surrounding the fetus. The procedure is recommended for women whose risk of producing babies with birth defects is greater than average (for example, women older than 35 years or women who have previously given birth to babies with birth defects). The moral question arises because if the test shows that the fetus will be deformed, mentally retarded, or seriously ill, the parents can choose to have an abortion rather than let the pregnancy run its course. Is it moral to take the risk (for example, of miscarriage) of having the test at all? Other issues are raised as well. For example, the sex of the fetus can be determined through amniocentesis. Is abortion moral when parents who have, say, four sons discover that their unborn child is a boy? Should the genes of an unborn baby be manipulated to conform with the parents'—or society's—idea of a superior human being? How much genetic manipulation is consistent with our ethical principles and values? As science becomes more sophisticated in this area, new ethical dilemmas arise.

Fetal Tissue Implantation

Parkinson's disease patients suffer tremors, muscular rigidity, and loss of balance as a result of a lack of the brain neurotransmitter dopamine. Research has discovered that fetal brain tissue, if implanted within the brain of Parkinson's patients, can produce enough dopamine to relieve many of the symptoms. However, the potential for abuse of this knowledge has prompted many groups and individuals to oppose the use of fetal tissue for implantation, or even for research purposes. One

Marital Age Around the World

It is not surprising that different countries with different cultures have different views of ethical issues. One of these issues is age at marriage. In the United States, it is believed to be immoral for a 13-year-old girl to marry, especially an older man. We even maintain legislation defining this as a violation of law. However, in other countries, the morality of early marriage, even to an older man, is not called into question. In developing countries, more than 60 million women aged 20–24 were married/in union before the age of 18. More than 31 million of them live in South Asia. In countries such as Bangladesh, Central African Republic, Chad, Guinea, Mali, and Niger, more than 60% of women entered into marriage or into a union before their eighteenth birthdays. Girls living in the poorest 20% of households are more likely to get married at an early age than those living in the wealthiest 20%. For example, in Peru, 45% of women were married by age 18 among the poorest 20% of the population, compared to 5% among the richest 20%. Women with primary education were significantly less likely to be married as children than those who received no education. In Zimbabwe, 48% of women who had attended primary school had been married by the age of 18, compared to 87% of those who had not attended school.

Parents choose to marry off their daughters early for a number of reasons. Poor families may regard a young girl as an economic burden and her marriage as a necessary survival strategy for her family. They may think that child marriage offers protection for their daughter from the dangers of sexual assault or, more generally, offers the care of a male guardian. Child marriage may also be seen as a strategy to avoid girls becoming pregnant outside of marriage. Gender discrimination can also underpin child marriage. Girls may be married young to ensure obedience and subservience within their husband's household and to maximize their childbearing.

UNICEF argues that child marriage can have serious harmful consequences for children, including *denial of education* (once married, girls tend not to go to school), *health problems* (including premature pregnancies, higher rates of maternal and infant mortality, and STIs, including HIV/AIDS), and *abuse* (a practice common in child marriages; children who refuse to marry or who choose a marriage partner against the wishes of their parents are often punished or even killed by their families in so-called honor killings).

Sources: UNICEF. Child protection from violence, exploitation and abuse: Child marriage. 2009. Available: http://www.unicef.org/protection/index_earlymarriage.html. UNICEF. *The state of the world's children 2009: Maternal and newborn health.* New York: Author, 2009. Available: http://www.unicef.org/sowc09/docs/SOWC09-Figure-2.4-EN.pdf.

of the concerns is that a woman will become pregnant with the intention to abort the fetus and use its brain tissue for a family member suffering from Parkinson's disease. Others argue that using human tissue in this manner defiles the sanctity of the human body.

Yet there are those who strongly support the use of fetal tissue to relieve Parkinson's and other diseases. They point to the socially acceptable practice of donating and transplanting organs such as hearts, livers, kidneys, lungs, and corneas.

In 1988, the federal government banned the use of federal funds for research involving aborted fetal tissue implantation. Believing this policy deprives certain patients from receiving adequate care, the American College of Obstetrics and Gynecology and the American Fertility Society in February 1991 established a private advisory body to guide scientists conducting fetal tissue and fertility research. This board, the National Advisory Board on Ethics in Reproduction, sets uniform standards, reviews proposed projects, advises researchers, and serves as a clearinghouse of information.

By 1993, the federal government's ban on research with fetal tissue implantation was lifted. Since then the National Institutes of Health (NIH) has awarded millions of dollars in grants for research involving the study, analysis, and use of human fetal tissue. Today research continues on the potential of fetal tissue in treatment of not only Parkinson's disease but also Alzheimer's disease, Huntington's disease, diabetes, multiple sclerosis, epilepsy, blindness, leukemia, hemophilia, sickle cell anemia, spinal-cord injuries, deficiencies of the immune system, birth defects, and pain (Kenney, Reinholtz, & Angellini, 1997). Supporting this research are the Alzheimer's Association, the Epilepsy Foundation of America, the Cystic Fibrosis Foundation, the Parkinson's Disease Foundation, and the Society for Pediatric Research.

Part of the remaining ethical issues regarding the use of human fetal tissue pertains to the finding

In 1990, Mary and Abe Ayala were told that the only chance to save their 17-year-old daughter Anissa from dying of leukemia was for her to have bone marrow transplantation. With no matching donors, the Ayalas decided to have another child (Marissa Eve) to use his or her bone marrow. Did the Ayalas act in a moral way? Did their physicians? What would you have done faced with such a dilemma?

Stem cell research has the potential to result in cures for debilitating diseases, but it is fraught with moral potholes. What do you think the policy ought to be regarding stem cell research and the appropriate source of stem cells?

that tissue from miscarriages and ectopic pregnancies appears rarely to be suitable for transplantation. However, tissue from induced abortions is effective when transplanted. Researchers argue that legal barriers to harvesting tissue from induced abortions stand in the way of building up the supply of usable fetal tissue.

Stem Cell Research

Stem cells are cells that can be found in embryos, fetuses, and adults. In adults, stem cells are specialized and can evolve into more cells of their own kind. In embryos, however, stem cells have the capacity to evolve into many different types of tissues and organs, depending on a complex of biological instructions. Embryonic stem cells are taken from embryos at the blastocyst stage of development (4 or 5 days after conception) when they are, in essence, a "blank page." Scientists are working on ways of instructing stem

cells to develop into specific tissue—for example, into insulin-producing pancreatic cells for implantation in diabetics.

The moral debate about stem cells involves a number of complex issues. For example, is it moral to use stem cells from aborted fetuses? Will this practice encourage more abortions? Is it moral to use stem cells from embryos created specifically for their stem cells? Is this the destruction of one human life to benefit another human life? Should scientific research, and consequently money that is devoted to scientific research, be concentrated on developing techniques for using adult stem cells rather than on embryonic stem cells? What should be the government's role in regulating and/or supporting stem cell research? Given the potential for stem cells to contribute to cures and/or treatments for Parkinson's disease, Alzheimer's disease, diabetes, heart disease, and arthritis, among others, should scientific research be entailed by governmental restrictions? Is that moral?

In 2001, President George W. Bush approved a regulation that would provide government funding for limited stem cell research. Bush, a conservative politician, tried to walk the fine line between what he believed to be morally justified and the potential for the enhancement of a large number of American lives—

 Did You Know . . .

Fetal brain tissue is not the only type of fetal cell that has potential for medical use. Early in development, the fetus's blood cells are produced by stem cells in the liver. Eventually these blood cells move into the fetus's bones and become bone marrow. Therefore, injecting fetal liver cells intravenously into patients is, in effect, giving them immune system transplantation.

Fetal liver transplants hold promise for such conditions as certain leukemias, sickle cell anemia, aplastic anemia, AIDS, and severe combined immunodeficiency disease.

Diabetics have also been given fetal insulin-producing pancreas cells, and fetal brain tissue's potential to aid in the treatment of Alzheimer's disease is very real.

another moral consideration. He decided that, on the one hand, stem cell research had a great deal of potential to cure diseases that affect large numbers of Americans. On the other hand, he believed that developing "human life" (embryos) to harvest their stem cells was immoral. Consequently, Bush decided that the government would provide funding for scientific research that used only adult stem cells or embryonic stem cells that had already been harvested. Bush estimated that there were about 60 of those groups of embryonic stem cells around the world. Staunch conservatives viewed this decision as immoral because it did not make a statement about the sanctity of life and allowed "immorally produced" embryonic stem cells to be used for research purposes. Scientists considered this decision immoral because it limited research to a small number of embryonic stem cells that were thought to be too homogenous to produce wide-scale cures (for example, many of these existing colonies of embryonic stem cells were obtained from white populations). Furthermore, scientists argued, adult stem cells do not have the capacity to develop into a range of tissue as do embryonic stem cells but are, instead, tissue specific. That limits their potential for a scientific breakthrough.

When Americans were surveyed, a majority supported stem cell research (Stem cell research, 2005). When asked if they favored or opposed stem cell research using embryonic stem cells, 58% were either strongly or somewhat in favor, 29% were either strongly or somewhat opposed, and 13% had no opinion. Of those opposed to the use of embryonic stem cells for research, 57% were opposed on religious grounds. Furthermore, 78% stated they thought the United States should be the global leader in medical and scientific research, in general. However, this is not the case when it comes to stem cell research. Whereas the federal government has restricted funding, several other countries have proceeded vigorously in stem cell research. They believe that, aside from developing techniques to cure many of the diseases plaguing humankind today, embryonic stem cell research is both moral and has tremendous economic potential for these countries' economies.

In 2009, bringing a different perspective to this issue, President Barack Obama lifted the restriction on federal funding of human embryonic stem cell research.

If you were the person deciding the role government ought to play in stem cell research, what would you decide? Which moral justifications would you offer to support that decision?

Prostitution

Prostitution is the selling of sexual gratification. Examples of prostitution were recorded even in ancient times, so contemporary society can take nei-ther credit nor blame for inventing this trade—only for the way in which it treats it.

People who consider prostitution immoral often argue that it degrades sexual intercourse, which is sanctified within marriage as an expression of love, into a mere animalistic act. Centuries ago Christianity adopted the Persian view, that the demands of the spirit and flesh were in conflict with each other, rather than the Greek view, which saw no conflict and allowed for prostitution (so long as the prostitutes were male). Nevertheless making some allowances for the flesh, Christianity developed incentives for marriage and deemed sexual intercourse within marriage appropriate and outside it sinful. Our culture has largely adhered to this view of who is a legitimate and morally acceptable sexual partner. To make a judgment about prostitution, a person must decide whether the desire for sexual services and sexual outlets is more important than the principle that coitus outside marriage is immoral.

In Vitro Fertilization

In 1980 the first "test-tube" baby clinic in the United States was approved by the state of Virginia. Located at the Norfolk General Hospital in Norfolk, Virginia, this clinic offers its services to couples who wish to conceive but are infertile as a result of blocked, missing, or damaged fallopian tubes of women. (It does not treat male infertility.) The clinic, officially named the In Vitro Clinic (for **in vitro fertilization**), had a waiting list of from 1 to 2 years just 1 week after gaining state approval.

> **in vitro fertilization**
> The creation of a pregnancy in a laboratory by uniting the sperm and egg outside the womb; sometimes termed the "test-tube" baby technique.

There are some who believe using in vitro fertilization to produce babies is immoral. For example, in March 1987 the Catholic Congregation for the Doctrine of the Faith issued "Instruction on Respect for Human Life in Its Origin and on the Dignity of Procreation," a document that defined generation of human life outside the body as "morally illicit." In addition to in vitro fertilization, other biomedical breakthroughs were condemned as immoral. Among these were genetic engineering, surrogate motherhood, cloning, and manipulations to produce human beings according to sex or other predetermined qualities. According to the document, the only approved method of human procreation is "the act of conjugal love."

Other ethical issues pertain to in vitro fertilization. For example, what will be its effect on the population of the world? Will it produce too many people for the available resources? What would that mean for the quality of life of the world's population? What should be done if the fetus develops defectively once

What is the appropriate and/or moral use of reproductive technologies such as in vitro fertilization? Should reproduction remain a natural phenomenon, or should medical advancements and techniques be used to enhance conception?

it has been implanted in the uterus? When choosing to have a baby by artificial means, should parents be allowed to select the baby's sex, eye color, intelligence, and so on? These issues need societal attention; we as citizens need to inform our representatives of our judgments regarding what is moral and immoral relative to in vitro fertilization.

Genetic Engineering

In vitro fertilization evokes images of genetic manipulation in the minds of some people. Of course, that is not its intent. However, as science progresses and reproductive technology develops new ways to manage and enhance reproduction, fears of Huxley's *Brave New World* emerge. There are hundreds of biotechnology companies devoted to identifying genes and their functions with the hope of obtaining patents for these genes and the ways in which they can be put to use. It is envisioned that these genes will lead to designer medicines, engineered foods, and eventually custom-made kids (Achenbach, 1998), and the companies that own these patents will make a lot of money. Even the U.S. government staked out a claim to this research by funding the largest scientific project, the Human Genome Project. The $3 billion Human Genome Project, in collaboration with the private firm Celera Genomics, decoded the entire human genetic code in 2003.

All this research raises the possibility that a new generation will be genetically manipulated so that parents will be able to select the color of their babies' eyes, height, athletic and intellectual abilities, and artistic tal-

ents. However, some experts are concerned about this possibility. Jeremy Rifkin, the eminent futurist, argues that in a few generations babies will be "engineered." The biologist Lee Silver believes that the human race will be divided into two distinct species, the "Naturals" and the "GenRich" (Achenbach, 1998).

However, there are other experts who disagree. They argue that although a sheep (Dolly) has been cloned, researchers are a long way from being able to clone humans. And, even if that were possible, scientists are too ethical to do that. However, it is disconcerting that there are groups of scientists who are attempting to clone a human as of the time of this writing. Finally, experts who do not see a *Brave New World* on the horizon expect that as we approach new and more sophisticated reproductive technological advancements, ethicists, clergy, philosophers, politicians, and others, will intervene to develop gene-technology protocols that are acceptable to our societal values and mores.

Whether we will have "designer babies" is still an open question. As citizens in a democratic society we need to keep abreast of the latest developments in this area, because the very nature of the human race may be at issue. The uses of this new technology may be as much a function of the will of the people as it is the interests of the scientists, and, if so, every person has a responsibility to become involved in some way.

The issue of bioethics is recognized throughout the world. The United Nations (UN) Commission on Human Rights adopted the first international guidelines on bioethics and the human genome. The "Universal Declaration on the Human Genome and Human Rights," cosponsored by 86 countries, sets standards for people researching and using genetic information and techniques. Although it specifically recognizes the rights to freedom of research and freedom of thought, it states that "practices which are contrary to human dignity, such as reproductive cloning of human beings, shall not be permitted." The United States is one of the countries that support the UN declaration.

Sexual Responsibility to a Partner

The last sexual ethical dilemma we discuss is, What degree of responsibility do we have, sexually, with respect to others? Should our sexual behavior achieve our own ends, regardless of the desires of our sexual partners? Conversely, are we under an obligation to subjugate our own sexual needs to the needs of our sexual partners? Given that two individuals are involved, just what is moral sexual behavior?

The issue of sexual responsibility, as are all the issues discussed so far, is complex. Certainly we are all responsible for ourselves and our own behavior, but when we take care of ourselves by involving someone else, the issue becomes clouded. As an example imagine that a typical couple, Paul and Paula, love each other and are engaged to be married. Paula wants to share coitus with Paul, but Paul considers sexual intercourse outside marriage immoral. Should Paula attempt to convince Paul that they should have intercourse? Would it be reasonable for her to threaten to date someone else if he refuses? Should Paul relegate his beliefs to second place and give in to Paula? What is their responsibility to themselves? To each other? To their future? To their relationship? These questions are not easy to answer. However, when sexual behavior involves someone else, there is always potential for manipulation or coercion. The moral nature of such behavior should be explored.

Even when a decision is the individual's alone, ethical dilemmas may arise. For example, should sexually active people use some means of contraception, even if their partners do not care? If not, are they behaving responsibly? What if one's religion opposes the use of contraception but one is sexually active and unwilling to risk pregnancy? As with all the issues we have explored, the means of resolving these questions is to rank the conflicting ethical principles according to our personal values.

Laws Regulating Sexual Behavior

Laws formalize moral decisions for a society. Our laws regarding sexual behavior developed from a general acceptance of specific ethical principles, values, and judgments about behaviors such as those we have explored. They have their roots in experience, in religious dogma, and in economics and politics.

Consensus—or general agreement—about which sexual actions should be considered permissible has not always been easily achieved. Indeed, communities have sometimes had to devise ingenious compromises to keep peace among their various moral factions. Consider, for example, the "Combat Zone" in Boston, Massachusetts. To meet the needs of people who frequented bars featuring topless dancers, attended X-rated movies, and so forth, but also to protect citizens opposed to such activities from exposure to them, the municipal government restricted the bars and theaters in question to a specific part of the city, nicknamed the "Combat Zone." The Combat Zone has subsequently been abolished. For similar reasons, some European countries have established red-light districts, in an attempt to limit prostitution to a single section of town.

However, even when consensus is achieved and codified into city, state, or federal law, it is by no

---

Myth vs Fact

Myth: Morality is morality. What is right is right, and what is wrong is wrong.
Fact: Most people agree that what is moral in one society may not be moral in another. Furthermore, what is considered moral in one situation may not be considered moral in another situation.

Myth: There is no systematic way in which to resolve ethical and moral issues. It is mostly a matter of intuition and subjective judgment.
Fact: Ethics is a system that uses ethical principles to determine the morality of a situation or decision. Ethical principles are valued according to many factors, including experience, religious teachings, cultural background, education, and family values.

Myth: In our diverse society, there are no commonly accepted ethical principles. Different groups have different values and different views of morality.

Fact: Although it is true that in a country with many different cultural groups living together there are many different views of morality, there are some ethical principles that we can all agree on. These include caring, respect for others, honesty, responsibility, and trustworthiness.

Myth: There are some situations about which there is no disagreement regarding morality. For example, there is no disagreement about HIV and AIDS, because AIDS is such a serious and deadly disease.
Fact: HIV and AIDS provide a good example of how complex moral decisions can be. For example, there is disagreement regarding whether condom advertisements should be allowed on television and whether needle-distribution programs for intravenous drug users should be developed.

---

means stable. State laws prohibiting prostitution, which were widely acceptable when they were enacted, are periodically under attack and may well someday be modified or rejected. Supreme Court rulings on abortion and on pornography have not settled those issues. Changes occur—albeit slowly—when there is a conflict between existing law and new morality. An illegal activity might begin to be seen as moral; a legal act, as immoral.

We will see in this discussion that sexual laws develop through a societal consensus of the valuing of ethical principles. The process of devising such laws involves identifying ethical principles, valuing them to define moral behavior, and then encoding laws to enforce that behavior (or prohibit it if defined as immoral). Because our values may change over time, however, we periodically reassess and change our laws governing sexual behavior.

Obscenity and Pornography

Some issues continue to be debated even in the face of definitive opinions from the Supreme Court. An example involves the definitions of **obscenity** and **pornography**. The Comstock Act of 1873, the first

Communication
DIMENSIONS

The Morality of Requesting a Variety of Sexual Behaviors

In some sexual relationships, one partner desires more variety in sexual activities than the other. For example, one partner may prefer anal sexual intercourse, and the other may object. Or one partner may be extremely excited by oral–genital sex, and the other may be turned off by it. One person may think of certain sexual activities as immoral, another as exciting. Too often, these conflicts result in anger and resentment, thereby interfering with other aspects of the relationship, not merely the sexual part. Consequently, partners should discuss differing sexual desires and resolve these issues. Fortunately, there are ways to do just that.

To begin, each person's thoughts and feelings should be expressed. A comment like "That's sick!" short-circuits any meaningful communication. The initial part of the conversation should be devoted to understanding the viewpoint of the other person, and that requires listening. There is time to express an opposing point of view, but not until one person has had the chance to be understood. Once one person has expressed his or her viewpoint, the other should. Refrain from arguing or disagreeing at this point. Merely listen.

Once both points of view have been aired, points of agreement should be identified. For example, both partners might agree that sex is a normal and desirable part of their relationship; that variety of sexual behaviors enhances the sexual relationship and thereby positively influences other aspects of their life together; that each cares about the other's feelings and sexual satisfaction; and that they want to make each other happy.

The part of communication regarding conflicts of ethics and morality that is most difficult is finding a compromise with which both persons are satisfied. Identifying areas of agreement provides a starting point in this process. Perhaps one partner is willing to try a particular sexual activity because he or she has identified a concern for making the other person happy. Perhaps the other is willing to forgo a particular sexual activity because it will make the other unhappy. The goal is to maintain the relationship as a stimulating one, not to engage in specific behaviors. The original focus on the behaviors is what is "wanted," whereas the real issue is the "need" for excitement and stimulation. That need can be met in ways that satisfy both partners with a little ingenuity and creativity.

Remember, though, no one should be forced, coerced, or manipulated to behave in any way that he or she considers immoral. That will result only in guilt, shame, or embarrassment and will not be healthy for the person or the relationship. If your partner is trying to manipulate you, the relationship is probably not worth saving.

---

obscenity
Something offensive to modesty or decency; often sexually related.

pornography
Sexually arousing music, art, literature, or films; a determination that may vary from individual to individual and from community to community.

major law concerning obscenity in the United States, prohibited the mailing of obscene or lewd material. The interpretation of what was obscene or lewd was left to the Postal Service. In 1957 the Supreme Court attempted to clarify the issue by ruling that sexuality-related material and obscene material were not one and the same. Rather, sexual material was ruled obscene (and therefore outside the protection of the First Amendment) only when sexual behavior was presented in a lewd and lascivious manner. But how was it to be determined whether some particular material was lewd or lascivious? The Supreme Court stated that the standard to

be applied was whether the average person would judge it as such.

Further rulings between 1957 and 1968 (55 separate legal opinions in 13 obscenity cases) attempted to define obscenity more explicitly. As a result, the phrase "utterly without redeeming social value" was added to the definition. In 1973 the Court rejected its own "utterly without redeeming social value" criterion and defined the standards of obscenity that are currently in effect:

1. Whether the average person applying contemporary community standards would find that the work, taken as a whole, appeals to the prurient (lustful) interests

2. Whether the work depicts or describes, in a patently offensive way, sexual conduct specified by state law

3. Whether the work, taken as a whole, lacks serious literary, artistic, political, or scientific value

Despite the history of legal activity, a consensus in the society as to the definition of obscenity has yet to be reached. With the advent of the Internet and the access it provides to sexually explicit material, the problem is exacerbated.

Rape

Although there is considerable debate about the psychological, sociological, and cultural causes of rape, the chief legal issue involves achieving consensus on a set of standards for enforcing the laws against rape. The legal definition of forcible rape is sexual intercourse against one's will, but because anyone might accuse another of rape, society has had to define acceptable evidence. Until recently a prosecutor had to prove that semen was present—on the woman's body or clothing—to gain a conviction of rape. However, many female victims do not have a medical exam after rape; others bathe or shower before being examined; and in many cases of true rape, the rapist fails to ejaculate. Because many rapists have been pronounced innocent because of a lack of such evidence, the presence of semen is no longer considered the sole evidence of forcible rape; bruises, the presence of a weapon, and even threats of force may now be accepted.

Defense attorneys have often focused on the victims, attempting to show that they were promiscuous and thus responsible for provoking sexual attacks. New laws reflect society's growing concern with protecting victims from unfair questioning, as well as with ensuring conviction when rape has actually occurred. These laws now prohibit questions regarding the victim's sexual experience during a rape trial. Thus the focus of the trial is on determining the guilt or innocence of the accused, not on the moral character of the victim.

Statutory Rape

Statutory rape is placed in a different legal category from forcible rape, and a situation ethicist might also put it in a different moral category. Statutory rape is sexual intercourse with a person below the legal age of consent, which varies from state to state. The statute is designed to protect children considered too immature to make sexual decisions for themselves. Even if boys or girls willingly participate in sexual intercourse, their consent is ignored for legal purposes. And even if they appear to be of age or lie about their age, the laws still apply, with few exceptions. In some states the exception is that a child

Myth vs Fact

Myth: As long as two adults agree, any sexual activity in which they engage is legal, as long as it is done in private.
Fact: Not long ago, most states had sodomy laws that made certain sexual activities illegal even though they were consensual and performed by adults. These laws have since been declared unconstitutional.

proved to be sexually promiscuous or a prostitute may be considered an adult.

Adultery

Adultery, or extramarital intercourse, is quite prevalent in the United States. Kinsey reported back in 1948 that more than one-third of the men in his study reported extramarital coitus; in 1953 he reported that half of the men and 26% of the women he studied had extramarital sexual intercourse by age 40 years. Many suspect that the incidence of extramarital coitus has increased since Kinsey's studies. However, Hicks and Leitenberg (2001) report that men are engaging in fewer instances of extramarital sexual intercourse. They report the incidence for men at 28%, similar to women (29%). Other researchers have found the prevalence of adultery to be even lower, between 20% and 25% (Atkins, Baucom, & Jacobson, 2001). Even so, our concept of morality vis-à-vis marriage still leads us to sustain the laws against it. Adultery is frequently a legal ground for divorce. When adultery is the basis of divorce and custody of children is challenged in court, the adulterous partner often loses custody.

Although it is illegal for a typical person to photograph and publish nude photos of minors, many "artists" seem to have few problems getting away with it. Many bookstores sell photo albums that contain full nudity of clearly underage boys and girls, without prosecution. Is it possible to distinguish ethically or legally between nude photos of minors that are taken for the purpose of arousal from those that are taken as "art"?

The practice of polygamy in the Mormon Church, which was a common occurrence until the mid-19th century, still continues in some small enclaves of Utah. In 2001, Tom Green, a fundamentalist Mormon, was convicted and sentenced to 5 years in prison in the most recent and biggest bigamy case in half a century. At the time of his trial, Green had a total of 5 wives and 30 children. Despite the fact that both the Mormon Church and the state of Utah are formally against the practice of polygamy as well as further charges that one of Green's wives was actually only 13 years old when he first had sexual intercourse with her, Green claims that he has been unfairly singled out. With an estimated total of 30,000 polygamists still existing in Utah and the western United States, Green maintains that he is only perpetuating a traditional religious practice.

Divorce

Laws involving divorce have been reformed over the years. Originally marriage and divorce laws in the United States were based on Judeo-Christian ethical principles involving the sanctity of the family and of parenthood. These laws reinforced the idea that the family was an economic necessity, both for the individual and for the society. Consequently divorce was granted by law only if misbehavior was proved in court. In other words, one of the marriage partners had to be at fault by being adulterous, mentally or physically cruel, and so on. When the number of divorces increased, and it became a common belief that people wishing to be free of each other should not be forced to remain married, many states adopted **no-fault divorce**. No-fault divorce statutes allow courts to dissolve marriages when no fault is cited and both partners agree to end the marriage.

Some people argue that no-fault divorce laws have led to more divorces (a bad thing); others say they have led to happier people (a good thing). Another way of looking at the prevalence of divorce—regardless of fault—is to argue that we should make marriage laws stricter, rather than making divorce laws looser. People would then have to work harder to get married, and those without a strong commitment to each other would be unlikely to follow through.

Alimony is money that a judge orders the partner who earns more to pay on the granting of a divorce to the partner who earns less or no money. As are other matters related to divorce, alimony is being reevaluated. Previously alimony was handled as punishment for divorce, and the husband was forced to make payments to his wife. Today judges are more likely to assess the particular circumstances in a case and award alimony to either the man or the woman, on the basis of their respective resources and contributions to the marriage.

no-fault divorce
The granting of divorce without either partner's proving the other was the cause of the marriage's failure.

alimony
Money a divorced person is instructed by the courts to pay regularly to his or her ex-spouse.

Exploring the
DIMENSIONS
of Human Sexuality

Our feelings, attitudes, and beliefs regarding sexuality are influenced by our internal and external environments. Go to sexuality.jbpub.com/dimensions/4e to learn more about the biological, psychological, and sociological factors that affect your sexuality.

Sociocultural Factors

- Religions often establish codes of ethics, which state for members beliefs on matters including abortion, premarital sexual activity, extramarital sexual activity, same-gender sexual relations, and nonintercourse sexual activities.
- Political beliefs often suggest ethical standards. Although there are exceptions, in general, Democrats and feminists generally take a pro-choice stance (not always), and Republicans and fundamentalist Christians take an antiabortion stance. Laws in the United States ban discrimination based on race, religion, gender, age, and sexual orientation for public organizations, but private organizations can still discriminate. In many Islamic countries, adultery is illegal—even punishable by death. Gender selection through female infanticide or amniocentesis coupled with abortion is tolerated in some countries.

Biological Factors

- Alcohol and drugs can blur decision-making ability.

Psychological Factors

- During the state of sexual arousal and response, it is often hard to make moral judgments that conflict with intense physiological feelings.

CASE STUDY

At the center of many ethical and moral dilemmas are cultural underpinnings—especially religious and political beliefs.

However, sometimes those cultural underpinnings clash. Consider the woman who unexpectedly finds herself pregnant. Raised as a member of the Roman Catholic religion—with its antiabortion doctrine—the woman has also been raised as a feminist, with a pro-choice doctrine. Further, consider the rights of her partner, who may have a different set of sociocultural doctrines to rely on for making moral decisions.

On a more personal level, it is important to make moral decisions regarding sexual relationships before becoming sexually involved. During a state of sexual arousal and response, it is often hard to put moral feelings ahead of intense physiological feelings.

States may pass specific laws dealing with sexuality; however, such laws must not conflict with federal laws and may be challenged for their constitutionality.

Summary

- Ethics is a system on which we base our moral decisions. Ethical principles provide guidelines for abstract questions, not solutions to individual cases.

- When ethical principles clash, we have an ethical dilemma. Ethical dilemmas are resolved by placing a value on the competing ethical principles, with the principle carrying the highest value being the one that guides the decision.

- Rule ethics uses ethical principles to guide decisions in all situations. Situation ethics is based on the premise that all situations are unique and, therefore, there are no ethical principles that can be used the same way to guide all moral decision.

- If a decision or action is moral, it is *good* or *right*. If a decision is immoral, it is *bad* or *wrong*.

- Laws represent the encoding of generally accepted societal views of morality. Laws regarding sexual behavior develop from a general consensus of specific ethical principles, values, and judgments about behavior. When laws are not representative of societal views of morality, they are not followed and often need to be changed.

- Sexual morality is a consideration in such sexually related areas as sexually transmitted infections, sexual activity among unmarried persons, emergency contraception, abortion, amniocentesis, fetal tissue implantation, stem cell research, prostitution, in vitro fertilization, genetic engineering, and sexual responsibility to a partner.

- Among laws pertaining to sexual behavior are those regarding obscenity and pornography, rape, statutory rape, adultery, and divorce.

Discussion Questions

1. Differentiate between ethics and morals. Apply the ethical principles of nonmaleficence, beneficence, autonomy/liberty, justice/fairness, and social utility to issues in human sexuality.

2. Discuss commonly accepted ethical principles and ways they can be applied in situations involving sexual behavior.

3. Which types of sexual behavior are regulated by laws? What is the basis of those laws?

Application Questions

Reread the chapter-opening story and answer the following questions.

1. Consider the ethical principles of nonmaleficence, beneficence, autonomy/liberty, justice/fairness, and social utility as they relate to the opening story. Which of the ethical principles did Wendy Weaver and the Nebo school district follow? Then explain how the case might have been affected if Weaver and the school district had followed other principles.

2. Was it ethical for Weaver to disclose her sexual orientation to a minor student? Should Weaver have considered the student's possible religious (70% of Utah residents are Mormon) objections to homosexuality before answering?

Critical Thinking Questions

1. Is practicing safer sex an ethical issue or a legal issue? For example, is it unethical not to have STI and HIV tests before starting a new relationship? Can this become a legal issue?

2. An unmarried woman who has been in a steady sexual relationship for 5 months discovers she is pregnant. Is it ethical, moral, or legal for the male to decide whether the female should have the child and keep it, give the child up for

adoption, or have an abortion? What if the couple breaks up before she finds out she is pregnant? What rights, if any, does the man have in relation to the baby he helped create?

3. The ethics and morality of creating (or re-creating) life sometimes reflect technological innovations of the times. As the age of electricity dawned in the 1800s, Mary Shelley's *Frankenstein* (1818) provoked ethical and moral concerns about the use of electricity. Today, the use of electricity in the defibrillator to save a heart attack patient is accepted as ethical, moral, and legal. In fact, it would be considered unethical, immoral, and illegal not to use a defibrillator when a life could be saved. During our current age of genetic research (beginning with the 1950s discovery of DNA), Michael Crichton's *Jurassic Park* provoked similar concerns about the misuse of genetic engineering. However, even as you read this question, new technological applications are being devised that can and will save lives. Do you think people in 200 years will look back at *Jurassic Park* and wonder why we feared genetic research?

Critical Thinking Case

The ability to select the gender of a child has for years been the source of ethical debate. In some countries, cultures approve of female infanticide or amniocentesis coupled with abortion. However, the cultural morals of the United States do not favor such methods.

Would the current U.S. culture accept a scientifically based method of gender selection? The Genetics and IVF Institute (Fairfax, Virginia) announced in September 1998 that it had found a way to separate male and female sperm cells. Using specialized technology, its personnel are able to sort out 85% of X-bearing sperm (females) and 65% of Y-bearing sperm (males). Using artificial insemination, the Institute can give parents potential for gender selection, in proportion to the sperm-sorting abilities.

The technique has been used for some time on animals, which are easier to sort by gender. Testing with humans began in 1998. Human applications include preventing the birth of children with rare genetic sex-linked diseases (such as X-linked hydrocephalus) or "balancing" families with an opposite-sex sibling. The Institute is not planning to market the sorting procedure to first-time parents who simply have a dream of a specific-gender child.

Do you think that sperm-sorting technology is ethically acceptable in the case of raising farm animals? How about in the name of protecting endangered species from extinction?

As far as human applications are concerned, do you find it ethical to use sperm sorting to prevent the birth of a child who has a genetic sex-linked disease? How about to have an additional child to provide needed bone marrow for transplantion to a current child? Finally, is it ethical to use sperm sorting to have a third or fourth child of the opposite gender?

Exploring Personal Dimensions

Determining Your Ethical Compass
Several ethical dilemmas are presented in this activity to help you determine which ethical principles you use to guide your behavior and your view of morality. Choose the one option for each dilemma that best represents your views, even though you might agree with more than one.

1. Juan and Maria decide to live together and share a sexual relationship. They are thinking that they may marry in the future, but not anytime soon.

   a. Juan and Maria should not move in together because we know that when men and women live together, they are not equals. Women tend to take on more of the household chores than men.

   b. Juan and Maria should be free to decide what is best for them.

c. Juan and Maria should not live together because Maria will suffer if she does not eventually marry Juan. She will be perceived as immoral by her family and her community.

d. No good will come of Juan and Maria's living together. In fact, it might harm society by encouraging sexual relations between people who are not married to each other.

2. Evan and Rhonda place their 2-year-old son in child care so they can both work outside the home.

a. This is unfair because Evan and Rhonda are placing their interests above the welfare of their son.

b. Each couple should be able to decide what is best for their family unit.

c. Without the direct and extensive contact with one of his parents, Evan and Rhonda's son will not grow and develop to his potential.

d. Society will suffer if this becomes a common practice because of the emotional cost and health effects that the community will eventually have to absorb.

3. Although Kevin and Latisha have a sexual relationship, Kevin has not disclosed to Latisha that he has herpes. Kevin argues that their relationship is not "serious" and, therefore, he should not have to divulge his STI to Latisha. Furthermore, Kevin states, he refrains from having intercourse with Latisha when he has noticeable sores.

a. Because Kevin knows about his STI and Latisha does not, Kevin is treating Latisha unfairly. He has more information than she, and that is not right.

b. Kevin has a right to decide to whom information about his health is released, as well as the nature of that information.

c. Lacking knowledge of Kevin's herpes, Latisha is likely to engage in behavior that can cause her harm.

d. If Kevin continues to withhold information about his health and infects other sexual partners, society will suffer, health premiums will be raised for the rest of us, and hospital and medical staff resources may have to be redirected from other health issues.

4. Frankie and Lynn had been married for 10 years when Frankie began a sexual relationship with his coworker Flo.

a. It is not fair that Frankie engages in sex outside his marriage whereas Lynn refrains because of her vows of fidelity. If Frankie engages in extramarital sex, why should Lynn not have affairs as well?

b. Frankie may have many reasons for deciding to have a sexual relationship with Flo. He is an adult and should be free to decide whether the risk outweighs the benefits he derives from the relationship with Flo.

c. If Lynn ever found out she would be devastated, and their marriage might end. If they have children, even more harm would be done.

d. Society cannot allow extramarital affairs to be unpunished; otherwise, we would have chaos, unstable families, and dysfunctional children growing into dysfunctional adults.

5. Rose and Amber are lovers who are often seen by their neighbors holding hands as they enter their apartment building. Several of the more conservative tenants have complained about being "confronted by two lesbians flaunting their relationship to everyone else."

a. It is not fair that heterosexual tenants can hold hands but gay couples are expected to refrain from doing so.

b. Rose and Amber should be able to do whatever they choose. It is a free world. The other residents are free to look away.

c. Raising this issue with Rose and Amber might make them self-conscious and lead to their questioning whether they are welcome in that apartment building. Furthermore, the strain of this confrontation might lead to stress that could harm their health.

   d. It is harmful to young children, who are impressionable and in the process of developing their own sexual orientation, to see outwardly gay couples' being accepted by society. For the good of the total society, gay couples should be more discreet.

If you found yourself selecting choice (a) more often than the other choices, you are predominantly guided by the ethical principle of *justice*, believing people ought to be treated fairly. If you selected choice (b) over the others, you are guided by *autonomy*, believing people ought to be free to make their own choices without interference from others. However, if you selected choice (c) most often, you are guided by the ethical principle of nonmaleficence, believing no harm ought to be done, and, when it is, the decision is immoral. And, if you found yourself most often selecting choice (d), you are guided by *social utility*, believing a decision needs to be considered in terms of the benefit or harm to society.

Suggested Readings

Aquinas, T., Regan, R. J., & Baumgarth, W. P., eds. *On law, morality, and politics*. Cambridge, MA: Hackett, 2003.

Arthur, J. *Morality and moral controversies: Readings in moral, social and political philosophy*, 8th Ed. Saddle River, NJ: Prentice Hall, 2008.

Bingham, C., & Gansler, L. L. *Class action: The landmark case that changed sexual harassment law*. New York: Alfred A. Knopf, 2003.

Blackburn, S. *Being good: A short introduction to ethics*. Oxford, UK: Oxford University Press, 2003.

Gerstmann, E. *Same-sex marriage and the constitution*. Cambridge, UK: Cambridge University Press, 2003.

Gert, B. *Common morality: Deciding what to do*. Oxford, UK: Oxford University Press, 2004.

Greenberg, J. *The code of ethics for the health education profession: A case study book*. Boston: Jones and Bartlett, 2001.

Mappes, T. A., & Zembaty, J. S. *Social ethics: Morality and social policy*. New York: McGraw-Hill Higher Education, 2002.

Mappes, T. A., & Zembaty, J. *Social ethics: Morality and social policy*. New York: McGraw-Hill Humanities, 2006.

Martin, M. W. *Everyday morality: An introduction to applied ethics*. Florence, KY: Wadsworth, 2006.

Web Resources

For links to the web sites below, visit *http://sexuality.jbpub.com/dimensions/4e* and click on Resource Links.

The Feminist Sexual Ethics Project
www.brandeis.edu/projects/fse

Explores sexual ethics within Judaism, Christianity, and Islam, and presents how the toleration of slavery in the early teachings of these religions affects the lives of women today. Among the links are those dealing with Jewish sexual ethics, Christian sexual ethics, and Muslim sexual ethics.

United Nations High Commissioner for Human Rights (UNHCHR)
www.ohchr.org/EN/Pages/WelcomePage.aspx

The Office of the High Commissioner for Human Rights (OHCHR) is a department of the United Nations Secretariat. It is mandated to promote and protect the enjoyment and full realization, by all people, of all rights established in the Charter of the United Nations and in international human rights laws and treaties. The mandate includes preventing human rights violations, securing respect for all human rights, promoting international cooperation to protect human rights, coordinating related activities throughout the United Nations, and strengthening and streamlining the United Nations system in the field of human rights. Among these rights are those that pertain to sexual issues—for example, female clitoral mutilation.

Sexual Ethics in Psychology
www.rotten.com/library/sex/sexual-ethics-in-psychology

Presents case studies to discuss the American Psychological Association's code of ethics that governs the interaction between therapists and patients. The sexual interaction between clinician and patient is emphasized.

Human Rights Campaign
www.hrc.org

The Human Rights Campaign is America's largest civil rights organization working to achieve gay, lesbian, bisexual, and transgender (GLBT) equality. HRC seeks to improve the lives of GLBT Americans by advocating for equal rights and benefits in the workplace, ensuring families are treated equally under the law, and increasing public support among all Americans through innovative advocacy, education, and outreach programs. The web site includes links to legislation, laws, work life, religion and faith, employment opportunities, and other subjects.

MayoClinic.com: Sex Therapy: Is It an Option for You?
www.mayoclinic.com/health/sex-therapy/MC00065

Answers questions about sex therapy to help people decide whether sex therapy is what they need and is what they are interested in. Questions answered are: How is sex therapy done? What kind of concerns do sex therapists address? Isn't it embarrassing to talk about sex? Does sex therapy ever involve sexual contact? How long does sex therapy take? How much does sex therapy cost? How do you find a sex therapist? Is sex therapy right for you?

Epilogue: Taking Responsibility for Your Sexual Health

THE SEXUAL FUTURE

It was a morning of unmatched brilliance; the sun shone brightly, the robins were singing, and the spring air was morning fresh. It was a typical morning in the year 2099 for Todd and his housemates Keri, Karen, and Jerry.

Excuse me. I am being impolite. I forgot that you were from another time. I should have introduced you to our way of life before mentioning my friends. Of course we have made lots of technological advances, as you will soon see. But given what was going on in your day, you could probably see that coming, even if you could not foresee the form. Beyond that, however, we have changed our attitudes and values, our ways of doing work, and our social, sexual, and family relationships. For example, in 2099 we are altogether more respectful of individual differences than you were in your time. Questions of morality do not dominate our way of life as they did yours, and much ignorance has been dispelled. Is it a good or bad time, you ask? Let me describe our ways to you and you can answer for yourself.

Keri, Karen, Jerry, and Todd range in age from 21 to 41 years, but they are not rushing off to work today. In fact they never rush off to work, because they all work at home. Most people do. It is the computer and all the other technological and communication advances, you see. Of course, as you did in the early part of this century, we all have computer terminals at home and we use them for work and play, as well as for banking, shopping, and communicating with one another over long and short distances. We play games on them and can program our terminals to play music for us. Our physicians even use them to diagnose illnesses and prescribe medication. (Wait until you hear about the medication we have!) Anyway, why do you think the morning air is so fresh? No cars to pollute it! In fact, there is very little transportation as you knew it. We have little need to go anywhere. Our computers meet most of our needs. Life really is easy.

Family life, as you can imagine, is also quite different from home life as you knew it. Long ago we realized that marriage was archaic—it just did not make sense in a rapidly changing society to expect two people to live together forever. People change as the society changes, but not all marriage partners change at the same pace. Once we understood this, we changed our laws to allow for a number of different marriage styles. The styles are not really new, but the legal and social ease of choosing and changing *is*. For example, we have repeating monogamous marriages

(RMMs), wherein one maintains only one partner at a time but, when the marriage becomes stale, one can dissolve the marriage easily and marry another partner. Some people marry 10 or more times in this manner. Polygamy (one person married to several people at the same time) is also common, as are multiple marriage partners (MMPs). MMPs allow several males to share several female marriage partners, and vice versa.

In spite of all our attempts to adapt marriage to our society, however, most people never marry. Rather they establish informal arrangements of convenience. Some live together, some raise children together (their own or those of others), and some just share particular events together. I, for example, have an informal arrangement with Betty for sexual play, with Tina for computer game play, and with Tasha for sharing of thoughts and important feelings.

By the way, we laugh when the computer tells us stories of your struggle with sexual equality. In 2099 we cannot imagine that males would be treated differently from females. I guess our attitude evolves partly because the need for physical strength continued to decrease, just as it was in your day, and that eliminated the male's biological advantage. You see, robots do all our strenuous work, and competitive sports (other than computer games) have long since been outlawed. They were thought to contribute to warlike attitudes that, with the existence of weapons that could destroy the world, were deemed intolerable. But really that only partly explains our sexual equality. We realize that people who are discriminated against eventually revolt. It is only a matter of time—treat a group unfairly and it eventually rebels, disturbing the peace. Furthermore, our scientists have discovered treatments that allow everyone, male and female, to feel however they wish and to acquire almost any trait they want or need. Because people can change themselves nearly at will, how could we believe any one or any group to be inferior?

Scientists have made other important advances, too. Most diseases are curable now—your dreaded cancer and heart diseases among them. But perhaps the single most significant advance has been the discovery of K25W. Added to our water supply by our leaders (all of whom are scientists rather than politicians), K25W is a chemical that prepares the mind to receive and accept subliminal messages.

What are subliminal messages, you ask? Just a little trick of the media trade. The subliminal messages are verbal messages delivered so quickly and at such a low volume that those who receive them are not even aware that messages have been conveyed. Subliminal messages can be visual, too, images relayed so quickly along with other broadcast material that viewers remain unaware of them. Your society experimented with a crude form of subliminal messages when, for instance, voices were hidden beneath the pleasant music that department store customers heard while shopping reminding customers to be polite and not to shoplift. But you did not have K25W in your water! We use subliminal messages to plant many ideas, one of which is sexual equality, in the minds of our citizens.

The one problem we are still wrestling with is how to solve the discontent of our elderly. Having eradicated many of the diseases that plagued you, plus eliminating traffic accidents, we have lengthened the life span of most people, and so the size of our elderly population has grown enormously. By the way, we do not think of 70-year-olds as elderly; people live now to the ages of 120, 130, even 140 years. Mind you, our old people are quite happy (remember K25W) and able to care for themselves (remember our medications). Still, they tell stories of their past, and young people wonder whether our society is really better than the one the old folks recall. There is much ambivalence in those recollections. The old ones speak of illness, on the one hand, and the joy of life, on the other hand; of cruelty and war, on the one hand, and the Peace Corps, on the other hand; of nursing homes, on the one hand, and growing old with families to care for you, on the other hand. No small wonder the younger ones are confused. But our scientists are working on this issue even as we speak. Before long it will be clear to all that our new society is developing in the right direction. After all, do we not live longer? Have we not eliminated sexual bias? Can we not take a pill and acquire just about any trait we want?

Well, that gives you a quick overview of some major areas of our life. Now let me tell you about my friends to show you examples of how some personal relationships work.

Todd is an Edibilist. His job relates to developing new strains of foods and nutrients. Because many of our citizens live to be 130 years old, world population has skyrocketed, and all the life-sustaining resources (food, energy, oxygen) are at a premium. Todd is married to Jerry (homosexual marriage is not uncommon among us, because people do not marry primarily to have babies). His recreational needs are met by Keri and his intellectual needs by Karen. Jerry is also Karen's sexual mate. As a matter of fact, they had a scare recently. No, not an unwanted pregnancy. That is no longer a problem. We have an enormous range of effective contraceptives (male contraceptives that prevent sperm development or immobilize sperm and female contraceptives are taken only once a year). Furthermore, someone who misuses reproductive privileges—by becoming pregnant without written approval from the Population and Parenthood

In *Demolition Man,* Sylvester Stallone plays a rogue cop put into cryogenic captivity and awakened in the year 2032. He is understandably perplexed by this strange new world, but when Sandra Bullock asks him to have sex and he realizes it involves a virtual reality helmet and no touching, he is outraged! What are the missing dimensions of sexuality in this scenario?

Screening Bureau—is liable to be sterilized by court order. As you can imagine, population control is a major concern, and reproductive control is therefore a governmental issue. At least we have no need for abortions!

No, Jerry and Karen's problem pertained not to pregnancy but to sexual dysfunction. We have eliminated the kinds of sexual dysfunction you were familiar with. Pills are available that eliminate inhibitions to sexual response. They can also lubricate vaginas, make penises erect, and even increase sexual desire. Jerry and Karen's problem arose when she popped a "desire" pill and Jerry did not want to take his. As yet it is not a matter of policy to add these chemicals to the water supply, as we do with K25W, to make people's sexual desires compatible. The controversy is ongoing as to whether controlling sexual desire should be left to individual discretion. At present the dysfunction of the sexual union, the term for our form of sexual dysfunction, is subject to the whims of the sexual partners. Opponents of adding desire chemicals to the water supply suggest that if one person drank a glass of water, felt a rush of desire, and could not find his or her partner, hysteria, frustration, violence, or a change of partner could ensue. Well, Jerry finally took his "desire" pill and the dysfunction was eliminated. It is my guess that if this incompatibility recurs, they will be looking for new mates.

Speaking of new mates, Keri is presently looking for one. Her old mate is raising her child and Keri would like a new mate with a drastically different endowment than the last. Keri's child was a dream come true, but only after some medical intervention. The Population and Parenthood Screening Bureau tested Keri both physiologically and psychologically to determine her qualifications for parenthood and approved her application. She chose John as the father because of his blond hair, blue eyes, impressive height, and high intelligence. Several months after conception, the amniotic fluid tests revealed that the fetus was male and had brown eyes and a cleft palate—not at all like John. You can imagine how quickly Keri ordered a genetic manipulation (GM)! When her daughter was born with blue eyes and devoid of any defects, Keri was elated and decided to keep her.

Keri's friend Josie is an interesting case. In fact, her situation would make a good riddle for you: How can someone be both the biological mother and the biological father of the same child? Well, Josie was not always Josie; she was once Joseph! Joseph was born a male and as a young adult deposited sperm in one of our neighborhood sperm banks. Joseph then decided that his maleness was unsuited to his disposition (unfortunately, his mother had not ordered a GM but had let nature take its course), and he had a sex-change operation. Joseph's male genitals were surgically removed and replaced with two ovaries, two fallopian tubes, a uterus, and a vagina. Once recuperated, Joseph, now Josie, used the deposited sperm to fertilize the ovum during her ovulation period. Hence when the baby was born, its mother and father were one and the same.

How important our genetic makeup may be in the future is explored in the film *Gattica.* Ethan Hawke plays a young man labeled an "invalid" because his parents decided not to undergo genetic engineering while he was in the womb. Barred from well-paying or respectable jobs, Ethan must take on the identity of a "valid" and risk his life to pursue his dreams. What possible effects do you think genetic engineering may have on sociocultural dimensions of sexuality?

But enough of unusual stories. Josie's situation is unique. Keri's case is more common. Perhaps she can soon choose another accurately genetically analyzed mate to make the kind of child she wants. If not, the GM people should be able to help, although, because they are in such demand, we encourage our citizens to do their genetic planning as much beforehand as possible (even though, as Keri's case indicates, this may result in something short of perfection).

By the way, the birthing process has changed much since your time. In 2099 women neither experience pain nor use unnatural chemicals during the delivery of babies. Instead we use endorphins. These substances were discovered more than a century ago but were not put to much use right away. Maybe you remember that endorphins are chemicals naturally produced by the human body that decrease pain and are related to relaxation. Since their discovery in the human brain, we have learned how to produce them synthetically. We administer these synthetic endorphins during childbirth (which, by the way, occurs in people's homes rather than in birthing factories—hospitals, I think you called them). Thus the birth of a baby involves nothing but joy—more joy than we have been able to develop with our medications.

For women too busy to carry the unborn for the 6 months required (we sped up the gestation process for convenience), surrogate mothers are available to do the job. A surrogate receives the fertilized ovum in her uterus and goes through the birth process as usual. The baby is then presented to the original parents and the surrogate is paid according to the birth weight and health of the baby (consequently surrogates do not smoke cigarettes, drink alcohol, or use drugs, and they monitor their nutrition carefully). Other options are available for parents of lesser financial means—animal uteruses serve as surrogate fetal development sites, as does the womb simulator (a machine in which a fetal development is maintained). These options allow the original mother to continue her usual routine unimpeded by pregnancy. However, the price she pays for this convenience is losing the joy of birthing. Moreover, a certain detachment often characterizes the mother–child relationship in such cases.

As you could probably guess, infertility does not exist today. We have so many ways of fertilizing ova and so many ways of organizing embryo and fetal development that our only problem is in restricting birth to a number that does not draw too heavily upon our society's resources.

Before you leave us, take with you the knowledge that sexual infections need not exist—it does not for us. As you can gather, I am sure, we are quite active sexually. And yet we managed to

eliminate sexually transmitted infections by the year 2047. We finally found the link among all the causative agents of STIs, including AIDS. We termed this link the *Syphgon factor*, after syphilis and gonorrhea, although a more appropriate name might be *basic biological matter–thwarting factor*. Soon after the link was found, a vaccine was developed to immunize people against STIs. Originally injected into the bloodstream, this chemical is now in pill form and is designed to dissolve under the tongue. Regarding cancer—breast, uterine, vaginal, testicular, and others—we have been able to teach people, using no medication, to control the flow of T lymphocytes to the cancerous area, thereby eliminating the cancer. Of course, to allow the technique to work, early detection is imperative; the required monthly screening (consisting only of passing through a sensitive doorway similar to that used by your generation to screen airline passengers) serves this purpose. Cancer has virtually been eliminated.

What? You want to know how we arrive at ethical and moral decisions? I am afraid you can only get into trouble asking these questions. Do you not remember the trouble they caused in your time? We leave ethical issues to our leaders. You ask why our leaders are scientists and not ethicists, philosophers, clergy, psychologists, or sociologists? Well, would you have nonscientists leading this highly technical society? We have to trust our leaders to do what is best for us.

To be honest, though, the questions you ask trouble me, too. For us, however, the opportunity to make some other choices has passed. Our society is what it is. It is, you might say, a snowball rolling downhill picking up more and more snow. But take a look at your time. Are not the seeds of our society already planted? Perhaps you still have the chance to nurture the humanizing aspects of your society and to prevent its dehumanizing aspects from developing and taking over your future.

■ Commentary

Interestingly, Greenberg and Bruess wrote the scenario you just read in the mid-1980s to promote discussion about the future and dimensions of sexuality (Greenberg & Bruess, 1986). As we reread this in preparation for its inclusion in this book, it struck us just how on target our predictions were. It made us think that we should be advising people on which stocks to invest in. Let us take a closer look at the future we projected two decades ago, at the characteristics of that future that already have come to pass and those that have not.

Social Dimensions

We described the year 2099 as one in which fewer people left their home and family to travel to work. Rather, they worked from home with the help of new technologies. We do not have to wait for 2099 for that to occur; it is already happening today. With the advent of the computer, paging systems, cell phones, and telecommunications capabilities, more people are "telecommuting" than ever before. As in the scenario, more and more people are shopping, banking, and communicating from home. If you want a book, you need only go to the web site of Amazon.com or Barnes and Noble. If you want to switch money from one bank account to another, you can hit a few keys on your home computer or a few numbers on your telephone and the transfer is completed. And, if you want to communicate with someone, you can do so by email, instant messaging, or iPhones and Blackberrys. The result should be more time for the family and for people about whom we care. However, this does not seem to be a social benefit we have as yet derived from technological advances. Too many people spend too much time at their computers, checking out Internet sites, receiving and sending email messages, or playing computer games.

Physical Dimensions

We also guessed right about the ability of physicians to use computers to treat patients better. Today, physicians can call on experts from afar, using computers and telecommunications to read X rays, computed tomography (CT) scans, and magnetic resonance imaging (MRI) results and make a diagnosis that a local physician may be incapable of making. Robots are even conducting surgeries managed from afar. This technology has tremendous potential for the diagnosis and treatment of sexually transmitted infections and other sexual illnesses.

In 2099, sexual dysfunction is not one of those matters about which citizens are concerned; they have a "desire pill." In a way, this is not much different from today's Viagra and other drugs that treat sexual dysfunctions. In addition, microsurgical techniques are available to alleviate some sexual dysfunctional problems.

However, in 2099 the reason the "desire pill" is not added to the water supply is that a person who took a drink and experienced sexual desire might form a "sexual union" with a stranger who happened to be nearby and available. Today, we have a different variable serving as a barrier to "haphazard" sexual unions: HIV and AIDS. The fear of con-

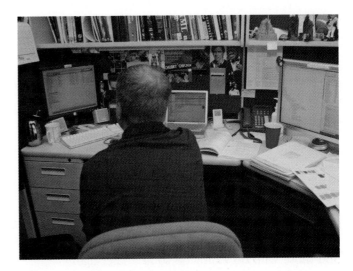

Many people telecommute, working from their homes with new technology. With decreased human contact, will our society change? For the better or for the worse?

tracting HIV has led to a decrease in casual sex and an increase in condom use when sexual activity does take place. Still, research to develop an HIV and AIDS vaccine, if successful, might once again lead to a more cavalier attitude toward sex and a reemergence of the sexually free attitude of the 1960s. And yet, many Americans and others around the world are not waiting for a vaccine. Too many refuse to adopt responsible sexual behavior and engage in safer-sex practices.

Marital Dimensions

In the year 2099, there is a new form of marriage—repeating monogamous marriage (RMM). Today, with the divorce and remarriage rates as they are, we have a de facto RMM system. We have even developed a name for the convoluted family structure possible when remarriage occurs (possibly several times

Blended families, as well as the large number of international adoptions, are having a dramatic effect on the families in the 21st century.

for the same parent): *blended families*. However, we have not institutionalized polygamy as was described in the scenario. We still believe in the fidelity of one marital partner to the other, although some might argue that the prevalence of extramarital sex provides evidence of a trend in the opposite direction. And today, as in the scenario, it is common for people to live together and not be married to each other. Young couples move in together to determine whether a long-term relationship is feasible for them. Gays live together as unmarried, in the eyes of the law at least, because legislators in many states have proscribed gay marriage. And elders cohabit because our society reinforces that arrangement through our tax codes and social welfare programs. Many Americans choose to remain unmarried, and those who do marry do so at a later age.

Gender Dimensions

We have discussed gender dimensions of sexuality throughout this book, and in 2099 attention is paid to this issue as well: Gender equality is a reality. In present-day society we have made great strides toward gender equality. It is no longer unusual for a female to be a physician or a lawyer. It is no longer unusual for a male to assume such household chores as cooking, cleaning, and child rearing. And yet, women are still paid less than men even when they do the same job; also, although men do more household chores when they and their spouses work full-time outside the home, women still assume a disproportionate share. And female genital mutilation is still practiced in many parts of the world. We have yet to discover a way to remedy the disparity in the way we treat our females and males in a manner that is best for women, men, children, and the rest of society, as they did in 2099 with the magical K25W. Still, we are headed in the right direction; the trend is toward greater gender equality and fairness. We hope that we will not have to wait until 2099 to see their full development.

Pregnancy and Childbearing Dimensions

In 2099, there are no unintended pregnancies. That is certainly not where we are today. More than half of all pregnancies in the United States are unintended, and our teenage pregnancy rate is one of the highest among developed countries. As in 2099, we have a wide range of effective contraceptives. The difference is that too few Americans use them or use them irregularly or incorrectly. That leads to a greater number of unwanted births, abortions, and adoptions than would otherwise be the case.

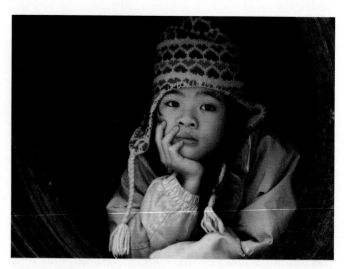

Some countries value male babies for their ability to support the family. This has resulted in infanticide in the form of female babies being aborted. How do you imagine females feel in such societies?

Perhaps our descendants in 2099 have the right idea with the Population and Parenthood Screening Bureau. Today, we have too many children who are abused and neglected. We have too many children who are taken from their birth parents and placed in foster care with the intent of having them adopted, although many never do get a stable family and remain in the foster care system until they become of emancipated age. Perhaps we need to pay as much attention to enhancing parenting skills as our descendants do in 2099.

One area in which we do not have to wait for 2099 is that of genetic manipulation. With medical scientific advances, it is possible to perform surgery on fetuses in the womb to remedy structural abnormalities. Soon we will be able to apply different genes to influence eye color, intelligence, or other traits. Researchers have already isolated stem cells from embryonic tissue that can eventually be used to grow human replacement parts for transplantation. People wonder, if Dolly the sheep has been cloned, will humans eventually be cloned? The ethical implications of rapidly developing scientific advances have outstripped our society's ability to develop laws that will assure that technology will be used to enhance our culture rather than diminish it.

Want a boy baby? No need to engage in abortion or infanticide, as in some countries. Just use sperm-separation techniques to improve the odds. No, this is not part of the 2099 scenario. This is occurring today. Want a child who is likely to be an athlete or a musician? Just be selective at the sperm bank, careful to choose sperm from a male who has the characteristics you want for your child. No, this is not part of the 2099 scenario. This is occurring today. The future is here!

■ Tonow

As the 21st-century narrator of our story implies, being aware of present trends and considering what personal and social agreements about sexuality may be like in the future can be fun, but it can also be a responsibility.

As our society evolves, we must not lose sight of our heritage and what we have learned from it. To that knowledge we must add new information—information filtered through ethical and moral awareness and values. As citizens of today and of the future, we can ill afford to shirk our responsibility to help shape our sexual society.

The physician Bernie Siegel works with cancer patients—"cancer survivors," he calls them. Knowing they probably have little time left to live, he helps them live "well" during the time left to them. This is a lesson that all of us could profit by learning. Siegel is fond of speaking of today, tomorrow, and "tonow." Using Siegel's terminology, many sexual futuristic issues are actually occurring tonow.

A woman is judged guilty of a criminal act and is considered to be a poor mother, so a judge prevents her from having other children. He offers her a choice of going to jail or having a contraceptive implant (Norplant) surgically placed on her arm. Tonow.

A society experiments on itself. Its children grow up with the majority of their mothers working full-time outside the home. In many cases, a male figure is absent from the home because of desertion, death, or divorce. What will the effects be? Tonow.

A country changes dramatically. What were once "minorities," when grouped together, become the majority. In many areas of the United States, Hispanic, Asian American, and African American populations have increased in numbers and in percentage of population. What will be the effects on sexuality? On attitudes toward sexual issues? On views of censorship, morality, abortion, and family life? Many believe the country will profit from this diversity. Will it? Tonow.

As people wrestle with a threat to their very lives, AIDS stalks all segments of the population. During the sexual revolution individuals fought for the right of free sexual expression; however, in this day there can be heavy consequences for such behavior. Will behavior change? How many deaths will occur before that happens? Will relationships ever be the same? Tonow.

It is our hope that this book helps to prepare you for your sexual tonow and your sexual tomorrow. Most likely your instructor hopes your sexuality course will have the same effect. No one can predict the future, but we can anticipate trends and prepare for them. How will you prepare? When will you start?

Discussion Questions

1. Vaccines were one of the greatest wonders of the 20th century and eradicated several major diseases. However, a small percentage of people contract the disease through the vaccine and are left disabled or dead. Would you be willing to take such a risk to be vaccinated for STIs or HIV? Would you subject your infant children to such vaccines to protect their future? Explain why or why not.

2. Over the time you have taken this course, you have undoubtedly heard news stories about current research that could affect your future sexuality. Relate some of the more interesting research projects, and discuss whether they are feasible, given the biological, psychological, and sociocultural dimensions of sexuality.

Application Questions

Reread the chapter-opening scenario and answer the following questions.

1. Would you prefer to live in your current world or in the world of 2099 described in the scenario? Explain your answer.

2. Allowing government control over subliminal messages (and lacing the drinking water with K25W) would give the government complete control of the population. How could government be regulated so that only positive messages (for example, gender equality) would be conveyed? What if the government decided to convey messages like "Don't vote for the opposing political party"—or worse?

Critical Thinking Questions

1. As our society continues to accept the ideal of diversity, we seem less and less likely to unify as a nation on any issue—especially sex! Consider the use of stem cells in the United States. Which sociocultural groups are likely to be in favor of their use? Which groups would be against it? Under which circumstances do you think the federal government would approve the use of embryonic stem cells?

2. Aldous Huxley, in *Brave New World,* portrayed a government that kept control of its people by granting them unrestrained sexual pleasures. George Orwell, in *1984,* took the opposite position: The government keeps control by discouraging sexual contact among spouses and forbidding it among nonmarried people. Compare and contrast these methods given what you know about the many dimensions of human sexuality.

Critical Thinking Case

What Is "Quality of Life"?

The year 2099 seems to have some attractive features. Diseases are curable. Computers do a lot of the work, and the remainder can often be done at home. Cars do not pollute air. People live longer and establish numerous relationships—each designed to meet a specific need.

And yet some of the citizens in the year 2099 seem disenchanted. Their marriages often do not last very long. They cannot have children whenever they want. They cannot engage in competitive sports. Their mind is manipulated as a result of K25W in their water supply.

Given these and the other conditions we have described, would you want to live in the year 2099? Why or why not?

What in life is important to you aside from *how long you live?*

What is present and what is absent in 2099 that you need to be happy sexually?

Exploring Personal Dimensions

The form below might be used in our fictional story set in 2099. In our story, those individuals wishing to conceive may have to answer questions very much like those in the form. Their answers determine whether they are given permission to have a child, as well as specifying the gender and appearance of the child. As you read through this form, consider whether it is ethical to ask such questions of potential parents. What would be the effects on the sociocultural dimensions of sexuality of applying such rules to parenting?

POPULATION AND PARENTHOOD SCREENING BUREAU

Parenthood Application

Name: _____
Mate's Name: _____
Address: _____
Computer Access Number: _____
Answer all of the following questions:

1. How long have you been mating? _____

2. List all illnesses/diseases experienced within the last year by the female mate: _____
_____
_____

3. List all illnesses/diseases experienced within the last year by the male mate: _____
_____
_____

4. On the breakup of your relationship, what do you plan for your child?
_____
_____
_____
_____

5. What time is best for you to be interviewed by our psychological team?
_____
_____
_____
_____

6. List those traits you want ensured in your child:
   a. Sex: _____
   b. Eye color: _____
   c. Hair color: _____
   d. Intelligence quotient: _____
   e. Height: _____
   f. Special abilities (for example, athletic, mathematical, artistic):
   _____
   _____

7. Which method of birth control do you employ? _____

8. Do you have any other children? _____

9. Which method of birthing do you plan? _____

10. How will your child be cared for during the workday? _____
_____
_____

11. List any parenting training you and your mate have received: _____
_____
_____

12. Will you agree to amniotic fluid screening during the pregnancy?
_____
_____

Special Note: Be aware that approval will not be granted to individuals who already have a child, who are untrained for parenthood, who do not agree to amniotic fluid screening, who have not planned for the daily care of their child-to-be, or who have not prepared for the breakup of their relationship.

References

101 ways to combat domestic violence. Feminists Against Violence Network, 2003. Available: www.geocities.com/Heartland/Meadows/7905/101.htm.

A woman's right to sue. *The Economist, 376, 8442* (September 3, 2005), 38–39.

Aamodt, A. Culture, in *Culture child-bearing health professionals*, Clark, A., ed. Philadelphia: F. A. Davis, 1978.

AARP. *American Association of Retired Persons/Modern Maturity sexuality study.* Washington, DC: Author, 1999.

Abbey, A., Buck, P.O., Zawacki, T., & Saenz, C. Alcohol's effects on perceptions of a potential date rape. *Journal of Studies on Alcohol, 64, no. 5* (September 2003), 668–677.

About SSSS: Mission statement: A special note about Sexual Harassment. Society for the Scientific Study of Sexuality (June 3, 2005). Available: http://www.sexscience.org.

About the Prison Rape Elimination Act of 2003. National Institute of Justice, 2007. Available: http://www.ojp.usdoj.gov/nij/topics/corrections/prison-rape/prea.htm.

Acevedo, B. P., & Aron, A. Does a long-term relationship kill romantic love? *Review of General Psychology, 13, 1* (2009), 59–65.

Achenbach, J. Splice of life. *The Washington Post Magazine* (November 29, 1998), 12–19, 27–30.

ACLU sues HHS over religious restrictions on funds for programs serving sex trafficking victims. *Daily Women's Health Report* (January 13, 2009). National Partnership for Women and Families. Available: http://nationalpartnership.org/.

ACOG. *Exercise during pregnancy.* Washington, DC: American College of Obstetricians and Gynecologists, 2003.

Adam, M. B., McGuire, J. K., Walsh, M., Basta, J., & LeCroy, C. Acculturation as a predictor of the onset of sexual intercourse among Hispanic and white teens. *Archives of Pediatric Adolescent Medicine, 159, no. 3* (March 2005), 261–265.

Adams, D. B., Gold, A. R., & Burt, A. D. Rise in female-initiated sexual activity at ovulation and suppression by oral contraceptives. *New England Journal of Medicine, 299* (1978), 1145–1150.

Addiego, F., Belzer, E., Perry, J., & Whipple, B. Female ejaculation: A case study. *Journal of Sex Research, 17* (1981), 13–21.

Adopting.org. *State regulations: Non-identifying & identifying information: Access to adoption records*, 2009. Available: http://www.adopting.org/adoptions/state-regulations-non-identifying-identifying-information-access-to-adoption-records-2.html.

Adult survivors of sex abuse in crisis. *Behavior Today, 21* (1990), 1–3.

Age at first menstruation continues to decline, especially among African Americans, study says. *Kaiser Daily Reproductive Health Report* (October 8, 2002). Available: www.kaisernetwork.org/daily reports.

Agency for Healthcare Research and Quality. U.S. preventive task force calls for chlamydia and lipid screening and issues two other recommendations. *Research Activities, no. 248* (2001), 23–24.

Agustin, L. Sex and the limits of enlightenment: The irrationality of legal regimes to control prostitution. *Sexuality Research & Social Policy, 5, 4* (December 2008), 73–85.

AIDS risk rising in older people. *Consumer Reports on Health, 15, no. 1* (January 2003), 7.

AIDS virus gets new name amid feuding, *Medical World News, 27* (1986), 14–15.

Airing it out. *Time, 160, no. 19* (November 4, 2002), 84.

Albert, Bill. *With one voice 2004: America's adults and teens sound off about teen pregnancy.* Washington, D.C.: National Campaign to Prevent Teen Pregnancy, December 2004.

Alcohol consumption among women who are pregnant or who might become pregnant—United States, 2002. *Morbidity and Mortality Weekly Report, 53* (2004), 1178–1181.

Aldrich, T., Becker, D., Garcia, S. G., & Lara, D. Mexican physicians' knowledge and attitudes about the human papillomavirus and cervical cancer: A national survey. *Sexually Transmitted Infections 81, no. 2* (2005), 135–141.

Altman, C. Gay and lesbian seniors: Unique challenges of coming out in later life, *SIECUS Report, 27, no. 3* (February/March 1999), 14–17.

Al Sabbah, H., Vereecken, C., Elgar, F. J., Nansel, T., Aasvee, K., Abdeen, Z., Ojaia, K., Ahiuwalia, N., & Maes, L. Body weight dissatisfaction and communication with parents among adolescents in 24 countries: International cross-sectional survey. *BMC Public Health, 9, 1* (February 6, 2009), 52.

Alzate, H., & Hoch, Z. The G spot and female ejaculation: A current appraisal. *Journal of Sex and Marital Therapy, 12* (1986), 211–220.

Alzate, H., & Londono, M. Vaginal erotic sensitivity. *Journal of Sex and Marital Therapy, 10* (1984), 49–56.

American Academy of Family Physicians. PMS: What you can do to ease your symptoms. *Family Doctor Org,* 2004. Available: http://familydoctor.org/141.xml?printxml.

American Academy of Pediatrics. *AAP releases revised breastfeeding recommendations* (2005). Available: http://www.aap.org/advocacy/releasers/feb05breastfeeding.htm.

American Academy of Pediatrics. Circumcision policy statement. *Pediatrics, 103* (1999), 686–693.

American Academy of Pediatrics. Pediatricians needed to make national breastfeeding awareness campaign successful. *Breastfeeding: Best for baby and mother: Section on breastfeeding* (2004), 1. Available: http://www.aap.org/advocacy/bf/8-27newsletter.pdf.

American Cancer Society. *American Cancer Society updates prostate cancer screening guidelines,* June 12, 1997.

American Cancer Society. *Breast cancer screening: The American Cancer Society and Living Well, October module,* 2007a.

American Cancer Society. *Cancer facts & figures 2008,* 2008a.

American Cancer Society. *Detailed guide: Cervical cancer—what are the key statistics?,* 2008b. Available: http://www.cancer.org/docroot/CRI/content/CRI_2_4_1X_What_are_the_key_statistics_for_cervical_cancer_8.asp.

American Cancer Society. *Mammogram rates dropping nation-wide: Experts worry about effect on breast cancer detection,* 2007b. Available: http://www.cancer.org/docroot/NWS/content/NWS_1_1x_Mammogram_Rates_Dropping_Nation-Wide.asp.

American College Health Association. *American College Health Association—National College Health Assessment: Reference group executive summary.* Baltimore, MD: Author, 2006.

American College Health Association. *American College Health Association—National College Health Assessment II: Reference group data report, fall 2008.* Baltimore, MD: Author, 2009, 8.

American College Health Association. National College Health Assessment. *Journal of American College Health, 56, 5* (March/April 2008), 469–479.

American College of Obstetricians and Gynecologists. *Dysmenorrhea.* San Francisco: Medem, 2006. Available: http://www.medem.com/medlib/article/ZZZH7MGV77C.

American College of Obstetricians and Gynecologists (ACOG). Private practice physicians perform episiotomy at higher rate than residents and hospital faculty. *ACOG News Release* (December 31, 2003). Available: http://www.acog.org/from_home/publications/press_releases/nr12-31-03.cfm

American fact finder. U.S. Bureau of the Census, 2009. Available: http://factfinder.census.gov/.

American Heart Association. *Sexual Activity and Heart Disease or Stroke,* 2009. Available: http://www.americanheart.org/presenter.jhtml?identifier=4714.

American Pregnancy Association. *Alcohol and pregnancy: What you should know,* 2008. Available: http://www.americanpregnancy.org/pregnancyhealth/alcohol.html.

American Pregnancy Association. *Ectopic pregnancy.* 2006. Available: http://www.americanpregnancy.org/pregnancycomplications/ectopicpregnancy.html.

American Psychiatric Association. *Diagnostic and Statistical Manual of Mental Disorders, Fourth Edition, Text Revision.* Washington, DC: American Psychiatric Association, 2000.

American Psychiatric Association. *Diagnostic and statistical manual of mental disorders.* Washington, DC: Author, 2005.

American Psychiatric Association. Statement: Diagnostic criteria for pedophilia (June 17, 2003).

American Psychological Association. *Report of the APA Taskforce on the Sexualization of Girls.* Washington, DC: Author, 2007.

American Psychological Association. Resolution on transgender, gender identity, and gender expression non-discrimination, August 2008. Available: http://www.apa.org/pi/lgbc/policy/transgender.pdf.

American Public Health Association. Condoms proven effective against HIV transmission. *The Nation's Health* (September 2001), 4.

American Society for Aesthetic Plastic Surgery. Quick facts, 2009. Available: http://www.surgery.org/download/2007QFacts.pdf.

American Society of Plastic Surgeons. Press kit, 2009. Available: http://www.plasticsurgery.org/media/Press_Releases/Plastic_Surgery_ProceduresMaintain_Steady_Growth_in_2007.html.

American Urological Association. Keep the heart strong by minding erectile health. Press release (February 1, 2005a).

American Urological Association. *Premature ejaculation: Guide on the pharmacologic management of premature ejaculation.* Linthicum, MD: Author, 2005b.

Ames, P. Belgian cabinet OKs gay marriages. *The Birmingham News* (June 24, 2001), 11A.

An arrangement of marriages. *Psychology Today, 26* (January/February 1993), 22.

An open letter to religious leaders on marriage equality. Religious Institute on Sexual Morality, Justice, and Healing 2004. Available: http://www.religiousinstitute.org.

Andersen, M. *Thinking about women: Sociological perspectives on sex and gender.* Boston: Allyn and Bacon, 2009, 54.

Andriole, G. L., et al. Mortality results from a randomized prostate-cancer screening trial. *New England Journal of Medicine, 360* (2009), 1310–1319.

Annon, J. S. *The behavioral treatment of sexual problems: Brief therapy.* New York: Harper & Row, 1976.

Antibiotic-resistant strains of *Neisseria gonorrheae:* Policy guidelines for detection, management and control. *MMWR Supplement 36* (1987), 1S–18S.

Apfelbaum, B. Why we should not accept sexual fantasies, in *Expanding the boundaries of sex therapy.* Berkeley, CA: Berkeley Sex Therapy Group, 1980.

Arafat, I., & Cotton, W. L. Masturbation practices of males and females. *Journal of Sex Research, 10* (1974), 293–307.

Archibald, G. Pro-gay group seeks support at PTA convention. *The Washington Times* (June 28, 2005).

Aries, P., & Bejin, A. *Western sexuality.* New York: Basil Blackwell, 1985.

Armour, Stephanie. When an employee switches gender, what's a company to do? *USA Today* (June 10, 2005), 1B–2B.

Aron, A., Fisher, H. A., Mashek, D. J., Strong, G., Li, H., & Brown, L. L. Reward, motivation and emotion systems associated with early-stage intense romantic love. *Journal of Neurophysiology, 94* (May 31, 2005), 327–337.

Arreola, S., Neilands, T., Pollack, L., Paul, J., & Datania, J. Childhood sexual experiences and adult health sequelae among gay and bisexual men: Defining childhood sexual abuse. *Journal of Sex Research, 45, 3* (July 2008), 246–252.

Artel, R., & W iswell, R. A. Exercise prescription in pregnancy, in *Exercise in pregnancy,* Artel, R., & Wiswell, R. A., eds. Baltimore: Williams & Wilkins, 1986, 225–228.

ASPSH. *Definitions of sexual health,* 2009. Available: http://aspsh.ca/definitions_of_sexual_health.

Association of Reproductive Health Specialists. Female sexual aversion disorder. *Clinical Proceedings,* 2005. Available: http://www.arhp.org/healthcareproviders/cme/onlinecme/NYNCP/aversion.cfm.

Association for Voluntary Sterilization. Estimate of the number of sterilizations performed in the United States, mimeo, December 1982.

Atkins, D. C., Baucom, D. H., & Jacobson, N. S. Understanding infidelity: Correlates in a national random sample. *Journal of Family Psychology, 15* (2001), 735–749.

Australian Herpes Management Forum. *Reducing the sexual transmission of genital herpes.* Westmead, Australia: Author, 2007. Available: http://www.ahmf.com.au/health_professionals/guidelines/reducing_gh_transmission.htm.

Avellar, S. The economic consequences of the dissolution of cohabiting unions. *Journal of Marriage and Family 67, no. 2* (May 2005), 315–327.

Avis, N. E., Zhao, X., Johannes, C. B., Ory, M., Brockwell, S., & Greendale, G. A. Correlates of sexual function among multi-ethnic middle-aged women: Results from the Study of Women's Health Across the Nation (SWAN). *Menopause, 12* (2005), 385–398.

Babwin, Don. Dove ads featuring "real women" meant to be an inspiration. *The Birmingham News* (August 3, 2005), 1G, 5G.

BabyCenter. *Great Pregnancy Exercise: Walking,* 2006. Available: http://www.babycenter.com/0_great-pregnancy-exercise-walking_7863.bc.

Bachu, A., & O'Connell, M. *Fertility of American women: June 2000.* Current Population Reports, P20-543RV. Washington, DC: U.S. Census Bureau, 2001.

Backman, T., Raumaro, I., Huhtala, S., & Koskenvuo. Pregnancy during the use of levonorgestrel intrauterine system. *American Journal of Obstetrics and Gynecology, 190* (2004), 50–54.

Bacon, C. G., Mittleman, M. A., Kawachi, I., et al. Sexual function in men older than 50 years of age: Results from the Health Professionals Follow-Up Study. *Annals of Internal Medicine, 139* (2003), 161–168.

Bailey, H. M., & Pillard, R. C., A genetic study of male sexual orientation. *Archives of General Psychiatry, 48* (1991), 1089–1086.

Bailey, J. M., Dunne, M. P., & Martin, N. G. Genetic and environmental influences on sexual orientation and its correlates in an Australian twin sample. *Journal of Personality & Social Psychology, 78, no. 3* (2000), 524–536.

Ballagh, S. A., & Heyl, A. Communicating with women about menstrual cycle symptoms. *Journal of Reproductive Medicine, 53* (2008), 837–846.

Bancroft, J., Herbenick, D., & Reynolds, M. Masturbation as a marker of sexual development, in *Sexual Development in Childhood,* J. Bancroft, ed. Bloomington, IN: Indiana University Press (2003), 438.

Bancroft, J., Janssen, E., Carnes, L., Goodrich, D., Strong, D., & Long, J. S. Sexual activity and risk taking in young heterosexual men: The relevance of sexual arousability, mood, and sensation seeking. *Journal of Sex Research 41, no. 2* (May 2004), 181–192.

Bancroft, J. & Vukadinovic, Z. Sexual addiction, sexual compulsivity, sexual impulsivity, or what? Toward a theoretical model. *Journal of Sex Research, 42, no. 3* (Aug. 2004), 225–234.

Banerjee, N. Lutherans recommend tolerance on gay policy. *The New York Times* (January 14, 2005).

Bangkok Post profiles group providing services for male commercial sex workers. *Kaiser Daily HIV/AIDS Report* (January 5, 2005). Available: http://www.kaisernetwork.org.

Banning, A. Mother–son incest: Confronting a prejudice. *Child Abuse and Neglect, 13* (1989), 563–570.

Barak, A. Sexual harassment on the Internet. *Social Science Computer Review 23, no. 1* (Spring 2005), 77–92.

Barbach, L. *For each other: Sharing sexual intimacy*. New York: New American Library, 2001.

Barbach, L. G. *For yourself: The fulfillment of female sexuality*. New York: Signet, 2000.

Barbach, L. G. *Women discover orgasm: A therapist's guide to a New Testament approach*. New York: Free Press, 1980.

Barbaro, M. In reversal, Wal-Mart will sell contraceptive. *The New York Times* (2006). Available: http://www.nytimes.com/2006/03/04/business/04walmart.html?_r=2&scp=1&sq=walmart%202006%20plan%20b&st=cse.

Barber, K. R., et al. Differences between African American and Caucasian men participating in a community-based prostate cancer screening program. *Journal of Community Health, 23* (1998), 441–451.

Bardes, B. A., Shelley II, M. C., & Schmidt, S. W. *American government and politics today: The essentials*. Belmont, CA: West/Wadsworth, 1998.

Barker, O. Victoria's Secret tones down suggestive displays. *USA Today* (October 10, 2005), p. 1D.

Barlett C. P., & Harris, R. J. The impact of body emphasizing video games on body image concerns in men and women. *Sex Roles, 59, 7–8* (October 2008), 586–601.

Barnard, N. D., Scialli, A. R., Hurlock, D., & Bertron, P. Diet and sex-hormone binding globulin, dysmenorrhea, and premenstrual symptoms. *Obstetrics and Gynecology, 95* (2000), 245–250.

Barnes, S. Individuals who don't follow the standard script of sex and romance find they are not alone. *Albany Times Union* (May 29, 2005), G1.

Baron, R. A. *Psychology*, 4th ed. Needham Heights, MA: Allyn & Bacon, 1998.

Barone, M. A., Johnson, C. H., et al. Characteristics of men receiving vasectomies in the United States, 1998–1999. *Perspectives on Sexual and Reproductive Health, 36, no. 1*, (January/February 2004), 27–33.

Bartley, N. The return of romance: Antidote to dreary reality of the 90s. *Watertown (NY) Daily Times* (February 13, 1994), 7.

Basile, K. C. Attitudes toward wife rape: Effects of social background and victim status. *Violence and Victims, 17, no. 3* (June 2002a), 341–354.

Basile, K. C. Prevalence of wife rape and other intimate partner sexual coercion in a nationally representative sample of women. *Violence and Victims 17, no. 5* (October 2002b), 511–524.

Basow, S. A., & Rubenfeld, K. "Troubles talk": Effects of gender and gender-typing. *Sex Roles, 48* (2003), 183–187.

Basson, R. The female sexual response: A different model. *Journal of Marital Therapy, 26* (2000), 51–65.

Basson, R. Sexual desire and arousal disorders in women. *New England Journal of Medicine, 354* (2006), 1497–1506.

Bates, G. On the nature of the hot flash. *Clinical Obstetrics and Gynecology, 24* (1981), 231–241.

Bauer, H. M., Ting, I., Greer, C. E., et al. Genital human papillomavirus infection in female university students as determined by a PCR-based method. *Journal of the American Medical Association, 265* (1991), 472–477.

Baumeister, R. F. The enigmatic appeal of sexual masochism: Why people desire pain, bondage, and humiliation in sex. *Journal of Social and Clinical Psychology, 16, no. 2* (1997), 133–150.

Baumeister, R., & Tice, D. *The social dimension of sex*. Boston: Allyn and Bacon, 2000.

Baxter, N. Preventive health care, 2001 update: Should women be routinely taught breast self-examination to screen for breast cancer? *Canadian Medical Association Journal, 164, no.13* (2001), 1837–1846.

Beal, C. R. *Boys and girls: The development of gender roles*. New York: McGraw-Hill, 1994.

Bechtel, L. S., Westerfield, C., & Eddy, J.-M. Autoerotic fatalities: Implications for health educators. *Health Education, 21* (1990), 38–40.

Beckman, N., Waern, M., Gustafson, D., & Skoog, I. Secular trends in self reported sexual activity and satisfaction in Swedish 70 year olds: Cross sectional survey of four populations, 1971–2001. *British Medical Journal, 337* (2008), a279.

Being a dad comes naturally: Hormone levels in new fathers versus men who are not fathers, *Science News* (July 8, 2000). Available: http://findarticles.com/p/articles/mi_m1200/is_2_158/ai_65132286/?tag=content;col1.

Beetz, A. M. Bestiality/zoophilia: A scarcely investigated phenomenon between crime, paraphilia, and love. *Journal of Forensic Psychology Practice, 4, no. 2* (2004), 1–36.

Bell, A. P., & Weinberg, M. S. *Homosexualities: A study of diversity among men and women*. New York: Simon & Schuster, 1978.

Bell, A. P., Weinberg, M. S., & Hammersmith, S. K. *Sexual preference: Its development in men and women*. Bloomington: Indiana University Press, 1981.

Bell, R. R. *Premarital sex in a changing society*. Englewood Cliffs, NJ: Prentice-Hall, 1966.

Belzer, E. G. Orgasmic expulsions of women: A review and heuristic inquiry. *Journal of Sex Research, 17* (1981), 1–12.

Belzer, E. G., Whipple, B., & Moger, W. On female ejaculation. *Journal of Sex Research, 20* (1984), 403–406.

Bem, S. L. Androgyny versus the tight little lives of women and chesty men. *Psychology Today* (September 1975), 58–62.

Benedetti, W. The naked truth: Junk and jubblies sell games. *MSNBC.com*, February 27, 2009. Available: http://www.msnbc.msn.com/id/29417313/.

Bergen, R. K. Marital rape: New research and directions. National Online Resource Center on Violence Against Women, 2009. Available: www.vawnet.org.

Bergen, R. K. The reality of wife rape: Women's experiences of sexual violence in marriage, in *Issues in intimate violence*, Bergen, R. K., ed. Thousand Oaks, CA: Sage, 1998.

Bergkvist, L., Adami, H. O., Persson, J., Hoover, R., & Schairer, C. The risk of breast cancer after estrogen and estrogen-progestin replacement. *New England Journal of Medicine, 321* (1989), 293.

Berk, L. E. *Exploring lifespan development*. Boston: Allyn and Bacom, 2008, 212.

Berkowitz, J. L., et al. Estrogen replacement therapy and fibrocystic disease in postmenopausal women. *American Journal of Epidemiology, 121* (1985), 238–245.

Berney, K. Hypoactive sexual desire disorder: "I'm not in the mood." *Discovery Health*, 2009. Available: http://health.discovery.com/centers/sex/articles/hypoactive.html.

Bernstein, A. C. *Flight of the stork*. Indiana: Perspectives Press, 1994.

Bestiality, Go ask Alice. Columbia University (2003). [Online]. Available: www.goaskalice.columbia.edu/0707.html.

Beware of penis-enlargement scams. MayoClinic.com (May 24, 2005). Available: http://www.mayoclinic.com/.

Bhutta, M. F. Sex and the nose: Human pheromonal response. *Journal of the Royal Society of Medicine, 100* (2007), 268–274.

Bieber, I., Dain, H., Dince, P., Drellich, M., Grand, H., Gundlach, R., Kremer, M., Rifkin, A., Wilbur, C., & Bieber, T. *Homosexuality: A psychoanalytic perspective*. New York: Basic Books, 1962.

Bilger, B. Muscle dysmorphia syndrome. *The Sciences, 38* (January/February 1998), 10.

Billowitz, M., & Kukke, S. Doing gender the "rights" way. *SIECUS Report, 32, no. 3* (Summer 2004), 5–10.

Birchard, K. Sex, please, we're british: Many students strip to pay bills, BBC reports. *Chronicle of Higher Education*, Today's News (May 2, 2001). Available: http://chronicle.com/daily/2001/05/2001050205n.htm

Birth control. *Encyclopaedia Britannica*, 2009. Available: http://www.britannica.com/EBchecked/topic/66704/birth-control.

Bivona, J., & Critelli, J. The nature of women's rape fantasies: An analysis of prevalence, frequency, and contents. *Journal of Sex Research, 45* (2008), 1–13.

Black, J., & Underwood, J. Young, female, and gay: Lesbian students and the school environment. *Professional School Counseling, 1, no. 3* (February 1998), 15–20.

Black journalists criticize media coverage of "down low" phenomenon, say articles wrongly link behavior to blacks, increase in AIDS cases. *Kaiser Daily HIV/AIDS Report*, August 9, 2005. Available: http://www.kaisernetwork.org

Bleakley, A., Hennessy, M., & Fishbein, M. Public opinion on sex education in US schools. *Archives of Pediatrics and Adolescent Medicine, 160* (November 2006), 1151–1156.

Blond, A. Impacts of exposure to images of ideal bodies on male body dissatisfaction: A review. *Body Image, 5, 3* (September 2008), 244–250.

Blonna, R., & Levitan, J. *Healthy sexuality.* Belmont, CA: Thompson Wadsworth, 2006. (427–b)

Blood supply grows safer, *FDA Consumer, 24* (1990), 5.

Blumstein, P., & Schwartz, P. *American couples.* New York: William Morrow, 1983.

Blumstein, P., & Schwartz, P. Intimate relationships and the creation of sexuality. In *Homosexuality/heterosexuality: Concepts of sexual orientation,* McWhirter, D. P., Sanders, S. A., & Reinisch, J. M., eds. New York: Oxford Press, 1990, pp. 307–320.

Bodo, C. Addicted to love. National Sexuality Resource Center, 2008. Available: http://nsrc.sfsu.edu/print/2835.

Body image. Planned Parenthood, 2009. Available: http://www.plannedparenthood.org/health-topics/body-image-23374.htm.

Boghosian, H. Gauntlet of change. National Lawyers Guild Foundation. *Guild Notes, 30, no. 2* (summer, 2005), 1–14.

The boomer sandwich. *Modern Maturity, 44w, no. 5* (September/October 2001), 94.

Bontempi, J. B., Mugno, R., Bulmer, S. M., Danvers, K., & Vancour, M. L. Exploring gender differences in the relationship between HIV/STD testing and condom use among undergraduate college students. *American Journal of Health Education, 40, 2* (March/April 2009), 97–105.

Boonstra, H. Condoms, contraceptives and Nonoxynol-9: Complex issues obscured by ideology. *Guttmacher Report on Public Policy, 8, no. 2,* (May 2005). Available: http://www.guttmacher.org/pubs/tgr/08/2/gr080204.html.

Boonstra, H. D. Advocates call for a new approach after the era of "abstinence-only" sex education. *Guttmacher Policy Review, 12, 1* (Winter 2009). Available: http://www.guttmacher.org/pubs/gpr/12/1/gpr120106.pdf.

Borenstein, S. The science of romance: Brains have a love circuit. *ajc.com: The Atlanta Journal Constitution* (February 13, 2009).

Boslett, L. Colleges decide how to comply with new sex-offender law. *The Chronicle of Higher Education, 49, no. 20* (January 24, 2003), A33–34.

Boston Women's Health Collective. *Our bodies, ourselves: For the new century.* New York: Simon & Schuster, 1998.

Boutigny, H., Boschin, F., & Delcourt-Debruyne, E. Periodontal diseases, tobacco and pregnancy. *Journal of Gynecological and Obstetrical Biological Reproduction 34* (2005), 74–83.

Bowen, F. Is there a case for an uneven playing field? *The Birmingham News* (January 9, 2003), 7E.

Bower, S. A., & Brower, G. *Asserting yourself: A practical guide for positive change.* Reading, MA: Perseus Books, 1976.

Bowes-Sperry, L., & O'Leary, A. M. To act or not act: The dilemma faced by sexual harassment observers. *Academy of Management Review 30, no. 2* (April 1, 2005), 288–306.

Boyer, D., & Fine, D. Sexual abuse as a factor in adolescent pregnancy and child maltreatment. *Family Planning Perspectives, 24, 1* (1992), 4–11.

Boylan, J. F. *She's not there: A life in two genders.* New York: Broadway Books, 2003.

Bradford, L. J. & Beck, K. H. Development and validation of a condom self-efficacy scale for college students, *Journal of American College Health, 39* (1991), 219–225.

Brannon, G. E., & Carroll, K. S. Paraphilias. *eMedicine Specialties—Psychiatry,* February 14, 2008. Available: http://emedicine.medscape.com/article/291419-print.

Brecher, E. *Love, sex, and aging.* Boston: Little, Brown, 1984.

Brennan, J. Reconciling immigrant values, in *Case studies in cultural diversity,* Ferguson, V. D., ed. Sudbury, MA: Jones and Bartlett, 1999, 185–189.

Bretschneider, J., & McCoy, N. Sexual interest and behavior in healthy 80–102 year olds. *Archives of Sexual Behavior, 17* (1988), 109–130.

Brinton, L. A., Richesson, D. A., Gierach, G. L., Lacey, J. V., Park, Y., Hollenbeck, A. R., & Schatzkin, A. Prospective evaluation of risk factors for male breast cancer. *Journal of the National Cancer Institute, 100* (2008), 1477–1481.

Briton, N. J., & Hall, J. A. Beliefs about female and male nonverbal communication. *Sex Roles, 32, nos. 1 & 2* (1995), 79–90.

Brody, J. E. Study identifies disorder afflicting body builders. *New York Times* (Late New York Edition), (January 6, 1998), F8.

Brooks, J., Ruble, D., & Clark, A. College women's attitudes and expectations concerning menstrual-related changes. *Psychosomatic Medicine, 39* (1977), 289–298.

Brooks, S. Exotic dancing and unionizing: The challenges of feminist and anti-racist organizing at the Lusty Lady Theater. *SIECUS Report 33, no. 2* (spring 2005), 12–15.

Brooks, S. B. Matchmaking ASAP. *The Birmingham News* (January 11, 2004), 1E & 8E.

Brooks-Gunn, J., & Furstenberg, F. F. Coming of age in the era of AIDS: Puberty, sexuality, and contraception. *The Millbank Quarterly, 68, suppl. 1* (1990).

Broom, S. Sex happens after 50, and so do sexually transmitted diseases. *SIECUS Report, 27, no. 3* (February/March 1999), 12–13.

Brosius, H. B., Weaver, J. B., & Staab, J. F. Exploring the social and sexual "reality" of contemporary pornography. *Journal of Sex Research, 30, no. 2* (1993), 161–170.

Brotto, L. A., Bitzer, J., Laan, E., Leiblum, S., & Luria, M. Women's sexual desire and arousal disorders. *Journal of Sexual Medicine, 7* (2010), 586–614.

Brotto, L. A., Heiman, J. R., & Tolman, D. L. Narratives of desire in mid-age women with and without arousal difficulties, *Journal of Sex Research, 46* (2009), 387–398.

Brower, V. Circumcision's back. *American Health* (September 1989), 126.

Brown, J., & Steele, J. R. Sexuality and the mass media: An overview. *SIECUS Report, 24, no. 4* (April/May 1996), 3–9.

Bruckner, H., Martin, A., & Bearman, P. S. Ambivalence and pregnancy: Adolescents' attitudes, contraceptive use and pregnancy. *Perspect Sex Reprod Health, 36, no. 6* (November/December 2004), 248–257.

Bruess, C. E., & Greenberg, J. S. *Sexuality education: Theory and practice,* 5th ed. New York: Macmillan, 2009.

Bruess, C. E., & Greenberg, J. S. *Sexuality education: Theory and practice.* Boston: Jones and Bartlett, 2009.

Bruess, C. E., & Richardson, G. *Decisions for health.* Dubuque, IA: Brown & Benchmark, 1995, 1.14–1.16.

Bryant, A. Hostile hallways: The AAUW survey on sexual harassment in American schools. *Journal of School Health, 63, no. 8* (October 1993), 355–357.

Bryla, K. Y. Effects of media on female body image: myth or reality? *Health Education Monograph Series, 19, no. 2* (2002), 13–16.

Budur, K., Mathews, M., & Mathews, M. Couvade syndrome equivalent? *Psychosomatics, 46* (2005), 71–72.

Bullivant, S. B., Sellergren, S. A., Stern, K., Spencer, N. A., Jacob, S., Mennella, J. A., & McClintock, M. K. Women's sexual experience during the menstrual cycle: Identification of the sexual phase by noninvasive measurement of luteinizing hormone. *Journal of Sex Research, 41* (2004), 82–93.

Bullough, V. L. Children and adolescents as sexual beings: A historical overview. *Child and Adolescent Psychiatric Clinics of North America, 13, no. 3* (2004), 447–459.

Bullough, V. L. *Sex, society & history.* New York: Science History Publications, 1976a.

Bullough, V. L. *Sexual variance in society and history,* New York: John Wiley & Sons, 1976b.

Bullough, V. L., & Bullough, B. *Human sexuality: An encyclopedia.* New York: Garland Press, 1994.

Burg, B. R. Masturbatory death and injury. *Journal of the Royal Society of Health, 107* (1987), 60–61.

Burgard, S. Factors associated with contraceptive use in late- and post-apartheid South Africa. *Studies in Family Planning, 35, no. 2* (June 2004), 91–104.

Burgess, A. W., & Morgenbesser, L. I. Sexual violence and seniors. *Brief Treatment and Crisis Intervention. 5, no. 2* (2005), 193–202.

Buss, D. *The evolution of desire: Strategies of human mating.* New York: Basic Books, 1994.

Buss, D., et al. International preferences in selecting mates. *Journal of Cross-Cultural Psychology, 21* (1990), 5–47.

Buvat, J., Buvat-Herbaut, M., Lemaire, A., Marcolin, G., & Quittelier, E. Recent developments in the clinical assessment and diagnosis of erectile dysfunction, in *Annual review of sex research, Vol. 1*, Bancroft, J., Davis, C. M., & Weinstein, D., eds. New York: Society for the Scientific Study of Sex Research, 1990, 265–308.

Cady, B. Breast cancer: Screening and diagnosis in a primary care practice. *Primary Care & Cancer*, 6 (1986), 23–38.

Cain, V. S., Johannes, C. B., Avis, N. E., Mohr, B., Schocken, M., Skurnick, J., & Ory, M. Sexual functioning and practices in a multi-ethnic study of midlife women: Baseline results from SWAN. *Journal of Sex Research, 40* (2003), 266–276.

Calefati, J. Gay high schools offer a haven from bullies. *U.S. News & World Report* (January 2, 2009). Available: http://www.usnews.com/articles/education/2008/12/31/gay-high-schools-offer-a-haven-from-bullies.

California Pacific Medical Center. *Breast cysts*. San Francisco, CA: Author, 2008. Available: http://www.cpmc.org/services/women/breast/breast_cyst.html.

Call, V., Sprecher, S., & Schwartz, P. The incidence and frequency of marital sex in a national sample. *Journal of Marriage and the Family 57, no. 3* (August 1995), 639–652.

Campbell, R., Sefl, T., & Alvons, C. The impact of rape on women's sexual health risk behaviors. *Health Psychology, 23, no. 1* (Jan. 2004), 67–74.

Campbell, R., & Wasco, S.M. Understanding rape and sexual assault. *Journal of Interpersonal Violence 20, no. 1* (January 2005), 127–131.

Can we raise gender-neutral children? in *Taking sides: Issues in family and personal relationships*, Schroeder, E., ed. Guilford, CT: McGraw-Hill/Dushkin, 2003.

Canavan, M., Meyer, W., & Higgs, D. The female experience of sibling incest. *Journal of Marital and Family Therapy, 18* (1992), 129–142.

Cancer in women this year. *USA Today* (August 5, 1998), 1A.

Canedy, D. Wal-Mart decides against selling a contraceptive. *The New York Times* (1999) Available: http://www.nytimes.com/1999/05/14/business/wal-mart-decides-against-selling-a-contraceptive.html.

Caron, S. L. *Cross-cultural perspectives on human sexuality*. Boston: Allyn & Bacon, 1998.

Caron, S. L., & Bertram, R. M. What college students want to know about sex. *Medical Aspects of Human Sexuality, 22* (April 1988), 18–20.

Carr, J. L., & VanDeusen, K. M. Risk factors for male sexual aggression on college campuses. *Journal of Family Violence, 19, no. 5* (Oct. 2004), 279–289.

Carson, C., & Gunn, K. Premature ejaculation: Definition and prevalence. *International Journal of Impotence Research, 18 suppl 1* (2006), S5–13.

Catalyst 2008 census of the *Fortune* 500 reveals women gained little ground advancing to business leadership positions. Catalyst, 2008. Available: http://www.catalyst.org/press-release/141/catalyst-2008-census-of-the-fortune-500-reveals-women-gained-little-ground-advancing-to-business-leadership-positions.

Cates, W., Grimes, D. A., & Schulz, K. F. The public health impact of legal abortion: 30 years later. *Perspectives on Sexual and Reproductive Health, 35, no. 1* (2003), 25.

Catholic Church. *Encyclical of Pope Paul VI, humanae vitae, on the regulation of birth, and Pope Paul VI's credo of the people of God*. Glen Rock, NJ: Paulist Press, 1968.

Cavanagh, S. E. The sexual debut of girls in early adolescence: The intersection of race, pubertal timing, and friendship group characteristics. *Journal of Research on Adolescence, 14, no. 3* (September 2004), 285–312.

Census: More elderly live together. *InteliHealth* (July 30, 2002). Available: www.intelihealth.com.

Census shows nearly 600,000 same-sex couple homes in most comprehensive count yet of gays and lesbians. Harvard Medical School's *Consumer Health Information* (August 21, 2001). Available: http://www.intellihealth.com.

Center for Families in Transition, Scottsdale, AZ. 2003. Available: www.centerforfamilies.net/index.htm.

Centers for Disease Control and Prevention. *Anti-resistant Gonorrhea*, 2009a. Available: http://www.cdc.gov/std/gonorrhea/arg/default.htm.

Centers for Disease Control and Prevention. Breastfeeding trends and updated national health objectives for exclusive breastfeeding—United States, birth years 2000–2004. *Morbidity and Mortality Weekly Report, 56* (2007a), 760–763.

Centers for Disease Control and Prevention. *Can I get HIV from mosquitoes?* 2006. Available: http://www.cdc.gov/hiv/resources/qa/qa32.htm.

Centers for Disease Control and Prevention. *Cases of HIV infection and AIDS in the United States and dependent areas*, 2006. Atlanta, GA: Author, 2008c, 18.

Centers for Disease Control and Prevention. *Chlamydia. STD fact sheets* (2005). Available: http://www.cdc.gov/std/healthcomm/fact_sheets.htm

Centers for Disease Control and Prevention. *FAQs for health professionals: Hepatitis B*, 2008. Available: http://www.cdc.gov/hepatitis/HBV/HBVfaq.htm#overview

Centers for Disease Control and Prevention. *Female sterilization: risk of ectopic pregnancy after tubal sterilization fact sheet* (2005). Available: http://www.cdc.gov/reproductivehealth/UnintendedPregnancy/EctopicPreg_factsheet.htm.

Centers for Disease Control and Prevention. *Fetal alcohol spectrum disorders*, 2006. Available: http://www.cdc.gov/ncbddd/fas/fasask.htm.

Centers for Disease Control and Prevention. *Genital herpes—CDC fact sheet*, 2008b. Available: http://www.cdc.gov/std/Herpes/STDFact-Herpes.htm.

Centers for Disease Control and Prevention. *Genital HPV infection—CDC fact sheet*. Atlanta, GA: Centers for Disease Control and Prevention, 2005.

Centers for Disease Control and Prevention. Heterosexual populations. Section 1: Core epidemiologic questions. Direct measure of risk behavior, in *Sample: Integrated epidemiologic profile for HIV/AIDS prevention and care planning—Louisiana, 2002*. Available: http://www.cdc.gov/hiv/topics/surveillance/resources/guidelines/epi-guideline/la_supp/section1q3_heterosexual.htm.

Centers for Disease Control and Prevention. *HIV/AIDS surveillance report, 15* (2004).

Centers for Disease Control and Prevention. *HIV/AIDS surveillance report, 2006, Vol. 18*. Atlanta: U.S. Department of Health and Human Services, Centers for Disease Control and Prevention, 2008d. Available: http://www.cdc.gov/hiv/topics/surveillance/resources/reports/.

Centers for Disease Control and Prevention. *HIV/AIDS and women*, 2007b. Available: http://www.cdc.gov/hiv/topics/women/.

Centers for Disease Control and Prevention. *HIV and AIDS in the United States: A picture of today's epidemic*. Atlanta, GA: Author, 2009. Available: http://www.cdc.gov/hiv/topics/surveillance/united_states.htm.

Centers for Disease Control and Prevention. *Rubella (German measles)*. Atlanta, GA: Centers for Disease Control and Prevention, 2005. Available: http://www.cdc.gov/nip/publications/Parents-Guide/pg-rubella.pdf.

Centers for Disease Control and Prevention. *Scabies—CDC fact sheet*. Atlanta, GA: Centers for Disease Control and Prevention, 2005.

Centers for Disease Control and Prevention. *Sexually transmitted diseases surveillance*, 2007c. Available: http://www.cdc.gov/std/stats07/toc.htm.

Centers for Disease Control and Prevention. *Sexually Transmitted Diseases Surveillance, 2008*, 2009b. Available: http://www.cdc.gov/STD/stats08/chlamydia.htm.

Centers for Disease Control and Prevention. Sexually transmitted diseases treatment guidelines, 2006. *Morbidity and Mortality Weekly Report, 55* (2006), 38.

Centers for Disease Control and Prevention (CDC). *Teen birth rates up slightly in 2007 for second consecutive year*, March 18, 2009. Available: http://www.cdc.gov/media/pressrel/2009/r090318.htm.

Centers for Disease Control and Prevention. *Youth Risk Behavior Survey*, 2003. Available: www.cdc.gov.

Central Intelligence Agency. *The 2008 world fact book*. Langley, VA: Author, 2009.

Cesarean section. 2005. Available: http://www.drkoop.com/encyclopedia/93/668.html.

Chan, E. C. Y., Vernon, S. W., O'Donnell, F. T., Ahn, C., Greisinger, A., & Aga, D. W. Informed consent for cancer screening with prostate-specific antigen: How well are men getting the message? *American Journal of Public Health, 93* (2003), 779–785.

Chandra, A., Martino, S. C., Collins, R. L., Elliott, M. N., Berry, S. H., Kanouse, D. E., & Miu, A. Does watching sex on television predict teen pregnancy? Findings from a national longitudinal survey of youth. *Pediatrics, 122, 5* (November 2008), 1047–1054.

Characteristics of freshmen, 2001. *Chronicle of Higher Education, 68, no. 1* (August 31, 2001), 22–23.

Chick, D., & Gold, S. R. A review of influences on sexual fantasy: Attitudes, experiences, guilt and gender. *Imagination and Cognitive Personality, 7* (1987–1988), 61–76.

Child sexual abuse, National Committee to Prevent Child Abuse, 1998.

Child Trends. Science says: Where and when teens first have sex. *Science Says, 1* (June 2003).

Child Welfare League of America. *A survey of 17 Florence Crittenton agencies serving minor mothers,* 1994.

Christensen, F. M. *Pornography: The other side.* New York: Praeger, 1990.

Chronology of significant legal and policy changes affecting women in the military: 1947–2003. Women's Research & Education Institute (2005). Available: http://www.wrei.org/projects/wiu/wim/wim_chron01.pdf.

Chuang, C. H., & Freund, K. M. Emergency contraception knowledge among women in a Boston community. *Contraception, 71, no. 2* (Feb. 2005), 157–160.

Clapp, D. Overview of assisted reproductive technologies. *Resolve Fact Sheet Series,* 1998.

Clark, T., & Epstein, R. Self-concept and expectancy for social reinforcement in noninstitutionalized male homosexuals. *Proceedings of the 77th Annual Convention of the American Psychoanalytical Association, 4* (1969), 575.

Clark, W. M., & Servivich, J. M. Twenty years and still in the dark? *Journal of Marital and Family Therapy, 23, no. 3* (July 1997), 239–253.

Clayton, A. H. Symptoms related to the menstrual cycle: Diagnosis, prevalence, and treatment. *Journal of Psychiatric Practice, 14* (2008), 13–21.

Cleland, J., & Ali, M. M. Reproductive consequences of contraceptive failure in 19 developing countries. *Obstetrics and Gynecology, 104, 2* (2004), 314–320.

Clement, U. Surveys of heterosexual behavior, in *Annual Review of Sex Research, Vol. 1,* Bancroft, J., Davis, C. M., & Weinstein, D., eds. New York: Society for the Scientific Study of Sex Research, 1990, 45–74.

Clements, M. Sex in America today. *Parade* (August 7, 1994), 4–6.

Cloud, J. The battle over gay teens. *Time, 166, no. 15* (October 10, 2005), 42–51.

Cluett, E. R., Pickering, R. M., Getliffe, K., & Saunders, N. J. Randomised controlled trial of labouring in water compared with standard of augmentation for management of dystocia in first stage of labour. *British Medical Journal, 328* (2004), 314.

Cocaine and pregnancy. *Medical Aspects of Human Sexuality, 25* (1991), 16.

Coen, S. Sexual interviewing, evaluation, and therapy: Psychoanalytic emphasis on the use of sexual fantasy. *Archives of Sexual Behavior, 7* (1978), 229–41.

Coffin, J. M., Baroody, S., Schneider, K., & O'Neill, J. Impaired cerebellar learning in children with prenatal alcohol exposure: A comparative study of eyeblink conditioning in children with ADHD and dyslexia. *Cortex, 41* (2005), 389–398.

Cohen, A. Harassment complaints ignored. *Herizons, 19, no. 1* (Summer 2005), 11–12.

Cohen, L. J., & Galynker, H. Clinical features of pedophilia and implications for treatment. *Journal of Psychiatric Practice, 8, no. 5* (September 2002), 276–289.

Cohen, P. Muscle mania. *New Scientist, 156* (November 22, 1997), 15.

Colditz, G. A., et al. The use of estrogen and progestins and the risk of breast cancer in postmenopausal women. *New England Journal of Medicine, 332* (1995), 1589–1593.

Coleman, E. What sexual scientists know...: About compulsive sexual behavior. Society for the Scientific Study of Sexuality (2005). Available: http://www.sexscience.org.

Collaborative Group on Hormonal Factors in Breast Cancer. Breast cancer and breastfeeding: Collaborative reanalysis of individual data from 47 epidemiological studies in 30 countries, including 50,302 women with breast cancer and 96,973 women without the disease. *Lancet, 360* (2002), 187–196.

Collins, D., Elliott, M., Berry, S., Kanouse, D., Kunkel, D., Hunter, S., & Miu, A. Watching sex on television predicts adolescent initiation of sexual behavior. *Pediatrics, 114, no. 3* (Sep. 2004), e280–e289.

Commission on Obscenity and Pornography. *The report of the Commission on Obscenity and Pornography.* New York: Bantam, 1970.

Common Sense Media. *Talking about "sexting,"* 2009. Available: http://www.commonsensemedia.org/talking-about-sexting.

Conde-Agudelo, A., Rosas-Bermúdez, A., & Karfury-Goeta, A. C. Birth spacing and risk of adverse perinatal outcomes. *Journal of the American Medical Association, 295* (2006), 1809–1823.

Confirmation of transmission of AIDS via artificial insemination. *Infectious Diseases* (January 1986), 19, 16.

Conklin, S. C., & Peters, R. *Sexual health not harm: Three lessons, three levels, student tested and prized.* Round Table Teaching Presentation at American Association of Sexuality Educators, Counselors and Therapists (AASECT), Chicago, IL, (May 15, 2004).

Connell, P., McKevitt, C., & Low, N. Investigating ethnic differences in sexual health: Focus groups with young people. *Sexually Transmitted Infections, 80, no. 4* (August 2004), 300–305.

Connolly, J. M., Slaughter, V., & Mealey, L. The development of preferences for specific body shapes. *Journal of Sex Research, 41, no. 1* (Feb. 2004), 5–15.

Contal, M., Masson, G., Boyer, C., Cazevielle, C., & Mares, P. Neonatal consequences of maternal smoking during pregnancy. *Journal of Gynecological and Obstetrical Biological Reproduction, 34* (2005), 215–222.

Contraceptive patch. *The Contraception Report, 12, no. 4* (2001), 12–14.

Cordell, K. *Vaginismus: Finding hope for unconsummated marriages and female sexual pain.* Featured Health Articles, February 2008. Available: http://www.womenshealth.gov/editor/2008/02/.

Corliss, R. Objects of our affection. *Time, 152, no. 8* (1998), 73–74.

Corliss, R. Sex, sex and rock 'n' roll. *Time, 166, no. 5* (August 1, 2005), 83.

Cornelius, M. D., & Day, N. L. The effects of tobacco use during and after pregnancy on exposed children. *Alcohol Research and Health, 24* (2000), 242–249.

Cotton-Houston, A., & Wheeler, K. Preorgasmic group treatment: Assertiveness, marital adjustment and sexual function in women. *Journal of Sex and Marital Therapy, 9* (1983), 296–302.

Courtwright, D. T. The neglect of female children and childhood: Sex ratios in nineteenth century America: A review of the evidence. *Journal of Family History, 15* (1990), 313–323.

Craig, M. E. Coercive sexuality in dating relationships: A situational model. *Clinical Psychology Review, 10* (1990), 395–423.

Crandell, S. Oh baby. *AARP The Magazine* (September/October, 2005), 108–117.

Crary, D. Abercrombie & Fitch's racy catalog draws odd coalition to call for boycott. *The Birmingham News* (June 22, 2001), 7C.

Crary, D. Health advocates tout new model of female condom. *Associated Press* (April 16, 2009).

Crepault, C. C., et al. Erotic imagery in women, in *Progress in sexuality.* Gemme, R., & C. C. Wheeler, ed. New York: Plenum, 1977.

Crime in the United States. U.S. Department of Justice, 2008. Available: http://www.fbi.gov/ucr/cius2007/data/table_01.html.

Crooks, R., & Baur, K. *Our sexuality,* 8th ed. Belmont, CA: Wadsworth, 2002.

Cullen, L. T. Cupid academy. *Time, 163, no. 7* (February 16, 2004), 67–68.

Curtis, K. California loses track of 33,000 sex offenders. *The Birmingham News* (January 8, 2003), 8A.

Cutler, W., Berg, G. P., Krieger, A., Huggins, G. R., Garcia, C. R., & Lawley, H. J. Human axillary secretions influence women's menstrual cycles: The role of donor extract from men. *Hormones and Behavior 20* (1986), 463–473.

Cybersex addiction checklist. Sexual Recovery Institute (2001). Available: http://www.sexualrecovery.com.

D'Augelli, A. R., Grossman, A. H., & Starks, M. T. Parents' awareness of lesbian, gay, and bisexual youths' sexual orientation, *Journal of Marriage and Family, 67, no. 2* (May 2005), 474–482.

Dahl, D. W., Gorn, G. J., & Weinberg, C. B. Condom-carrying behavior among college students. *American Journal of Public Health, 87* (1997), 1059.

Dailard, C. Recent findings from the "Add Health" survey: Teens and sexual activity. *The Guttmacher Report, 4, no. 4* (August 2001), 1–3, 2–4.

Dailard, C. Understanding "abstinence": Implications for individuals, programs and policies. *The Guttmacher Report, 6, no. 5* (December 2003).

Dalal, A. Sexual stereotypes stop females from feeling pleasure. *Sex, Etc.* (2005).

Dalton, K. *Once a month.* Ramona, CA: Hunter House, 1979.

Daneback, K, Cooper, A., & Mansson, S. An Internet study of cybersex participants. *Archives of Sexual Behavior, 34, no. 3* (June 2005), 321–328.

Daniel, E. L., & Levine, C. *Taking sides: Clashing views on controversial issues in health and society,* 5th ed. Guilford, CT: McGraw-Hill Dushkin, 2001.

Date.com is so 2004. *Time, 165, no, 25* (June 20, 2005), 19.

Date rape drugs. The National Women's Health Information Center, 2005. Available: www.4woman.gov.

Date rape drugs. U.S. Department of Health and Human Services, Office on Women's Health, 2008. Available: http://www.womenshealth.gov/faq/date-rape-drugs.cfm.

Dating and domestic violence. Rape, Abuse & Incest National Network, 2009. Available: http://www.rainn.org/get-information/types-of-sexual-assault/dating-and-domestic-violence.

Davidson, J. K. The utilization of sexual fantasies by sexually experienced university students. *Journal of American College Health, 34* (1985), 24–32.

Davies, M. Correlates of negative attitudes toward gay men: Sexism, male role norms, and male sexuality. *Journal of Sex Research, 42, no. 3* (August, 2004), 259–266.

Davis, D. M. Portrayals of women in prime time network television: Some demographic characteristics. *Sex Roles, 23* (1990), 325–332.

Davis, K. E. Near and dear: Friendship and love compared. *Psychology Today, 22* (February 1985).

Davis, S. R., Moreau, M., Kroll, R., et al. Testosterone for low libido in postmenopausal women not taking estrogen. *New England Journal of Medicine, 359* (2008), 2005–2017.

Daw, J. Is PMDD real? *Monitor on Psychology, 33* (2002). Available: http://www.apa.org/monitor/oct02/pmdd.html.

Dawood, K., Pillard, R. C., Horvath, C., Revelle, W., & Bailey, J. M. Familial aspects of male homosexuality. *Archives of Sexual Behavior, 29, no. 2* (2000), 155–163.

DeBeauvoir, S. *The coming of age.* New York: Warner Books, 1973.

Decker, M. R., Silverman, J. G., & Raj, A. Dating violence and sexually transmitted disease/HIV testing and diagnosis among adolescent females. *Pediatrics, 116, no. 2* (Aug. 2005), 272–276.

Deckers, P., & Ricci Jr., A. Pain and lumps in the female breast. *Hospital Practice* (February 28, 1992), 67–94.

Degler, C. N. *At odds: Women and the family in America from the revolution to the present.* New York: Oxford University Press, 1980.

Degrees conferred by degree-granting institutions, by level of degree and sex of student. *Digest of Education Statistics* (2009). Available: http://nces.ed.gov/programs/digest/d07/tables/dt07_258.asp.

Deirmenjian, J. M. Pedophilia on the Internet. *Journal of Forensic Sciences, 47, no. 5* (Sep. 2002), 1090–1092.

Dekeyser-Boccara, J., & Milliez, J. Smoking and ectopic pregnancy: Is there a causal relationship? *Journal of Gynecological and Obstetrical Biological Reproduction, 34* (2005), 119–123.

DeLamater, J. D., & Friedrich, W. N. Human sexual development. *The Journal of Sex Research, 39* (2002), 10–14.

Demir, E., & Dickson, B. J. Fruitless splicing specifies male courtship behavior in Drosophila. *Cell, 121* (June 3, 2005), 785–794.

Denizet-Lewis, B. Friends, friends with benefits and the benefits of the local mall. *The New York Times* (May 30, 2004).

Dennis, J. Theater's pass cards let teens see films rated R. *The Birmingham News* (June 9, 2004), p. 1G.

Dennison, R. P., & Russell, S. T. Positive perspectives on adolescent sexuality: Contributions of the National Longitudinal Study of Adolescent Health. *Sexuality Research & Social Policy, 2, 4* (December 2005), 54–59.

DePaulo, B. M., Kirkendol, S. E., Kashy, S. E., Wyer, M. M., & Epstein, J. A. Lying in everyday life. *Journal of Personality and Social Psychology, 70, no. 5* (1996), 979–997.

DeQuine, J. Out of the closet and on to fraternity row. *Time, 161, no. 11* (March 17, 2003), 8.

Derby, C. A., Mohr, B. A., Goldstein, I., et al. Modifiable risk factors and erectile dysfunction: Can lifestyle changes modify risk? *Urology, 56* (2000), 302–306.

Dew, M. The effects of attitudes on inferences of homosexuality and perceived physical attractiveness in women. *Sex Roles, 12* (1985), 143–155.

Dewan, S. United Church of Christ backs gay marriage. *The Birmingham News* (July 5, 2005), p. A1.

Dickson, A. Men friends. *Time, 155, no. 4* (January 17, 2000), 89

Diken, B., & Laustsen, C. B. Becoming abject: Rape as a weapon of war. *Body & Society, 11, no. 1* (2005), 111–128.

Dinh, T. H., Sternberg M., Dunne E. F., & Markowitz L. E. Genital warts among 18- to 59-year-olds in the United States, National Health and Nutrition Examination Survey, 1999–2004. *Sexually Transmitted Diseases, 35* (2008), 357–360.

Discovery Health: Paraphilia 2005. Available: http://health.discovery.com/centers/sex/sexpedia/paraphilia_print.html.

Ditmore, M. New U.S. funding policies on trafficking affect sex work and HIV-prevention efforts worldwide. *SIECUS Report 33, no. 2* (Spring 2005), 26–29.

Division of Sexually Transmitted Diseases. Sexually transmitted diseases treatment guidelines 2002. *Morbidity and Mortality Weekly Report, 51* (2002). Available: http://www.cdc.gov/STD/treatment/62002TG.htm#HumanPapillomavirusInfection.

Division of STD Prevention. *Sexually transmitted disease surveillance, 2003.* Atlanta, GA: Centers for Disease Control and Prevention, 2004.

Divorce and children. American Academy of Pediatrics, 2001. Available: http://www.aap.org/family/divorce.htm

Do women and men communicate differently? In *Taking sides: Issues in family and personal relationships,* Schroeder, E., ed. Guilford, CT: McGraw-Hill/Dushkin, 2003.

Do men and women lead differently? *Leadership Strategies 3, no. 10* (October 2000): 8.

Do men and women speak different languages? in *Taking sides: Clashing views on controversial issues in family and personal relationships,* Vail, A. ed. Guilford, CT: Dushkin/McGraw-Hill, 1999.

Dodge, B, Reece, M, Cole, S. L., & Sandfort, T. G. Sexual compulsivity among heterosexual college students. *Journal of Sex Research, 41 no. 4* (November 2004), 343–350.

Doell, R. G. Sexuality in the brain. *Journal of Homosexuality, 28, nos. 3–4* (1995), 345–354.

Does divorce create long-term negative effects for children? In *Taking sides: Issues in family and personal relationships,* Schroeder, E., ed. Guilford, CT: McGraw-Hill/Dushkin, 2003.

Dolan, B. No sex please, we're ignorant. *Time* (September 17, 1990), 71.

Dolance, S. A whole stadium full: Lesbian community at Women's National Basketball Association games. *Journal of Sex Research, 42, no. 1* (February 2005), 74–83.

Dolgov, A. Russian women enslaved for sex. *The Birmingham News* (May 17, 2001), 10A.

Doll, H., Vessey, M., & Painter, R. Return of fertility in nulliparous women after discontinuation of the intrauterine device: Comparison with women discontinuing other methods of contraception. *British Journal of Obstetrics and Gynecology, 108, 3* (March 2001), 304–314.

Domestic homicides. Domestic violence is a serious, widespread social problem in America: The facts 2005. Family Violence Prevention Fund. Available: http://endabuse.org.

Domestic violence and children. Domestic violence is a serious, widespread social problem in America: The facts 2005. Family Violence Prevention Fund. Available: http://endabuse.org.

Donaghue, N. Body satisfaction, sexual self-schemas, and subjective well-being in women. *Body Image, 6, 1* (January 2009), 37–42.

Dorner, G. Hormonal induction and prevention of female homosexuality. *Journal of Endocrinology, 42* (1968), 162–163.

Dorner, G., Rohde, W., Stahl, F., Krell, L., & Masius, W. A neuroendocrine predisposition for homosexuality in men, *Archives of Sexual Behavior, 4* (1975), 1–8.

Dowie, M. Teratology: The loneliest science. *American Health* (June 1990) 59–67.

Downey, L. International change in sex behavior: A belated look at Kinsey's males. *Archives of Sexual Behavior, 9* (1980), 267–317.

Doyle, J., Stern, L., Hagan, M., Hao, J., & Gricar, J. Advances in contraception: IUDs from a managed care perspective. *Journal of Women's Health, 17, 6* (July 2008), 987–992.

Drummond, T. A win for gays. *Time, 155, no. 12* (March 27, 2000), 38.

Ducret, L. What are the epidemiological data on smoking and co-addictions during pregnancy? *Journal of Gynecological and Obstetrical Biological Reproduction, 34* (2005), 55–66.

Duff-Bell, B. Same-sex marriage bill passes in Canada's House. *The Birmingham News* (June 29, 2005), 14A.

Dunn, P. C., Knight, S. M., & Glascoff, M. A. Gender-specific changes in students' sexual behaviors and attitudes at a southeastern university between 1973 and 1988. *Journal of American College Health, 41, no. 3* (1992), 99–104.

Dunne, E. F., Unger, E. R., Sternberg M., McQuillan, G., Swan, D. C., Patel, S. S., & Markowitz, L. E. Prevalence of HPV infection among females in the United States. *Journal of the American Medical Association, 297* (2007), 813–819.

Durban, M., DiClemente, R., & Siegel, D. Factors associated with multiple sex partners among junior high school students. *Journal of Adolescent Health, 14, 3* (1993), 292–207.

Durex condom maker using "humor" ads to sell condoms in Europe. *Kaiser Network Daily HIV/AIDS Report.* Henry J. Kaiser Family Foundation. Available: www.kaisernetwork.org.

Dyspareunia. Medical-Library.org, 2009. Available: http://www.medical-library.org/journals4a/sexual_dysfunction_2.htm.

Dyspareunia. Merck Manuals Online Medical Library, 2003. Available: http://www.merck.com/mmhe/sec22/ch250/ch250b.html.

Eagly, A. H. Transformational, transactional, and laissez-faire leadership styles: A meta-analysis comparing women and men. *Psychological Bulletin, 129, no. 4* (July 2003), 569–591.

Eastwood, K. L., et al. Abortion training in United States obstetrics and gynecology residency programs. *Obstetrics and Gynecology, 108* (2006), 303–308.

Eaton, D. K., Kann, L., Kinchen, S., et al. Youth Risk Behavior Surveillance—United States, 2007. *Morbidity and Mortality Weekly Report, 57, SS-4* (June 6, 2008), 1–131.

The ecology of birth control. Chicago: G. D. Searle, 1971.

Edelman, M. W. *Families in peril: An agenda for social change.* Cambridge, MA: President and Fellows of Harvard College, 1987.

Edwards, M. We have a responsibility to dialogue with the media. *SIECUS Report, 24, no. 5* (June/July 1996), 5.

Ehrhardt, A. A., Evers, K., & Money, J. Influence of androgen and some aspects of sexual dimorphic behavior in women with the late-treated adrenogenital syndrome. *Johns Hopkins Medical Journal, 123* (1968), 115–122.

Ehrhardt, A. A., Myer-Bahlburg, H. F. L., Rosen, L. R., Feldman, J. F., Veridiano, J. F., Zimmerman, N. P., & McEwen, B. S. Sexual orientation after exposure to exogenous estrogen. *Archives of Sexual Behavior, 14, no. 1* (1985), 57–77.

Eisen, M., Zellman, G. L., & McAlister, A. L. Evaluating the impact of a theory-based sexuality and contraceptive education program. *Family Planning Perspectives, 21* (January/February 1990), 4–5.

El Hadi, A. A Step forward for opponents of female genital mutilation in Egypt. *Lancet, 349* (1997), 129–130.

Elder, S. Sexual foreplay: What's in it for men? *WebMD,* 2009. Available: http://men.webmd.com/guide/sexual-foreplay-whats-for-men.

Ellingson, L. Lesbian health issues: A ten year review. *Health Education Monograph Series, 19, no. 1* (2002), 40–45.

Elliott, S., & Umberson, D. The performance of desire: Gender and sexual negotiation in long-term marriages. *Journal of Marriage and Family, 70, 2* (April 2008), 391–406.

Ellis, A. Healthy and disturbed reasons for having extramarital relations, in *Encounter with family realities,* Powers, E. A. & Lees, M.-W., eds. St. Paul, MN: West, 1977, 374–375.

Ellis, A., & Harper, R. *A guide to rational living.* North Hollywood, CA: Melvin Powers, Wilshire Book Company, 1975.

Ellis, A., & Harper, R. *A new guide to rational living.* Englewood Cliffs, NJ: Prentice-Hall, 1979.

Ellis, B. J., & Symons, D. Sex differences in sexual fantasy: An evolutionary psychological approach. *Journal of Sex Research, 27* (1990), 527–555.

Elmer-Dewitt, P. Now for the truth about Americans and sex. *Time* (October 17, 1994), 64.

Empower Health Corporation. Sexual dysfunction overview, 1998.

Ende, J., Rockwell, S., & Glasgow, M. The sexual history in general medical practice. *Archives of Internal Medicine, 44* (1984), 55.

Endocrinology Society. *Endocrinology and impotence (erectile dysfunction),* 1998.

Endometriosis Association. What is endometriosis? *Endo-Online* (2005). Available: http://www.endo-online.org/endo.html.

Eng, T. R., & Butler, W. T., eds. *The hidden epidemic: Confronting sexually transmitted diseases.* Washington, DC: Institute of Medicine, 1996.

Erickson, E. H. *Childhood and society.* New York: Norton, 1950.

Erlik, Y., et al. Association of waking episodes with menopausal hot flash. *Journal of the American Medical Association, 245* (1981), 1741–1744.

Escobar-Chaves, S., Tortolero, S., Markham, C., Low, B., Eitel, P., & Thickstun, P. Impact of the media on adolescent sexual attitudes and behaviors. *Pediatrics, 116, no. 1* (July 2005), 303–326.

Esposito, K., Giuliano, F., Di Palo, C., Giugliano, G., Marfella, R., D'Andrea, F., D'Armiento, M., & Giugliano, D. Effects of lifestyle changes on erectile dysfunction in obese men. *Journal of the American Medical Association, 291* (2004), 2978–2984.

Espry, E., et al. Abortion education in medical schools: A national survey. *American Journal of Obstetrics and Gynecology, 192* (2005), 640–643.

Estelles, J., Rodriguez-Arias, M., Maldonado, C., Aguilar, M. A., & Minarro, J. Prenatal cocaine exposure alters spontaneous and cocaine-induced motor and social behaviors. *Neurotoxicology and Teratology, 27* (2005), 449–457.

Evenson, K. R., Savitz, D. A., & Huston, S. L. Leisure-time physical activity among pregnant women in the US. *Paediatric Perinatal Epidemiology, 18* (2004), 400–407.

Exhibitionism. Psychology Today's Conditions Center (2005). Available: http://cms.psychologytoday.com/conditions/index.php?term=exhibitionism&print=1.

Fackelmann, K. Booze and babies: How much danger? New research finds potential risk in even light drinking. *USA Today* (November 20, 2002), D9.

Facts about trauma. APA Online (2005). Available: http://www.apa.org/.

Facts for features. U.S. Census Bureau, September 11, 2008. Available: http://www.census.gov/Press-Release/www/releases/archives/facts_for_features_special_editions/.

The facts on international gender-based violence. Family Violence Prevention Fund (2005). Available: www.endabuse.org.

The facts on the military and violence against women. Family Violence Prevention Fund (2005). Available: www.endabuse.org.

The facts on the workplace and domestic violence. Family Violence Prevention Fund (2005). Available: www.endabuse.org.

Fast-tracking the first AIDS drug. *FDA Consumer* (October 1987), 13–15.

FDA nears OK on silicone breast implants. *Intellihealth* (July 29, 2005). Available: http://www.intellihealth.com.

FDA news. FDA updates labeling for Ortho Evra contraceptive patch, U.S. Food and Drug Administration, P05-90 (November 10, 2005). Available: http://www.fda.gov/bbs/topics/news/2005/NEW01262.html.

FDA OKs hormonal implant. *Family Planning Perspectives, 20, no. 6* (November/December 1990), 1–4.

Feldman, H. A., Johannes, C. B., Derby, C. A., et al. Erectile dysfunction and coronary risk factors. *Preventive Medicine, 30* (2000), 328–338.

Female orgasmic disorder. *The Merck manual of diagnosis and treatment*, 2005. Available: http://www.merck.com/mrkshared/mmanual/section18/chapter243/243c.jsp.

Feminist wire daily newsbriefs, September 30, 2005. *Ms. Magazine*. Available: http://www.msmagazine.com/.

Fergusson, D. M., Horwood, L. J., & Lynskey, M. T. Childhood sexual abuse, adolescent sexual behaviors and sexual revictimization. *Child Abuse and Neglect, 21, no. 8* (1997), 789–803.

Fernandez-Ruiz, J., Gomez, M., Hernandez, M., de Miguel, R., & Ramos, J. A. Cannabinoids and gene expression during brain development. *Neurotoxological Research, 6* (2004), 389–401.

Fetishism. Discovery Health (2005). Available: http://health.discovery.com/centers/sex/sexpedia/fetishism_print.html

Fetishism. Sinclair Intimacy Institute (2001). Available: http://www.intimacyinstitute.com.

Fetishism. University of Iowa Health Care (2001). Available: www.uihealthcare.com/topics/mentalemotionalhealth/ment3145.html.

Fields, J. America's families and living arrangements: 2003. *Current Population Reports*, U.S. Census Bureau, 2004.

Files, J. Number of gays discharged from services drops again. *The New York Times* (February 13, 2005).

Filomeno, A. H. Promoting parent–adolescent communication to facilitate healthy sexual socialization of youth. *Health Education Monograph Series, 19, no. 2* (2002),17–21.

Finkelhor, D. Early and long-term effects of child sexual abuse: An update. *Professional Psychology: Research and Practice, 21* (1990), 325–330.

Finkelhor, D. *A sourcebook on child sexual abuse*. Thousand Oaks, CA: Sage, 1986.

Finkelhor, D., Ormrod, R., Turner, H., & Hamby, S. L. The victimization of children and youth: A comprehensive, national survey. *Child Maltreatment, 10, no. 1* (February 2005), 5–25.

First marriage, dissolution, divorce, and remarriage in the United States. National Center for Health Statistics, U.S. Centers for Disease Control (2001). Available: http://www.cdc.gov.nchs

Fisch, H. Older men are having children, but the reality of a male biological clock makes this trend worrisome. *Geriatrics, 64* (2009), 14–17.

Fisher, H. E. *Anatomy of love*. New York: W. W. Norton, 1992.

Fiumara, N. J. Gonorrhea. Part I. Acute infection. *Medical Aspects of Human Sexuality, 21* (1987), 65–72.

Fiumara, N. J. Herpes simplex infection. *Medical Aspects of Human Sexuality, 20* (1986a), 72–73.

Fontaine, J. H. Experiencing a need: School counselors' experiences with gay and lesbian students. *Professional School Counseling, 1, no. 3* (February 1998), 9–14.

Food and Drug Administration. Female condom, 1993. Available: http://www.fda.gov/ForConsumers/ByAudience/ByPatientAdvocates/HIVandAIDSActivities/ucm126373.htm.

Food and Drug Administration. New warning for Nonoxynol 9 OTC contraceptive products re: STDs and HIV/AIDS, 2007. Available: http://www.fda.gov/ForConsumers/ByAudience/ForPatientAdvocates/HIVandAIDSActivities/ucm124023.htm.

Ford, K., Woosung, S., & Lepowski, J. Characteristics of adolescents' sexual partners and their association with use of condoms and other contraceptive methods. *Family Planning Perspectives, 33, no. 3* (May/June 2001), 100–105, 132.

Fraley, S. S., Mona, L. P., & Theodore, P. S. The sexual lives of lesbian, gay, and bisexual people with disabilities: Psychological perspectives. *Sexuality Research & Social Policy, 4, 1* (March 2007), 15–26.

Frank, D. A., Rose-Jacobs, R., Beeghly, M., Wilbur, M., Bellinger, D., & Cabral, H. Level of prenatal cocaine exposure and 48-month IQ: importance of preschool enrichment. *Neurotoxicology and Teratology, 27* (2005), 15–28.

Frankowski, B. L. American Academy of Pediatrics Clinical Report: Guidance for the clinician in rendering pediatric care. *Pediatrics, 113* (June 2004), 1827–1832.

Freeman, C. E. Trends in educational quality of girls and women: 2004. National Center for Education statistics. *Education Statistics Quarterly, 6, no. 4* (November 23, 2005).

French prostitutes protest crackdown. *The Birmingham News* (November 6, 2002), 9A.

Frequently asked questions. Ashley Madison Agency, 2005. Available: http://www.ashleymadison.com.

Friday, N. *Forbidden flowers*. New York: Pocket Books, 1975.

Friedrich, W. N., Fisher, J., Broughton, D., Houston, M., & Shafran, C. R. Normative sexual behavior in children: A contemporary sample. *Pediatrics, 101, no. r* (April 1998), e9.

Friedrich, W. N., Whiteside, S. P., & Talley, N. J. Noncoercive sexual contact with similarly aged individuals: What is the impact? *Journal of Interpersonal Violence, 19, no. 9* (September 2004), 1075–1084.

Frisco, M. Parental involvement and young women's contraceptive use. *Journal of Marriage and Family, 67, no. 1* (February 2005), 110–121.

Fromm, E. *The art of loving*. New York: Harper and Row, 1956.

Frost, J. J., Darroch, J. E., & Remez, L. Improving contraceptive use in the United States. *Guttmacher—In Brief, 1* (2008).

Frye, M. Lesbian sex, in *Through the prism of difference: Readings on sex and gender*, Zinn, M. B., Hondagneu-Sotelo, P., & Messner, M. A., eds. Boston: Allyn & Bacon, 1997.

Fung, M. M., Bettencourt, R., & Barrett-Conner, E. Heart disease risk factors predict erectile dysfunction 25 years later. *Journal of the College of Cardiology, 43* (2004), 1405–1411.

Galdas, P. M., Cheater, F., & Marshall, P. Men and health help-seeking behavior: Literature review. *Journal of Advanced Nursing, 49* (2005), 616–622.

Gallup. Religion, politics inform Americans' view on abortion, 2006. Available: http://www.gallup.com/poll/22222/Religion-Politics-Inform-Americans-Views-Abortion.aspx.

Gardner, J., & Miller, L. Promoting the safety and use of hormonal contraceptives. *Journal of Women's Health, 14, no. 1*, (2005), 53–60.

Garner, D. *The 1997 Psychology Today Body Image Survey*. Available: http://www.psychologytoday.com/print/25283.

Garshasbi, A., & Faghih, Z. S. The effect of exercise on the intensity of low back pain in pregnant women. *International Journal of Gynaecology and Obstetrics, 88* (2005), 271–275.

Gauthier, T. W., Drews-Botsch, C., Falek, A., Coles, C., & Brown, L. A. Maternal alcohol abuse and neonatal infection. *Alcohol and Clinical and Experimental Research, 29* (2005), 1035–1043.

Gay, lesbian, and bisexual adolescents. SIECUS fact sheet, 1998. Available: www.siecus.org/pubs/fact/fact0013.html.

Gearon, C. The search for a female Viagra, *Discovery Health*, July 25, 2005. Available: http://health.discovery.com/centers/womens/viagra/viagra_print.html.

Geddes, L. Ultrasound nails location of the elusive G spot. *Independent* (February 20, 2008). Available: http://www.sensualism.com/sex/g-spot.html.

Geiger, B., Fischer, M., & Eshet, Y. Date-rape supporting and victim-blaming attitudes among high school students in a multiethnic society. *Journal of Interpersonal Violence, 19, no. 4* (April 2004), 406–426.

Geissbuehler, V., Stein, S., & Eberhard, J. Waterbirths compared with landbirths: An observational study of nine years. *Journal of Perinatal Medicine, 32* (2004), 308–314.

Gerressu, M., Mercer, C. H., Graham, C. A., Wellings, K., & Johnson, A. M. Prevalence of masturbation and associated factors in a British national probability survey. *Archives of Sexual Behavior, 37* (2008), 266–278.

Gerschick, T. J., & Miller, A. S. Coming to terms: Masculinity and physical disability, in *Men's lives*, 4th ed., Kimmel, M. S., & Messner, M. A., eds. Needham Heights, MA: Allyn & Bacon, 1998.

Gerstman, B. B., Burke, L., Delaney, J., & McLellan, B. Steroidal contraceptive use update, United States, 1989–1994. *Pharmacoepidemiology and Drug Safety, 5* (1996), 141–147.

Giedd, J. Teen brains: Still under construction. Parents play important role. *NIH News in Health* (September 2005). Available: http://newsinhealth.nih.gov.

Gillath, O., Mikulincer, M., Birnbaum, G. E., & Shaver, P. R. Does subliminal exposure to sexual stimuli have the same effects on men and women? *Journal of Sex Research, 44, 2* (April, 2007), 111–121.

Gladu, R. H. Female sexual dysfunction: Classification, physiology, diagnosis and treatment. *Journal of Sexual and Reproductive Health Medicine, 2* (2002), 21–27.

Gladue, R., Green, R., & Hellman, R. Neuroendocrine response to estrogen and sexual orientation. *Science, 225* (1983), 1496–1499.

Gold, A. R., & Adams, D. B. Motivational factors affecting fluctuations of female sexual activity at menstruation. *Psychology of Women Quarterly, 5* (1981), 670–680.

Goldberg, D. C., Whipple, B., Fishkin, R., Waxman, H., Fink, P., & Weisberg, M. The Grafenberg spot and female ejaculation: A review of initial hypotheses. *Journal of Sex and Marital Therapy, 9* (1983), 27–37.

Goldschmidt, L., Richardson, G. A., Cornelius, M. D., & Day, N. L. Prenatal marijuana and alcohol exposure and academic achievement at age 10. *Neurotoxicology and Teratology, 26* (2004), 521–532.

Goldstein, H. Making movies, mastering the media. *Teenwire.com*, (November 18, 2005).

Gonzales, L. The biology of attraction. *Men's Health, 20, no. 6* (September 2005), 186–193.

Goodale, K. R., Watkins, P. L., & Cardinal, B. J. Muscle dysmorphia: A new form of eating disorder? *American Journal of Health Education, 32, no. 5* (September/October 2001), 260–266.

Goodman, A. The long wait for male birth control. *Time* (August 3, 2008). Available: http://www.time.com/time/health/article/0.8599.1829107.00.html.

Goodnough, A., & Davey, M. Effort to track sex offenders draws resistance. *The New York Times* (February 9, 2009). Available: http://www.nytimes.com/2009/02/09/us/09offender.html?hp.

Goodson, P., McCormick, D., & Evans, A. Searching for sexually explicit materials on the Internet: An exploratory study of college students' behavior and attitudes. *Archives of Sexual Behavior, 30* (2001), 101–118.

Goodwill ambassador and former "Spice Girl" Geri Halliwell to launch British sex education web site. *Kaiser Daily Reproductive Health Report* (October 25, 2001). Available: www.kaisernetwork.org.

Gottesman, N. HIV over 50. *AARP the Magazine* (July–August 2005), 62.

Grafenberg, E. The role of urethra in female orgasm. *International Journal of Sexology, 3* (1950), 145–148.

Graham, J. The thinking woman's guide to liposuction. *American Health for Women, 16, no. 3* (April 1997), 70–75.

Grant, J. E., & Potenza, M. N. *Textbook of men's mental health.* Arlington, VA: American Psychiatric Publishing, 2006, 175.

Grant, P. Face time. *Modern Maturity, 44, no. 2* (March/April 2001): 60–69.

Gravina, G. L., Brandetti, F., Martini, P., Carosa, E., Di Stasi, S. M., Morano, S., Lenzi, A., & Jannini, E. A. Measurement of the thickness of the urethrovaginal space in women with or without vaginal orgasm. *Journal of Sexual Medicine, 5* (2008), 610–618.

Graziottin, A. Female sexual dysfunction: Clinical approach. *Urodinamica, 14* (2004), 105–111.

Greenberg, J. A. Hysteroscopic sterilization: History and current methods. *Reviews in Obstetrics and Gynecology, 1, 3* (Summer 2008), 113–121.

Greenberg, J. S. A study of the self-esteem and alienation of male homosexuals. *Journal of Psychology 83* (1973), 137–43.

Greenberg, J. S. *Comprehensive stress management,* 11th ed. New York: McGraw-Hill Higher Education, 2009.

Greenberg, J. S., Bruess, C. E., & Mullen, K. D. *Sexuality: Insights and issues.* Madison, WI: WCB Brown & Benchmark, 1986.

Greenhouse, L. Court blocks law regulating Internet access to pornography. *The New York Times* (June 30, 2004).

Greenhouse, L. Justices back law to make libraries use Internet filters. *New York Times* (June 24, 2003). Available: www.nytimes.com.

Greenwood, S. Women's health: Menstrual cramps. *Medical Self-Care* (November/December 1986), 20–21.

Grimes, D. A. Intrauterine device and upper genital-tract infection. *Lancet, 356, 9234* (September 16, 2000), 1013–1019.

Grimsley, K. Father to get $665,000 in Maryland leave case. *The Washington Post* (August 29, 2002), EO1.

Grismaijer, S., & Singer, S.R. *Dressed to kill.* Pahoa, HI: ISCD Press, 2002.

Grossman, L. Grow up? Not so fast. *Time, 165, no. 4* (January 24, 2005), 42–53.

Grummer-Strawn, L. M., Scanlon, K. S., & Fein, S. B. Infant feeding and feeding transitions during the first year of life. *Pediatrics, 122 suppl* (2008), S36–S42.

Grunbaum, J., et. al. Youth Risk Behavior Surveillance—United States, 2003. *Surveillance Summaries, Morbidity and Mortality Weekly Report, 53.SS-2* (May 21, 2004), 1–95. Available: http://www.cdc.gov/nccdphp/dash/yrbs/.

Grunbaum, J., Kann, L., Kinchen, S., Ross, J., Hawkins, J., Lowry, R., Harris, W. A., McManus, T., Chyen, D., & Collins, J. Youth risk behavior surveillance—United States, 2003. In: *Surveillance Summaries, May 21, 2004. MMWR, 53, no. SS-2* (2004), 1–20.

Grunebaum, A., & Chervenak, F. The baby or the bathwater: Which should be discarded? *Perinatal Medicine, 32* (2004), 306–307.

Guffey, M. E. *Business communication: Process and product,* 3rd ed. Belmont, CA: Wadsworth, 1999.

Gullette, D. L., & Turner, J. G. Pros and cons of condom use among gay and bisexual men as explored via the Internet. *Journal of Community Health Nursing, 20* (2003), 161–177.

Gunasekera, H., Chapman, S., & Campbell, S. Sex and drugs in popular movies: An analysis of the top 200 films. *Journal of the Royal Society of Medicine, 98* (2005), 464–470.

Guptka, G. Gender, sexuality, and HIV/AIDS: The what, the why, and the how. *SIECUS Report, 29, no. 5* (June/July 2001), 6–12.

Guttmacher Institute. Can more progress be made? Teenage sexual and reproductive health behaviors in developed countries. In *Executive summary.* New York: Author, 2001, 1–6.

Guttmacher Institute. *Facts brief: Induced abortion in the United States.* New York: Author, 2005.

Guttmacher Institute. *Facts on contraceptive use,* January 2008a. Available: http://www.guttmacher.org/pubs/fb_contr_use.html.

Guttmacher Institute. *Facts on induced abortion in the United States,* 2009a. Available: http:///www.guttmacher.org/pubs/fb_induced_abortion.html.

Guttmacher Institute. *Sex and America's teenagers,* 1994.

Guttmacher Institute. *State facts on induced abortion in the United States,* July 2008b. Available: http:///www.guttmacher.org/pubs/fb_induced_abortion.html.

Guttmacher Institute. *State policies in brief: Abortion reporting requirements,* January 1, 2009b.

Guttmacher Institute. *State policies in brief: Bans on "partial-birth" abortion,* January 1, 2009c.

Guttmacher Institute. *State policies in brief: Counseling and waiting periods for abortion,* January 1, 2009d.

Guttmacher Institute. *State policies in brief: Parental involvement in minors' abortions,* January 1, 2009e.

Guttmacher Institute. *State policies in brief: Protecting access to clinics,* January 1, 2009f.

Guttmacher Institute. *State policies in brief: Restricting insurance coverage of abortion,* January 1, 2009g.

Guttmacher Institute. *State policies in brief: State funding for abortion under medicaid,* January 1, 2009h.

Guttmacher Institute. *State policies in brief: State policies on later-term abortions,* January 1, 2009i.

Haas, A., & Haas, K. *Understanding sexuality.* St. Louis: Times Mirror/Mosby, 1990.

Haffner, D., & Casselman, M. Toy story. *SIECUS Report, 24, no. 4.* (1996), 3–4.

Haffner, D. W. *Beyond the big talk: Every parents' guide to raising sexually healthy teens.* New York: Newmarket Press, 2001.

Haffner, D. W., & Goldfarb, E. S. But, does it work? Improving evaluations of sexuality education. Sexuality Information and Education Council of the United States, 1988.

Haffner, D. W., & Schwartz, P. *What I've learned about sex.* New York: Perigee Books, 1998.

Haffner, D. W., & Stayton, W. R. Sexuality and reproductive health, *Contraceptive technology,* 7th revised ed., Hatcher, R. A., et al. New York: Ardent Media, 1998.

Halderman, B. L., Zelhart, P. F., & Jackson, T. T. The study of fantasy: Determinants of fantasy function and content. *Journal of Clinical Psychology, 41* (1984), 325–330.

Halpern-Felsher, B. L., Cornell, J. L., Kropp, R. Y., & Tschann, J. M. Oral versus vaginal sex among adolescents: Perceptions, attitudes, and behavior. *Pediatrics, 115, no. 4* (April 2005), 845–851.

Hamer, D. H., Hu, S., Magnuson, V. L., & Spencer, T. L. A linkage between DNA markers on the X-chromosome and male sexual orientation. *Science, 261, no. 5119* (1993), 321–327.

Hamilton, B. E., Martin, J. A., & Ventura, S. J. Births: Preliminary data for 2007. *National Vital Statistics Reports, 57, 12* (March 18, 2009), 1–23.

Hammer, S. M., et al. A trial comparing nucleoside monotherapy and combination therapy in HIV-infected adults with CD4 cell count from 200 to 500 per cubic millimeter. *New England Journal of Medicine, 335* (1996), 1081–1099.

Hamson, S. The passive/active divide: What the village is teaching our children about gender. *SIECUS Report, 32, no. 3* (Summer 2004), 14–16.

Hans, J. D. Do love styles predict lifetime number of sex partners? *American Journal of Sexuality Education, 3, 2* (2008), 149–159.

Harawa, N. T., et al., Associations of race/ethnicity with HIV prevalence and HIV-related behaviors. *Journal of Acquired Immune Deficiency Syndrome, 35, no. 5* (March 2004), 526–536.

Hariton, B. E. The sexual fantasies of women. In *Psychology Today* (editors). *The female experience.* Del Mar, CA: Communications/Research/Machines, 1973.

Harmon, A. Online activity sheds its stigma as losers. *Com. New York Times* (June 29, 2003).

Harrell, G. D., & Frazier, G. L. *Marketing: Connecting with customers.* Upper Saddle River, NJ: Prentice Hall, 1999, 26.

Harris Interactive. Only a small majority still support *Roe v. Wade* and opposition is at its highest in 20 years. *Harris Poll,* March 3, 2005. Available: http://www.harrisinteractive.com/harris_poll/index.asp?PID=547.

Harris, M. B. Coming out in a school setting: Former students' experiences and opinions about disclosure, in *School experiences of gay and lesbian youth: The invisible minority,* Harris, M. B., ed. New York: Harrington Park Press/Haworth Press, 1997, 85–100.

Harvey, S. M., Beckman, L. J., & Satre, S. J. Choice of and satisfaction with methods of medical abortion among U.S. clinic patients. *Family Planning Perspectives, 33, no. 5* (2001), 212–216.

Hatcher, R. A., Trussell, J., Nelson, A. L., Stewart, F. H., & Kowal, D. *Contraceptive technology,* 19th revised ed. New York: Ardent Media, 2007.

Hatcher, R. A., Trussell, J., Stewart, F. H., Nelson, A. L., Cates, W., Guest, F., & Kowal, D. *Contraceptive technology,* 18th revised ed. New York: Ardent Media, 2004.

Hatcher, R. A., Zieman, M., et al. *A pocket guide to managing contraception.* Tiger, GA: Bridging the Gap Foundation, 2004.

Hatfield, E. Passionate and compassionate love. In *The psychology of love,* Sternberg, R., & Barnes, M., eds. New Haven: Yale University Press, 1988.

Hayes, R. D., Dennerstein, L., Bennett, C. M., & Fairley, C. K. What is the "true" prevalence of female sexual dysfunctions and does the way we assess these conditions have an impact? *Journal of Sexual Medicine, 5* (2008), 777–787.

Healthy aging for older adults. Centers for Disease Control and Prevention, 2009. Available: http://cdc.gov/print.do?url=http://www.cdc.gov/aging/.

Heath, D. An investigation into the origins of a copious vaginal discharge during intercourse—enough to wet the bed—that is not urine. *Journal of Sex Research, 20* (1984), 194–215.

Heffelfinger, J., et al. *Estimates of the number of cases of primary and secondary syphilis occurring among men who have sex with men in the United States, 1999–2002.* Presented at the 2004 National STD Prevention Conference, March 8–11, 2004. Philadelphia, PA, 2004.

Heiman, J. R. Treating low sexual desire: New findings for testosterone in women. *New England Journal of Medicine, 359* (2006), 2047–2049

Help end domestic violence, National Resource Center on Domestic violence. n.d.

Henderson, M. Scientist may be first man to find the female G-spot. *The Times* (February 21, 2008). Available: http://www.timesonline.co.uk/tol/news/uk/science/article3406113.ece.

Henshaw, S. K. *U.S. teenage pregnancy statistics with comparative statistics for women aged 20–24.* New York: Alan Guttmacher Institute, 2004.

Henshaw, S. K., & Finer, L. B. The accessibility of abortion services in the United States, 2001. *Perspectives on Sexual and Reproductive Health, 35* (2003), 16–24.

Henshaw, S. K., & Kost, K. *Trends in characteristics of women obtaining abortions, 1974–2004.* New York: Alan Guttmacher Institute, 2008.

Henslin, J. M. *Sociology,* 2nd ed. Needham Heights, MA: Allyn & Bacon, 1995.

Herdt, G. H., & Kertzner, R. I do, but I can't: The impact of marriage denial on the mental health and sexual citizenship of lesbians and gay men in the United States. *Sexuality Research & Social Policy, 3, no. 1* (March 2006), 33–44.

Herman, J. Father–daughter incest, in *Rape and sexual assault,* Burgess, A. W., ed. New York: Garland, 1985.

Heston, L., & Shields, J. Homosexuality in twins. *Archives of General Psychiatry, 18* (1968), 149–160.

Hicks, T., & Leitenberg, H. Sexual fantasies about one's partner versus someone else: Gender differences in incidence and frequency. *Journal of Sex Research, 38* (2001), 43–50.

High court to hear arguments on child porn amendment. *The Birmingham News* (October 28, 2001), 20A.

Hill, Z. E., Cleland, J., & Ali, M.M. Religious affiliation and extramarital sex among men in Brazil. *International Family Planning Perspectives, 30, no. 1* (2004), 20–26.

Hillis, S. D., Anda, R. F., Felitti, V. J., & Marchbanks, P. A. Adverse childhood experiences and sexual risk behaviors in women: A retrospective cohort study. *Family Planning Perspectives, 33, no. 5* (September/October 2001), 206–211.

History of sex surveys: Factors in the sex life of 2200 women. Trivia-Library.com (2005). Available: www.trivia-library.com.

Hitchens, C. Cardinal's law: Two questions for the pope, *Slate,* April 14, 2008. Available: http://www.slate.com/id/2188971.

Hite, S. *The Hite report.* New York: Macmillan, 1976.

Hite, S. *The Hite report on male sexuality.* New York: Alfred Knopf, 1981.

Hite, S. *Women and love: A cultural revolution in progress.* New York: Alfred Knopf, 1987.

HIV/AIDS in the United States. Atlanta, GA: U.S. Centers for Disease Control and Prevention, 2008. Available: http://www.cdc.gov/hiv/resources/factsheets/us.htm.

Hock, R. R. *Human sexuality,* 2nd ed. New York: Prentice Hall, 2007.

Hoff, C. C., McKusisk, L., Hilliard, B., & Coates, T. J. The impact of HIV antibody status on gay men's partner preferences: A community perspective. *AIDS Education and Prevention, 4* (1992), 197–204.

Hoffman, R. M. Conceptualizing heterosexual identity development: Issues and challenges. *Journal of Counseling and Development, 82* (2004), 375–380.

Hollender, M. H. Women's wish to be held: Sexual and nonsexual aspects. *Medical Aspects of Human Sexuality,* (October 1970), 12–26.

Hollywood madam caters for ladies. *BBC News* (November 11, 2005).

Holmes, M., et al. Association of dietary intake of fat and fatty acids with risk of breast cancer. *Journal of the American Medical Association, 281* (1999), 914–920.

Hoover, E. Freshmen's views: Politics, admissions, and marijuana. *Chronicle of Higher Education, 45, 21* (January 20, 2009), A18–A19.

Hoover, E. Policing public sex. *Chronicle of Higher Education, 49, no. 19* (January 17, 2003), A31.

Horgan, T. G., Mast, M. S., & Hall, J. A. Gender differences in memory for the appearance of others. *Personality and Social Psychology Bulletin, 30, no. 2* (2004), 185–196.

Hortobagyi, G. N., McLelland, R., & Reed, F. M. Your key role in breast cancer screening. *Patient Care, 24* (1990), 82–113.

Horvath, K. J., Beadnell, B., & Bowen, A. M. Sensation seeking as a moderator of Internet use on sexual risk taking among men who have sex with men. *Sexual Research and Social Policy, 3, 4* (2006), 77–90.

Hostile hallways: Bullying, teasing, and sexual harassment in school. *American Journal of Health Education, 32, no. 5* (September/October 2001), 307–309.

How popular is Danni Ashe compared to other stars? (2003). Available: www.billiondownloadwoman.com/pop.html.

How to approach treatment of the sexual addict. Sexual Recovery Institute (2001). Available: http://www.sexualrecovery.com.

Howard, D. W., & Wang, M. Q. Risk profiles of adolescent girls who were victims of dating violence. *Adolescence 3, no. 149* (2003), 1–14.

Huang, V., Munarriz, R., & Goldstein, I. Bicycle riding and erectile dysfunction: An increase in interest (and concern). *Journal of Sexual Medicine, 2* (2005), 594–595.

Hubacher, D., Lara-Ricalde, R., Taylor, D. J., Guerra-Infante, F., & Guzman-Rodriguez, R. Use of copper intra-uterine devices and the risk of tubal infertility among nulligravid women. *New England Journal of Medicine, 345, 8* (August 23, 2001), 561–567.

Hughes, Z. Dying to be thin. *Ebony* (July 2005), 72–76.

Humphreys, T. Perceptions of sexual consent: The impact of relationship history and gender. *Journal of Sex Research, 44, 4* (October 2007), 307–315.

Hunt, M. *Sexual behavior in the 1970's.* Chicago: Playboy Press, 1974.

Hunter, J. Violence against lesbian and gay male youths. *Journal of Interpersonal Violence, 5* (1990), 295–300.

Hurd, Y. L., Wang, X., Anderson, V., Beck, O., Minkoff, H., & Dow-Edwards, D. Marijuana impairs growth in midgestation fetuses. *Neurotoxicology and Teratology, 27* (2005), 221–229.

Hurt, H., Brodsky, N. L., Roth H., Malmud, E., & Giannetta, J. M. School performance of children with gestational cocaine exposure. *Neurotoxicology and Teratology, 27* (2005), 203–211.

Hutchinson, J. B., ed. *Biological determinants of sexual behavior.* New York: John Wiley & Sons (1978).

Hymowitz, C., & Weissman, M. *A history of women in America: From the founding mothers to feminists—how women shaped the life and culture of America.* New York: Bantam Books, 1978.

Hypoxyphilia/auto-erotic asphyxia. Psych-Direct 2005. Available: http://www.psychdirect.com/forensic/Criminology/para/aea.htm.

Imbornoni, A. A women's rights movement in the U.S. Available: www.infoplease.com/spot/womenstimeline3.html.

In their own right: Addressing the sexual and reproductive health needs of American men. Alan Guttmacher Institute (2002). Available: www.agi-usa.org/pubs/exs_men.html.

Increasing number of Cambodian "beer girls" selling sex. *Kaiser Daily HIV/AIDS Report* (January 15, 2003). Available: www.kaisernetwork.org/daily_reports.

India-based company to begin selling female condoms. *Kaiser Daily HIV/AIDS Report* (August 31, 2005). Available: http://www.kaisernetwork.org/daily_reports/rep_index.cfm?hint=1&DR_ID=31728.

Inki, P. Long-term use of the levonorgestrel-releasing intrauterine system. *Contraception, 75, suppl 6* (2007), s161–166.

Innala, S. M., & Ernulf, K. E. Asphyxiophilia in Scandinavia. *Archives of Sexual Behavior, 18* (1989), 181–189.

International Foundation for Gender Education (2005). Available: http://www.ifge.org/.

Intimacy and aging: Tips for sexual health and happiness. *MayoClinic.com* (November 18, 2003). Available: www.mayoclinic.com/invoke.cfm?id=HA00035.

Jacobson, J. The loneliest athletes. *Chronicle of Higher Education, 49, no. 10* (November 1, 2002a), A36–A38.

Jacobson, J. Rice U. football coach chastised for comments on gay athletes. *Chronicle of Higher Education, 49, no. 11* (November 18, 2002b), A32.

Jacoby, S. Sex in America 2005. *AARP the Magazine, 48, no. 4b* (July/August 2005), 57–62+.

James, M. S. Museum of Sex to debut in New York (2002). Available: www.ABCnews.com.

Jamieson, D. J., & Steege, J. F. The prevalence of dysmenorrhea, dyspareunia, pelvic pain, and irritable bowel syndrome in primary care practices. *Obstetrics and Gynecology, 87* (1996), 55–58.

Jamison, P. L., & Gebhard, P. H. Penis size increases between flaccid and erect states: An analysis of the Kinsey data. *Journal of Sex Research, 24* (1988), 177.

Janicek, M. F., & Averette, H. E. Cervical cancer: Prevention, diagnosis, and therapeutics. *CA: Cancer Journal for Clinicians, 51* (2001), 92–114.

Janus, S., & Janus, C. *The Janus report on sexual behavior.* New York: John Wiley & Sons, 1993.

Jarrow, J. P., & Amawalt, B. D. Two perspectives on the etiology and treatment of erectile dysfunction: A matter of the heart and the brain. *Endocrinology News, January 2006.* Chevy Chase, MD: Endocrinology Society, 2006.

Jenner, L., & Ferguson, R. 2008 Catalyst census of women corporate officers and top earners of the FP500. Catalyst, March 2009. Available: http://www.catalyst.org/publication/295/2008-catalyst-census-of-women-corporate-officers-and-top-earners-of-the-fp500.

Jensen, J. M. The evolution of Margaret Sanger's *Family Limitation* pamphlet, 1914–1921. *Journal of Women in Culture and Society, 6, 3* (Spring 1981), 548–567.

Jesdanun, A. Internet porn district clears hurdle with initial approval of .xxx domain. *The Birmingham News* (June 13, 2005), 9C.

Jimenez, J. A., & Abreu, J. M. Race and sex effects on attitudinal perceptions of acquaintance rape. *Journal of Counseling Psychology, 50, no. 2* (April 2003), 252–256.

Johnson, E. H., & Jackson, L. A. What is the significance of black–white differences in risky sexual behavior? *Journal of the National Medical Association, 86, no. 10* (October 2004), 745–759.

Johnson, K. C., & Davis B. Outcomes of planned home births with certified professional midwives: Large prospective study in North America. *British Medical Journal, 330* (2005), 1416–1422.

Johnson, R. E., Nahmias, A. J., Magder, L. S., et al. A seroepidemiologic survey of the prevalence of herpes simplex virus type 2 infection in the United States. *New England Journal of Medicine, 321* (1989), 7–12.

Johnston, J. Economy taking a toll on marriages. *Cincinnati Enquirer* (January 11, 2009).

Johnston, L. D., O'Malley, P. M., Bachman, J. G., & Schulenberg, J. E. *Monitoring the Future national results on adolescent drug use: Overview of key findings, 2008.* Bethesda, MD: National Institute of Drug Abuse, 2009.

Johnston, M. W., & Bell, A. P. Romantic emotional attachment: Additional factors in the development of the sexual orientation of men. *Journal of Counseling and Development, 73, no. 6* (July/August 1995), 621–625.

Joint United Nations Programme on HIV/AIDS. Global summary of the AIDS epidemic, December 2004. *AIDS Epidemic Update* (December 2004). Available: http://www.unaids.org/wad2004/report_pdf.html

Joint United Nations Programme on HIV/AIDS. *2004 report on the global AIDS epidemic.* Geneva, Switzerland, 2004.

Jones, J. C., & Barlow, D. H. Self-reported frequency of sexual urges, fantasies, and masturbatory fantasies in heterosexual males and females. *Archives of Sexual Behavior, 19* (1990), 269–279.

Jones, M. A. A few statistics on LGBT issues. *Gay Rights* (2009). Available: http://gayrights.change.org/blog/view/a_few_statistics_on_lgbt_issues.

Jones, R. K., Zolna, M. R. S., Henshaw, S. K., & Finer, L. B. Abortion in the United States: Incidence and access to services, 2005. *Perspectives on Sexual and Reproductive Health, 40* (2008), 6–16.

Joseph, C. Scarlet wounding: Issues of child prostitution. *Journal of Psychohistory, 23, no. 1* (1995), 2–17.

Joseph, J. Singing the push-up blues, *ABCNews.com* (September 7, 1998).

Joyce, J. *Ulysses.* New York: Random House, 1934.

Judge voids same-sex marriage ban in Nebraska. *The New York Times* (May 13, 2005).

Just the facts about sexual orientation and youth. Washington, DC: American Psychological Association, 2000.

Kahn, A. The estrogen dilemma: Osteoporosis forces hard choices on older women. *Medical Self-Care* (Winter 1984), 40–45.

Kaiser Family Foundation and *Seventeen* magazine release latest SexSmarts survey on teen sexual behavior. Kaiser Family Foundation (July 9, 2002). Available: www.kaisernetwork.org/daily_reports.

Kaiser Family Foundation. *U.S. teen sexual activity,* 2005. Available: http://www.kff.org/youthhivstds/upload/U-S-Teen-Sexual-Activity-Fact-Sheet.pdf.

Kakuchi, S. Japan only now confronting rising HIV rate—women in sex trade most at risk. *San Francisco Chronicle* (March 17, 2003), A8.

Kalant, H. Adverse effects of cannabis on health: An update of the literature since 1996. *Progress in Neuropsychopharmacology and Biological Psychiatry, 28* (2004), 849–863.

Kalichman, S. C., & Cherry, C. Male polyurethane condoms do not enhance brief HIV-STD risk reduction interventions for heterosexually active men: Results from a randomized test of concept. *International Journal of STD & AIDS, 10, 8* (1999), 548–553.

Kallman, F. J. Comparative twin study on the genetic aspects of male homosexuality. *Journal of Nervous and Mental Disease, 115* (1952), 283–298.

Kalmus, D., Davidson, A., Cohall, A., Laraque, D., & Cassell, C. Preventing sexual risk behaviors and pregnancy among teenagers: Linking research and programs. *Perspectives on Sexual and Reproductive Health, 35, no. 2* (March/April 2003).

Kanin, E. J. False rape allegations. *Archives of Sexual Behavior, 32, no. 1* (1994), 81–92.

Kaplan, H. S. *Disorders of sexual desire.* New York: Simon & Schuster, 1979.

Kaplan, H. S. *The evaluation of sexual disorders.* New York: Brunner/Mazel, 1983.

Kaplan, H. S. *How to overcome premature ejaculation.* New York: Brunner/Mazel, 1989.

Kaplan, H. S. *The new sex therapy: Active treatment of sexual dysfunction.* New York: Brunner/Mazel, 1974.

Kaplan, H. S. *Sexual aversion, sexual phobias, and panic disorder.* New York: Brunner/Mazel, 1989.

Kardel, K. R. Effects of intense training during and after pregnancy in top-level athletes. *Scandinavian Journal of Medicine in Science and Sports, 15* (2005), 79–86.

Karofsky, P. F. Relationship between adolescent–parental communication and initiation of first intercourse by adolescents. *Journal of Adolescent Health, 28, no. 1* (January 2001), 41–45.

Kasindorf, M., Bayles, F., & Grossman, C. L. Boston church scandal starts chain reaction. *USA Today* (December 19, 2002), 13A.

Katz, J. E. Empirical and theoretical dimension of obscene calls to women in the United States. *Human Communication Research, 21* (1994), 155–182.

Katzenstein, D. A., et al. The relation of virologic and immunologic markers to clinical outcomes after nucleoside therapy in HIV-infected adults with CD4 cell count from 200 to 500 per cubic millimeter. *England Journal of Medicine, 335* (1996), 1091–1098.

Kaufman, M. Impotence drugs will get blindness warning. *Washington Post* (July 9, 2005) p. A6.

Kaufman, M. Morning-after pill study contradicts claim by foes: Easy access did not lead to riskier behavior. *Washington Post* (January 5, 2005), p. A09.

Keeping kids sexually safe. *Families Are Talking 3, no. 3* (2004),1–4.

Kegel, A. Sexual functions of the pubococcyngeus muscle. *Western Journal of Surgery, Obstetrics, and Gynecology, 60* (1952), 521–524.

Kemper, M., & Rodriguez, M. Talk about sex. SIECUS, 2005. Available: http://www.siecus.org/_data/global/images/TalkAboutSex.pdf.

Kempner, M. E. Marriage: Institution or relationship? *SIECUS Report, 33, no. 1* (winter 2005), 2–4.

Kempner, M. E. Sex workers: A glimpse into public health perspectives. *SIECUS Report, 33, no. 2* (Spring 2005), 2.

Kendall-Tackett, K., & Marshall, R. Sexual victimization of children: Incest and child sexual abuse, in *Issues in intimate violence,* Bergen, R. K., ed. Thousand Oaks, CA: Sage, 1988.

Kenney, J. W., Reinholtz, C., & Angellini, P. J. Ethnic differences in childhood and adolescent sexual abuse and teenage pregnancy. *Journal of Adolescent Health 21, no. 1* (1997), 3–10.

Kerber, L. K. Moving beyond stereotypes of feminism. *Chronicle of Higher Education, 45, no. 33* (April 23, 1999), B6–B8.

Kershaw, S. A life as a Live! Nude! Girl! has a few strings attached. *The New York Times* (June 2, 2004).

Keverne, E. B. Importance of olfactory and vomeronasal systems for male sexual function. *Physiology and Behavior, 83* (2004), 177–187.

Key, W. B. *Subliminal seduction.* Englewood Cliffs, NJ: Prentice Hall, 1973.

Khanobdee, C., Sukratanachaiyakul, V., & Gay, J. T. Couvade syndrome in expectant Thai fathers. *International Journal of Nursing Studies, 30* (1993), 125–131.

Kiecolt-Glaser, J. The risks of marital discord. *U.S. News & World Report* (January 28 2009). Available: http://researchnews.osu.edu/archive/fighting.htm.

Kiehl, S. I can't go on like this. *The Birmingham News* (July 17, 2005), 1E+.

King, V. A Comparison of cohabiting relationships among older and younger adults. *Journal of Marriage & Family, 67, no. 2* (January 2005), 271–285.

Kingston, D. A., Malamuth, N. M., Federoff, P., & Marshall, W. L. The importance of individual differences in pornography use: Theoretical perspectives and implications for treating sexual offenders. *Journal of Sex Research, 46, 2 & 3* (March 2009), 216–232.

Kinsey, A. C., Pomeroy, W. B., & Martin, C. E. *Sexual behavior in the human female.* Philadelphia: Saunders, 1953.

Kinsey, A. C., Pomeroy, W. B., & Martin, C. E. *Sexual behavior in the human male.* Philadelphia: Saunders, 1948.

The Kinsey Institute. *The history and concept of sexology,* 1998.

Kirby, D. *Do abstinence-only programs delay the initiation of sex among young people and reduce teen pregnancy?* Washington, DC: National Campaign to Prevent Teen Pregnancy, 2002a.

Kirby, D. Effective approaches to reducing adolescent unprotected sex, pregnancy, and childbearing. *Journal of Sex Research, 39, no. 7* (2002b), 51–58.

Kirby, D. *Emerging answers: Research findings on programs to reduce sexual risk-taking and teen pregnancy.* Washington, DC: National Campaign to Prevent Teen Pregnancy, 2001.

Kirby, D. *Emerging answers 2007: Research findings on programs to reduce teen pregnancy and sexually transmitted diseases.* Washington, DC: National Campaign to Prevent Teen and Unplanned Pregnancy, 2007.

Kirby, D., & Coyle, K. Changing risk-taking behavior: Preliminary conclusions from research, in *The sexuality education challenge,* Drolet, J. C., & Clark, K., eds. Santa Cruz, CA: ETR Associates, 1994.

Kirby, D., Lepore, G., & Ryan, J. Executive summary: Sexual risk and protective factors, in *Putting what works to work,* ETR Associates (September 2005).

Klach, D. *Woman plus woman: Attitudes toward lesbianism.* New York: Simon & Schuster, 1974.

Klein, H. Couvade syndrome: Male counterpart to pregnancy. *International Journal of Psychiatry Medicine, 21* (1991), 57–69.

Klitsch, M. Subgroups of U.S. women differ widely on exposure to sexual intercourse. *Family Planning Perspectives, 22* (1990), 94–95.

Kluger, J. What's sex got to do with it? *Time, 161, no. 3* (January 20, 2003), 35.

Knafo, G., & Jaffe, Y. Sexual fantasizing in males and females. *Journal of Research in Personality 19* (1984), 451–62.

Knopik, V. S., Sparrow, E. P., Madden, P. A., Bucholz, K. K., Hudziak, J. J., Reich, W., Slutske, W. S., Grant, J. D., McLaughlin, T. L., Todorov, A., Todd, R. D., & Heath, A. C. Contributions of parental alcoholism, prenatal substance exposure, and genetic transmission to child ADHD risk: A female twin study. *Psychological Medicine, 35* (2005), 625–635.

Koch grants benefits for domestic partners. *Washington Post* (August 8, 1989), A6.

Koch, P. B. Women's bodies as a "puzzle" for college men: Grounded theory research. *American Journal of Sexuality Education, 1, 3* (2006), 51–72.

Koernig, S. K., & Granitz, N. Progressive yet traditional: The portrayal of women compared to that of men in e-commerce magazine advertisements. *Journal of Advertising, 35, 2* (2006), 81–98.

Kolata, G. Deadliness of breast cancer in blacks defies easy answer. *The New York Times* (August 3, 1994), C10.

Kolodny, R. C., Masters, W. H., & Johnson, V. E. *Textbook of sexual medicine.* Boston: Little, Brown, 1979.

Koss-Feder, L. Bunking in with mom and dad. *Time, 173, 8* (March 2, 2009), 537.

Koutedakis, Y., & Jamurtas A. The dancer as a performing athlete: Physiological considerations. *Sports Medicine, 34* (2004), 651–661.

Kraemer, B., Delsignore, A., Schnyder, U., & Hepp, U. Body image and transsexualism. *Psychopathology, 41, 2* (December 2008), 96–100.

Krans, E. E., Gearhart, J. G., Dubbert, P. M., Klar, P. M., Miller, A. L., & Replogle, W. H. Pregnant women's beliefs and influences regarding exercise during pregnancy. *Journal of the Mississippi Medical Association, 46* (2005), 67–73.

Krilov, L. R. What do you know about genital warts? *Medical Aspects of Human Sexuality, 25* (1991), 43–45.

Kristof, N. Cambodia, where sex traffickers are king. *The New York Times* (January 15, 2005).

Kronenberg, F., & Fugh-Berman, A. Complementary and alternative medicine for menopausal symptoms: A review of randomized, controlled trials. *Annals of Internal Medicine, 137* (2002), 805–813.

Kuchment, A., & Springen, K. The tangled web of porn in the office. *Newsweek* (December 8, 2008), 14.

Kuck, D. L., & Johnson, B. E. *Criminal sanctions in context: A date rape scenario.* Presented at the Southern Sociological Society, 2003.

Kurdek, L. A. Are gay and lesbian cohabiting couples really different from heterosexual married couples? *Journal of Marriage & Family, 66, no. 4* (November 2004), 880–900.

Kuriansky, J. Sexuality and television advertising: An historical perspective. *SIECUS Report, 24, no. 5* (June/July 1996), 13.

Kuyoh, M. A., Toroitich-Ruto, C., Grimes, D. A., Schulz, K. F., & Gallo, M. F. Sponge versus diaphragm for contraception: a Cochrane review. *Contraception, 67, no. 1* (2003). 15–18.

LaFraniere, S. Entrenched epidemic: Wife-beatings in Africa. *The New York Times* (August 11, 2005).

Lanuza, E., Novejarque, A., Martinez-Hernandez, J., Agustin-Pavon, C., & Martinez-Garcia, F. Sexual phero-mones and the evolution of the reward system of the brain: The chemosensory function of the amygdala. *Brain Research Bulletin, 75* (2008), 460–466.

Larsen, D. What are some signs of incest? About incest abuse 2005b. Available: http://incestabuse.about.com/cs /incestrecovery/f/incestafraid_p.htm.

Larsen, D. Why would children be afraid to tell about incest? About incest abuse 2005a. Available: http://incestabuse. about.com/cs/incestrecovery/f/ incestafraid_p.htm.

Larsson, L. L. Low-impact exercise during pregnancy—a study of safety. *ACTA Obstetricia et Gynecologica Scandinavica, 84* (2005), 34–38.

Laumann, E. O., Gagnon, J. H., Michael, R. T., & Michaels, S. *The social organization of sexuality: Sexual practices in the United States.* Chicago: University of Chicago Press, 1994.

Laumann, E. O., Michael, R. T., & Gagnon, J.-H. A political history of the National Sex Survey of Adults. *Family Planning Perspectives, 26, no. 1* (January/February 1994), 634–638.

Laumann, E. O., Paik, A., & Rosen, R. C. Sexual dysfunction in the United States: Prevalence and predictors. *Journal of the American Medical Association, 281* (1999), 537–544.

Lee, J. Love-styles, in *The psychology of love,* Sternberg, R., & Barnes, M., eds. New Haven: Yale University Press, 1988.

Lee, J., Pomeroy, E. C., Yoo, S. K., & Rheinboldt, K. T. Attitudes toward rape—a comparison between Asian and Caucasian college students. *Violence Against Women, 11, no. 2* (February 2005), 177–196.

Lee, U. J., & Jones, J. S. Incidence of prostate cancer in male breast cancer patients: A risk factor for prostate cancer screening. *Prostate Cancer and Prostatic Diseases* (May 27, 2008).

Leff, L. Court rules country club treated lesbians unfairly. *The Birmingham News* (August 2, 2005), 4A.

Lefkowitz, E. S., Gillen, M. M., Shearer, C. L., & Boone, T. L. Religiosity, sexual behaviors, and sexual attitudes during emerging childhood. *Journal of Sex Research, 41, no. 2* (May 2004), 150–159.

Lehfeldt, H. Margaret Sanger and the modern contraceptive techniques. *Journal of Sex Research, 3, 4* (November 1967), 253–255.

Leiblum, S. Sex-starved marriages sweeping the US. *Sexual & Relationship Therapy, 18* (2003), 427–428.

Leiblum, S. R., & Pervin, L. A. *Principles and practice of sex therapy.* New York: Guilford Press, 1980.

Leitenberg, H., Greenwald, E., & Tarran, M. The relation between sexual activity among children during preadolescence and/or early adolescence and sexual behavior and sexual adjustment in young adulthood. *Archives of Sexual Behavior, 18, no. 4* (1989), 299–313.

Leitenberg, H., & Henning, K. Sexual fantasy. *Psychological Bulletin, 117* (1995), 469–496.

Lescano, C. M., Houck, C. D., Brown, L. K., Doherty, G., DiClemente, R. J., Fernandez, M. I., Pugatch, D., Schlenger, W. E., & Silver, B. J. Correlates of heterosexual anal intercourse among at-risk adolescents and young adults. *American Journal of Public Health, 99* (2009), 1131–1136.

LeVay, S. A difference in hypothalmic structure between heterosexual and homosexual men. *Science, 253* (1991), 1034–1037.

Levin, R., & Levin, A. Sexual pleasure: The surprising preferences of 100,000 women. *Redbook* (September 1975), 38.

Lewis, J. E., Malow, R. M., & Ireland, S. J. HIV/AIDS risk in heterosexual college students: A review of a decade of literature. *Journal of American College Health, 45, no. 4* (1997), 147–158.

Lewis, R. Genetic screening—fetal signposts on a journey of discovery. *FDA Consumer, 24* (1990), 17–23.

Lewis, R. W., Fugl-Meyer, K. S., Bosch, R., Fugl-Meyer, A. R., Laumann, E. O., E. Lizza, E., & Martin-Morales, A. Epidemiology/risk factors of sexual dysfunction. *Journal of Sexual Medicine, 1* (2004), 35–39.

Liebowitz, M. *The chemistry of love.* Boston: Little, Brown, 1983.

Linberg, L. D., & Singh, S. Sexual behavior of single adult American women. *Perspectives on Sexual and Reproductive Health, 40* (2008), 27–33.

Lindau, S. T., Schumm, L. P., Laumannm, E. O., Levinson, W., O'Muircheartaigh, C. A., & Waite, L. J. A study of sexuality and health among older adults in the United States. *New England Journal of Medicine, 357, 8* (August 23, 2007), 762–774.

Link, A., & Copeland, P. Sexual magnetism: Pheromones—the scent of sex. *Urban Male Magazine* (Winter 2001), 38–39.

Lipka, S. Feminine critique. *Chronicle of Higher Education, 50, no. 37* (May 21, 2004), A35–36.

Lipman, J. J. A qualitative analysis of women's relational and sexual functioning following date rape. *Dissertation*

Abstracts International, 63, no. 3-B (September 2002), 1567.

Lips, H. The gender wage gap: Debunking the rationalizations. Center for Gender Studies (2005). Available: http:// www.womensmedia.com/new/ Lips-Hilary-gender-wage-gap.shtml.

Liptak, A. California ruling expands same-sex parental rights. *The New York Times* (August 23, 2005). Available: http://www.nytimes.com/2005/08/23/ national/23gay.html.

Listening to understand. *The Pryor Report Success Workshop,* a supplement to *The Pryor Report Management Newsletter* (August 1998).

Litman, R. E. Bondage and sadomasochism, in *Sexual dynamics of anti-social behavior,* 2nd ed., Schlesinger, L. B. & Revitch, E., eds. Springfield, IL: Charles C. Thomas, 1997.

Little, K. Sexual assault nurse examiner (SANE) programs: Improving the community response to sexual assault victims. *OVC Bulletin* (2005). Available: http://www.ojp.usdoj.gov/.

Liu, C. Does quality of marital sex decline with duration? *Archives of Sexual Behavior, 32, no. 1* (February 2003), 55–60.

Living together before marriage may hurt—not help—chances of successful match. *InteliHealth* (July 25, 2002). Available: www.intelihealth.com.

Lohr, S. In video game, a download unlocks hidden sex scenes. *The New York Times* (July 11, 2005).

Long, C. Female magazines evolve to feature flabby. *Intelihealth.* Harvard Medical School's Consumer Health Information (2005). Available: http://www. intelihealth.com.

LoPiccolo, J. Direct treatment of sexual dysfunction in the couple, in *Handbook of sexology,* Money, J., & Masaph, H., eds. Amsterdam: Elsevier/North-Holland, 1977, 1227–1244.

Lotozo, E. Pair seek to give true picture of young gay America. *Knight Ridder Newspapers* (June 4, 2003). Available: www.glsen.org.

Louis Harris and Associates, Inc. *In their own words: Adolescent girls discuss health and health care issues.* New York: Commonwealth Fund, 1997.

Lowe, B. D., Schrader, S. M., & Breitenstein, M. J. Effect of bicycle saddle designs on the pressure to the perineum of the bicyclist. *Medicine and Science in Sports and Exercise, 36* (2004), 1055–1062.

Luscombe, B. Pumping it up, *Time, 58, no. 11* (September 3, 2001), Y26.

Lynch, A., McDuffie, R., Murphy, J., et al. Preeclampsia in multiple gestation: The role of assisted reproductive technologies. *Journal of Obstetrics and Gynecology, 93* (2002), 445–451.

MacGeorge, E. L., Graves, A. R., Feng, B., & Gillihan, S. J. The myth of gender cultures: Similarities outweigh differences in men's and women's provision of and responses to supportive communication. *Sex Roles, 50* (2004), 143–175.

MacWilliams, B. Turning tricks for tuition. *Chronicle of Higher Education, 49, no. 11* (November 8, 2002), A48.

Magann, E. F. Antepartum, intrapartum, and neonatal significance of exercise on healthy low-risk pregnant working women, *Obstetrics and* Gynecology, *99* (2002), 466–472.

Mahoney, P., & Williams, L. M. Sexual assault in marriage: Prevalence, consequences, and treatment of wife rape, in *U.S. Air Force domestic violence literature review,* 1998.

Males, females and evolution: An interview with Helen Fisher. *Family Life Matters 43* (Spring 2001), 1, 4–5.

Mallon, R. *Demonstration of vestigial prostate tissue in the human female.* (October 1984). Paper presented at the Annual Regional Conference of the American Association of Sex Educators, Counselors, and Therapists, Las Vegas, NV.

Maltz, W., & Boss, S. *Private thoughts.* Novalo, CA: New World Library, 2001.

Mancini, J., & Orthner, D. Recreational sexuality preferences among middle-class husbands and wives. *Journal of Sex Research, 14* (1978), 95–106.

Manlove, J., Ikramullah, E., & Terry-Humen, E. Condom use and consistency among male adolescents in the United States. *Journal of Adolescent Health, 43, 4* (October 2008), 325–333.

Manusov, V., Floyd, K., & Kerssen-Griep, J. Yours, mine, and ours. *Communication Research, 24, no. 3* (1997), 234–260.

Many people with HIV don't tell partners and don't use condoms, study shows. *The Nation's Health* (March 1998), 2.

Marceau, L., Kleinman, K., Goldstein, I., & McKinlay, J. Does bicycling contribute to the risk of erectile dysfunction? Results from the Massachusetts Male Aging Study (MMAS). *International Journal of Impotence Research, 13* (2001), 298–302.

March of Dimes. *Birth defects,* 2006a. Available: http://search.marchofdimes.com/cgi-bin/MsmGo.exe?grab_id=6&page_id=10027264&query=birth+defects&hiword=BIRTHED+BIRTHING+BIRTHS+DEFECT+DEFECTIVE+DEFECTOS+birth+defects+.

March of Dimes. *HIV and AIDS in pregnancy.* White Plains, NY: March of Dimes, 2005. Available: http://search.marchofdimes.com/cgi-bin/MsmGo.exe?grab_id=532&page_id=5966592&query=HIV&hiword=HIV+.

March of Dimes. *Illicit drug use during pregnancy,* 2006b. Available: http://www.marchofdimes.com/professionals/14332_1169.asp.

Marelich, W. D., Lundquist, J., Painter, K., & Mechanic, M. B. Sexual deception as a social exchange process: Development of a behavior-based deception scale. *Journal of Sex Research, 45, 1* (January 2008), 27–35.

Marinoble, R. M. Homosexuality: A blind spot in the school mirror. *Professional School Counseling, 1, no. 3* (February 1998), 4–7.

Marital rape. Indiana Coalition Against Sexual Assault, 2000. Available: http://www.incasa.org/PDF/Brochures/Marital_Rape.pdf.

Marks, G., et al. Self-disclosure of HIV infection to sexual partners. *American Journal of Public Health, 81* (1991), 1321–1323.

Marret, S. Effects of maternal smoking during pregnancy on fetal brain development. *Journal de Gynecologie, Obstetrique et Biologie de la Reproduction, 34* (2005), 230–233.

Marriages and divorces, 1900–2004. *Infoplease.* Available: http://print.infoplease.com/ipa/A0005044.html.

Marsh, R., Steinglass, J. E., Gerber, A. J., O'Leary, K. G., Wang, Z., Murphy, D., Walsh, T., & Peterson, B. S. Deficient activity in the neural systems that mediate self-regulatory control in bulimia nervosa. *Archives of General Psychiatry, 66, 1* (2009), 51–63.

Martin, D., & Lyon, P. *Lesbian-woman.* New York: Bantam (1972).

Martin, J. A., et al. Births: Final data for 2006. *National Vital Statistics Reports, 57* (2009).

Martin, J. A., Hamilton, B. E., Sutton, P. D., Ventura, S. J., Menacker, F., Kirmeyer, S., & Mathews, T. J. Births: Final data for 2006. *National Vital Statistics Reports, 57, 7* (January 7, 2009), 102.

Martin, J. A., Hamilton, B. E., & Ventura, S. J. Births: Preliminary data for 2000. *National Vital Statistics Report, 49, no. 5* (2001), 1–20.

Martins, Y., Tiggemann, M., & Churchett, L. The shape of things to come: Gay men's satisfaction with specific body parts. *Psychology of Men and Masculinity, 9, 4* (October 2008), 248–256.

Marx, B. P. Lessons learned from the last twenty years of sexual violence research. *Journal of Interpersonal Violence, 20, no. 2* (February 2005), 225–230.

Maslow, A. H. *Toward a psychology of being,* 2nd ed. Princeton, NJ: Van Nostrand, 1968.

Masochism. University of Iowa Health Care (2001). Available: www.uihealthcare.com/topics/mentalemotionalhealth/ment3155.html.

Mason, G. E., & Riger, S. The impact of past sexual experiences on attributions of responsibility for rape, *Journal of Interpersonal Violence, 19, no. 10* (October 2004), 1157–1171.

Masoni, S., Maio, A., Trimarchi, G., de Punzio, C., & Fioretti, P. The couvade syndrome, *Journal of Psychosomatic Obstetrics and Gynaecology, 15* (1994), 125–131.

Masters, W. H., & Johnson, V. E. *Homosexuality in perspective.* Boston: Little, Brown, 1979.

Masters, W. H., & Johnson, V. E. *Human sexual inadequacy.* Boston: Little, Brown, 1970.

Masters, W. H., & Johnson, V. E. *Human sexual response.* Boston: Little, Brown, 1966.

Masters, W. H., Johnson, V. E., & Kolodny, R. C. *Human sexuality.* Boston: Little, Brown, 1982.

Masters, W. H., Johnson, V. E., & Kolodny, R. C. *Human sexuality,* 2nd ed. Boston: Little, Brown, 1985.

Matteo, S., & Rissman, E. Increased sexual activity during the midcycle portion of the human menstrual cycle. *Hormones and Behavior, 18* (1984), 249–255.

Mayer Laboratories. Mayer labs acquires Today sponge distribution rights, April 6, 2009. Available: http://www.mayerlabs.com/images/pdf/today-media-kit.pdf.

Maynard, R. A., Trenholm, C., Devaney, B., Johnson, A., Clark, M. A., Homrighausen, J., & Kalay, E. *First-year impacts of four Title V, Section 510 abstinence education programs.* Princeton, NJ: Mathematica Policy Research, June 2005.

Mayo Clinic. *Ask a Women's Health Specialist: Premenstrual dysphoric disorder (PMDD): A severe form of PMS.* Rochester, MN: Author, 2008. Available: http://www.mayoclinic.com/health/pmdd/AN01372.

Mayo Clinic. *Sex education: Talking to toddlers and preschoolers about sex,* 2009. Available: http://www.mayoclinic.com/health/sex-education/HQ00547.

Mayo Clinic. *Women's health: Amenorrhea.* Rochester, MN: Author, 2007a. Available: http://www.mayoclinic.com/health/amenorrhea/DS00581/DSECTION=causes.

Mayo Clinic. *Women's health: Premenstrual syndrome (PMS).* Rochester, MN: Author, 2007b. Available: http://www.mayoclinic.com/health/premenstrual-syndrome/DS00134.

Mayo Health Clinic. *Dietary suggestions for premenstrual syndrome,* 1998.

Mayo Clinic Staff. *Genital herpes. MayoClinic.com,* 2008a. Available: http://www.mayoclinic.com/health/genital-herpes/DS00179/DSECTION=treatments-and-drugs.

Mayo Clinic Staff. *Infertility: Causes,* 2007a. Available: http://www.mayoclinic.com/health/infertility/ds00310/dsection=causes.

Mayo Clinic Staff. *Pregnancy nutrition: Essential nutrients when you're eating for two,* 2007b. Available: http://www.mayoclinic.com/health/pregnancy-nutrition/PR00110.

Mayo Clinic Staff. *Premature ejaculation. MayoClinic.com,* 2007c. Available: http://www.mayoclinic.com/health/premature-ejaculation/DS00578/DSECTION=causes.

Mayo Clinic Staff. *Vaginal yeast infections: Are home remedies effective? MayoClinic.com,* 2008b. Available: http://www.mayoclinic.com/print/vaginal-yeast-infection/AN01308/METHOD=print.

McCabe, M. P., & Wauchope, M. Behavioral characteristics of men accused of rape: Evidence for different types of rapists. *Archives of Sexual Behavior, 34, no. 2* (April 2005), 241–253.

McCarthy, B. W., Ryan, M., & Johnson, F. A. *Sexual awareness: A practical approach.* San Francisco: Boyd & Fraser, 1975.

McCarthy, P. Ageless sex, *Psychology Today* (March 1989), 62.

McClain, D. L. Sex and chess: Is she a queen or a pawn? *The New York Times* (November 27, 2005).

McConaghy, N. Pedophilia: A review of the evidence. *Australian and New Zealand Journal of Psychiatry, 32, no. 2* (1998), 252–265.

McCormack, W., ed. *Chlamydia.* Chicago: Abbott Laboratories Diagnostic Division, 1984.

McDonald, T. W., & Kline, L. M. Perceptions of appropriate punishment for committing date rape: Male college students recommend lenient punishments. *College Student Journal, 38, no. 1* (March 2004), 44–57.

McEwan, S. L., DeMan, A. F., & Simpson-Housley, P. Acquaintance rape, ego-identity achievement, and locus of control. *Social Behavior and Personality, 33, no. 6* (2005), 587–592.

McFarland, M. B., & Kaminski, P. L. Men, muscles, and mood: The relationship between self-concept, dysphoria, and body image disturbances. *Eating Behavior, 10, 1* (January 10, 2009), 68–70.

McGee, R. Don't look at me. National Sexuality Resource Center, April 17, 2007. Available: http://nsrc.sfsu.edu/print/2641.

McGuire, T. R. Is homosexuality genetic? A critical review and some suggestions. *Journal of Homosexuality, 28, nos. 1–2* (1995), 115–145.

McKeen, C. A. Gender roles: An examination of the hopes and expectations of the next generation of managers in Canada and China. *Sex Roles, 52, nos. 7–8* (April 2005), 533–546.

McKinley, J. Gay marriage ban inspires new wave of activists. *The New York Times* (December 10, 2008).

McLennen, J. C. Domestic violence between same-gender partners: Recent findings and future research. *Journal of Interpersonal Violence, 20, no. 2* (February 2005), 149–154.

McMillan, M. Cervical scanner. *Washington Post* (September 14, 2004), HE2.

McQueen, A. Study: Debt, anxiety sway women from college, *AP/AOL* (June 10, 1999).

Meckler, L. American family becomes more traditional, complex. *The Birmingham News* (April 13, 2001), 5A.

Meckler, L. Bush-era abortion rules face possible reversal. *The Wall Street Journal* (December 17, 2008), A5.

Meese, M. Backlash: Women bullying women at work. *The New York Times* (May 10, 2009). Available: http://www.nytimes.com/2009/05/10/business/10women.html.

Meilman, P. W., Riggs, P., & Turco, J. H. A college health services' response to sexual assault issues. *Journal of American College Health, 39* (1990), 145–147.

Memmott, M. Slavery, related abuses growing worldwide, report says. *USA Today* (May 25, 2001), 13A.

Men suffer from phantom pregnancy. *BBC Home,* 2007. Available: http://news.bbc.co.uk/1/hi/health/6751709.stm.

Men, women more different than thought. *Intelihealth* (September 27, 2004), Available: http://www.intelihealth.com.

Menopause. National Institute on Aging, 2008. Available: http://www.nia.nih.gov/HealthInformation/Publications/menopause.htm.

Michael, R., Gagnon, J., Laumann, E., & Kolata, G. *Sex in America.* Boston: Little, Brown, 1994.

Michael, R. T., Gagnon, J. H., Laumann, E. O., & Kolata, G. *Sex in America: A definitive survey.* New York: Warner Books, 1995.

Michaels, M. A church plan on sex abuse. *Time, 160, no. 22* (November 25, 2002), 25.

Michels, T. M., Kropp, R. Y., Eyre, S. L., & Halpern-Felsher, B. L. Initiating sexual experiences: How do young adolescents make decisions regarding early sexual activity? *Journal of Research on Adolescence, 15* (2005), 583–607.

Middleton, D. R. *Exotics and erotics: Human cultural and sexual diversity.* Long Grove, IL: Waveland Press, 2002.

MIDIRS. *Informed choice: The use of water during childbirth.* Bristol, UK: Author, 2005.

Military "don't tell" policy hushes up rape and sexual assault. National Organization for Women (2003). Available: http://www.now.org.

Miller, D. W., & Sharlet, J. The Adonis complex studies men's obsession with a "male body ideal": Physicist examines "the soul-battering system" that envelops professionals. *Chronicle of Higher Education,* Research & Publishing section, May 26, 2000. Available: http://chronicle.com/.

Miller, M. More men turning to implants to enhance pecs. *The Birmingham News* (November 26, 2002), 1D, 3D.

Miller, S. A., & Byers, E. S. Actual and desired duration of foreplay and intercourse: Discordance and misperceptions within heterosexual couples. *Journal of Sex Research, 41, no. 3* (August 2004), 301–309.

Miller-Loncar, C., Lester, B. M., Seifer, R., Lagasse, L. L., Bauer, C. R., Shankaran, S., Bada, H. S., Wright, L. L., Smeriglio, V. L., Bigsby, R., & Liu, J. Predictors of motor development in children prenatally exposed to cocaine. *Neurotoxicology and Teratology, 27* (2005), 213–220.

Mind on the Media. Inspiring independent thinking and fostering critical analysis of media messages, 2009. Available: http://www.mindonthemedia.org/index.php?type=static&page=shocking.

Mind over fatter: The bulk of bigorexia (2005). Available: http://www.mindoverfatter.co.za/html/bigorexia.htm.

Minnes, S., Singer, L. T., Arendt, R., & Satayathum, S. Effects of prenatal cocaine/polydrug use on maternal-infant feeding interactions during the first year of life. *Journal of Developmental Behavioral Pediatrics, 26* (2005), 194–200.

Mitchell, K. J., Finkelhor, D., & Wolak, J. The Internet and family and acquaintance sexual abuse. *Child Maltreatment, 10, no.1* (February 2005), 49–60.

Moelker, W. Treatment of aversion. *Web4Health* (2003). Available: http://web4health.info/en/answers/sex-dislike-treat.htm.

Money, J. *Gay, straight, and in-between.* New York: Oxford University Press, 1988.

Money, J. Paraphilias: Phenomenology and classification. *American Journal of Psychotherapy, 38, no. 2* (April 1984), 164–179.

Money, J. Pornography in the home, in *Contemporary sexual behavior,* Zubin, J., & Money, J., eds. Baltimore: Johns Hopkins Press, 1973.

Money, J. Sin, sickness, or status: Homosexual gender identity and psychoneuroendocrinology. *American Psychologist, 42* (1987), 384–399.

Money, J., & Athanasiou, R. Pornography: Review and bibliographic annotations. *American Journal of Obstetrics and Gynecology, 115* (January 1973), 130–146.

Money, J., & Ehrhardt, A. E. *Man and woman, boy and girl.* Baltimore: Johns Hopkins Press, 1972.

Money, J., & Schwartz, M. Dating, romantic and nonromantic friendships and sexuality in 17 early-treated androgenital females, aged 16–25, in *Congenital adrenal hyperplasia,* Lee, P. A., et al., eds. Baltimore: University Park Press, 1977.

Monk-Turner, E., Wren, K., McGill, L., Matthiae, C., Brown, S., & Brooks, D. Who is gazing at whom? A look at how sex is used in magazine advertisements. *Journal of Gender Studies, 17, 3* (September 2008), 201–209.

Monro, F., & Huon, G. Media-portrayed idealized images, body shame, and appearance anxiety. *International Journal of Eating Disorders, 38, 1* (July 2005), 85–90.

Monroe, L. M., Kinney, L. M., Weist, M. D., Dafeamekpor, D. S., Dantzler, J., & Reynolds, M. W. The experience of sexual assault. *Journal of Interpersonal Violence, 20, no. 7* (July 2005), 767–776.

Montenegro, X. P. Lifestyles, dating and romance: A study of midlife singles. *AARP the Magazine* (September 2003). Available: www.aarp.org.

Moore, K. *Drop in teen birth rate not cause for complacency.* Washington, DC: Child Trends, 2001.

Moore, K. A. *Teen births: Examining the recent increase.* National Campaign to Prevent Teen and Unplanned Pregnancies, October 2008.

More than 1,200 alleged incidents of human trafficking reported in the U.S. U.S. Department of Justice, January 15, 2009. Available: http://www.ojp.usdoj.gov/bjs/pub/press/cshti08pr.htm.

Morgan, R. Bisexual students face tension with gay groups. *Chronicle of Higher Education, 49, no. 14* (November 29, 2002), A31.

Morgan, R. The men in the mirror. *Chronicle of Higher Education, 49, no. 5* (September 27, 2002), A53–A54.

Morrison, M. M., & Shaffer, D. R. Gender-role congruence and self-referencing as determinants of advertising effectiveness. *Sex Roles, 48, 5–6* (September 2003), 265–275.

Morse, B. J. Beyond the conflict tactics scale: Assessing gender differences in partner violence. *Violence and Victims, 10, no. 4* (1995), 251–272.

Mortenson, T. G. *Demographics and demographic change in American higher education.* Pell Center for the Study of Opportunity in Higher Education (2005). Available: http://www.brevard.edu/fyc/listserv/remarks/mortenson.htm.

Mosher, W. D., Chandra, A., & Jones, J. Sexual behavior and selected health measures: Men and women 15–44 years of age, United States, 2002. *Advance Data from Vital and Health Statistics, 362* (September 15, 2005), 1–17.

Mosher, W. D., Martinez, G. M., Chandra, A., Abma, J. C., & Wilson, S. J. Use of contraception and use of family planning services in the United States: 1982–2002. *Advanced Data, 350* (2004).

Most sexually active teens first had sex at home, late at night, survey shows. Henry J. Kaiser Family Foundation (September 26, 2002). Available: www.kaisernetwork.org/daily_reports.

Mouzon, L. D., Battle, A., Clark, K. P., Coleman, S., & Ogletree, R. J. African-American college students' perceptions of sexual coercion. *Health Educator, 37, no. 1* (Spring 2005), 16–21.

MTV launches new gay cable TV channel. *ABC News* (June 28, 2005). Available: http://abcnews.go.com.

Mulcahy, J. J. Penile implant infections: Prevention and treatment. *Current Urology Reports, 9* (2008), 487–491.

Mulhauser, D. Dating among college students is all but dead, survey finds. *Chronicle of Higher Education, 47, no. 48* (August 10, 2001), A51.

Munjack, D. J., & Kanno, P. H. Retarded ejaculation: A review. *Archives of Sexual Behavior, 8* (1979), 139–150.

Murphy, D. E. Gays celebrate, and plan for broader rights. *The New York Times* (June 27, 2003). Available: www.nytimes.com.

Murstein, B. L. *Love, sex, and marriage.* New York: Springer, 1974.

Myers, J. Nonmainstream body modification: Genital piercing, branding, burning, and cutting. *Journal of Contemporary Ethnography, 21* (1992), 267–306.

Nagao, K., Ishii, N., Kamidono, S., & Osada, T. Vardenafil (Levitra) clinical trial group: Safety and efficacy of vardenafil in patients with erectile dysfunction: Result of a bridging study in Japan. *International Journal of Urology, 11* (2004), 515–524.

Nagel, B., Matsuo, H., McIntyre, K. P., & Morrison, N. Attitudes toward victims of rape. *Journal of Interpersonal Violence, 20, no. 6* (June 2005), 725–737.

Nahleh, Z. A., Srikantiah, R., Safa, M., Jazieh, A. R., Muhleman, A., & Komrokji, R. Male breast cancer in the Veterans Affairs population: A comparative analysis. *Cancer, 109* (2007), 1471–1477.

NARAL Pro-Choice America. Roe v. Wade *and the right to choose* (2005). Available: http://www.prochoiceamerica.org.

Natali, A., Bartolini, M., Lucarini, S., Vignolini, G., Nelli, F., & Menchi, I. Statistical evaluation of hemodynamic effects of regular use of sildenafil on the human corpora cavernosa. *Urologia Internationalis, 82* (2009), 53–60.

Nathan, S. The epidemiology of the *DSM-III* psychosexual dysfunctions. *Journal of Sex and Marital Therapy, 12* (1986), 267.

The nation: Attitudes and characteristics of freshmen. *Chronicle of Higher Education, 49, no. 1* (August 30, 2002), 26.

National Abortion Federation. *Violence statistics.* Washington, DC: Author, 2009. Available: http://www.prochoice.org/about_abortion/violence/violence_statistics.html.

National Abortion Federation. *What is medical abortion?* Washington, DC: Author, 2008. Available: http://www.prochoice.org/about_abortion/facts/medical_abortion.html.

National Academy of Sciences. *Dietary reference intakes* (2004). Available: http://www.iom.edu/project.asp?id=4574.

National Campaign to Prevent Teen and Unplanned Pregnancy. *Fast facts: Teen sexual behavior and contraceptive use: Data from the Youth Risk Behavior Survey, 2007,* 2008. Available: http://www.thenationalcampaign.org/resources/pdf/fast-facts-yrbs-2007.pdf.

National Campaign to Prevent Teen and Unplanned Pregnancy. *Kiss and tell: What Teens Say About Love, Trust, and Other Relationship Stuff survey results,* 2007. Available: http://www.thenationalcampaign.org/resources/pdf/pubs/kiss_tell.pdf.

National Campaign to Prevent Teen Pregnancy. The general facts and stats. *teenpregnancy.org* (May 2005).

National Cancer Institute. *Breast cancer screening modalities: Mammography.* Washington, DC: Author, 2008a. Available: http://www.cancer.gov/cancertopics/pdq/screening/breast/HealthProfessional/page5.

National Cancer Institute. *Cervical cancer.* Washington, DC: Author, 2008b. Available: http://www.cancer.gov/cancertopics/types/cervical.

National Cancer Institute. *Surveillance epidemiology and end results: SEER stat fact sheets, Cancer, corpus and uterus.* Washington, DC: Author, 2008c. Available: http://seer.cancer.gov/statfacts/html/corp.html.

National Center for Complementary and Alternative Medicine. *10 things to know about evaluating medical resources on the Web,* 2009. Available: http://nccam.nih.gov/health/webresources/.

National Center for Health Statistics. *Health, United States, 2006.* Hyattsville, MD: Author, 2006.

National Center for Health Statistics. *Health, United States, 2008.* Hyattsville, MD: Author, 2008.

National Center for Health Statistics. National Ambulatory Medical Care Survey (2004). Available: http://www.cdc.gov/nchs/about/major/ahcd/ahcd1.htmData%20Highlights.

National Council on the Aging. *Half of older Americans report they are sexually active: 4 in 10 want more sex, says new survey.* Press release, September 28, 1998.

National Guidelines Task Force. *Guidelines for comprehensive sexuality education: Kindergarten–12th grade,* 3rd ed. New York: Sexuality Information and Education Council of the United States, 2004.

National Institute of Diabetes and Digestive and Kidney Disorders. *Erectile dysfunction,* 2005. Available: http://kidney.niddk.nih.gov/kudiseases/pubs/impotence/.

National Institute on Aging. Menopause: Age page (2005). Available: http://www.niapublications.org/engagepages/Menopause.pdf.

National Institute on Aging. *The menopause of life.* Washington, DC: Department of Health and Human Services, 1986.

National Institutes of Health. Osteoporosis. *Medline Plus: Medical encyclopedia* (2005). Available: http://www.nlm.nih.gov/medlineplus/ency/article/000360.htm#Causes,%20incidence,%20and%20risk%20factors.

National Kidney and Urologic Diseases Information Clearinghouse. *Erectile dysfunction.* Bethesda, MD: National Kidney and Urologic Diseases Information Clearinghouse, 2003. Available: http://kidney.niddk.nih.gov/kudiseases/pubs/impotence/#cause.

National Kidney and Urological Diseases Information Clearinghouse. *Urinary incontinence in men.* Bethesda, MD: Author, 2007. Available: http://kidney.niddk.nih.gov/kudiseases/pubs/uimen/#kegel.

National Library of Medicine. Lindane. *MedlinePlus,* 2008. Available: http://www.nlm.nih.gov/medlineplus/druginfo/meds/a682651.html.

National Library of Medicine. Orgasmic dysfunction. *Medline Plus,* 2009a. Available: http://www.nlm.nih.gov/medlineplus/ency/article/001953.htm.

National Library of Medicine. Sildenafil. *Medline Plus* (2005a). Available: http://www.nlm.nih.gov/medlineplus/druginfo/medmaster/a699015.html.

National Library of Medicine. Tadalafil. *Medline Plus* (2005b). Available: http://www.nlm.nih.gov/medlineplus/druginfo/uspdi/500491.html.

National Library of Medicine. Vaginismus. *Medline Plus,* 2009b. Available: http://www.nlm.nih.gov/medlineplus/ency/article/001487.htm.

National Library of Medicine. Vardenafil. *Medline Plus* (2005c). Available: http://www.nlm.nih.gov/medlineplus/druginfo/medmaster/a603035.html.

National survey of adolescents and young adults: Sexual health knowledge, attitudes, and experiences. Menlo Park, CA: Henry J. Kaiser Family Foundation, 2003.

National Victims Center and Crime Victims Research and Treatment Center. *Rape in America.* Arlington, VA: National Victims Center, 1992.

Navarro, M. Long silent, oldest profession gets vocal and organized. *The New York Times* (December 18, 2004).

Navarro, M. Women tailor sex industry to their eyes. *The New York Times* (Feb. 20, 2004).

Nearly 2 in 10 young teens sexually active: NBC News, *People* magazine commission landmark national poll. *NBC News* (January 19, 2004, updated January 31, 2005). Available: http://www.msnbc.msn.com/id/6839072.

Nelson, J. B. *Embodiment: An approach to sexuality and Christian theology.* Minneapolis: Augsburg, 1978.

Nemours Foundation. *Toxic shock syndrome.* Jacksonville, FL: Author, 2007. Available: http://kidshealth.org/teen/sexual_health/girls/tss.html.

Ness, Carol. PBS shies from show. *San Francisco Examiner* (June 6, 1999).

New contraceptive choices. *Population Reports, Series M, no. 19* (April 2005); Baltimore, MD: INFO Project, Johns Hopkins Bloomberg School of Public Health, 2005.

New federal law on computer porn upheld despite vagueness concerns, 1998.

New study shows women own 20% of businesses with revenues exceeding $1 million. Center for Women's Business Research, December 3, 2008. Available: www.womensbusinessresearch.org.

Newman, A. L., & Peterson, C. Anger of women incest survivors. *Sex Roles, 34, nos. 7–8* (1996), 463–474.

NIDUS Information Services. *Ask NOAH about: Impotence (erectile dysfunction),* 1998. Available: http://noah.cuny.edu/wellconn/impotence.html

Noden, M. Dying to win. *Sports Illustrated* (August 8, 1994), 52–60.

Noland, J. S., Singer, L. T., Short, E. J., Minnes, S., Arendt, R. E., Lester Kirchner, H., & Bearer, C. Prenatal drug exposure and selective attention in preschoolers. *Neurotoxicology and Teratology, 27* (2005), 429–38.

Nordstrom B. B., Sood, B. G., Sokol, R. J., Ager, J., Janisse, J., Hannigan, J. H., Covington, C., & Delaney-Black, V. Gender and alcohol moderate prenatal cocaine effects on teacher-report of child behavior. *Neurotoxicology and Teratology, 27* (2005), 181–189.

North American Menopause Society. The role of testosterone therapy in postmenopausal women: Position statement of the North American Menopause Society. *Menopause, 12* (2005), 497–511.

NOT-2-LATE.com, 2009. Available: http://ec.princeton.edu/.

Notes from the research. *SIECUS Development* (Summer/Fall 2002), 2.

Notice to readers: Sexual Assault Awareness Month—April 2005. U.S. Centers for Disease Control. Available: http://www.cdc.gov/mmwr/preview/mmwrhtml/mm5412a8.htm.

Number of married U.S. teens increased by 50% in 1990s; some attribute to abstinence education. *Kaiser Daily Reproductive Health Report* (November 11, 2002). Available: www.kaisernetwork.org/daily_reports.

Nutter, D., & Condron, M. Sexual fantasy and activity patterns of females with inhibited sexual desire versus normal controls. *Journal of Sex and Marital Therapy, 9* (1983), 276–282.

O'Keefe, M. The times are trying politicians' souls. *The Oregonian* (April 20, 1995), A1.

O'Neill, A. Altered states. *People Weekly, 50, no. 16* (November 2, 1998), 110–120.

O'Sullivan, L. F., & Brooks-Gunn, J. The timing of changes in girls' sexual cognitions and behaviors in early adolescence: A prospective, cohort study. *Journal of Adolescent Health, 37, no.3* (2005), 211–219.

Office of the Surgeon General. *The Surgeon General's call to action to promote sexual health and responsible sexual behavior.* Rockville, MD: United States Department of Health and Human Services, 2001.

Okami, P., Olmstead, R., Abrahamson, P. R., & Pendleton, L. Early childhood exposure to parental nudity and scenes of parental sexuality ("primal scenes"): An 18-year longitudinal study of outcome. *Archives of Sexual Behavior, 27, no. 2* (1998), 361–384.

Okie, S. RU-486 joining methotrexate in reshaping abortion. *Washington Post* (October, 13, 2000), A3.

On Equal Pay Day NOW calls attention to persistent gender wage gap. National Organization for Women, April 27, 2009. Available: http://www.now.org/press/04-09/04-27.html.

Oncalem, R. & King, B. Comparison of men's and women's attempts to dissuade sexual partners from the couple using condoms. *Archives of Sexual Behavior, 30, no. 4* (August 2001), 379–391.

Ontario Consultants on Religious Tolerance. Brief descriptions of the sex belief systems, 2009. Available: http://www.religioustolerance.org/hom6beli1.htm.

Ontario Consultants on Religious Tolerance. Homosexuality and bisexuality: All sides to the issue (2005). Available: http://www.religioustolerance.org/homosexu.htm.

Orecklin, M. Stress and the superdad. *Time, 164, no. 8* (August 23, 2004), 38–39.

Orgasmic dysfunction. *Medical-Library.org,* 2009. Available: http://www.medical-library.org/journals4a/sexual_dysfunction_2.htm.

Osborne, D. Sexual health: An interview with a Mayo clinic specialist. MayoClinic.com (December 2004). Available: http://www.mayoclinic.com/invoke.cfm?id=HQ01363.

Overcoming sexual victimization of boys and men. *Male Survivor* (2005). Available: http://www.malesurvivor.org/10%20Facts.htm.

Overland, M. A. In Kashmir, militant group threatens to shoot female Muslim students who do not wear veil. *The Chronicle of Higher Education,* Today's News (September 17, 2001). Available: http://chronicle.com/daily/2001.

Overview of the status of women in the states. Washington, DC: IWPR, 2001. Available: www.iwpr.org/.

Owen, C. The importance of sexual communication. *suite101.com,* July 2008. Available: http://improving-relationships.suite101.com.

Padgett, P. M. Personal safety and sexual safety for women using online personal ads. *Sexuality Research & Social Policy, 4, 2* (June 2007), 27–37.

Padgett, T. A welcome mat for gays? *Time, 165, no. 23* (June 6, 2005), 20.

Painter, A. *Tantric sex techniques to reinvigorate lovemaking.* Discovery Health. Sexual Health Center: Tantric Sex, 2009. Available: http://health.discovery.com/centers/sex/tantric/tantricsex.html.

Paraphilias. *MedicineNet.com,* 2009. Available: http://www.medicinenet.com/paraphilia/article.htm.

Paraphilias. *Psychology Today's* Conditions Center, 2005. Available: http://cms.psychologytoday.com/conditions/index.php?term=paraphilias&print=1.

Pardun, C. J., & Forde, K. R. Sex in the media: Do condom ads have a chance? *SIECUS Report, 31, no. 2* (December 2002/January 2003), 22–23.

Parental advisory. The Recording Industry of America 2003. Available: http://www.riaa.com/issues/parents/advisory.asp

Partner notification for preventing human immunodeficiency virus (HIV) infection: Colorado, Idaho, South Carolina, Virginia. *Morbidity and Mortality Weekly Report, 37* (1988), 393, 401.

Pastor's column hits the growth of porn. *The Birmingham Post Herald* (September 1, 2001), D9.

Patterson, J. Killer cramps. *Shape* (August 1990), 20–22.

Peacock, P. Marital rape, in *Issues in intimate violence,* Bergen, R. K., ed. Thousand Oaks, CA: Sage, 1998.

Pearson, J. C. *Gender and communication.* Dubuque, IA: William C. Brown, 1985.

Pedophilia: Who are the men who "love" children in intolerable ways? *Harvard Mental Health Letter, 20, no. 7* (January 2004), 1–4.

Penhollow, T. M., Young, M., & Denny, G. Predictors of quality of life, sexual intercourse, and sexual satisfaction among active older adults. *American Journal of Health Education, 40, 1* (January/February 2009), 14–22.

Penhollow, T., Young, M., & Denny, G. The impact of religiosity on the sexual behaviors of college students. *American Journal of Health Education, 36, no. 2* (March/April 2005), 75–83.

Peplau, L. A. Human sexuality: How do men and women differ? *Current Directions in Psychological Research, 12, no. 2* (April 2003), 37–40.

Peplau, L. A., & Cochran, S. D. A relationship perspective on homosexuality, in *Homosexuality/heterosexuality: Concepts of sexual orientation,* McWhirter, D. P., Sanders, S. A., & Reinisch, J. M., eds.. New York: Oxford Press, 1990, pp. 321–349.

Perry, J. D. Treating vaginismus with Perry brand sensors, 1992.

Perry, J. D., & Whipple, B. Pelvic muscle strength of female ejaculators: Evidence in support of a new theory of orgasm, *Journal of Sex Research, 17* (1981), 22–39.

Person, E. S., Terestman, N., Myers, W. A., & Goldberg, E. L. Gender differences in sexual behaviors and fantasies in a college population. *Journal of Sex and Marital Therapy, 15, no. 3* (1989), 187–214.

Pfafflin, F., & Eher, R. What to do with sexual offenders? *International Journal of Offender Therapy and Comparative Criminology, 47, no. 4* (2003), 361–365.

Phalen, K. F. PMS: Pretty miserable symptoms. *Washington Post Health* (August 1, 2000b), 19.

Phalen, K. F. Your own personal heat wave. *Washington Post Health* (June 12, 2001), 19.

Philadelphoff-Puren, N. Contextualising consent: The problem of rape and romance. *Australian Feminist Studies, 20, no. 46* (March 2005), 31–42.

Pitts, M., Smith, A., Grierson, J., O'Brien, M., & Mission, S. Who pays for sex and why? An analysis of social and motivational factors associated with male clients of sex workers. *Archives of Sexual Behavior, 33, no. 4* (Aug. 2004), 353–358.

Planned Parenthood. Safer sex, 2009. Available: http://www.plannedharenthood.org.

Planned Parenthood Federation. *Thinking about adoption,* 2009. Available: http://www.plannedparenthood.org/health-topics/pregnancy/adoption-21520.htm.

Planned Parenthood Federation of America. *Birth control: The condom* (2003). Available: http://www.plannedparenthood.org/bc/Condom.htm#Female.

Plotnik, R. *Introduction to psychology,* 3rd ed. Pacific Grove: CA: Brooks/Cole, 1993, 27–28.

Plous, S., & Neptune, D. Racial and gender biases in magazines and advertising. *Psychology of Women Quarterly, 21, no. 4* (December 1997), 627–644.

Polinski, M. Preparing for fatherhood: The male pregnancy experience, feeling her pregnancy pain. *Pregnancy Today,* 2009. Available: http://www.pregnancytoday.com/articles/fatherhood/feeling-her-pain-2045.

Polit, D. F., White, C. M., & Morgan, T. D. Child sexual abuse and premarital intercourse among high-risk adolescents. *Journal of Adolescent Health Care, 11* (1990), 231.

Poniewozik, J. Hot tubs and cold shoulders. *Time, 160, no. 7* (August 12, 2002), 56–58.

Pope, E. When illness takes sex out of a relationship. *SIECUS Report, 27, no. 3* (February/March 1999), 8–11.

Pope, V. Trafficking in women. *U.S. News and World Report* (April 7, 1997), 38.

Popenoe, D. Cohabitation, marriage and child wellbeing. National Marriage Project, 2008. Available: http://marriage.rutgers.edu/Publications/2008cohabreport.html.

Popenoe, D. The future of marriage in America. National Marriage Project, 2007. Available: http://marriage.rutgers.edu/Publications/SOOU/TEXTSOOU2007.htm.

Popenoe, D., & Whitehead, B. D. The state of our unions 2000. The National Marriage Project. 2001 Available: http://marriage.rutgers.edu/state_of_our_union%202000%20text%20only.htm.

Popenoe, D., & Whitehead, B. D. The state of our unions 2005. The National Marriage Project, Rutgers, the State University of New Jersey, 2005. Available: http://marriage.rutgers.edu.

Popp, D., Donovan, R. A., Crawford, M., Marsh, K. L., & Peele, M. Gender, race, and speech style stereotypes. *Sex Roles, 48* (2003), 317–325.

Population Reference Bureau. *The world's youth 2000.* Washington, DC: Author, 2000.

Porche, D. J. Men are victims of sexual violence. *American Journal of Men's Health, 2, 3* (September 2008), 217.

Preidt, R. TV commercials color gender choices for careers. *MedicineNet.com,* May 28, 2008. Available: http://www.medicinenet.com.

Preti, G., Winnifred, C., Celso, R., Garcia, G. Huggins, R., & Lawley, H. J. Human axillary secretions influence women's menstrual cycles: The role of donor extract of females. *Hormones and Behavior, 20* (1986), 474–482.

Prevalence of domestic violence. Domestic violence is a serious, widespread social problem in America: The facts 2005. Family Violence Prevention Fund. Available: http://endabuse.org.

Prime, J., & Moss-Racusin, C. A. Engaging men in gender initiatives: What change agents need to know. Catalyst, May 2009. Available: http://www.catalyst.org/publication/323/engaging-men-in-gender-initiatives-what-change-agents-need-to-know.

Prison rape. National Institute of Justice, 2007. Available: http://www.ojp.usdoj.gov/nij/topics/corrections/prison-rape/welcome.htm.

Proctor, F., Wagner, N., & Butler, J. The differentiation of male and female orgasm: An experimental study, in *Perspectives on human sexuality,* Wagner, N., ed. New York: Behavioral Publications, 1974.

Prostitutes are people too. *Lancet Online, 365* (May 7, 2005), 1618.

Prostitution in the United States—the statistics, 1998.

Psychiatric Disorders.com. *Sexual aversion disorder,* 2008. Available: http://www.psychiatric-disorders.com/articles/Sexual-dysfunctions/sexual-aversion-disorder.php.

Ptacek, J. Why do men batter their wives?, in *Issues in intimate violence,* Bergen, R. K., ed. Thousand Oaks, CA: Sage, 1998.

PTC study: Broadcast TV family hour fare filthier than ever. Parents' Television Council, September 5, 2007. Available: http://parentstv.org.

Pulsifer, M. B., Radonovich, K., Belcher, H. M., & Butz, A. M. Intelligence and school readiness in preschool children with prenatal drug exposure. *Neuropsychology, Development, and Cognition, 10* (2004), 89–101.

Putman, A. G., College students' perception of date rape: The relationship between personal relevance and victim empathy. *Dissertation Abstracts International, 65, no. 5-B* (Dec. 2002), 2599.

Quinacrine sterilization: Introduction and overview (2002). Available: http://www.quinacrine.com/intro.html.

Quindlen, A. *Thinking out loud.* New York: Random House, 1988.

Ramchandran, D., & Salem, R. M. New findings on contraceptives. *Population Reports, Series M (20)* (June 2008). Baltimore, MD: INFO Project, Johns Hopkins Bloomberg School of Public Health.

Ransom, S., & Moldenhauer, J. Premenstrual syndrome: Systematic diagnosis and individualized therapy. *The Physician and Sportsmedicine, 26* (1998).

Rape trauma syndrome—what everyone should know. *Male Survivor, 2005.* Available: http://malesurvivor.org/Professionals/Articles/rts.htm

Rathus, S. A., Nevid, J. S., & Fichner-Rathus, L. *Human sexuality in a world of diversity.* Boston, MA: Pearson, 2008.

Redfearn, S. Hormone questions linger: Experts address women's issues. *Washington Post* (July 7, 2002), F1, F4.

Redfearn, S. A new ring cycle: Contraceptive woos the way. *Washington Post* (August 6, 2002), F1, F4.

Redfield, R. R., & Burke, D. S. HIV infection: The clinical picture, in *The science of AIDS: Readings from* Scientific American *magazine.* New York: W. H. Freeman, 1989.

Redfran, S. Pap plus: Some ob-gyns are adding a visual screen to aid cancer detection. *Washington Post* (April 4, 2002), F1.

Reeder, H. M. Exploring male–female communication: Three lessons on gender. *Journal of School Health, 75, no. 3* (March 2005), 115–117.

Reinberg, S. Childbirth at home as safe as hospital delivery: Study review finds no increased problems for low-risk women. *HealthDay News* (June 16, 2005).

Reinisch, J., & Beasley, R. *The Kinsey Institute new report on sex.* New York: St. Martin's, 1991.

Reinisch, J. M., Hill, C. A., Sanders, S. A., & Zembia-Davis, M. High-risk sexual behavior at a Midwestern university—a confirmation survey. *Family Planning Perspectives, 27, no. 2* (March/April 1995), 79–82.

Reiss, I. L. Changing trends, attitudes and values on premarital sexual behavior in the U.S., in *Human sexuality and the mentally retarded,* de la Cruz, F. F., & La Vock, G. D., eds. New York: Brunner/Mazel, 1973, 286–289.

Remafedi, G., et al. Demography of sexual orientation in adolescents. *Pediatrics, 89, no. 4* (1992), 714–721.

Rempala, D. M., & Bernien, F. J. The consideration of rape: The effect of target information disparity on judgments of guilt. *Journal of Applied Social Psychology, 35, no. 3* (March 2005), 536–550.

Rempel, J. K., & Burris, C. T. Let me count the ways: An integrative theory of love and hate. *Personal Relationships, 12, no. 2* (June 2005), 297–313.

Rensberger, R. Pheromones discovered in humans: Substances help regulate female reproductive cycle. *Washington Post* (November 1986) A1, A7.

Renzetti, C. M., & Curren, D. J. *Living sociology*. Needham Heights, MA: Allyn & Bacon, 1998.

Research Forecasts, Inc. *The Tampax report: A summary of survey results on a study of attitudes toward menstruation*. New York: Tampax, 1981.

Rescued from sex slavery. *CBS News, 48 Hours* (July 22, 2005).

Resolve conflict in four steps. *Communication Briefings, 14, no. 3* (January 1995), 2.

Resuming sexual activity later in life. *MayoClinic.com* (November 19, 2004). Available: http://www.mayoclinic.com/invoke.cfm?id=AN00951.

Reuters. Study again clears silicone, *Washington Post* (June 22, 1999), A2.

Reynolds, K. *Pregnancy and birth: Your questions answered*. New York: DK Publishing, 1997.

Rich, G. Midnight callers. *Psychology Today Here to Help*, 2004. Available: http://www.psychologytoday.com/articles/pto-19990701-000010.html.

Rich, M. *The influence of entertainment media on sexual attitudes and behavior: Managing the media monster*. Washington, DC: National Campaign to Prevent Teen and Unplanned Pregnancy, 2008.

Rickert, V. I., Sanghvi, R., & Wiemann, C. M. Is lack of sexual assertiveness among adolescent and young adult women a cause for concern? *Perspectives on Sexual and Reproductive Health, 34, no. 4* (July/August 2002), 16–28.

Rideout, V., & Hoff, T. *Sex, kids, and the family hour: A three party study of sexual context on television*. California: Children Now and the Henry J. Kaiser Family Foundation, 1996.

Rimm, M. Marketing pornography on the information superhighway. *Georgetown Law Journal* (1998).

Ripley, A. Who says a woman can't be Einstein? *Time, 165, no. 10* (March 7, 2005), 51–60.

Risch, H. A., & Howe, G. R. Menopausal hormone usage and breast cancer: A record linkage cohort study. *American Journal of Epidemiology, 139* (1994), 670–683.

Robbins, L. Swoopes says she is gay, and exhales. *The New York Times* (October 27, 2005).

Rodgers, J. New contraceptive device developed by Weill Cornell Researchers is designed to prevent sexual transmission of HIV, May 19, 2009. Available: http://news.med.cornell.edu/wcmc/wcmc_2009/05_19_09.shtml).

Rodriguez, C., Patel, A. V., Calle, E. E., Jacob, E. J., & Thun, M. Estrogen replacement therapy and ovarian cancer mortality in a large prospective study of US women. *Journal of the American Medical Association, 285, no. 11* (2001), 1460–1465.

Rodruguez, A. Kidnapped, forced to wed. *The Chicago Tribune* (July 24, 2005).

Rolfe, D. Wal-Mart sells "sanitized" music, film—censorship or public service? The Dove Foundation, 2005. Available: http://www.dove.org.

Rooney, M. Freshmen show rising political awareness and changing social views. *The Chronicle of Higher Education, 49, no. 21* (January 31, 2003), A35–A38.

Roper Starch Worldwide. *Teens talk about sex: Adolescent sexuality in the 90s*. New York: Sexuality Information and Education Council of the United States, 1994.

Rosaria, M. The psychosexual development of urban lesbian, gay, and bisexual youth. *Journal of Sex Research, 33, no. 2* (1996), 113–126.

Rose, E., DiClemente, R. J., Wingood, G. M., Sales, J. M., Lathan, T. P., Crosby, R. A., Zenilman, J., Melendez, J., & Hardin, J. The validity of teens' and young adults' self-reported condom use. *Archives of Pediatrics & Adolescent Medicine, 163, 1* (2009), 61–64.

Rosen, R. C. Prevalence and risk factors of sexual dysfunction in men and women. *Current Psychiatry Reports, 2* (2000), 189–195.

Rosenbaum, J. E. Patient teenagers? A comparison of the sexual behavior of virginity pledgers and matched nonpledgers. *Pediatrics, 123, 1* (January 2009), e110–e120. Available: http://pediatrics.aappublications.org/cgi/reprint/123/1/e11o.

Rosenberg, L. Hormone replacement therapy: The need for reconsideration. *American Journal of Public Health, 83* (1993), 1670–1673.

Rosenberg, M. J., Waugh, M. S., Solomon, H. M., & Lyszkowski, A. L. The male polyurethane condom: A review of current knowledge. *Contraception, 53, 3* (March 1996), 141–146.

Rospenda, K. M., Richman, J. A., Ehmke, J. L. Z., & Zlatoper, K. W. Is workplace harassment hazardous to your health? *Journal of Business and Psychology, 20, no. 1* (September 2005), 95–110.

Ross, M. W. Situating sexuality electronically: The Internet and sexual expression. *Sexuality Research & Public Policy, 4, 2* (June 2007), 1–4.

Rovner, S. A reversal on circumcision. *Washington Post Health* (May 15, 1990).

Rowland, D. L., Strassberg, D. S., de Gouveia Brazao, C. A., & Slob, A. K. Ejaculatory latency and control in men with premature ejaculation: An analysis across sexual activities using multiple sources of information. *Journal of Psychosomatic Research, 48* (2000), 69–77.

Rubinson, L., & Rubertis, L. D. Trends in sexual attitudes and behaviors of a college population over a 15-year period. *Journal of Sex Education and Therapy, 17, no. 1* (1991), 32–41.

Rubinstein, S., & Caballero, B. Is Miss America an undernourished role model? *Journal of the American Medical Association*, Research Letter, 283, no. 12 (March 22/29, 2000), 1569.

Ruble, D., & Brooks-Gunn, J. Menstrual myths. *Medical Aspects of Human Sexuality, 13* (June 1979), 110–127.

Rumbough, T. B. *Controversial uses of the Internet by college students*, 2001. Available: http://www.eucuase.edu/ir/library/pdf/C5D1618.pdf.

Ruscombe-King, R. Homophobia, prejudice and attitudes to gay men and lesbians. *AVERT* (an international AIDS charity), 2009. Available: http://avert.org/homophobia.htm.

Russell, S. T. LGBTQ youth are at risk in U.S. school environment. *SIECUS Report, 29, no. 4* (April/May 2001), 19–22.

Russo, F. Bridal vows revisited. *Time, 156, no. 4* (July 24, 2000), G1–G3.

Russo, N. F., & Zierk, K. L. Abortion, childbearing, and women's well-being. *Professional Psychology: Research and Practice, 23* (1992), 269.

Ryan, C., & Futterman, D. Social and developmental challenges for lesbian, gay, and bisexual youth. *SIECUS Report, 29, no. 4* (April/May 2001), 5–18.

Ryan, C., Huebner, D., Diaz, R. M., & Sanchez, J. Family rejection as a predictor of negative health outcomes in white and Latino lesbian, gay, and bisexual young adults. *Pediatrics, 123, 1* (January 2009), 346–352.

Saad, L. Abortion views hold steady over past year: Public makes sharp distinction about abortion circumstances. *Gallup News Service* (June 2, 2003). Available: http://www.gallup.com/poll/content/default.aspx?ci=8521

Saad, L. Americans evenly divided on morality of homosexuality. Gallup, Inc., 2008. Available: http://www.gallup.com/poll/108115/Americans-Evenly-Divided-Morality-Homosexuality.aspx.

Sachs, A. Work's bad girls. *Time, 158, no. 11* (September 3, 2001), Y7–Y8.

Sadism. University of Iowa Health Care (2001). Available: www.uihealthcare.com/topics/mentalemotionalhealth/ment3168.html.

Sadler, A. G., Booth, B. M., Cook, B. L., & Doebbeling, B. N. Factors associated with women's risk of rape in the military environment. *American Journal of Industrial Medicine, 43* (2003), 262–273.

Sadker, D., & Zittleman, K. Gender bias lives, for both sexes. *Education Digest, 70, no. 8* (April 2005), 27–30.

Sadock, B. J., Kaplan, H. I., & Freedman, A. M. *The sexual experience*. Baltimore: Williams & Wilkins, 1973.

Sadomasochism. Sinclair Intimacy Institute (2001). Available: http://www.intimacyinstitute.com.

Sadowski, M. Sexuality minority students benefit from school-based support—where it exists. *Harvard Education Letter, Research Online* (September/October, 2001). Available: http.//www.edletter.org/current/.

Saewyc, E. M., Homma, Y., Skay, C. L., Bearinger, L. H., Resnick, M. D., & Reis, E. Protective factors in the lives of bisexual adolescents in North America. *American Journal of Public Health, 99, 1* (January 2009), 110–117.

Saewyc, E. M., Taylor, D., Homma, Y., & Ogilvie, G. Trends in sexual health and risk behaviours among adolescents students in British Columbia. *Canadian Journal of Human Sexuality, 17, 1–2* (2008), 1–13.

Safer sex guidelines. Information. Education. Action (2009). Available: http://www.aids.org/factSheets/151-Safer-Sex-Guidelines.html.

Saigal, C. S. Obesity and erectile dysfunction: Common problems, common solution? *Journal of the American Medical Association, 291* (2004), 3011–3012.

Saigal, C. S., Wessells, H., & Wilt, T. Predictors and prevalence of erectile dysfunction in a racially diverse population. *Archives of Internal Medicine, 166* (2006), 207–212.

Salter, D., McMillan, D., Richards, M., Talbot, T., Hodges, J., Bentovim, A., Hastings, R., Stevenson, J., & Skuse, D. Development of sexually abusive behavior in sexually victimized males: A longitudinal study. *Lancet, 361, no. 9356* (February 8, 2003), 471–476.

Sample lesson plan using JSR. Allentown, PA: Society for the Scientific Study of Sexuality, 2005. Available: http://www.sexscience.org/publications.

Sampson, O., Navarro, S. K., Khan, A., Hearst, N., Raine, T. R., Gold, M., Miller, S., & Thiel de Bocanegra, H. Barriers to adolescents' getting emergency contraception through pharmacy access in California: Differences by language and region. *Perspectives on Sexual and Reproductive Health, 41, 2* (June 2009), 110–118.

Samuels, M., & Samuels, N. All about circumcision. *Medical Self-Care* (Spring 1983), 20–23.

Sanchez, D. T., & Kiefer, A. K. Body concerns in and out of the bedroom: Implications for sexual pleasure and problems. *Archives of Sexual Behavior, 36, 6* (December 2007), 808–820.

Sanchez, R. Oregon ignites revolution in adoption. *The Washington Post* (November 26, 1998), A1.

Sanchez-Flores, H. Everything I do, a man does. *SIECUS Report* 32, no. 3 (summer 2004), 17–20.

Sanders, S. A. Midlife sexuality: The need to integrate biological, psychological, and social perspectives. *SIECUS Report, 27, no. 3* (February/March 1999), 3–7.

Santelli, J. S., Abma, J., Ventura, S., Lindberg, L., Morrow, B., Anderson, J. E., Lyss, S., & Hamilton, B. Can changes in sexual behaviors among high school students explain the decline in teen pregnancy rates in the 1990s? *Journal of Adolescent Health, 35* (2004), 80–90.

Santelli, J. S., Lindberg, L. D., Finer, L. B., & Singh, S. Explaining recent declines in adolescent pregnancy in the United States: The contribution of abstinence and improved contraceptive use. *American Journal of Public Health, 97* (2007), 150–156.

Santelli, J. S., Orr, M., Lindberg, L. D., & Diaz, D. C. Changing behavioral risk for pregnancy among high school students in the United States, 1991–2007. *Journal of Adolescent Health, 45, 1* (July 2009), 25–32.

Sarkar, N. N. The combined contraceptive vaginal device (NuvaRing(R)): A comprehensive review. *European Journal of Contraception & Reproductive Health Care, 10, no. 2* (June 2005), 73–78.

Sarrel, P., & Sarrel, L. The *Redbook* report on sexual relationships, part I. *Redbook* (October 1980), 73–80.

Satcher, D. *Surgeon General's call to action to promote sexual health and responsible sexual behavior.* United States Department of Health and Human Services, July 9, 2001.

Sato, S., et al. Transvaginal ultrasonography screening detects early-stage ovarian cancer. *Cancer 2000, 89* (2000), 582–587.

Savage, D. "Conscience" rule for doctors may spark abortion controversy. *Los Angeles Times* (December 2, 2008).

Savage, J., Brodsky, N. L., Malmud, E., Giannetta, J. M., & Hurt, H. Attentional functioning and impulse control in cocaine-exposed and control children at age ten years. *Journal of Developmental Behavioral Pediatrics, 26* (2005), 42–47.

Savic, I., Berglund, H., & Lindstrom, P. Brain response to putative pheromones in homosexual men. *Proceedings of the National Academy of Sciences, 102, no. 20* (May 17, 2005), 7356–7361.

Saxe, L. Lying: Thoughts of an applied social psychologist. *American Psychologist, 46, no. 4* (1991), 409–415.

Sayer, L. C. Gender, time and inequality: Trends in women's and men's paid work, unpaid work and free time. *Social Forces, 84* (2005), 285–303.

Scheidlower, J. Sex talk, *Esquire, 127* (January 1997), 29.

Schmid, R. E. Unmarried couples top 4 million. *AP/AOL* (July 27, 1998).

Schmidt, G. The dilemma of the male pedophile. *Archives of Sexual Behavior, 31, no. 6* (Dec. 2002), 473–477.

Schnarch, D., & Morehouse, R. Online sex, dyadic crises, and pitfalls for MFTs. *Family Therapy Magazine, 1, no. 5* (September/October 2002), 14–19.

Schoenstadt, A. Bulimia statistics. *MedTV,* January 29, 2007. Available: http://bulimia.emedtv.com/bulimia/bulimia-statistics.html.

Schover, L., Friedman, J., Weiler, S., Heiman, J., & LoPiccolo, J. Multiaxial problem-oriented system for sexual dysfunctions. *Archives of General Psychiatry, 39* (1982), 614–619.

Schrader, S. M., Breitenstein, M. J., & Lowe, B. D. Cutting off the nose to save the penis. *Journal of Sexual Medicine, 5* (2008), 1932–1940.

Schroder, F. H., et al. Screening and prostate-cancer mortality in a randomized European study. *New England Journal of Medicine, 360* (2009), 1320–1328.

Schuklenk, U., & Ristow, M. The ethics of research into the cause(s) of homosexuality. *Journal of Homosexuality 31, no. 3* (1996), 5–30.

Schuler, J., & Curtis, G. B. Pregnancy and baby: All change. *iVillage.co.uk,* 2009. Available: http://www.ivillage.co.uk/pregnancyandbaby/parent/postnatal/articles/0,,36_163114,00.html.

Schwartz, M. F., & Bauman, J. E. *Hyperprolactinemia and sexual dysfunction in men.* Paper presented at the Annual Meeting of the Society for Sex Therapy and Research, New York, March 1981.

Schwartz, P., & Rutter, V. *The gender of sexuality.* Walnut Creek, CA: AltaMira Press, 2000.

Schwarz, E. B., Ray, R. M., Stuebe, A. M., Allison, M. A., Ness, R. B., Freiberg, M. S., & Cauley, J. A. Duration of lactation and risk factors for maternal cardiovascular disease. *Obstetrics and Gynecology, 113* (2009), 974–982.

Schwebke, J. R. Gonorrhea in the '90s. *Medical Aspects of Human Sexuality, 25* (1991), 42–46.

Schweitzer, S. Connecticut approves gay civil unions. *The Boston Globe* (April 21, 2005).

Segal, J. Nonverbal communication. *Helpguide Newsletter,* October 2008. Available: http://www.helpguide.org/mental/eq6_nonverbal_communication.htm.

Selverstone, R. Adolescent sexuality: Developing self-esteem and mastering developmental tasks. *SIECUS Report, 18, 1* (1989), 1–5.

Semans, J. Premature ejaculation: A new approach. *Southern Medical Journal, 49* (1956), 353–358.

Senbel, A. M., & Mostafa, T. Yohimbine enhances the effect of sildenafil on erectile process in rats. *International Journal of Impotence Research, 20* (2008), 409–417.

Sepillian, V. P., & Wood, E. *Ectopic pregnancy,* 2007. Available: http://emedicine.medscape.com/article/258768-overview.

Sevely, J., & Bennett, J. Concerning female ejaculation and the female prostate. *Journal of Sex Research,* 14 (1978), 1–20.

Sex and Tech. Washington, DC: National Campaign to Prevent Teen and Unplanned Pregnancy, 2008. Available: http://www.thenationalcampaign.org/sextech/PDF/SexTech_Summary.pdf.

Sexual activity and heart disease or stroke. American Heart Association, 2005. Available: http://www.americanheart.org/presenter.jhtml?identifier=4714.

Sexual addiction. *MedicineNet.com,* 2009. Available: http://www.medicinenet.com/sexual_addiction/article.htm.

Sexual and reproductive health: Women and men, 2002, Guttmacher Institute. Available: www.agi-usa.org/pubs/fb_10-02.html.

Sexual assault of young children as reported to law enforcement. U.S. Dept. of Justice (2005). Available: http://www.ojp.usdoj.gov/bjs/abstract/saycrle.htm.

Sexual attitudes and behavior of male teens. *Science Says, 6,* (Oct. 2003).

Sexual behavior among high school students—United States, 1990. *Morbidity and Mortality Weekly Report, 40, no. 51–52* (1992), 885–888.

Sexual behavior of young adolescents. *Science Says, 3* (Sep. 2003).

Sexual harassment. U.S. Equal Employment Opportunity Commission, 2005. Available: www.eeoc.gov/types/sexual_harassment.html

Sexual harassment. U.S. Equal Employment Opportunity Commission, 2009. Available: http://www.eeoc.gov/types/sexual_harassment.html.

Sexual harassment charges. U.S. Equal Employment Opportunity Commission, 2009. Available: http://www.eeoc.gov/stats/harass.html.

Sexual harassment on campus: Drawing the line. American Association of University Women Educational Foundation, 2005. Available: http://www.aauw.org/research/dtl.cfm.

Sexual health coverage in women's, men's, and teen magazines. Henry J. Kaiser Family Foundation (2000). Available: www.kff.org.

Sexual problems overview, 2005. Available: http://www.drkoop.com/ency/93/001951.html.

Sexual sadism. PsychDirect 2005. Available: http://www.psychdirect.com/forensic/Criminology/para/sadism.htm.

Sexual violence: Fact sheet. National Center for Injury Prevention and Control, U.S. Centers for Disease Control, 2005. Available: http://www.cdc.gov/ncipc/factsheets/svfacts.htm.

Sexuality update: Women with type 2 herpes at risk of cervical cancer. *Medical Aspects of Human Sexuality, 21* (1987), 17.

Sexually transmitted diseases treatment guidelines, 2006. Atlanta, GA: Centers for Disease Control and Prevention, 2006. Available: http://www.cdc.gov/mmwr/preview/mmwrhtml/rr5511a1.htm.

Shainess, N., & Greenwald, H. Debate: Are fantasies during sexual relations a sign of difficulty? *Sexual Behavior, 1* (1971), 38–54.

Shankaran, S., Das, A., Bauer, C. R., Bada, H. S., Lester, B., Wright, L. L., & Smeriglio, V. Association between patterns of maternal substance abuse and infant birth weight, length, and head circumference. *Pediatrics, 114* (2004), 226–234.

Shealy, K. R., Scanlon, K. S., Labiner-Wolfe, J., Fein, S. B., & Grummer-Strawn, L. M. Characteristics of breastfeeding practices among us mothers. *Pediatrics, 122 suppl* (2008), S50–S55.

Sheehy, G. *Passages.* New York: Bantam, 1976.

Sheehy, G. *Understanding men's passages: Discovering the new map of men's lives.* New York: Random House, 1998.

Sheeran, P. *Women, society, the state and abortion: A structuralist analysis.* New York: Prager, 1987.

Shier, D., Butler, J., & Lewis R. *Hole's Essentials of human anatomy and physiology.* New York: McGraw-Hill, 2003.

Shipman, C., & Kay, K. Women will rule business. *Time, 173, 20* (May 25, 2009), 46–47.

Should lesbian and gay couples be allowed to adopt? In *Taking sides: Issues in family and personal relationships,* Schroeder, E., ed. Guilford, CT: McGraw-Hill/Dushkin, 2003.

Should parents surgically alter their intersex infants? In *Taking sides: Issues in family and personal relationships,* Schroeder, E., ed. Guilford, CT: McGraw-Hill/Dushkin, 2003.

Should people not cohabit before getting married? In *Taking sides: Issues in family and personal relationships,* Schroeder, E., ed. Guilford, CT: McGraw-Hill/Dushkin, 2003.

Should prostitution be legal? In *Taking sides: Issues in family and personal relationships,* Schroeder, E., ed. Guilford, CT: McGraw-Hill/Dushkin, 2003.

Should same-sex couples be allowed to marry legally? In *Taking sides: Issues in family and personal relationships,* Schroeder, E., ed. Guilford, CT: McGraw-Hill/Dushkin, 2003.

SIECUS Policy and Advocacy. Statement of Sexuality Information and Education Council of the United States (SIECUS) on the public health and ethical concerns regarding abstinence-only-until-marriage programs and the need for comprehensive sexuality education, 2008a. Available: http://www.siecus.org/index.cfm?fuseaction=feature.showFeature&FeatureID=1156&varuniqueuserid=75184022109.

SIECUS Policy and Advocacy. A portrait of sexuality education and abstinence-only-until-marriage programs in the states (fiscal year 2008 edition), 2008b. Available: http://www.siecus.org/index.cfm?fuseaction=Page.ViewPage&PageID=1164.

SIECUS position statement on human sexuality, 2009. Available: http://siecus.org/index.cfm.

SIECUS position statements on sexuality issues, 2005.

SIECUS position statements on sexuality issues, 2009a. Available: www.siecus.org.

SIECUS questions and answers: LGBTQ youth issues, 2009b. Available: www.siecus.org.

Silverberg, C. Are male and female orgasms different? *About.com: Sexuality,* 2008. Available: http://sexuality.about.com/od/sexualhealthqanda/f/sex_question41.htm.

Silverberg, C. How to talk with your kids about sex. *About.com Sexuality,* March 2008. Available: http://sexuality.about.com/od/sexeducationforparent1/a/talk_sex_kids.htm?p=1.

Silverberg, C. Sexual communication ground rules. *About.com Sexuality,* January 2009. Available: http://sexuality.about.com/od/improvingsexcommunication/a/ground_rules.htm.

Simons, J. S., & Carey, M. P. Prevalence of sexual dysfunctions: Results from a decade of research. *Archives of Sexual Behavior, 30* (2001), 177–219.

Singer, J., & Singer, I. Types of female orgasms. *Journal of Sex Research 8* (1972), 255–267.

Singh, D. Female mate value at a glance: Relationship of waist-to-hip ratio to health, fecundity, and attractiveness. *Human Ethology & Evolutionary Psychology, 23* (December 2002), 81–91.

Single parenting and today's family. American Psychological Association, 1998. Available: http://helping.apa.org/family/single.html

Skene, A. Two important glands of the urethra. *American Journal of Obstetrics,* 265 (1980), 265–270.

Slob, A. K., Ernste, M., & Van der Werff ten Bosch, J. J. Menstrual cycle phase and sexual arousability in women. *Archives of Sexual Behavior, 20* (1991), 567–577.

Sloss, C., & Harper, G. When street sex workers are mothers. *Archives of Sexual Behavior, 33, no. 4* (August 2004), 329–341.

Small operators can make a real killing on the Web. *USA Today* (August 20, 1997), 1.

Smith, A. M., Fried, P. A., Hogan, M. J., & Cameron, I. Effects of prenatal marijuana on response inhibition: An fMRI study of young adults. *Neurotoxicology and Teratology, 26* (2004), 533–542.

Smith, G. L., Greenup, R., & Takafuji, E. T. Circumcision as a risk factor for urethritis in racial groups. *American Journal of Public Health, 77* (1987), 452–454.

Smith, L., Schoonover, S., Lauver, D., & Allen, Jr., P. Sexually transmitted diseases, in *Sexual health promotion,* Fogel, C. I., & Lauver, D., eds. Philadelphia: Saunders, 1990.

Smith, M. D., & Morra, N. N. Obscene and threatening telephone calls to women: Data from a Canadian national survey. *Gender and Society, 8, no. 4* (1994), 584–596.

Smith, T. W. *American sexual behavior: Trends, socio-demographic differences, and risk behavior.* Chicago: National Opinion Research Center, 2003.

Smock, P. J., Bergstrom, C., Huang, P., & Manning, W. Why shack up? Motivations to cohabit among young adults in the U.S. Presented at 37th World Congress of the International Institute of Sociology, Stockholm, Sweden, July 5–9, 2005.

Snegroff, S. The stressors of non-marital sexual intercourse. *Health Education, 17* (1986), 21–23.

Snyder, M., & Ickes, W. Personality and social behavior, in *The handbook of social psychology,* Lindzey, G., & Aronsen, E., eds. New York: Random House, 1985, 883–937.

Soderlund, G. Journalist or panderer? Framing underage webcam sites. *Sexuality Research & Social Policy, 5, 4* (December 2008), 62–72.

Sommerfield, J. Lifting the curse: Should monthly periods be optional? *MSNBC Online.*

Sonenstein, F. What teenagers are doing right: Changes in sexual behavior over the past decade. *Journal of Adolescent Health, 35* (2004), 77–78.

Sonenstein, F. L. Can we afford to be complacent about teens' use of condoms. *Journal of Adolescent Health, 43* (October 2008), 313–314.

Sonfield, A., Gold, R. B., Frost, J. J., & Darroch, J. E. U.S. insurance coverage of contraceptives and the impact of contraceptive coverage mandates, 2002. *Perspectives on Sexual and Reproductive Health, 36* (2004), 72–79.

Song, S. Starvation on the Web. *Time, 166, no. 3* (July 18, 2005), 57.

Sonnenberg, F. A., Burkman, R. T., et al. Cost-effectiveness and contraceptive effectiveness of the transdermal contraceptive patch. *American Journal of Obstetrics and Gynecology, 192* (2005), 1–9.

South, S. J., Haynie, D. L., & Bose, S. Residential mobility and the onset of adolescent sexual activity. *Journal of Marriage and Family, 67, no. 2* (May 2005), 499–514.

South African anti-rape condom could reduce risk of pregnancy, HIV, STDs. *Kaiser Daily HIV/AIDS Report* (September 02, 2005). Available: http://www.kaisernetwork.org.

Spaise, T. L. Necrophilia and SM: The deviant side of *Buffy the Vampire Slayer*. *Journal of Popular Culture, 38, 4* (May 2005), 744–762.

Spake, A. The truth about "The Silent Scream." *Ms.* (July 1985), 88, 91–92, 112–114.

Spalding, L. R., & Peplau, L. A. The unfaithful lover: Heterosexuals' perceptions of bisexuals and their relationships. *Psychology of Women Quarterly, 21* (1997), 611–625.

Spark, R. F. Patient information: Sexual problems in men. *UpToDate, 16* (2008), 3. Available: http://www.uptodate.com/patients/content/topic.do?topicKey=~nXT881SoKLFIS2T&selectedTitle=2~150&source=search_result.

Spector, I., & Carey, M. Incidence and prevalence of sexual dysfunctions: A critical review of the empirical literature. *Archives of Sexual Behavior, 19* (1990), 389–408.

Speroff, L., & Darney, P. D. *A clinical guide for contraception, 4th ed.* Philadelphia, PA: Lippincott Williams & Wilkins, 2005.

Speroff, L., et al. The comparative effect on bone density, endometrium, and lipids of continuous hormones as replacement therapy (CHART study). *Journal of the American Medical Association, 276* (1996), 1397–1403.

Sperry, S., Thompson, J. K., Sarwer, D. B., & Cash, T. F. Cosmetic surgery reality TV viewership: Relations with cosmetic surgery attitudes, body image, and disordered eating. *Annals of Plastic Surgery, 62, 1* (January 2009), 7–11.

Spielvogel, J. J. *Western civilization*, 3rd ed. St. Paul, MN: West, 1997.

Spitz, I., et al. The safety and efficacy of early pregnancy termination with mifepristone and misoprostol: Results from the first multicenter U.S. trial. *New England Journal of Medicine, 338* (1998), 1241–1247.

Spors, H., & Sobel, N. Male behavior by knockout. *Neuron, 55* (2007), 689–693.

Spousal rape laws: 20 years later. National Center for Victims of Crime, 2004. Available: http://www.ncvc.org/ncvc/main.aspx?dbName=DocumentViewer&DocumentID=32701.

Staley, M., Hussey, W., Roe, K., Harcourt, J., & Roe, K. In the shadow of the rainbow: Identifying and addressing health disparities in the lesbian, gay, bisexual, and transgender population—a research and practice challenge. *Health Promotion Practice, 2, no. 3* (July 2001) 207–211.

Stalking: domestic violence is a serious, widespread social problem in America: The facts. Family Violence Prevention Fund, 2005. Available: http://endabuse.org.

Stanton, A. Affairs, part 2: Understanding what went wrong. Health and age. Novartis Foundation for Gerontology, 2001. Available: www.healthandage.com/Home/gid2=1258.

State politics & policy. *Daily Women's Health Policy Report*, National Partnership for Women & Families, May 18, 2009. Available: http://www.nationalpartnership.org/site/News.

Startling new study shows one in six women incestuously abused before age 18. *Sexuality Today, 9, nos. 37–38* (1986), 2

Statistics on women in the military. Women in Military Service for America Memorial Foundation, April 7, 2009. Available: http://www.womensmemorial.org/PDFs/StatsonWIM.pdf.

Stein, R. Caesarean births hit high mark. *Washington Post* (December 16, 2002), A1.

Steiner-Adair, C., & Sjostrom, L. *Full of ourselves: A wellness program to advance girl power, health, and leadership.* New York: Teachers College Press, 2006.

Stem cell research: What Americans think. *Parade* (July 10, 2005), p. 5.

Stermac, L., Del Bove, G., & Addison, M. Stranger and acquaintance sexual assault of adult males. *Journal of Interpersonal Violence, 19, no 8* (Aug. 2004), 901–915.

Sternberg, R. *The triangle of love: Intimacy, passion, commitment.* New York: Basic Books, 1988.

Sternberg, R. A triangular theory of love. *Psychological Review, 93* (1986), 119–135.

Sternberg, S. U.S. AIDS threat rebounds. *USA Today* (August 14, 2001), 1A.

Stipp, D. Better prognosis: Research on impotence upsets idea that it is usually psychological. *Wall Street Journal* (April 14, 1987), 1, 25.

Stone, A. Gay troops kept in uniform despite "telling," report says, and report says harassment of military's gays doubles. *USA Today* (March 9, 2000): 4A–5A.

Strassberg, D. S., & Lockerd, L. K. Force in women's sexual fantasies. *Journal of Sexual Behavior, 27* (1998), 403–414.

Strauss, L. T., Herndon, J., Chang, J., Parker, W. Y., Bowens, S. V., Zane, S. B., & Berg, C. J. Abortion surveillance—United States, 2001. *Morbidity and Mortality Weekly Report, 53* (2004).

Striegel-Moore, R. H., Rosselli, F., Perrin, N., Debar, L., Wilson, G. T., May, A., & Kraemer, H. C. Gender differences in the prevalence of eating disorder symptoms. *International Journal of Eating Disorders* (December 23, 2008).

Strong, B., DeVault, C., Sayad, B. W., & Yarber, W. L. *Human sexuality: Diversity in contemporary America*, 5th ed. New York: McGraw-Hill, 2005.

Strovny, D. The importance of foreplay. *AskMen.com*, 2009. Available: http://www.askmen.com/dating/love_tip/sextip18.html.

Stubblefield, P. G., Carr-Ellis, S., & Borgatta, L. Methods for induced abortion. *Obstetrics and Gynecology, 104* (2004), 174–185.

Student sexuality: How can and should schools respond? *Alabama School Boards, 25, no. 3* (September–October 2004), 6–7+.

Suárez, I., Bodega, G., Rubio, M., Fernández-Ruiz, J. J., Ramos, J. A., & Fernández, B. Prenatal cannabinoid exposure down-regulates glutamate transporter expressions (GLAST and EAAC1) in the rat cerebellum. *Developmental Neuroscience, 26* (2004, 45–53.

Substance use and risky sexual behavior: Attitudes and practices among adolescents and young adults. *American Journal of Health Education, 33, no. 5* (September/October 2002), 278–281.

Sudden cardiac death gender gap closing in on women. *InteliHealth* (December 20, 2002). Available: www.intelihealth.com.

Sue, D. Erotic fantasies of college students during coitus. *Journal of Sex Research, 15* (1979), 299–305.

Suicide Prevention Resource Center. Suicide risk and prevention for lesbian, gay, bisexual, and transgender youth. Newton, MA: Education Development Center, 2008.

Summers, N. Podcasting: Talking dirty on your iPod. *Newsweek Periscope* (August 1, 2005). Available: http://msnbc.msn.com/id/8681666/site/newsweek/?rf=technorati.

Surgery may be hasty for unclear gender. *Intelihealth* (2005). Available: http://www.intelihealth.com/.

Survey finds gaps between safe-sex claims, behavior among U.S. adults. *Kaiser Daily Reproductive Health Report*, (April 7, 2004). Available: http://www.kaisernetwork.org

Survey USA public opinion poll (1998). Available: www.surveyusa.com.

Surveys show change in attitudes toward sex among high school and college students, higher incidences of "casual" and oral sex. *Kaiser Daily Reproductive Health Report* (January 21, 2003). Available: www.kaisernetwork.org.

Sussman, J. R., & Levitt, B. B. *Before you conceive: The complete prepregnancy guide.* New York: Bantam Books, 1989.

Swami, V. An examination of the love-is-blind bias among gay men and lesbians. *Body Image* (February 3, 2009).

Swartz, M. Buzz and Alan. *The New Yorker* (August 24 & 31, 1998), 66–78.

Tai, Y. C., Domchek, S., Parmigiani, G., & Chen, S. Breast cancer risk among male BRCA1 and BRCA2 mutation carriers. *Journal of the National Cancer Institute, 99* (2007), 1811–1814.

Tan, C. L. Latest hot accessory for successful women: The lesser boyfriend. *The Birmingham News* (April 22, 2001), 1E, 5E.

Tanfer, K., & Aral, S. Sexual intercourse during menstruation and self-reported sexually transmitted disease history among women. *Sexually Transmitted Diseases, 23* (1996), 395–401.

Tang, M-X. Effects of estrogen during menopause on risk and age at onset of Alzheimer's disease. *Lancet, 348* (1996), 429–432.

Tannahill, R. *Sex in history.* New York: Stein & Day, 1980.

Tannen, D. *You just don't understand.* New York: Ballantine Books, 1991.

Tardif, M., & Van Gijseghem, H. The gender identity of pedophiles: What does the outcome data tell us? *Journal of Child Sex Abuse, 14, no. 1* (2005), 57–74.

Tavris, C. Are girls really as mean as books say they are? *Chronicle of Higher Education, 48, no. 43* (July 5, 2002), B7–B9.

Taylor, C. B., Bryson, S., Luce, K. H., Cunning, D., Doyle, A. C., Abascal, L. B., Rockwell, R., Dev, P., Winzelberg, A. J., & Wilfley, D. E. Prevention of eating disorders in at-risk college-age women. *Archives of General Psychiatry, 63, 8* (August 2006), 881–888.

Tecson, B. J. Are women smarter than men? *MTV News,* May 23, 2005. Available: http://www.mtv.com/news/articles/1502764/05232005/id_0.jhtml?headlines=true.

Teen girls help FBI nab cyber stalkers. *ABC News,* June 28, 2005. Available: http://abcnews.go.com/WNT/print?id=889662

Teen sexual behavior. National Campaign to Prevent Teen and Unplanned Pregnancy. *Science Says, 36* (June 2008). Available: http://www.thenationalcampaign.org/resources/pdf/pubs/WOV2007_fulltext.pdf.

Teens and oral sex. *Science Says, 17* (September 2005).

Teens unsatisfied with sex ed classes. *Kaiser Daily Reproductive Health Report* (September 11, 2001). Available: www.kaisernetwork.org.

Tests confirm condoms block AIDS virus. *Medical World News, 27* (1986), 31–32.

Thayton, W. R. A theology of sexual pleasure. *SIECUS Report, 30* (2002), 393–400.

The American freshman: National norms for fall 2007. *Chronicle of Higher Education, 54, 24* (February 1, 2008), A34.

The social health of marriage in America: Updates of social indicators. National Marriage Project, Rutgers, the State University of New Jersey, February 2009.

This year's freshmen at 4-year colleges: A statistical profile. *Chronicle of Higher Education, 51, no. 22* (February 4, 2005), A34.

This year's freshmen at 4-year colleges: A statistical profile. *Chronicle of Higher Education, 55, 21* (January 30, 2009), A19.

Thomas, C. B. A new scarlet letter. *Time, 157, no. 23* (June 11, 2001), 82.

Thompson, E. Reform rabbis get OK to preside at same-sex commitments. *The Birmingham News* (2000).

Thompson, S. C., Anderson, K., Freedman, D., & Swan, J. Illusions of safety in a risky world: A study of college students' condom use. *Journal of Applied Social Psychology, 26* (2006), 189–210.

Thoni, A., & Moroder, L. Waterbirth: A safe and natural delivery method: Experience after 1355 waterbirths in Italy. *Midwifery Today, 70* (2004), 44–48.

Thought police recruited in new child porn law, 1998.

Tiefer, L. *Sex is not a natural act.* Boulder, CO: Westview Press, 1995.

Tiefer, L. Three crises facing sexology. *Archives of Sexual Behavior, 23, no. 4* (1994), 361–373.

TieMeyer, M. Eating disorders: Bulimia statistics. *About.com Eating Disorders,* 2007. Available: http://eatingdisorders.about.com/od/whatisbulimianervosa/p/bulimiastats.htm?p=1.

Tiggemann, M., Martins, Y., & Churchett, L. Beyond muscles: Unexplored parts of men's body image. *Journal of Health Psychology, 13, 8* (November 2008), 1163–1172.

Timeline—the pill. The American Experience by PBS, 2002. Available: http://www.pbs.org/wgbh/amex/pill/timeline/index.html.

Toner, J. P., & Flood, J. T. Fertility after the age of 40. *Obstetrics and Gynecology Clinics of North America, 20* (1993), 261–272.

Torstveit, M. K., & Sundgot-Borgen, J. Low bone mineral density is two to three times more prevalent in non-athletic premenopausal women than in elite athletes: A comprehensive controlled study. *British Journal of Sports Medicine, 39* (2005), 282–287.

Toshiyasu, A., Tetsuya, I., Katsurou, T., et al. Comparative study for the treatment of erectile dysfunction with sildenafil and vardenafil: Multi-centric research in Nagano City. *Nippon Hinyokika Gakkai Zasshi, 100* (2009), 1–6.

Tower Urology Group. *The new miracle in male genital health,* 1998.

Transvestic fetishism. *PsychDirect* (2005). Available: http://www.psychdirect.com/forensic/Criminology/para/transfetishism.htm.

Transvestism. University of Iowa Health Care (2001). Available: www.uihealthcare.com/topics/mentalemotionalhealth/ment3174.html.

Transvestism. University of Iowa Health Care (2005). Available: http://www.uihealthcare.com.

Trebay, G. The secret power of lesbian style. *The New York Times* (June 27, 2004).

Trends in sexual risk behaviors among high school students—United States, 1991–2001. *Morbidity and Mortality Weekly Report, 51, no. 38* (September 27, 2002), 856–859.

Trenholm, C., Devaney, B., Fortson, K., Quay, L., Wheeler, J., & Clark, M. *Impacts of four Title V, Section 510 abstinence education programs, final report.* Princeton, NJ: Mathematica Policy Research, 2007. Available: http://aspe.hhs.gov/hsp/abstinence07/report.pdf.

Tripp, C. A. *The homosexual matrix.* New York: New American Library, 1976.

Trussell, J. Contraceptive efficacy, *Contraceptive Technology,* 19th revised ed., Hatcher, R. A., et al., eds. New York: Ardent Media, 2007.

Tucker, P., & Irwin, J. D. University students' satisfaction with, interest in improving, and receptivity to attending programs aimed at health and well-being. *Health Promotion Practice* (February 5, 2009).

Tullman, G., Gilner, F., Kolodny, R., Dornbush, R., & Tullman, G. The pre- and post-therapy measurement of communication skills of couples undergoing sex therapy at the Masters and Johnson Institute. *Archives of Sexual Behavior, 10* (1981), 95–99.

Turkey says only virgins can be nurses. *The Birmingham News* (July 20, 2001), 8A.

TV sexual scenes nearly double since 1998. Kaiser Family Foundation, *Kaiser Daily Women's Health Policy* (November 10, 2005). Available: http://kaisernetwork.org.

Tyson, A. S. Sexual abuse is found rife in guard and reserves. *Washington Post* (September 30, 2005), A2.

Uhlman, M. Many children trade sex to survive, study says. *The Birmingham News* (September 11, 2001), 1A.

UNAIDS. HIV prevention hampered by homophobia, 2009. Available: http://www.unaids.org/en/KnowledgeCentre/Resources/FeatureStories/archive/2009/20090113_MSMLATAM.asp.

UNICEF. *Female genital manipulation/cutting: A statistical exploration.* New York: Author, 2005.

United States Code Annotated Title 47. U.S. Department of Justice (March 3, 2003). Available: www.usdoj.gov/criminal/cybercrime/47usc223NEW.htm.

"Unusual" FDA order requiring corrections to Yaz ad campaign. National Partnership for Women & Families, *Daily Women's Health Policy Report* (February 11, 2009).

Upadhyay, U. D. New contraceptive choices. *Population Reports, Series M, 19* (April 2005). Baltimore, MD: Johns Hopkins Bloomberg School of Public Health, INFO Project. Available: http://www.populationreports.org/m19/.

U.S. abortion rate declines overall but increases among low-income women, report says. Henry J. Kaiser Family Foundation (October 9, 2002). Available: www.kaisernetwork.org/daily_reports.

U.S. Census Bureau. American community survey: Earnings in the past twelve months, 2007. Available: http://factfinder.census.gov/servlet/STTable?-geo_id=01000US&-qr_name=ACS_2005_EST_G00_S2001&-ds_name=ACS_2005_EST_G00_.

U.S. Census Bureau. *U.S. population projections: National population projections, 2008,* 2008. Available: http://www.census.gov/population/www/projections/summarytables.html.

U.S. Census Bureau. *Statistical abstracts of the United States: 2002.* Washington, DC: U.S. Census Bureau, 2002.

U.S. Department of Health and Human Services. *Adoption and foster care statistics.* Washington, DC: Administration for Children and Families, 2008a. Available: http://www.acf.hhs.gov/programs/cb/stats_research/afcars/trends.htm.

U.S. Department of Health and Human Services. Depression during and after pregnancy. *Womenshealth.gov*, 2009. Available: http://www.womenshealth.gov/FAQ/depression-pregnancy.cfm#d.

U.S. Department of Health and Human Services. *Healthy People 2010: Understanding and improving health*, 2nd ed. Washington, DC: U.S. Government Printing Office, 2000.

U.S. Department of Health and Human Services, Health Resources and Services Administration, Maternal and Child Health Bureau. *Child Health USA 2007*. Rockville, MD: U.S. Department of Health and Human Services, 2008.

U.S. Department of Health and Human Services. *Women's health.gov: Frequently asked questions: Polycystic ovary syndrome*. Washington, DC: Author, 2007b. Available: http://womenshealth.gov/faq/polycystic-ovary-syndrome.cfm#a.

U.S. Department of Health and Human Services. *Women's health.gov: Frequently asked questions: Premenstrual syndrome*. Washington, DC: Author, 2007a. Available at: http://womenshealth.gov/faq/premenstrual-syndrome.cfm.

U.S. Preventive Services Task Force. Screening for breast cancer: U.S. Preventive Services Task Force recommendation statement. *Annals of Internal Medicine, 151* (2009), 716–726.

U.S. Preventive Services Task Force. Screening for prostate cancer: U.S. Preventive Services Task Force recommendation statement. *Annals of Internal Medicine, 149* (2008), 185–191.

U.S. Requirement that AIDS groups sign pledge against commercial sex work "harms" AIDS work. *Daily HIV/AIDS Report*, Kaiser Family Foundation, 2005. Available: http://www.kaisernetwork.org/daily_reports/rep_index.cfm?hint=1&DR_ID=32372

U.S. Surgeon General issues first call to action on disability. United States Department of Health and Human Services, July 26, 2005. Available: www.surgeongeneral.gov.

Use of AZT expanded. *FDA Consumer, 24* (1990), 17.

Van Goozen, S. H. M., Wiegart, V. M., & Helmond, F. A. Psychoendocrinological assessment of the menstrual cycle: The relationship between hormones, sexuality, and mood. *Archives of Sexual Behavior, 26* (1997), 359–382.

Van Wagner, K. Top 10 nonverbal communication tips. *About.com Psychology*, 2009. Available: http://psychology.about.com/od/nonverbalcommunication/tp/nonverbaltips.htm.

Van Wijk, A., van Horn, J., Bullens, R., Bijleveld, C., & Doreleijers, T. Juvenile sex offenders: A group on its own? *International Journal of Offender Therapy and Criminology, 49, no. 1* (February 2005), 25–36.

Viewership: Relations with cosmetic surgery attitudes, body image, and disordered eating. *Annals of Plastic Surgery, 62, no. 1* (January 2009), 7–11.

Vitagliano, E. Malevolent bargains. *American Family Association Journal* (April 2004).

Vlassoff, M., Singh, S., Darroch, J. E., Carbone, E., & Bernstein, S. Assessing costs and benefits of sexual and reproductive health interventions. New York: Guttmacher Institute, 2004.

Vo, K. Universities reach out to gay, lesbian students. *San Jose Mercury News* (May 25, 2003), A7.

Vobejda, B. Web site to list foster children for adoption. *Washington Post* (November 25, 1998), A5.

von Krafft-Ebing, R. *Psychopathia sexualis*. Stuttgart, Germany, 1902.

Voracek, M., & Fisher, M. L. Shapely centrefolds? Temporal changes in body measures: Trend analysis. *British Medical Journal, 325* (December 21, 2002), 1447–1448.

Voyeurism. Health topics: University of Iowa Health Care 2005. Available: http://www.uihealthcare.com.

Waddell, L. Florida county ending official support of gay events. *The New York Times* (June 26, 2005), sect 1, p. 15.

Wald, A., Koutsky, L., Ashley, R. L., et al. Genital herpes in a primary care clinic: Demographic and sexual correlates of herpes simplex type 2 infections. *Sexually Transmitted Diseases, 24* (1997), 149–155.

Waldo, C. R., & Kemp, J. L. Should I come out to my students? *Journal of Homosexuality, 14, no. 2* (1997), 79–94.

Walen, S. R., & Roth, D. A cognitive approach to sex therapy, in *Theories of human sexuality*, Geer, J. H. & O'Donohue, W. T., eds. New York: Plenum, 1987.

Walker, J., Archer, J., & Davies, M. Effects of rape on men: A descriptive analysis. *Archives of Sexual Behavior 34, no. 1* (February 2005), 69–80.

Wallerstein, E. *Circumcision*. New York: Springer, 1980.

Wallerstein, J. S. *Nine "psychological tasks" needed for a good marriage*. American Psychological Association, 1996.

Wallick, M. M. Homophobia and heterosexism: Out of the medical school closet. *North Carolina Medical Journal, 58, no. 2* (March–April 1997), 123–125.

Walling, A. D. Exercise during pregnancy is associated with thinner babies. *American Family Physician* (May 15, 2002). Available: http://www.aafp.org/afp/20020515/tips/12.html.

Walsh, A. *The science of love: Understanding love and its effects on mind and body*. Buffalo, NY: Prometheus, 1991.

Walsh, M. Riley restates rules against harassment. *Education Week, 17, no. 4* (July 8, 1998), 1, 30.

Warren, A. K. Cascading gender biases, compounding effects: An assessment of talent management systems. Catalyst, February 2009. Available: http://www.catalyst.org/publication/292/cascading-gender-biases-compounding-effects-an-assessment-of-talent-management-systems.

Waterbirth International. *Known benefits of water labor and waterbirth*, 2008. Available: http://www.waterbirth.org/mc/page.do?sitePageId=45768.

Waters, R. Estrogen to prevent Alzheimer's. *Health, 11* (1997), 40–42.

Wax, E. In Sudan, sitting in one prison to escape another. *The Washington Post* (August 3, 2005), A16.

The way we live now. *New York Times* (May 7, 2000), p. 18.

We want to live as humans. *Human Rights Watch, 14, no 11* (December 2002), 1–52.

WebMD. Genital herpes guide: All about genital herpes: Treatment options, 2007. Available: http://www.webmd.com/genital-herpes/guide/genital-herpes-treatment-options.

Weinberger, D. R., Elvevåg, B., & Giedd, J. N. *The adolescent brain: A work in progress*. National Campaign to Prevent Teen Pregnancy, June 2005. Available: http://www.teenpregnancy.org/resources/reading/pdf/BRAIN.pdf.

Weinstein, E., & Rosen, E. *Teaching about human sexuality and family: A skills-based approach*. Belmont, CA: Thomson Wadsworth, 2006.

Weiss, K. G. *Never calling it rape: An interpretive exploration of unacknowledged date rape and their accounts*. Presented at the Society for the Study of Social Problems (SSSP), 2002.

Weiss, R. E. Couvade syndrome: Sympathetic pregnancy. *About.com*, 2009. Available: http://pregnancy.about.com/cs/forfathersonly/a/couvade.htm.

Weissgerber, T. L., Wolfe, L. A., & Davies, G. A. The role of regular physical activity in preeclampsia prevention. *Medical Science and Sports Exercise, 36* (2004), 2024–2031.

West, S. L., D'Aloisio, A. A., Agans, R. P., Kalsbeek, W. D., Borisov, N. N., & Thorp, J. M. Prevalence of low sexual desire and hypoactive sexual desire disorder in a nationally representative sample of US women. *Archives of Internal Medicine, 168* (2008), 1441–1449.

What families won't tell. *UAB Medical Center Magazine, 2* (Fall 1986), 19–21.

What gender gap? *Kiplinger's, 55, no. 2* (February 2001), 22, 24.

What is sexual addiction? Sex Addicts Anonymous, 2003. Available: www.sexaa.org/addict.htm.

What is sexual assault? National Women's Health Information Center, 2005. Available: www.4woman.gov.

What scientists know about pornography. Allentown, PA: Society for the Scientific Study of Sexuality, 2007.

Whatley, M. A. The effect of participant sex, victim dress, and traditional attitudes on causal judgments for marital rape victims. *Journal of Family Violence 20, no. 3* (June 2005), 191–200.

Where do babies come from? *Family Life Educator* (Winter 1987), 5–7.

Whitehead, B. D., & Popenoe, D. Life without children: The social retreat from children and how it is changing America. National Marriage Project, Rutgers, the State University of New Jersey, 2008.

Whitman, F., & Diamond, M. *A preliminary report on the sexual orientation of homosexual twins.* Paper presented at the Western Region Annual Conference of the Society for the Scientific Study of Sex, Scottsdale, AZ, January 1986.

Whitty, M. T. The realness of cybercheating: Men's and women's representations of unfaithful Internet relations. *Social Science Computer Review, 23, no. 1* (Spring 2005), 57–67.

Who are the victims? Rape, Abuse & Incest National Network, 2009. Available: http://www.rainn.org/get-information/statistics/sexual-assault-victims.

Why don't we hear others? *Communication Briefings, 22, no. 1* (July 2005), 1.

Why it's important to talk about sexual orientation. *Families Are Talking 3, no. 2* (2004), 1–3.

Why men die younger than women. *Consumer Reports on Health, 14, no. 12* (December 2002), 1,3–4.

Wickelgren, I. Estrogen: A new weapon against Alzheimer's. *Science, 276* (1997), 676–677.

Wiest, W. Semantic differential profiles of orgasm and other experiences among men and women. *Sex Roles, 3* (1977), 399–403.

Williams, L. J., Correa, A., & Rassmussen, S. Maternal lifestyle factors and risk for ventricular septal defects. *Birth Defects Research. Part A, Clinical and Molecular Teratology, 70* (2004), 59–64.

Wilson, G. D. Gender differences in sexual fantasy: An evolutionary analysis. *Personality and Individual Differences, 22* (1997): 27–31.

Wilson, G. T., Nathan, P. E., O'Leary, K. D., & Clark, L. A. *Abnormal psychology: Integrating perspectives.* Needham, MA: Allyn & Bacon, 1996.

Wilson, R. Second sex. *Chronicle of Higher Education, 52, no. 7* (October 10, 2005), A10–A12.

Winikoff, B., et al. Acceptability and feasibility of early pregnancy termination by mifepristone-misoprostol. *Archives of Family Medicine, 7* (1998), 360–366.

Winship, E. *Reaching your teenager.* New York: Houghton Press, 1983.

Wiswell, T. E., Smith, F. R., & Bass, J. W. Decreased incidence of urinary tract infections in circumcised male infants. *Pediatrics, 75* (1985), 901–903.

Woellert, L. An all-out assault on sexual content. *Business Week* (November 21, 2005), 118.

Wolak, M. A., Finkelhor, D., & Mitchell, K. Online sex abuse cases not characterized by deception, abduction and force, research shows. APA Online, 2004. Available: http://www.apa.org/releases/online_sexabuse.html.

Wolak, J., Finkelhor, D., & Mitchell, K. *Trends in arrests of "online predators."* Durham, NH. Crimes Against Children Research Center, March 31, 2009.

Wolpe, J. *Psychotherapy by reciprocal inhibition.* Stanford: Stanford University Press, 1958.

Women in American history. *Bitannica Online.* Available: http://www.britannica.com.

Women in the military. National Organization for Women, 1990. Available: http://www.now.org/issues/military/policies/wim.html.

Women, too, may benefit from Viagra. *CNN.com* (May 1, 2000). http://www.archives.cnn.com/2000HEALTH/women/05/01/women.sex.fnction/

Women up to 10 times more likely to have poor body image than men, *InteliHealth: Women's Health* (May 14, 2001). Available: www.intelihealth.com.

Wong, N. C. Study: 1 in 5 kids pressed for sex online. *The Birmingham News* (June 21, 2001), 7A.

Worthington, R. L., Savoy, H. B., Dillon, F. R., & Vernaglia, E. R. Heterosexual identity development: A multidimensional model of individual and social identity. *The Counseling Psychologist, 30,* (2002), 496–531.

Woods, N. F. *Human sexuality in health and illness.* St. Louis: Mosby, 1979.

Worden, M., & Worden, B. D. *The gender dance in couples therapy.* Pacific Grove, CA: Brooks/Cole, 1998.

Working moms turn traditional when they're home. American Psychological Association, 1998.

World Health Organization. *Fact sheet: Female genital mutilation.* Geneva, Switzerland: Author, 2008. Available: http://www.who.int/mediacentre/factsheets/fs241/en/print.html.

World Health Organization (WHO) Department of Reproductive Health and Research & Johns Hopkins Bloomberg School of Public Health/Center for Communication Programs (CCP), INFO Project. *Family planning: A global handbook for providers (2008 update).* Baltimore & Geneva: CCP & WHO, 2008.

World Health Organization Task Force on Post-ovulatory Methods of Fertility Regulation. Comparison of two doses of mifepristone in combination with misoprostol for early medical abortion: A randomized trial, *British Journal of Obstetrics and Gynecology, 107, no. 4* (2000), 524–530.

Wosick-Correa, K. R., & Joseph, L. J. Sexy ladies sexing ladies: Women as consumers in strip clubs. *Journal of Sex Research, 45, 3* (July 2008), 201–216.

Wright, V. C., Schieve, L. A., Reynolds, M. A., & Jeng, G. Assisted reproductive technology surveillance, United States, 2002. *Morbidity and Mortality Weekly, 54* (2005), 1–24.

Writing Group for the PEPI Trial. Effects of hormone therapy on bone mineral density: Results from the postmenopausal estrogen/progestin interventions (PEPI) trial. *Journal of the American Medical Association, 276* (1996), 1389–1396.

Writing Group for the Women's Health Initiative Randomized Controlled Trial. Risks and benefits of estrogen plus progestin in healthy postmenopausal women. *Journal of the American Medical Association, 288* (2002), 321–333.

Wylie, K. R. Sex and relationship education is more than the facts of life. *Sexual & Relationship Therapy, 17* (2002), 317–319.

Xu, F., et al. Repeat chlamydia trachomatis infection in women: Analysis through a surveillance case registry in Washington State, 1993–1998. *American Journal of Epidemiology, 152, no. 12* (2000), 1164–1170.

Xu, X, Zhu, F., O'Campo, P. Koenig, M. A., Mock, V., & Campbell, J. Prevalence of and risk factors for intimate partner violence in China. *American Journal of Public Health 95, no. 1* (2005), 78–85.

Young, J. R. Gay student is forced out of a campus leadership post at an Iowa college. *Chronicle of Higher Education, 49, no. 13* (November 22, 2002), A58.

Young Americans more likely than their parents' generation to oppose abortion, surveys. *Kaiser Daily Reproductive Health Report* (September 26, 2002). Available: www.kaisernetwork.org/daily_reports.

Younis J. S., Jadaon, J., Izhaki, I., Haddad, S., Radin, O., Bar-Ami, S., & Ben-Ami, M. A simple multivariate score could predict ovarian reserve, as well as pregnancy rate, in infertile women. *Fertility and Sterility* (April 13, 2009).

Youssef, H. The history of the condom. *Journal of the Royal Society of Medicine, 86* (April 1993), 266–228.

Youth Risk Behavior Surveillance System. *Trends in the prevalence of sexual behaviors national YRBS: 1991–2007,* 2008. Available: http://www.cdc.gov/HealthyYouth/yrbs/pdf/yrbs07_us_sexual_behaviors_trend.pdf.

Yudt, S. Masturbation myths. *Teenwire.com.* Planned Parenthood Federation of America (November 9, 2004).

Zaidi, I. F., Crepaz, N., Song, R., et al. Epidemiology of HIV/AIDS among Asians and Pacific Islanders in the United States. *AIDS Education and Prevention, 17* (2005), 405–417.

Zanghellini, A. Scientific positivism and the controversy over research into lesbian and gay parenting. *Sexuality Research & Social Policy, 4, 3* (September 2007), 100–114.

Zaslow, J. Premarital survey may help couples choose a right mate. *The Birmingham News* (February 2, 2003), D1, D3.

Zaviacic, M., Zaviacicova, A., Holoman, I. K., & Molcan, J. Female urethral expulsions evoked by local digital stimulation of the G-spot: Differences in the response patterns. *Journal of Sex Research, 24* (1988), 311.

Zhang, X., Sliwowska, J. H., & Weinberg, J. Prenatal alcohol exposure and fetal programming: Effects on neuroendocrine and immune function. *Experimental Biological Medicine, 230* (2005), 376–388.

Zidovudine for children. *FDA Consumer, 24* (1990), 5.

Zieman, M., Hatcher, R. A., Cwlak, C., Darney, P. D., Creinin, M. D., & Stosure, H. R. *The pocket guide to managing contraception, 2007–2009 edition.* Tiger, GA: Bridging the Gap Foundation, 2007. Available: http://www.managingcontraception.com/shopping/mcpocket.pdf.

Zilbergard, B., & Ellison, C. R. Desire discrepancies and arousal problems in sex therapy, in *Principles and practices of sex therapy*, Lieblum, S. R., & Pervin, L. A., eds. New York: Guilford, 1980.

Zilbergeld, B., & Kilmann, P. The scope and effectiveness of sex therapy. *Psychotherapy, 21* (1984), 319–326.

Zimmer, D. E., Borchardt, E., & Fischle, C. Sexual fantasies of sexually distressed and nondistressed men and women: An empirical comparison. *Journal of Sex and Marital Therapy, 9* (1983), 38–50.

Zimmerman, A., & Dahlberg, J. The sexual objectification of women in advertising: A contemporary cultural perspective. *Journal of Advertising Research, 48, 1* (March 2008), 71–79.

Zorpette, G. You see brawny; I see scrawny. *Scientific American, 278* (March 1998), 24–25.

Zucker, K. J., & Bradley, S. J. Gender identity and psychosexual disorders. *American Psychiatric Association Focus, 3* (2005), 598–617.

Zukerman, Z., & Orvieto, R. Letter to the editor. *Journal of Andrology, 28, 5* (September/October 2007), 635.

Zuger, B. Monozygotic twins discordant for homosexuality: Report of a pair and significance of the phenomenon. *Comprehensive Psychiatry, 17* (1976), 661–669.

Glossary

69 Two partners' simultaneous stimulation of each other's genitalia orally. The numerals 6 and 9 visually describe the body positions.

abortifacient A medical method that causes an embryo or fetus to die.

abortion Purposeful termination of a pregnancy.

abstinence Avoidance of any type of sexual intercourse.

acquaintance rape Rape by a friend, acquaintance, or date; also known as *date rape*.

acquired immune deficiency syndrome (AIDS) A syndrome caused by the human immunodeficiency virus (HIV), characterized by a depressed immune system and the presence of one or more opportunistic diseases.

active listening Paraphrasing what someone has said to demonstrate interest and understanding.

adipose Pertaining to fat tissue in the body.

afterbirth The delivery of the placenta.

aggressiveness Standing up for one's basic rights, but at the expense of someone else's basic rights.

alimony Money a divorced person is instructed by the courts to pay regularly to his or her ex-spouse.

amenorrhea The absence of menstruation in a woman who should be menstruating.

amniocentesis Withdrawal by syringe of amniotic fluid to determine the presence of fetal abnormalities.

amniotic fluid The fluid inside the amniotic sac in which the fetus floats; it acts as a shock absorber, maintains the fetus at a constant temperature, and serves as a nutrient.

amniotic sac A fluid-filled membrane that surrounds the developing infant in the uterus.

ampulla The enlarged portion of the vas deferens where sperm are provided nutrients from the seminal vesicles; also, the part of the fallopian tube of women containing the cilia.

anal intercourse Insertion of the penis into the anus.

analgesics Substances that decrease pain locally, such as topical creams.

analingus Licking of the anus.

androgens Male sex hormones.

androgynous Exhibiting a combination of masculine and feminine traits as defined by the society.

anesthetics Substances that elicit unconsciousness and thereby relieve pain.

annular Type of hymen that surrounds the vaginal opening.

anorexia nervosa A condition in which the individual severely limits caloric intake.

antiandrogen drugs Chemicals that reduce the sex drive by lowering the testosterone level in the bloodstream.

antibodies A class of proteins secreted by the immune system that bonds with antigens. Antibodies fight off disease-causing organisms.

areola The darkened part of the breast immediately surrounding the nipple.

arousal phase The second stage of Kaplan's model of sexual response, which consists of physiological arousal and changes and, possibly, orgasm.

artificial insemination Introduction of semen into the uterus by noncoital means.

asphyxiophilia Desire for a state of oxygen deficiency to enhance sexual excitement.

assertiveness Standing up for one's basic rights without violating anyone else's rights.

assigned gender Intentional decision to raise a child as a boy or a girl, usually made at birth based on the child's genital appearance.

aversion therapy Pairing an undesirable sexual behavior with a painful response.

bar girls Sex workers who are supposed to act available so customers will buy them drinks.

Barbach's technique A method of treating orgasmic dysfunction and sexual unresponsiveness developed by Lonnie Barbach that focuses on awareness of feelings and sensations through self-exploration and stimulation.

Bartholin's glands Small glands located within the labia minora that secrete a few drops of fluid during sexual arousal.

basal body temperature A woman's body temperature immediately upon waking.

basal body thermometer A special thermometer used to measure changes in basal body temperature.

behavior therapy Applying learning principles to help people change behavior.

bestiality Sexual contact with animals—also called *zoophilia*.

binge-eating disorder (BED) Eating disorder characterized by recurrent binge eating but not by inappropriate weight-control measures.

biopsy (open biopsy) Usually referred to as an open biopsy, a minor surgical procedure during which tissue of a tumor is removed and examined for presence of cancer.

birthing room A homelike birth setting now available in some hospitals.

bisexual One whose erotic, romantic, and affectional attraction is toward both genders.

blended orgasm An orgasm in a female in which there are contractions of the muscles in the outer third of the vagina as well as breath holding; a combination of the vulval and uterine orgasms.

bloody show The expelling of the mucus plug (often streaked with blood) that has closed off the cervix during pregnancy.

body composition The percentage of fat versus lean tissue.

body image The mental image we have of our own physical appearance

body mass index (BMI) Weight in kilograms divided by the square of the height in meters.

bondage perversion Getting sexual pleasure from being bound, tied up, or otherwise restricted.

bonding A process of developing a close physical and psychological relationship with one's caregiver. A sense of close emotional attachment.

Braxton-Hicks contractions Weak and slow uterine contractions that occur during the last few months of pregnancy.

breast abscess Infection of the breast characterized by redness, swelling, and a painful or tender mass.

breast budding First stage of breast development in females, whereby breast tissue elevates as a small mound.

breast cancer The second most common type of cancer in women.

breast self-examination (BSE) A periodic self-care procedure that involves feeling the breast for any abnormalities. The test is performed once every menstrual cycle or every month after menopause.

breech delivery A delivery in which the infant is born with another body part first, rather than head first. This form of delivery can be hazardous for both mother and infant.

bulbocavernosus muscle A muscle that encircles and supports the vagina.

bulimia nervosa A condition in which the individual periodically binges and purges, with an obsessive fear of becoming fat.

bypassing When misunderstandings result from missed meanings.

calendar method Charting of the length of a woman's periods for several months to determine the days she is most likely to be fertile.

call girls Highly paid female sex workers who work by appointment only.

candidiasis A common form of vaginitis, sometimes called a yeast infection, which is caused by the fungus *Candida albicans*.

carcinoma A type of cancer emanating from epithelial cells.

case study In-depth study of individual(s) or small groups.

causation A relationship in which one event causes another event to occur.

cerebral cortex The part of the brain called the gray matter that controls higher-order functioning such as language and judgment.

cervical cap Shallow rubber cap, smaller than a diaphragm, that covers the cervix to prevent sperm from entering the uterus.

cervical secretions Normal fluids from the cervix that change consistency during the month.

cervix The mouth of the uterus, through which the vagina extends.

cesarean section (C-section) Surgical intervention to deliver the fetus, placenta, and membranes through an incision in the walls of the abdomen and uterus.

chancre A painless lesion that is symptomatic of the primary stage of syphilis and appears at the site of contact.

change-of-life baby A baby born to a menopausal woman who, in spite of not menstruating regularly, ovulated.

chemotherapy Use of chemicals (medication) to treat disease may be oral, intravenous, intramuscular, or topical.

child pornography Use of minors in sexually explicit media.

child sexual abuse Any sexual abuse involving fondling, erotic kissing, oral sexual activity, or genital penetration between an adult and a child, including pedophilia and incest.

chlamydia A term that encompasses several major diseases caused by *Chlamydia trachomatis*, including genitourinary tract infection, a type of conjunctivitis in newborns, a type of pneumonia in infants, lymphogranuloma venereum, and trachoma.

Chlamydia trachomatis An intracellular parasite that causes chlamydial infections.

chloasma A yellow to brown patch of skin pigmentation that may appear on the faces of pregnant white women; sometimes referred to as the "mask of pregnancy."

chorionic villi sampling (CVS) A technique for prenatal detection of genetic defects that involves removal of some of the villi growing on the outer surface of the chorion and examining their chromosomes.

chromosomally mediated–resistant *N. gonorrhoeae* **(CMRNG)** Strain of gonorrhea resistant to penicillin because its DNA makes its cell membrane impermeable to penicillin.

cilia Hairlike structures that guide objects, such as ova, moving past them.

ciprofloxacin-resistant *N. gonorrhoeae* Strain of gonorrhea resistant to the drug ciprofloxacin.

circumcision The surgical removal of the foreskin covering the glans penis.

clinical breast exam A breast examination conducted by a physician to detect any abnormalities.

clitoral hood The skin covering the clitoris.

clitoridectomy Surgical removal of the clitoris.

clitoris The structure located at the upper part of the labia minora that is homologous to the penis and is very sensitive to stimulation.

cognitive development Explains the ability to think concretely or abstractly.

cohabitation Situation in which people who live together and share a sexual relationship are not married.

coitus interruptus The Latin term for *withdrawal*, which means "interrupted intercourse."

colostrum The yellow fluid secreted by the breasts just before and after childbirth until milk production begins.

colposcopy An examination of the vagina and cervix using an instrument—a colposcope—to detect abnormal tissue growth.

combined pill (COC) Oral contraceptive containing estrogen and progestin.

come out Accept and make homosexual orientation public.

common-law marriage The recognition by some states that heterosexual couples who have lived together for a specified period and have represented themselves as married are in fact legally married.

conception The union of the sperm and ovum; also called *fertilization*.

conceptual identity Who am I in my world?

conceptus The fertilized ovum; the product of conception.

condom A sheath that covers the penis.

conformity with peers Desire to be like everyone else.

consensual In this context, a married person's engaging in extramarital sexual activity with the knowledge and permission of the spouse.

contraception Means of preventing pregnancy in spite of sexual intercourse.

contraction The shortening or tension of uterine muscles during labor.

control group In an experiment, the group not subjected to a particular event or condition.

coprophilia Sexual pleasure associated with feces.

coronal ridge (corona) The raised ridge where the glans penis ends and the penile shaft begins.

corpora cavernosa A cavernous structure located within the clitoris and the penis that fills with blood during sexual excitement, causing erection.

corpus The upper two-thirds of the uterus.

corpus luteum A yellowish structure that develops in the Graafian follicle at the discharge of an ovum and that produces progesterone and estrogen.

corpus spongiosum A spongy body in the penis that contains a network of blood vessels and nerves.

correlation A relationship between two events; a statistical measure that shows how variables are naturally related to each other.

cosmetic surgery Surgery done for the sole purpose of improving the appearance.

Cowper's glands Two pea-sized glands adjacent to the urethra that secrete a lubricating fluid before ejaculation.

cribriform Type of hymen that creates a sievelike covering for the vaginal opening.

critical thinking Thinking that avoids blind acceptance of conclusions or arguments and closely examines all assumptions.

crowning The presentation of the baby's head at the vaginal opening.

cunnilingus The stimulation of the female genitalia by the mouth, lips, and/or tongue of the sexual partner.

cystic mastitis Known also as fibrocystic disease, a condition characterized by fluid-filled lesions (cysts) that are tender and believed to be related to estrogen activity.

date-rape drugs Sedative hypnotic drugs used to incapacitate victims who are then sexually molested or raped.

decoding Translating the message from its symbol form into meaning.

delivery The stage of childbirth characterized by the expulsion of the infant and the placenta.

Depo-Provera (DPMA) An injectable progestin-only contraceptive.

dermoid cyst A type of benign ovarian cyst commonly found in young women.

desire phase The first stage of the sexual response cycle, as described in Helen Singer Kaplan's model, which consists of psychologically becoming interested in sex before any physical changes occur.

diaphragm Shallow rubber cap that covers the cervix and prevents sperm from entering the uterus.

digital rectal examination (DRE) A rectal examination whereby a physician inserts a finger into the rectum of a male patient to check for any abnormalities of the prostate.

dilation In childbirth, the gradual opening of the cervix during labor.

dilation and evacuation (D&E) Surgical procedure that involves dilating the cervix, scraping the walls of the uterus, and removing the endometrial lining with suction.

dildos Artificial penises.

douche Cleansing of the vagina by inserting a nozzle that secretes a recommended cleansing substance, a controversial procedure.

duration How long something occurs or has occurred.

dysmenorrhea Painful menstruation.

dyspareunia Pain in the genital area during sexual intercourse.

early adolescence First stage of adolescence, defined by pubertal changes—usually ages 9–13 years for females and ages 11–15 years for males.

eclampsia Pregnancy-induced hypertension accompanied by swelling of the face, neck, and upper extremities, plus convulsions or coma, which may be fat.

ectopic pregnancy The attachment and development of the zygote in a location other than in the uterus.

ejaculation The ejection of semen from the penis during orgasm.

ejaculatory incompetence A condition in which a male is unable to ejaculate in the vagina; sometimes referred to as retarded ejaculation.

Electra complex Freud's theory that 3- to 5-year-old girls want to take their father away from their mother.

electronic fetal monitoring A technique used during labor whereby a physician places an electrode on the woman's abdomen to monitor the fetal heart rate for signs of fetal distress.

embryo The developing fetus during the 2 months after conception.

embryonic stage The stage of prenatal development that includes the first 8 weeks of pregnancy.

emergency contraception The use of oral contraceptives after unprotected sex has occurred at midcycle.

encoding Converting an idea into words or gestures to convey meaning.

endocrine glands Glands that secrete their products into the bloodstream.

endometriosis The growth of the endometrium uterine lining at a location other than in the uterus.

endometrium The innermost layer of the uterus, to which the fertilized egg attaches and by which it is nourished as it develops before birth, which is partly discharged (if pregnancy does not occur) with the menstrual flow.

epididymis The location where sperm are stored in the testes and where nutrients are provided to help the sperm develop.

episiotomy Incision between the vulva and anus to enlarge the vaginal opening at the time of birth.

erectile dysfunction The inability of a man to maintain an erection long enough to have sexual intercourse; commonly known as *impotence*.

erection The extension of the penis and its engorgement with blood when the male is sexually stimulated.

erotica Sexually oriented material that may be artistically produced or motivated.

essentialism Belief that once the cultural and historical aspects are taken away, the essence of sexuality is biological.

estrogen A hormone produced by the ovaries whose level in the blood helps control the menstrual cycle.

ethical dilemma When two or more ethical principles work in opposing fashion in a particular situation, resulting in bewilderment regarding what is moral and what is immoral.

ethical principles Guides by which we can judge an action or decision as moral or immoral.

ethics A system that uses ethical principles to make decisions about morality.

ethnicity The degree of identification an individual feels with a particular ethnic group.

excitement phase The second stage of Kaplan's model of sexual response, which consists of physiological arousal and changes and, possibly, orgasm.

exhibitionism Achievement of sexual gratification by exhibiting the genitals to observers.

expected date of confinement (EDC) Due date for normal pregnancy that is usually estimated by Nägele's rule.

experiment Observation of behavior (or effects) under controlled conditions.

experimental group In an experiment, the group subjected to a particular event or condition.

external urethral sphincter The valve that closes during the emission stage, resulting in a buildup of semen, and that opens during the ejaculation stage, allowing semen to be expelled.

fallopian tubes (oviduct) The routes through which eggs leave the ovaries on their way to the uterus, in which fertilization normally occurs.

feedback When the receiver responds verbally or nonverbally.

fellatio Oral contact with a male's penis.

female condom A polyurethane or synthetic rubber sheath with flexible inner and outer rings worn inside the vagina.

femininity Those qualities characteristic of and suitable for girls and women according to the rules and expectations of a society.

fertility-awareness methods Methods used to determine fertile days.

fertility-awareness-combined methods Calculation of a woman's fertile times and use of a barrier or withdrawal on fertile days.

fetal alcohol spectrum disorders (FASD) The full spectrum of birth defects that are caused by prental alcohol exposure.

fetal alcohol syndrome (FAS) Impaired psychological and physical characteristics common in infants born to alcoholic women.

fetal stage Period from the ninth week of pregnancy to birth.

fetishism Paraphilia in which an inanimate object elicits sexual arousal.

fetus The developing child from the ninth week after conception until birth.

fibroadenoma A benign (noncancerous) tumor that is firm, round, and somewhat movable.

fimbriae The fingerlike ends of the fallopian tubes that catch the ova when they are discharged from the ovaries.

flaccid The relaxed, unerect state of the penis.

flooding Experiencing something so frequently that you no longer are aroused by it. This is a technique used to become more comfortable with sexual terminology.

focus group A form of research where a group of 6 to 10 people are asked about a topic and then discuss related issues.

follicle-stimulating hormone (FSH) A hormone, secreted by the anterior portion of the pituitary gland, that "instructs" the ovaries to prepare an egg to be released from a follicle.

follicular phase The part of the menstrual cycle during which menstruation occurs and the pituitary increases the production of FSH so the follicles mature: a combination of the menstrual and proliferative phases.

foreplay Physical contact preceding sexual intercourse.

foreskin (prepuce) The covering of the glans penis, which is removed during circumcision.

frequency How often something occurs or has occurred.

frottage Obtaining of sexual pleasure from rubbing or pressing against another person.

functional cyst An ovarian cyst that occurs on the follicle or corpus luteum, usually caused by the failure of the follicle to rupture and release an egg.

functional identity What adult roles will I play in the world?

fundus The upper end of the uterus, closest to the opening of the fallopian tubes.

gay Male or female homosexual. (*Gay* used alone probably refers to a male, though it is acceptable to refer to a *gay female*.)

gender constancy The concept that people's gender does not change—even if they change their dress or behavior.

gender dysphoria Feeling trapped in the body of the "wrong" sex.

gender identity The awareness and acceptance of one's gender.

gender role Complex groups of ways males and females are expected to behave in a given culture.

gender-role stereotyping Expectation that individuals will behave in certain ways because they are male or female.

gender schema A grouping of mental representations about male and female physical qualities, behaviors, and personality traits.

gender stereotypes Beliefs about how each gender should behave, which may be over-generalized or rigidly held.

gender typing The process whereby children develop behavior that is appropriate to their gender.

generalization The ability to conclude that the same results would be obtained outside the study.

genital herpes An STI characterized by tiny fluid-filled blisters that appear on the genitals and in the genital tract.

gigolo A man who is paid to provide escort and sexual services, usually for wealthy, middle-aged women.

glans penis The head of the penis.

gonadotropins Sexual hormones secreted by the pituitary that stimulate the gonads to produce their hormones.

gonads The male testes and the female ovaries, which produce gonadotropin hormones responsible for the development of secondary sexual characteristics.

gonorrhea An STI that commonly starts with inflammation of the mucous membrane lining of the openings of the body (e.g., mouth, vagina).

Graafian follicle A part of the ovary from which a mature egg ruptures, allowing the corpus luteum to develop in the location where the egg was released.

Grafenberg spot (G spot) An area located along the anterior wall of the vagina, several inches into the vaginal canal, that when stimulated in some women may result in sexual excitement and/or orgasm.

gynecologist A physician specializing in women's reproductive health.

gynecomastia Glandular tissue development in the breasts of boys.

herpes simplex virus (HSV) The virus that causes oral and genital herpes infections.

heterosexist An attitude that reinforces heterosexuality as the privileged and powerful norm.

heterosexual One whose primary erotic, romantic, and affectional attraction is toward members of the other gender.

homologous Organs that differ but that developed from the same tissue—for example, the glans penis and clitoris.

homophobia An irrational fear of homosexuality.

homosexual One whose primary erotic, romantic, and affectional attraction is toward members of one's own gender.

hormone A chemical substance secreted by a ductless gland, which is carried to an organ or tissue where it has a specific effect.

hormone therapy Form of treatment for cancer that uses hormones to combat cancer cell growth.

hot flashes Intermittent sensations of heat reported by menopausal women, possibly caused by decreased estrogen production.

house (brothel) prostitutes Sex workers who work in brothels.

human chorionic gonadotropin (HCG) A hormone secreted by the placenta whose presence in a woman's urine is the most common medical method of determining pregnancy.

human immunodeficiency virus (HIV) A retrovirus that causes AIDS.

human papillomavirus (HPV) A persistent STI caused by any of a group of viruses associated with the development of cervical cancer and/or genital warts.

human sexuality A part of your total personality. It involves the interrelationship of biological, psychological, and sociocultural dimensions.

hustler A male sex worker who performs homosexual acts for pay.

hymen A thin connective tissue covering the opening of the vagina.

hyperthyroidism Excessive functional activity of the thyroid gland.

hyperventilation Deep and rapid breathing that occurs during sexual excitation.

hypogonadism Decreased activity of the gonads that may result in retardation of growth and sexual development.

hypothalamus A structure in the brain that controls the pituitary gland and is directly connected by nerve pathways to various organs of the body.

hypothesis Tentative proposal or an educated guess about the results of a research study.

hypothyroidism A deficiency of thyroid activity.

"I" statement Statement that begins with an "I" to express personal feelings.

imaginary audience Belief in early adolescence that other people are looking at you as if you are onstage.

immoral What is judged to be wrong according to a system of ethics.

impotence Difficulty in achieving and maintaining an erection.

incest Sexual behavior between relatives who are too closely related to be married.

infants Babies from birth to 1 year old.

infertility The inability to reproduce.

informed consent Document required to participate in a research study after the purposes, risks, and benefits of the study have been explained.

inhibited sexual desire (ISD) A lack of interest in sexual activity of various sorts; also called *hypoactive sexual disorder (HSD)*.

internal urethral sphincter The valve that prevents urine from entering the urethra and sperm from entering the bladder during ejaculation.

intersexuality A condition in which a person has reproductive organs of both sexes.

interstitial cells The cells (sometimes called Leydig's cells) between the seminiferous tubules, where testosterone is produced.

interstitial-cell-stimulating hormone (ICSH) A hormone, secreted by the anterior portion of the pituitary gland in males, that stimulates the production of sperm.

interview Oral research method designed to gather information.

intrauterine device (IUD) Synthetic device that is inserted into the uterus to prevent the sperm from fertilizing the ovum.

intrauterine system (IUS) Synthetic device placed in the uterus that releases a continuous amount of hormone (levonorgestrel) to prevent ovulation, fertilization, or implantation.

introitus The vaginal entrance.

invasive cervical cancer Cancer that has invaded a wide area of cervical tissue.

in vitro fertilization The creation of a pregnancy in a laboratory by uniting the sperm and egg outside the womb; sometimes termed the "test-tube" baby technique.

Kamasutra Ancient sex manual from India.

Kegel exercises Exercises to help women develop greater control of muscles supporting the genitalia.

klismaphilia Sexual arousal produced by the use of enemas.

labia majora Two large folds of skin whose main function is to protect the external genitalia and the opening of the vestibule (defined later).

labia minora Two folds of skin lying inside the labia majora, which contain numerous blood vessels and nerve receptors.

labor The process of expelling a child by uterine contractions, dilation of the cervix, and bearing-down pressure.

lactation Production of breast milk.

lactobacilli Bacteria in the vagina that aid in keeping it healthy; also called *Doderlein bacilli*.

lactogen A hormone that stimulates the production of milk, the principal one being prolactin.

Lamaze method An approach to childbirth in which exercise and breath control are central to reducing anxiety and discomfort.

laparoscopy Female sterilization procedure that involves inserting a narrow viewing instrument—a laparoscope— through an incision in the abdomen and then performing ligation or applying clips or rings to block the fallopian tubes.

late adolescence Period of transition to adulthood, beginning usually at age 16 years for females and age 17 years for males.

late luteal phase dysphoric disorder (LLPDD) A type of premenstrual syndrome in which mental and emotional symptoms occur the week before menstruation. This is the name given to that condition by the American Psychiatric Association.

latency period Outdated Freudian theory that children aged 6–12 years old have no sexual feelings or interest.

latent herpes genitalis The stage of genital herpes characterized by inactivity of the herpesvirus, during which an infected individual is asymptomatic and transmission of the virus is rare.

latent syphilis A stage of syphilis that may last for years: early latent (about 1 to 4 years in duration) and late latent (may last for years); it may be symptom free or cause degenerative complications.

latex A synthetic rubber.

lesbian Female homosexual.

letdown The tingling sensation in the breasts when milk is forced out about 30 to 60 seconds after the infant begins to suckle.

libido Sexual desire, or drive.

ligation The tying of the fallopian tubes to prevent the sperm–egg union.

limbic system The part of the brain referred to as the "seat of emotions," which produces emotions in response to physical and psychological signals.

liposuction A technique for removing adipose tissue with a suction-pump device.

locus of control Refers to an individual's perception of the main causes of events in life. More simply, is life's destiny controlled by the self (*internal locus*) or by external forces such as fate or other people (*external locus*)?

lumpectomy Removal of a lesion, benign or malignant.

luteal phase The same phase of the menstrual cycle as the secretory phase, which includes ovulation and the production of LH from the corpus luteum.

luteinizing hormone (LH) A hormone, secreted by the anterior portion of the pituitary gland, that stimulates ovulation.

male climacteric Sometimes termed the "male menopause," which occurs at about the same age that women experience menopause, when men experience slightly decreased testosterone production and begin to question the directions in which their lives are headed.

mammary glands Milk-secreting glands located in the female breast.

mammography An X ray of the breasts to detect any abnormality before it is visible or palpable.

manual vacuum aspiration (MVA) A variation of vacuum aspiration that uses nonelectric suction instruments and can be used from detection of pregnancy through 12 weeks.

masculinity Those qualities characteristic of and suitable for boys and men according to the rules and expectations of a society.

massage parlors Places where sex workers can be hired to perform sexual acts under the guise of giving a massage.

masturbation Self-stimulation of the genitals.

meatus The opening of the urethra in the head of the penis, where both seminal fluid and urine are passed.

medical abortion A procedure that uses drugs to induce abortion.

menarche The time when a female begins her first menstrual cycle, usually at 8 to 16 years of age.

menopause The time when a woman's menstrual cycle ceases, usually between 40 and 55 years of age.

menstrual phase The part of the menstrual cycle during which the endometrial lining is sloughed off as the menstrual flow.

menstruation The cyclical emission of the blood-enriched endometrium when pregnancy does not occur.

metastasis Spread of cancer from a primary site to other parts of the body.

methotrexate A drug that blocks the hormone progesterone, which is needed to maintain a pregnancy.

middle adolescence The typical "teenage years," usually ages 13–16 years for females and ages 14–17 years for males.

midlife crisis A time of life, usually between 40 and 50 years of age, during which men question the path their lives have taken and make plans for changing their goals.

midwifery The practice by nonphysicians of assisting in the process of pregnancy and childbirth. Lay midwives are not trained health care professionals; nurse midwives are registered nurses who have received advanced training and often certification in the techniques of the birthing process.

mifepristone A drug that blocks the hormone progesterone, which is needed to maintain a pregnancy.

minilaparotomy Female sterilization procedure that involves a small incision in the abdomen through which the fallopian tubes are pulled so they can be blocked.

minipill (POP) A progestin-only pill.

misoprostol A prostaglandin that causes uterine contractions.

mons pubis (mons veneris, mount of Venus) The rounded, soft area above the vaginal opening that becomes covered with hair at puberty.

moral What is judged to be right according to a system of ethics.

morning sickness The condition of nausea and vomiting that is common in early pregnancy; thought to be caused by hormonal changes.

motility The ability to move spontaneously, which is required for fertilization.

multiple orgasms Orgasms that occur without the need for a refractory, or recovery, period.

muscle dysmorphia A disorder whereby a bodybuilder in top shape considers himself or herself to be puny.

myometrium The middle layer of the uterus, consisting of smooth muscle that aids in the pushing of the newborn through the cervix.

myotonia Muscle tension occurring during sexual arousal.

natural childbirth Drug-free childbirth; sometimes called *prepared childbirth*.

natural family planning (NFP) Calculation of a woman's fertile times and abstention from intercourse on fertile days.

necrophilia Sexual relations with a dead person.

needle biopsy Insertion of a needle into a lump in a breast to see whether fluid (which indicates a cyst rather than a tumor) can be removed.

Neisseria gonorrhoeae The bacterium that causes gonorrhea; also known as *gonococcus*. Street names include "clap" and "drip."

no-fault divorce The granting of divorce without either partner's proving the other was the cause of the marriage's failure.

nonassertiveness Giving up one's basic rights so others may achieve theirs.

nonconsensual In this context, a married person's engaging in sexual intercourse without the consent of the spouse.

nongonococcal urethritis (NGU) Inflammation of the urethra caused by *Chlamydia trachomatis*, and *Ureaplasma urealyticum, Mycoplasma hominis, Trichomonas vaginalis*, herpes simplex virus, and unknown organisms.

Nonoxynol 9 (N-9) The major spermicidal ingredient in U.S.-made products.

nuclear family A married couple and their children.

nymphomania An excessive, insatiable sexual drive in women.

objectivity Being sure the results are the same no matter who asks the questions or records the answers.

obscenity Personal or societal judgment that something is offensive. Something offensive to modesty or decency; often sexually related.

observation Watching subjects in a particular setting.

obstetrical analgesia A nondrug pain reliever used in delivery (e.g., hypnosis).

obstetrician A physician who specializes in the care of pregnant women and the process of childbirth. Because these physicians are also gynecologists, they are often referred to as obstetrician–gynecologists or OB–GYNs.

Oedipus complex A development stage in which the boy wants to possess his mother sexually and sees the father as a rival (similar to the female *Electra complex*).

open marriage A marriage in which partners allow each other to have intimate and emotional relationships with others.

opportunistic diseases A major manifestation of AIDS, diseases that occur in the presence of a suppressed immune system.

oral contraceptive (OC) A daily pill taken to prevent ovulation.

orgasm The peak release of sexual tension, accompanied by sensory pleasure and involuntary rhythmic muscular contractions; ejaculation in the male.

orgasmic dysfunction The consistent or frequent inability of a woman to achieve an orgasm.

orgasmic platform The narrowing of the outer third of the vagina during orgasm caused by contractions of the muscles in that area.

orgasmic reconditioning Increasing sexual arousal to socially appropriate stimuli.

os The opening to the uterus.

osteoporosis A condition of weakened bones resulting from decalcification (loss of calcium) of bone that increases in the absence of estrogen and is of particular concern in postmenopausal women.

ovarian cancer Cancer of the ovaries that causes more cancer deaths than any other cancer of the female reproductive system.

ovary A structure of the female genitalia that houses ova before their maturation and discharge and that produces estrogen and progesterone.

Ovist Adherent to the 17th-century belief that the preformed baby was contained within the female body and that the male's sperm simply activated its development.

ovulation The part of the menstrual cycle when the ovum is discharged from the ovary.

ovulation methods Observation of signs of ovulation to calculate fertile days.

oxytocin A pituitary hormone that stimulates the breasts to eject milk so that breastfeeding may occur after childbirth.

Pap smear A test of the tissue of the cervix for cervical cancer (named after its founder, Dr. Papanicolaou).

paracervical block An anesthetic used during childbirth that blocks pain sensations in the pelvic area, in which injections are given at positions around the cervix.

paraphilia Literally meaning "love (*philia*) beyond the usual (*para*)," this term refers to various sexual behaviors previously referred to as deviant.

partial ejaculatory incompetence A condition in which, during ejaculation, only a seepage of semen occurs, and orgasm lacks pleasurable sensations.

partialism Paraphilia in which sexual arousal is associated with a particular body part.

parturition The process of giving birth.

pediculosis lice Also known as crabs, of three common types: *Pediculus corporis*, a body louse; *Pediculus capitis*, a head louse; and *Pediculus pubis*, a pubic louse.

pedophilia Sexual behavior in which a child is the sexual object.

peer marriage Relationship in which partners have equal status.

pelvic inflammatory disease (PID) Infection of the reproductive organs, particularly the uterus, fallopian tubes, and pelvic cavity.

penetrative behaviors Any behavior whereby penetration occurs—for example, penile–vaginal intercourse, oral sex, or anal intercourse.

penicillinase-producing *N. gonorrhoeae* (PPNG) Strain of gonococcus resistant to all forms of penicillin.

penile strain gauge A wire or cuff placed around the penis to measure physiological changes over time.

penis Structure of the male external genitalia consisting of the root, shaft, and glans; also contains the urethra, through which urine is excreted.

perfect use The ability of a method of contraception to prevent pregnancy as measured by consistent and correct use.

perimenopause (climacteric) The period just before menopause when the production of estrogen and progesterone is decreasing, usually a 5- to 10-year period.

perimetrium The outermost layer of the uterus, sometimes termed the *serosa*, a very elastic layer that allows the uterus to accommodate a growing embryo and fetus.

pheromones Substances that when secreted have a specific scent found to be sexually arousing.

phimosis Condition resulting when penile erection causes pain because the foreskin is too tight.

pimps Individuals who set up female sex workers with clients.

pituitary The "master gland," an endocrine gland located at the base of the brain that stimulates the other endocrine glands to produce their hormones.

placenta An organ of interchange between mother and fetus; oxygen, nutrients, and waste are exchanged through its cells.

plethysmograph A laboratory measuring device that charts physiological changes over time.

PLISSIT A model of sexual therapy that consists of moving through the stages of giving permission, limited information, specific suggestion, and, if that does not work, intensive therapy.

polyurethane A type of plastic.

population The group being studied in a research project.

pornography Visual and written materials used for the purpose of sexual arousal.

postmenopause hormone therapy (PHT) Treatment of menopausal women who have insufficient estrogen production with synthetic estrogen supplements.

precocious puberty Pubertal development before the age of 7 years.

preeclampsia Pregnancy-induced hypertension; symptoms include swelling of the face, neck, and upper extremities; and excess levels of protein in the urine.

premature Type of birth in which an infant is born before the complete term of gestation but late enough in the pregnancy that it has a chance to survive.

premature ejaculation The inability of a man to control ejaculation for a sufficient length of time during coitus.

premenstrual syndrome (PMS) Marked mood fluctuation during the week before menstruation, accompanied by physical symptoms.

prenatal care Care given to an expectant mother before the birth of her child that typically consists of monitoring fetal development, screening for high-risk pregnancy, and providing education for pregnancy and childbirth.

primary amenorrhea A condition in which a woman of age 18 years or older has never menstruated.

primary dysmenorrhea Painful menstruation, the cause of which is unknown.

primary erectile dysfunction A condition in which an adult male has never had an erection sufficient to engage in sexual intercourse.

primary herpes genitalis The first stage of a genital herpes infection; it begins with infection by the herpesvirus and the formation of antibodies. Common symptoms include painful lesions in or around the genital area, a sluggish feeling, fever, and possibly swollen lymph nodes. Up to 75% of infected persons may be asymptomatic in the primary stage.

primary ISD A condition in which a person has always been uninterested in sexual activity.

primary syphilis The first stage of syphilis most generally manifested by the appearance of a painless lesion called a *chancre*.

procreation Sexual intercourse for the purpose of reproduction.

prodrome Itching, tingling, or burning sensations that occur where a herpes lesion will appear.

progesterone A hormone secreted by the corpus luteum signaling the endometrium to develop in preparation for a zygote.

prolactin A pituitary hormone that stimulates the production of milk from the mammary glands.

proliferative phase The first part of the menstrual cycle, during which FSH production is increased and the follicles are maturing.

prostaglandins Hormonelike substances produced by body tissue that may cause dysmenorrhea.

prostate gland A structure of the male internal genitalia that secretes a fluid into the semen before ejaculation to aid sperm motility and prolong sperm life.

prostatitis Infection of the prostate gland.

prostitution Participating in sexual activity for pay or profit.

prurient Characterized by lustful thoughts or wishes.

psychosexual development The blending of sexual aspects of one's development with other psychological factors.

pubic lice A parasite, commonly referred to as crabs, a louse that grips the pubic hair and feeds on tiny blood vessels of the skin.

pubococcygeal muscle A muscle that encircles the vagina and supports it.

questionnaire Written instrument designed to gather information.

quickening Movements of the fetus felt by the mother; usually occurs about the fourth month of pregnancy.

radiation therapy A form of treatment for cancer that uses carefully directed radiation to destroy cancer cells.

random sample A sample that represents the larger population and that is chosen without bias, so that every member of the larger population had an equal chance to be selected.

rape Forcible sexual intercourse with a person who does not give consent.

rape trauma syndrome A two-phase reaction to rape. An acute phase involves intense emotional responses for several weeks. The long-term phase may last several years and involves reorganization and establishment of control.

recurrent herpes genitalis The fourth stage of a genital herpes infection, which is characterized by a reactivation of the virus and the appearance of blisters on the skin. Not all people with herpes have recurrences.

refractory (recovery) period The time needed by males for recovery between orgasms.

releasing factors Chemicals released from the hypothalamus that affect the function of various body parts.

resolution phase A stage of the sexual response cycle consisting of a return to the prearoused state.

retarded ejaculation A condition in which penile erection occurs during sexual intercourse but ejaculation does not; sometimes termed ejaculatory incompetence.

reticular activating system (RAS) A network of nerves that connect the cortex and the subcortex—the connection between mind and body.

retroviruses A group of viruses consisting of ribonucleic acid (RNA) surrounded by a protein coat that can convert their RNA into deoxyribonucleic acid (DNA) once they have invaded a living cell, allowing them to take over the cell and reproduce themselves.

Rh factor The presence of Rh agglutinogens (antigens) in the blood, which indicates that a person is Rh positive, whereas its absence designates the person as Rh negative.

rhinoplasty Surgery done to change the shape of the nose.

rule ethics Guiding principles used in all situations to arrive at moral decisions, which are considered applicable to all situations.

saddle (epidural) block An anesthetic used during childbirth that blocks pain sensations in the buttocks, perineum, and inner thigh.

sample A segment of the larger population.

satyriasis An excessive, insatiable sexual drive in men—also called *Don Juanism*.

scabies Skin irritation caused by a tiny mite that is transferred from one person to another by close contact, sexual or otherwise.

scientific method Research conducted in an atmosphere free from bias.

scrotum (scrotal sac) A sac of skin that contains the testes and spermatic cords.

secondary amenorrhea A condition in which a woman has ceased menstruating after menarche.

secondary dysmenorrhea Painful menstruation caused by some identifiable condition such as endometriosis.

secondary erectile dysfunction A condition in which an adult male has previously had an erection sufficient to engage in sexual intercourse but no longer has.

secondary ISD A condition in which a person was at one time interested in sexual activity but is no longer interested.

secondary sexual characteristics Changes occurring during adolescence—such as growth of pubic hair, breast development, and testes and penile development.

secondary syphilis The second stage of syphilis, characterized by a rash.

secretory phase The second part of the menstrual cycle, during which ovulation occurs and the production of LH stimulates the development of the corpus luteum.

self-esteem Sense of personal worth.

self-report data The respondents' descriptions of something.

Semans stop–start method A method of controlling premature ejaculation (developed by James Semans) in which the man tells his partner to stop stimulating him when he feels ejaculation approaching.

semen The male ejaculate, which contains sperm and other secretions.

semenarche First ejaculation of semen for boys.

seminal vesicles Two sacs of the male internal genitalia that secrete nutrients to nourish sperm.

seminiferous tubules The structures located within the testes that actually produce the sperm.

sensate focus A method of alleviating sexual unresponsiveness by procedures designed to encourage erotic feelings and sexual pleasuring.

septate Type of hymen that bridges the vaginal opening.

seronegative The result of a blood test for antibodies to HIV that indicates no presence of such antibodies.

seropositive The result of a blood test for antibodies to HIV that indicates that such antibodies have been found in the blood.

sexism The prejudgment that because of gender a person will possess negative traits.

sexology The study of sexuality.

sexual aversion An irrational fear of sexual activity.

sexual cognition Attitudes, expectations, beliefs, and values framing one's sexual experiences.

sexual dysfunction A specific, chronic disorder involving sexual performance.

sexual fantasies Thoughts, images, and daydreams of a sexual nature.

sexual harassment Unwelcome verbal, physical, or sexual conduct that has the effect of creating an intimidating, hostile, or offensive environment.

sexual identity Inner sense of oneself as a sexual being, including one's identification in terms of gender and sexual orientation.

sexual masochism Sexual gratification that results from experiencing pain.

sexual orientation One's erotic, romantic, and affectional attraction to the same gender, to the opposite gender, or to both.

sexual preference Term formerly used to describe sexual orientation that is now outdated, because sexual orientation is no longer commonly considered to be a conscious individual preference or choice, but to be formed by a complicated network of factors.

sexual response cycle The sequence of physiological and psychological reactions as a result of sexual arousal.

sexual sadism Sexual gratification that results from inflicting pain on another person.

sexual self-concept Who am I as a sexual being?

sexual unresponsiveness Commonly referred to as *frigidity* or female sexual arousal disorder, a sexual dysfunction that causes a woman to experience little or no erotic pleasure through sexual stimulation.

sexually healthy relationship Consensual, non-exploitative, honest, mutually pleasurable, safe and protected from unwanted pregnancy, STIs, and other harm (National Guidelines Task Force, 2004).

sexually related diseases (SRDs) Diseases of the reproductive system that can occur in either sexually active or sexually inactive individuals.

sexually transmitted infections (STIs) Infections that are primarily contracted through sexual contact.

shedding herpes genitalis The third stage of a genital herpes infection, during which virus is excreted from the body even though an infected individual experiences no signs or symptoms.

silent infection A stage of HIV infection characterized by no symptoms other than the presence of HIV antibodies.

single-parent family For whatever reason, only one parent who is living with a child or children.

situation ethics A belief that no one set of rules can apply to all situations and each specific situation must be analyzed to determine which ethical principles are applicable.

situational homosexuality Homosexual behavior limited to circumstances in which members of the same gender are deprived of contact with the other gender.

Skene's glands Glands located along the walls of the vagina that are thought to be analogous to the male prostate gland and the site from which some women eject a fluid during orgasm.

smegma A cheeselike substance secreted by the glans penis that must be removed from below the foreskin of uncircumcised males to prevent irritation and/or infection.

social cognition Ability to see a situation from another person's point of view.

social constructionism The belief that sexual identities are acquired from and influenced and modified by an ever-changing social environment.

social training Improving a person's social skills.

socialization The process of guiding people into socially acceptable behavior by providing information, rewards, and punishments.

sodomy A term that specifically refers to anal intercourse, but is often used to refer to almost any sexual behavior someone might not consider normal.

sonogram A diagnostic picture revealing the fetal outline. In ultrasonography, sound waves are bounced off the fetus. With a scanner, the image is then projected onto a computer screen, revealing whether certain defects are present.

speculum A metal (or plastic) instrument that is inserted into the vagina to hold the walls apart, allowing for medical examination.

spermatic cord The cord from which the testicle is suspended that contains the vas deferens, blood vessels, nerves, and muscle fibers.

spermatocytes Cells that develop through several stages to form sperm.

spermatogenesis The manufacturing of sperm in the seminiferous tubules.

spermatorrhea (wet dreams, or nocturnal emissions) Emission of semen during sleep.

spermatozoa (sperm) The mature male sperm cell.

spermicide Chemical detergent compound that immobilizes or kills sperm on contact; as a barrier, prevents sperm from entering the uterus through the cervical os.

spirochete A spiral-shaped bacterium, one of which, *Treponema pallidum*, causes syphilis.

spontaneous abortion (miscarriage) The natural termination of a pregnancy.

squeeze technique A method of helping men control premature ejaculation whereby the penis is gently squeezed when the man senses ejaculation is imminent.

statistical significance The likelihood that a study's results are due to the relationship uncovered between the study's variable as opposed to chance.

statutory rape Intercourse with a person younger than the legal age of consent.

Stein–Leventhal syndrome Reproductive malfunction in women; a syndrome of endocrine origin that involves ovarian cysts, amenorrhea, and infertility.

stepfamily A family with children that is formed as a result of remarriage.

stereotyping The expectation that individuals will exhibit certain characteristics or behaviors.

sterilization A procedure that makes a person biologically incapable of reproducing.

steroids Synthetic versions of the male hormone testosterone that promote tissue growth.

stranger rape Rape of a person by an unknown person.

streetwalkers Sex workers who work on the streets.

survey Research in which people complete questionnaires or are personally interviewed.

swinging Swapping of mates for sexual activities.

symptomatic infection The second stage of HIV infection, characterized by HIV antibodies as well as general signs and symptoms such as swollen lymph glands, fatigue, unexplained weight loss, night sweats, persistent fever, and diarrhea.

symptothermal method A combination of natural family planning methods, in which both temperature and signs of ovulation are observed and charted.

syphilis An STI caused by the spirochete *Treponema pallidum*.

systematic desensitization A means of overcoming anxiety by approaching the anxiety-provoking stimulus in small steps.

tachycardia An increase in heart rate that occurs during sexual activity.

Tanner scale Scale developed by Dr. John Tanner for measuring pubertal development in boys and girls.

teratology The study of causative factors of birth defects.

testes Male gonads contained within the scrotal sacs that produce sperm cells and the male sex hormone testosterone. Singular form: testicle.

testicular cancer Cancer of the testicles; the most common form of cancer in men aged 29 to 35 years.

testosterone The male sex hormone produced in the testes that is responsible for the development of male secondary sexual characteristics.

tetracycline-resistant *N. gonorrhoeae* (TRNG) Strain of gonorrhea that produces a substance that inactivates tetracycline.

thriving Normal physical and psychological pattern of weight gain, neuromuscular development and other developmental attributes of infants.

toxemias of pregnancy Hypertensive conditions, subdivided into preeclampsia and eclampsia.

toxic shock syndrome (TSS) A syndrome caused by *Staphylococcus aureus* bacteria in which symptoms include high fever, nausea, vomiting, diarrhea, and a drop in blood pressure; a potentially fatal syndrome that has been linked with the use of superabsorbent tampons.

transgender A general term used when one's identity does not match one's physical/genetic sex. It includes such diverse categories as transsexualism and transvestism.

transsexual A person whose gender identity does not match her or his biological sex; also a person who wishes to have, or has had, his or her gender surgically altered to conform to his or her gender identity.

transudation The process of vaginal lubrication resulting from engorgement of blood that creates pressure that forces moisture to seep from the spaces between the cells.

transvestite A person who achieves sexual satisfaction from wearing clothes usually worn by the other gender.

tribadism Rubbing genitals against someone's body or genital area.

trichomoniasis (trick) A type of vaginitis that can be an STI or an SRD. Symptoms include a foul-smelling, foamy white or yellow-green discharge that irritates the vagina and vulva. Urethritis may also be present.

troilism Having sexual relations with another person while a third person watches.

true labor Characterized by regularly spaced contractions of the uterus, thinning and dilation of the cervix, and a descending of the presenting part of the fetus into the vagina.

tummy tuck Extensive surgical procedure that removes excess skin and fat from the abdomen.

typical use The ability of a method of contraception to prevent pregnancy as actually used at home by people not being monitored.

umbilical cord The lifeline between mother and fetus, which contains two arteries and one vein. Food, oxygen, and chemicals are transported to the child through the arteries, and waste is returned to the mother through the vein.

urethra The tube through which the bladder empties urine outside the body and through which the male ejaculate exits.

urine The body-waste product stored in the bladder and eliminated through the urethra.

urophilia Sexual pleasure associated with urine.

uterine orgasm An orgasm in a female that can occur only in the presence of penile penetration and that involves a woman's holding her breath just before orgasm and then exhaling when the climax occurs.

uterus A pear-shaped hollow structure of the female genitalia in which the embryo and fetus develop before birth.

vacuum aspiration Surgical procedure that uses a suction tube to evacuate the contents of the uterus, which can be used through the first weeks of the second trimester.

vagina A hollow, tunnellike structure of the female internal genitalia whose reproductive functions are to receive the penis and its ejaculate, serve as a route of exit for the newborn, and provide an exit for menstrual flow.

vaginal plethysmography Insertion of a probe into a woman's vagina to measure changes in blood volume.

vaginismus The involuntary contraction of the muscles surrounding the vaginal entrance so that entry of the penis is prevented.

validity, validation Demonstration that tests measure what they are designed to measure.

values Those beliefs to which we attach the most worth.

variable A measurable event that varies or is subject to change.

vas deferens The duct, through which sperm stored in the epididymis is passed, that is cut or blocked during vasectomy.

vasa efferentia The duct through which sperm produced in the seminiferous tubules travel to the epididymis.

vasectomy Cutting or cauterizing of the vas deferens to prevent sperm from being ejaculated; a means of sterilization.

vasocongestion Increased blood flow to an area of the body; which occurs in the pelvic area during sexual arousal.

vasovasectomy Reversal of a vasectomy, so that sperm can be ejaculated.

vestibule The area containing the vaginal and urethral openings.

volunteer bias Characteristics of volunteers that are likely to influence research results.

voyeurism Obtaining of pleasure from watching people who are undressing or engaging in sexual behavior.

vulva The female external genitalia.

vulval orgasm An orgasm in a female that includes the contractions of the orgasmic platform, which is not sexually satisfying and, as a result, allows another orgasm to occur almost immediately.

withdrawal Removing the penis from the vagina before ejaculation.

zidovudine The first drug (brand name Retrovir; also known as AZT) approved by the FDA for the treatment of AIDS. This antiviral drug slows the replication of the AIDS virus, thus slowing the course of the syndrome.

zoophilia Sexual contact with animals—also called *bestiality*.

zygote A fertilized egg.

Index

condoms, 181, 182
confinement, expected date of, 218
conflicts, resolving, 82–84
  active listening, 84
  alternative solutions, 84
  identifying position, 84
conformity with peers, 400
consensual extramarital sexual activity,
    447–448
consent, informed, 38
constructionism, social, 6
consumers of sexual information, 20
contemplating adoption, 284–285
contraception, 16, 54–55, 174–213, 691
  abstinence, 177–179, 580–581
    effectiveness, 177–179
    reversibility, 179
  BioRing, 208
  cervical cap, 201–202
  combined contraceptive patch, 196–197
    effectiveness, 196–197
  combined injectables, 197
    effectiveness, 197
    reversibility, 197
  combined vaginal ring, 202–203
    effectiveness, 202
    reversibility, 202
  contraceptive sponges, 186
  in developing countries, 208–209
  diaphragm, 200–201
    effectiveness, 201
    reversibility, 201
  effectiveness, 176–177
  emergency, 185, 195, 206
  female condom, 184–186
    effectiveness, 186
  female sterilization, 204–207
  fertility awareness methods, 188–190
    effectiveness, 190
    reversibility, 190
  future of, 207–209
  implants, 198
    effectiveness, 198
    reversibility, 198
  intrauterine devices, 198–200
    effectiveness, 199
  laparoscopy, 205
  male condom, 181–184
    consistent use, 181
    correct use, 181–183
    effectiveness, 183
  male contraceptive methods, 207
  male sterilization, 203–204
  minilaparotomy, 205
  Nesterone, 208–209
  nonprescription methods, 177–190
  nonsurgical female sterilization, 206
  oral contraceptives, 190–196
    effectiveness, 194, 196
    emergency contraception, 195–196
    reversibility, 194
  permanent methods, 203–207
  prescription methods, 190–203
  reversibility, 207
  safer sex, contrasted, 177
  spermicides, 187–188
    effectiveness, 187
    reversibility, 187
  sterilization, 203
    effectiveness, 203
    reversibility, 203

transcervical methods, 205–206
  withdrawal, 180–181
    effectiveness, 180–181
contraceptive sponges, 186
contractions, 240
control, locus of, 397
control group, 34
controlling sex work, 672–674
coprophilia, 506
corona, 132
coronal ridge, 132
corpora cavernosa, 95, 137
corpus, 99
corpus luteum, 101
corpus spongiosum, 137
correlation, 19, 36
  causation, distinguished, 19–20
cosmetic surgery, 344–347
Cowper's glands, 139
cribriform, 96
crisis, midlife, 458
critical thinking, 18–20
  correlation vs. causation, 19–20
  sexual information, 20
crowning, 242
C-section. *See* Cesarean section
cultural influences on sexuality, 11–18
  conception, 15–16
  contraception, 16–17
  control of sexual behavior, 13–15
  gender roles, 17–18
  sexual revolution, 12–13
culture life behaviors, 402–403
cunnilingus, 482
CVS. *See* Chorionic villi sampling
cyberspace, 656
cyst
  dermoid, 121
  functional, 121
cystic mastitis, 119

D

D&E. *See* Dilation and evacuation
date rape, 74, 515, 519–521
date-rape drugs, 524–525
Davis, Katherine, 41
decision-making model, 22
  evaluation, 22
  implementation, 22
  recognition, 22
  review, 22
decision-making process, 22
decoding, 69
delivery, 239, 241–243
  breech, 242
delivery date, 221
delivery of placenta, 243
Department of Health and Human
    Services, 589
Department of Justice, Office on
    Violence Against Women, 555
Depo-Provera, 197
derailer, 80
  sexual communication and, 80
dermoid cysts, 121
DES. *See* diethylstilbestrol
desensitization, systematic, 636
desire dysfunctions, 624–626
  frequency, 625–626
  inhibited sexual desire, 624–625
  sexual aversion, 626

desire phase, 161
desires, discussing, 167
diabetes, 236
diaphragm, 200–201
  effectiveness, 201
  reversibility, 201
diet, 338
diethylstilbestrol, 235
dieting, 343
digital rectal examination, 143
dilation, 240
dilation and evacuation, 263, 264
dildos, 484
dimensions of communication, 23
dimensions of human sexuality,
    4–11
  biological dimension, 5
  interactive nature of sexual dimen-
      sions, 4
  psychological dimensions, 5–6
  sociocultural dimensions, 6–11
    ethical influences, 9
    medial influences, 9–10
    multicultural influences, 7–8
    political influences, 10–11
    religious influences, 6–7
    socioeconomic influences, 8–9
direct observation, 35
disability decision making, 378
Discovery Health: Paraphilia, 511
diseases, 235–237
dissatisfaction with body parts, 333
diversity, 335–336
Division of STD Prevention, 589
divorce, 448–452, 700
  no-fault, 700
Don Juanism, 508
donor eggs, 460
*Double Your Dating: Sexual Communica-
    tion Workbook*, 91
douching, 121
Dove Foundation, 681
DRE. *See* Digital rectal examination
dreamer, 80
  sexual communication and, 80
drug therapy, 507–509
drugs, 233–235
  childbirth, 243
due date, 221
duration, 34
dysfunction, 614
  discussing, 619
dysmenorrhea, 107–108
  primary, 107
  secondary, 108
dyspareunia, 620, 636
dysphoria, gender, 313

E

early adolescence, 405
early developers, 399
early sexuality researchers, 40–42
  Davis, Katherine, 41
  Ellis, Henry Havelock, 40
  Freud, Sigmund, 40–41
  Hirschfeld, Magnus, 41
  Mosher, Clelia, 42
  von Krafft-Ebing, Richard, 40
Eating Disorder Referral and Informa-
    tion Center, 351
eating disorders, 339–342

tummy tuck, 346
twentieth-century sexuality researchers,
    42–62
  Beasley, Ruth, 49
  contraception, 54–55
  ethnic differences, 53–54
  Hite, Shere, 47–48
  homosexual activity, 44
  Johnson, Virginia, 44–46
  Kaiser Family Foundation, 49–50
  Kinsey, Alfred C., 43–44
  Masters, William, 44–46
  masturbation, 43
  National Health and Social Life
    Survey, 46–47
  National Survey of Young Teens Sexual
    Attitudes and Behavior, 50–51
  nocturnal dreams, 43
  popular literature, 47–51
  premarital intercourse, 43–44
  premarital sexual attitudes, 51–53
  Reinisch, Jane, 49
  Sarrel, Lorna and Philip, 48–49
  scientific literature, 43–47
  Seventeen Magazine, 49–50
  sexuality education, 57–58
types of adoptions, 284
types of orgasm, 166–167
types of relationships, 432–434

U
ultrasonography, 253
umbilical cord, 217
unexpected pregnancy, 260–291
UNHCHR. *See* United Nations High
    Commissioner for Human Rights
United Nations High Commissioner for
    Human Rights, 705
urethra, 137
urethral opening, 96

urethral sphincter, 156
urethritis, nongonococcal, 565
  incidence, 565
  symptoms, 565
  treatment, 565
urine, 137
urophilia, 506
U.S. Census Bureau, 471
U.S. Department of Justice, Office on
    Violence Against Women, 555
uterine orgasm, 167
uterus, 99–100

V
vacuum aspiration, 262
  manual, 262
vagina, 97–98, 121–122
vaginal infections, 576–578
  candidiasis, 577–578
  trichomoniasis, 576–577
vaginal plethysmography, 38
vaginismus, 622, 636
validity, 39
variance of sexual differentiation, 250–251
vas deferens, 137
vasa efferentia, 138
vasectomy, 203
vasocongestion, 157
vasovasectomy, 203
Veronica's Voice, 681
vesicles, seminal, 138
vestibule, 96
video games, 652–653
videotapes, 652–653
viral infections, 568–576
  genital warts, 568–569
    cervical cancer, 570–571
    diagnosis, 570
    treatment, 570

hepatitis B, 575–576
  complications, 575
  diagnosis, 575–576
  symptoms, 575
  treatment, 575–576
herpes genitalis, 571–575
  complications, 572–573
  diagnosis, 573–575
  symptoms, 572–573
  treatment, 573–575
human papillomavirus, 568–571
volunteer bias, 33
vomiting, 239
von Krafft-Ebing, Richard, 40
voyeurism, 499–500
vulval orgasm, 166

W
Walen and Roth model, 161–162
warts, genital, 568–569
  cervical cancer, 570–571
  diagnosis, 570
  treatment, 570
weight, 229–230, 336
wet dreams. *See* Nocturnal emissions
withdrawal, 180–181
  effectiveness, 180–181
women, oppression of, 308
women's movement, 318–322
WomensMedia.com-Expert Advice for
    Working Women, 327

Z
zidovudine, 599
Zilbergeld and Ellison's model, 161
zoophilia, 504
zygote, 105, 216

Credits

Inc.; **page 247** © Kari Weatherly/Photodisc/Getty Images; **page 253** © Jiang JingJie/ShutterStock, Inc.

Unexpected Pregnancy Outcomes
page 265 (top) © Larry Downing/Reuters /Landov; **(bottom)** © Brendan Smialowski/EPA/Landov; **page 283** © Varina Hinkle/ShutterStock, Inc.

Chapter 9
page 295 © prism68/ShutterStock, Inc.; **page 297** © Anita Patterson Peppers/ShutterStock, Inc.; **page 298** © David Buffington/Photodisc/Getty Images; **page 299** © LiquidLibrary; **page 301** © WENN/Landov; **page 303** © Photos.com; **page 304** © Jennifer Hogan/Dreamstime.com; **page 307** © Dan Thomas Brostrom/ShutterStock, Inc.; **page 309** © AP Photos; **page 311** © Photos.com; **page 313** © Domenech Castello/EPA/Landov; **page 316** © Thinkstock LLC; **page 317 (top)** © Stephen Coburn/ShutterStock, Inc.; **(bottom)** © Bartomeu Amengual/age fotostock; **page 318** Courtesy of Library of Congress, Prints & Photographs Division, [reproduction number LC-USZ62-25812]; **page 320** © Jeff Greenberg/PhotoEdit, Inc.; **page 321** © Kim Ludbrook/EPA/Landov

Body Image
page 330 (top) © Gabi Moisa/ShutterStock, Inc.; **(bottom)** © Kzenon/ShutterStock, Inc.; **page 331** © Patricia Malina/ShutterStock, Inc.; **page 334** © Bjorn Svensson/Alamy Images; **page 335** © Michael Germana/SSI Photo/Landov; **page 336** © Eriko Sugita /Reuters/Landov; **page 337** © Photodisc; **page 339** © Photodisc; **page 340 (left)** © AP Photos; **(right)** © Kelley Chin, The *Kansas City Star*/AP Photos; **page 341** © Banana Stock/age fotostock; **page 343 (left)** © Rick Maiman, *Bloomberg News*/Landov; **(right)** © Ira Mark Gostin/AP Photos; **page 344** © Noel Hines/Landov; **page 346** © Alex Grimm/Reuters/Landov

Chapter 10
page 357 © Photos.com; **page 358** © Photos.com; **page 360** © Paige Falk/ShutterStock, Inc.; **page 362** © Liang Wen You/ShutterStock, Inc.; **page 364** © Joe Gough/ShutterStock, Inc.; **page 369** © Photos.com; **page 370** © LiquidLibrary; **page 373** © Kevin Dietsch/Landov; **page 374** © Scott Anderson, *Racine Journal Times*/AP Photos; **page 376** © Chris Haston/NBC/The Kobal Collection; **page 378** © Terry Schmitt/UPI Photo/Landov; **page 379** © Galina Barskaya/ShutterStock, Inc.

Chapter 11
page 388 © Thinkstock LLC/Jupiterimages; **page 392** © LiquidLibrary; **page 394** © Andrey Stratilatov/ShutterStock, Inc.; **page 396** © Dennis MacDonald/age fotostock; **page 397** © Family Communications/Reuters/Landov; **page 400 (left)** © Photos.com; **(right)** © Mark E. Stout/ShutterStock, Inc.; **page 402** © Jason Stitt/ShutterStock, Inc.; **page 407** © Stephen Coburn/

ShutterStock, Inc.; **page 417** © Richard Hutchings/Photo Researchers, Inc.

Chapter 12
page 427 © Photos.com; **page 429** © Photos.com; **page 431** © Photos.com; **page 433** © Photos.com; **page 434** © Directphoto.org/Alamy Images; **page 435** © AbleStock; **page 437** © Avava/ShutterStock, Inc.; **page 439** © PhotoCreate/ShutterStock, Inc.; **page 440** © WizData, Inc./ShutterStock, Inc.; **page 442 (top)** © Photos.com; **(bottom)** © WizData, Inc./ShutterStock, Inc.; **page 443** © Photos.com; **page 444** © Photos.com; **page 446** © Graca Victoria/ShutterStock, Inc.; **page 448** © Suzanne Tucker/ShutterStock, Inc.; **page 450** © Dhannte/ShutterStock, Inc.; **page 451** © Lori Carpenter/ShutterStock, Inc.; **page 452** © Photos.com; **page 453** © Sylvia Corday Photo Library Ltd./Alamy Images; **page 454** © Sandy Schaeffer/MAI/Landov; **page 456 (left)** © Zdenka Micka/ShutterStock, Inc.; **(right)** © Diane Critelli/ShutterStock, Inc.; **page 457** © Simone van den Berg/ShutterStock, Inc.; **page 459** © Photodisc; **page 461** © Monkey Business Images/Dreamstime.com; **page 462** © Photodisc/Getty Images; **page 463** © Photos.com; **page 465** © Mark Richards/PhotoEdit

Chapter 13
page 475 Courtesy of AIDS Action Committee of Massachusetts, Inc.; **page 481** © Photos.com; **page 482** © Gertjan Hooijer/ShutterStock, Inc.

Alternative Sexual Behavior
page 500 © Darren Baker/ShutterStock, Inc.; **page 502** © Karen Struthers/ShutterStock, Inc.; **page 503** © Rusian/ShutterStock, Inc.; **page 504** © Figaro Magahn/Photo Researchers, Inc.; **page 508** © Vlad Mereuta/ShutterStock, Inc.

Chapter 14
page 515 © Courtesy of The Violence Against Women Coalition/Junior League Minneapolis; **page 518 (left)** © The Kobal Collection; **(right)** © Tim Harman/ShutterStock, Inc.; **page 519** © Luba V. Nel/ShutterStock, Inc.; **page 522** © www.imagesource.com/Jupiterimages; **page 524** Courtesy of DEA; **page 525** © Joseph/ShutterStock, Inc.; **page 527** © Charles Rex Arbogast/AP Photos; **page 528** © Hader Glang/ShutterStock, Inc.; **page 535** © Goldenkb/Dreamstime.com; **page 538** © Photos.com; **page 539** © The Kobal Collection; **page 541** Courtesy of The National Coalition Against Domestic Violence; www.ncadv.org; **page 545** © Andres Rodriguez/ShutterStock, Inc.; **page 546** © Louis Lanzano/AP Photos; **page 547** © Jaimie Duplass/ShutterStock, Inc.; **page 550** © BananaStock/Jupiterimages

Chapter 15
page 563 (top) Courtesy of Joe Miller/CDC; **(middle)** © Mediscan/Visuals Unlimited; **(bottom)** Courtesy of CDC; **page 566** Courtesy of CDC; **page 567** Courtesy

of CDC; **page 568 (top)** Courtesy of Bill Schwartz/CDC; **(bottom)** Courtesy of J. Pledger, BSS/VD/CDC; **page 570 (left)** Courtesy of Susan Lindsley/CDC; **(right)** Courtesy of Joe Millar/CDC; **page 571** Courtesy of Dr. Herrmann/CDC; **page 572** Courtesy of Susan Lindsley/CDC; **page 574** Courtesy of Dr. N.J. Flumara, Dr. Gavin Hart/CDC; **page 575** Courtesy of National Cancer Institute; **page 576** Courtesy of Tom Watanabe/U.S. Navy; **page 577** Courtesy of CDC; **page 578** © Ken Greer/Visuals Unlimited; **page 579** Courtesy of W.H.O/CDC; **page 580** Courtesy of Susan Lindsley/CDC; **page 581** © Elena Ray/ShutterStock, Inc.

HIV and AIDS
page 595 © Timothy E. Goodwin/ShutterStock, Inc.; **page 597** © Roger L. Wollenberg/UPI/Landov; **page 601** © *Fort Worth Star-Telegram*/MCT/Landov; **page 602** © Landov; **page 603** © LiquidLibrary; **page 604** © Corbis; **page 606** © Jeff Christensen/Reuters/Landov

Chapter 16
page 615 © Christine Gonsalves/ShutterStock, Inc.; **page 617** © AbleStock; **page 620** © Galina Barskaya/ShutterStock, Inc.; **page 622** © Photodisc; **page 624** © JJJ/ShutterStock, Inc.; **page 626** © Creatas; **page 627** © Photos.com; **page 629** © Ryan McVay/Photodisc/Getty Images; **page 633** © Laura Cavanaugh/UPI Photo/Landov

Chapter 17
page 646 © Mike Segar/Reuters/Landov; **page 647** © Andrey Burmakin/ShutterStock, Inc.; **page 651**

© The Kobal Collection; **page 652** © Jacqueline Abromeit/ShutterStock, Inc.; **page 655** © TOSP Photo/ShutterStock, Inc.; **page 657** Courtesy of Persian Kitty; **page 659 (right)** © Ismael Montero Verdu/ShutterStock, Inc.; **page 663** © Photos.com; **page 664** © Rob Marmion/ShutterStock, Inc.; **page 667** Sam Mircovich/Reuters/Landov; **page 669** © Robert J. Beyers II/ShutterStock, Inc.; **page 675** © Kuzma/ShutterStock, Inc.

Chapter 18
page 684 © Stuart Johnson, *Desert News*/AP Photos; **page 688** © Leah-Anne Thompson/ShutterStock, Inc.; **page 688** © AbleStock; **page 690** © Photos.com; **page 694 (left)** © Julie Markes/AP Photos; **(right)** Courtesy of Linda Bartlett/National Cancer Institute; **page 696** © Antonio Petrone/ShutterStock, Inc.; **page 699** © Dynamic Graphics/Jupiterimages; **page 700** © Tom Green Defense Team/AP Photos

Epilogue: Taking Responsibility for Your Sexual Health
page 709 (top) © Andrew Cooper/The Kobal Collection; **(bottom)** © Columbia/TriStar Motion Picture Companies/The Kobal Collection; **page 711 (bottom)** © Darren Baker/ShutterStock, Inc.; **page 712** © jean schweitzer/ShutterStock, Inc.

Unless otherwise indicated, all photographs and illustrations are under copyright of Jones and Bartlett Publishers, LLC, or have been provided by the authors.

Rhina Acosta